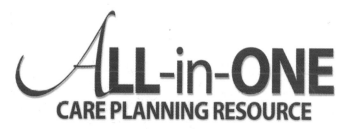

ALL-in-ONE
CARE PLANNING RESOURCE

*Medical-Surgical, Pediatric, Maternity,
and Psychiatric Nursing Care Plans*

See what nursing students have to say about
All-in-One Care Planning Resource . . .

"The care plans are extremely thorough and well-organized. The rationale feature is a great asset to nursing students developing critical thinking skills and good, sound clinical judgment."
Jeffrey Waddell Pittsburgh State University, Pittsburgh, Kansas

"Wonderful! Love the introductions that give you a complete picture of the signs and symptoms, assessments, and diagnostic tests you need to care for patients in clinicals."
Yvonne Gubersky, University of Arizona, Tucson, Arizona

"Rationales are clear and easy to read. It has lab values, and the teaching is specific to each diagnosis. It has everything! A great way to see the whole picture."
Brianna Chavez, Belmont University, Nashville, Tennessee

"I don't have to carry around four books anymore! This is one book with everything in it."
Leshia Gann, Belmont University, Nashville, Tennessee

"WOW!! Very thorough and complete in all aspects of patient care. I especially like the description of the condition with expected signs and symptoms and lab values."
James Green, Columbus State University, Columbus, Georgia

"The rationales that follow the interventions are great for planning your care and knowing why you are doing your interventions. Interventions and rationales are awesome! Patient and family teaching and discharge planning are very beneficial for clinical teaching."
Hattie McDowell, Truman State University, Kirksville, Missouri

"Well organized and easy to read. The student's best guide through nursing school!"
Jennifer Marler, Jacksonville University, Jacksonville, Florida

"An excellent source for not only completing accurate care plans, but providing holistic care for patients in prioritizing their health needs. I wish I had been able to utilize such a fantastic resource like this during my long care-plan-making nights!"
Nicole Colline, Quinnipiac University, Hamden, Connecticut

"More detail in the rationales makes the interventions more understandable! I definitely got my money's worth—covered all areas of nursing in one care plan book."
Ashley Zerwekh, Gateway Community College, Phoenix, Arizona

"I love how this book includes labs for specific disorders. It includes everything . . . a lot of good information! I wish I had this when I was a sophomore."
Vanessa Lincoln, Truman State University, Kirksville, Missouri

"Very thorough. Covered all aspects of the physiologic and psychosocial problems as well as listing of resources to refer patients to."
Cindy Green, Columbus State University, Columbus, Georgia

"I like the 'related-to' feature. And it's nice to have the lists of resources to send home with the families at discharge."
Suzanne Brown, Oklahoma State University, Oklahoma City, Oklahoma

"It's very handy to have a book that's all-in-one!"
Tanya Hentges, Truman State University, Kirksville, Missouri

"I wish I had this book for my first semester of clinicals. The material . . . pulls together related information that would usually be found in several separate textbooks. Nursing students can lighten their backpack for clinicals with this one book that includes it all."
Julie Wilner, University of Michigan, Ann Arbor, Michigan

All-in-ONE
CARE PLANNING RESOURCE

Medical-Surgical, Pediatric, Maternity, and Psychiatric Nursing Care Plans

Pamela L. Swearingen, RN
Special Project Editor

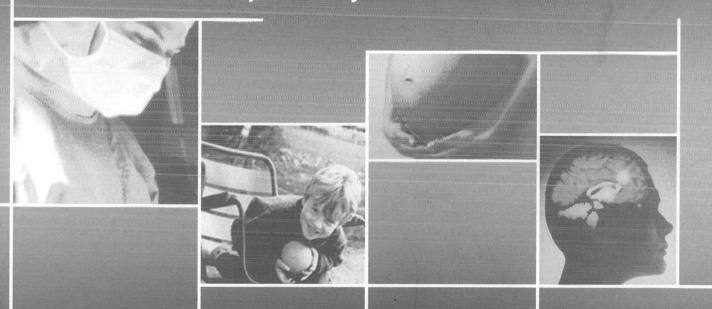

Mosby
An Affiliate of Elsevier

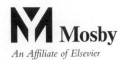
Mosby
An Affiliate of Elsevier

11830 Westline Industrial Drive
St. Louis, Missouri 63146

NOTICE

Nursing is an ever-changing field. Standard safety precautions must be followed, but as new research and
clinical experience broaden our knowledge, changes in treatment and drug therapy may become necessary
or appropriate. Readers are advised to check the most current product information provided by the
manufacturer of each drug to be administered to verify the recommended dose, the method and duration of
administration, and contraindications. It is the responsibility of the licensed health care provider, relying on
experience and knowledge of the patient, to determine dosages and the best treatment for each individual
patient. Neither the publisher nor the editor assumes any liability for any injury and/or damage to persons
or property arising from this publication.

Library of Congress Cataloging-in-Publication Data

All-in-one care planning resource: medical-surgical, pediatric, maternity, and psychiatric nursing
care plans/Pamela L. Swearingen, special project editor.
     p.; cm.
Includes bibliographical references and index.
ISBN 0-323-01953-6
     1. Nursing care plans. 2. Surgical nursing. 3. Pediatric nursing. 4. Maternity nursing.
5. Psychiatric nursing. I. Swearingen, Pamela L.
     [DNLM: 1. Nursing Process—organization & administration. 2. Nursing Care-methods.
3. Patient Care Planning. WY 100 A437 2004]
RT49.A45 2004
610.73—dc21
                                     2003051230

Executive Publisher: Robin Carter
Developmental Editor: Kristin Geen
Publishing Services Manager: Melissa Lastarria
Project Manager: Joy Moore
Senior Book Designer: Amy Buxton

Printed in the United States

Last digit is the print number: 9 8 7 6 5 4 3

Contributors

Medical-Surgical Nursing Care Plans

Lolita M. Adrien, RN, MS, CNS, CWOCN
Nursing Learning Specialist
Contra Costa College
San Pablo, California
★Contributed care plans for Crohn's Disease, Fecal
   Diversions, and Ulcerative Colitis.

Nancy Arnold, RN, MN, CRRN, CIRS
Vice President
Numotech, Inc.
Northridge, California
★Contributed care plan for Managing Wound Care.

Linda S. Baas, RN, PhD, CCRN
Associate Professor of Nursing
College of Nursing and Health
University of Cincinnati
Cincinnati, Ohio
★Contributed care plan for Prolonged Bedrest.

Marianne Saunorus Baird, RN, MN
Case Manager
Saint Joseph's Hospital of Atlanta
Atlanta, Georgia
★Contributed Endocrine Care Plans.

Marie Bakitas, RN, ARNP, CHPN
Palliative Care Nurse Practitioner
Dartmouth-Hitchcock Medical Center
Lebanon, New Hampshire
★Contributed care plan for Palliative and End-of-Life Care.

Susan A. Bethel, RN, MS, CNRN
Director of Nursing
Greenville Hospital System
Greenville, South Carolina
★Contributed Neurologic Care Plans.

Cheryl L. Bittel, RN, MSN, CCRN
Clinical Nurse Specialist
Saint Joseph's Hospital of Atlanta
Atlanta, Georgia
★Contributed Cardiovascular Care Plans.

Michelle T. Bott, RN, BScN, MN
Professional Practice Coordinator
Guelph General Hospital
Guelph, Ontario
★Contributed care plans for Acute Renal Failure, Chronic
   Renal Failure, Hemodialysis, Peritoneal Dialysis, and
   Normal Laboratory Values appendix.

Paula A. Caron, RN, MS, ARNP, AOCN
Advanced Practice Nurse
Norris Cotton Cancer Center, Dartmouth-Hitchcock
   Medical Center
Lebanon, New Hampshire
★Contributed care plans for Cancer Care, Psychosocial
   Support, and Psychosocial Support of the Patient's Family
   and Significant Others.

Christine DiGeronimo, RN, BSN
Clinical Educator
Dartmouth-Hitchcock Medical Center
Lebanon, New Hampshire
★Contributed care plans for Perioperative Care and Care of
   the Renal Transplant Recipient.

Patti G. Eisenberg, RN, MSN, CS
Medical-Surgical Clinical Nurse Specialist
Community Hospitals Indianapolis
Indianapolis, Indiana
★Contributed care plan for Providing Nutritional Support.

Linda Frank, RN, PhD, ACRN
Assistant Professor, Department of Infectious Diseases
Graduate School of Public Health, University of Pittsburgh
Pittsburgh, Pennsylvania
★Contributed care plan for Caring for Individuals with
   Human Immunodeficiency Virus Disease.

Karen Goff, RN, BSN
Case Manager, Gastrointestinal Services
Saint Joseph's Hospital of Atlanta
Atlanta, Georgia
★Contributed care plans for Appendicitis; Cholelithiasis,
   Cholecystitis, and Cholangitis; Cirrhosis; Hepatitis;
   Pancreatitis; Peptic Ulcers; and Peritonitis.

Cheri Goll, RN, MSN
Senior Consultant
Cardiovascular Service Line
Saint Vincent Hospital
Indianapolis, Indiana
★Contributed Respiratory Care Plans.

Marguerite Jackson, RN, PhD, FAAN
Director, Department of Education, Development
 and Research
University of California San Diego Medical Center
Associate Clinical Professor of Family and Preventive Medicine
University of California San Diego School of Medicine
San Diego, California
★Contributed Infection Prevention and Control appendix.

Patricia Jansen, RN, MS, APRN, CS
Geriatric Clinical Nurse Specialist
San Jose Medical Center
San Jose, California
★Contributed care plans for Care of the Older Adult, Benign
 Prostatic Hypertrophy, Ureteral Calculi, Urinary Diversions,
 and Urinary Tract Obstruction.

Ingrid B. Mroz, RN, MS, CCRN, CS
Clinical Nurse Specialist, Intensive Care Unit
Dartmouth-Hitchcock Medical Center
Lebanon, New Hampshire
★Contributed care plan for Pain.

Dottie Roberts, RN, BC, MSN, MACI, ONC
Clinical Nurse Specialist, Rehabilitative & Medical Services
Palmetto Health Baptist
Columbia, South Carolina
★Contributed Musculoskeletal Care Plans.

Nancy A. Stotts, RN, EdD, FAAN
Professor
University of California San Francisco
San Francisco, California
★Contributed care plan for Managing Wound Care.

Carol Monlux Swift, RN, BSN, CNRN
El Camino Hospital
Mountain View, California
★Contributed Neurologic Care Plans.

S. Michele Vanet, RN,C, BSN
Resource Nurse and Nursing Supervisor
Louis A. Johnson VA Medical Center
Clarksburg, West Virginia
★Contributed Hematologic Care Plans.

Mary Young, RN, MSN, ARNP, CS
Adult Nurse Practitioner
Dartmouth-Hitchcock Medical Center
Lebanon, New Hampshire
★Contributed care plan for Abdominal Trauma.

Pediatric Nursing Care Plans

Sherry D. Ferki, RN, MSN
Adjunct Faculty, Pediatric Clinical Instructor
College of the Albemarle, ADN Program
Elizabeth City, North Carolina

Maternity Care Plans

Deborah E. Swenson, RN, BSN, ARNP
Perinatal Nurse Practitioner
OBSTETRIX Medical Group of Washington, Inc.
Seattle, Washington

Psychiatric Nursing Care Plans

Verna Benner Carson, PhD, APRN/PMH
National Director of RESTORE Family Behavioral Health
Tender Loving Care—Staff Builders Home Health Care
Fallston, Maryland

Preface

All-in-One Nursing Care Planning Resource is a one-of-a-kind book featuring nursing care plans for all four core clinical areas. The inclusion of pediatric, maternal, and psychiatric nursing *in addition* to medical-surgical nursing care plans allows students to use one book throughout the nursing curriculum. This unique presentation—combined with solid content, an open and accessible format, and clinically relevant features—makes this a must-have care plans book for nursing students.

ORGANIZATION

This book is organized into four separate sections for medical-surgical, pediatric, maternal, and psychiatric care plans. Within each section, care plans are listed alphabetically by disorder or condition (the medical-surgical nursing care plans are organized alphabetically within each body system). General information that applies to more than one disorder can be found in the *General Care Plans* section, where nursing diagnoses and interventions for perioperative care, pain, prolonged bedrest, cancer care, psychosocial support for patients, psychosocial support for the patient's family and significant others, older adult care, and end-of-life care are discussed.

Each disorder uses the following consistent format:

- **Overview,** *including a review of pathophysiology, where appropriate*
- **Health Care Setting,** *such as hospital, primary, community, or long-term care*
- **Assessment,** *covering Signs and Symptoms and Physical Assessment*
- **Diagnostic Tests**
- **Nursing Diagnoses with Desired Outcomes**
- **Nursing Interventions and Rationales** *in a clear two-column format*
- **Related NIC Interventions and NOC Outcomes**
- **Patient-Family Teaching and Discharge Planning**

FEATURES

The care plans in this book were written by clinical experts in each subject area to ensure the most current and accurate information. In addition to reliable content, the book offers the following special features:

- A **consistent, easy-to-use format** facilitates quick and easy retrieval of information.
- The **Health Care Setting** is specified for each care plan, since these conditions are treated in various settings such as hospital, primary care, long-term care facility, community, and home care.
- **Outcome criteria with specific timelines** assist in setting realistic goals for nursing outcomes and providing quality, cost-effective care.
- **Detailed, specific rationales** for each nursing intervention apply concepts to clinical practice.
- The **Patient-Family Teaching and Discharge Planning** section highlights key patient education topics, as well as resources for further information.
- The new **NANDA Taxonomy II** nursing diagnoses are included in each care plan.
- Related **NIC (Nursing Interventions Classification) interventions and NOC (Nursing Outcomes Classification) outcomes** are listed for each nursing diagnosis.
- Separate care plans on **Pain** and **End-of-Life Care** focus on palliative care for patients with terminal illnesses, as well as relief of acute and chronic pain.
- The **newest infection prevention and control guidelines** from the Centers for Disease Control and Prevention (CDC) are included in the appendix.
- Normal laboratory values are listed in the appendix, including separate tables for Complete Blood Count; Serum, Plasma, and Whole Blood Chemistry; and Urine Chemistry.

This book was carefully prepared to meet the needs of today's busy nursing student. We welcome comments on how we can enhance its usefulness in subsequent editions.

Pamela L. Swearingen

Reviewers

Janet Brown, RN, MSN, CNS
Associate Professor
School of Nursing
California State University, Chico
Chico, California

Kitty Cashion, RN, BC, MSN
Clinical Nurse Specialist
Department of OB/GYN
University of Tennessee Health Science Center
Memphis, Tennessee

Monica Kwong Gilliam, RN, MSN, FNP
Former Nursing Instructor
Merritt College
Oakland, California

Trish Goudie, RN, CNM, MSN
Dean and Associate Professor
College of Nursing
Montana State University–Northern
Havre, Montana

Judith E. Kuczek, RN, MS
Learning Laboratory Coordinator
School of Nursing
Northern Illinois University
DeKalb, Illinois

Karol Burkhart Lindow, RN,C, CNS, MSN
Associate Professor of Nursing
Kent State University, Tuscarawas Campus
New Philadelphia, Ohio

Kenneth J. A. Lown, RN, MSN, CPNP
Pediatric Nurse Practitioner;
Associate Clinical Director, HIV/Primary Care
Mount Sinai/New York University Health System
New York, New York

Dottie Mathers, RN, MSN
Associate Professor
Department of Nursing
Pennsylvania College of Technology

Julie S. Snyder, RN,C, MSN
Adjunct Faculty
School of Nursing
Old Dominion University
Norfolk, Virginia

Lisa South, RN, DSN
Assistant Professor
University of Alabama
Huntsville, Alabama

Harriet Wichowski, RN, PhD
Associate Professor
School of Nursing
University of Tennessee at Chattanooga
Chattanooga, Tennessee

Contents

Cancer Care

The term *cancer* refers to several disease entities, all of which have in common the proliferation of abnormal cells. To varying degrees these cells have lost their ability to function and divide in an organized fashion. As a result they may develop new functions not characteristic of their site of origin, spread and invade uncontrollably, and cause death of other cells. Cancers can cause local disease and dysfunction, metastasize and cause problems at other body sites, and eventually cause systemic destruction and failure.

HEALTH CARE SETTING

Medical or surgical floor in acute care, primary care, hospice, home care

CARE OF PATIENTS WITH CANCER

Lung cancer

Lung cancer remains the most common cause of cancer deaths among men and women in the United States. Despite more recent treatment advances in surgery, chemotherapy, and radiation therapy, the cure rate remains low. Although exposure to certain known carcinogens such as radon and asbestos may cause lung cancer, the greatest number of lung cancer cases are linked to tobacco smoking.

Most cases of lung cancer are consistent with four major cell types: small cell, adenocarcinoma, squamous, and large cell. A small portion of lung cancer cases are mesothelioma, bronchial gland tumors, or carcinoids. The cell type determines the appropriate treatment. Depending on the stage of lung cancer at presentation, surgery, chemotherapy, and/or radiation therapy may be part of the medical treatment plan.

Screening: Currently none exists for lung cancer, although studies are in process for evaluating efficacy of routine computed tomography (CT) scanning for individuals at high risk for developing lung cancer.

See also: "Perioperative Care" for appropriate nursing diagnoses, outcomes, and interventions and **Activity Intolerance,** p. 15, in this section.

Nervous system tumors

These tumors may be primary or secondary tumors of the brain or spinal cord. They are classified according to their cell of origin and graded according to their malignant behavior. Although histologically the tumor may be benign, the enclosed nature of the central nervous system (CNS) may result in tumor effects causing significant damage or even death. Treatment is initially surgical if the tumor site is accessible. For some tumors, complete resection is tantamount to cure. Radiation therapy and chemotherapy also may be implemented postoperatively. Metastatic CNS tumors may be removed surgically but are more often treated with radiation therapy. Chemotherapy also may be an option for control.

See also: "Perioperative Care" for appropriate nursing diagnoses, outcomes, and interventions and "Head Injury" for **Deficient Knowledge:** Craniotomy procedure, p. 345.

Gastrointestinal malignancies

Malignancies of the gastrointestinal (GI) system include carcinomas of the stomach, esophagus, bowel, anus, rectum, pancreas, liver, and gallbladder. Each disease site has its own staging criteria and prognostic factors. Most early stage tumors of all sites are treated with a plan that includes chemotherapy and surgery. Many treatment plans now begin with preoperative chemotherapy in the weeks preceding surgery. Anorectal-sparing approaches include preoperative radiation therapy and chemotherapy. Radiation therapy is used less frequently with gastric, colon, and liver tumors.

Screening: Currently the only GI site with recommended screening parameters is the colon. The American Cancer Society (ACS) recommends individuals over age 50 yr have a flexible sigmoidoscopy every 5 yr. When a family history exists of first-degree relatives with colorectal cancer, the ACS recommends that screening colonoscopy begin at age 40 yr. Although commonly performed, the value of fecal occult blood testing to detect occult tumors is somewhat controversial as a reliable screening tool; the ACS recommends one annually.

See also: "Perioperative Care," p. 47, "Fecal Diversions," p. 475, and "Managing Wound Care," p. 583, for appropriate nursing diagnoses, outcomes, and interventions.

Neoplastic diseases of the hematopoietic system

Hematopoietic system cancers include lymphoma, leukemia, plasma cell disorders, and myeloproliferative disorders.

Lymphomas, classified as Hodgkin's and non-Hodgkin's, depending on cell type, are characterized by abnormal proliferation of lymphocytes. In addition to characteristic lymph node enlargement, involvement of other lymphoid organs such as the liver, spleen, and bone marrow does occur. Treatment is predicated by the stage of the disease on presentation. Patients with Hodgkin's lymphoma often may be given a favorable prognosis, whereas patients with non-Hodgkin's lymphoma may be faced with treatment decisions for the remainder of their lives. Currently there is no routine screening done for lymphoma.

Leukemia is the abnormal proliferation and accumulation of white blood cells (WBCs). Divided into two categories, leukemia presents as either acute or chronic, depending on cellular characteristics. Acute leukemia is characterized by abnormal proliferation of immature precursor or progenitor WBCs. Classification depends on cell type involved. Although the optimum treatment is still unknown, it is predominantly chemotherapy, with radiation therapy involved when CNS prophylaxis is indicated.

Chronic leukemia is characterized by abnormal proliferation of mature differentiated WBCs, and its treatment is chemotherapy. In some cases the question is *when* to start treatment because some forms may be indolent for a long time.

In both types of leukemia the abnormal cells may interfere with normal production of other WBCs, red blood cells (RBCs), and platelets. Immunity may be compromised, resulting in frequent and possibly fatal infections.

Screening: No programs exist for leukemia, and diagnosis usually occurs when the patient has symptoms such as fever, malaise, bruising or bleeding, infections, adenopathy, hepatosplenomegaly, weight loss, or night sweats. Diagnosis is usually confirmed with a complete blood count (CBC), followed by bone marrow aspiration.

See also: "Hematologic Disorders," pp. 515-568, for appropriate nursing diagnoses, outcomes, and interventions related to care of patients with abnormal blood cells.

Breast cancer

The incidence of breast cancer in the United States continues to rise. On diagnosis, several factors are considered to determine treatment planning and prognosis. Very important is the stage of disease. Tumor differentiation is also a prognostic factor, with poorly differentiated tumors foreboding a worse prognosis. Other factors considered in treatment and prognosis are the rate of tumor growth (S-phase), DNA characteristics (ploidy), estrogen and progesterone receptors, other biochemical changes (e.g., HER-2/*neu*), lymph node metastases, and distant metastases. Treatment may include any, all, or a combination of the following: surgery, chemotherapy, radiation therapy, hormonal treatment, or biologic therapy. Because breast cancer is considered a chronic disease, therapy may span several years.

Screening: The ACS recommends that all women over 40 yr have an annual mammogram and annual breast examination by a clinician and perform monthly breast self-examination (BSE). Women between 20 and 30 yr should have a breast examination by a clinician every 3 yr and do monthly BSE.

See also: "Perioperative Care," p. 47, for appropriate nursing diagnoses, outcomes, and interventions and **Risk for Disuse Syndrome,** p. 5, in this section.

Genitourinary cancers

Genitourinary cancers for men include malignancies of the bladder, prostate gland, testicle, and kidneys.

Bladder cancer is classified as superficial or invasive. Treatment is chosen based on extent of disease and may include surgery, local or systemic chemotherapy, laser, or radiation. Metastases occur commonly in bone, liver, and lungs.

Screening: No standards currently exist for screening for bladder cancer; however, survival may depend on prompt evaluation of early symptoms.

Prostate cancer occurs more commonly in men over 50 yr of age. Treatment may consist of a combination of interstitial or external radiation therapy, chemotherapy, surgery, or hormonal therapy. Choice of treatment is determined in part by the stage of disease and cellular histology at diagnosis and by clinician preference. In general, prostate cancers tend to grow slowly and metastasize late, thus patients may live several years with the disease.

Screening: The ACS recommends digital rectal examination (DRE) and prostate-specific antigen (PSA) annually for men over 50 yr and younger for men at increased risk.

Testicular cancer occurs most often in men between ages 20 and 40. Tumors generally are classified as seminomas and nonseminomas, depending on their cellular line of differentiation, with many being of a mixed cell type. Nonseminomas tend to grow and metastasize more aggressively. Treatment nearly always begins with surgery and may be followed by chemotherapy and radiation therapy, depending on histology, blood tumor markers, and bulk of disease.

Screening: Because cryptorchidism significantly increases the risk of later development of testicular cancer, surgical correction is recommended before age 6. Screening programs are not routinely conducted. Any scrotal mass should be evaluated promptly.

Renal cell carcinomas occur in about 2% of all malignant diagnoses and are most predominantly classified as adenocarcinomas with histologic variants. Surgery is nearly always the treatment of choice for early stage renal cell cancers, and radiation therapy is usually recommended only for control of symptoms with more advanced disease. Chemotherapy has a limited role in management of renal cell cancer. Biologic response modifiers are used to manage more advanced disease.

Screening: No screening programs exist to detect renal cell cancer, and the incidence might be lowered if the predominance of cigarette smoking could be reduced. Any reports of hematuria should be investigated thoroughly. Patient presentation with any other symptoms compatible with renal cell carcinoma usually forebodes more advanced disease.

See also: "Perioperative Care," p. 47, "Urinary Diversions," p. 279, and "Benign Prostatic Hypertrophy," p. 231, for appropriate nursing diagnoses, outcomes, and interventions. Also see **Stress Urinary Incontinence,** p. 6 and **Sexual Dysfunction,** p. 12, in this section.

Sites of neoplasms of the female pelvis include the vulva, vagina, cervix, uterus, and ovaries. Bladder and kidney cancers are discussed earlier.

With increased use of the Papanicolaou (Pap) smear as a screening tool for *cervical cancer,* the incidence of invasive cervical cancer has decreased, while the incidence of preinvasive carcinoma in situ (CIS) has increased. Treated early, usually with surgery and sometimes with radiation therapy, cervical cancer is a curable disease. Advanced stages may be treated with surgery, chemotherapy, and radiation.

Ovarian tumors may be detected during an annual pelvic exam; however, they are more commonly occult until the patient has symptoms of advanced disease. Treatment is initially surgical, which is a vital step for proper tumor staging. Survival is directly related to proper treatment, which can only be determined by proper staging. Chemotherapy is commonly given after surgery.

Endometrial cancer usually is treated with surgery, and in all but the earliest stages, this is followed by radiation therapy. Chemotherapy is usually reserved for advanced stages in which a surgical cure is not feasible and invasion of local or more distant tissues has occurred.

Screening: The ACS recommends an annual Pap smear and pelvic examination for all women over age 18 and younger for women who are sexually active. Women at high risk for endometrial cancer should have a uterine biopsy at menopause.

See also: "Perioperative Care," p. 47, for appropriate nursing diagnoses, outcomes, and interventions.

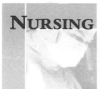

NURSING DIAGNOSES AND INTERVENTIONS FOR GENERAL CANCER CARE

Note: *The following nursing diagnoses, outcomes, and interventions relate to generalized cancer care. Those for care specific to chemotherapy, immunotherapy, and radiation therapy follow this section.*

Nursing Diagnosis:

Risk for Activity Intolerance

related to interrupted blood flow secondary to pericardial tamponade

Desired Outcome: During activity, patient rates perceived exertion at ≤3 on a 0-10 scale and exhibits cardiac tolerance to activity, as evidenced by systolic BP within 20 mm Hg of resting BP, RR ≤20 breaths/min, HR ≤20 bpm above resting HR, and absence of chest pain or new dysrhythmia.

INTERVENTIONS	RATIONALES
Monitor for evidence of activity intolerance and ask patient to rate perceived exertion. For further information see "Prolonged Bedrest" for **Activity Intolerance,** p. 67.	Declining activity tolerance may signal deterioration of patient's condition. Pericardial tamponade, if present, may be caused by an accumulation of fluid in the pericardial space, tumor, invasion of the mediastinum, pericardial fibrosis, or effusion from radiotherapy. Patients at increased risk for pericardial tamponade include those with corresponding cancers, such as mesothelioma, sarcoma, leukemia, lymphoma, melanoma, primary GI cancer, and metastatic lung and breast tumors.
Monitor VS for decreasing BP and increasing HR and RR outside of acceptable parameters as noted in "desired outcome." If noted, report them immediately.	Indicators of cardiopulmonary decompensation, which signals need for prompt treatment.
Make sure patient maintains bedrest during febrile period and understands rationale for doing so.	Febrile episodes require increased metabolic activity. Increased physical activity during this time may present an energy demand the heart is unable to meet.

Continued

INTERVENTIONS	RATIONALES
Anticipate patient's needs by placing personal articles within easy reach.	To decrease patient's energy expenditure and hence demand on the heart.
Advise patient about importance of frequent rest periods during convalescence.	Energy expenditure during the recovery phase without corresponding rest cycles can result in setbacks and patient frustration.

●●● **Related NIC and NOC labels:** *NIC:* Energy Management; Environmental Management; Vital Signs Monitoring *NOC:* Energy Conservation; Activity Tolerance

Nursing Diagnosis:

Ineffective Breathing Pattern

related to decreased lung expansion secondary to fluid accumulation in the lungs (pleural effusion), pulmonary fibrosis, pneumonectomy, or lobectomy

Desired Outcome: Immediately following intervention, patient's breathing pattern moves toward eupnea.

INTERVENTIONS	RATIONALES
Auscultate breath sounds q2-4h (or as indicated by patient's condition).	Decreasing breath sounds or the presence of a pleural friction rub could signal impending deterioration of pulmonary status.
Monitor oximetry readings; report O_2 saturation ≤92%.	Many patients with altered pulmonary function receive supplemental oxygen at this saturation level, on either a continuous or prn basis.
Ensure patency of chest drainage system (see guidelines, p. 147, in "Pneumothorax/Hemothorax").	A malfunctioning chest drainage system can lead to respiratory distress.
Position patient in semi-Fowler's position.	Promotes maximum chest expansion by decreasing compression on the lungs by abdominal organs to facilitate respiratory function.
If hyperinflation therapy is prescribed, instruct patient in its use. Reinforce teaching and document patient's progress.	Expanding the alveoli during prolonged inspiration phase aids in preventing atelectasis and pulmonary consolidation and promotes oxygenation.
For patients with gross pleural effusion, provide the following instructions for apical expansion breathing exercises: - Sit upright. - Position fingers just below the clavicles. - Inhale and attempt to push upper chest wall against the pressure of the fingers. - Hold breath for a few seconds and then exhale passively.	Patients at increased risk for pleural effusion are those with corresponding cancers, including lymphoma, leukemia, mesothelioma, lung and breast cancers, and metastasis to the lung from other primary cancers. When performed at frequent intervals, this exercise will help expand involved lung tissues, minimize flattening of the upper chest, and mobilize secretions.

●●● **Related NIC and NOC labels:** *NIC:* Respiratory Monitoring; Positioning; Teaching; Procedure/Treatment; Oxygen Therapy *NOC:* Respiratory Status: Ventilation

Nursing Diagnosis:

Constipation

related to treatment with certain chemotherapy agents, narcotic analgesics, tranquilizers, and antidepressants; less than adequate intake of food and fluids because of anorexia, nausea, or dysphagia; hypercalcemia; spinal cord compression; mental status changes; decreased mobility; or colonic disorders

Note: For desired outcomes and interventions, see "Prolonged Bedrest," p. 75, for **Constipation;** and "General Care of Patients with Neurologic Disorders" for **Constipation,** p. 302.

Note: Patients with cancer should not go more than 2 days without having a bowel movement. Patients receiving Vinca alkaloids are at risk for ileus in addition to constipation. Preventive measures, such as use of senna products (Senokot) or docusate calcium with casanthranol, especially for patients taking narcotics, are highly recommended. In addition, all individuals taking narcotics should receive a prophylactic bowel regimen.

Nursing Diagnosis:

Diarrhea

related to chemotherapeutic drugs; antacids containing magnesium; radiation therapy to the abdomen or pelvis; enteral feedings; food intolerance; and bowel dysfunction, such as tumors, Crohn's disease, ulcerative colitis, and fecal impaction

Note: For desired outcomes and interventions, see "Ulcerative Colitis" for **Risk for Impaired Perineal/Perianal Skin Integrity** related to prolonged diarrhea, p. 000, and "Caring for Patients with Human Immunodeficiency Virus Disease" for **Diarrhea,** p. 574. For patients receiving chemotherapy with potential for causing diarrhea (e.g., 5-fluorouracil, CPT-11), instruct patient about the need for having an appropriate antidiarrheal medication (loperamide) available and other methods used to combat the effects of diarrhea (fluid replacement, addition of psyllium to the diet to provide bulk to stool, careful perineal hygiene). Advise patient to notify health care provider if experiencing more than three loose stools per day.

Nursing Diagnosis:

Risk for Disuse Syndrome

related to upper extremity immobilization secondary to discomfort, lymphedema, treatment-related injury, or infection after mastectomy or breast surgery

Desired Outcomes: Within the 24-hr period before surgery, patient verbalizes knowledge about importance of and rationale for upper extremity movements and exercises. On recovery, patient has full range of motion (ROM) of the upper extremity

INTERVENTIONS	RATIONALES
Consult surgeon before the breast surgery. Consider such factors as wound healing, suture lines, and extent of the surgical procedure.	To determine type of surgery anticipated and to develop an individualized exercise plan with the surgeon specific to patient's needs.
Encourage finger, wrist, and elbow movement.	To aid circulation, help minimize edema, and help maintain mobility in the involved extremity.
Elevate extremity as tolerated.	To decrease edema.
Have patient use affected arm for personal hygiene and activities of daily living (ADL). Add other exercises (clasping hands behind head and "walking" fingers up the wall) as soon as patient is ready.	To promote progressive exercise. After drains and sutures have been removed (usually 7-10 days postoperatively), patient should begin exercises that will enhance external rotation and abduction of the shoulder. Ultimately patient should be able to achieve maximum shoulder flexion by touching fingertips together behind the back.
For patients who have had an axillary dissection (with lumpectomy or radical mastectomy) avoid giving injections, measuring BP, or taking blood samples from affected arm. Remind patient about her lowered resistance to infection and importance of promptly treating any breaks in the skin.	Loss of lymph nodes alters lymph drainage, which may result in edema of the arm and hand, and increases risk of infection as well.
Advise patient to treat minor injuries with soap and water and to notify health care provider if signs of infection occur.	To help prevent infection or receive prompt treatment if it occurs.

INTERVENTIONS	RATIONALES
Advise patient to wear a Medic-Alert bracelet that cautions against injections and tests in involved arm.	To promote patient safety/infection prevention.
Advise patient to wear a thimble when sewing and a protective glove when gardening or doing chores that require exposure to harsh chemicals, such as cleaning fluids. Explain that cutting cuticles should be avoided and lotion should be used to keep the skin soft. An electric razor should be used for shaving the axilla.	To promote skin integrity and protect hand and arm from injury and subsequent infection.

●●● **Related NIC and NOC labels:** *NIC:* Exercise Therapy: Joint Mobility; Exercise Therapy: Muscle Control; Exercise Promotion; Teaching: Prescribed Activity/Exercise *NOC:* Mobility Level

Nursing Diagnosis:

Incontinence, Stress Urinary

related to temporary loss of muscle tone in the urethral sphincter after radical prostatectomy

Desired Outcome: Immediately following patient teaching, patient relates understanding of the cause of the temporary incontinence and the regimen that must be observed to promote bladder control. Within the 24-hr period following interventions, patient verbalizes understanding of bladder incontinence and reports attainment of better incontinence management.

INTERVENTIONS	RATIONALES
Explain to patient that there is potential for urinary incontinence after prostatectomy but that it should resolve within 6 mo. Describe the reason for the incontinence (temporary loss of muscle tone in urethral sphincter), using aids such as anatomic illustrations.	A knowledgeable patient is not only less anxious but more likely to comply with the treatment regimen.
Encourage patient to maintain adequate fluid intake of at least 2-3 L/day (unless contraindicated by an underlying cardiac dysfunction or other disorder).	Dilute urine is less irritating to the prostatic fossa, as well as less likely to result in incontinence. Paradoxically, patients with urinary incontinence often reduce their fluid intake to avoid incontinence.
Educate patient about dietary irritants that may increase stress incontinence and the importance of avoiding them.	Caffeine and alcoholic beverages are examples of irritants that may increase stress incontinence.
Establish a bladder routine with patient.	
Assess and document voiding pattern. Teach patient to keep a voiding diary that incorporates this information.	Documenting time, amount voided, amount of fluid intake, timing of fluid intake followed by voiding, and related information such as degree of wetness experienced (e.g., number of incontinence pads used in a day, degree of underwear dampness) and exertion factor causing the wetness (e.g., laughing, sneezing, bending, lifting) may help patient manage incontinence.
Determine amount of time between voidings. Establish a voiding schedule that does not exceed this time period.	This helps estimate amount of time patient can hold his urine and avoid incontinence episodes.
Assist patient with scheduling times for emptying bladder, such as (initially) q1-2h when awake and q4h at night. Provide patient and significant other with written copy of the schedule.	If successful, patient can then attempt to lengthen time intervals between voidings. **Note:** Patients need to empty their bladders at least q4h to reduce risk of urinary tract infection (UTI) caused by urinary stasis.
Teach patient Kegel exercises and their importance.	Kegel exercises strengthen pelvic area muscles, which will help regain bladder control.

Continued

INTERVENTIONS	RATIONALES

Assist patient with identifying the correct muscle groups.
 	
   To strengthen proximal muscle: Instruct patient to attempt to shut off urinary flow after beginning urination, hold for a few seconds, and then start the stream again. Explain that if this can be accomplished, the correct muscle is being exercised.
 	
   To strengthen distal muscle: Teach patient to contract the muscle around the anus as though to stop a bowel movement. **Note:** A common error when attempting to identify the correct muscle group is contraction of the buttocks, quadriceps, and abdominal muscles.
	The patient must first identify the correct muscle groups in order to perform Kegel exercises correctly.

Teach patient to repeat these exercises 10-20 times, 4 times/day.	These exercises require diligent effort to reverse incontinence and in fact may need to be done for several months before any benefit is obtained.
Remind patient to discuss any incontinence problems with health care provider during follow-up examinations.	To ensure follow-up treatment for this problem.

●●● **Related NIC and NOC labels:** *NIC:* Pelvic Muscle Control; Urinary Elimination Management; Urinary Habit Training *NOC:* Urinary Continence

Nursing Diagnosis:

Deficient Knowledge:

Side effects of antiandrogen therapy or bilateral orchiectomy

Desired Outcome: Immediately following patient education, patient verbalizes accurate knowledge about the extent and duration of body changes that result from antiandrogen therapy or bilateral orchiectomy.

INTERVENTIONS	RATIONALES
Inform patient of side effects of estrogen therapy and orchiectomy (e.g., breast enlargement, breast tenderness, loss of sexual desire, impotence). As indicated, teach him about the side effects of hormone therapy (e.g., luteinizing hormone–releasing hormone [LHRH] agonists, antiandrogens), including hot flashes, impotence, or diarrhea.	A knowledgeable patient likely will have less stress about his treatment, comply with the treatment regimen accordingly, and report side effects promptly for timely treatment.
For patients taking estrogen therapy, provide instruction about symptoms related to complications of heart failure, thrombophlebitis, and myocardial infarction, which should be reported to health care provider. Provide reassurance that most side effects will disappear after therapy has been discontinued.	Shortness of breath; orthopnea; dyspnea; pedal edema; unilateral leg swelling or pain; and left arm, left jaw, or chest pain can occur during estrogen therapy. A knowledgeable patient will be more likely to report these symptoms promptly to his health care provider for early treatment.
If appropriate, explain to patient that before initiating estrogen therapy, health care provider may prescribe radiation therapy to areolae of the breasts.	To minimize painful gynecomastia. However, this procedure will not decrease other side effects.
Assure patient undergoing orchiectomy that the procedure will not affect his ability to have an erection and orgasm but that he will not ejaculate.	This knowledge may bring some reassurance to the patient.

●●● **Related NIC and NOC labels:** *NIC:* Teaching: Procedure/Treatment *NOC:* Knowledge: Treatment Regimen

Nursing Diagnosis:

Deficient Knowledge:

Purpose, type, and management of venous access device (VAD)

Desired Outcome: Immediately following patient education, patient and significant other/caregiver verbalize accurate understanding about the VAD, including its purpose, appropriate management measures, and reportable complications.

INTERVENTIONS	RATIONALES
Determine patient's and caregiver's level of understanding of the purpose of a VAD.	A VAD can be used for venipunctures and administration of drugs, fluids, and blood products. Determining patient's and caregiver's current knowledge base will help the nurse devise an individualized teaching plan.
Provide a model of the device and explain the insertion procedure.	Visual aids augment understanding. Three types of VADs are generally used: tunneled catheters, nontunneled catheters, and implanted ports.
	Nontunneled catheters can be inserted at the bedside or in the clinic under local anesthesia. Tunneled central venous catheters and implanted ports are inserted in the operating room under sterile conditions and local anesthesia.
Explain that there may be mild discomfort, similar to a toothache, for 48 hr after the procedure. Reassure patient that discomfort responds readily to pain medication.	Explaining expected sensations and likely amelioration with analgesics reduces anxiety and provides patient with guidelines for reportable symptoms.
If possible, introduce patient and caregiver to another individual who has the device so that they may discuss their concerns with someone who has experienced insertion and care of a VAD.	Conversing with someone who has already undergone a procedure may increase knowledge, decrease anxiety, and provide another avenue of support.
Teach VAD maintenance care. Provide both verbal and written instructions, including educational materials provided by VAD manufacturer.	Maintenance care likely will be done while patient is at home, where written materials will serve as a reference.
If the VAD is not implanted, have patient or caregiver demonstrate maintenance care of the device. Provide 24-hr emergency number to call in the event of problems.	Patient/family should demonstrate dressing care, flushing technique, and cap-changing routine before hospital discharge. This demonstration will reinforce previous teaching and when done correctly provide emotional support that this care can be done when at home.
Teach patient about the type of catheter used.	*Nontunneled catheters:* inserted by venipuncture into the vessel of choice, usually basilic, cephalic, or medial cubital vein near or at the antecubital area or jugular or subclavian vein in the upper thorax. A peripherally inserted central catheter (PICC) is an example of a nontunneled catheter. Maintenance involves flushing daily and after each use with normal saline and heparinized solution and performing sterile dressing and cap changes. Refer to institutional policies for specific instructions. Nontunneled catheters usually are indicated for short-term therapy (1 wk to a few months). Patients and families in a home care setting may need to care for this catheter.
	Tunneled central venous catheters: inserted into a central vein with a portion of the catheter tunneled through subcutaneous tissue and exiting the body at a convenient area, usually the chest. Examples include Broviac, Hickman, and Groshong. Maintenance involves flushing daily or after each use with saline or heparinized saline solution

Continued

INTERVENTIONS	**RATIONALES**
	(Groshong catheters are flushed weekly or after use with plain saline; no heparinized solution is used); sterile dressing changes until insertion site is healed; and sterile cap changes. Refer to institutional policies for specific instructions.
Explain that a Dacron cuff encircles the catheter about 2 inches from the exiting end of the catheter.	Tissue grows into this cuff, helping to prevent catheter dislodgement and decreasing risk of microorganisms migrating along catheter surface and entering the bloodstream.
Explain purpose of multi-lumen catheter if one is used.	Multi-lumen catheters enable simultaneous infusions of medications, blood products, etc.
If patient's VAD is implanted, describe the port and explain its purpose.	Implanted ports are commonly inserted when long-term therapy is anticipated or lack of venous access is expected to be a chronic issue. An implanted port consists of a catheter inserted into a central or peripheral vein attached to a plastic or metal port sutured in place in a surgically created subcutaneous pocket, most commonly on the chest. Venous access ports are completely embedded under the skin and may have single or multiple access ports. Access to the port may be from the top or side, depending on port style. Because catheter components are internal, risk for infection is reduced and attention required from patients is minimal when the port is not accessed.
Caution that noncoring needles *must* be used to access the port.	Noncoring needles allow the system to reseal when the needle is removed and prevent damage to the port system.
Explain that the catheter should not be flushed with any syringe smaller than 10 ml.	Excess pressures are generated by smaller syringes.
Demonstrate applying pressure to sides of the port when removing needle.	This promotes ease of removal and hence patient comfort.
Explain and demonstrate maintenance procedures with implanted ports.	Maintenance involves preparation of the site for access with an antibacterial preparation solution (e.g., povidone-iodine solution) and flushing at least monthly or after each use with normal saline and heparinized solution. Refer to institutional policies for specific instructions. Implanted ports may be Hickman or Groshong type. (It may be necessary for the nurse to know the type the patient has to ensure that the catheter is flushed with the correct solution.)
Have patient return demonstration.	This demonstration will reinforce previous teaching and when done correctly will provide emotional support that this care can be done when at home.
Discuss potential complications associated with VADs, along with appropriate self-management measures.	A knowledgeable patient likely will identify and self-manage complications that arise or report them to health care provider as appropriate for timely treatment.
Infection: Teach how to assess exit site for erythema, swelling, local increased temperature, discomfort, purulent drainage, and fever >38° C (>100.4° F).	Infection at the catheter site may necessitate antibiotic therapy.
Bleeding: Teach how to apply pressure to the site. Instruct patient and caregiver to notify health team member if bleeding does not stop in 5 min.	A properly prepared patient is less likely to panic and more likely to act appropriately if bleeding occurs.
Clot in the catheter: Teach how to flush catheter without using excessive pressure.	Excessive pressure could damage or dislodge the catheter (particularly an implanted port).

Continued

INTERVENTIONS	RATIONALES
If flushing does not dislodge the clot, instruct patient and caregiver to notify health team member.	Both fibrin sheaths and small blood clots respond readily to urokinase therapy. The usual dose of urokinase is 5000-10,000 U. Suggested dwell time in the catheter is 30-60 min. It is not unusual for small blood clots or fibrin sheaths to develop on the end of the catheter. The most common manifestation of a fibrin sheath is the ability to infuse fluids with the inability to aspirate blood.
Disconnected cap: Teach how to tape all connections and importance of always carrying hemostats or alligator clamps with padded blades to prevent catheter tearing. Teach measures to take if the cap becomes disconnected (i.e., clamp the tubing and go to a local health care institution for cleansing of the catheter).	Catheters usually are clamped beyond the cap, so risk of life-threatening air embolus is unlikely.
Extravasation: Instruct patient to report pain, burning, and stinging in the chest, clavicle, or port pocket or along the subcutaneous tunnel during drug administration.	Although this is a relatively rare complication, it can cause severe damage if a chemotherapeutic vesicant is involved.

●●● **Related NIC and NOC labels:** *NIC:* Teaching: Procedure/Treatment *NOC:* Knowledge: Treatment Regimen

Nursing Diagnosis:

Acute Pain

related to disease process, surgical intervention, or treatment effects

Note: For desired outcome and interventions, see this nursing diagnosis in "Pain," p. 41.

Nursing Diagnosis:

Chronic Pain

related to direct tumor involvement; infiltration of tumor into nerves, bones, or hollow viscus; or postchemotherapy or postradiotherapy syndrome

Desired Outcome: Patient participates in a prescribed pain regimen and reports that pain associated with direct involvement or infiltration of the tumor and side effects associated with the prescribed therapy are reduced or at an acceptable level within 1-2 hr of intervention, based on a pain assessment tool (e.g., descriptive, numeric [on a scale of 0-10], or visual scale).

INTERVENTIONS	RATIONALES
After patient has undergone a complete medical evaluation of the physiologic cause of the pain, whether it is acute or chronic, and the most effective strategies for pain relief, review the evaluation and pain relief strategies with patient and significant other/caregiver.	To determine patient's level of understanding and reinforce findings, thereby promoting knowledge and compliance with pain relief strategies.

Continued

INTERVENTIONS	RATIONALES
Ensure ongoing assessment of pain at regularly scheduled intervals. Promptly report any change in pain pattern or new complaints of pain to health care provider.	Pain is dynamic, and competent management requires frequent assessment.
Include the following in pain assessment:	
- *Characteristics* (e.g., "burning" or "shooting" often describes nerve pain).	Not all types of pain are managed solely by opioid therapy. Characterizing pain accurately will result in better pharmacologic intervention and assist nurse in developing a customized plan that incorporates nonpharmacologic measures as well.
- *Location and sites of radiation.*	
- *Onset and duration.*	Determining precipitating factors (as with onset) may assist in preventing or alleviating pain.
- *Severity:* Use a pain scale that is appropriate and comfortable for patient (e.g., descriptive, numeric, or visual scale). For example, use of a numeric scale would require patient to rate pain from 0 (none) to 10 (worst).	Severe pain can signal complications such as internal bleeding or leaking of visceral contents. Using a pain scale provides an objective measurement that enables the health care team to assess effectiveness of pain management strategies. Optimally, patient's rated pain on a 0-10 scale is ≤4.
- *Aggravating and relieving factors.*	May assist in preventing or alleviating pain.
- *Previous use of strategies that have worked to relieve pain.*	Strategies that have worked in the past may work for current pain.
Assess patient's and caregiver's attitudes and knowledge about the pain medication regimen.	It is important to dispel any misperceptions about narcotic-induced addiction when chronic pain therapy is necessary. Many patients and their families have fears related to patient's ultimate addiction to narcotics. Fears of addiction may result in ineffective pain management.
Incorporate the following principles of pharmacologic management:	Pharmacologic management of pain is often the mainstay of treatment of chronic cancer pain.
- Administer opioid and nonopioid analgesics in the correct dose, at the correct frequency, and via the correct route.	Chronic cancer analgesia is more effective when given around the clock (at scheduled intervals) rather than as needed.
- Recognize and treat side effects of opioid analgesia early.	Side effects include nausea and vomiting, constipation, sedation, itching, and respiratory depression. The presence of these side effects does not necessarily preclude continued use of the drug.
- Use prescribed adjuvant medication, including tricyclic antidepressants, antihistamines, dextroamphetamines, steroids, phenothiazines, and anticonvulsants.	Adjuvant medications help increase efficacy of opioids and may minimize their objectionable side effects as well.
- Monitor for signs and symptoms of tolerance, and when it occurs discuss treatment with health care provider.	Patients with chronic pain often require increasing doses of opioids. Respiratory depression occurs rarely in these patients.
- Recognize the potential for physical dependence in patients taking opioids for a prolonged period. Reassure patient that this dependence is physiologic, not psychologic.	Opioids should not be stopped abruptly in these patients, but rather should be tapered gradually because withdrawal discomfort may occur.
- Use nonpharmacologic approaches, such as acupressure, biofeedback, massage, etc., when appropriate.	Adjuvant therapies are often very effective in enhancing effects of opioid therapy.

●●● **Related NIC and NOC labels:** *NIC:* Medication Management; Pain Management; Acupressure; Biofeedback; Simple Massage *NOC:* Comfort Level; Pain Control; Pain: Disruptive Effects

Nursing Diagnosis:

Sexual Dysfunction

(erectile dysfunction, body changes, impaired sexual self-concept, and infertility) *related to* the disease process; psychosocial issues; radiation therapy to the lower abdomen, pelvis, and gonads; chemotherapeutic agents, especially actinomycin D, alkylating agents, amsacrine, bleomycin, cytarabine, daunorubicin, epirubicin, methotrexate, mitomycin, procarbazine, and vinblastine; or surgery

Desired Outcome: Immediately following patient education, patient identifies potential treatment side effects on sexual and reproductive function and acceptable methods of contraception during treatment.

INTERVENTIONS	RATIONALES
Determine patient's readiness to discuss sexual concerns.	Gentle, sensitive, open-ended questions allow patients to signal their readiness to discuss concerns.
As appropriate, initiate discussion about effects of treatment on sexuality and reproduction.	The PLISSIT model provides an excellent framework for discussion. This four-step model includes the following: (1) **P**ermission—give the patient permission to discuss issues of concern; (2) **L**imited **I**nformation—provide patient with information about expected treatment effects on sexual and reproductive function, without going into complete detail; (3) **S**pecific **S**uggestions—provide suggestions for managing common problems that occur during treatment; and (4) **I**ntensive **T**herapy—although most individuals can be managed by nurses using the first three steps in this model, some patients may require referral to an expert counselor.
Assess impact of diagnosis and treatment on patient's sexual functioning and self-concept.	Sexual dysfunction affects every individual differently. It is important not to assume its meaning but rather explore it with the individual and allow him or her to give meaning to the changes.
If relevant, determine possibility of pregnancy before treatment is initiated.	Pregnancy will cause a delay in treatment. If treatment cannot be delayed, a therapeutic abortion may be recommended.
Discuss possibility of decreased sexual response or desire.	May result from side effects of therapy. Informing patient may allay unnecessary anxiety.
Encourage patient to maintain open communication with partner about needs and concerns. In the presence of symptoms related to therapy, suggest such interventions as taking a nap before sexual activity or using pain or antiemetic medication to help decrease symptoms. Other suggestions include using a water-based lubricant if dyspareunia or fatigue is a problem, changing the usual time of day for intimacy, or using supine or side-lying positions, which require the least expenditure of energy.	The nurse might use this discussion to suggest exploration of alternate methods of sexual fulfillment, such as hugging, kissing, talking quietly together, or massage. Encouraging open dialogue promotes intimacy and helps prevent ill feelings or emotional withdrawal by either partner.
Discuss possibility of temporary or permanent sterility, which can be a result of treatment.	This discussion could open the door to explaining possibility of sperm banking for men before chemotherapy treatment or oophoropexy (surgical displacement of ovaries outside the radiation field) for women undergoing abdominal radiation therapy.
Teach importance of contraception during treatment if relevant. Discuss issues related to timing of pregnancy after treatment. Suggest patient have genetic counseling before becoming a parent, as indicated.	Healthy offspring have been born from parents who have received radiation therapy or chemotherapy, but long-term effects have not been clearly identified.

Continued

INTERVENTIONS	RATIONALES
For patient undergoing lymphadenectomy for testicular cancer, explain that ejaculatory failure may occur if the sympathetic nerve is damaged but that erection and orgasm will be possible.	If ejaculatory failure does occur, patient should know that artificial insemination is possible because the semen flows back into the urine, from which it can be extracted, enabling the ovum to become impregnated artificially.
If appropriate, explain that a silicone prosthesis may be placed in the scrotum after orchiectomy. Consult health care provider about the potential for this procedure.	This will help the scrotum achieve a normal appearance.

●●● **Related NIC and NOC labels:** *NIC:* Sexual Counseling; Self-Esteem Enhancement; Reproductive Technology Management *NOC:* Sexual Functioning

Nursing Diagnosis:

Impaired Skin Integrity

related to pigmentation changes (malignant skin lesions)

Desired Outcomes: Patient's skin lesions do not exhibit evidence of infection. Immediately following patient education, patient verbalizes and demonstrates measures that promote skin comfort, healing, and infection management.

INTERVENTIONS	RATIONALES
Identify populations at risk for malignant lesions.	Individuals with primary tumors of the breast, lung, colon/rectum, ovary, or oral cavity and individuals with malignant melanoma, lymphoma, or leukemia are at risk for malignant skin lesions and should be told about this potential.
Identify common sites of cutaneous metastases.	These sites include anterior chest, abdomen, head (scalp), and neck and should be assessed in patients at risk.
Inspect skin lesions.	Their presence necessitates being alert to and documenting general characteristics, location and distribution, configuration, size, morphologic structure (e.g., nodule, erosion, fissure), drainage (color, amount, character), and odor so that changes can be detected and reported promptly.
Monitor for local warmth, swelling, erythema, tenderness, purulent drainage.	Indicators of infection, which can occur as a result of nonintact skin.
Perform the following skin care for nonulcerating lesions and teach these interventions to patient and significant other, as indicated:	Maintaining skin integrity reduces risk of infection.
- Wash affected area with tepid water and pat dry.	Excessively warm temperatures damage healing tissue.
- Avoid pressure on the area.	To prevent further damage to friable tissue.
- Apply dry dressing.	Protects area from exposure to irritants and mechanical trauma (e.g., scratching, abrasion).
- Apply occlusive dressings, such as Telfa, using paper tape.	To enhance penetration of topical medications.
- Teach patient to avoid wearing wool and corduroy.	These fabrics are irritating to the skin.
Perform the following skin care for ulcerating lesions and teach these interventions to patient and significant other, as indicated.	

Continued

INTERVENTIONS	RATIONALES
For cleansing and debriding:	
Use ½-strength hydrogen peroxide and normal saline solution, followed by a rinse with normal saline.	To irrigate and debride the lesion. Rinsing removes peroxide and residual wound debris.
Use cotton swabs or sponges to apply gentle pressure.	Using gentle pressure with these swabs or sponges debrides the ulcerated area and protects granulation tissue.
As necessary, gently irrigate using only a syringe.	If the ulcerated area is susceptible to bleeding, gentle pressure protects delicate granulation tissue.
Use soaks (wet dressings) of saline, water, Burow's solution (aluminum acetate), or hydrogen peroxide.	Methods of debridement.
Be sure to rinse hydrogen peroxide or aluminum acetate off the skin.	Failure to do so could result in further skin breakdown.
As necessary, use wet-to-dry dressings.	For gentle debridement.
For prevention and management of local infection:	
Irrigate and scrub with antibacterial agents, such as acetic acid solution or povidone-iodine.	To prevent/manage local infection.
Collect wound cultures as prescribed.	To determine presence of infection and optimal antibiotic therapy.
Apply topical antibacterial agents (e.g., sulfadiazine cream, bacitracin ointment) as prescribed.	For open areas susceptible to infection.
Administer systemic antibiotics as prescribed.	For wound that is more extensively infected.
To maintain hemostasis:	
Use silver nitrate sticks for cautery.	To maintain hemostasis in the presence of capillary oozing.
Use oxidized cellulose or pack the wound with Gelfoam or similar product.	For bleeding in larger surface areas.
To control odor:	
Cleanse wound and change dressings as frequently as necessary.	To control odor and promote patient comfort.
Collect specimens for culture and sensitivity of the wound drainage, as prescribed.	To determine presence of infection and optimal antibiotic therapy.
Use antiodor agents (e.g., open a bottle of oil of peppermint or place a tray of activated charcoal).	To control pervasive odor in patient's room.
Collaborate with an enterostomal therapy (ET) or wound care nurse as needed.	When wounds fail to respond to more traditional interventions, an ET or wound care nurse may provide alternate suggestions that may be more effective.
Also see "Providing Nutritional Support," p. 589, and "Managing Wound Care," p. 583.	Wound healing depends on adequate intake of nutrients for tissue synthesis.

●●● **Related NIC and NOC labels:** *NIC:* Skin Surveillance; Infection Protection; Medication Administration: Skin; Skin Care: Topical Treatments; Wound Care: Closed Drainage; Wound Irrigation *NOC:* Tissue Integrity: Skin and Mucous Membranes; Wound Healing: Secondary Intention

Nursing Diagnosis:

Ineffective Peripheral Tissue Perfusion

related to interrupted blood flow secondary to lymphedema

Desired Outcome: Within the 24-hr period following intervention/treatment, patient exhibits adequate peripheral perfusion as evidenced by peripheral pulses >2+ on a 0-4+ scale, normal skin color, decreasing or stable circumference of edematous site, bilaterally equal sensation, and ability to perform ROM in the involved extremity.

INTERVENTIONS	RATIONALES
Assess involved extremity for degree of edema, quality of peripheral pulses, color, circumference, sensation, and ROM.	To determine presence/degree of lymphedema and potential threat to limb from hypoxia. Patient populations at risk include those who have had a radical mastectomy, lymph node dissection (upper and lower extremities), blockage of the lymphatic system from tumor burden, radiation therapy to the lymphatic system, or any combination of these.
Elevate and position involved extremity on a pillow in slight abduction.	This position will decrease edema.
Encourage wearing loose-fitting clothing.	Tight-fitting clothing may cause areas of constriction, reducing lymph and blood flow, as well as creating potential areas for impaired skin integrity.
Consult physical therapist (PT) and health care provider about development of exercise plan.	To ensure mobility, which helps decrease edema by promoting lymph flow.
Suggest use of elastic bandages.	To promote a decrease of edema in mild, chronic cases.
Suggest use of compressive bandages or sequential compression devices.	To promote a decrease of edema in more severe cases.

●●● **Related NIC and NOC labels:** *NIC:* Circulatory Precautions; Positioning; Skin Surveillance
NOC: Tissue Perfusion: Peripheral

NURSING DIAGNOSES AND INTERVENTIONS SPECIFIC TO PATIENTS UNDERGOING CHEMOTHERAPY, IMMUNOTHERAPY, AND RADIATION THERAPY

Nursing Diagnosis:
Activity Intolerance

related to decreased oxygen-carrying capacity of the blood secondary to anemia occurring with some chemotherapeutic drugs, radiation therapy, chronic disease, or surgery; or related to decreased oxygenation secondary to chronic lung changes, lobectomy, or pneumonectomy

Desired Outcome: During ADL, patient rates perceived exertion at ≤3 on a 0-10 scale and exhibits tolerance to ADL as evidenced by RR 12-20 breaths/min with normal depth and pattern (eupnea), HR ≤100 bpm, and absence of dizziness and headaches.

INTERVENTIONS	RATIONALES
As patient performs ADL, be alert for dyspnea on exertion, dizziness, postural hypotension, palpitations, headaches, and verbalization of increased exertion level.	These are signs of activity intolerance and decreased tissue oxygenation. If these signs are present, patient may be at risk for falls, which necessitates implementation of safety measures.
Ask patient to rate perceived exertion (see "Prolonged Bedrest" for **Risk for Activity Intolerance,** p. 67).	A rate of perceived exertion (RPE) >3 is a sign of activity intolerance and usually necessitates stopping the activity.

Continued

INTERVENTIONS	RATIONALES
As prescribed, administer erythropoietin.	Epoetin alfa (Epogen, Procrit) is a synthetic form of erythropoietin that stimulates production of RBCs to treat anemia associated with cancer chemotherapy.
Teach importance of taking vitamin and iron supplements and intake of foods high in iron such as liver and other organ meats, seafood, green vegetables, cereals, nuts, and legumes.	To reverse the effects of anemia.
Teach relationship of fatigue and activity intolerance to patient's therapy.	Fatigue and activity intolerance are temporary side effects of chemotherapy or radiation therapy and will abate gradually when therapy has been completed. Understanding this relationship likely will help the patient cope better with the treatment.
Facilitate coordination of care providers to provide rest periods as needed between care activities.	Undisturbed rest periods of at least 90 min in duration will help regain energy stores. Frequent activity periods without associated rest periods may result in depleted energy stores and emotional exhaustion.
As indicated, monitor oximetry with patient at rest and during activity; report O_2 saturation ≤92%. Administer oxygen as prescribed and encourage deep breathing.	Saturation at this level indicates need for oxygen supplementation and may be necessary only during periods of activity.
Administer blood components as prescribed.	Infusing RBCs increases hemoglobin level and corrects anemia.
Double-check type and crossmatching with a colleague and monitor for and report signs of transfusion reaction.	To ensure accuracy and prevent life-threatening transfusion reactions.
Using mutually agreed-on goals (e.g., "Could you walk up and down the hall once, or twice?" or appropriate amount, depending on patient's tolerance), encourage gradually increasing activities to tolerance as patient's condition improves.	Mutually agreed-on goals likely will enhance compliance with activity, which will increase patient's activity tolerance.

●●● **Related NIC and NOC labels:** *NIC:* Activity Therapy; Energy Management; Mutual Goal Setting; Nutrition Management; Oxygen Therapy *NOC:* Activity Tolerance; Endurance; Energy Conservation

Nursing Diagnosis:

Disturbed Body Image

related to alopecia secondary to radiation therapy to the head and neck or administration of certain chemotherapeutic agents

Desired Outcome: Immediately following patient education about alopecia, patient discusses the effects alopecia has on self-concept, body image, and social interaction and identifies measures to prevent, minimize, or enable adaptation to alopecia.

INTERVENTIONS	RATIONALES
Discuss potential for hair loss with patient before treatment as follows:	Patient needs to be informed about expected hair loss, depending on type of therapy, to develop strategies for coping and adaptation.
- Radiation therapy of 1500-3000 cGy to the head and neck will produce either partial or complete hair loss, but it is temporary.	It may be reassuring for patient to know that hair loss is temporary and onset usually occurs within 5-7 days, with regrowth beginning 2-3 mo after the final treatment.

Continued

INTERVENTIONS	RATIONALES
- Radiation therapy >4500 cGy usually results in permanent hair loss.	Patient may need to develop strategies for permanent hair loss.
- Hair loss associated with chemotherapy is commonly delayed until about 2 wk after administration of chemotherapy.	Hair loss is temporary and related to specific agent, dose, and duration of administration. Patient should understand that regrowth usually begins 1-2 mo after the last treatment and often temporarily grows back a different texture. Common chemotherapeutic agents that cause alopecia include actinomycin D, amsacrine, bleomycin, cyclophosphamide, daunomycin, docetaxel, doxorubicin, epirubicin, etoposide (VP-16), topotecan (Hycamtin), idarubicin, ifosfamide, irinotecan (CPT-11), paclitaxel, teniposide, vinblastine, and vincristine.
Explore the impact hair loss has on patient's self-concept, body image, and social interaction.	Alopecia is an extremely stressful side effect for most people. For some men, beard loss is disturbing as well.
Caution patient about inadvisability of scalp hypothermia and tourniquet applications.	These measures during IV chemotherapy have not proved to be effective in minimizing hair loss and are contraindicated with some malignancies.
Suggest the following adaptive measures: cut hair short before treatment; select a wig before hair loss occurs, which will enable patients to match color and style of their own hair; wear a hair net or turban during hair loss to collect hair that falls out; use scarves, hats, caps, and turbans to cover the head; use makeup and accessories to enhance self-concept.	These measures may help minimize the psychologic impact of hair loss. Being prepared by having head coverings available when hair loss actually occurs may reduce anxiety surrounding the event. **Note:** Wigs are tax deductible and often are reimbursed by insurance with the appropriate prescription. Some centers and communities have wig banks that provide used and reconditioned wigs at no cost.
Inform patient that hair loss may occur on body parts other than the head.	Areas such as the axillae, groin, legs, eyes (eyelashes and eyebrows), and face also may lose hair. Loss of facial hair makes it difficult for makeup to stay on.
Instruct patient to keep head covered.	To minimize sunburn during summer and prevent heat loss during winter. Certain chemotherapy agents and radiation therapy may sensitize skin to sun exposure.
Provide information about alopecia available through community resources, such as the American Cancer Society's "Look Good, Feel Better" national program.	These are resources that promote adaptation to alopecia.

●●● **Related NIC and NOC labels:** *NIC:* Body Image Enhancement; Coping Enhancement; Counseling; Emotional Support; Self-Esteem Enhancement; Support Group *NOC:* Body Image; Self-Esteem

Nursing Diagnosis:

Risk for Infection

related to inadequate defenses secondary to myelosuppression that occurs with chemotherapy, radiation therapy, immunotherapy, or malignancy

Desired Outcomes: Patient is free of infection as evidenced by normothermia, BP ≥90/60 mm Hg, and HR ≤100 bpm. Immediately following patient education, patient identifies risk factors for infection, verbalizes early signs and symptoms of infection and reports them promptly to health care professional if they occur, and demonstrates appropriate self-care measures to minimize the risk of infection.

INTERVENTIONS	RATIONALES
Before administering chemotherapy, ensure that blood counts and other related laboratory studies are within accepted parameters per institutional policy.	Chemotherapy causes predictable drops in WBC, RBC, and platelet counts. Administering chemotherapy to individuals with counts below specified parameters may put them at risk for infection, bleeding, or worsening anemia.
Obtain the absolute neutrophil count (ANC) by using the following formula: ANC = (% of segmented neutrophils + % of bands) $\times$ Total WBC count - ANC of 1500-2000/mm^3 = no significant risk - ANC of 1000-1500/mm^3 = minimal risk - ANC of 500-1000/mm^3 = moderate risk - ANC of <500/mm^3 = severe risk	The ANC may be used to determine if patient is at unacceptable risk for infection when administering chemotherapy. Neutropenic precautions need to be initiated. Neutropenic precautions need to be initiated.
Assess each body system thoroughly.	To determine potential for and actual sources of infection.
Monitor VS, temperature, and invasive sites q4h.	Temperature $\geq$38° C (100.4° F), increased HR, decreased BP, and the following clinical signs: tenderness, erythema, warmth, swelling, and drainage at invasive sites; chills; and malaise are signs of infection. **Note:** Signs of infection may be absent in the presence of neutropenia. A fever of $\geq$38° C ($\geq$100.4° F) may be the *only* sign of infection in the neutropenic patient.
Assess for subtle changes in mental status: restlessness or irritability; warm and flushed skin; chills, fever, or hypothermia; increased urine output; bounding pulse; tachypnea; and glycosuria.	These are signs of impending sepsis, which often precede the classic signs of septic shock: cold, clammy skin; thready pulse; decreased BP; and oliguria. These signs should be reported promptly for timely intervention.
Avoid invasive procedures when possible.	To decrease risk of infection.
Place sign on patient's door indicating that neutropenic precautions are in effect for patients with ANC $\leq$1000/mm^3.	These patients are very vulnerable to infection.
Instruct all persons entering patient's room to wash hands thoroughly.	Washing hands is an important form of infection prevention.
Restrict individuals from entering who have transmissible illnesses.	Individuals with colds, influenza, chickenpox, or herpes zoster can transmit these illnesses to the patient.
Encourage patient to practice good personal hygiene.	To decrease risk of infection.
Notify health care provider immediately if patient's temperature is >38° C (>100.4° F).	A possible sign of infection necessitating an emergent CBC.
Initiate antibiotic therapy as prescribed within 1 hr when ANC is $\leq$500/mm^3 and patient is febrile.	Inasmuch as the only sign of infection in a neutropenic patient is fever, initiation of antibiotic therapy in a timely fashion is imperative.
Implement oral care routine: -Teach patient to use a soft-bristle toothbrush after meals and before bed (bristles may be softened even more by running them under hot water). -Inspect oral cavity daily, noting presence of white patches on the tongue or mucous membrane. -Administer nystatin (Mycostatin) swish and swallow or swish and spit as prescribed to prevent development of oral candidiasis. -Monitor for vesicles, crusted lesions that may signal herpes simplex; administer acyclovir if it is prescribed.	 To prevent injury to oral mucosa that could result in infection. To minimize risk of infection associated with nonintact oral mucosa. Individuals with prolonged neutropenia are at risk for candidiasis and other fungal, bacterial, and viral infections. To prevent or minimize herpetic infections in patients with prolonged neutropenia who are at risk for herpes.

Continued

INTERVENTIONS	RATIONALES
Encourage coughing, deep breathing, and turning.	To minimize risk of pneumonia and skin breakdown, which can lead to infection.
Avoid use of rectal suppositories, rectal temperature, or enemas. Caution patient to avoid straining at stool. Suggest use of stool softener.	To minimize risk of traumatizing rectal mucosa, thereby decreasing risk of infection. Patients with prolonged neutropenia are at increased risk for perirectal infection.
Teach patient to use electric shaver rather than razor blade; avoid vaginal douche and tampons; use emery board rather than clipper for nail care; check with health care provider before dental care; avoid all invasive procedures; use antimicrobial skin preparations before injections; change IV sites q48-72h or per protocol.	These measures help maintain skin integrity, thereby minimizing risk for infection.
Instruct patient to use water-soluble lubricant before sexual intercourse and avoid oral and anal manipulation during sexual activities. Patients should abstain from sexual intercourse during periods of severe neutropenia.	These measures decrease risk of introducing infection because of nonintact skin.
If indicated, advise patient to avoid the following: foods with high bacterial count (raw eggs, raw fruits and vegetables, foods prepared in a blender that cannot adequately be cleaned); bird, cat, and dog excreta; plants, flowers, and sources of stagnant water.	Although scientifically unproved, tradition holds that patient be taught these measures to avoid these potential sources of infection during periods of neutropenia.
As prescribed, administer colony-stimulating factors.	To minimize risk of myelosuppression associated with chemotherapy, especially for patients with a history of neutropenia with infections in the past.
For more information, see Appendix for "Infection Prevention and Control," p. 831.	

●●● **Related NIC and NOC labels:** *NIC:* Infection Protection; Medication Administration; Risk Identification; Teaching: Disease Process; Environmental Management; Skin Surveillance; Chest Physiotherapy; Nutrition Management; Oral Health Maintenance *NOC:* Immune Status; Infection Status

Nursing Diagnosis:

Risk for Injury

(to staff, patients, and environment) *related to* preparation, handling, administration, and disposal of chemotherapeutic agents

Desired Outcome: Chemotherapy exposure to staff and environment is minimized at all times by proper preparation, handling, administration, and disposal by individuals familiar with these agents.

INTERVENTIONS	RATIONALES
Implement the following measures: use a biologic safety cabinet (laminar flow hood); absorbent, plastic-backed pad placed on the work area; latex gloves (powder free and a minimum of 0.007-inch thick); full-length impervious (nonabsorbent) gown with cuffed sleeves and back closure; and goggles. Wear gloves and gowns during all handling and disposing of these agents.	These measures minimize potential for aerosolization with resultant inhalation and direct skin contact with chemotherapeutic drugs during preparation.

Continued

INTERVENTIONS	RATIONALES
Ensure that chemotherapy is prepared by pharmacists or specially trained and supervised personnel and administered by nurses familiar with the agents.	A chemotherapy administration certification course inclusive of clinical mentoring is highly recommended for nurses planning to administer chemotherapeutics to ensure safe preparation and handling of chemotherapy agents and management of complications such as spills and individual contact with these drugs.
Limit exposure to chemotherapy to individuals who are not pregnant or planning pregnancy.	Although no information is available regarding reproductive risks of handling chemotherapy drugs in workers who use a biologic safety cabinet and wear protective clothing, employees who are pregnant, planning a pregnancy (male or female), or breastfeeding or who have other medical reasons prohibiting exposure to chemotherapy may elect to refrain from preparing or administering these agents or caring for patients during their treatment and up to 48 hr after completion of therapy (OSHA, 1995).
Prime IV tubing with diluent, not with fluid containing the chemotherapy agent.	This enables the nurse to challenge the vein before infusing potentially tissue-irritating or damaging agents.
Use syringes and IV administration sets with Luer-Lok fittings.	To prevent accidental dislodgement of needles or tubing and an accidental chemotherapy spill.
When removing IV administration set, wear latex gloves and wrap sterile gauze around needle before removing it.	To prevent direct or aerosol contact with the drug.
Place all needles (which have not been crushed, clipped, or recapped), drugs, drug containers, and related material in a puncture-proof container that is clearly marked *Biohazardous Waste*. **Note:** Follow this procedure for disposal of immunotherapy waste as well.	Proper disposal of waste prevents accidental exposure to other workers and the environment.
Wear latex gloves (and impermeable gown and goggles if splashing is possible) when handling all body excretions for 48 hr after chemotherapy.	The drug is excreted through urine and feces and present in blood and body fluids for approximately 48 hr after chemotherapy.
Ensure that only specially trained personnel clean a chemotherapy spill using a spill kit.	Chemotherapy spills could result in inadvertent exposure to other health care workers, the public, other patients, and the environment, and therefore only staff properly trained in handling these agents should be allowed to manage a spill. Double-gloves, eye protection, and an appropriate, full-length gown will be worn. Absorbent pads are used to absorb liquid; solid waste is picked up with moist absorbent gauze; glass fragments are collected with a small scoop—never with hands. These areas are cleansed three times with a detergent solution. All waste is put in a biohazardous waste container.
Avoid any activity in which the hand goes to the mouth (e.g., eating, drinking, smoking) in any area in which the chemical is given or prepared.	Inadvertent ingestion of chemotherapeutic drug may occur.
In the event of skin contact with the drug, wash affected area with soap and water. Notify health care provider for follow-up care. If eye contact occurs, irrigate eye with water for 15 min and notify health care provider for follow-up care.	Chemotherapeutic drugs may be absorbed through skin and mucous membranes.

●●● **Related NIC and NOC labels:** *NIC:* Environmental Management: Worker Safety; Risk Identification; Area Restriction *NOC:* Safety Status: Physical Injury

Nursing Diagnosis:

Risk for Injury

(to staff, other patients, and visitors) *related to* risk of exposure to sealed sources of radiation, such as cesium-137 (^{137}Cs), iridium-192 (^{192}Ir), iodine-125 (^{125}I), or samarium-153 (^{153}Sm); or unsealed sources of radiation, such as iodine-131 (^{131}I) or phosphorus-32 (^{32}P)

Desired Outcome: Staff and visitors verbalize understanding about the potential dangers of radiation therapy and measures that must be taken to ensure safety.

INTERVENTIONS	RATIONALES
Assign patient a private room (with private bathroom) and place an appropriate radiation precaution sign on patient's chart, door, and ID bracelet.	To minimize radiation exposure risk to employees, other patients, and visitors. Most institutions have a radiation safety committee that assists in providing and enforcing guidelines to minimize radiation risks to employees and the environment (committee guidelines should be kept readily available). The committee approves certain rooms that may be used for patients undergoing radioactive treatment to minimize exposure to employees and other patients.
Follow radiologist or agency protocol for visitor restrictions.	To minimize radiation exposure risk to visitors. Visitors usually are restricted to 1 hr/day and should stand 6 ft from the bed.
Ensure that pregnant women and children younger than 18 yr do not enter the room.	Rapidly dividing cells (e.g., those of a fetus) are more susceptible to effects of radiation
Implement the two major principles involved in care of patients with radiation source: time and distance.	To ensure optimal care planning and staff and visitor safety. This will minimize amount of time spent in room of patients with radiation sources, thus reducing exposure time, and maximize distance from implant (e.g., if the implant is in patient's prostate, stand at head of bed [HOB]).
	Time: Staff members should not spend more than 30 min/shift with patient and should not care for more than two patients with implants at the same time. Staff should perform non-direct care activities in the hall (e.g., opening food containers, preparing food tray, opening medications). Linen should be changed only when it is soiled, rather than routinely, and complete bed baths should be avoided.
	Distance: Radiation exposure is greater the closer one is to the source.
Wear gloves when in contact with secretions and excretions of all patients treated with unsealed radiation sources. Flush toilet several times after depositing urine or feces from commode.	Fluids from patients with unsealed radiation sources are a source of radiation exposure.
	Note: Urine from individuals with sealed radiation is not a source of radiation exposure and can be discarded in the usual manner. However, patients with implanted ^{125}I seeds should save all urine so that it may be assessed for presence of seeds.
Save all linen, dressings, and trash from patients with sealed sources of radiation.	They will be analyzed by the safety committee representative before being discarding to ensure seeds have not been misplaced, which could result in accidental exposure to people or the environment.
Keep long, disposable forceps and a sealed box in the room at all times.	For their protection from radiation exposure in the event seeds are displaced, all staff members must use forceps but never hands to pick up the seeds.
Use disposable products for all patients with unsealed radiation. Cover all articles in the room with paper.	To prevent inadvertent radiation exposure via body fluids.

Continued

INTERVENTIONS	RATIONALES
Attach a radiation badge (dosimeter) to your clothing before entering the room.	To monitor amount of personal radiation exposure. According to federal regulations, radiation should not exceed 400 mrem/mo. Nurses who care for patients with radiation implants rarely receive this much exposure.

●●● **Related NIC and NOC labels:** *NIC:* Environmental Management: Safety; Area Restriction *NOC:* Safety Status: Physical Injury

Nursing Diagnosis:

Deficient Knowledge:

Type of, procedure for, and purpose of radiation implant (internal radiation) and measures for preventing and managing complications

Desired Outcome: Before radiation implant is inserted, patient and significant other/caregiver verbalize accurate understanding of implant type and procedure and identify measures for preventing and managing complications.

INTERVENTIONS	RATIONALES
Determine patient's and caregiver's level of understanding of the radiation implant. Explain afterloading or preloading, as indicated.	Knowledge level will determine content of the individualized teaching plan.
	Afterloading: The implant carrier is inserted in the operating room, and the radioactive source is inserted later.
	Preloading: Radioactive source is implanted with the carrier.
Explain that the implant is used to provide high doses of radiation therapy to one area.	This method spares normal tissue from radiation.
Explain that radiation precautions (see **Risk for Injury,** earlier) are necessary.	To protect health care team, other patients, and visitors.
Gynecologic implants: Explain that the following may occur: vaginal drainage, bleeding, or tenderness; impaired bowel or urinary elimination; and phlebitis. Instruct patient to report any of these or associated signs and symptoms.	An informed patient likely will report untoward signs and symptoms promptly to ensure timely treatment.
Explain that complete bedrest is required.	To prevent displacement of the implants. The HOB may be elevated to 30-45 degrees, and the patient may log roll from side to side. A urinary catheter is placed to facilitate urinary elimination.
Advise that a low-residue diet and medications may be prescribed.	To prevent bowel movements during implant period. Generally a bowel clean-out (oral cathartics and/or enemas until clear) is prescribed.
Teach patient to perform isometric exercises while on bedrest.	To minimize risk of contractures or muscle atrophy and promote venous return during bedrest.
Encourage patient to take analgesics routinely for pain or to request analgesic before pain becomes severe.	To keep pain at a minimal level. Prolonged stimulation of pain receptors results in increased sensitivity to painful stimuli and will increase amount of drug required to relieve pain.

Continued

INTERVENTIONS	RATIONALES
Explain importance and rationale for wearing antiembolism hose and performing calf-pumping and ankle-circling exercises while on bedrest. If prescribed, describe rationale for and use of sequential compression devices or pneumatic foot pumps.	To prevent the lower extremity venostasis, thrombophlebitis, and emboli that can occur during enforced bedrest.
Explain that ambulation will be increased gradually when bedrest no longer is required (see "Prolonged Bedrest," p. 67, for guidelines after prolonged immobility).	Gradual increments in ambulation will promote return to normal body function without undue stress on the body.
Explain that after radiation source has been removed, patient should dilate vagina via sexual intercourse or a vaginal dilator.	To prevent vaginal fibrosis or stenosis.
Head and neck implants:	
After a complete nutritional assessment, discuss measures for nutritional support during the implantation, such as a soft or liquid diet, a high-protein diet, and optimal hydration (>2500 ml/day). Explain that a nutritional consult may be necessary.	Irradiated tissues may be swollen, irritated, and painful, which may interfere with nutritional intake. A high-protein diet promotes healing.
Teach signs and symptoms of infection at the site of implantation.	Fever, pain, swelling, local increased warmth, erythema, and purulent drainage at the implantation site may occur. Patient should report these indicators promptly to ensure timely treatment
When appropriate, advise need for careful and thorough oral hygiene while the implant is in place.	Irradiated tissues are vulnerable to infection by bacteria, yeast, and viruses.
	Note: When implants are placed within tongue, palate, or other structures of the buccal cavity, patient should not perform oral hygiene. Oral hygiene will be specifically prescribed by health care provider and generally accomplished by the nurse. Improper mouth care could result in dislodgement of the device, pain, or improper cleansing.
Encourage patient to take analgesics routinely for pain or to request analgesic before pain becomes severe.	To ensure optimal pain management. Prolonged stimulation of pain receptors results in increased sensitivity to painful stimuli and will increase amount of drug required to relieve pain.
Advise patient to use a humidifier.	To aid in maintaining moist mucous membranes and secretions.
Teach alternative means for communication if patient's speech deteriorates. Consult speech therapist as appropriate.	Patient should be aware that cards, Magic Slate, pencil and paper, and picture boards are potential communication measures. Preparing patient before impairment likely would reduce anxiety.
Breast implants:	
Teach signs of infection that may appear in the breast.	Patient should be aware that pain, fever, swelling, erythema, warmth, and drainage at insertion site are indicators of infection and should be reported immediately for timely treatment.
Teach importance of avoiding trauma at implant site and keeping skin clean and dry.	To help maintain skin integrity, prevent infection, and promote healing.
Encourage patient to take analgesics routinely for pain or to request analgesic before pain becomes severe.	Pain is more efficiently managed when pain medications are administered promptly and before it becomes severe.
Prostate implants:	
Explain need for patient to use a urinal for voiding.	To ensure that urinary output is measured every shift and enable inspection of urine for presence of radiation seeds.

Continued

INTERVENTIONS	RATIONALES
Instruct patient or caregiver to report dysuria, decreasing caliber of stream, difficulty urinating, voiding small amounts, feelings of bladder fullness, or hematuria.	Localized inflammation from radiation may cause urinary obstruction.
Caution that patient's linen, dressings, and trash will be saved.	To enable examination for presence of seeds.
Encourage patient to take analgesics routinely for pain or to request analgesic before pain becomes severe.	Pain is more efficiently managed when pain medications are administered promptly and before it becomes severe. Prolonged stimulation of pain receptors results in increased sensitivity to painful stimuli and will increase amount of drug required to relieve pain.

●●● **Related NIC and NOC labels:** *NIC:* Preparatory Sensory Information; Teaching: Procedure/ Treatment; Radiation Therapy Management; Learning Readiness Enhancement *NOC:* Knowledge: Treatment Procedures; Knowledge: Treatment Regimen

Nursing Diagnosis:

Deficient Knowledge:

Chemotherapy drugs, appropriate self-care measures for minimizing side effects, and available community and educational resources

Desired Outcome: Before specific chemotherapeutic drugs are administered, patient and significant other/caregiver verbalize accurate knowledge about potential side effects and toxicities, appropriate self-care measures for minimizing side effects, reportable side effects, and available community and educational resources.

INTERVENTIONS	RATIONALES
Establish patient's and caregiver's current level of knowledge about patient's health status, goals of therapy, and expected outcomes.	Understanding knowledge level of patient and caregiver will facilitate development of an individualized teaching plan.
Assess patient's cognitive and emotional readiness to learn.	Teaching must be tailored to patient's comprehensive abilities. The denial process may prevent comprehension of teaching content.
Recognize barriers to learning. Define all terminology as needed. Correct any misconceptions about therapy and expected outcomes.	Barriers, including ineffective communication, inability to read, neurologic deficit, sensory alterations, fear, anxiety, or lack of motivation will affect patient's learning and the teaching plan.
Assess patient's and caregiver's learning needs and establish short-term and long-term goals with these individuals.	Identifying preferred methods of learning and amount of information they would like to receive enables the nurse to develop a teaching plan based on this information.
Use individualized verbal and audiovisual strategies. Give simple, direct instructions; reinforce this information frequently.	To promote learning and comprehension. Because anxiety may interfere with comprehension, repetition will help reinforce teaching.
Provide an environment free from distractions and conducive to teaching and learning.	A quiet setting free of distraction facilitates learning and retention.
Discuss drugs patient will receive. Provide both written and verbal information.	Patient should be able to verbalize accurate knowledge about route of administration, duration of treatment, schedule, frequency of laboratory tests, most common side effects and toxicities, follow-up care, and appropriate self-care.

Continued

INTERVENTIONS

RATIONALES

INTERVENTIONS	RATIONALES
Provide emergency phone numbers.	In the event patient develops fever or side effects of chemotherapy that require emergent intervention.
Provide educational materials from resources such as the American Cancer Society, National Cancer Institute, and pharmaceutical companies.	This information reinforces teaching.
Identify appropriate community resources that assist with transportation, costs of care, and skilled care as appropriate.	Community resources may provide comfort for families under stress and prevent psychosocial issues from interfering with the plan of care.

●●● **Related NIC and NOC labels:** *NIC:* Teaching: Procedure/Treatment; Learning Facilitation; Learning Readiness Enhancement; Chemotherapy Management *NOC:* Knowledge: Treatment Regimen; Knowledge: Treatment Procedures

Nursing Diagnosis:

Deficient Knowledge:

Purpose and procedure for external beam radiation therapy, appropriate self-care measures after treatment, and available educational and community resources

Desired Outcome: Before external radiation beam therapy is initiated, patient and significant other/caregiver identify its purpose and describe the procedure, appropriate self-care measures, goals of treatment, side effects, and available educational and community resources.

INTERVENTIONS

RATIONALES

INTERVENTIONS	RATIONALES
See first six interventions under **Deficient Knowledge: Chemotherapy, p. 24.**	
Provide information about treatment schedule, duration of each treatment, and number of treatments planned.	Outlining the plan of care reduces anxiety and assists patient and family with planning their lives and activities accordingly.
	Radiation therapy usually is given 5 days/wk, Monday through Friday. The treatment itself lasts only a few minutes; the majority of the time is spent preparing patient for treatment. Immobilization devices and shields are positioned before treatment.
Explain that the skin will be marked with permanent pinpoint dots called tattoos.	Tattoos assist technician in positioning radiation beam accurately.
However, if gentian violet is used, explain the importance of not washing the marks (see **Impaired Skin/Tissue Integrity, p. 35,** for more information).	
Caution patient that it is important not to use skin lotions or soaps unless approved by the radiation therapy provider.	Some products are not appropriate for use with radiation.
Discuss side effects that may occur with radiation treatment and appropriate self-care measures. See subsequent nursing diagnoses and interventions for more detail about local side effects and self-care measures.	Patient should be aware that systemic side effects include fatigue and anorexia; however, the most commonly occurring side effects appear locally (e.g., those associated with head and neck radiation include mucositis, xerostomia, altered taste sensation, dental caries, sore throat, hoarseness, dysphagia, headache, and nausea and vomiting).

Continued

INTERVENTIONS	RATIONALES
Provide a written copy of side effects specific to patient's site of radiation therapy. Explain that the National Cancer Institute has a booklet entitled "Radiation and You" that lists side effects and side effect management.	Supplemental written materials enhance knowledge and understanding.
Provide information about community resources for transportation to and from the radiation center and for skilled nursing care, as needed.	Stress associated with travel to a radiation center may interfere significantly with the lives of family members and may even give patient cause to terminate treatment. Home care nurses can assist patient and family at home as treatment progresses and side effects become more pronounced.

●●● **Related NIC and NOC labels:** *NIC:* Preparatory Sensory Information; Teaching: Procedure/Treatment; Radiation Therapy Management; Learning Readiness Enhancement *NOC:* Knowledge: Treatment Procedures; Knowledge: Treatment Regimen

Nursing Diagnosis:

Deficient Knowledge:

Immunotherapy and its purpose, potential side effects and toxicities, appropriate self-care measures to minimize side effects, and available community and education resources

Desired Outcome: Before immunotherapy is administered, patient and significant other/caregiver verbalize understanding of its purpose, potential side effects and toxicities, appropriate self-care measures to minimize side effects, reportable symptoms, and available community and education resources.

INTERVENTIONS	RATIONALES
See first seven interventions under **Deficient Knowledge:** Chemotherapy, p. 24.	
Discuss treatment plan and goals of treatment with patient and significant other. Provide verbal and written information, as well as educational materials.	A knowledgeable patient likely will feel less anxious and comply with the treatment plan. A knowledgeable family likely will support patient, provide encouragement, and assist with patient compliance.
Teach proper injection technique and site rotation schedule. Teach importance of recording site of injection, time of administration, side effects, self-management of side effects, and any medications taken, as well as proper disposal of needles. Teach proper handling and storage of medication (e.g., refrigeration).	These patients often give their own injections of interferon. A diary or log will facilitate self-care.
As appropriate, arrange for community nursing follow-up for additional supervision and instruction.	Home care nursing support may reinforce teaching, assist with patient monitoring, and provide emotional support to patient and family.
Teach expected side effects of interferon.	Fever, chills, and flulike symptoms are expected side effects of interferon.
Suggest that patient take acetaminophen, with health care provider's approval, to manage these symptoms.	Usual management strategy.

Continued

INTERVENTIONS	RATIONALES
Teach patient to monitor and record temperature 2 times/day and drink 2000 to 3000 ml fluid/day.	To detect fever, an expected interferon side effect, and replace fluid losses that can occur as a result.
Provide information about nutritional supplementation.	Dose-related anorexia and weight loss are other common side effects of interferon.

●●● **Related NIC and NOC labels:** *NIC:* Teaching: Procedure/Treatment; Learning Facilitation; Learning Readiness Enhancement; Medication Management; Teaching: Prescribed Medication *NOC:* Knowledge: Treatment Regimen; Knowledge: Treatment Procedures

Nursing Diagnosis:

Imbalanced Nutrition: Less than body requirements

related to nausea and vomiting or anorexia occurring with chemotherapy, radiation therapy, or disease; fatigue; or taste changes

Desired Outcomes: Immediately following patient education, patient and significant other/caregiver verbalize accurate understanding of basic nutritional principles and strategies to prevent weight loss and promote tissue healing. Within 7 days following interventions, patient reports improved appetite and/or increased nutritional intake and exhibits weight gain.

INTERVENTIONS	RATIONALES
For anorexia: Monitor for clinical signs of malnutrition. See "Providing Nutritional Support" for **Imbalanced Nutrition,** p. 592. Weigh patient daily.	Nausea, vomiting, anorexia, and taste changes all may contribute to weight loss.
Assess patient's food likes and dislikes, as well as cultural and religious preferences related to food choices.	Providing foods on patient's "like" list as often as feasible and avoiding foods on "dislike" list optimally will promote sufficient intake. However, foods previously enjoyed may become undesirable, whereas previously disliked foods may appeal.
Explain that anorexia can be caused by pathophysiology of cancer, surgery, and side effects of chemotherapy and radiation therapy.	Taste and olfactory receptors have a high rate of cell growth and may be sensitive to chemotherapy and radiation therapy.
Teach importance of increasing caloric intake.	To increase energy, minimize weight loss, and promote tissue repair.
Teach importance of increasing protein intake.	To facilitate repair and regeneration of cells.
Suggest that patient eat several small meals at frequent intervals throughout the day.	Smaller, more frequent meals are usually better tolerated than larger meals.
Encourage use of nutritional supplements.	To promote nutritional intake that will meet body requirements.
Consider use of megestrol acetate, thalidomide, or prednisone. Consult patient's health care provider accordingly.	These agents have proved to have a positive influence on appetite stimulation and weight gain in individuals with cancer.
For nausea and vomiting: Assess patient's pattern of nausea and vomiting: onset, frequency, duration, intensity, and amount and character of emesis.	Knowledge about the pattern of nausea and vomiting enables use of proper medication, route, and timing.

Continued

INTERVENTIONS	RATIONALES
Explain that nausea and vomiting may be side effects of chemotherapy and radiation therapy. (Nausea and vomiting also may occur with advanced cancer, bowel obstruction, some medications, or metabolic abnormalities.)	The pathophysiology of nausea and vomiting is complex and involves transmission of impulses to receptors in the brain. Various antiemetics work at different points in the nausea/vomiting cycle.
Teach patient to take antiemetic 1-2 hr before chemotherapy as directed and to continue to take the drug as prescribed; also consider duration of previous nausea and vomiting episodes following chemotherapy. Explain that antiemetics are most effective if taken at nausea onset.	To cover the expected emetogenic period of the chemotherapy agent given. Nausea is better controlled when the goal is prevention.
Teach patient to eat cold foods or food served at room temperature.	The odor of hot food may aggravate nausea.
Suggest intake of clear liquids and bland foods.	Strong odors and tastes can stimulate nausea or suppress appetite.
Teach patient to avoid sweet, fatty, highly salted, and spicy foods, as well as foods with strong odors.	Same as above.
Minimize stimuli such as smells, sounds, or sights.	Previous stimuli associated with nausea may provoke anticipatory nausea.
Encourage patient to eat sour or mint candy.	To decrease unpleasant, metallic taste.
If not contraindicated, teach patient to take oral chemotherapy at bedtime.	To minimize incidence of nausea.

Encourage patient to explore various dietary patterns:
 	
    - Avoid eating or drinking for 1-2 hr before and after chemotherapy if anticipatory nausea occurs.
 	
    - Follow a clear liquid diet for 1-2 hr before and 1-24 hr after chemotherapy if nausea is present.
 	
    - Avoid contact with food while it is being cooked; avoid being around people who are eating.
 	
    - Eat small, light meals at frequent intervals (5-6 times/day).
	Some patients become nauseated in anticipation of chemotherapy. Reducing food intake at this time may lessen this symptom.
	
	Prolonged exposure to smells can extinguish appetite or promote nausea.
	
	Presenting large volumes of food can be overwhelming, thereby extinguishing the appetite or causing nausea.

Suggest that patient sit near an open window.	Breathing fresh air when feeling nauseated may relieve nausea.
Help patient find an appropriate distraction technique (e.g., music, television, reading).	Helping patient focus on things other than nausea may be helpful in nausea management.
Teach patient to use relaxation techniques. See **Health-Seeking Behaviors:** Relaxation technique effective for stress reduction, p. 183.	This technique may help prevent anticipatory nausea and vomiting.
For fatigue: If patient is easily fatigued, encourage eating small meals frequently. Document intake.	The energy required to consume and digest a large meal may exacerbate fatigue and discourage further nutritional intake.
Provide foods that are easy to eat.	"Finger foods" (e.g., crackers with cheese or peanut butter, nuts, chunks of fruit, smoothies) require less energy expenditure to eat and enable patient to eat in a position of comfort rather than sitting at a table, which requires more energy.
If patient uses supplemental oxygen during periods of exertion, encourage using it while eating.	Food consumption requires energy. A fatigued, hypoxic person likely will consume less food.
Avoid offering meals immediately after exertion.	A fatigued person will be less likely to want to eat and will tire quickly while eating, which also requires energy expenditure.

Continued

INTERVENTIONS	RATIONALES
For taste changes: Suggest that patient try foods not previously enjoyed.	Previously enjoyed foods may no longer seem attractive, whereas foods that were once undesirable may now seem pleasant.
Encourage good mouth care; assess mucous membrane for thrush, lesions, or stomatitis.	Thrush infections can cause taste alterations yet are easily treated. A coated tongue may interfere with ability to taste.
Suggest that patient try strongly flavored foods.	Patients often report that usual foods taste like sawdust.

●●● **Related NIC and NOC labels:** *NIC:* Fluid Monitoring; Nutrition Monitoring; Teaching: Prescribed Diet; Weight Gain Assistance; Sustenance Support *NOC:* Nutritional Status: Nutrient Intake; Nutritional Status: Food and Fluid Intake

Nursing Diagnosis:

Impaired Oral Mucous Membrane

related to treatment with chemotherapy agents (especially antitumor antibiotics), antimetabolites, and Vinca alkaloids; radiation therapy to head and neck; ineffective oral hygiene; gingival diseases; poor nutritional status; and thrush infection secondary to treatment

Desired Outcomes: Patient complies with therapeutic regimen within 12-24 hr of instruction. Patient's oral mucosal condition improves within 3 days following interventions as evidenced by intact oral mucous membrane; moist, intact tongue and lips; and absence of pain and lesions.

INTERVENTIONS	RATIONALES
In the presence of myelosuppression, caution patient not to floss teeth or use a stiff toothbrush.	The oral cavity is a prime site for infection in a myelosuppressed patient. Actions such as brushing with a stiff toothbrush and flossing could affect integrity of the oral mucous membrane and place patient at risk for infection.
For patient with moderate to severe stomatitis, administer parenteral analgesics, such as morphine, as prescribed.	To relieve pain and promote adequate nutritional intake.
For patients with xerostomia (dryness of the mouth from a lack of normal salivary secretion) caused by radiation, suggest chewing sugarless gum; sucking sugarless candy, frozen fruit juice pops, or sugar-free popsicles; or taking frequent sips of water. Saliva substitutes are another option, although they are expensive and do not last long.	To replenish oral hydration and promote mucous membrane integrity. A dry mouth also interferes with nutritional intake.
Advise patient that close dental follow-up is essential.	Lack of or decrease in salivary fluid predisposes patient to dental caries. Fluoride treatment is recommended for these patients for this reason.

●●● **Related NIC and NOC labels:** *NIC:* Oral Health Restoration; Chemotherapy Management; Fluid Management; Pain Management; Oral Health Maintenance *NOC:* Oral Health; Tissue Integrity: Skin and Mucous Membranes

Nursing Diagnosis:

Ineffective Protection

related to risk of bleeding/hemorrhage secondary to thrombocytopenia (for all patients receiving chemotherapy and radiation therapy, as well as those with cancer, particularly involving the bone marrow)

Desired Outcome: Patient is free of signs and symptoms of bleeding as evidenced by negative occult blood tests, HR ≤100 bpm, and systolic BP ≥90 mm Hg.

INTERVENTIONS	RATIONALES
Identify platelet counts that place individuals at increased risk for bleeding.	Platelets 150,000-300,000/mm³ = normal risk for bleeding. Platelets <50,000/mm³ = moderate risk for bleeding. Initiate thrombocytopenic precautions. Platelets <20,000/mm³ = severe risk of bleeding. Patient may develop spontaneous bleeding; initiate thrombocytopenic precautions. Platelets <10,000/mm³ = **critical** risk of bleeding.
Perform a baseline physical assessment, monitoring for evidence of bleeding.	Petechiae, ecchymosis, hematuria, coffee ground emesis, tarry or bloody stools, hemoptysis, heavy menses, epistaxis, headaches, somnolence, mental status changes, confusion, and blurred vision signal evidence of bleeding and should be reported promptly for timely intervention.
Also monitor VS every shift or with each appointment if patient is not hospitalized.	Hypotension and tachycardia are signs that signal bleeding and should be reported promptly for timely intervention.
Report systolic BP >140 mm Hg.	Patient may be at risk for intracranial bleeding caused by higher blood pressure.
Avoid use of rectal thermometer (use a tympanic thermometer when available).	To prevent inadvertent injury that would result in bleeding.
Test all secretions and excretions.	They may contain occult blood.
Perform a psychosocial assessment, including patient's past experience with thrombocytopenia; the effect of thrombocytopenia on patient's lifestyle; and changes in patient's work pattern, family relationships, and social activities.	To help identify learning needs and necessity of skilled care after hospital discharge. It also provides nurse with information regarding patient's coping skills and possible need for psychosocial support.
Place a sign on patient's door, indicating that thrombocytopenia precautions are in effect for patients with platelet count <50,000/mm³.	For patient's safety to notify all who enter that patient is at risk for bleeding.
In the presence of bleeding, begin pad count for heavy menses (discourage use of tampons); measure quantity of vomiting and stool; elevate (when possible).	Tampons may cause inadvertent trauma during placement with resultant bleeding.
Apply direct pressure and ice to site of bleeding (VAD, venipuncture); and deliver platelet transfusion as prescribed.	To ensure that bleeding has ceased after venipuncture or port access before leaving patient.
Initiate oral care at frequent intervals. Advise patient to brush with soft-bristle toothbrush after meals and before bed (hot water run over bristles may soften them further). In the presence of gum bleeding, teach patient to use sponge-tipped applicator rather than toothbrush, avoid dental floss, and avoid mouthwash with more than 6% alcohol content.	To promote integrity of gingiva and mucosa, which will prevent unnecessary bleeding and reduce risk of infection.
Suggest use of normal saline solution mouthwashes 4 times/day and water-based ointment for lubricating lips.	Alcohol may irritate impaired oral tissues.

Continued

INTERVENTIONS	**RATIONALES**
Implement bowel program and check with patient daily for bowel movement.	Daily monitoring of bowel pattern promotes early intervention for constipation. If patient's platelet level is critically low, straining at stool must be avoided to prevent intraabdominal bleeding.
Assess need for stool softeners or psyllium.	To prevent constipation and straining, which could lead to bleeding.
Encourage adequate hydration (at least 2500 ml/day) and high-fiber foods.	To promote stools that are soft and with added bulk, both of which will facilitate bowel movements.
Avoid use of rectal suppositories, enemas, or harsh laxatives.	To minimize risk of bleeding/infection from inadvertent trauma to rectal mucosa.
Teach patient measures that reduce risk of bleeding.	Patient should use electric shaver rather than razor; apply direct pressure and elevation for 3-5 min after injections and venipuncture; and avoid vaginal douche and tampons, constrictive clothing, aspirin or aspirin-containing products (because of aspirin's antiplatelet action), alcohol ingestion, anticoagulants, and nonsteroidal antiinflammatory drugs (NSAIDs). In addition, patient should perform gentle nose blowing, use emery board rather than clippers for nail care, check with health care provider before seeking dental care, and avoid bladder catheterization if possible.
When appropriate, instruct patient to abstain from sexual intercourse when the platelet count is <50,000/mm^3. Instruct patient to use water-soluble lubrication during sexual intercourse.	To maintain integrity of vaginal tissue and prevent bleeding.
Caution patient to remove hazardous objects or furniture from environment. Advise caretaker to assist with ambulating if patient's physical mobility is impaired.	To reduce possibility of trauma or injury that could result in bleeding.
When platelet count is <20,000/mm^3, teach patient to avoid moving up in bed, straining at stool, bending at the waist, and lifting heavy objects (>10 lb). Suggest bedrest if patient's platelet count is <10,000/mm^3.	To prevent Valsalva's and other maneuvers that increase intracranial pressure and therefore place patient at increased risk for intracerebral bleeding.
Avoid invasive procedures when possible. Use smaller-gauge needles if punctures are necessary and apply gentle pressure at puncture site until bleeding stops.	To minimize risk of bleeding.
See "Thrombocytopenia," p. 525, for more information.	

●●● **Related NIC and NOC labels:** *NIC:* Bleeding Precautions; Hemorrhage Control *NOC:* Coagulation Status

Nursing Diagnosis:

Disturbed Sensory Perceptions: Auditory, Tactile, and Kinesthetic

related to use of chemotherapeutic drugs such as cisplatin, cytarabine, 5-fluorouracil, high–dose methotrexate, nitrosoureas, paclitaxel, or Vinca alkaloids

Desired Outcome: Patient reports early signs and symptoms of ototoxicity and peripheral neuropathy; measures are implemented promptly to minimize these side effects.

INTERVENTIONS	RATIONALES
Explain that tinnitus or decreased hearing can occur with use of cisplatin.	These problems usually are dose related and a result of cumulative side effects. Most commonly, high-frequency hearing loss occurs, although with cumulative doses, speech-frequency hearing range also may be affected but is less common.
Suggest that patient face the speaker and watch speaker's lips during conversation.	Teaches patient skills with which to cope with hearing loss and maintain communicative skills.
Suggest patient use hearing aids for a trial before purchase.	A hearing aid may be helpful, or it may amplify background noise and worsen speech comprehension.
In instances of hearing loss from cisplatin, refer patient to community resources for hearing-impaired persons.	Hearing loss from cisplatin is usually irreversible.
Monitor patient for development of peripheral neuropathy. Inform patient that severity of symptoms may abate when treatment is halted; however, recovery can be slow and usually is incomplete.	Peripheral neuropathy can occur with several antineoplastic agents. Neurotoxicity is cumulative with some chemotherapy drugs, and therefore assessment of symptoms is done before delivery of each dose. The first symptom usually is numbness and tingling of the fingers and toes, which can progress to difficulty with fine motor skills, such as buttoning shirts or picking up objects. The most severely affected individuals may lose sensation at hip level and have difficulty with balance and ambulation.
Instruct patient to report early signs and symptoms.	The earlier the patient reports these signs and symptoms, the more timely will be the interventions to minimize them.
Suggest consultation with PT or occupational therapist (OT).	To evaluate and maximize functional capacity, as well as assist with environmental modifications.
Monitor bowel elimination daily in individuals at risk for paralytic ileus associated with neuropathy.	Patients taking vincristine or vinblastine are at risk and require monitoring for this problem.
Administer stool softeners, psyllium, or laxatives daily if patient has not had a bowel movement within a 48-hr period or as prescribed. As indicated, instruct patient to increase fluid intake to 2000-3000 ml/day.	If constipation is a problem, patient should be placed on a bowel regimen. Prevention of constipation is easier than treating constipation.

●●● **Related NIC and NOC labels:** *NIC:* Communication Enhancement: Hearing Deficit; Environmental Management: Safety; Peripheral Sensation Management; Exercise Therapy: Balance; Exercise Therapy: Ambulation *NOC:* Communication: Receptive Ability; Sensory Function: Proprioception; Sensory Function: Cutaneous; Balance

Nursing Diagnoses:

Impaired Skin Integrity and Impaired Tissue Integrity

(or risk for same) *related to* treatment with chemical irritants (chemotherapy)

Desired Outcomes: Before chemotherapy is initiated, patient identifies potential side effects of chemotherapy on the skin and tissue and measures that will maintain skin/tissue integrity and promote comfort. After chemotherapy has been initiated, patient relates the presence of intact or improving skin and tissue integrity.

Note: Skin reactions include the following: transient erythema/urticaria, hyperpigmentation, telangiectasis, photosensitivity, hyperkeratosis, acnelike reaction, ulceration, and radiation recall. Finger-nails may develop half-moon markings called "Beau's lines," which are clinically insignificant.

INTERVENTIONS	RATIONALES
Transient erythema/urticaria: Perform and document pretreatment assessment of patient's skin.	Pretreatment assessment will enable a more accurate assessment of the posttreatment reaction. Alterations of skin or nails that occur in conjunction with chemotherapy are a result of destruction of the basal cells of the epidermis (general) or of cellular alterations at the site of chemotherapy administration (local). Transient erythema/urticaria may be generalized or localized at the site of chemotherapy administration. It may be caused by several agents, including doxorubicin hydrochloride (Adriamycin), bleomycin, L-asparaginase, mithramycin, and mechlorethamine.
Assess onset, pattern, severity, and duration of the reaction after treatment.	Reactions are specific to the agent used and vary in onset, severity, and duration. Usually they occur soon after chemotherapy is administered and disappear in several hours.
Hyperpigmentation: Inform patient before treatment that this reaction is to be expected and will disappear gradually when the course of treatment is finished.	Hyperpigmentation is believed to be caused by increased levels of epidermal melanin-stimulating hormone. It can occur on the nail beds, on the oral mucosa, or along the veins used for chemotherapy administration, or it can be generalized. Hyperpigmentation is associated with many chemotherapeutic agents, but incidence is highest with alkylating agents and antitumor antibiotics. In addition, it can occur with tumors of the pituitary gland.
Caution patient to wear sunscreen with a high SPF ($\geq$15) and to cover exposed areas.	Sunlight may exacerbate hyperpigmentation.
Telangiectasis (spider veins): Inform patient that this reaction is permanent but that the vein configuration will become less severe over time	Telangiectasis is believed to be caused by destruction of the capillary bed and occurs as a result of applications of topical carmustine and mechlorethamine.
Photosensitivity: Assess onset, pattern, severity, and duration of the reaction.	Photosensitivity can occur during the time the agent is administered, or it can reactivate a skin reaction caused by sun exposure when the agent is administered in close proximity to sun exposure. It may be caused by bleomycin, dacarbazine, dactinomycin, daunorubicin, doxorubicin hydrochloride, fluorouracil, methotrexate, and vinblastine.
Teach patient to avoid exposing skin to the sun. Advise patient to wear protective clothing and use an effective sun-screening agent (SPF of 15 or greater). Caution patient regarding tanning booths as well.	Photosensitivity is enhanced when skin is exposed to ultraviolet light. Acute sunburn and residual tanning can occur with short exposure to the sun.
In the event that burning takes place, advise patient to treat it like a sunburn.	Such measures as taking a tepid bath and using moisturizing cream are usually effective.
Hyperkeratosis: For patients taking bleomycin, assess for presence of skin thickening and loss of fine motor function of the hands.	Hyperkeratosis presents as a thickening of the skin, especially over hands, feet, face, and areas of trauma. It is disfiguring and causes loss of fine motor function of the hands.
In the presence of skin thickening, assess for fibrotic lung changes: dyspnea, cough, tachypnea, crackles.	Hyperkeratosis may be an indicator of more severe fibrotic changes in the lungs that usually are not reversible.
Reassure patient that skin thickening is usually reversible when bleomycin has been discontinued.	Patient will be less anxious knowing the condition is reversible.

Continued

INTERVENTIONS	RATIONALES
Acnelike reaction: Explain cause of the skin reaction and reassure patient that it is temporary.	An acnelike reaction presents as erythema, especially of the face, and progresses to papules and pustules, which are characteristic of acne and will disappear when the drug is discontinued.
Suggest that patient use a commercial preparation, such as benzoyl peroxide lotion, gel, or cream.	To treat and conceal blemishes.
Teach patient about proper skin care:	
- Avoid hard scrubbing.	Scrubbing can cause skin breaks that enable bacterial entry.
- Avoid use of antibacterial soap. Use a plain soap, such as Ivory or Camay.	Removal of nonpathogenic bacteria on the skin results in replacement by pathogens, which are implicated in the genesis of acne.
- Avoid oil-based cosmetics.	Oil can clog pores and trap bacteria.
Ulceration: Assess for ulceration.	Ulceration presents as a generalized, shallow lesion of the epidermal layer and may be caused by several chemotherapeutic agents.
Treat ulcers with a solution of $\frac{1}{4}$-strength hydrogen peroxide and $\frac{3}{4}$-strength normal saline q4-6h; rinse with normal saline solution.	To cleanse the lesions.
Expose the ulcer to the air, if possible.	A dark, moist, warm environment may promote bacterial growth and delay healing.
Be alert to presence of infection at the ulcerated site.	Local warmth, swelling, tenderness, erythema, and purulent drainage may be present at the site of ulceration and should be reported to health care provider for treatment.
Radiation recall reaction: Explain why radiation recall can occur and its signs and symptoms.	Radiation recall reaction occurs when chemotherapy is given at the same time as or after treatment with radiation therapy. It presents as erythema and may be followed by dry desquamation at the radiation site. More severe reactions can progress to vesicle formation and wet desquamation. After the skin heals, it is permanently hyperpigmented. This reaction is most often associated with dactinomycin and doxorubicin.
Teach patient preventive measures that may lessen severity of radiation recall reaction.	Preventive strategies that may lessen severity of radiation recall reaction include the following: - Avoiding wearing tight-fitting clothes, harsh fabrics, excess heat or cold exposure to the area, salt water or chlorinated pools, deodorants, perfumed lotions, cosmetics, and shaving of the area. - Using mild detergents, such as Ivory Snow. - For pruritus, using corticosteroid cream (triamcinolone acetonide 0.1%). Diphenhydramine (25 mg q6h) may be prescribed for severe pruritus.

●●● **Related NIC and NOC labels:** *NIC:* Skin Surveillance; Bathing; Medication Administration: Skin; Chemotherapy Management; Skin Care: Topical Treatments; Wound Care; Infection Protection; Infection Control; Teaching: Procedure/Treatment *NOC:* Tissue Integrity: Skin and Mucous Membranes; Wound Healing: Secondary Intention

Nursing Diagnoses:

Impaired Skin Integrity and Impaired Tissue Integrity

related to radiation therapy

Desired Outcomes: Before radiation therapy, patient identifies potential skin reactions and the management interventions that will promote comfort and skin integrity. After initiation of radiation therapy, patient relates the presence of intact or improving skin/tissue integrity.

INTERVENTIONS	RATIONALES
Assess degree and extensiveness of the skin reaction.	Severe skin reactions may necessitate a delay in radiation treatments.
	The degree and extensiveness of the skin reaction are described by the following stages:
	- **Stage I:** inflammation, mild erythema, slight edema.
	- **Stage II:** inflammation; dry desquamation; dry, scaly, itchy skin.
	- **Stage III:** inflammation, edema, wet desquamation, blisters, peeling.
	- **Stage IV:** skin ulceration and necrosis, permanent loss of hair in the treatment field, suppression of sebaceous glands. *Late effects:* fibrosis and atrophy of the skin, fibrosis of the lymph glands.
Teach patient the following skin care measures for the treatment field:	Enables patient to self-treat or obtain specialized help for skin reaction stage.
- Cleanse skin gently and in a patting motion, using a mild soap, tepid water, and a soft cloth. Rinse the area and pat it dry.	Stage I reactions often do not require special interventions other than gentle, normal skin care.
- Apply cornstarch, A&D ointment, ointments containing aloe or lanolin, or mild topical steroids as prescribed.	Care for skin with stage II reaction.
- Cleanse area with ½-strength hydrogen peroxide and normal saline, using an irrigation syringe. Rinse with saline or water and pat dry gently	Care for skin with stage III reaction.
- Use nonadhesive absorbent dressings, such as Telfa or Adaptic and an ABD pad for draining areas. Be alert to indicators of infection.	
- Use moisture-permeable and vapor-permeable dressings, such as hydrocolloids and hydrogels, on noninfected areas. Care for skin with stage III reaction.	
- Apply topical antibiotics (e.g., sulfadiazine cream, bacitracin ointment) to open areas prone to infection.	Care for skin with stage IV reaction.
- Debride wound of eschar (necessary before healing can occur).	
- After removing eschar (results in yellow-colored wound), keep the wound clean. Wet-to-moist dressings often are used to keep the wound clean and prevent infection.	
- Collaborate with an ET nurse as needed on wound-healing techniques.	

●●● **Related NIC and NOC labels:** *NIC:* Skin Surveillance; Bathing; Medication Administration: Skin; Radiation Therapy Management; Skin Care: Topical Treatments; Wound Care; Infection Protection; Teaching: Procedure/Treatment *NOC:* Tissue Integrity: Skin and Mucous Membranes; Wound Healing: Secondary Intention

Nursing Diagnosis:

Impaired Swallowing

related to esophagitis secondary to radiation therapy to the neck, chest, and upper back or use of chemotherapy agents, especially the antimetabolites; obstruction (tumors); or thrush

Desired Outcomes: Before food or fluids are given, patient exhibits the gag reflex and is free of symptoms of aspiration as evidenced by RR 12-20 breaths/min with normal depth and pattern (eupnea), normal skin color, and the ability to speak. Immediately following instruction, patient verbalizes accurate knowledge of the early signs and symptoms of esophagitis, alerts health care team as soon as they occur, and identifies measures for maintaining nutrition and comfort.

INTERVENTIONS	RATIONALES
Monitor patient for evidence of impaired swallowing with concomitant respiratory difficulties.	Esophagitis can occur with radiation therapy to the neck, chest, and upper back or be caused by chemotherapy agents, tumors, or thrush. Impaired swallowing places patient at risk for aspiration and necessitates aspiration precautions.
Teach patient early signs and symptoms of esophagitis.	Sensation of lump in the throat with swallowing, difficulty with swallowing solid foods, and discomfort or pain with swallowing occur early in esophagitis. Patient should report these indicators promptly to staff if they occur so that timely interventions can be made.
Monitor patient's dietary intake and provide the following guidelines:	Impaired swallowing predisposes patient to nutritional deficits. Dietary intake should be monitored closely to evaluate early weight loss trends.
- Maintain a high-protein diet.	To promote healing.
- Eat foods that are soft and bland.	To minimize pain while swallowing.
- Add milk or milk products to the diet (for individuals without excessive mucous production); add sauces and creams to foods.	An efficient way to add protein, fat, and calories to the diets of patients with swallowing difficulties.
Ensure adequate fluid intake of at least 2 L/day.	Patients with impaired swallowing are at risk for dehydration because they may avoid drinking and eating to prevent pain.
Implement the following measures and discuss them with patient accordingly:	
- Use a local anesthetic, as prescribed. Lidocaine 2% and diphenhydramine may be taken via swish and swallow before eating.	Reducing pain associated with swallowing will assist in maintaining adequate nutritional intake. **Caution:** These anesthetics may decrease patient's gag reflex.
- Suggest that patient sit in an upright position during meals and for 15-30 min after eating.	Esophageal reflux may occur with obstructions and can be distressing.
- Administer mild analgesics, such as liquid ASA or acetaminophen, as prescribed.	Discomfort may prevent patient from maintaining adequate nutritional intake. If pain is unrelieved with mild analgesics, an opioid such as oxycodone or morphine may be necessary.
- If prescribed, give patient sucralfate	Sucralfate helps protect esophageal mucosa from further destruction.
- Encourage frequent oral care with normal saline or sodium bicarbonate solution.	Impaired mucous membranes are at risk for infection with bacteria, yeast, and viruses.
- Teach patient to avoid irritants such as alcohol, tobacco, and alcohol-based commercial mouthwashes.	Irritants exacerbate discomfort and may prevent intake of adequate nutrients.

Continued

INTERVENTIONS	RATIONALES
Suction mouth as needed, using low, continuous suction equipment.	To manage secretions and prevent aspiration.
Teach patient to expectorate saliva into tissues and dispose of tissues in nearby waste cans.	Intervention to manage oral secretions using proper infection control measures.

●●● **Related NIC and NOC labels:** *NIC:* Aspiration Precautions; Airway Suctioning; Positioning; Risk Identification; Nutrition Management *NOC:* Aspiration Control; Swallowing Status

Nursing Diagnosis:

Impaired Tissue Integrity

(or risk for same) *related to* extravasation of vesicant or irritating chemotherapy agents

Desired Outcomes: After chemotherapy administration, patient's tissue remains intact without evidence of inflammation or pain along the injection site. If, however, extravasation does occur, it is treated as quickly as possible with minimal damage to patient's tissue.

INTERVENTIONS	RATIONALES
Ensure that vesicant chemotherapy is administered by a nurse who is experienced in venipuncture and knowledgeable about chemotherapy.	Vesicant agents have the potential to produce tissue damage and therefore should be administered by a nurse skilled in venipuncture. Vesicant agents include dactinomycin, daunomycin, doxorubicin, mitomycin C, epirubicin, estramustine, idarubicin, mechlorethamine, mitoxantrone, paclitaxel, vinblastine, vincristine, vindesine, and vinorelbine. The following irritants have the potential to produce pain along the injection site with or without inflammation: amsacrine, bleomycin, carmustine, dacarbazine, doxorubicin liposome, etoposide, ifosfamide, plicamycin, streptozocin, docetaxel, and teniposide.
Select IV site carefully, using a new site if possible.	Ideally the IV site will be newly accessed for vesicant administration. A site >24 hr old should be avoided because it is difficult to ensure vessel integrity.
Avoid sites such as the antecubital fossa, wrist, or dorsal side of the hand.	In these sites there is increased risk of damage to underlying tendons or nerves if extravasation occurs.
Assess patency of IV line before and during administration of the drug. Instruct patient to report burning, itching, or pain immediately.	Extravasation of vesicants often causes immediate symptoms. Prompt reporting of these symptoms by the patient will enable early intervention to minimize tissue damage.
Assess entry site at frequent intervals. Instruct patient to report discomfort at the site promptly.	Erythema and swelling around the needle site and patient discomfort are common with extravasation. Early intervention at the site of extravasation minimizes tissue damage.
Caution: Do not use blood return solely as an indicator that extravasation has not occurred.	Blood return is possible in the presence of extravasation.
Ensure that extravasation kit is readily available, along with institutional guidelines for extravasation management.	Not all vesicants have antidotes. When administering vesicants with known antidotes, the antidote should be readily available in combination with the extravasation kit. Because time is of the essence to minimize tissue destruction when extravasation occurs, institutional guidelines or extravasation kit must be readily accessible before initiating drug delivery.

Continued

INTERVENTIONS	RATIONALES
In the event of extravasation, follow these general guidelines:	
- Stop infusion immediately and aspirate any remaining drug from the needle. To do this, first attach syringe to the tubing and aspirate the drug.	To remove as much drug as possible from extravasated site and thereby limit tissue exposure.
- Consult health care provider.	To obtain directions for extravasation management.
- Leave needle in place if indicated.	For access if an antidote is to be used with the extravasated drug.
- Attach syringe containing the recommended antidote and instill antidote per procedural guidelines. Remove IV needle from the site.	The antidote neutralizes any remaining drug, which ideally will prevent tissue damage. However, not all vesicant drugs have known antidotes.
- If recommended, inject extravasated site with the antidote, using a tuberculin (TB) syringe and a 25- to 27-gauge needle.	Procedure to follow if IV catheter already has been removed.
- Do not apply pressure to the site. Apply a sterile occlusive dressing, elevate site, and apply heat or cold as recommended.	Pressure may cause added tissue damage.
- Document incident, noting date, time, needle insertion site, VAD type and size, drug, drug concentration, approximate amount of drug that extravasated, patient symptoms, extravasation management, and appearance of the site. Check institutional guidelines regarding necessity of photo documentation. Monitor the site at frequent intervals.	Documentation of actions taken ensures accuracy should questions arise later about how the extravasation was managed. Photos provide a reference point for evaluation.
- Provide patient with information about site care and follow-up appointments for evaluation of extravasation. If appropriate, collaborate with health care provider regarding a plastic surgery consultation.	Tissue damaged by extravasation may take a long time to heal or may deteriorate so much that plastic surgery may be necessary. Patient needs to understand these possibilities to ensure optimum extravasation management.

●●● **Related NIC and NOC labels:** *NIC:* Chemotherapy Management; Medication Management
NOC: Tissue Integrity: Skin and Mucous Membranes

Nursing Diagnosis:

Impaired Urinary Elimination

related to hemorrhagic cystitis secondary to cyclophosphamide/ifosfamide treatment; oliguria or renal toxicity secondary to cisplatin or high-dose methotrexate administration; renal calculi secondary to hyperuricemia; or dysuria secondary to cystitis

Desired Outcomes: Patients receiving cyclophosphamide/ifosfamide test negative for blood in their urine, and patients receiving cisplatin exhibit urine output of ≥100 ml/hr 1 hr before treatment and 4-12 hr after treatment. Patients with leukemia and lymphomas and those taking methotrexate exhibit urine pH ≥6.5 before infusion.

INTERVENTIONS	RATIONALES
Ensure adequate hydration during treatment and for at least 24 hr after treatment for patients taking cyclophosphamide (Cytoxan), ifosfamide, methotrexate, and cisplatin. Teach patient importance of drinking at least 2-3 L/day. (IV hydration also may be required, especially with high-dose chemotherapy.)	Adequate hydration ensures sufficient dilution of the drug by urine in the urinary system and prevents exposure of renal cells to high drug concentrations and possible toxicity. Renal failure also may ensue when cellular breakdown products deposit in the renal tubules when patient has been inadequately hydrated before chemotherapy given for leukemia or lymphoma.

Continued

INTERVENTIONS	**RATIONALES**
Administer cyclophosphamide early in the day. Encourage patients to void q2h during the day and before going to bed.	To minimize retention of metabolites in the bladder during the night.
Test urine for presence of blood and report positive results to health care provider.	Hemorrhagic cystitis can occur in patients taking cyclophosphamide/ifosfamide and should be reported promptly to ensure timely intervention.
Monitor I&O q8h during high-dose treatment for 48 hr after treatment. Be alert to decreasing urinary output.	Most chemotherapy drugs are eliminated from the body within a 48-hr period. Maintaining adequate urine output for 48 hr prevents high drug metabolite concentrations in the kidneys and bladder.
Ensure that mesna is administered before ifosfamide and then 4 hr and 8 hr after the infusion (or via a continuous infusion).	To minimize risk of hemorrhagic cystitis with ifosfamide or cyclophosphamide.
Test all urine for the presence of blood.	Ifosfamide and cyclophosphamide can cause hemorrhagic cystitis.
Promote fluid intake to maintain urine output at approximately 100 ml/hr. Monitor I&O during infusion and for 24 hr after therapy to ensure that this level of urinary output is attained.	Adequate fluid intake and resultant urinary output ensure that drug metabolites in high concentrations do not stay within the urinary system for prolonged periods.
For patients receiving cisplatin, prehydrate with IV fluid (150-200 ml/hr). Monitor I&O hourly for 4-12 hr after therapy.	To ensure that urine output is maintained at ≥100-150 ml/hr, which decreases potential for nephrotoxicity, a potential side effect of cisplatin. Patients may require diuretics to maintain this output. Cisplatin can be administered as soon as urine output is 100-150 ml/hr.
Promote fluid intake for at least 24 hr after treatment, especially for patients taking diuretics. Notify health care provider promptly if urine output drops to <100 ml/hr in the hospitalized patient.	Continual flushing of the urinary system prevents concentration of cisplatin metabolites in the kidneys and potential associated nephrotoxicity. Urine output should be kept at a relatively high level.
In patients with leukemia or lymphoma, monitor I&O q8hr, being alert to a decreasing output, and test urine pH with each voiding to ensure that it is >6.5.	If cellular breakdown products that occur from the chemotherapy effect on tumor cells are allowed to concentrate in the renal tubules, renal failure can occur. Proper hydration prevents this potential cause of renal failure. Alkaline urine will promote excretion of the uric acid that results from tumor lysis associated with treatment of leukemia and lymphoma.
Administer sodium bicarbonate or acetazolamide (Diamox) as prescribed.	These agents alkalinize the urine.
Administer allopurinol as prescribed.	Allopurinol prevents uric acid formation and is often administered before chemotherapy for patients with leukemia or lymphoma.
Monitor leukemia and lymphoma patients for the presence of urinary calculi. For more information, see "Ureteral Calculi," p. 273.	Urinary calculi can occur as a result of hyperuricemia caused by chemotherapy treatment of leukemia and lymphoma, which causes rapid cell lysis and increased excretion of uric acid.
Teach patient signs of cystitis: fever, pain with urination, malodorous or cloudy urine, and urinary frequency and urgency. Instruct patient to notify health care provider if these signs and symptoms occur.	Cystitis can occur as a result of cyclophosphamide and ifosfamide treatment and should be reported to patient's health care provider for timely intervention.

●●● **Related NIC and NOC labels:** *NIC:* Urinary Elimination Management; Fluid Management; Medication Management *NOC:* Urinary Elimination

Pain

Nursing Diagnosis:

Acute Pain or Chronic Pain

related to disease process, injury, or surgical procedure

Desired Outcome: Subjective report of pain, use of a pain scale (e.g., report of ≤4 on a 0-10 scale), behavioral indicators, report of family, and/or physiologic indicators reflect an acceptable level of pain within 1-2 hr of intervention (depending on drug, route of administration, and peak action of the drug used).

Note: The right drug is the one that works with the fewest side effects.

INTERVENTIONS	RATIONALES
Obtain a thorough pain history, including previous/ongoing pain experiences, previously used methods of pain control and what was/was not effective, patient's attitude toward pain medication, and the effect of pain on activities of daily living (ADL).	A pain history enables development of a systematic approach to pain management for each patient, using information gathered from pain history and the hierarchy of pain measurement (self-report, pathologic conditions or procedures that usually cause pain, behavioral indicators, report of family, and physiologic indicators). Agency for Health Care Policy and Research (AHCPR) and American Pain Society (APS) state self-report of pain is the single most reliable indicator of pain.
Teach patients that pain management is part of their treatment.	Patients have the right to appropriate assessment and management of their pain (JCAHO, 2002).
Assess for pain at frequent intervals. Use a formal patient-specific method of assessing self-reported pain when possible, including description, location, intensity, and aggravating/alleviating factors. Use the selected scale consistently. Educate patient about pain assessment tools as appropriate.	The first step of effective pain management is accurate assessment of pain. Numerical rating scales of 0 (no pain) to 10 (worst possible pain) and descriptive scales are commonly used for adults who are cognitively intact. The FACES pain rating scales may be useful for children and elderly and cognitively impaired adults.
Assess for behavioral and physiologic responses to pain.	Behavioral and physiologic responses are potential indicators of pain in patients who are unable to self-report.
	Behavioral responses: Examples include facial expression (grimacing, facial tension), vocalization (moaning, groaning,

INTERVENTIONS	RATIONALES
	sighing, crying), verbalization (praying, counting), body action (rocking, rubbing, restlessness), and behaviors (massaging, guarding, short-attention span, irritability, sleep disturbance). Behavioral examples may be seen in patients with impaired communication, including those who are cognitively impaired, unconscious, or conscious but unable to communicate.
	Physiologic responses: Examples include diaphoresis, vasoconstriction, increased or decreased BP (≥15% from baseline), increased pulse rate (≥15% from baseline), pupillary dilation, change in respiratory rate (usually increased to >20 breaths/min), muscle tension or spasm, and decreased intestinal motility (evidenced by nausea, vomiting). Physiologic indicators may reflect pain as a result of autonomic stimulation of the sympathetic and parasympathetic responses.
Evaluate patient's health history for evidence of alcohol and drug (prescribed and nonprescribed) use. Ensure that surgeon, anesthesiologist, and other health care providers are aware of any significant findings. Consult a pain management team if available.	Other drug use could affect effective doses of analgesics. All care providers must be consistent in setting limits while providing effective pain control through pharmacologic and nonpharmacologic methods. Psychiatric or clinical pharmacology consultation may be necessary.
Administer analgesics according to the World Health Organization (WHO) three-step analgesic ladder.	The WHO analgesic ladder focuses on selecting analgesics and adjuvants based on pain intensity. The WHO analgesic ladder has been endorsed by the AHCPR Guidelines (1994) and the American Pain Society (1999).
	The three steps include:
	- Level one: nonopioid +/– adjuvant
	- Level two: opioid for mild to moderate pain, +/– nonopioid, +/– adjuvant
	- Level three: opioid for moderate to severe pain, +/– nonopioid, +/– adjuvant
Recognize that choice of agents is based on three general considerations: therapeutic goal, patient's medical condition, and drug cost. Additional considerations are patient's previous experience with a specific agent and recall of side effects experienced with a specific agent.	Individualized therapeutic goal and the stage of illness/disease process are important factors in agent selection to maximize pain relief and minimize potential of adverse side effects. The difference in cost of different drugs used to accomplish the same goal may be large. Where there is no proven or expected benefit of using one drug in preference to another to accomplish a desired goal, the less costly drug should be considered.
As indicated/prescribed, titrate the dose to achieve the desired effect.	Initial effect and duration of action may differ vastly from very low in the elderly and acutely ill to very high in the young adult or chronic alcohol/drug user. The goal is to develop a safe and effective pain management plan.
Recognize that the preferred route is the one that is least invasive while achieving adequate relief:	Aversion to painful routes of delivery (e.g., SC, IM) may lead to underreporting of pain by patients and to undermedication by nurses. Choice of route may be based on convenience, anticipated analgesic requirements, side effects, and cost.
- Oral: often optimal.	Oral route is convenient and flexible and produces relatively steady analgesia.
- IV: alternative for those unable to take PO medications or for quick onset. Consider patient-controlled analgesia (PCA).	IV route is used for agents with quick time to onset of analgesia and for severe pain.

Continued

INTERVENTIONS	RATIONALES
- IM analgesia: APS suggests that this route be used rarely, and AHCPR Acute Pain Practice Guidelines suggest that it be avoided when possible.	IM analgesia is inconsistent, is less titratable, and can cause complications such as hematoma, granuloma, infection, aseptic tissue necrosis, and nerve injury.
- Transdermal, subcutaneous, and epidural: other routes that may be considered.	
As prescribed, administer nonopioid agents.	For relief of mild-to-moderate pain that may be associated with surgery, trauma, soft tissue injury, and inflammatory conditions.
	Nonopioid agents include salicylates (acetylsalicylic acid [Aspirin]), para-aminophenol derivatives (acetaminophen [Tylenol]), nonsteroidal antiinflammatory drugs (NSAIDs: ibuprofen [Motrin, Advil, Nuprin], naproxen [Naprosyn, Anaprox], ketorolac [Toradol]), and indoleacetic acids (indomethacin [Indocin]).
Assess for return of gastrointestinal (GI) function (presence of bowel sounds, absence of vomiting) before administering oral agents.	To ensure optimal absorption of the drug.
Recognize that NSAIDs are very effective when combined or used with centrally acting opioid analgesics.	NSAIDs have peripheral effects and a different mechanism of action compared with centrally acting opioid analgesics. They also have a dose-sparing effect and may contribute to reduction of opioid side effects. Unless contraindicated, APS recommends use of nonopioid agents even if pain is severe enough to require addition of an opioid. NSAIDs offer varying degrees of antipyretic, antiinflammatory, and analgesic actions.
As prescribed, administer opioid (e.g., morphine) analgesic.	For pain of greater severity that may be associated with major trauma, major surgery, and cancer. Morphine is the standard of comparison for opioid analgesics.
Administer meperidine (Demerol) with caution.	Normeperidine, a metabolite of meperidine, is a central nervous system (CNS) excitotoxin, which with repetitive dosing may produce anxiety, muscle twitching, and seizures. Patients with impaired renal function and patients taking monoamine oxidase (MAO) inhibitors are particularly at risk. Recommended use is for <48 hr for acute pain in patient without renal or CNS dysfunction or dose <600 mg/24 hr (APS, 1999).
Caution: Do not use naloxone to attempt to reverse normeperidine toxicity.	Naloxone does not reverse normeperidine toxicity and may potentiate hyperexcitability.
Administer mixed agonist-antagonist agents as prescribed in patients who are unable to tolerate other opioids.	Mixed agonist-antagonist agents such as butorphanol (Stadol) and pentazocine (Talwin) produce analgesia by binding to the opioid receptors while blocking or remaining neutral to the mu receptors. To date, there is no convincing evidence that agonist-antagonists offer any advantage over morphine-like agonists in the treatment of acute pain (Hoskin & Hanks, 1991).
Caution: Do not administer mixed agonist-antagonist analgesics concurrently with morphine or other pure agonists.	Reversal of analgesic effects may occur.
Reassess pain level frequently and assess for side effects: • Routinely at scheduled intervals (i.e., q2-4h with VS). • With each report of pain. • Following pain medication administration based on time of onset and duration of action of prescribed and administered agents.	To monitor for level of pain relief and evidence of side effects, including sedation and respiratory depression. More opioid is required to produce respiratory depression than to produce sedation. Sedative effects precede respiratory depression. Close monitoring of the level of sedation and respiratory status may prevent respiratory depression.

Continued

INTERVENTIONS	RATIONALES
In the presence of an increasing level of sedation, increase the frequency of monitoring and reduce the amount or frequency of the dose as prescribed.	To decrease the level of sedation and risk of respiratory depression.
Have naloxone (Narcan) readily available.	To reverse severe respiratory depression.
If use of naloxone is necessary, titrate with caution.	Too much too fast can precipitate severe pain, hypertension, tachycardia, and even cardiac arrest (Brimacombe et al., 1991).
Caution: Monitor older adults and individuals with chronic obstructive pulmonary disease (COPD), asthma, and other respiratory disorders closely when they are receiving opioid analgesics. Consider using reduced doses and titrate carefully.	Elderly who are opioid naïve and patients with coexisting conditions are at higher risk of respiratory depression (Pasero & McCaffrey, 1994).
Check analgesic record for the last dose and amount of medication given during surgery and in postanesthesia recovery room. Be careful to coordinate timing and dose of postoperative analgesics with previously administered medication.	To manage pain effectively without overdosing or underdosing.
Administer prn analgesics before pain becomes severe. Consider conversion to scheduled dosing with supplemental prn analgesics when pain exists for ≥12 hr out of 24 hr.	Prolonged stimulation of pain receptors results in increased sensitivity to painful stimuli and will increase the amount of drug required to relieve pain. **Note:** Addiction to opioids occurs infrequently in hospitalized patients.
Administer intermittently scheduled analgesics $\frac{1}{2}$ hr before painful procedures and ambulating and at bedtime.	This ensures that peak effect of analgesic is achieved at inception of the activity or procedure.
As prescribed, consider using analgesic adjuvants, such as anticonvulsants, antihistamines, and benzodiazepines.	These agents are used to augment and prolong analgesia, not specifically to treat isolated anxiety, depression, etc.
Administer tricyclic antidepressant agents as prescribed.	Tricyclic antidepressant agents produce analgesia while improving mood and sleep. Amitriptyline has the best documented analgesia but is the least well tolerated owing to its anticholinergic effects.
Caution: Use caution if administering with opioids.	Concomitant use with opioids may lead to sedation and orthostatic hypotension.
Administer benzodiazepines as prescribed.	Benzodiazepines are anxiolytic sedatives with little to no analgesic effect. They are useful for decreasing recall, treating acute anxiety, and decreasing muscle spasm associated with acute pain. They may decrease opioid requirement by decreasing pain perception. If administered without an analgesic, patient's perception of pain may increase.
Administer anticonvulsants as prescribed.	Anticonvulsants may be prescribed for pain associated with nerve injury from tumor or other destructive process.
Administer antihistamines as prescribed.	Antihistamines potentiate the effect of opioid analgesics. **Note:** Phenergan may increase perceived pain intensity and increase restlessness.
Avoid substituting sedatives and tranquilizers for analgesics.	Sedatives and tranquilizers are not analgesics.
Wean patient from opioid analgesics by decreasing dose or frequency. Convert to oral therapy as soon as possible.	In general, doses should be reduced by no more than 10%-20% per day with vigilant assessment for withdrawal signs and symptoms.
When changing route of administration or medication, be certain to use equianalgesic doses of the new drug.	Changing route of medication administration often results in inadequate pain relief because of ineffective equianalgesic conversion.

Continued

INTERVENTIONS	RATIONALES
Implement use of nonpharmacologic methods of pain control, such as acupressure, reflexology, cold/heat administration, massage, range-of-motion (ROM) exercises, transcutaneous electrical nerve stimulation (TENS), relaxation, distraction, hypnosis, and/or biofeedback.	Some patients may benefit from reducing drug therapy, and others may have unsatisfactory relief from pharmacologic interventions. Nonpharmacologic methods may augment action of pharmacologic interventions. Many of these techniques may be taught to and implemented by patient and significant other.
Maintain a quiet environment and plan nursing activities to enable long periods of uninterrupted rest at night.	To promote rest and sleep, which may decrease level of pain.
Evaluate for and correct nonoperative sources of discomfort.	Such sources as uncomfortable position, full bladder, and infiltrated IV site can be readily corrected without drug use.
Position patient comfortably and reposition at frequent intervals.	To relieve discomfort caused by pressure and improve circulation.
Carefully evaluate patient and notify health care provider immediately if pain increases unexpectedly.	Sudden or unexpected changes in pain intensity can signal complications such as internal bleeding or leakage of visceral contents.
Document pain assessments and efficacy of analgesics and other pain control interventions, using the pain scale or other formalized method.	Communicates level of pain relief, interventions, effectiveness of the interventions, and ongoing follow-up to meet the analgesic goal.

●●● **Related NIC and NOC labels:** *NIC:* Medication Management; Pain Management; Analgesic Administration; Medication Administration; Positioning; Acupressure; Biofeedback; Simple Massage; Simple Relaxation Therapy; Transcutaneous Electrical Nerve Stimulation (TENS); Distraction; Heat/Cold Application; Hypnosis *NOC:* Comfort Level; Pain Control; Pain: Disruptive Effects; Pain Level

Perioperative Care

Nursing Diagnosis:

Deficient Knowledge:

Surgical procedure, preoperative routine, and postoperative care

Desired Outcome: Patient verbalizes knowledge about the surgical procedure, including preoperative preparations and sensations and postoperative care and sensations, and demonstrates postoperative exercises and use of devices within the 24-hr period before surgical procedure or during immediate postoperative period for emergency surgery.

INTERVENTIONS	RATIONALES
Preoperatively:	
Evaluate patient's desire for knowledge about diagnosis and procedure.	Some individuals find detailed information helpful; others prefer very brief and simple explanations.
Assess for factors that would affect patient's ability to learn.	A well-developed teaching plan would be useless if patient is unable or unwilling to process information. Barriers to learning include ineffective communication, neurologic deficit, sensory alterations, fear, anxiety, and lack of motivation.
Assess patient's understanding about the diagnosis, surgical procedure, preoperative routine, and postoperative regimen. Determine past surgical experiences and their positive or negative effect on patient. Assess nature of any concerns or fears related to surgery. Document and communicate these assessment data to others involved in patient's care.	Assessing patient's knowledge, past experiences, and concerns about the surgical procedure will enable nurse to focus on individual areas in need of greatest intervention.
Based on your assessment, clarify and explain diagnosis and surgical procedure accordingly. When possible, emphasize associated sensations (i.e., dry mouth, thirst, muscle weakness). Determine patient's knowledge about informed consent. Provide ample time for instruction and clarification and reinforce health care provider's explanation of the procedure.	This information provides a knowledge base from which patient can make informed therapy choices and consent for procedures and presents an opportunity to clarify misconceptions.

Continued

INTERVENTIONS	RATIONALES
Use anatomic models, diagrams, and other audiovisual aids when possible. Provide simply written information based on patient's individual needs. Provide written and verbal information in patient's native language for non–English-speaking patients. If needed, arrange for an interpreter. **Note:** Evaluate patient's reading comprehension before providing written materials.	Because individuals learn differently, using more than one teaching modality will provide teaching reinforcement of verbal information given.
Explain perioperative course of events, reviewing the following with patient and significant other:	To increase patient's knowledge of surgical procedure, which optimally will promote compliance and minimize stress.
- Where patient will be before, during, and immediately after surgery.	Patient may be in postanesthesia care unit (PACU), intensive care unit (ICU), or specialty unit.
- Sounds and other sensations that the patient may experience during the immediate postoperative period.	Including sensory information in patient teaching is consistent with current nursing research that has determined patient outcomes are improved when expected sensations are explained.
- Preoperative medications and timing of surgery (scheduled time, expected duration).	
- If indicated, preoperative bowel preparation.	
- Pain management, including sensations to expect and methods of relief. If patient-controlled analgesia (PCA) or patient-controlled epidural anesthesia (PCEA) will be prescribed, have patient return demonstration of use of delivery device.	Increases likelihood of successful pain management. Some patients mistakenly expect to be pain free; others fear becoming addicted to narcotics.
- Placement of perioperative surgical devices used for patient's surgery. Enable patient to see these devices when possible.	Patients may be unfamiliar with use and purpose of tubes, catheters, drains, cooling systems (Cryocuff), continuous passive motion (CPM) units, oxygen delivery systems, and similar devices. Learning about them and seeing them in advance of surgery may help decrease patient's fears and anxieties perioperatively.
- Use of antiembolism stockings, sequential compression devices (SCDs), pneumatic foot pumps, or similar devices.	To prevent venous stasis and decrease risk of thrombus formation.
- Expected dietary alterations and progression, including NPO status followed by clear liquids until return of full gastrointestinal (GI) function.	Traditionally, health care providers have progressed patients from clear liquids to a regular diet after surgery for a variety of reasons, including ease of swallowing and digestion and being more readily tolerated in the presence of an ileus. However, practitioners are questioning the scientific basis of this diet advancement. Recent studies are indicating that a clear liquid diet may not always be indicated.
- Need to refrain from smoking during the perioperative period.	Inhalation of toxic fumes/chemical irritants can damage lung tissue by decreasing cilia, which line the respiratory tract and carry particles to the lower pharynx. Damaged lung tissue increases likelihood of hypoxemia and lung infections, including pneumonia.
- Visiting hours and location of waiting room.	Families may feel less anxious when they are aware of a designated area where they can wait and receive updates on progress of the surgery. Knowledge of visiting hours likely will reassure them that they will have access to patient after surgery.
- Restrictions of activity and positions, as indicated by specific surgical procedure.	For example, patients undergoing total hip arthroplasty will have specific positional limitations.

Continued

INTERVENTIONS	RATIONALES
Postoperatively: Explain postoperative activities, exercises, and precautions. Have patient return demonstration of the following devices and exercises, as appropriate:	Compliance is enhanced when patients are knowledgeable about activities, exercises, and precautions. Patients gain confidence when they practice new skills before surgery and gain feedback on their technique.
- Deep-breathing and coughing exercises (see **Ineffective Airway Clearance,** p. 51).	To prevent atelectasis, pneumonia, and other respiratory disorders that can occur during the postoperative period.
- Splinting of abdominal and thoracic incisions.	To reduce pain and stress on incision line, thereby increasing effectiveness of bronchial hygiene.
Caution: Individuals for whom increased intracranial, intrathoracic, or intraabdominal pressure is contraindicated should not cough.	Coughing increases intracranial, intrathoracic, and intraabdominal pressure. Patients undergoing intracranial surgery, spinal fusion, eye and ear surgery, and similar procedures should avoid vigorous coughing because it raises intracranial pressure, which could cause harm. Coughing after a herniorrhaphy and some thoracic surgeries should be done in a controlled manner, with the incision supported carefully, to avoid raising intraabdominal and intrathoracic pressure dramatically.
- Use of incentive spirometry and other respiratory devices.	This device, when used with coughing and deep breathing, expands alveoli and mobilizes secretions, which will help prevent atelectasis, pneumonia, pulmonary embolism, and other respiratory disorders.
Use of PCA/PCEA device.	To reduce pain. Adequate pain management increases mobility, which decreases risk of nosocomial pneumonia.
- Calf-pumping, ankle-circling, and footboard-pressing exercises.	To promote circulation and prevent thrombophlebitis in lower extremities (see "Venous Thrombosis/Thrombophlebitis," p. 217, for more information).
- Movement in and out of bed.	Logrolling, raising self by using a trapeze device, and gradual movement are techniques that may be required to reduce strain on operative site.
Before patient is discharged, teach prescribed activity precautions.	To prevent excessive strain on operative site. A patient who has a total hip replacement, for example, will need to follow activity precautions to prevent dislocation of the new joint.
Recommend planned, progressive exercise.	Increasing exercises gradually to tolerance, avoiding heavy lifting (>10 lb), and avoiding driving a car (often for as long as 4-6 wk) are precautions given to most surgical patients for safety because of potential for decreased attention span and impaired reflexes resulting from opioid use. Lifting precautions may reduce stress on surgical incisions. Restrictions on sexual activity are indicated by the surgical procedure. Returning progressively to preoperative activity level promotes physical and psychosocial well-being.
Explain importance of scheduling adequate rest.	Prevention of fatigue and getting adequate rest promote healing.
Review and have patient or significant other demonstrate wound/tube/drain care. Provide written instructions appropriate to learning level and identify means for obtaining supplies.	Fosters safety, independence, and self-care.
Discuss discharge medications, including use of prescribed and over-the-counter (OTC) medications.	A knowledgeable individual is likely to follow the therapeutic regimen. This information also decreases chance of adverse medication reactions by alerting patient in advance to reportable side effects.

Continued

INTERVENTIONS	RATIONALES
Review importance of adequate diet and fluid intake.	Adequate intake of fluids and nutrients decreases risk of dehydration and electrolyte imbalance, promotes tissue healing, and helps decrease fatigue.
Identify parameters for notifying health care provider if problems develop before return appointment: nausea/vomiting, difficulty voiding, temperature >38.3° C (101° F), symptoms of wound infection, inadequate pain relief, or abrupt change in pain characteristics.	Early treatment of symptoms may prevent progression to more serious or life-threatening symptoms.
Identify resources for patient on return to home: for example, visiting nurse, Meals-on-Wheels, primary care provider, and outpatient rehabilitation center. Provide phone numbers.	This knowledge may decrease anxiety by identifying potential support systems, and it provides a means of continuity of care and follow-up after discharge.
Review importance of postoperative return to clinic appointment.	Provides evaluation of healing and progress.
Provide time for patient to ask questions and express feelings of anxiety; be reassuring and supportive.	Expressing feelings of anxiety and having questions answered are essential ways of reducing anxiety while learning new information.

●●● **Related NIC and NOC labels:** *NIC:* Teaching: Preoperative; Preparatory Sensory Information; Teaching: Procedure; Anxiety Reduction; Teaching: Prescribed Activity/Exercise *NOC:* Knowledge: Treatment Procedures; Knowledge: Prescribed Activity; Knowledge: Treatment Regimen

Nursing Diagnosis:

Risk for Injury

related to exposure to pharmaceutical agents and other external factors during the perioperative period

Desired Outcome: Patient does not exhibit injury or untoward effects of pharmacotherapy or other external factors following surgery.

INTERVENTIONS	RATIONALES
Assess need for holding, administering, or adjusting patient's maintenance medications before or immediately after surgery. Consult health care provider as necessary.	Some medications, such as anticonvulsants and cardiac medications, should be continued throughout perioperative period. Sometimes patient needs to be weaned from medications such as baclofen (Lioresal) for the perioperative period. Other medications may require increased dosages during surgery or alternative routes (i.e., hydrocortisone [Solu-Cortef] in place of prednisone and with increased dosage for steroid-dependent patients).
Reinforce importance of NPO time.	Reduces risk of aspiration postoperatively. Frequently, clear liquids are allowed up to 2 hr before surgery.
Verify completion of preoperative activities and procedures and document on preoperative checklist or medical record.	Documentation on patient's preoperative checklist or in patient's medical record helps ensure communication among health care team members, continuity, and optimum patient outcomes.
Verify site of surgery, allergies, wounds, dressings, or drains.	Decreases risk of untoward outcomes. Noting patient's pre-existing wounds, dressings, and drains also helps ensure appropriate intraoperative positioning.

Continued

INTERVENTIONS	RATIONALES
Ensure that consent has been signed and witnessed and that patient understands what the procedure involves. Answer questions or call health care provider to answer patient's questions. Ensure that patient's ID bracelet, blood transfusion bracelet, and allergy alert bracelets are in place.	To ensure all appropriate documentation is present and that all steps have been taken to provide for patient's safety and well-being.
Determine whether patient is usually addressed with a nickname or name other than that on the medical record; document this finding on the preoperative checklist.	Patient may more readily respond to a nickname while recovering from anesthesia.
Review medical record; report untoward findings to health care provider.	Health care provider may not be aware of recent abnormal electrocardiogram (ECG), suspicious chest radiograph, or abnormal laboratory findings.
Prepare surgical site as prescribed and perform additional preoperative procedures as indicated.	Preoperative preparations may include showering with antimicrobial agent, clipping of hair, or use of depilatory agent (shaving is not usually recommended). Additional procedures may include douche, enema, or eye drop administration.
Administer preoperative analgesia, sedation, or other medications as prescribed. Give all medications, especially antibiotics, in a timely manner.	To ensure adequate serum levels. Giving antibiotics preoperatively may decrease risk of infection postoperatively.
Following administration of medications, keep bed in lowest position and side rails up and remind patient not to get out of bed without assistance.	Sedatives administered preoperatively may alter mental status and coordination, increasing patient's risk for injury.

●●● **Related NIC and NOC labels:** *NIC:* Risk Identification; Environmental Management: Safety; Surgical Precautions; Fall Prevention *NOC:* Risk Control; Safety Status: Physical Injury

Nursing Diagnosis:

Ineffective Airway Clearance

related to increased tracheobronchial secretions secondary to effects of anesthesia; ineffective coughing secondary to central nervous system (CNS) depression or pain and muscle splinting; and possible laryngospasm secondary to endotracheal tube or allergic reaction to anesthetics

Desired Outcome: Patient's airway is clear as evidenced by normal breath sounds to auscultation, RR 12-20 breaths/min with normal depth and pattern (eupnea), normothermia, normal skin color, and O_2 saturation >92% on room air.

INTERVENTIONS	RATIONALES
Assess respiratory status, including breath sounds, q1-2h during immediate postoperative period and q8h during recovery.	To be alert to and report presence of rhonchi that do not clear with coughing, labored breathing, tachypnea (RR >20 breaths/min), mental status changes, restlessness, cyanosis (a late sign), and presence of fever (≥38.3° C [101° F]), which are all signs of respiratory system compromise.
Use oximetry as indicated and report saturation ≤92% to health care provider.	Pulse oximetry is a noninvasive measure of arterial oxygen saturation. Values ≤92% are consistent with hypoxia and probably signal the need for oxygen supplementation or workup to determine cause of desaturation. Oximetry is especially indicated in patients with chronic obstructive

Continued

INTERVENTIONS	RATIONALES
	pulmonary disease (COPD), respiratory or cardiovascular disease, cardiothoracic surgery, major surgery, prolonged general anesthesia, and surgery for a fractured pelvis or long bone, as well as in debilitated patients and older adults. These individuals are at increased risk for desaturation.
Turn patient q2h. Encourage deep breathing and coughing q2h or more often for the first 72 hr postoperatively. Assist patient into Fowler's position or sitting on side of bed for pulmonary toilet. Support upper extremities with pillows.	To expand alveoli and mobilize secretions. The effects of anesthesia and immobility may collapse alveoli and place patient at risk for nosocomial pneumonia, atelectasis, and pulmonary embolism. Proper positioning promotes chest expansion and ventilation of basilar lung fields.
In the presence of fine crackles and if not contraindicated, have patient cough.	To clear the bronchial tree of secretions.
Demonstrate how to splint abdominal and thoracic incisions with hands or a pillow.	To ease discomfort and facilitate deep breathing and coughing.
If indicated, medicate ½ hr before deep breathing, coughing, or ambulation.	To decrease pain and promote compliance with deep-breathing exercises and full lung expansion.
If indicated, teach patient the "step-cough" technique. Coach patient to cough in rapid succession.	A step cough may be indicated for patients with a weak cough or poor reserve. A few weak coughs in a row may stimulate a stronger productive cough at the end of the cycle. This method is also less fatiguing than regular coughing exercises.
Consider whether patient may be more motivated to perform pulmonary toilet with an incentive spirometer or positive expiratory pressure (PEP) device.	Devices may be a motivating factor because patient has a visual indicator of effectiveness of the breathing effort.
	Caution: Vigorous coughing may be contraindicated for some individuals. Patients undergoing intracranial surgery, spinal fusion, eye and ear surgery, and similar procedures should avoid vigorous coughing because it raises intracranial pressure, which could harm the individual. Coughing after a herniorrhaphy and some thoracic surgeries should be done in a controlled manner, with the incision supported carefully, to avoid dramatic increase in intraabdominal and intrathoracic pressures.
Be alert to progression of airway compromise and ensure that emergency airway equipment (i.e., intubation tray, endotracheal tubes, suctioning equipment, tracheostomy tray) is readily available.	For use in the event of sudden airway obstruction or ventilatory failure.
Administer humidified oxygen as prescribed.	To supplement oxygen and prevent further drying of respiratory passageways and secretions via added humidity.
Encourage hydration of at least 2500 ml/day if not contraindicated.	To loosen secretions, making them easier to expectorate, while also promoting adequate hydration.

●●● **Related NIC and NOC labels:** *NIC:* Respiratory Monitoring; Vital Signs Monitoring; Chest Physiotherapy; Airway Suctioning; Oxygen Therapy; Aspiration Precautions *NOC:* Respiratory Status: Gas Exchange; Respiratory Status: Airway Patency

Nursing Diagnosis:

Risk for Aspiration

related to entry of secretions, food, or fluids into the tracheobronchial passages secondary to CNS depression, depressed cough and gag reflexes, decreased GI motility, abdominal distention, recumbent position, presence of gastric tube, and possible impaired swallowing in individuals with oral, facial, or neck surgery

Desired Outcome: Patient's upper airway remains unobstructed as evidenced by clear breath sounds, RR 12-20 breaths/min with normal depth and pattern (eupnea), normal skin color, and O_2 saturation >92%.

INTERVENTIONS	RATIONALES
See interventions under **Ineffective Airway Clearance**, earlier.	
Monitor respiratory rate, depth, and effort q4h or more frequently as needed. Note signs of aspiration: dyspnea, cough, cyanosis, wheezing, or fever.	To detect early signs of aspiration quickly to initiate prompt, life-saving treatment and prevent respiratory compromise.
	Caution: Patients with dysphagia are at high risk for aspiration because of potential for oral residue and pooling in the larynx, but they may not cough or exhibit signs of choking.
If sedated patient experiences nausea or vomiting, turn immediately into a side-lying, flat position. Fully alert patients may remain in an upright position.	To minimize potential for aspiration.
Treat nausea promptly with antiemetics. Give histamine H_2-receptor blocking agents, omeprazole (Prilosec), metoclopramide (Reglan), and similar agents as prescribed.	To decrease nausea, vomiting, and acidity of gastric contents and stimulate GI motility. H_2-receptor antagonists increase gastric pH, and nonparticulate antacids (e.g., Bicitra, Citra pH, and Alka Seltzer Gold) act as aspiration pneumonitis prophylaxis. Neutralizing gastric acidity may reduce severity of pneumonia if aspiration occurs.
As necessary, suction oropharynx with a Yankauer or similar suction device.	For immediate removal of vomitus, which could be aspirated. Patients at high risk for aspiration should have suctioning apparatus immediately available for this life-saving intervention.
Confirm placement of feeding tube with x-ray before initiating feeding. Check placement and patency of gastric tubes before initiation of intermittent feedings and medications.	To prevent instilling anything into patient's airway.
Check gastric tube feeding residuals q4h in patients having continuous feedings. Hold tube feeding if >100 ml residual in gastric tube or >200 ml residual in nasogastric (NG) tube, or per institution protocol.	High gastric tube residuals can predispose patient to regurgitation and aspiration.
Keep head of bed (HOB) elevated during feeding and for at least 30 min afterward.	Maintaining a sitting position after meals decreases risk of aspiration by facilitating gravity drainage from the stomach to the small bowel. An upright position also helps prevent reflux.
Assess abdomen q4-8h by inspection, auscultation, palpation, and percussion for increasing size, firmness, increased tympany, and decreased or high-pitched bowel sounds.	A distended and rigid abdomen along with increased or absent bowel sounds may indicate an ileus, which places patient at increased risk for vomiting and aspiration. Increased tympany or high-pitched bowel sounds may signal mechanical obstruction, which also places patient at increased risk for vomiting and aspiration.
Encourage early and frequent ambulation.	To improve GI motility and reduce abdominal distention caused by accumulated gases.

Continued

INTERVENTIONS	RATIONALES
Before initiating oral feeding, check gag reflex and ability to swallow.	Assessing patient's swallowing ability by gently touching both sides of larynx with thumb and forefinger while patient swallows is essential before beginning oral feedings. Even patients with intact gag reflex may aspirate.
Introduce oral fluids cautiously, especially in patients with oral, facial, and neck surgery.	These patients may be at increased risk for aspiration because of potential disruption of muscles and tissues involved with mastication and swallowing.
If indicated, arrange for a speech/swallowing evaluation, especially if patient has a tracheostomy.	Aspiration occurs frequently in patients with tracheostomies. Evaluation with a consult/swallowing study will determine whether tracheostomy cuff should be inflated or deflated during oral feeding. Having the cuff inflated impairs swallowing and increases risk for aspiration in some patients; in others the opposite is true.
If patient requires feeding, allow adequate time for chewing and swallowing food.	Eating hurriedly increases risk of aspiration because of incomplete chewing and inattention to careful swallowing.
For additional information, see "Providing Nutritional Support" for **Risk for Aspiration,** p. 594. Also see **Risk for Aspiration,** p. 101, in "Care of Older Adults."	

●●● **Related NIC and NOC labels:** *NIC:* Aspiration Precautions; Vomiting Management; Positioning; Postanesthesia Care; Respiratory Monitoring; Vital Signs Monitoring; Gastrointestinal Intubation
NOC: Aspiration Control

Nursing Diagnosis:

Impaired Gas Exchange

(or risk of same) *related to* decreased lung expansion secondary to CNS depression, pain, muscle splinting, recumbent position, and effects of anesthesia; and related to decreased ventilatory function secondary to disease process

Desired Outcome: Within 12 hr of intervention, patient exhibits effective ventilation as evidenced by relaxed breathing, clear breath sounds, normal color, appearance of adequate oxygenation, and $PaO_2 \geq 80$ mm Hg or within patient's normal or baseline parameters.

INTERVENTIONS	RATIONALES
Perform preoperative baseline assessment of patient's respiratory system, noting rate, rhythm, degree of chest expansion, quality of breath sounds, cough, and sputum production, as well as smoking history and current respiratory medications. Note preoperative O_2 saturation and arterial blood gas (ABG) values if available.	Baseline assessment enables rapid detection of subsequent postoperative problems and timely intervention for same.
Encourage patient to refrain from smoking for at least 1 wk after surgery. Explain effects of smoking on the body.	Inhalation of toxic fumes/chemical irritants can damage lung tissue, increasing likelihood of hypoxemia and respiratory infection.
Auscultate breath sounds at least q4-8h.	Crackles and wheezes may indicate airway obstruction leading to hypoxemia.

Continued

INTERVENTIONS	RATIONALES
Monitor O_2 saturation continuously via oximetry in high-risk patients (e.g., those who are heavily sedated or have pre-existing lung disease, older adults) and at periodic intervals in other patients as indicated. Notify health care provider if O_2 saturation is ≤92%.	Pulse oximetry is a noninvasive method of measuring saturated hemoglobin in tissue capillaries. Oxygen saturation ≤92% may signal need for supplemental oxygen.
Note blood gas results as available. Assess patient for signs of hypoxia. Administer humidified oxygen as prescribed.	Declining Pao_2 may signal hypoxemia and need for supplemental oxygen. Early signs of hypoxia include restlessness, dyspnea, tachycardia, tachypnea, and confusion. Cyanosis, especially of the tongue and oral mucous membranes, and extreme lethargy or somnolence are late signs of hypoxia.
Watch for onset of hypoventilation, especially in patients with chronic lung disease, as evidenced by increased somnolence after initiating or increasing oxygen therapy.	Patients with chronic lung disease may need the hypoxic drive to breathe and may hypoventilate with oxygen therapy.
Position patient in high Fowler's position as tolerated. Assist patient with turning and deep-breathing exercises q2h for the first 72 hr postoperatively.	To promote expansion of lung alveoli and prevent pooling of secretions, which could lead to nosocomial pneumonia.
If patient has an incentive spirometer or PEP device, provide instructions and ensure compliance with its use q2h or as prescribed.	Deep breathing expands alveoli and aids in mobilizing secretions to the airways, and subsequent coughing further mobilizes and clears secretions.
Unless contraindicated, assist patient with ambulation by second postoperative day.	To promote circulation and ventilation, which may prevent formation of deep vein thrombosis and pulmonary embolism.
Administer analgesics as prescribed.	To reduce pain, which optimally will facilitate patient's ease with coughing and deep-breathing exercises and ambulation.
When appropriate, teach methods of splinting wounds or painful areas.	To decrease discomfort, which will enable effective cough.
Instruct patients who are unable to cough effectively in "step" cough, that is, a succession of short exhalations that may stimulate a more forceful cough.	To promote coughing and increase sputum clearance in patients who are unable to raise secretions. Controlled cough uses the diaphragm muscles, making the cough more forceful and effective.
If patient is dyspneic, teach how to use pursed-lip breathing.	Pursed-lip breathing uses intercostal muscles, decreases the respiratory rate, increases tidal volume, and increases oxygen saturation to reverse effects of dyspnea.
As indicated, suggest patient with dyspnea lean over a bedside table.	In this position, patient may have less dyspnea because pressure on the gastric area allows better contraction of the diaphragm.
When not contraindicated, instruct patient to increase fluid intake (>2.5 L/day).	To decrease viscosity of pulmonary secretions and facilitate their mobilization.

●●● **Related NIC and NOC labels:** *NIC:* Respiratory Monitoring; Vital Sign Monitoring; Fluid Management; Medication Management; Pain Management; Postanesthesia Care; Teaching: Prescribed Activity; Teaching: Procedure/Treatments; Cough Enhancement; Oxygen Therapy; Acid-Base Monitoring
NOC: Vital Signs Status; Respiratory Status: Airway Patency; Respiratory Status: Ventilation

Nursing Diagnosis:

Risk for Deficient Fluid Volume

related to postoperative bleeding/hemorrhage

Desired Outcomes: Patient remains normovolemic as evidenced by BP ≥90/60 mm Hg (or within patient's preoperative baseline), HR 60-100 bpm, RR 12-20 breaths/min with normal depth and pattern (eupnea), brisk capillary refill (<2 sec), warm extremities, distal pulses >2+ on a 0-4+ scale, urinary output ≥30 ml/hr, and urine specific gravity <1.030. Patient verbalizes orientation to person, place, and time and does not demonstrate significant mental status changes.

INTERVENTIONS	RATIONALES
Monitor VS q4h during first 24 hr of the postoperative period.	There is greater potential for postoperative bleeding/hemorrhage during this period. Decreasing pulse pressure (difference between systolic and diastolic BP), decreasing BP, increasing HR, and increasing RR are indicators of internal hemorrhage and impending shock.
Assess patient at frequent intervals during first 24 hr for presence of pallor, diaphoresis, cool extremities, delayed capillary refill, diminished intensity of distal pulses, restlessness, agitation, mental status changes, and disorientation. Also note subjective complaints of thirst, anxiety, or a sense of impending doom.	Indicators of internal hemorrhage and impending shock.
Monitor and measure urinary output q4-8h during initial postoperative period. Report average hourly output <30 ml/hr. Assess urinary specific gravity and report specific gravity ≥1.030 to health care provider.	Urine volumes <30 ml/hr and specific gravity ≥1.030 are indicators of deficient fluid volume, which can signal bleeding/hemorrhage.
Inspect surgical dressing for rapid saturation of dressing with bright red blood. Record saturated dressings and report significant findings to health care provider.	Evidence of frank bleeding, which necessitates prompt intervention.
If initial postoperative dressing becomes saturated, reinforce it and notify health care provider.	Health care provider may want to perform the initial dressing change.
Monitor wound drains and drainage systems for drainage >50 ml/hr for 2-3 hr and report findings to health care provider.	This is excessive drainage and should be reported promptly for timely intervention.
Note amount and character of drainage from gastric and other tubes at least q8h. **Note:** After gastric and some other GI surgeries, patient will have small amounts of bloody or blood-tinged drainage for the first 12-24 hr. Be alert to large or increasing amounts of bloody drainage.	If drainage appears to contain blood (e.g., bright red, burgundy, or dark coffee ground appearance), it will be necessary to perform an occult blood test (may be performed in the laboratory). If test is newly or unexpectedly positive, results should be reported to health care provider for timely intervention.
Review complete blood count (CBC) values.	Elevated Hct and Hgb can occur with dehydration. Evidence of bleeding may be indicated by decreases in Hgb from normal (male 14-18 g/dl; female 12-16 g/dl) and decreases in Hct from normal (male 40%-54%; female 37%-47%). Significant decreases occur with active bleeding, an emergency situation.
Maintain a patent 18-gauge or larger IV catheter. See "Cardiac and Noncardiac Shock," p. 171, for management.	For use if hemorrhagic shock develops.

●●● **Related NIC and NOC labels:** *NIC:* Bleeding Precautions; Blood Products Administration; Hemorrhage Control; Shock Prevention; Venous Access Devices Maintenance; Vital Signs Monitoring; Laboratory Data Interpretation *NOC:* Fluid Balance

Nursing Diagnosis:

Risk for Deficient Fluid Volume

related to active loss secondary to presence of indwelling drainage tubes, wound drainage, or vomiting; *inadequate intake of fluids* secondary to nausea, preoperative and postoperative NPO status, CNS depression, or lack of access to fluids; or *failure of regulatory mechanisms* with third spacing of body fluids secondary to the effects of anesthesia, endogenous catecholamines, blood loss during surgery, and prolonged recumbency

Desired Outcome: Patient remains normovolemic as evidenced by BP ≥90/60 mm Hg (or within patient's preoperative baseline), HR 60-100 bpm, clear breath sounds, distal pulses >2+ on a 0-4+ scale, balanced I&O, urine specific gravity ≤1.030, serum electrolytes and Hct within normal limits, stable or increasing weight, good skin turgor, warm skin, moist mucous membranes, and normothermia.

INTERVENTIONS	RATIONALES
Monitor VS q4-8h during recovery phase.	Decreasing BP, increasing HR, and slightly increased body temperature are indicators of deficient fluid volume.
Assess patient's physical status q4-8h.	Dry skin, dry mucous membranes, excessive thirst, diminished intensity of peripheral pulses, and alteration in mental status are indicators of deficient fluid volume.
Assess skin turgor by lifting a section of skin along forearm, abdomen, or calf. Release skin and watch its return to original position.	With good hydration, skin will return quickly; with dehydration, skin will remain in lifted position (tenting) or return slowly.
	Note: This test may be less reliable in older adults; older adults have decreased skin elasticity and decreased subcutaneous fat.
Monitor urinary output and check specific gravity q4-8h.	Concentrated urine (specific gravity >1.030) and low or decreasing output (average normal output is 60 ml/hr or 1400-1500 ml/day) are indicators of deficient fluid volume.
Use catheter bag with urometer as indicated.	Provides mechanism for accurate monitoring of urinary output.
Measure, describe, and document any emesis. Assess for and document excessive perspiration. Include your assessment of both with documentation of urinary, fecal, and other drainage for a total estimation of patient's fluid balance.	Both sensible and insensible losses need to be determined to ensure complete picture of patient's fluid volume status.
Measure and record output from drains, ostomies, wounds, and other sources. Ensure patency of gastric and other drainage tubes. Record quality and quantity of output.	Same as above.
Report significant findings to health care provider.	Replacement fluids likely will be indicated.
Monitor patient's weight daily. Always weigh patient at the same time every day, using same scale and same type and amount of bed clothing.	Daily weight measurement is an effective means of evaluating hydration status. Weighing patient at the same time and under the same conditions avoids discrepancies that could reflect inaccurate losses or gains.
If means is present, check central venous pressure (CVP).	Although weight is the most accurate reflection of patient's overall fluid status, CVP is an indication of circulating blood volume. Normal value is 2-6 mm Hg.
Assess for potential causes of nausea and vomiting.	Causes such as opioid analgesics, loss of gastric tube patency, and environmental factors (e.g., unpleasant odors or sights) can be reversed.
Administer antiemetics (e.g., hydroxyzine, ondansetron, prochlorperazine, promethazine), metoclopramide (Reglan), or similar agents as prescribed.	To combat nausea and vomiting, which may impair intake and add to fluid losses.
Instruct patient to request medication *before* nausea becomes severe.	It is easier to control nausea if it is treated before it gets severe.
Administer antacids as prescribed if nausea and vomiting are present.	Antacids neutralize gastric acidity and may reduce severity of pneumonia if aspiration occurs.
Monitor serum electrolytes.	Fluid loss may cause significant electrolyte imbalances.
Be alert to low potassium levels (K^+ <3.5 mEq/L) and lethargy, irritability, anorexia, vomiting, muscle weakness and cramping, paresthesias, weak and irregular pulse, and respiratory dysfunction.	Signs and symptoms of hypokalemia, which when detected and reported promptly may prevent potentially life-threatening cardiac dysrhythmias.
Also assess for low calcium levels (Ca^{++} <8.5 mg/dl) and tetany, muscle cramps, fatigue, irritability, personality changes, and Trousseau's or Chvostek's sign.	Signs and symptoms of hypocalcemia. If detected and reported promptly, cardiac emergency may be prevented.

Continued

INTERVENTIONS	RATIONALES
	Trousseau's sign is elicited by applying a BP cuff to the arm, inflating it to slightly higher than systolic BP, and leaving it inflated for 1-4 min. Carpopedal spasms are indicative of hypocalcemia.
	Chvostek's sign is assessed by tapping the face just below the temple (where the facial nerve emerges). The sign is positive if twitching occurs along side of nose, lip, or face.
Administer and regulate IV fluids and electrolytes as prescribed until patient is able to resume oral intake. When IV fluids are discontinued, encourage intake of oral fluids, at least 2-3 L/day in the nonrestricted patient.	Oral fluids usually are restricted until peristalsis returns (72-96 hr postoperatively) and NG tube is removed. However, ice chips or small sips of clear liquids may be allowed.
Provide oral hygiene.	NPO status and deficient fluid volume cause dry mouth.
Monitor for signs of paralytic ileus: absent bowel sounds, flatus and abdominal distention.	Intraoperative manipulation of internal organs, stress, and the depressive effects of some anesthetics and narcotics on peristalsis may cause paralytic ileus, usually between post-operative days 3 and 5. Abdominal pain may be localized, sharp, or intermittent.
Begin fluids slowly and in small amounts. Monitor patient's response.	If nausea, emesis, or increased distention occur, decrease or stop oral foods/fluids and assess need to restart IV fluids.
As possible, respect patient's preference in oral fluids and keep them readily available in patient's room.	Patient will more likely comply with increased oral fluid intake if it is better tolerated and readily available.

●●● **Related NIC and NOC labels:** *NIC:* Fluid/Electrolyte Management; Hypovolemia Management; Vital Signs Monitoring; Electrolyte Management: Hypocalcemia; Electrolyte Management: Hypokalemia
NOC: Electrolyte & Acid/Base Balance; Hydration

Nursing Diagnosis:

Excess Fluid Volume

related to presence of cardiac, renal, or chronic liver disease; sodium intake with intraoperative IV fluid; or perioperative activation of the neuroendocrine system secondary to the physiologic stress response and release of antidiuretic hormone (ADH), aldosterone, and glucocorticoids

Desired Outcome: Within the 24-hr period after intervention/treatment, patient becomes normo-volemic as evidenced by BP within patient's normal range or preoperative baseline, distal pulses <4+ on a 0-4+ scale, absence of jugular-venous distention or galloping heart rhythm, presence of eupnea, clear breath sounds, absence of or barely detectable edema, 24-hr I&O within normal limits, and body weight at or near preoperative baseline.

INTERVENTIONS	RATIONALES
Assess for and report increase or drop in BP, bounding pulses, dyspnea, crackles, S_3 heart sound, and pretibial or sacral edema.	A drop in BP and an S_3 galloping rhythm may indicate impending heart failure. Crackles and dyspnea may signal a shift of fluid from the vascular space to the pulmonary interstitial space and alveoli causing pulmonary edema.
Measure extremity edema with a measuring tape.	A tape measure is more accurate than a 0-4+ edema scale.
With HOB elevated 30-45 degrees, note presence of distended neck and peripheral veins.	This could signal excess fluid volume, which could occur with cardiac decompensation or heart failure.

Continued

INTERVENTIONS	RATIONALES
Maintain record of 8-hr and 24-hr I&O. Note and report significant imbalance.	Normal 24-hr output is 1400-1500 ml, and normal 1-hr output is 60 ml/hr. Decreased urinary output could be a sign of fluid volume excess.
Monitor serum osmolality (normal range is 280-300 mOsm/kg H_2O), serum glucose, serum electrolytes such as Na^+ (normal range is 137-147 mEq/L) and K^+ (normal range is 3.5-5 mEq/L), BUN (normal range is 6-20 mg/dl), creatinine (normal range is 0.6-1.5 mg/dl), and Hct (normal ranges are male 14-18 g/dl and female 12-16 g/dl).	With the physiologic stress response to surgery, the neuroendocrine system produces ADH and aldosterone. Na^+ is retained and K^+ is lost. Glucocorticoids are also produced, causing glucose values to rise and protein to break down. The result is fluid retention (excess fluid volume), which is manifested by an alteration in electrolytes and hemodilution of Hct.
Weigh patient daily, using same scale and same type and amount of bed clothing. Note significant weight gain.	Weight changes reflect changes in body fluid volume. One L of fluid equals approximately 2.2 lb. Weighing patient at the same time and under the same conditions avoids discrepancies that could reflect inaccurate losses or gains.
Anticipate postoperative diuresis approximately 48-72 hr after surgery.	This may occur because of mobilization of third-space (interstitial) fluid.
Administer diuretics such as furosemide (Lasix) as prescribed.	To mobilize interstitial fluid and decrease excess fluid volume.
Also be alert to signs of hypokalemia (see discussion of hypokalemia and hyponatremia in **Risk for Deficient Fluid Volume**, p. 56).	Diuretic therapy may cause dangerous K^+ depletion that could result in cardiac dysrhythmias. As well, diuretic therapy can lead to hyponatremia because of sodium losses.
Be aware that older adults and individuals with cardiac or renal disease are at increased risk for developing postoperative fluid volume excess.	Older adults have age-related changes of decreased glomerular filtration rate (GFR). Decreased kidney function and increased probability of chronic illness such as cardiac disease may signal higher risk of postoperative excessive fluid volume.
Monitor for restlessness, anxiety, or confusion, particularly in elders or in patients with cardiac and renal disease. Use safety precautions if symptoms are present.	With excessive fluid volume compromising cardiac output, hypoxia may occur, which manifests as restlessness and agitation and places patient at increased risk for injury. Hyponatremia from excess fluid volume may cause similar symptoms with cerebral edema and mental status changes.

●●● **Related NIC and NOC labels:** *NIC:* Fluid/Electrolyte Management; Vital Signs Monitoring; Electrolyte Management: Hypokalemia *NOC:* Fluid Balance; Electrolyte and Acid/Base Balance

Nursing Diagnosis:

Risk for Infection

related to inadequate primary defenses (broken skin, traumatized tissue, decrease in ciliary action, stasis of body fluids), invasive procedures, or chronic disease

Desired Outcome: Patient is free of infection as evidenced by normothermia; HR ≤100 bpm; RR ≤20 breaths/min with normal depth and pattern (eupnea); negative cultures; clear and normal-smelling urine; clear and thin sputum; no significant mental status changes; orientation to person, place, and time; and absence of unusual tenderness, erythema, swelling, warmth, or drainage at the surgical incision.

INTERVENTIONS	RATIONALES
Monitor for and report signs of infection such as increased body temperature; erythema, warmth, or induration of skin; and foul discharge from wounds or drains.	With onset of infection the immune system is activated, causing symptoms of infection to appear. Sustained temperature elevation after surgery may signal presence of pulmonary complications, urinary tract infection, wound infection, or thrombophlebitis.
Assess temperature with an electronic thermometer.	Presence of a fever affects treatment decisions. Electronic thermometers have established accuracy, whereas tympanic thermometers recently have been deemed to have questionable accuracy. Mercury thermometers have been eliminated in many institutions for safety reasons.
Note and report significant laboratory values such as white blood cell (WBC) count and differential and culture results.	Increased total WBC counts signal infection. Cultures of urine, respiratory secretions, blood, wounds, and indwelling devices identify pathogens and guide antibiotic therapy. **Note:** Effects of aging on the hypothalamus may decrease fever response to infection.
Evaluate mental status, orientation, and level of consciousness (LOC) q4-8h or more frequently as indicated.	Consider infection the likely cause if altered mental status or LOC is unexplained by other factors, such as age, medication, or disease process.
Encourage and assist patient with coughing, deep breathing, incentive spirometry, and turning q2-4h and note quality of breath sounds, cough, and sputum.	To expand alveoli in the lung and mobilize secretions, which will decrease the potential for respiratory infection/pneumonia.
Evaluate IV and tube/drain sites for erythema, warmth, swelling, tenderness, and unusual drainage.	These are signs of infection. The body may be mounting a response to ward off offending pathogens.
Change IV line and site if evidence of infection is present and do so according to agency protocol (q48-72h).	Infection control guidelines.
Assess stability of tubes/drain.	Movement of improperly secured tubes and drains enables access of pathogens at insertion site.
Maintain dependent gravity drainage of indwelling catheters, tubes, and irrigation lines. Evaluate patency of all surgically placed tubes or drains. Irrigate, gently "milk," or attach to low-pressure suction as prescribed. Promptly report unrelieved loss of patency.	Prevents stasis and reflux of body fluids, which can result in infection.
Note color, character, amount, and odor of all drainage. Report presence and amount.	Foul-smelling, creamy, and abnormal drainage are indicators of infection.
Evaluate incisions and wound sites for unusual erythema, warmth, tenderness, induration, swelling, delayed healing, and purulent or excessive drainage.	Signs of infection that signal the body may be mounting a response to ward off offending pathogens.
Wash hands before and after caring for patient and wear gloves when contact with blood, drainage, or other body substance is likely.	Handwashing is an effective means of preventing microbial transmission. Wearing gloves protects caregiver from patient's body substances.
Change dressings as prescribed, using "no touch" and sterile techniques. Prevent cross-contamination of wounds in same patient by changing one dressing at a time and washing hands between dressing changes.	Infection control guidelines.
Be alert to patient complaints of a feeling of "letting go" or a sudden profusion of serous drainage on the dressing or a bulge in the dressing.	It is likely a wound dehiscence evisceration has occurred. Wound infection and poor wound healing puts patient at risk for wound dehiscence.
If patient develops evisceration, do not reinsert tissue or organs. Place a sterile, saline-soaked gauze over eviscerated tissues and cover with a sterile towel until wound can be evaluated by health care provider.	Keeping viscera moist with a sterile towel increases viability of tissues and reduces risk of contamination and further infection.

Continued

INTERVENTIONS

RATIONALES

INTERVENTIONS	RATIONALES
Maintain patient on bedrest, usually in semi-Fowler's position with knees slightly bent. Keep patient NPO and anticipate need for IV therapy and a return to operating room.	To provide comfort, prevent further evisceration, and prepare patient for surgical repair.
When appropriate, encourage use of intermittent catheterization q4-6h instead of indwelling catheter.	In most cases there is less risk of infection with intermittent than with indwelling catheterization, especially in patient's own home. Emptying the bladder routinely prevents stasis of urine and decreases presence of pathogens.
Keep drainage collection container below bladder level.	To prevent reflux of urine (and potential pathogens) into bladder, which could lead to infection.
Avoid kinks or obstructions in drainage tubing; ensure free flow of urine.	To help prevent urinary stasis. An "air lock" or other obstruction of the drainage system may cause urinary distention or bladder stretch injury.
Do not open closed urinary drainage system unless absolutely necessary; Irrigate catheter only with health care provider's prescription and when obstruction is the known cause.	Keeping the system closed decreases risk of contamination and infection.
Assess for chills; fever (>37.7° C [100° F]); dysuria; urgency; frequency; flank, low back, suprapubic, buttock, inner thigh, scrotal, or labial pain; and cloudy or foul-smelling urine.	Indicators of urinary tract infection (UTI), which signal the body is mounting a response to ward off offending pathogens.
Encourage intake of 2-3 L/day in nonrestricted patients.	To minimize potential for UTI by diluting the urine and maximizing urinary flow.
Ensure that perineum and meatus are cleansed during daily bath and perianal area is cleansed after bowel movements. Do not hesitate to remind patient of these hygiene measures.	Microorganisms can be introduced into the body via the catheter. Good hygiene decreases the number of microorganisms.
Be alert to swelling, purulent drainage, and persistent meatal redness. Intervene if patient is unable to perform self-care.	Indicators of meatal infection and potential UTI.
Ensure foreskin is drawn down over the glans in uncircumcised male patients.	Uncircumcised males are at risk for balanitis (inflammation of the glans penis), especially with fluid shifts after surgery and improper care of the foreskin.
Change catheter according to established protocol or sooner if sandy particles can be felt in distal end of catheter or if patient develops UTI. Change drainage collection container according to established protocol or sooner if it becomes foul smelling or leaks.	Because the catheter can be a source of infection, changing the system per protocol (usually every month) is customary.
Obtain cultures of suspicious drainage or secretions (e.g., sputum, urine, wound) as prescribed. For urine specimens, be certain to use sampling port, which is at proximal end of drainage tube.	To determine if an infection is present and direct therapy with an appropriate antibiotic if it is.
Cleanse area with an antimicrobial wipe and use a sterile syringe with 25-gauge needle to aspirate urine.	Larger-gauge needles form larger puncture holes that increase risk of compromising the sterile system.

●●● **Related NIC and NOC labels:** *NIC:* Infection Control; Infection Protection; Environmental Management; Incision Site Care; Infection Control: Intraoperative; Laboratory Data Interpretation; Respiratory Monitoring; Skin Surveillance; Specimen Management; Wound Care; Chest Physiotherapy; Perineal Care; Tube Care; Urinary Retention Care *NOC:* Infection Status; Wound Healing: Primary Intention

Nursing Diagnosis:

Constipation

related to functional factors such as immobility, inadequate toileting, disrupted abdominal musculature or weakness; psychologic factors such as stress of surgery or mental confusion; pharmacologic factors such as anesthesia and use of opioids, diuretics, and other medications; mechanical factors such as intraoperative manipulation of abdominal viscera, ileus, and bowel obstruction; and physiologic factors such as poor eating habits, lack of fiber or fluid intake, dehydration and electrolyte imbalances, and decreased motility of GI tract

Desired Outcome: Patient returns to his or her normal bowel elimination pattern as evidenced by return of active bowel sounds within 48-72 hr after most surgeries, absence of abdominal distention or sensation of fullness, and the elimination of soft, formed stools.

INTERVENTIONS	RATIONALES
Monitor for and document elimination of flatus or stool.	Signals return of intestinal motility.
Review current medications.	Many medications affect normal bowel function and cause constipation. Examples are antidepressants, iron supplements, opiate analgesics, muscle relaxants, and anticholinergics.
Assess for abdominal distention or tenderness; absent, hypoactive, or high-pitched bowel sounds; and sensation of fullness.	Gross distention, extreme tenderness, and prolonged absence of bowel sounds are signs of decreased GI motility and possible ileus. High-pitched bowel sounds may indicate impending bowel obstruction.
Encourage in-bed position changes, exercises, and ambulation to patient's tolerance unless contraindicated.	To stimulate peristalsis, which promotes bowel elimination.
When NG tube is removed, monitor patient for abdominal distention, nausea, and vomiting.	Signs that GI motility is still decreased and requires further intervention.
Monitor and document patient's response to diet advancement from clear liquids to a regular or other prescribed diet. Report significant findings.	Poor response to diet advancement as evidenced by abdominal distention, nausea, and vomiting may signal continued decreased GI motility and should be reported for timely intervention. Postoperatively, decreased GI motility can result from stress (autonomic), surgical manipulation of the intestine, immobility, and effects of medications.
If not contraindicated, encourage oral fluid intake (≥2500 ml/day).	To promote soft stools that will minimize need to strain.
Offer prune juice and administer stool softeners, mild laxatives, senna-based herbal teas, and enemas as prescribed.	To promote bulk and softness in stools.
As appropriate, encourage a high-fiber diet (fresh vegetables and fruits, bran cereals). Monitor and record results.	High-fiber foods promote bulk in stools, which helps prevent constipation.
Encourage physical activity as soon as it is allowed.	Activity improves abdominal muscle tone and stimulates appetite and peristalsis.
Arrange periods of privacy during patient's attempts at bowel elimination.	Privacy can promote relaxation and success with defecation.

●●● **Related NIC and NOC labels:** *NIC:* Bowel Management; Diet Staging; Exercise Promotion; Fluid Management; Medication Management; Enteral Tube Feeding *NOC:* Bowel Elimination; Hydration; Symptom Control

Nursing Diagnosis:

Disturbed Sleep Pattern

related to preoperative anxiety, stress, postoperative pain, noise, and altered environment

Desired Outcome: Within the 24-hr period following intervention/treatment, patient relates minimal or no difficulty with falling asleep and describes a feeling of being well rested.

INTERVENTIONS	RATIONALES
Implement measures such as providing eye shields, dimming lights, reducing pain, using patient's own pillow, and maintaining a quiet environment.	Behavioral interventions are the preferred method for insomnia because of their established efficacy and absence of drug side effects.
If behavioral interventions are ineffective, administer sedative/hypnotic as prescribed.	To promote sleep.
Use special care when administering these drugs to patients who are also taking opioid analgesics, as well as to older adults.	Sedative/hypnotics may cause CNS depression and contribute to respiratory depressant effects of opioid analgesics. Active metabolites of many of the benzodiazepines may accumulate and result in greater physiologic effects or toxicity. As well, there is a greater incidence of sleep disruption in older adults with chronic illnesses who take this combination of drugs.
After administering sedative/hypnotic, be certain to raise side rails, lower bed to its lowest position, and caution patient not to smoke in bed.	Patient will become drowsy, which necessitates these safety measures.
Administer analgesics at bedtime.	To reduce pain and augment effects of hypnotic.
Be certain that consent for surgery is signed before administering sedative/hypnotic.	Patient should sign legal document only when alert and cognizant of its contents.

●●● **Related NIC and NOC labels:** *NIC:* Sleep Enhancement; Environmental Management; Medication Administration; Pain Management *NOC:* Sleep

Nursing Diagnosis:

Impaired Physical Mobility

related to postoperative pain, decreased strength and endurance secondary to CNS effects of anesthesia or blood loss, musculoskeletal or neuromuscular impairment secondary to disease process or surgical procedure, perceptual impairment secondary to disease process or surgical procedure (e.g., ocular surgery, neurosurgery), or cognitive deficit secondary to disease process or effects of opioid analgesics and anesthetics

Desired Outcome: Optimally, by hospital discharge (depending on type of surgery), patient returns to preoperative baseline physical mobility as evidenced by the ability to move in bed, transfer, and ambulate independently or with minimal assistance.

INTERVENTIONS	RATIONALES
Assess patient's preoperative physical mobility by evaluating coordination and muscle strength, control, and mass.	Preoperative/baseline assessments enable accurate measurements of postoperative mobility problems.
Assess for medically imposed restrictions against movement, especially with conditions or surgeries that are orthopedic, neurosurgical, or ocular.	Restricted movement and positioning can prevent exacerbation of preexisting condition.
Evaluate and correct factors that limit physical mobility.	Factors such as oversedation with opioid analgesics, failure to achieve adequate pain control, and poorly arranged physical environment can be corrected.
Initiate movement from bed to chair and ambulation as soon as possible after surgery, depending on postoperative prescriptions, type of surgery, and patient's recovery from anesthetics (usually 12-24 hr after surgery).	Patient usually can tolerate a graduated progression in activity and ambulation.
Assist patient with moving slowly to a sitting position in bed and then standing at bedside before attempting ambulation. For more information, see **Ineffective Cerebral Tissue Perfusion**, p. 73.	Many anesthetic agents depress normal vasoconstrictor mechanisms and can result in sudden hypotension with quick changes in position.
Encourage frequent movement and ambulation by postoperative patients. Provide assistance as indicated and explain importance to patient.	To reduce potential for postoperative complications, including atelectasis, pneumonia, thrombophlebitis, skin breakdown, muscle weakness, and depressed GI motility.
Teach in-bed exercises.	Exercises such as gluteal and quadriceps muscle sets (isometrics) and ankle circling and calf pumping promote muscle strength, increase venous return, and prevent stasis.
For additional information, see "Prolonged Bedrest" for **Risk for Activity Intolerance**, p. 67, and **Risk for Disuse Syndrome,** p. 69.	

●●● **Related NIC and NOC labels:** *NIC:* Exercise Promotion: Ambulation; Energy Management; Fall Prevention; Pain Management *NOC:* Mobility Level

Nursing Diagnoses:

Risk for Falls/Risk for Injury

related to physiologic factors such as visual or auditory deficit, arthritis, sleeplessness, syncope, orthostatic hypotension, anemia, vascular disease, hypoglycemia, neuropathy, poor balance, or fatigue; cognitive factors such as diminished mental status; pharmacologic factors such as anesthesia or use of opioids, sedatives, and hypnotics; and environmental factors such as slippery floors, cluttered walkway, unfamiliar or poorly lighted room, and use of restraints

Desired Outcome: Patient does not fall and remains free of injury as evidenced by absence of bruises, wounds, or fractures.

INTERVENTIONS	RATIONALES
Orient and reorient patient to person, place, and time during initial postoperative period.	Orientation and repeated explanations increase mental awareness and alertness, which decrease risk of injury caused by disorientation. These measures also help patient cope with unfamiliar surroundings.
Maintain side rails on stretchers and beds in upright and locked positions.	Prevents injury to head and extremities. Some individuals experience agitation and thrash about as they emerge from anesthesia.

Continued

INTERVENTIONS	RATIONALES
Secure all IV lines, drains, and tubing.	To prevent dislodgement.
Maintain bed in its lowest position when leaving patient's room.	To protect patient in the event of a fall.
Be certain call mechanism is within patient's reach; instruct patient about its use.	Patient can call for help when it is needed, for example, when needing to toilet.
Keep path to bathroom clear.	Increases safety for patients who attempt to ambulate to bathroom.
Identify patients at risk for falling. Correct or compensate for risk factors.	To reduce risk of falling in susceptible individuals. Risk factors include: - *Time of day:* night shift, peak activity periods such as meals, bedtime. - *Medications:* opioid analgesics, sedatives, hypnotics, and anesthetics. - *Impaired mobility:* individuals requiring assistance with transfer and ambulation. Use assistive devices and provide nonskid footwear. - *Sensory deficits:* diminished visual acuity caused by disease process or environmental factors; changes in kinesthetic sense because of disease or trauma. Ask patient to wear glasses and hearing aids. - *Postural hypotension:* Ask patient to change positions slowly. - *Age-related factors:* Older adults have decreased baroreceptor sensitivity causing decreased compensatory mechanisms for maintaining BP when standing up. This may cause postural hypotension. Instruct patient to change positions slowly.
Communicate patient's risk for falling/injury to health care staff as appropriate.	All staff members need to be aware of risk factors so that they may initiate appropriate interventions to maintain patient's safety.
Use restraints and protective devices if necessary and prescribed.	For patient's protection during emergent stage. However, because they can cause agitation, their use should be infrequent and as a last resort. Behavioral intervention or a patient sitter is preferred.

●●● **Related NIC and NOC labels:** *NIC:* Environmental Management: Safety; Fall Prevention; Risk Identification *NOC:* Safety Status: Physical Injury

Nursing Diagnosis:

Risk for Impaired Skin Integrity

related to presence of secretions/excretions around percutaneous drains and tubes

Desired Outcome: Patient's skin around percutaneous drains and tubes remains intact and nonerythematous.

INTERVENTIONS	RATIONALES
Change dressings as soon as they become wet. (Health care provider may prefer to perform the first dressing change at the surgical incision.) Use sterile technique for all dressing changes.	To protect wound from contamination and accumulation of fluids that may cause excoriation.
Keep area around drains as clean and dry as possible. Use sterile normal saline, soap and water, or other prescribed solution to clean around drain site.	Intestinal secretions, bile, and similar drainage can lead quickly to skin excoriation.
If some external drainage is present, position a pectin-wafer skin barrier around drain or tube or use ointments, such as zinc oxide, petrolatum, and aluminum paste.	Skin barriers and ointments are used to protect the skin from drainage that could cause breakdown because of caustic enzymes, especially from the small bowel.
If indicated, consult enterostomal therapy (ET) nurse or wound care nurse. For additional information, see "Managing Wound Care," p. 583.	For intervention if drainage is excessive, skin excoriation develops, or a collection bag can be placed over drains and incisions.

●●● **Related NIC and NOC labels:** *NIC:* Skin Surveillance; Incision Site Care; Infection Control; Infection Protection; Skin Care: Topical Treatments; Wound Care *NOC:* Tissue Integrity: Skin & Mucous Membranes

Nursing Diagnosis:

Impaired Oral Mucous Membrane

related to NPO status and/or presence of NG or endotracheal tube

Desired Outcome: At time of hospital discharge, patient's oral mucosa is intact, without pain or evidence of bleeding.

INTERVENTIONS	RATIONALES
Provide oral care and oral hygiene q4h and prn. Arrange for patient to gargle, brush teeth, and cleanse the mouth with sponge-tipped applicators as necessary.	For comfort and to prevent excoriation and excessive dryness.
Use a moistened cotton-tipped applicator to remove encrustations. Carefully lubricate lips and nares with water-soluble lubricant, antimicrobial ointment, petroleum jelly, or emollient cream as appropriate.	For comfort and to decrease risk of tissue breakdown caused by dry tissues.
Obtain a prescription for lidocaine gargling solution or spray.	If patient's throat tissue is irritated from presence of an NG tube.

●●● **Related NIC and NOC labels:** *NIC:* Oral Health Maintenance *NOC:* Tissue Integrity: Skin & Mucous Membranes

ADDITIONAL NURSING DIAGNOSES/ PROBLEMS:

Prolonged Bedrest

Patients on prolonged bedrest face many potential physiologic problems. Some are short term and easily corrected. Others, such as joint contractures, may result in permanent disability. This section reviews the most common physiologic and psychosocial problems that may occur. With early discharge from the hospital, many of these problems now are seen when the patient is transferred to a long-term care facility or when discharged to home.

HEALTH CARE SETTING

Extended care, acute care, home care

Nursing Diagnosis:

Risk for Activity Intolerance

related to deconditioned status

Desired Outcomes: Patient exhibits cardiac tolerance to activity or exercise as evidenced by HR ≤20 bpm over resting HR, systolic BP ≤20 mm Hg over or under resting systolic BP, RR ≤20 breaths/min with normal depth and pattern (eupnea), normal sinus rhythm, warm and dry skin, and absence of crackles (rales), new murmurs, new dysrhythmias, gallop, or chest pain. During exercise, patient rates perceived exertion (RPE) at ≤3 on a scale of 0 (none) to 10 (maximal).

INTERVENTIONS	RATIONALES
Perform range-of-motion (ROM) exercises 2-4 times/day on each extremity. Individualize the exercise plan based on the following guidelines:	To build stamina by increasing muscle strength and endurance and prevent physiologic problems such as contractures and pressure damage to skin caused by inactivity. **Caution:** Avoid isometric exercises in cardiac patients. These exercises can increase systemic arterial blood pressure.
- *Mode or type of exercise:* begin with passive exercises, moving the joints through the motions of abduction, adduction, flexion, and extension. Progress to active-assisted exercises in which you support the joints while the patient initiates muscle contraction. When patient is able, supervise active isotonic exercises. Have patient repeat each exercise 3-10 times.	Beginning with passive movement, progressing to active-assisted, and continuing with active isotonic takes the patient from the least exerting to the most exerting exercises over a period of time, thus enabling gradual tolerance.

Continued

INTERVENTIONS	RATIONALES
Stop any exercise that results in muscular or skeletal pain. Consult a physical therapist (PT) about necessary modifications.	To prevent an injury to a joint too inflamed or diseased to tolerate the type or intensity of exercise.
- *Intensity:* begin with 3-5 repetitions as tolerated by the patient.	Starting with minimal intensity and progressing step-by-step to more intensity enables gradual tolerance.
Measure HR and BP at rest, peak exercise, and 5 min after exercise.	These assessments will help determine tolerance to the exercise. If HR or systolic BP *increases* >20 bpm or >20 mm Hg over the resting level, this is a sign of intolerance, which means the number of repetitions needs to be decreased.
	If HR or systolic BP *decreases* >10 bpm or >10 mm Hg at peak exercise, this could be a sign of left ventricular failure, denoting that the heart cannot meet this workload.
- *Duration:* begin with 5 min or less of exercise. Gradually increase the exercise to 15 min as tolerated.	Starting with minimal duration and progressing to greater duration enables gradual tolerance.
- *Frequency:* begin with exercises 2-4 times/day.	As duration increases, frequency can be reduced.
- *Assessment of exercise tolerance:* monitor for excessive shortness of breath.	Excessive shortness of breath may occur if (1) transient pulmonary congestion occurs secondary to ischemia or left ventricular dysfunction; (2) lung volumes are decreased; (3) oxygen-carrying capacity of the blood is reduced; or (4) there is shunting of blood from the right to the left side of the heart without adequate oxygenation.
Assess BP, skin, heart rhythm, and breath sounds.	If cardiac output does not increase to meet the body's needs during modest levels of exercise, systolic BP may fall; the skin may become cool, cyanotic, and diaphoretic; dysrhythmias may be noted; crackles (rales) may be auscultated; or a systolic murmur of mitral regurgitation may occur.
- If patient tolerates the exercise, increase the intensity or number of repetitions each day.	Tolerance is a sign that cardiovascular and respiratory systems are able to meet the demands of these low-level ROM exercises.
Ask patient to rate perceived exertion experienced during exercise, basing it on the following scale developed by Borg (1982): 0 = Nothing at all 1 = Very weak effort 2 = Weak (light) effort 3 = Moderate 4 = Somewhat stronger effort 5 = Strong effort 7 = Very strong effort 9 = Very, very strong effort 10 = Maximal effort	Exercises to prevent deconditioning should be performed at low levels of effort. The patient should not experience an RPE >3 while performing ROM exercises. Intensity of the exercise should be reduced and the frequency increased until an RPE of ≤3 is attained.
As the patient's condition improves, increase activity as soon as possible to include sitting in a chair.	To promote optimal conditioning, activity should be increased to correspond to patient's increased tolerance.
Assess for orthostatic hypotension. Prepare patient for this change by increasing amount of time spent in high Fowler's position and moving patient slowly and in stages.	Orthostatic hypotension can occur as a result of decreased plasma volume and difficulty in adjusting immediately to postural change. For more information about orthostatic hypotension, see **Ineffective Cerebral Tissue Perfusion,** later.
Progress activity in hospitalized patients as follows:	

Continued

INTERVENTIONS

RATIONALES

Level I: Bedrest: Flexion and extension of extremities 4 times/day, 15 times each extremity; deep breathing 4 times/day, 15 breaths; position change from side to side q2h.

Level II: Out of bed to chair: As tolerated, 3 times/day for 20-30 min; may perform ROM exercises 2 times/day while sitting in chair.

Level III: Ambulate in room: As tolerated, 3 times/day for 3-5 min in room.

Level IV: Ambulate in hall: Initially, 50-200 ft 2 times/day; progressing to 600 ft 4 times/day; may incorporate slow stair climbing in preparation for hospital discharge.

Monitor for signs of activity intolerance.	Activity intolerance is evidenced by a decrease in BP >20 mm Hg and an increase in heart rate to >120 bpm (or >20 bpm above resting HR in patients receiving β-blocker therapy).
Have patient perform self-care activities as tolerated.	Self-care activities such as eating, mouth care, and bathing may increase patient's activity level.
Teach significant other the purpose and interventions for preventing deconditioning. Involve him or her in patient's plan of care.	Significant others can promote and participate in patient's activity/exercises once they understand the rationale and are familiar with the interventions.
Provide emotional support to patient and significant other as patient's activity level is increased.	To help allay fears of failure, pain, or medical setbacks.

●●● **Related NIC and NOC labels:** *NIC:* Energy Management; Exercise Promotion: Strength Training; Exercise Therapy: Ambulation; Exercise Therapy: Joint Mobility; Exercise Therapy: Muscle Control; Vital Signs Monitoring; Emotional Support; Teaching: Prescribed Activity/Exercise *NOC:* Activity Tolerance; Endurance

Nursing Diagnosis:

Risk for Disuse Syndrome

related to paralysis, mechanical immobilization, prescribed immobilization, severe pain, or altered LOC

Desired Outcome: Patient exhibits complete ROM of all joints without pain, and limb girth measurements are congruent with or increased over baseline measurements.

Note: ROM exercises should be performed at least twice per day for all immobilized patients with *normal* joints. Modification may be required for patient with flaccidity (i.e., immediately after cerebrovascular accident [CVA] or spinal cord injury [SCI]) to prevent subluxation or for patient with spasticity (i.e., during the recovery period for patient with CVA or SCI) to prevent an increase in spasticity. Consult PT or occupational therapist (OT) for assistance in modifying the exercise plan for these patients. Recognize that ROM exercises are restricted or contraindicated for patients with rheumatologic disease during the inflammatory phase and for joints that are dislocated or fractured.

INTERVENTIONS

RATIONALES

During assessment of patient's joints, pay special attention to the following areas: shoulders, fingers, hips, knees, and feet.	These areas are especially susceptible to joint contracture. Shoulders can become "frozen" to limit abduction and extension; wrists can "drop," prohibiting extension; fingers can develop flexion contractures that limit extension;

Continued

INTERVENTIONS	RATIONALES
	hips can develop flexion contractures that affect the gait by shortening the limb or develop external rotation or adduction deformities that affect the gait; knees may have flexion contractures that can develop to limit extension and alter the gait; and feet can "drop" as a result of prolonged plantar flexion, which limits dorsiflexion and alters the gait.
Ensure that patient changes position at least q2h. Post a turning schedule at patient's bedside.	Position changes not only will maintain correct body alignment, thereby reducing strain on the joints, but also prevent contractures, minimize pressure on bony prominences, decrease venostasis, and promote maximal chest expansion.
- Place patient in proper body alignment. Maintain this position with pillows, towels, or other positioning aids.	A position in which the head is neutral or slightly flexed on the neck, hips are extended, knees are extended or minimally flexed, and feet are at right angles to the legs achieves proper standing alignment, which helps promote ambulation when patient is ready to do so.
- Ensure patient is prone or side lying with hips extended for the same amount of time spent in the supine position or, at a minimum, 3 times/day for 1 hr.	This position helps prevent hip flexion contracture.
- When head of bed (HOB) must be elevated 30 degrees, extend patient's shoulders and arms, using pillows to support the position. **Caution:** Ensure that patient spends time with hips in extension (see preceding intervention).	This position maintains proper spinal posture. Elevating HOB promotes hip flexion.
- Allow fingertips to extend over edge of the pillows.	Maintains normal arching of the hands.
- When patient is in the side-lying position, extend lower leg from the hip.	To help prevent hip flexion contracture.
- When able to place patient in prone position, move patient to end of the bed and allow feet to rest between mattress and footboard.	This will prevent not only plantar flexion and hip rotation but also injury to heels and toes.
- Place thin pads under angles of the axillae and lateral aspects of the clavicles.	To prevent internal rotation of the shoulders and maintain anatomic position of the shoulder girdle.
Use positioning devices liberally.	Using pillows, rolled towels, blankets, sandbags, antirotation boots, splints, and orthotics helps maintain joints in neutral position, which will help ensure that they remain functional when activity is increased.
When using adjunctive devices, monitor involved skin at frequent intervals.	To assess for alterations in skin integrity and implement measures to prevent skin breakdown.
Assess patient's feet for footdrop. Document this assessment daily.	Footdrop may occur with prolonged plantar flexion. However, because feet lie naturally in plantar flexion, assess for patient's inability to dorsiflex (pull the toes up toward the head). This is a sign of footdrop, and it requires prompt intervention to prevent or ameliorate permanent damage.
Teach patient and significant other the rationale and procedure for ROM exercises and have patient return the demonstrations. Review **Risk for Activity Intolerance,** earlier, to ensure patient does not exceed his or her tolerance. Explain importance of exercising more stringently joints that are especially prone to contracture.	To facilitate compliance with exercise program and prevent contracture formation.

Continued

INTERVENTIONS	RATIONALES
Provide patient with a handout that reviews exercises and lists repetitions for each. Instruct significant other to encourage patient to perform exercises as required.	Facilitates learning and compliance.
Perform and document limb girth measurements, dynamography, and ROM and establish exercise-baseline limits.	To assess existing muscle mass, strength, and joint motion for subsequent evaluation.
Explain to patient how muscle atrophy occurs. Emphasize importance of maintaining or increasing muscle strength and tissue elasticity around the joint via exercise.	Muscle atrophy occurs because of disuse or failure to use the joint, often caused by immediate or anticipated pain. This explanation encourages patient to perform exercises inasmuch as disuse eventually may result in decreased muscle mass and blood supply and a loss of periarticular tissue elasticity, which in turn can lead to increased muscle fatigue and joint pain with use.
Explain need to participate maximally in self-care as tolerated. For noncardiac patients needing greater help with muscle strength, assist with resistive exercises. For patients in beds with Balkan frames, provide means for resistive exercise by implementing a system of weights and pulleys.	To help maintain muscle strength and promote a sense of participation and control.
First determine patient's baseline level of performance on a given set of exercises and then set realistic goals with patient for repetitions.	Well-planned goals provide markers for assessing effectiveness of the exercise plan and progress made.
If the joints require rest, implement isometric exercises to help achieve endurance.	In these exercises, patient contracts a muscle group and holds the contraction for a count of 5 or 10. The sequence is repeated for increasing counts or repetitions until an adequate level of endurance has been achieved. Thereafter, maintenance levels are performed.
Provide a chart to show patient's progress; give patient positive reinforcement.	Attaining progress and having positive reinforcement promote continued compliance.
Post the exercise regimen at the bedside. Teach exercise regimen to significant other and elicit his or her support and encouragement for patient's performance of these exercises.	To ensure consistency by all health care personnel and involvement and support of significant other.
As appropriate, teach transfer or crutch-walking techniques and use of a walker, wheelchair, or cane. Include significant other in the demonstrations and stress importance of good body mechanics.	To ensure patient can maintain highest possible level of mobility
Provide periods of uninterrupted rest between exercises/activities.	To enable patient to replenish energy stores.
Seek a referral to a PT or OT as appropriate.	For patient who has special needs or who is not in a care facility.

●●● **Related NIC and NOC labels:** *NIC:* Activity Therapy; Energy Management; Exercise Promotion; Risk Identification; Sleep Enhancement; Teaching: Prescribed Activity/Exercise; Exercise Therapy: Joint Mobility; Exercise Therapy: Muscle Control; Exercise Therapy: Ambulation; Positioning *NOC:* Endurance; Immobility Consequences: Physiological; Mobility Level

Nursing Diagnosis:

Ineffective Peripheral Tissue Perfusion

related to interrupted venous flow secondary to prolonged immobility

Desired Outcomes: At least 24 hr before discharge from care facility (or within the 48-hr period following this diagnosis), patient performs exercises independently, adheres to the prophylactic regimen, and maintains an intake of 2-3 L/day of fluid unless contraindicated. Within 3 days of this diagnosis, patient has adequate peripheral perfusion as evidenced by normal skin color and temperature and adequate distal pulses (>2+ on a 0-4+ scale) in peripheral extremities.

INTERVENTIONS	RATIONALES
Teach patient that pain, redness, swelling, and warmth in the involved area and coolness, edema, unnatural color or pallor, and dilated veins distal to the involved area should be reported to staff member promptly if they occur.	These are indicators of deep vein thrombosis (DVT). A knowledgeable patient is likely to report these indicators promptly for timely intervention.
Monitor for indicators just listed, along with routine VS checks and laboratory test results.	Additional signs of DVT may include fever, tachycardia, and elevated erythrocyte sedimentation rate (ESR).
Perform passive ROM or encourage active ROM exercises.	To increase circulation, which will promote peripheral tissue perfusion.
Teach patient calf-pumping (ankle dorsiflexion–plantar flexion) and ankle-circling exercises.	Same as above. Patient should repeat each movement 10 times, performing each exercise hourly during extended periods of immobility, provided that patient is free of symptoms of DVT.
Encourage deep breathing.	Deep breathing increases negative pressure in the lungs and thorax to promote emptying of large veins and thus increase peripheral tissue perfusion.
When not contraindicated by peripheral vascular disease (PVD), ensure that patient wears antiembolism hose, pneumatic foot pump devices, or pneumatic sequential compression stockings.	To prevent venous stasis, the precursor to DVT. The pneumatic devices, which provide more compression than antiembolism hose, are especially useful in preventing DVT in patients who are mostly immobile.
Remove antiembolism hose or device for 10-20 min q8h. Reapply hose after elevating patient's legs at least 10 degrees for 10 min.	To inspect underlying skin for evidence of irritation or breakdown. Elevating the legs before reapplying the hose promotes venous return and decreases edema, which otherwise would remain and cause discomfort when the hose are reapplied.
Instruct patient not to cross feet at the ankles or knees while in bed.	May cause venous stasis.
If patient is at risk for DVT, elevate foot of bed 10 degrees.	To increase venous return.
In nonrestricted patient, increase fluid intake to at least 2-3 L/day. Educate patient about need to drink large amounts of fluid (9-14 8-oz glasses). Monitor I&O to ensure compliance.	To reduce hemoconcentration, which can contribute to development of DVT.
Administer anticoagulant agents as prescribed and monitor appropriate laboratory values (e.g., prothrombin time [PT], partial thromboplastin time [PTT]).	Patients at risk for DVT, including those with chronic infection and history of PVD and smoking, as well as patients who are older, obese, and anemic, may require anticoagulants to minimize risk of clotting. Drugs such as aspirin, sodium warfarin, phenindione derivatives, heparin, or low-molecular-weight heparin (LMWH, e.g., enoxaparin sodium) may be given. Many patients are taught how to self-administer LMWH injections after hospital discharge. Optimal laboratory values are 10-13.5 sec for PT and 60-70 sec or 1.5-2.5 × control value if on anticoagulant therapy for PTT. Values higher than these signify that patient is at increased risk for bleeding.
Teach patient to self-monitor for and report bleeding.	Anticoagulant drugs increase risk of bleeding. It is important that patient know signs of bleeding so that he or she can report them as soon as they are noted to ensure timely intervention. Possible types of bleeding include epistaxis, bleeding gums, hematemesis, hemoptysis, melena, hematuria, hematochezia, menometrorrhagia, and ecchymoses.
Teach medication and food interactions that can affect warfarin.	To reduce possibility of drug and/or food interactions in patients taking warfarin. Examples include foods high in vitamin K (interfere with anticoagulation) and drugs such as aspirin (enhance response to warfarin) and diuretics (decrease response to warfarin).

Continued

INTERVENTIONS	RATIONALES
In patients prone to DVT, acquire bilateral baseline measurements of midcalf, knee, and midthigh and record them on patient's Kardex. Monitor these measurements daily and compare them with baseline measurements.	To assess for extremity enlargement caused by DVT.

●●● **Related NIC and NOC labels:** *NIC:* Circulatory Care: Venous Insufficiency; Skin Surveillance; Bed Rest Care; Circulatory Precautions; Positioning; Pressure Management; Fluid Management; Pneumatic Tourniquet Precautions; Embolus Care: Peripheral *NOC:* Tissue Integrity: Skin and Mucous Membranes; Tissue Perfusion: Peripheral

Nursing Diagnosis:

Ineffective Cerebral Tissue Perfusion

(orthostatic hypotension) or risk for same *related to* interrupted arterial flow to the brain secondary to prolonged bedrest

Desired Outcome: When getting out of bed, patient has adequate cerebral perfusion as evidenced by HR <120 bpm and BP ≥90/60 mm Hg (or within 20 mm Hg of patient's normal range), dry skin, normal skin color, and absence of vertigo and syncope immediately after position change, with return of HR and BP to resting levels within 3 min of position change.

INTERVENTIONS	RATIONALES
Assess patient for recent diuresis, diaphoresis, or change in vasodilator therapy.	These are factors that increase risk of orthostatic hypotension because of fluid volume changes. For example, bedrest incurs a diuresis of about 600-800 ml during the first 3 days. Although this fluid decrease is not noticed when the patient is supine, the lost volume will be evident (i.e., with orthostatic hypotension) when the body tries to adapt to sitting and standing.
Also be alert for diabetic cardiac neuropathy, denervation after heart transplant, advanced age, or severe left ventricular dysfunction.	These are factors that increase risk of orthostatic hypotension because of altered autonomic control.
Explain cause of orthostatic hypotension and measures for preventing it.	Patients who are informed as to cause and ways of preventing orthostatic hypotension are more likely to avoid it. Measures to prevent orthostatic hypotension are discussed in subsequent interventions.
For patients who continue to have difficulty with orthostatic hypotension, apply antiembolism hose.	Used to prevent DVT, antiembolism hose also may be useful in preventing orthostatic hypotension by promoting venous return once the patient is mobilized. It may be necessary to supplement the hose with elastic wraps to the groin when the patient is out of bed. These wraps should encompass the entire surface of the legs.
When patient is in bed, provide instructions for leg exercises as described under **Risk for Activity Intolerance**, p. 67. Encourage patient to perform leg exercises immediately before mobilization.	To promote venous return.
Prepare patient for getting out of bed by encouraging position changes within necessary confines.	To reacclimate patient to upright position. It is sometimes possible and advisable to use a tilt table.

Continued

INTERVENTIONS	RATIONALES
Follow these guidelines for mobilization:	
- Check BP in any high-risk patient for whom this will be the first time out of bed. Instruct patient to immediately report symptoms of lightheadedness or dizziness.	Low BP, lightheadedness, and dizziness are signs of orthostatic hypotension and necessitate a return to the supine position.
- Have patient dangle legs at the bedside.	Provides for a gradual adjustment to the possible effects of venous pooling and related hypotension in the person who has been supine or in Fowler's position for some time. Dangling of the legs may be necessary until intravascular fluid volume is restored. It also provides an opportunity for leg exercise that can reduce risk of venous stasis.
- Be alert to diaphoresis, pallor, tachycardia, hypotension, and syncope. Question patient about presence of lightheadedness or dizziness.	Indicators of orthostatic hypotension.
- Again, encourage performance of leg exercises.	To promote venous return.
- If indicators of orthostatic hypotension occur, check VS.	A drop in systolic BP of 20 mm Hg and an increased pulse rate, combined with symptoms of vertigo and impending syncope, signal need for return to a supine position.
- If leg dangling is tolerated, have patient stand at the bedside with two staff members in attendance. If no adverse signs or symptoms occur, have patient progress to ambulation as tolerated.	To ensure patient's safety in the event of a fall.

●●● **Related NIC and NOC labels:** *NIC:* Circulatory Care: Arterial Insufficiency; Cerebral Perfusion Promotion; Positioning; Vital Signs Monitoring; Circulatory Care: Venous Insufficiency *NOC:* Circulation Status; Tissue Perfusion: Cerebral

Nursing Diagnosis:

Ineffective Breathing Pattern

related to decreased lung expansion secondary to inactivity or omission of deep breathing

Desired Outcomes: Patient demonstrates deep breathing and effective coughing at least hourly and is eupneic (RR 12-20 breaths/min with normal depth and pattern) at all other times. Auscultation of patient's lungs reveals no adventitious sounds.

INTERVENTIONS	RATIONALES
Auscultate breath sounds at least q2-4h (or as indicated by patient's condition) and during hyperinflation therapy. Report significant findings.	To assess for any decrease in breath sounds or presence of/increase in adventitious breath sounds, which can signal ineffective breathing pattern.
Instruct patient in use of hyperinflation device (e.g., an incentive spirometer).	To expand the lungs maximally. The emphasis of this therapy is on inhalation. Patient inhales slowly and deeply 2 × normal tidal volume and holds the breath at least 5 sec at the end of inspiration to maintain adequate alveolar inflation. Deep breathing expands the alveoli and aids in mobilizing secretions to the airways, and coughing further mobilizes and clears the secretions. The recommended number of inspirations/hr is 10.

Continued

INTERVENTIONS	RATIONALES
Administer analgesics as prescribed.	To reduce pain, which may facilitate patient's ease with coughing and deep-breathing exercises.
When appropriate, teach methods of splinting wounds or painful areas.	To enable cough.
Instruct patients who are unable to cough effectively in cascade cough.	To clear the airway when usual cough is not possible. Cascade cough is a succession of shorter and more forceful exhalations than in usual coughing.
Encourage activity as prescribed.	To help mobilize secretions and promote effective airway clearance.
When not contraindicated, instruct patient to increase fluid intake (>2.5 L/day).	To decrease viscosity of pulmonary secretions and facilitate their mobilization and removal.
When appropriate, coordinate deep breathing and coughing exercises with peak effectiveness of bronchodilator therapy.	To maximize potential for mobilization of secretions.

●●● **Related NIC and NOC labels:** *NIC:* Airway Management; Respiratory Monitoring; Positioning; Cough Enhancement; Exercise Promotion *NOC:* Respiratory Status: Ventilation

Nursing Diagnosis:

Constipation

related to less than adequate fluid, dietary intake, and bulk; immobility; lack of privacy; positional restrictions; and use of opioid analgesics

Desired Outcomes: Immediately following this diagnosis, patient verbalizes knowledge of measures that promote bowel elimination. Patient relates the return of normal pattern and character of bowel elimination within 3-5 days of this diagnosis.

INTERVENTIONS	RATIONALES
Assess patient's bowel history.	To determine normal bowel habits and interventions that are used successfully at home.
Monitor and document patient's bowel movements, diet, and I&O.	To track bowel movements and factors that promote or prevent constipation.
Assess for indicators of constipation and fecal impaction.	Indications of constipation include fewer than patient's usual number of bowel movements, abdominal discomfort or distention, straining at stool, and patient complaints of rectal pressure or fullness. Fecal impaction may be manifested by oozing of liquid stool and confirmed via digital examination.
Auscultate for bowel sounds in each abdominal quadrant for at least 1 min.	Bowel sounds are gurgles occurring normally at a rate of 5-32/min. Bowel sounds are decreased or absent with paralytic ileus. High-pitched rushing sounds or "tinkles" may be heard during abdominal cramping and may signal intestinal obstruction.
If a rectal impaction is suspected, use a gloved, lubricated finger to remove stool from the rectum; administer oil retention enemas as indicated.	Digital stimulation may be adequate to promote bowel movement. Oil retention enemas may soften impacted stool.

Continued

INTERVENTIONS	RATIONALES
Teach importance of a high-fiber diet.	To increase peristalsis and likelihood of normal bowel movements. High-fiber foods include bran, whole grains, nuts, and raw and coarse vegetables and fruits with skins.
Advise a fluid intake of at least 2-3 L/day (unless this is contraindicated by a renal, hepatic, or cardiac disorder).	Good hydration softens the stool, making it easier to evacuate. Patients with renal, hepatic, or cardiac disorders may be on fluid restrictions.
Maintain patient's normal bowel habits whenever possible.	Offering bedpan, ensuring privacy, and timing medications, enemas, or suppositories so that they take effect at the time of day patient normally has a bowel movement may facilitate regularity of bowel movements.
Provide warm fluids before breakfast and encourage toileting at that time.	Takes advantage of gastrocolic and duodenocolic reflexes.
Maximize activity level within limitations of patient's endurance, therapy, and pain.	To promote peristalsis, which helps prevent constipation.
Request pharmacologic interventions from health care provider when necessary, starting with the most gentle.	Starting with the gentlest interventions helps prevent rebound constipation and ensures minimal disruption of patient's normal bowel habits.
	The following is a suggested hierarchy of interventions: - Bulk-building additives (psyllium), bran - Mild laxatives (apple or prune juice, Milk of Magnesia) - Stool softeners (docusate sodium, docusate calcium) - Potent laxatives and cathartics (bisacodyl, cascara sagrada) - Medicated suppositories - Enemas
Discuss the role that opioid analgesics and other medications have in constipation.	Opioids, antidepressants, anticholinergics, iron supplements, diuretics, and muscle relaxants are known to cause constipation.
Teach alternative methods of pain control (such as massage, cold/heat application, acupressure, Reiki, ROM exercises).	Alternative, nontoxic methods of pain control may decrease need for opioid analgesics and hence likelihood of constipation caused by opioid analgesics.

●●● **Related NIC and NOC labels:** *NIC:* Bowel Management; Constipation/Impaction Management; Exercise Promotion; Fluid Management; Medication Management; Nutrition Management; Self-Care Assistance: Toileting *NOC:* Bowel Elimination; Hydration

Nursing Diagnosis:

Deficient Diversional Activity

related to prolonged illness and hospitalization

Desired Outcome: Within 24 hr of intervention, patient engages in diversional activities and relates the absence or decrease of boredom.

INTERVENTIONS	RATIONALES
Be alert to patient wishing for something to read or do, daytime napping, and expressed inability to perform usual hobbies of confinement.	These are indicators of boredom.

Continued

INTERVENTIONS	RATIONALES
Assess patient's activity tolerance as described on p. 67.	Activity tolerance will determine amount of activity the patient can engage in within limits of his or her diagnosis.
Collect a database by assessing patient's normal support systems and relationship patterns with significant other. Question patient and significant other about patient's interests.	This will enable nurse to explore diversional activities that may be suitable for the health care setting and patient's level of activity tolerance.
Personalize patient's environment with favorite objects and photographs of significant others.	To provide visual stimulation.
Provide low-level activities commensurate with patient's tolerance.	To promote mental stimulation and reduce boredom. Examples include books or magazines pertaining to patient's recreational or other interests, computer games, television, and writing for short intervals.
Initiate activities that require little concentration and proceed to more complicated tasks as patient's condition allows.	Initially patient may find difficult tasks frustrating. Physiologic problems such as anemia and pain may make concentration difficult.
Encourage discussion of past activities or reminiscence.	This could serve as a substitute for performing favorite activities during convalescence.
Encourage significant other to visit within limits of patient's endurance and to involve patient in activities that are of interest to him or her, such as playing cards or board games. Encourage significant other to stagger visits throughout the day.	Visiting and partaking in activities with loved ones likely would reduce boredom.
Suggest that significant other bring a radio, or, if appropriate, rent a television or radio from the care facility if not part of the standard room charge.	Watching TV and listening to radio often are good diversions.
If appropriate for patient, arrange for health care facility volunteers to visit, play cards, read books, or play board games.	To reduce boredom.
As appropriate for patient who desires social interaction, consider relocation to a room in an area of high traffic.	People watching can be a good diversion.
As patient's condition improves, assist with sitting in a chair near a window so that outside activities can be viewed. When patient is able, provide opportunities to sit in a solarium so that he or she can visit with other patients. If the physical condition and weather permit, take patient outside for brief periods.	New scenery, whether within the same room or in another area, can reduce boredom, as can meeting and speaking with other people.
Increase patient's involvement in self-care.	Performing in-bed exercises (e.g., deep breathing, ankle circling, calf pumping), keeping track of I&O, and similar activities can and should be accomplished routinely by patients to provide a sense of purpose, accomplishment, and control, which likely will diminish boredom.

●●● **Related NIC and NOC labels:** *NIC:* Activity Therapy; Socialization Enhancement; Therapeutic Play; Bibliotherapy; Reminiscence Therapy; Role Enhancement; Support System Enhancement
NOC: Social Involvement

Nursing Diagnosis:

Sexual Dysfunction

(or risk for same) *related to* actual or perceived physiologic limitations on sexual performance secondary to disease, therapy, or prolonged hospitalization

Desired Outcome: Within 72 hr of this diagnosis, patient relates satisfaction with sexuality and/or understanding of the ability to resume sexual activity.

INTERVENTIONS	RATIONALES
Assess patient's normal sexual function, including importance placed on sex in the relationship, frequency of interaction, normal positions used, and the couple's ability to adapt or change to meet requirements of patient's limitations.	To determine patient's normal sexual function and adaptations that will be necessary under current conditions.
Identify patient's problem diplomatically and clarify it with patient.	To determine if patient suffers from sexual dysfunction resulting from lack of privacy, current illness, or perceived limitations. Indicators of sexual dysfunction can include regression, acting-out with inappropriate behavior such as grabbing or pinching, sexual overtures toward staff members, self-enforced isolation, and similar behaviors.
Encourage patient and significant other to verbalize feelings and anxieties about sexual abstinence, having sexual relations in the care facility, hurting the patient, or having to use new or alternative methods for sexual gratification. Develop strategies in collaboration with patient and significant other.	To promote patient's understanding of ways to achieve sexual satisfaction.
Encourage acceptable expressions of sexuality.	Examples of positive and acceptable behaviors may eliminate inappropriate behaviors. Examples for a woman could include wearing makeup and jewelry and for a man, shaving and wearing own shirts and shorts.
Inform patient and significant other that it is possible to have time alone together for intimacy. Provide that time accordingly by putting a "Do Not Disturb" sign on the door, enforcing privacy by restricting staff and visitors to the room, or arranging for temporary private quarters.	Facilitates intimacy by ensuring patient's privacy.
Encourage patient and significant other to seek alternate methods of sexual expression when necessary.	Accustomed methods of sexual expression may not work under current circumstances. Alternate methods may include mutual masturbation, altered positions, vibrators, and identification of other erotic areas for the partner.

●●● **Related NIC and NOC labels:** *NIC:* Sexual Counseling; Self-Esteem Enhancement *NOC:* Sexual Functioning

Nursing Diagnosis:

Ineffective Role Performance:

Dependence vs. independence

Desired Outcome: Within 24 hr of this diagnosis, patient collaborates with caregivers in planning realistic goals for independence, participates in own care, and takes responsibility for self-care.

INTERVENTIONS	RATIONALES
Encourage patient to be as independent as possible within limitations of endurance, therapy, and pain.	To facilitate independence as much as feasible. Recognize, however, that temporary periods of dependence are appropriate because they enable the individual to restore energy reserves needed for recovery.
Ensure that all health care providers are consistent in conveying their expectations of eventual independence.	To ensure that all health care providers promote independence as much as possible.
Alert patient to areas of excessive dependence and involve him or her in collaborative goal setting to achieve independence.	Although there are times when dependence is needed and desired, it is healthy to begin to foster a degree of independence as recovery progresses.
Allow patient to express emotions, but provide support, understanding, and realistic hope for a positive role change. Provide positive reinforcement when patient meets or advances toward goals.	Minimizing patient's expressed feelings of depression can add to anger and depression. Offering realistic hope and encouragement can provide needed emotional support in movement toward independence.
If indicated, provide self-help devices.	To increase patient's independence with self-care.

●●● **Related NIC and NOC labels:** *NIC:* Coping Enhancement; Counseling; Role Enhancement; Body Image Enhancement; Emotional Support; Normalization Promotion *NOC:* Coping; Role Performance

ADDITIONAL NURSING DIAGNOSES/ PROBLEMS:

"Psychosocial Support"	p. 81
"Pneumonia" for interventions related to prevention of same	p. 135
"Pressure Ulcers" for **Impaired Tissue Integrity** (for patients without pressure ulcers who are at risk because of immobility)	p. 586

Psychosocial Support

Nursing Diagnosis:

Deficient Knowledge:

Current health status and therapies

Desired Outcome: Before invasive procedure, surgical procedure, initiation of medications, or hospital discharge (as appropriate), patient verbalizes understanding about his or her current health status and therapies.

INTERVENTIONS	RATIONALES
Assess patient's current level of knowledge about his or her health status and therapies.	Assessing patient's level of knowledge enables development of an individualized teaching plan, as well as correction of misperceptions and misinformation.
Assess cognitive and emotional readiness to learn.	A well-developed teaching plan of care is worthless if the patient is unable or unwilling to process information. Barriers to learning include ineffective communication, neurologic deficit, sensory alterations, fear, anxiety, or lack of motivation.
Assess learning needs and establish short-term and long-term goals.	Well-planned goals provide markers for assessing effectiveness of the teaching plan and progress made.
Use individualized verbal or written information. Give simple, direct instructions. As indicated, use audiovisual tools as supplemental information.	Because individuals learn differently, using more than one teaching modality will provide more opportunities to assimilate information.
Encourage significant other to reinforce correct information about diagnosis and therapies to patient.	Anxiety often filters the information given. Involving a spouse or other family member provides teaching reinforcement as the patient processes the information provided.
Encourage patient's interest in health care information by planning care collaboratively. Explain rationale for care and therapies.	Involving patient in his or her own care planning promotes compliance with the treatment plan and engenders a sense of control and ownership.
Talk frequently with patient.	Frequent patient interaction enables evaluation of comprehension and provides opportunities for reinforcement. Many individuals may not understand seemingly simple medical terms (e.g., *terminal, malignant, constipation*).

Continued

INTERVENTIONS	RATIONALES
Request that patient repeat what he or she has been told. Tell patient to ask you any questions and reassure him or her that lack of comprehension/retention during illness is to be expected.	Anxiety may interfere with reception, comprehension, and retention. Individuals in crisis often need repeated explanations before information can be understood. Creating an environment of permission in which patient feels comfortable asking questions and revealing knowledge deficits facilitates learning.
Provide written materials about therapies.	To reinforce teaching and enable review at a later time.
As appropriate, assess understanding of informed consent. Assist patient to use information he or she receives to make informed health care decisions (e.g., about invasive procedures, surgery, resuscitation).	Assessing patient's level of comprehension assists nurse in determining whether consent is truly informed. Patients sometimes need to discuss previous teaching to assimilate the information given.

●●● **Related NIC and NOC labels:** *NIC:* Teaching: Disease Process; Health System Guidance; Learning Readiness Enhancement; Active Listening; Teaching: Procedure/Treatment; Preparatory Sensory Information; Decision-Making Support; Patient Rights Protection *NOC:* Knowledge: Disease Process; Knowledge: Illness Care; Knowledge: Treatment Regimen

Nursing Diagnosis:

Anxiety

related to actual or perceived threat of death, change in health status, threat to self-concept or role, unfamiliar people and environment, or the unknown

Desired Outcome: Within 1-2 hr of intervention, patient's anxiety has resolved or decreased as evidenced by patient's verbalization of same, HR ≤100 bpm, RR ≤20 breaths/min, and absence of or decreased irritability and restlessness.

INTERVENTIONS	RATIONALES
Engage in honest communication with patient; provide empathetic understanding. Listen closely.	To establish an atmosphere that allows free expression.
Be alert to verbal and nonverbal cues about patient's anxiety level.	Being cognizant of patient's level of anxiety enables nurse to provide appropriate interventions, as well as modify the plan of care accordingly. Levels of anxiety include: - *Mild:* restlessness, irritability, increased questions, focusing on the environment. - *Moderate:* inattentiveness, expressions of concern, narrowed perceptions, insomnia, increased HR. - *Severe:* expressions of feelings of doom, rapid speech, tremors, poor eye contact. Patient may be preoccupied with the past or unable to understand the present and may have tachycardia, nausea, and hyperventilation. - *Panic:* inability to concentrate or communicate, distortion of reality, increased motor activity, vomiting, tachypnea.
For patients with severe anxiety or panic state, refer to psychiatric clinical nurse specialist, case manager, or other health team members as appropriate.	Patients in severe anxiety or panic state may require more sophisticated interventions or pharmacologic management.
If patient is hyperventilating, encourage slow, deep breaths by having patient mimic your own breathing pattern.	Modeling provides patient with a focal point for learning effective breathing technique.

Continued

INTERVENTIONS	**RATIONALES**
Validate nursing assessment of anxiety with patient.	Validating patient's anxiety level provides confirmation of nursing assessment, as well as openly acknowledges patient's emotional state. In so doing, patient is given permission to share feelings. For example, "You seem distressed. Are you feeling uncomfortable now?"
Encourage patient to express fears, concerns, and questions.	Encouraging questions gives patient an avenue in which to share concerns. For example, "I know this room looks like a maze of wires and tubes. Please let me know when you have any questions."
After an episode of anxiety, review and discuss with patient the thoughts and feelings that led to the episode.	To validate with patient the cause of the anxiety and explore interventions that may avert another episode.
Identify patient's maladaptive coping behaviors. Review coping behaviors that patient has used in the past. Assist patient with using adaptive coping to manage anxiety.	Identifying maladaptive coping behaviors (e.g., denial, anger, repression, withdrawal, daydreaming, or dependence on narcotics, sedatives, or tranquilizers) helps establish a proactive plan of care to promote healthy coping skills. For example, "I understand that your wife reads to you to help you relax. Would you like to spend a part of each day alone with her?"
Provide an organized, quiet environment (see **Disturbed Sensory Perception,** p. 84).	To reduce sensory overload that may contribute to anxiety.
Introduce self and other health care team members; explain each individual's role as it relates to patient's care.	Familiarity with staff and their individual roles may increase patient's comfort level and decrease anxiety.
Teach patient relaxation and imagery techniques. See **Health-Seeking Behaviors:** Relaxation technique effective for stress reduction, p. 183.	Teaching relaxation and imagery skills empowers patient to manage anxiety-provoking episodes more skillfully and fosters a sense of control.
Enable support persons to be in attendance whenever possible.	Many people benefit from the support of others and find that it reduces their stress level.

●●● **Related NIC and NOC labels:** *NIC:* Anxiety Reduction; Active Listening; Behavior Management; Calming Technique; Coping Enhancement; Presence; Environmental Management; Progressive Muscle Relaxation; Simple Relaxation Therapy; Support Group *NOC:* Anxiety Control; Coping

Nursing Diagnosis:

Impaired Verbal Communication

related to neurologic or anatomic deficit, psychologic or physical barriers (e.g., tracheostomy, intubation), or cultural or developmental differences

Desired Outcome: At the time of intervention, patient begins to communicate needs and feelings and reports decreased or absent feelings of frustration over communication barriers.

INTERVENTIONS	**RATIONALES**
Assess cause of impaired communication (e.g., tracheostomy, cerebrovascular accident, cerebral tumor, Guillain-Barré syndrome).	Determining cause of communication impairment will enable nurse to develop a customized plan of care that incorporates communication skills the patient can use, given his or her disability.

Continued

INTERVENTIONS	RATIONALES
Involve patient and significant other/caregiver in assessing patient's ability to read, write, and understand English. If patient speaks a language other than English, collaborate with English-speaking family member or an interpreter.	To establish effective communication and ensure teaching materials provided are at a level appropriate for patient.
When communicating with patient, face him or her, make direct eye contact, and speak in a clear, normal tone of voice.	A visual- or hearing-impaired person often develops compensatory methods, for example, lip reading for a person who is hearing-impaired.
When communicating with a deaf person about the treatment plan, arrange to have an interpreter present if possible.	To facilitate effective communication, promote informed consent, and enable patient to ask questions.
If patient cannot speak because of a physical barrier (e.g., tracheostomy, wired mandibles), provide reassurance and acknowledge his or her frustration.	To decrease frustration caused by inability to communicate verbally. For example, "I know this is frustrating for you, but please do not give up. I want to understand you."
Provide slate, word cards, pencil and paper, alphabet board, pictures, or other device. Adapt call system to meet patient's needs. Document meaning of signals used by patient to communicate.	To enable effective communication, promote continuity of care, and lessen patient's anxiety.
Explain source of patient's communication impairment to caregiver; teach caregiver effective communication alternatives (see above).	Inability to communicate with ease may cause feelings of isolation that can be intensified if patient has difficulty communicating with caregiver.
Monitor for nonverbal messages. Validate their meaning with patient.	Nonverbal expression, such as facial expressions, hand movements, and nodding of the head, is a valid means of communication, and its meaning must be validated to facilitate understanding.
Encourage patient to communicate needs; reinforce independent behaviors.	Inability to speak may foster maladaptive behaviors, and this reinforces need for patient to be understood.
Be honest with patient; do not pretend to understand if you are unable to interpret patient's communication.	Pretending to understand patient will only add to his or her frustration and diminish trust.

●●● **Related NIC and NOC labels:** *NIC:* Active Listening; Communication Enhancement: Hearing Deficit; Communication Enhancement: Speech Deficit; Communication Enhancement: Visual Deficit; Presence; Environmental Management; Cognitive Stimulation; Cultural Brokerage; Reality Orientation *NOC:* Communication Ability; Communication: Expressive Ability; Communication: Receptive Ability

Nursing Diagnosis:

Disturbed Sensory Perception

related to therapeutically or socially restricted environment; psychologic stress; altered sensory reception, transmission, or integration; or chemical alteration

Desired Outcome: At the time of intervention, patient verbalizes orientation to person, place, and time; reports some ability to concentrate; and expresses satisfaction with the degree and type of sensory stimulation being received.

INTERVENTIONS	RATIONALES
Assess factors contributing to patient's sensory-perceptual alteration.	Some factors may be readily reversible. Others will require palliative measures. Modifying environmental stimulation and intervening for physiologic factors as much as feasible

Continued

INTERVENTIONS	RATIONALES
	may reduce patient stress, promote normal sleep patterns, and assist in maintaining orientation.
	- *Environmental factors:* excessive noise in the environment; constant, monotonous noise; restricted environment (immobility, traction, isolation); social isolation (restricted visitors, impaired communication); therapies
	- *Physiologic factors:* altered organ function, sleep or rest pattern disturbance, medication, previous history of altered sensory perception
Avoid constant lighting; maintain day/night patterns. Reduce noise whenever possible by decreasing alarm volumes, avoiding loud talking, keeping room door closed, providing earplugs.	Manages or ameliorates factors contributing to environmental stimulus overload.
As determined by patient's needs, provide sensory stimulation in the following ways:	To enable a plan of care suitable for patient's needs.
- As needed, orient patient to surroundings. Display clocks, large calendars, and meaningful photographs and objects from home. Direct patient to reality as necessary.	Helps patient attain/maintain orientation.
- Depending on patient preference, provide a radio, music, reading materials, and tape recordings of family and significant other. Earphones help to block out external stimuli.	Provides stimuli that help distract patient from illness-related concerns and may assist with orientation for disoriented patient.
- Position patient to look toward window when possible.	Assists with maintaining day/night pattern and provides external stimuli for orientation and diversion.
- Discuss current events, time of day, holidays, and topics of interest during patient care activities.	Another avenue for promoting orientation. For example, "Good morning, Mr. Smith. I'm Ms. Stone, your nurse for the afternoon and evening, 3 PM to 11 PM. It's sunny outside. Today is the first day of summer."
- Establish personal contact by touch to help promote and maintain patient's contact with the real environment.	Touch—other than that required to deliver care—meets a basic human need and is often overlooked in a busy health care facility.
- Encourage significant other to communicate with patient frequently, using a normal tone of voice.	Families may require encouragement and direction to be comfortable interacting with their loved one who has been changed by illness or its treatment.
- Convey concern and respect for patient. Introduce yourself and call patient by name.	Assists in maintaining basic human dignity while providing orientation.
- Stimulate patient's vision with mirrors, colored decorations, and pictures.	Provides visual diversions.
- Stimulate patient's sense of taste with sweet, salty, and sour substances as allowed.	Provides gustatory sensations.
- Encourage use of eyeglasses and hearing aids.	Promotes accurate perception of external stimuli.
Inform patient before initiating therapies and using equipment.	Helps patient process events, as well as anticipate uncomfortable noises or sensations.
Assess patient's sleep/rest pattern. Make sure patient attains at least 90 min of uninterrupted sleep as often as possible. For more information, see next nursing diagnosis.	Sleep deprivation causes increased stress that can lead to irritability and disorientation.

●●● **Related NIC and NOC labels:** *NIC:* Cognitive Stimulation; Reality Orientation; Communication Enhancement: Hearing Deficit; Communication Enhancement: Visual Enhancement; Speech Deficit; Environmental Management; Sleep Enhancement *NOC:* Cognitive Orientation; Communication: Receptive Ability; Hearing Compensation Behavior; Sensory Function: Vision

Nursing Diagnosis:

Disturbed Sleep Pattern

related to environmental changes, illness, therapeutic regimen, pain, immobility, psychologic stress, or hypoxia

Desired Outcomes: Immediately after assessment, patient identifies factors that promote sleep. Within 8 hr of intervention, patient shows progress toward attaining 90-min periods of uninterrupted sleep and verbalizes beginning satisfaction with his or her ability to rest.

INTERVENTIONS	RATIONALES
Assess patient's usual sleeping patterns (e.g., bedtime routine, hours of sleep per night, sleeping position, use of pillows and blankets, napping during the day, nocturia).	Some or all of patient's usual sleep pattern may be incorporated into the plan of care. A routine as similar to patient's normal routine as possible will help promote sleep.
Explore relaxation techniques with patient.	Imagining relaxing scenes, listening to soothing music or taped stories, and using muscle relaxation exercises are relaxation techniques that are known to promote rest/sleep.
Identify causative factors and activities that contribute to patient's insomnia, awaken patient, or adversely affect sleep pattern.	Factors such as pain, anxiety, hypoxia, therapies, depression, hallucinations, medications, underlying illness, sleep apnea, respiratory disorder, caffeine, and fear may contribute to sleep pattern disturbance. Some may be ameliorated, and others may be modified.
Organize procedures and activities to allow for 90-min periods of uninterrupted rest/sleep. Limit visiting during these periods.	Ninety minutes of sleep allows complete progression through the normal phases of sleep.
Provide a quiet and dimly lighted environment to promote sleep/rest.	Excessive noise and light can cause sleep deprivation. Providing earplugs, reducing alarm volume, and using white noise (i.e., low-pitched, monotonous sounds: electric fan, soft music) may facilitate sleep. Dimming the lights for a period of time, drawing the drapes, and providing blindfolds are other ways of promoting sleep.
If appropriate, put limitations on patient's daytime sleeping. Attempt to establish regularly scheduled daytime activity (e.g., ambulation, sitting in chair, active range of motion [ROM]).	Physical activity causes fatigue and may facilitate nighttime sleeping. Napping less during the day will promote a more normal nighttime pattern.
Investigate usefulness of and provide such measures as earplugs, pain and anxiety reduction, and use of patient's own bedclothes and pillows.	Nonpharmacologic comfort measures that are likely to promote patient's sleep.
Also see this nursing diagnosis in "Perioperative Care," p. 63.	

●●● **Related NIC and NOC labels:** *NIC:* Energy Management; Sleep Enhancement; Exercise Promotion; Environmental Management: Comfort; Music Therapy; Progressive Muscle Relaxation; Simple Relaxation Therapy; Simple Guided Imagery *NOC:* Rest; Sleep

Nursing Diagnosis:

Fear

related to separation from support systems, unfamiliarity with environment or therapeutic regimen, loss of sense of control, or uncertainty about the future

Desired Outcome: Immediately following interventions patient expresses fears and concerns and within 8 hr of interventions reports feeling greater psychologic and physical comfort.

INTERVENTIONS	RATIONALES
Assess patient's perceptions of his or her surroundings and health status. Evaluate patient's verbal and nonverbal responses.	To determine factors contributing to patient's feelings of fear.
Acknowledge patient's fears.	Acknowledging feelings encourages communication and hence reduces fear. Empathy lessens sense of isolation and fear. For example, "I understand this equipment frightens you, but it is necessary to help you breathe."
Provide opportunities for patient to express fears and concerns.	An empathic response promotes expression of fears and provides reassurance that concerns are acknowledged. For example, "You seem very concerned about receiving more blood today."
Listen closely to patient.	Expressions of anger, denial, occasional withdrawal, and demanding behaviors may be coping responses.
Encourage patient to ask questions and gather information about the unknown. Provide information about equipment, therapies, and routines according to patient's ability to understand.	Increasing knowledge level about therapies and procedures reduces/eliminates fear of the unknown and affords a sense of control.
Encourage patient to participate in and plan care whenever possible.	To promote increased sense of control, which will help decrease fears.
Provide continuity of care by establishing a routine and arranging for consistent caregivers whenever possible. Appoint a case manager or primary nurse and associate nurses.	Consistency in care providers promotes familiarity and trust.
Discuss with health care team members the appropriateness of medication therapy for patients with disabling fear or anxiety.	Pharmacologic interventions are sometimes necessary in assisting patients to cope with fears/anxieties about treatment, diagnosis, and prognosis.
When there is a question of the patient surviving the illness or surgery, consult with health care provider about a visit by another individual with the same disorder or situation who has survived the surgery or disorder.	Many people benefit from outside sources of support in decreasing fears. Interaction with another person who has had a similar experience provides hope and encouragement.
Explore patient's desire for spiritual or psychologic counseling.	Exploring spiritual dimension of the current experience may assist patient to cope with fear and stress.

●●● **Related NIC and NOC labels:** *NIC:* Anxiety Reduction; Active Listening; Coping Enhancement; Presence; Support System Enhancement; Support Group *NOC:* Anxiety Control: Fear Control

Nursing Diagnosis:

Ineffective Coping

related to health crisis, sense of vulnerability, or inadequate support systems

Desired Outcome: Within the 24-hr period after this diagnosis is made, patient verbalizes feelings, identifies strengths and coping behaviors, and demonstrates fewer ineffective coping behaviors.

INTERVENTIONS	RATIONALES
Assess patient's perceptions and ability to understand current health status.	Evaluation of patient's comprehension enables development of an individualized care plan.

Continued

INTERVENTIONS	RATIONALES
Establish honest communication with patient.	To promote effective therapeutic communication. For example, "Please tell me what I can do to help you."
Help patient identify previous methods of coping with life problems.	How patient has handled problems in the past may be a reliable predictor of how he or she will cope with current problems.
Support positive coping behaviors.	Identifies, reinforces, and facilitates positive coping behaviors. For example, "I see that reading that book seems to help you relax."
Help patient identify or develop a support system.	Many people benefit from outside support systems in helping them cope.
Arrange community referrals, as appropriate.	Support in the home environment promotes healthier adaptations and may avert crises.
Identify factors that inhibit patient's ability to cope.	Enables patient to identify areas such as unsatisfactory support system, deficient knowledge, grief, and fear that may contribute to anxiety and ineffective coping and to consider modification of same.
Assess for maladaptive coping behaviors.	Examples of maladaptive behaviors include severe depression; dependence on narcotics, sedatives, or tranquilizers; hostility; violence; and suicidal ideation. Patient may have used substances and other maladaptive behaviors in controlling anxiety. This pattern can interfere with ability to cope with current situation. If appropriate, nurses should discuss these behaviors with patient. For example, "You seem to be requiring more pain medication. Are you having more physical pain, or does it help you cope with your situation?"
Refer patient to psychiatric liaison, clinical nurse specialist, case manager, or clergy as appropriate.	Professional intervention may assist with altering maladaptive behaviors.
As patient's condition allows, assist with reducing anxiety. See **Anxiety**, p. 82.	Anxiety makes effective coping more difficult to achieve.
Maintain an organized, quiet environment. See **Disturbed Sensory Perception**, p. 84.	To help reduce patient's sensory overload to help with coping.
Encourage regular visits by family and caregiver. Encourage them to talk with patient.	To help minimize patient's emotional and social isolation, which will promote coping behaviors.
As appropriate, explain to family and caregiver that increased dependency, anger, and denial may be adaptive coping behaviors used by patient in early stages of crisis until effective coping behaviors are learned.	Lack of understanding about patient's maladaptive coping can lead to unhealthy interaction patterns and contribute to anxiety within the family.

●●● **Related NIC and NOC labels:** *NIC:* Coping Enhancement; Anxiety Reduction; Emotional Support; Support System Enhancement; Family Involvement Promotion; Referral *NOC:* Coping; Social Support

Nursing Diagnosis:

Anticipatory Grieving

related to perceived potential loss of physiologic well-being (e.g., expected loss of body function or body part, changes in self-concept or body image, illness, death)

Desired Outcome: Within the 24-hr period after intervention, patient and significant other/caregiver begin to express grief, participate in decisions about the future, and discuss concerns with health care team members and each other.

INTERVENTIONS	RATIONALES
Encourage patient to discuss feelings associated with antici-pated losses.	Conveys message that grief is a normal and expected reaction to loss of physiologic well-being.
Assess factors contributing to anticipated loss.	Misperceptions about contributing factors may result in unneces-sary fear/stress/grief. Dialogue may allay some anxieties.
Assess and accept patient's behavioral response.	Reactions such as disbelief, denial, guilt, anger, and depression are normal reactions to grief.
Determine patient's stage of grieving.	Comprehension of patient's stage of grief enables more effective therapeutic interventions. It is normal for a person to move from one stage to another and then revert to a previous stage. The time required to do so varies from individual to individual. If a person is unable to move into the next stage, referral for professional intervention may be indicated. - *Protest stage:* denial, disbelief, anger, hostility, resentment, bargaining to postpone loss, appeal for help to recover loss, loud complaints, altered sleep and appetite - *Disorganization stage:* depression, withdrawal, social isolation, psychomotor retardation, silence - *Reorganization stage:* acceptance of loss, development of new interests and attachments, restructuring of lifestyle, return to preloss level of functioning
Assess spiritual, religious, and sociocultural expectations related to loss.	Helping patient find meaning in his or her experience may facilitate the grieving process. For example, "Is religion an important part of your life? How do you and your family deal with serious health problems?"
Refer to the clergy or community support groups as appropriate.	Reinforces that there are support systems and resources to help work through grief.
Demonstrate empathy. Encourage patient and significant other to share their concerns.	Empathetic communication (including respecting desire not to communicate) promotes a trusting relationship and open dialogue. For example, "This must be a very difficult time for you and your family" or "Is there anything you'd like to talk about today?"
In selected circumstances, explain the grieving process.	This approach may help patient and family better understand and acknowledge their feelings and help family members better understand behaviors and verbalizations expressed by patient.
Assess grief reactions of patient and significant other and identify those individuals with potential for dysfunctional grieving reactions (e.g., absence of emotion, hostility, avoidance). If potential for dysfunctional grieving is present, refer the individual to psychiatric clinical nurse specialist, case manager, clergy, or other source of counseling as appropriate.	To identify and reduce dysfunctional grieving, if present. Promoting normal progression through the grieving stages may allay unnecessary emotional suffering.
When appropriate, assess patient's wishes about tissue donation.	If patient is grieving an expected death, tissue donation may assist with finding meaning in the death.

●●● **Related NIC and NOC labels:** *NIC:* Coping Enhancement; Grief Work Facilitation; Anticipatory Guidance; Emotional Support; Family Support; Hope Installation; Spiritual Support *NOC:* Coping; Family Coping; Psychosocial Adjustment: Life Change

Nursing Diagnosis:

Powerlessness

related to health care environment or illness–related regimen

Desired Outcome: Within 24 hr of this diagnosis, patient begins to make decisions about care and therapies and reports a beginning attitude of realistic hope and a sense of self-control.

INTERVENTIONS	RATIONALES
Assess patient's personal preferences, needs, values, and attitudes.	To help develop a care plan individualized for patient's needs, which optimally will decrease sense of powerlessness.
Assess for expressions of fear, lack of response to events, and lack of interest in information.	These are signals of patient's feelings of powerlessness.
Evaluate caregiver practices and adjust them to support patient's sense of control.	To increase patient's sense of control. For example, if the patient always bathes in the evening to promote relaxation before bedtime, modify the care plan to include an evening bath rather than follow the hospital routine of giving a morning bath.
Ask patient to identify activities he or she can perform independently.	Self-care activities likely will promote sense of control.
Whenever possible, offer alternatives related to routine hygiene, diet, diversional activities, visiting hours, and treatment times.	To promote sense of control and power over daily routine.
When distant relatives and casual acquaintances request information about patient's status, check with patient and family members before sharing that information.	To ensure privacy and preserve patient's territorial rights whenever possible.
Avoid overprotection and parenting behaviors toward patient. Instead, act as an advocate for patient and significant other.	To discourage patient's dependency on staff and promote independent behaviors.
Assess support systems; involve significant other in patient care whenever possible. Refer to clergy and other support persons or systems as appropriate.	Many people feel empowered by outside support systems. Promoting family involvement reduces their feelings of powerlessness as well.
Offer realistic hope for the future. On occasion, encourage patient to direct his or her thoughts beyond the present.	This likely will increase sense of control and power and promote hopefulness.
Determine patient's wishes about end-of-life decisions and document advanced directives as appropriate.	To promote sense of control and power about these decisions.

●●● **Related NIC and NOC labels:** *NIC:* Decision-Making Support; Family Involvement Promotion; Patient Rights Protection; Active Listening; Coping Enhancement; Referral *NOC:* Family Participation in Professional Care; Participation: Health Care Decisions

Nursing Diagnosis:

Spiritual Distress

related to separation from religious ties or cultures or challenged belief and value system

Desired Outcome: Within 24 hr of this diagnosis, patient begins to verbalize his or her religious beliefs and express hope for the future, attainment of spiritual well-being, and resolution of conflicts.

INTERVENTIONS	RATIONALES
Assess patient's spiritual or religious beliefs, values, and practices.	To determine patient's spiritual needs, which will assist in development of an individualized care plan. For example, "Do you have a religious preference? How important is it to you? Are there any religious or spiritual practices in which you wish to participate while in the hospital?"
Inform patient of the availability of spiritual resources, such as a chapel or volunteer chaplain.	To increase awareness of available spiritual resources and promote a sense of acceptance of patient's spirituality.
Display a nonjudgmental attitude toward patient's religious or spiritual beliefs and values.	To create an environment that is conducive to free expression.
Identify available support persons or systems that may assist in meeting patient's religious or spiritual needs (e.g., clergy, fellow church members, support groups).	Many people derive an increased sense of hope from religious and spiritual counselors.
Be alert to comments related to spiritual concerns or conflicts.	Comments such as "I don't know why God is doing this to me" and "I'm being punished for my sins" suggest that patient is feeling some degree of spiritual distress.
Listen closely and ask questions.	Helps patient resolve conflicts related to spiritual issues and helps nurse plan how best to assist patient. For example, "I understand that you want to be baptized. We can arrange to do that here."
Provide privacy and opportunities for religious practices, such as prayer and meditation.	Many people find prayer and meditation difficult in a nonprivate setting.
If spiritual beliefs and therapeutic regimens are in conflict, provide patient with honest, concrete information.	To encourage informed decision making. For example, "I understand your religion discourages receiving blood transfusions. We respect your position; however, it does not allow us to give you the best care possible."
Refer patient or significant other to an ethics committee.	To assist in resolving care dilemmas, if appropriate.

●●● **Related NIC and NOC labels:** *NIC:* Spiritual Support; Emotional Support; Referral; Support System Enhancement *NOC:* Spiritual Well-Being

Nursing Diagnosis:

Social Isolation

related to altered health status, inability to engage in satisfying personal relationships, altered mental status, body image change, or altered physical appearance

Desired Outcome: Within 24 hr of this diagnosis, patient begins to demonstrate interaction with others.

INTERVENTIONS	RATIONALES
Assess factors contributing to patient's social isolation.	To determine causes of social isolation and modify those factors that can be altered. Examples include: - Restricted visiting hours - Absence of or inadequate support system - Inability to communicate (e.g., presence of intubation/tracheostomy)

Continued

INTERVENTIONS	RATIONALES
	- Physical changes that affect self-concept - Denial or withdrawal - Hospital environment
Be especially alert to the social needs of older adults and disabled, chronically ill, or economically disadvantaged persons.	These individuals are most at risk for social isolation.
Help patient identify feelings associated with loneliness and isolation.	To facilitate intervention based on individual need. For example, "You seem very sad when your family leaves the room. Can you tell me more about your feelings?"
Determine patient's need for socialization and identify available and potential support person or systems. Explore methods for increasing social contact.	Assessing need for interaction and developing a care plan accordingly will reduce sense of isolation surrounding the illness. Methods for increasing social contact include TV, radio, tapes of loved ones, intercom system, more frequent visitations, and scheduled interaction with nurse or support staff.
Provide positive reinforcement for socialization that lessens patient's feelings of isolation and loneliness.	To reduce sense of isolation and promote healthy socialization. Encouraging interaction gives patient permission to ask for social interaction from the nurse while decreasing sense of isolation. For example, "Please continue to call me when you need to talk to someone. Talking will help both of us to better understand your feelings."
Facilitate patient's ability to communicate with others (see **Impaired Verbal Communication**, p. 83).	Impaired communication may be the cause of social isolation.

●●● **Related NIC and NOC labels:** *NIC:* Socialization Enhancement; Support System Enhancement; Active Listening; Emotional Support; Presence; Visitation Facilitation; Communication Enhancement; Family Involvement Promotion *NOC:* Social Involvement; Social Support; Well-Being

Nursing Diagnosis:

Disturbed Body Image

related to loss or change in body parts or function or physical trauma

Desired Outcomes: Within 24 hr of this diagnosis, patient acknowledges or begins to acknowledge body changes and demonstrates movement toward incorporating changes into self-concept. Patient does not demonstrate maladaptive response, such as severe depression.

INTERVENTIONS	RATIONALES
Establish open, honest communication with patient.	To promote an environment conducive to free expression in which patient is comfortable talking about body image concerns. For example, "Please feel free to talk to me whenever you have any questions."
Assess for verbal and nonverbal indicators suggesting body image disturbance.	Patient may exhibit nonverbal indicators (avoidance of looking at or touching body part, hiding or exposing body part) or verbal indicators (expression of negative feeling about body, expression of feelings of helplessness, personalization or depersonalization of missing or mutilated part, or refusal to acknowledge change in structure or function of body part).

Continued

INTERVENTIONS	RATIONALES
When planning patient's care, be aware of therapies that may influence patient's body image (e.g., medications or invasive procedures and monitoring).	Various drugs and surgical procedures can cause body changes. Monitoring equipment and invasive procedures can cause a diminished image of self and feelings of helplessness.
Assess patient's knowledge of the pathophysiologic process that has occurred and his or her present health status. Clarify any misconceptions.	To promote patient's understanding of health status and clarify misconceptions that may be contributing to disturbed body image.
Discuss the loss or change with patient. Recognize that what may seem to be a small change may be of great significance to the patient (e.g., arm immobilizer, catheter, hair loss, ecchymoses, facial abrasions).	Loss of any type has meaning of differing magnitudes for each individual. Talking about these issues may be a first step in accepting changes.
Explore with patient concerns, fears, and feelings of guilt.	Some body changes may reverse with time, and this information may lessen stress and concern. Assessing emotional reactions to the loss may help the nurse provide therapeutic support. For example, "I understand you are frightened. Your face looks different now, but you will see changes and it will improve. Gradually you will begin to look more like yourself."
Encourage patient and significant other to interact with one another. Help family to avoid reinforcement of their loved one's unhappiness over a changed body part or function.	Support and encouragement from loved ones help many people cope better with body changes. Guiding family members appropriately in their dealings with patients promotes healthy interactions that foster well-being. For example, "I know your son looks very different to you now, but it would help if you speak to him and touch him as you would normally."
Encourage patient to participate gradually in self-care activities as he or she becomes physically and emotionally able.	Self-care activities and a sense of getting back to normal can contribute to a sense of wholeness and control. Assisting patient with resuming a sense of normalcy promotes progression through the stages of grief.
Allow for some initial withdrawal and denial behaviors.	This is normal. For example, when changing dressings over traumatized part, explain what you are doing but do not expect patient to watch or participate initially.
Discuss opportunities for reconstruction of the loss or change.	To promote a realistic sense of hope and help patient plan for the future. Examples include surgery, prosthesis, grafting, physical therapy, cosmetic therapies, modified clothing, and organ transplant.
Recognize manifestations of severe depression (e.g., sleep disturbances, change in affect, change in communication pattern). As appropriate, refer to psychiatric clinical nurse specialist, case manager, clergy, or support group.	To assess patient for risk for self-harm, including suicide. See **Risk for Suicide,** p. 806, in "Major Depression."
Offer choices and alternatives whenever possible. Emphasize patient's strengths and encourage activities that interest patient.	To help patient attain a sense of autonomy and control.
If possible, refer patient to a support group or another patient who has had a similar experience (e.g., Reach to Recovery volunteer for a breast surgery patient).	Many people benefit from outside support systems and sharing experiences with another person who has had a similar experience.
Be aware that touch may enhance a patient's self-concept and reduce sense of isolation.	Touch may mitigate a sense that patient is hideous or unattractive because of the body change.

●●● **Related NIC and NOC labels:** *NIC:* Body Image Enhancement; Active Listening; Coping Enhancement; Self-Care Assistance; Support Group; Self-Esteem Enhancement *NOC:* Body Image; Psychosocial Adjustment: Life Change; Self-Esteem

ADDITIONAL NURSING DIAGNOSES/ PROBLEMS:

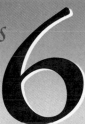

Psychosocial Support for the Patient's Family and Significant Others

Nursing Diagnosis:

Interrupted Family Processes

related to situational crisis (patient's illness)

Desired Outcome: Within the 24-hr period following intervention, family members begin demonstrating effective adaptation to change/traumatic situation as evidenced by seeking external support when necessary and sharing concerns within the family unit.

INTERVENTIONS	RATIONALES
Assess family's character: social, environmental, ethnic, and cultural factors; relationships; and role patterns.	Having this information will assist nurse in developing an individualized care plan.
Identify family developmental stage.	The family may be dealing with other situational or maturational crises, such as an elderly parent or a teenager with a learning disability
Assess previous adaptive behaviors.	How the family has dealt with problems in the past may be a reliable predictor of how they will adapt to current issues. For example, "How does your family react in stressful situations?"
Discuss observed conflicts and communication breakdown.	Awareness of this information will assist with development of an individualized plan of care, including referral for specialized care if appropriate. For example, "I noticed that your brother would not visit your mother today. Has there been a problem we should be aware of? Knowing about it may help us better care for your mother."

Continued

INTERVENTIONS	RATIONALES
Acknowledge family's involvement in patient care and promote strengths. Encourage family to participate in patient care conferences. Promote frequent, regular patient visits by family members.	This reinforces positive ways of dealing with the crisis and promotes a sense of involvement and control for the family. For example, "You were able to encourage your wife to turn and cough. That is very important to her recovery."
Provide family with information and guidance related to the critically ill patient. Acknowledge the stresses of hospitalization and encourage family to discuss feelings of anger, guilt, hostility, depression, fear, and sorrow. Refer to clergy, clinical nurse specialist, or social services as appropriate.	Encouraging expressions of emotion assists family members in beginning the process of grieving. For example, "You seem to be upset since being told that your husband is not leaving the hospital today." Acknowledging their feelings promotes acceptance and facilitates therapeutic communication.
Evaluate patient and family responses to one another. Encourage family to reorganize roles and establish priorities as appropriate.	To facilitate family's adaptation to the situation regarding patient and prevent unnecessary conflict. Assisting family members to redefine their roles may reduce confusion and provide direction. For example, "I know your husband is concerned about his insurance policy and seems to expect you to investigate it. I'll ask the financial counselor to talk with you."
Encourage family to schedule periods of rest and activity outside the hospital and to seek support when necessary.	Persons undergoing stress sometimes require guidance of others to promote their own self-care. For example, "Your neighbor volunteered to stay in the waiting room this afternoon. Would you like to rest at home? I'll call you if anything changes."

●●● **Related NIC and NOC labels:** *NIC:* Coping Enhancement; Family Support; Emotional Support; Grief Work Facilitation; Respite Care *NOC:* Family Coping

Nursing Diagnosis:

Readiness for Enhanced Family Coping

related to use of support persons or systems, referrals, and choosing experiences that optimize wellness

Desired Outcomes: Within 24 hr of patient's diagnosis, family members express intent to use support persons or systems and resources and identify alternative behaviors that promote family communication and strengths. Family members express realistic expectations and do not demonstrate ineffective coping behaviors.

INTERVENTIONS	RATIONALES
Assess family relationships, interactions, support persons or systems, and individual coping behaviors.	To facilitate development of an individualized care plan using existing family structure.
Permit movement through stages of adaptation.	Allows family members to process events surrounding patient's illness in a healthy manner.
Acknowledge family expressions of hope, future plans, and growth among family members.	A sense of hopefulness is essential to process painful events in a healthy manner.
Provide opportunities in a private setting for family interactions, discussions, and questions.	To encourage development of open, honest communication within the family and promote sharing of emotions in a nonpublic forum. For example, "I know the waiting room is very crowded. Would your family like some private time together?"

Continued

INTERVENTIONS	RATIONALES
Refer family to community or support groups (e.g., ostomy support group, head injury rehabilitation group).	Many people benefit from support of other people who have had similar experiences in learning new coping strategies.
Encourage family to explore outlets that foster positive feelings.	Provides direction in practicing effective coping skills. Examples of outlets that foster positive feeling include periods of time outside the hospital area, meaningful communication with patient or support individuals, and relaxing activities such as showering, eating, exercising.

●●● **Related NIC and NOC labels:** *NIC:* Family Support; Normalization Promotion; Coping Enhancement; Support Group; Support System Enhancement *NOC:* Family Coping; Caregiver Well-Being

Nursing Diagnosis:

Compromised Family Coping

related to inadequate or incorrect information or misunderstanding, temporary family disorganization and role change, exhausted support persons or systems, unrealistic expectations, fear, or anxiety

Desired Outcome: Within 24 hr of this diagnosis, family members begin to verbalize feelings, identify ineffective coping patterns, identify strengths and positive coping behaviors, and seek information and support from nurse or other support persons or systems outside the family.

INTERVENTIONS	RATIONALES
Establish open, honest communication within the family. Assist family in identifying strengths, stressors, inappropriate behaviors, and personal needs.	To promote positive, effective communication among family members. This also enables family to examine areas that contribute both to effective and ineffective coping in a nonthreatening environment. For example, "I understand your mother was very ill last year. How did you manage the situation?" "I know your loved one is very ill. How can I help you?"
Assess family members for ineffective coping and identify factors that inhibit effective coping.	Ineffective methods of coping (e.g., depression, chemical dependency, violence, withdrawal) can interfere with ability to deal with the current situation. Awareness of barriers to effective coping (e.g., inadequate support system, grief, fear of disapproval by others, and deficient knowledge) is the first step toward promoting changes and healthy adaptation. For example, "You seem to be unable to talk about your husband's illness. Is there anyone with whom you can talk about it?"
Assess family's knowledge about patient's current health status and treatment. Provide information frequently and allow sufficient time for questions. Reassess family's understanding at frequent intervals.	To increase family's knowledge of patient's health status and promote more effective coping. By providing information frequently and answering questions, stress, fear, and anxiety can be attenuated.
Provide opportunities in a private setting for family to talk and share concerns with nurses. If appropriate, refer family to psychiatric clinical nurse specialist for therapy.	Family may need additional assistance in working through family issues.
Offer realistic hope. Help the family to develop realistic expectations for the future and to identify support persons or systems that will assist them with planning for the future.	To foster realistic expectations about patient's future health status and promote adaptation to impending changes.

Continued

INTERVENTIONS	RATIONALES
Encourage diversional activities (e.g., time outside the hospital) and interaction with support persons or systems outside the family.	Promoting respite enhances coping and assists family members in remaining focused and supportive of patient. For example, "I know you want to be near your son, but if you would like to go home to rest, I will call you if any changes occur."

●●● **Related NIC and NOC labels:** *NIC:* Coping Enhancement; Caregiver Support; Family Support; Respite Care *NOC:* Family Coping

Nursing Diagnosis:

Disabled Family Coping

related to unexpressed feelings, ambivalent family relationships, or disharmonious coping styles among family members

Desired Outcome: Within 24 hr of this diagnosis, family members begin to verbalize feelings, identify sources of support as well as ineffective coping behaviors that create ambivalence and disharmony, and begin to develop realistic goals, plans, and actions.

INTERVENTIONS	RATIONALES
Establish open, honest communication and rapport with family members.	To promote an atmosphere in which family will express honest feelings and needs and move toward healthy coping and adaptation. For example, "I am here to care for your mother and to help your family as well."
Identify ineffective coping behaviors. Refer to psychiatric clinical nurse specialist, case manager, clergy, or support group as appropriate.	Ineffective coping behaviors (e.g., violence, depression, substance misuse, withdrawal) can interfere with learning effective strategies. Awareness of ineffective or destructive coping behaviors is the first step toward promoting change. For example, "You seem to be angry. Would you like to talk to me about your feelings?"
Identify perceived or actual conflicts.	Enables family to examine areas that require change in a nonthreatening environment and identify potential sources of support. For example, "Are you able to talk freely with your family members?" "Are your brothers and sisters able to help and support you during this time?"
Assist in quest for healthy functioning and adaptations within the family unit.	Facilitating open communication among family members and encouraging behaviors that support family cohesiveness promote skill acquisition in a nonthreatening environment and identify existing coping strengths.
Assist family members in developing realistic goals, plans, and actions. Refer them to clergy, psychiatric nurse, social services, financial counseling, and family therapy as appropriate.	Helps provide direction in making necessary changes and adaptations.
Encourage family members to spend time outside the hospital and to interact with support individuals. Respect family's need for occasional withdrawal.	A life out of balance adds to stress and promotes maladaptive coping.

Continued

INTERVENTIONS	RATIONALES
Include family members in patient's plan of care. Offer them opportunities to become involved in patient's care.	Becoming involved in patient's care (e.g., ROM exercises, patient hygiene, and comfort measures such as back rubs) may decrease feelings of powerlessness, thereby increasing coping ability.

●●● **Related NIC and NOC labels:** *NIC:* Coping Enhancement; Family Support; Family Integrity Promotion; Respite Care; Support System Enhancement; Referral; Spiritual Support *NOC:* Caregiver Emotional Health; Caregiver-Patient Relationship; Family Coping

Nursing Diagnosis:

Fear

related to patient's life-threatening condition and deficient knowledge about same

Desired Outcome: Immediately following intervention, significant others/family members report that fear has lessened or exhibit less fear in a nonverbal manner.

INTERVENTIONS	RATIONALES
Assess family's fears and their understanding of patient's clinical situation.	Some fears may be realistic, and others may not be and will necessitate clarification.
Evaluate verbal and nonverbal responses.	Some family members may not readily verbalize their fears but may give nonverbal cues such as withdrawing emotionally (evidenced by body position, facial expression, attitude of disinterest), refusing to be present during the discussion, or disrupting the discussion.
Acknowledge family's fear.	Simple acknowledgement and giving more information can go a long way toward decreasing fear. For example, "I understand these tubes must frighten you, but they are necessary to help nourish your son."
Assess family's history of coping behavior.	How a family has coped with fear in the past often is a reliable predictor of how they will cope in the current situation. For example, "How does your family react to difficult situations?" Awareness of maladaptive responses may assist nurse in fostering more productive methods of coping.
Determine resources and significant others available for support.	When under stress, family may not recall sources of support without being reminded. For example, "Who usually helps your family during stressful times?"
Provide opportunities for family members to express fears and concerns.	Verbalizing feelings in a nonthreatening environment can help them deal with unresolved/unrecognized issues that may be contributing to the current stressor.
Be alert to adaptive coping responses during initial period of crisis.	Anger, denial, withdrawal, and demanding behavior may be adaptive coping responses during the initial period of crisis.
Provide information at frequent intervals about patient's status, treatments, and equipment used. Demonstrate a caring attitude.	To increase family's knowledge of patient's health status and thereby alleviate fear of the unknown.
Encourage family to identify fears.	Identifying fears allows the nurse to dispel inaccuracies, which will help the family cope with the situation as it exists.

Continued

INTERVENTIONS	RATIONALES
Recognize fear/anxiety and encourage family members to describe their feelings.	Before family members can learn coping strategies, they must first clarify their feelings. For example, "You seem very uncomfortable tonight. Can you describe your feelings?"
Be alert to maladaptive responses to fear. Provide referrals to psychiatric clinical nurse specialist or other staff member as appropriate.	Violence, withdrawal, severe depression, hostility, and unrealistic expectations for staff or of patient's recovery are maladaptive responses to fear, and they require expert guidance.
Offer *realistic* hope, even if it is hope for the patient's peaceful death.	Even though family members may have feelings of hopelessness, it sometimes helps to hear realistic expressions of hope.
Explore family's desire for spiritual or other counseling.	People often derive hope and experience a decrease in fear and dread from spiritual counseling.
For other interventions, see **Interrupted Family Processes** and **Disabled Family Coping,** listed earlier.	

●●● **Related NIC and NOC labels:** *NIC:* Anxiety Reduction; Active Listening; Coping Enhancement; Support System Enhancement; Counseling *NOC:* Anxiety Control; Fear Control

Nursing Diagnosis:

Deficient Knowledge:

Patient's current health status or therapies

Desired Outcome: Immediately following teaching, family members/significant others begin to ask appropriate questions and verbalize accurate understanding of patient's current health status or treatment.

INTERVENTIONS	RATIONALES
At frequent intervals, inform family about patient's current health status, therapies, and prognosis. Use individualized verbal, written, and audiovisual strategies.	To promote family's accurate understanding of patient's health status. Providing information frequently allays unnecessary anxiety and enables family members to process and plan.
Evaluate family at frequent intervals for understanding of information that has been provided. Assess factors for misunderstanding and adjust teaching as appropriate.	Some individuals in crisis need repeated explanations before comprehension can be ensured (e.g., "I have explained many things to you today. Would you mind summarizing what I've told you so that I can be sure you understand your husband's status and what we are doing to care for him?").
Encourage family to relay correct information to patient.	This will reinforce comprehension for both the family and patient and promote open communication.
Encourage family to seek information and express feelings, concerns, and questions.	This promotes an atmosphere in which family members have permission to ask for more information and express concerns.
Ask family members if their needs for information are being met.	Reinforces understanding by family members and assures them that the information/support they desire will be met. For example, "Do you have any questions about the care your mother is receiving or about her condition?"
If indicated, help family members use the information they receive to make health care decisions about patient.	Family members may require assistance in processing information and applying it appropriately (e.g., regarding surgery, resuscitation, organ donation).

●●● **Related NIC and NOC labels:** *NIC:* Teaching: Disease Process; Learning Readiness Enhancement; Teaching: Procedure/Treatment *NOC:* Knowledge: Disease Process; Knowledge: Illness Care; Knowledge: Treatment Procedures

Care of the Older Adult

Nursing Diagnosis:

Risk for Aspiration

related to decreased masticatory muscle function secondary to age-related changes

Desired Outcomes: Patient swallows independently without choking. Patient's airway is patent and lungs are clear to auscultation both before and after meals.

INTERVENTIONS	RATIONALES
Perform a baseline assessment of patient's ability to swallow by asking if he or she has any difficulty swallowing or if any foods or fluids are difficult to swallow or cause gagging. If patient is unable to answer, consult patient's caregiver or significant other. Document findings.	To determine patient's ability to swallow without choking. This assessment should be compared with subsequent assessments to determine improvements or deficits.
Assess patient's ability to swallow by placing thumb and index finger on either side of the laryngeal prominence and asking patient to swallow. Check for the gag reflex by *gently* touching one side and then the other of the posterior pharyngeal wall using a tongue blade. Document both findings.	Ability to swallow and an intact gag reflex are necessary before patient takes foods or fluids orally.
Place patient in an upright position while he or she is eating or drinking, and support this position with pillows on patient's sides.	To minimize the risk of choking and aspirating. This position facilitates gravitational flow of foods and fluids into the stomach and through the pylorus.
Monitor patient when he or she is swallowing.	To determine ability to swallow without choking. Deficits may necessitate aspiration precautions.
Watch for drooling of saliva or food or an inability to close lips around a straw.	These are signs of limited lip, tongue, or jaw movement.
Check for retention of food in sides of mouth.	Indication of poor tongue movement.

Continued

INTERVENTIONS	RATIONALES
Monitor patient for coughing or choking before, during, and after swallowing.	This likely signals aspiration of material into the airway. It may occur up to several minutes following placement of food or fluid in the mouth.
Monitor patient for changes found during lung auscultation (e.g., crackles, wheezes, rhonchi), shortness of breath, dyspnea, increasing temperature, and cyanosis.	These are signs of silent aspiration. Elders have increased risk for silent aspiration.
Be alert to decreasing level of consciousness (LOC).	This is a sign that patient is at increased risk for aspiration or in fact already has aspirated.
Monitor patient for a wet or gurgling sound when talking after a swallow.	This indicates aspiration into the airway and signals a delayed or absent swallow reflex and a delayed or absent gag reflex.
For patients with poor swallowing reflex, tilt their head forward 45 degrees during swallowing. **Note:** For patients who have hemiplegia, tilt head toward the unaffected side.	This will help prevent inadvertent aspiration by closing off the airway.
As indicated, request evaluation by speech therapist.	For further assessment of gag and swallow reflex.
Anticipate videofluoroscopy of swallowing in evaluation of patient's gag and swallow reflex.	This procedure is used to determine whether patient is aspirating, consistency of materials most likely to be aspirated, and cause of the aspiration. Using four consistencies of barium, the radiologist and speech therapist watch for the presence of reduced or ineffective tongue function, reduced peristalsis in the pharynx, delayed or absent swallow reflex, and poor or limited ability to close the epiglottis that protects the airway.
Thicken patient's fluids if this has been prescribed, based on results of the swallowing video.	Agents are added to the fluid to make it more viscous and easier for patient to swallow. Similarly, mechanical soft, pureed, or liquid diets may be prescribed to enable patient to ingest food with less potential for aspiration.
Provide adequate rest periods before meals.	Fatigue increases risk of aspiration.
Remind patients with dementia to chew and swallow with each bite. Check for retained food in sides of mouth.	Patients with dementia might forget to chew and swallow.
Ensure that patient has dentures in place, if appropriate, and that they fit correctly.	Chewing well minimizes risk of choking.
Ensure that someone stays with patient during meals or fluid intake.	For added safety in the event of choking or aspiration.
Provide patient with adequate time to eat and drink.	Generally, patients with swallowing deficits require twice as much time for eating and drinking as those whose swallowing is adequate.
Be aware of location of suction equipment to be used in the event of aspiration.	If patient is at increased risk for aspiration, suction equipment should be available at the bedside.
If patient aspirates, implement the following:	
Follow American Heart Association (AHA) standards if patient displays characteristics of complete airway obstruction (i.e., choking).	This is an emergency situation.
For partial airway obstruction, encourage patient to cough as needed.	To clear airway.
For partial airway obstruction in the unconscious or nonresponsive individual who is not coughing, suction airway with a large-bore catheter such as the Yankauer or tonsil suction tip.	To clear airway.
For either a complete or partial aspiration, inform health care provider and obtain prescription for chest x-ray.	To determine if food/fluid remains in airway.

Continued

INTERVENTIONS	RATIONALES
Implement NPO status until diagnosis is confirmed.	To prevent further risk to patient.
Monitor breathing pattern and RR q1-2h after a suspected aspiration for alterations (i.e., tachypnea).	To assess for change in patient's condition.
Anticipate use of antibiotics.	There is risk for infection/pneumonia after aspiration.
Encourage patient to cough and deep breathe q2h while awake and q4h during the night.	To prevent infection and promote expansion of available lung tissue.

●●● **Related NIC and NOC labels:** *NIC:* Aspiration Precautions; Respiratory Monitoring; Vital Signs Monitoring; Airway Suctioning *NOC:* Aspiration Control; Swallowing Status

Nursing Diagnosis:

Constipation

related to changes in diet, activity, and psychosocial factors secondary to hospitalization or prolonged bedrest

Desired Outcomes: Patient states that bowel habit has returned to normal pattern within 3–4 days of this diagnosis. Stool appears soft, and patient does not strain in passing stools.

INTERVENTIONS	RATIONALES
On admission, assess and document patient's normal bowel elimination pattern. Include frequency, time of day, associated habits, and successful methods used to correct constipation in the past. Consult patient's caregiver or significant other if patient is unable to provide this information.	To establish baseline and determine patient's normal bowel elimination pattern.
Inform patient that changes occurring with hospitalization may increase potential for constipation. Urge patient to institute successful nonpharmacologic methods used at home as soon as this problem is noticed or prophylactically as needed.	Constipation is easier to treat preventively than it is when present and/or prolonged.
Teach patient the relationship between fluid intake and constipation. Unless otherwise contraindicated, encourage fluid intake that exceeds 2500 ml/day.	A high fluid intake promotes soft stool and decreases risk/degree of constipation. A high fluid volume may be contraindicated in patients with renal, cardiac, or hepatic disorders who may have fluid restrictions.
Teach patient the relationship between types of foods consumed and constipation.	To educate patient on how to avoid constipation.
When possible, encourage patient to include roughage as a part of each meal (e.g., raw fruits and vegetables, whole grains, nuts, fruits with skins). For the patient unable to tolerate raw foods, encourage intake of bran via cereals, muffins, and breads.	Eating roughage reduces potential for constipation by promoting bulk in the stool.
Titrate amount of roughage to the degree of constipation.	Too much roughage taken too quickly can cause diarrhea, gas, and distention.
Teach patient the relationship between constipation and activity level. Encourage optimum activity for all patients. Establish and post an activity program to enhance participation; include devices necessary to enable independence.	To increase patient's understanding that exercise can prevent or decrease constipation by promoting peristalsis.

Continued

INTERVENTIONS	RATIONALES
Advise patient about the need to maintain usual bowel elimination pattern/schedule. Provide materials or support measures that patient normally uses (e.g., cup of coffee on arising, privacy, short walk).	Scheduling interventions that coincide with patient's bowel habit are more likely to promote bowel movements. If patient's bowel movement occurs in the early morning, using patient's gastrocolic or duodenocolic reflex promotes colonic emptying. Drinking hot liquids in the morning, for example, also promotes peristalsis. If patient's bowel movement occurs in the evening, it may be effective to ambulate patient just before the appropriate time.
Ask patient if toilet seat height seems the same as that at home. If the toilet is too low, provide a high-rise toilet seat or a footstool to raise patient's feet off the floor comfortably.	For comfort, to facilitate bowel movements, and prevent falls that could occur if patient were to lower self to toilet that is too low.
Attempt to use methods that patient has used successfully in the past.	Older persons tend to focus on loss of habit as an indicator of constipation rather than on the number of stools. Aggressive interventions may result in rebound constipation and interfere with patient's subsequent bowel movements.
Do not intervene pharmacologically until patient has not had a stool for 3 days. When requesting a pharmacologic intervention, use more benign, oral methods first.	Intervening slowly, using more benign methods first, helps avoid rebound constipation. The following hierarchy is suggested: - Bulk-building additives such as psyllium or bran - Mild laxatives (apple or prune juice, Milk of Magnesia) - Stool softeners (docusate sodium, docusate calcium) - Potent laxatives or cathartics (bisacodyl, cascara sagrada) - Medicated suppositories (glycerin, bisacodyl) - Enema (tap water, saline, sodium biphosphate/phosphate)
After diagnostic imaging of the gastrointestinal (GI) tract with barium, ensure that patient receives postexamination laxative. Emphasize diet, fluid, activity, and resumption of routines. If no bowel movement occurs in 3 days, begin with mild laxatives to try to regain normal pattern.	To facilitate removal of the barium. After any procedure involving a bowel clean-out, there may be rebound constipation from the severe disruption of bowel habit.
Monitor hydration status for signs of dehydration.	Dehydration can occur as a result of osmotic agents used. Deficient fluid volume can result in hard stools, which are more difficult to evacuate.
See also "Prolonged Bedrest" for **Constipation,** p. 75.	

●●● **Related NIC and NOC labels:** *NIC:* Constipation Management; Fluid Management; Exercise Promotion; Nutrition Management *NOC:* Bowel Elimination; Hydration; Symptom Control

Nursing Diagnosis:

Risk for Deficient Fluid Volume

related to inability to obtain fluids by self secondary to illness, placement of fluid, or presence of chronic illness; or related to use of osmotic agents during radiologic tests

Desired Outcomes: Patient's mental status, VS, and urine color, consistency, and concentration remain within normal limits for patient. Patient's mucous membranes remain moist, and there is no "tenting" of skin. Patient's intake equals output.

INTERVENTIONS	RATIONALES
Monitor fluid intake. In nonrestricted individuals, encourage fluid intake of 2-3 L/day. Specify intake goals for day, evening, and night shifts.	To ensure patient's hydration status is adequate.
Monitor for presence of urinary incontinence. If present, correlate to intake. If intake is low, encourage intake of noncaffeinated fluids.	Fear of incontinence leads to decreased intake. However, decreased intake leads to more highly concentrated urine, which in turn irritates the bladder and can result in incontinence.
Assess and document skin turgor. Check hydration status by pinching skin over sternum or forehead.	Skin that remains in the lifted position (tenting) and returns slowly to its original position indicates dehydration. A furrowed tongue is a signal of severe dehydration.
Assess and document color, amount, and frequency of any fluid output, including emesis, urine, diarrhea, or other drainage.	Enables comparison of intake to output amounts. Urine that is dark in color signals concentration and thus dehydration.
Monitor patient's orientation, ability to follow commands, and behavior.	Loss of ability to follow commands, decrease in orientation, and confused behavior can signal a dehydrated state.
Weigh patient daily at the same time of day (preferably before breakfast) using the same scale and bed clothing. Be alert to wide variations in weight (e.g., ≥2.5 kg [5 lb]).	Using comparable measurements ensures more accurate comparisons. Wide variations can signal increased or decreased hydration status.
Monitor laboratory tests for elevations in serum Na^+, blood urea nitrogen (BUN), and serum creatinine levels.	These elevations often occur with dehydration.
If patient is receiving IV therapy, monitor cardiac and respiratory systems for signs of overload. Assess radial and apical pulses and listen to lung fields during every VS assessment.	Overload could precipitate heart failure or pulmonary edema. Rising HR, crackles, and bronchial wheezes can be signals of heart failure or pulmonary edema.
Carefully monitor I&O when patient is receiving dyes for contrast.	These agents act osmotically to pull fluid into the interstitial tissue. Evidence of third spacing of fluids, including increasing peripheral edema, especially sacral; output significantly less than intake (1:2); and urine output <30 ml/hr, may be present.
Offer patient fluid whenever in the room. Offer a variety of drinks that patient enjoys.	Older persons have a decreased sense of thirst and need encouragement to drink.
Limit caffeine.	Caffeine tends to act as a diuretic.
Assess patient's ability to obtain and drink fluids by self. Place fluids within easy reach. Use cups with tops to minimize concern over spilling.	Removes barriers to adequate fluid intake.
Ensure access to toilet, urinal, commode, or bedpan at least q2h when patient is awake and q4h at night. Answer call light quickly.	The time between recognition of the need to void and urination decreases with age.

●●● **Related NIC and NOC labels:** *NIC:* Fluid/Electrolyte Management; Intravenous Therapy; Vital Signs Monitoring; Cardiac Care: Acute; Urinary Elimination Management; Self-Care Assistance: Feeding
NOC: Nutritional Status: Food & Fluid Intake; Hydration; Fluid Balance Electrolyte & Acid/Base Balance

Nursing Diagnosis:

Impaired Gas Exchange

(or risk for same) *related to* decreased functional lung tissue secondary to age-related changes

Desired Outcomes: Patient's respiratory pattern and mental status remain normal for patient. Patient's arterial blood gas (ABG) or pulse oximetry values are within patient's normal limits.

INTERVENTIONS	RATIONALES
Assess and document the following on admission and routinely thereafter: respiratory rate, pattern, and depth; breath sounds; cough; sputum; and sensorium. If available, monitor oxygenation status via ABG findings (optimally Pao_2 >80%-95%) or pulse oximetry (optimally >94%).	To establish a baseline for subsequent assessments.
Assess for subtle changes in mentation.	Mentation changes such as increased restlessness, anxiety, disorientation, and presence of hostility can signal decreased oxygenation.
Assess lungs for the presence of adventitious sounds, while recognizing that crackles may not signal respiratory problems.	The aging lung has decreased elasticity. The lower part of the lungs is no longer adequately aerated. As a result, crackles commonly are heard in individuals ≥75 yr. This sign alone does not mean that a pathologic condition is present. Crackles that do not clear with coughing in an individual with no other clinical signs (e.g., fever, increasing anxiety, changes in mental status, increasing respiratory depth) are considered benign.
Encourage patient to cough and breathe deeply. When appropriate, instruct patient in the use of incentive spirometry.	To promote alveolar expansion and clear secretions from the bronchial tree, thereby helping to ensure better gas exchange.
Unless contraindicated, encourage fluid intake >2.5 L/day.	To ensure less viscous pulmonary secretions, which are more easily mobilized.
Treat fevers promptly, manage pain, minimize pacing activity, and lessen anxiety.	Interventions that reduce the potential for increased oxygen consumption.

●●● **Related NIC and NOC labels:** *NIC:* Vital Signs Monitoring; Laboratory Data Interpretation; Oxygen Therapy; Respiratory Monitoring; Chest Physiotherapy; Cough Enhancement *NOC:* Vital Signs Status; Tissue Perfusion: Pulmonary; Respiratory Status: Gas Exchange

Nursing Diagnosis:

Hopelessness

related to slow recovery from illness or surgery secondary to decreased physiologic reserve

Desired Outcome: Within 2-4 days of interventions, patient verbalizes knowledge of his or her strengths, feelings about health, and understanding of a potentially long recovery.

INTERVENTIONS	RATIONALES
Monitor patient for signs of hopelessness/depression.	Behavior such as refusal to participate in own care; refusal to eat or marked decline in appetite or intake; refusal to answer questions; and statements such as "I don't care," "Leave me alone," and "Let me die." are signs of hopelessness and depression.
Encourage patient to verbalize feelings of despair, frustration, fear, and anger and concerns regarding hospitalization and health. Reassure patient and significant other that such feelings and concerns are normal.	Verbalization of feelings and the knowledge that these feelings are normal often help minimize feelings of despair.
Discuss normal age-related changes with patient and significant other.	Recovery periods are longer for older adults because of decreased physiologic reserve.

Continued

INTERVENTIONS	RATIONALES
Encourage short-term goals and praise small steps, such as participation in own care.	To help decrease frustrations caused by slow recovery.
Educate patient about how the aging process slows recovery.	Decrease in physiologic reserve increases recovery time.
Arrange a care conference to discuss discharge requirements specific to the patient. Involve patient and significant other in the conference. Set realistic goals based on patient's condition and desires.	Reassurance about continuity of care may help diminish feelings of frustration and hopelessness.

●●● **Related NIC and NOC labels:** *NIC:* Active Listening; Emotional Support; Mutual Goal Setting; Family Support; Role Enhancement *NOC:* Quality of Life; Hope; Decision Making; Depression Control

Nursing Diagnosis:

Hypothermia

(or risk for same) *related to* age-related changes in thermoregulation and/or environmental exposure

Desired Outcome: Patient's temperature returns to patient's normal limits at a rate of 1° F/hr after interventions.

INTERVENTIONS	RATIONALES
Monitor patient's temperature, using a low-range thermometer if possible.	To determine if patient has hypothermia. Older adults can have a normal temperature of 35.5° C (96° F).
Assess temperature orally by placing thermometer far back in patient's mouth.	This method provides the most accurate assessment of patient's core temperature.
If necessary, assess temperature rectally.	Axillary temperature measurement should be avoided in older adults because they have decreased peripheral circulation and loss of subcutaneous fat in the axillary area, resulting in formation of a pocket of air that may make readings inaccurate.
Assess and document patient's mental status.	Increasing disorientation, mental status changes, or presence of atypical behavior can signal hypothermia.
Monitor carefully the following patients who are at risk for environmental hypothermia: those taking sedatives, hypnotics (including anesthetics), and muscle relaxants.	These drugs decrease shivering. In addition, all older adults are at risk for environmental hypothermia at ambient temperatures of 22.22°-23.89° C (72°-75° F).
Ensure that patients going for testing or x-ray examinations are sent with enough blankets to keep warm.	To prevent hypothermia.
If patient is mildly hypothermic, initiate slow rewarming.	To reverse mild hypothermia, one method of slow rewarming is raising room temperature to at least 23.89° C (75° F). Other methods of external warming include use of warm blankets, head covers, and warm circulating air blankets.
If patient's temperature falls below 35° C (95° F), warm patient internally.	To reverse moderate to severe hypothermia, patient is warmed internally by administering warm oral or IV fluids. Warmed saline gastric or rectal irrigations or introduction of warmed humidified air into the airway are other methods of internal warming.

Continued

INTERVENTIONS	RATIONALES
Assess for signs of too rapid rewarming.	Signs of too rapid rewarming include irregular HR, dysrhythmias, and very warm extremities caused by vasodilation in the periphery, which causes heat loss from the core.
If patient's temperature fails to rise 1° F/hr using these techniques, anticipate laboratory tests, including white blood cell (WBC) count for possible sepsis, thyroid test for hypothyroidism, and glucose level for hypoglycemia.	Causes other than environmental ones may be responsible for the hypothermia.
As prescribed, administer antibiotics for sepsis, initiate thyroid therapy, or administer glucose for hypoglycemia.	The patient's temperature likely will not return to normal unless the underlying condition has been treated.

●●● **Related NIC and NOC labels:** *NIC:* Hypothermia Treatment; Vital Signs Monitoring; Environmental Management; Heat Application; Fluid Management *NOC:* Thermoregulation

Nursing Diagnosis:

Risk for Infection

related to age-related changes in immune and integumentary systems; suppressed inflammatory response secondary to long-term medication use (e.g., antiinflammatory agents, steroids, analgesics); slowed ciliary response; or poor nutrition

Desired Outcome: Patient remains free of infection as evidenced by orientation to person, place, and time and behavior within patient's normal limits; respiratory rate and pattern within patient's normal limits; urine that is straw colored, clear, and of characteristic odor; core temperature and HR within patient's normal limits; sputum that is clear to whitish in color; and skin that is intact and of normal color and temperature for patient.

INTERVENTIONS	RATIONALES
Assess patient's baseline VS, including LOC and orientation. Also be alert to HR >100 bpm and RR >24 breaths/min. Auscultate lung fields for adventitious sounds, recognizing that crackles may be a normal finding when heard in the lung bases.	A change in mentation is a leading sign of infection in older patients. Other signs of infection include tachycardia and tachypnea. Adventitious breath sounds may or may not be seen until late in the course of illness.
Monitor patient's temperature, using a low-range thermometer if possible.	Older adults may run lower temperatures. A temperature of 35.5° C (96° F) may be normal, whereas a temperature of 36.67°-37.22° C (98°-99° F) may be considered febrile.
Obtain temperature readings rectally if the oral reading does not match the clinical picture (i.e., patient's skin is very warm, patient is restless, mentation is depressed), or if the temperature reads ≥36.11° C (97° F).	To ensure that patient's core temperature is accurately determined. If temperature measurement is done using a tympanic thermometer, reliability of the electronic tympanic thermometer may be inconsistent because of improper use.
Assess patient's skin for tears, breaks, erythema, or ulcers. Document condition of patient's skin on admission and as an ongoing assessment (refer to **Risk for Impaired Skin Integrity,** p. 110).	Skin that is not intact is susceptible to infection.
Assess quality and color of patient's urine. Document changes when noted and report findings to health care provider. Also be alert to urinary incontinence.	Urinary tract infections (UTIs), as manifested by cloudy, foul-smelling urine without painful urination, and urinary incontinence are the most common infection in older adults.

Continued

INTERVENTIONS	RATIONALES
Avoid insertion of urinary catheters when possible.	Urinary catheter use increases risk of infection.
Obtain drug history in reference to use of antiinflammatory or immunosuppressive drugs or long-term use of analgesics or steroids.	These drugs mask fever, a sign of infection.
If infection is suspected, anticipate initiation of IV fluid therapy.	To maintain optimal hydration. Fluids also will replace losses caused by fever and help thin secretions for easier expectoration.
Anticipate need for blood cultures, urinalysis, and urine culture.	To isolate bacteria type.
Anticipate need for WBC count.	To determine immune response. WBC count $\geq 11,000/mm^3$ can be a late sign of infection in older patients because the immune system is slow to respond to insult.
Expect a chest x-ray examination if patient's chest sounds are not clear.	To rule out pneumonia.
If infection is present, prepare for initiation of broad-spectrum antibiotic therapy and oxygen therapy.	To eliminate infection and promote oxygenation. Fever increases cardiac workload (i.e., HR rises) as the body responds to infection. Because of decreased physiologic reserve, elders may have increased risk of heart failure or pulmonary edema from prolonged tachycardia.
Prepare for use of acetaminophen to treat fever.	Acetaminophen decreases temperature and cardiac output, which will decrease cardiac load.
For more information, see Appendix for "Infection Prevention and Control," p. 831.	

●●● **Related NIC and NOC labels:** *NIC:* Respiratory Monitoring; Vital Signs Monitoring; Skin Surveillance; Specimen Management *NOC:* Infection Status

Nursing Diagnosis:

Powerlessness

related to hospital environment

Desired Outcome: Within 2-4 days after interventions, patient participates in care and verbalizes feelings of control over his or her environment.

INTERVENTIONS	RATIONALES
Encourage patient to verbalize feelings about hospitalization and illness.	To determine if patient is experiencing feelings of powerlessness.
Assist patient in identifying factors that contribute to feelings of powerlessness.	Identifying causative factors is the first step in eliminating them.
Encourage patient to participate in activities of daily living (ADL) as much as possible. Provide adequate time for patient to complete ADL.	Participating in self-care will help decrease feelings of powerlessness.
As often as possible, enable patient to participate in scheduling of activities.	Having a "say so" in scheduling may decrease feelings of powerlessness.
Discuss with patient and significant other realistic goals of care and encourage patient's participation in care planning.	Participating in care planning helps promote some sense of control and power.

Continued

INTERVENTIONS	RATIONALES
Explain procedures and routines. Inform patient when changes in the plan of care are necessary.	Staying well informed decreases sense of powerlessness.
Provide flexibility in patient's plan of care when possible (e.g., if patients want to wear their own clothes, enable them to do so).	Having flexibility promotes a sense of having some control and power.

●●● **Related NIC and NOC labels:** *NIC:* Active Listening; Decision-Making Support; Self-Responsibility Facilitation; Mutual Goal Setting *NOC:* Participation: Health Care Decisions

Nursing Diagnosis:

Risk for Impaired Skin Integrity

related to decreased subcutaneous fat and decreased peripheral capillary networks secondary to age–related changes in the integumentary system

Desired Outcome: Patient's skin remains nonerythemic and intact.

INTERVENTIONS	RATIONALES
Assess patient's skin on admission and routinely thereafter.	To provide a baseline for subsequent assessments of patient's skin integrity.
Note any areas of erythema or any breaks in the skin surface.	Redness or breaks in skin integrity necessitate aggressive skin care interventions to prevent further breakdown and infection.
Ensure that patient turns frequently (at least q2h).	To alternate sites of pressure relief.
Lift or roll patient across sheets when repositioning.	Pulling, dragging, or sliding patient across sheets can lead to friction and shear (cutaneous or subcutaneous tissue) injury.
Monitor skin over bony prominences for presence of erythema.	Skin that lies over the sacrum, scapulae, heels, spine, hips, pelvis, greater trochanter, knees, ankles, costal margins, occiput, and ischial tuberosities is at increased risk for breakdown because of excessive external pressure.
Use pillows or foam wedges.	To maintain alternative positions and pad bony prominences.
Use lotions on dry skin.	To promote moisture and suppleness. Lanolin-containing lotions are especially useful.
Use alternating-pressure mattress, air-fluidized mattress, waterbed, air bed, or other pressure-sensitive mattress for older patients who are on bedrest or unable to get out of bed.	To protect skin from injury caused by prolonged pressure.
Avoid placing tubes under patient's limbs or head. Place pillow or pad between patient and tube for cushioning.	Excess pressure from tubes can create a pressure ulcer.
Get patient out of bed as often as possible. Liberally use mechanical lifting devices to aid in safe patient transfers.	Promotes blood flow, which helps prevent skin breakdown.
If patient is unable to get out of bed, assist with position changes q2h.	To alternate sites of pressure relief.
Establish and post a turning schedule on the patient care plan and at the bedside.	To increase awareness of staff and patient/family to turning schedule.

Continued

INTERVENTIONS	RATIONALES
Ensure that patient's face, axillae, and genital areas are cleansed daily.	Complete baths dry out older adults' skin and should be given every other day instead.
Use tepid water (90°-105° F [32.2°-40.5° C]) and super-fatted, nonperfumed soaps	These measures help to prevent dry skin.
Avoid hot water.	Can burn skin of older adults, who have decreased pain and temperature sensitivity.
Minimize use of plastic protective pads under patient. When used, place at least one layer of cloth (drawsheet) between patient and plastic pad to absorb moisture.	These pads trap moisture and heat and can lead to skin breakdown.
Use skin protectant on patients with urinary or fecal incontinence.	A light barrier on the skin helps prevent skin breakdown from chemical irritants.
Avoid use of adult incontinence pads (i.e., diapers).	These pads keep moisture trapped against the skin and must be changed q2h.
For other interventions, see "Providing Nutritional Support," p. 589, and "Managing Wound Care," p. 583.	Good nutrition and skin care help prevent skin breakdown.

●●● **Related NIC and NOC labels:** *NIC:* Skin Surveillance; Positioning; Circulatory Precautions; Pressure Management; Skin Care: Topical Treatments; Bathing *NOC:* Tissue Integrity: Skin & Mucous Membranes; Immobility Consequences: Physiologic

Nursing Diagnosis:

Disturbed Sleep Pattern

related to unfamiliar surroundings and hospital routines

Desired Outcome: Within 24 hr of interventions, patient reports attainment of adequate rest. Mental status remains normal for the patient.

INTERVENTIONS	RATIONALES
Assess and document patient's sleeping pattern, obtaining information from patient or patient's caregiver or significant other.	Elders typically sleep less than they did when they were younger and often awaken more frequently during the night.
Ask questions about naps and activity levels.	Individuals who take naps and have a low level of activity frequently sleep only 4-5 hr/night.
Determine patient's usual nighttime routine and attempt to emulate it.	Following patient's usual nighttime rituals may facilitate sleep.
Attempt to group together activities such as medications, VS, and toileting.	To reduce the number of interruptions and facilitate rest and sleep.
Provide pain medications, back rub, and conversation at bedtime.	To provide comfort measures and facilitate sleep.
Monitor patient's activity level. Involve patient in daytime care or activities.	To ensure adequate rest and facilitate sleep. If patient complains of being tired after activities or displays behaviors such as irritability, yelling, or shouting, encourage napping after lunch or early in the afternoon. Otherwise, discourage daytime napping, especially in the late afternoon, because it can interfere with nighttime sleep.

Continued

INTERVENTIONS	RATIONALES
Avoid stimulants such as coffee, cola, and tea after 6 PM.	Stimulants can make it difficult to fall and stay asleep.
Decrease fluid intake after 8 PM. Administer diuretics in the morning.	To decreases nighttime awakenings to urinate.
Provide a quiet and peaceful environment as much as possible.	Excessive noises, bright overhead lights, noisy roommates, and loud talking can cause sleep deprivation. Use of sound generators (e.g., of ocean waves) or white noise (e.g., fan) may promote sleep.

●●● **Related NIC and NOC labels:** *NIC:* Energy Management; Sleep Enhancement; Exercise Promotion; Environmental Management: Comfort; Simple Massage; Pain Management *NOC:* Rest; Sleep

Nursing Diagnosis:

Disturbed Thought Processes

related to decreased cerebral perfusion secondary to age-related decreased physiologic reserve or cardiac dysfunction; electrolyte imbalance secondary to age-related decreased renal function; altered sensory/perceptual reception secondary to poor vision or hearing; or decreased brain oxygenation secondary to illness state and decreased functional lung tissue

Desired Outcomes: Patient's mental status returns to normal for the patient within 3 days of treatment. Patient sustains no evidence of injury or harm as a result of mental status.

INTERVENTIONS	RATIONALES
Assess patient's LOC and mental status on admission. Obtain preconfusion functional and mental status abilities from significant other. Ask patient to perform a three-step task (e.g., "Hold this piece of paper in your left hand, fold it in half, and put it by your side.").	To provide a baseline for subsequent assessments of patient's confusion.
Test short-term memory by showing patient how to use the call light, having the patient return the demonstration, and then waiting at least 5 min before having patient demonstrate use of call light again. Document patient's response in behavioral terms (describe the "confused" behavior).	Inability to remember beyond 5 min indicates poor short-term memory.
Identify cause of acute confusion (e.g., consult health care provider regarding oximetry or ABG values to assess oxygenation levels; serum glucose or fingerstick glucose to determine glucose level; and electrolytes and complete blood count (CBC) to ascertain imbalances and/or presence of elevated WBC count as a determinant of infection). Assess hydration status by pinching skin over the sternum or forehead for turgor and checking for dry mucous membranes and furrowed tongue.	Acute confusion is caused by physical or psychosocial conditions and not by age alone.
Assess for pain using a rating scale from 0-10. If patient is unable to use a scale, assess for behavioral cues such as grimacing, clenched fists, frowning, and hitting. Ask family/significant other to assist in identifying pain behaviors.	Acute confusion can be a sign of pain.
Treat patient for pain, as indicated, and monitor behaviors.	If pain caused the confusion, patient's behavior should change accordingly.

Continued

INTERVENTIONS	RATIONALES
Review cardiac status. Assess apical pulse, and notify health care provider of an irregular pulse that is new to the patient. If patient is on a cardiac monitor or telemetry, watch for dysrhythmias; notify health care provider accordingly.	Dysrhythmias and other cardiac dysfunctions may result in decreased oxygenation, which can lead to confusion.
Review current medications, including over-the-counter (OTC) drugs, with the pharmacist.	Certain medications, such as digoxin or theophylline, cause acute confusion. Drugs that are anticholinergic also can cause confusion, as can drug interactions.
Monitor I&O at least q8h.	Optimally, output should match intake. Dehydration and certain drugs can result in acute confusion.
Anticipate/encourage a creatinine clearance test.	Renal function plays an important role in fluid balance and is the main mechanism of drug clearance. BUN and serum creatinine are affected by hydration status and in the elderly reveal only part of the picture. Therefore, to fully understand and assess renal function in elders, creatinine clearance has to be tested.
Have patient wear glasses and hearing aid or keep them close to the bedside and within easy reach for patient use.	To decrease sensory confusion.
Keep urinal and other routinely used items within easy reach for the patient. Establish a toileting schedule and post it on the care plan and, inconspicuously, at the bedside. Offer to assist with toileting or offer patient urinal or bedpan q2h while awake and q4h during the night.	A confused patient may wait until it is too late to seek assistance with toileting. A patient with a short-term memory problem cannot be expected to use the call light.
Check on patient at least q30min and every time you pass the room. Place patient close to nurses' station if possible. Provide an environment that is nonstimulating and safe.	A confused patient requires extra safety precautions.
Provide soothing music but not TV.	Patients who are confused regarding place and time often think the action on TV is happening in the room.
Keep a clock with large numerals and large print calendar at the bedside, and verbally remind patient of the date and day as needed.	Reorienting patient to surroundings may decrease confusion.
Tell patient in simple terms what is occurring. For example, "It's time to eat breakfast," "This medicine is for your heart," "I'm going to help you get out of bed."	Sentences that are more complex may not be understood.
Encourage patient's significant other to bring items familiar to patient, including blanket, bedspread, pictures of family and pets.	To promote orientation while providing comfort.
If patient becomes belligerent, angry, or argumentative while you are attempting to reorient, *stop this approach.* Do not argue with patient or patient's interpretation of the environment. State, "I can understand why you may (hear, think, see) that."	To prevent escalation of anger in a confused person.
If patient displays hostile behavior or misperceives your role (e.g., nurse becomes thief, jailer), leave the room. Return in 15 min. Introduce yourself as though you had never met. Begin dialogue anew. When you return, enable patient to share feelings about the previous encounter as appropriate.	Patients who are acutely confused have poor short-term memory and may not remember the previous encounter or that you were involved in that encounter.
If patient attempts to leave the hospital, walk with patient and ask him or her to tell you about the destination (e.g., "That sounds like a wonderful place! Tell me about it."). Keep tone pleasant and conversational. Continue walking with patient away from exits and doors around the unit. After a few	Distraction is an effective means of reversing a behavior in the patient who is confused.

Continued

INTERVENTIONS	RATIONALES
minutes, attempt to guide patient back to the room. Offer refreshments and a rest (e.g., "We've been walking for a while and I'm a little tired. Why don't we sit and have some juice while we talk?").	
If patient has a permanent or severe cognitive impairment, check on her or him at least q30min and reorient to base-line mental status as indicated; however, do not argue with patient about his or her perception of reality.	Arguing can cause a cognitively impaired person to become aggressive and combative.
If patient tries to climb out of bed, he or she may need to use the toilet; offer the urinal or bedpan or assist to the com-mode. Alternately, if patient is not on bedrest, place him or her in chair or wheelchair at nurses' station for added supervision.	To promote patient's safety.
Bargain with patient. Try to establish an agreement to stay for a defined period, such as until the health care provider, breakfast or lunch, or significant other arrives.	This is a delaying strategy to defuse anger. Because of poor memory and attention span, patient may forget he or she wanted to leave.
Have patient's significant other talk with patient by phone or come in and sit with patient if his or her behavior requires checking more often than q30min.	To promote patient's safety.
If patient is attempting to pull out tubes, hide the tubes (e.g., under blankets). Put stockinette mesh dressing over IV lines. Tape feeding tubes to the side of the face using paper tape and drape the tube behind patient's ear.	Remember: out of sight, out of mind.
Evaluate continued need for therapy that no longer may be necessary.	Such therapies may become irritating stimuli. For example, if patient is now drinking, discontinue IV line; if patient is eating, discontinue feeding tube.
Use restraints with caution.	Patients can become more agitated when wrist and arm restraints are used.
Use medications cautiously for controlling behavior.	Follow the maxim "start low and go slow" with medications because elders can respond to small amounts of drugs.
	Neuroleptics, such as haloperidol, can be used successfully in calming patients with dementia or psychiatric illness (con-traindicated for individuals with parkinsonism). However, if patient is experiencing acute confusion or delirium, short-acting benzodiazepines (e.g., lorazepam) are more effective in reducing anxiety and fear. Anxiety or fear usually triggers destructive or dangerous behaviors in the acutely confused older patient. A short-acting benzo-diazepine, such as lorazepam, will decrease feelings of anxiety and calm the patient after 1 or 2 doses. **Note:** Neu-roleptics can cause akathisia, an adverse drug reaction evidenced by increased restlessness.
Also see "Dementia—Alzheimer's Type," p. 793, as appropriate.	

●●● **Related NIC and NOC labels:** *NIC:* Dementia Management; Reality Orientation; Cerebral Perfusion Promotion; Environmental Management: Safety; Neurologic Monitoring *NOC:* Information Processing; Identity; Distorted Thought Control; Decision Making; Cognitive Orientation; Cognitive Ability

Palliative and End-of-Life Care

According to the World Health Organization (1990), palliative care is the active total care of patients whose disease is not responsive to curative treatment. Control of pain and other symptoms and of psychologic, social, and spiritual problems is paramount. The goal of palliative care is achievement of the best quality of life for patients and their families. The following nursing diagnoses relate specifically to issues, outcomes, and interventions that are common across medical diagnoses for patients receiving a palliative care approach in the terminal phase of illness.

HEALTH CARE SETTING

Primary care, hospitalization, hospice or palliative care, home health care

Nursing Diagnosis:

Deficient Knowledge:

Choices regarding disease management when cure is unrealistic

Desired Outcome: Patient and family express accurate knowledge about advanced directives and complete documents in accordance with state laws before hospitalization for acute crisis or within weeks of diagnosis of life-limiting illness.

INTERVENTIONS	RATIONALES
Advise patient and family of need for prompt legal preparations (will, trusts, Durable Power of Attorney for Health Care [DPOA-HC]). Assist patient with identifying appropriate DPOA-HC. Discuss role/limitations of DPOA-HC.	Ensures that patient and family are aware of legal preparations and promotes understanding of ability to make choices and have control when illness becomes advanced.
Discuss meaning of Do Not Resuscitate (DNR) Order or other Limitations of Therapy.	Ensures that patient and family/significant others understand what will occur during this phase of care.
Explain what is meant by Comfort Measures Only. Explain process of care related to withholding and/or withdrawing artificial food and fluids.	This information will help patient make decisions regarding care and nutrition outlined in Advanced Directives.

Continued

INTERVENTIONS	RATIONALES
Discuss and document patient's wishes. Ensure that patient's preferences for hydration and nutrition are addressed specifically in DPOA-HC or Living Will documents as required by state law.	Makes patient's wishes regarding autopsy, organ donation/transplantation, hydration and feeding tubes, use of antibiotics, chemotherapy, radiation therapy, diagnostic procedures, blood transfusions, and IVs known to family members and health care providers and ensures that those wishes are clear.
Assist patient in completion of Advanced Directives documents, including "Five Wishes" if available.	"Five Wishes," a program currently available in most states, is a style of advanced directives that outlines the type of care a patient desires, not just what should be withheld.
Secure copies of legal documents and place in patient's medical record.	
Encourage professional counseling if any of the above cause discord within the family.	Patients should select a DPOA-HC that is capable of carrying out their wishes. The patient's wishes may not be the wishes of the person who is the closest relative.

●●● **Related NIC and NOC labels:** *NIC:* Teaching: Disease Process; Teaching: Procedure/Treatment; Patients Rights Protection; Decision-Making Support *NOC:* Knowledge: Treatment Procedure(s)

Nursing Diagnosis:

Deficient Knowledge:

Progressive disease process and expectations as death approaches

Desired Outcome: Within 24 hr of educational process, patient and family relate accurate under-standing of the palliative care approach to management of disease progression and express preferences for care, care goals, and preferred site of death.

INTERVENTIONS	RATIONALES
Describe principles of palliative care to patient and family.	Promotes understanding that palliative care is not "giving up" but rather focuses on achieving the best possible quality of life for patient and family when the disease is no longer curable.
Discuss interventions for managing symptoms as death approaches.	Aggressive symptom management and ensuring best quality of life are very active treatments that can be provided. For example, "You should not feel 'there is nothing more to be done' because curative treatment is no longer effective."
Refer patient to palliative care or hospice care providers, while maintaining relationships with family/primary care physicians, community, and specialist care providers as appropriate.	Helps ensure that patient and family do not feel abandoned as care shifts to a palliative focus.
Understand the practical insurance and financial issues related to hospice care vs. home care.	There is a wide variation of reimbursement for hospice and palliative care provided by private insurers and HMOs. For example, Medicare hospice benefits provide a package of services via approved hospice programs; whereas the "plain" Medicare plan (Parts A & B) does not cover these services unless the patient is homebound.
Provide information for calling hospice or palliative care team for home visit and/or symptom management suggestions when death is imminent.	These are alternatives to calling for emergency care (e.g., calling 911). However, calling 911 for an individual receiving home care can enable emergency personnel to provide comfort measures rather than resuscitation interventions.

●●● **Related NIC and NOC labels:** *NIC:* Teaching: Disease Process; Health System Guidance *NOC:* Knowledge: Disease Process; Knowledge: Treatment Regimen

Nursing Diagnosis:

Chronic Pain

related to progressive disease state, immobility, chronic pain states, obstructions, organ failure, or neuropathy

Desired Outcomes: Within 4 hr of this nursing diagnosis, patient expresses or exhibits acceptable level of physical comfort with minimal side effects from analgesics. Family assists patient with maintaining, responding to, and titrating analgesia as patient's condition changes.

INTERVENTIONS	RATIONALES
Distinguish between physical pain and suffering.	Consider the cause of distress to be other than physical suffering if rapid, appropriate titration of analgesics does not relieve distress. In this case, sedation may be the only means to relieve suffering.
Assess regularly and use behavioral cues for patients who are unable to communicate.	Many patients are unable to communicate as death nears.
Allow patient to define balance between discomfort and analgesics.	Many symptoms (e.g., dry mouth) cause discomfort and are managed in ways other than by using analgesics.
Address addiction concerns of patient and family.	Pain is an appropriate indication for use of opioids, and under these circumstances, patients are not "addicted" to medications.
Address fears of respiratory depression from increasing opioid use.	Most patients receive opioid analgesics at end of life. Decreasing levels of consciousness and respirations are expected as part of the dying process and are not a toxicity of opioids.
See "Pain," p. 41, for more information.	

♦♦♦ **Related NIC and NOC labels:** *NIC:* Pain Management; Dying Care *NOC:* Comfort Level

Nursing Diagnosis:

Ineffective Breathing Pattern (Dyspnea)

related to progression of disease process

Desired Outcome: Within 1 hr of this nursing diagnosis, patient states that he or she does not perceive difficulty with breathing.

INTERVENTIONS	RATIONALES
Assess patient's perception of dyspnea. Consider use of a 0-10 intensity scale.	Patient's perception should guide treatment interventions.
Realize that objective parameters may not coincide with patient's perception of dyspnea.	Patient may have low oxygen saturation as measured by pulse oximetry but not feel dyspneic and vice versa.
Assess for treatable causes of dyspnea.	Anemia, heart failure, pleural effusion, ascites, and pneumonia, for example, are causes of ineffective breathing pattern (other than simply end of life) that can be treated.
Consider least invasive interventions first to relieve underlying pathologicy condition causing dyspnea (e.g. antibiotics, steroids, diuretics). Carefully evaluate risk vs. benefit of more invasive techniques such as thoracentesis, paracentesis, and radiation therapy; consider imminence of death.	To ensure that invasive therapies will have time to offer relief, not simply cause undue discomfort during dying process.

Continued

INTERVENTIONS	RATIONALES
Advise family that although breathing changes are common and distressing, they are manageable.	Breathing changes in the patient can be upsetting to the family.
Maintain room at cool temperature.	To minimize feelings of suffocation.
Administer oxygen by nasal cannula only if this offers subjective relief of dyspnea. Use lowest flow rate possible and offer humidification if technically possible.	To provide comfort.
Avoid face mask.	A face mask can interfere with ability to communicate with significant others.
Administer morphine or other opioid regularly by available route to relieve dyspnea.	The oral route (pills or elixir) is preferred, but if this is not possible, use rectal, sublingual, nebulized, SC, or IV route.
Place fan close to patient's face.	The face contains baroreceptors that respond to air movement and can effectively relieve perception of dyspnea.
Position patient with head/upper body elevated. Suggest sleeping in chair, if needed.	Elevation of the head may make breathing easier and provide comfort.
Administer nebulized bronchodilators, steroids, and/or opioids.	To relieve dyspnea.
Teach relaxation breathing techniques to patient and family. Encourage physical touch/massage as a calming technique.	To relieve anxiety, which may improve breathing pattern.
Consider need for pharmacologic management of anxiety (e.g., use of anxiolytics).	To alleviate fear and concomitant breathlessness.
Discuss principle of "double effect" of medications. Elicit patient preferences and values about alertness vs. sedation to relieve discomfort if both goals cannot be achieved. Honor patient's choices for symptom management.	Some medicines may relieve symptoms but at the expense of the unintended side effect of sedation or hastened death.

●●● **Related NIC and NOC labels:** *NIC:* Positioning; Respiratory Monitoring; Anxiety Reduction; Oxygen Therapy; Teaching: Prescribed Activity/Exercise *NOC:* Respiratory Status: Ventilation; Vital Signs Status

Nursing Diagnosis:

Ineffective Airway Clearance

related to increased pulmonary secretions and congestion secondary to diminishing level of consciousness as death approaches

Desired Outcomes: Patient does not show signs of struggle or discomfort when "death rattle" is present. Immediately following explanation, the family expresses understanding that these noisy respirations are more distressing to them than to the (unconscious) patient.

INTERVENTIONS	RATIONALES
Explain the cause of the noisy breathing.	It is a result of secretions in the upper airway in patients who are too weak to cough effectively.
Assure family and significant others that patient's breathing, though noisy, is peaceful and unlabored. Point out signs that indicate patient is not exhibiting distress.	Noisy breathing can be distressing to family and friends of the patient.
Attempt to position patient laterally and recumbent rather than supine.	To maintain as patent an airway as possible.
Use oxygen only if it enables patient to have unlabored respirations.	To promote comfort by minimizing labored respirations.

Continued

INTERVENTIONS	RATIONALES
Avoid suctioning, other than in the oral cavity.	Aggressive, deep suctioning will increase, not decrease, secretions.
Maintain patient in a relatively dehydrated state.	To minimize accumulation of pulmonary secretions.
If death rattle persists despite dehydration, administer prescribed anticholinergics via least invasive route.	Anticholinergics decrease secretions and are much more effective when administered early in the onset of this symptom. Effective agents include scopolamine patch, glycopyrrolate (IV, SC, PO), atropine, and hyoscine butylbromide.
Reassure family that patients are often unaware of discomfort at this point.	To relieve anxiety of family and significant others about possible discomfort resulting from dehydration to manage pulmonary secretions.

●●● **Related NIC and NOC labels:** *NIC:* Airway Management; Positioning *NOC:* Aspiration Control; Respiratory Status: Airway Patency

Nursing Diagnosis:

Disturbed Thought Processes: Delirium

related to disease progression, infection, altered metabolic state, or symptom management side effects

Desired Outcomes: Reversible etiologies of delirium are treated within hours of onset. When delirium is irreversible, agitation is reduced or minimized, optimally within 1 hr of intervention.

INTERVENTIONS	RATIONALES
Assess for causes of delirium in the terminally ill.	Common causes of delirium in the terminally ill that may be reversed or treated with relatively noninvasive measures include brain metastasis, steroid use, opioid toxicity, anticholinergics, benzodiazepines, withdrawal from drug/ethanol, unrelieved pain, itching, constipation, urinary retention, infection, hepatic encephalopathy, hypo/hyperglycemia, hypoxia, hypercalcemia, and dehydration.
Correct metabolic abnormalities, empty the bladder, relieve constipation, provide gentle hydration. As prescribed, decrease/eliminate medications that are not directed at comfort.	Interventions for potentially reversible causes of delirium.
Maintain a quiet, well-lighted environment.	To relieve anxiety, which optimally will reduce agitation.
Role-model soft-spoken language for family.	Patient likely maintains sense of hearing even when other senses are impaired. A quiet environment will help reduce agitation.
Use padded side rails, put bed in low position, and avoid physical restraints. Use patient companion or other environmental safety measures, for example, bed alarms.	To ensure physical safety for patient who has delirium, while avoiding measures such as restraints that promote agitation.
Administer medications alone or in conjunction with benzodiazepines as prescribed.	To manage delirium and control agitation. Benzodiazepines alone can cause paradoxical effect and my increase agitation.
Reorient patient frequently. Have large-faced clocks and calendars within sight.	Reminding patient of person, place, and time may help reorient and mitigate delirium.
Advise family that delirium may signal imminent death.	To prepare family for death.

Continued

INTERVENTIONS	RATIONALES
Consider sedation if this is consistent with patient and family preferences and values. Avoid use of phrase "terminal sedation" rather than "sedation in imminently dying."	The former phrase implies sedation to end patient's life rather than intent of sedation for symptom management and alleviation of distress in patient who is dying.

●●● **Related NIC and NOC labels:** *NIC:* Reality Orientation; Delirium Management; Medication Management; Calming Technique; Environmental Management; Decision-Making Support; Counseling; Patients Rights Protection; Family Support *NOC:* Cognitive Orientation; Decision Making

Nursing Diagnosis:

Risk for Imbalanced Fluid Volume: Dehydration or edema

related to inability to regulate food and fluid intake and output secondary to disease progression

Desired Outcomes: Patient's desires for fluid intake are determined by subjective feelings of thirst. Patient receives hydration according to stated preferences. Hydration goals are realistic with appropriate endpoints such as correction of a metabolic disorder that results in decreased delirium and enhanced subjective well-being. Immediately following explanation, patient and/or significant others verbalize understanding that artificial hydration does not alleviate thirst.

INTERVENTIONS	RATIONALES
Do not attempt to manage perception of dry mouth by achieving normal hydration.	This perception is often the result of mouth breathing or other cause that is unresponsive to oral hydration.
Be aware of peripheral edema, urinary incontinence, pleural effusion, ascites, pulmonary congestion, enhanced "death rattle."	Signs and symptoms of uncomfortable fluid overload.
Address issue of nutrition, hydration, and feeding tubes on Advanced Directive.	To ensure that patient's wishes are followed.
Advise and encourage family not to insist that patient eat.	It is normal to eat and drink less at end of life. Dehydration results in a peaceful, painless death.
Administer rectal acetaminophen regularly.	To reduce discomfort of dehydration-related fever.
Perform meticulous oral care using mouth/lip moisturizers.	To minimize discomfort of dry mouth.
If family wishes to continue oral feedings, encourage frequent meals, small portions, use of small plates, and companionship during meals.	Recognizes cultural/ethnic implications of foods/beverages and eating/drinking while providing for smaller portions that are more realistic for patients at end of life.
Prepare soft, easily swallowed substances such as soups, milk shakes, yogurt, custards, ice cream. Prepare foods away from patient's sight/smell.	To promote comfort during the feeding process.
Provide nonirritating liquids that are pleasing to patient. Administer fluids if patient/family so request using least invasive route (e.g., via hypodermoclysis or IV as last resort).	To treat negative effects of dehydration (e.g., delirium).
Advise family to expect urine to become scant and dark in color.	To relieve family's anxiety about urine color and output.

●●● **Related NIC and NOC labels:** *NIC:* Fluid Management; Medication Administration; Nutrition Management; Feeding; Oral Health Restoration *NOC:* Fluid Balance; Nutritional Status: Food & Fluid Intake

Nursing Diagnosis:

Risk for Imbalanced Nutrition: Less than body requirements

related to anorexia, nausea and vomiting, cachexia, intestinal obstruction, impaired swallowing, and aspiration risk secondary to disease progression

Desired Outcomes: Patient does not report the presence of hunger. Family honors patient's wishes regarding artificial nutrition.

INTERVENTIONS	RATIONALES
Remind family that eating will not reverse the underlying disease state. Identify other ways family can express love.	Many families see food as an expression of love and will become distressed when patient is no longer able to have a "normal" nutritional intake.
Help patient and family understand that a normal nutritional status is unrealistic as the disease progresses and the body no longer processes ingested nutrients.	Loss of interest in food is normal near death. Artificial nutrition such as parenteral nutrition does not relieve feelings of hunger, nor does it prolong survival in a terminal state. The body only takes in and uses what it needs.
If appropriate, obtain a nutritional consult.	A nutritional consult will determine the most digestible feedings, given the patient's underlying disease. Oral nutrition is the method of choice for patients who can swallow and have intact GI systems. Enteral routes include nasogastric, gastrostomy, and jejunostomy tubes. However these routes can result in harm if the GI system cannot absorb and digest nutrients.
Avoid giving commercial nutritional supplements.	Supplements may result in an inability to ingest foods that patient likes and enjoys, and they may be unpalatable.

●●● **Related NIC and NOC labels:** *NIC:* Nutrition Management; Sustenance Support *NOC:* Nutritional Status

Nursing Diagnosis:

Impaired Oral Mucous Membrane: Dry mouth/xerostomia

related to reduced saliva, mouth breathing, oral infections, mucositis, and/or dehydration

Desired Outcome: Patient's oral mucous membrane becomes moist within 1 hr of this diagnosis.

INTERVENTIONS	RATIONALES
Encourage topical interventions to relieve a dry mouth. Use a misting spray bottle with saline to moisten oral mucous membrane. Use emollients on lips.	Studies have shown that dry mouth is the most common and distressing symptom of a conscious person at end of life. IV fluids and interventions directed at a normal hydration status rarely relieve dry mouth.
Encourage family to assist with mouth care.	Involves family in patient care when possible.
If patient is on oxygen, add humidifier.	To relieve dry oral mucous membranes.
Rule out oral thrush, herpes; treat if necessary.	Potential causes of dry or painful mouth.
Encourage fluid intake via frequent sips of water, popsicles, ice chips. Encourage soups, sauces, gravies, ice cream, and frozen yogurt in patients able to eat.	To provide comfort and relieve oral dryness.

Continued

INTERVENTIONS	RATIONALES
Avoid substances such as caffeine, alcohol, and alcohol-based products, for example, mouthwash and cough syrups.	These substances can cause oral dryness.
Offer spray bottle filled with water and a few drops of vegetable oil. Suggest use of lemon drops or other sour candy if patient can tolerate without aspiration. Administer saliva substitutes.	To keep mucous membranes moist.
Encourage good dental hygiene (soft toothbrush, regular brushing and flossing).	Relieves unpleasant tastes while helping maintain oral mucous membrane.

●●● **Related NIC and NOC labels:** *NIC:* Oral Health Maintenance; Fluid Management; Dying Care
NOC: Oral Health

Nursing Diagnoses:

Fear/Anxiety

related to life-threatening condition, pain, the unknown (death), and patient's concern that he or she will be forgotten

Desired Outcomes: Patient's fears and anxieties are acknowledged and addressed immediately following this diagnosis. Within 1 hr of this diagnosis, patient (and family) state that fear and anxiety have been lessened.

INTERVENTIONS	RATIONALES
Distinguish between anxiety and fear. Identify appropriate interventions (see **Death Anxiety,** which follows).	Anxiety is a state of apprehension and dread whose source the patient cannot identify. Fear often has a realistic, definable cause. Distinguishing between the two will enable appropriate interventions.
Reassure patient that pain and other discomforts will be managed.	To relieve anxiety and fear.
Identify and address family's fears and concerns. Keep family informed of physical symptoms to expect as death approaches (e.g., changes in breathing, decreased level of consciousness, coolness and mottling of skin).	Physical symptoms of death can be distressing to the family. Knowing what to expect may help them cope with their anxieties and fears related to patient's approaching death.
Encourage patient and family to seek support from pastoral counselors in addressing religious beliefs about the meaning of suffering, death, and afterlife if appropriate.	Spiritual guidance can help the family cope with anxieties and fears about loss of their loved one and for the patient may help resolve anxieties and fears related to spiritual concerns and conflicts.
Assist patient and family with creating videos or audios and scrapbooks.	Recalled memories can help facilitate the grieving process and mitigate fears for the patient that he or she will be forgotten.

●●● **Related NIC and NOC labels:** *NIC:* Anxiety Reduction; Active Listening; Counseling; Support System Enhancement; Support Group; Emotional Support; Dying Care *NOC:* Anxiety Control; Fear Control

Nursing Diagnosis:

Death Anxiety

related to impending death, fear of unmanaged physical symptoms, and fear of unknown

Desired Outcomes: Immediately following interventions, patient states (or exhibits) that he or she is free of physical discomforts and emotional distress. Family members verbalize understanding of the dying process.

INTERVENTIONS	RATIONALES
Provide aggressive symptom management of physical discomforts before attempting to assess anxiety.	Physical symptoms can cause anxiety.
Help patient recognize early physical manifestations of anxiety, for example, racing heart, sweating, feeling flushed, wheezing.	To minimize escalation of anxiety.
Support patient and family in expressing fears and anxieties related to previous experiences with the dying. Listen carefully to stories to anticipate special needs during current death event. Encourage them to say or write down what they most want the dying patient to know, even if the patient is not conscious.	Discussion may help to reduce anxiety.
Review age-appropriate guidelines for child participation in care and presence with dying family member and encourage family to allow children to be present consistent with these guidelines. Include pets if possible in patient visitation.	To help them cope with their fears and anxieties about the death of their family member.
Obtain referrals or guidance of specific religious counselors to support patient through anxiety regarding this issue.	Encourages patient to share impressions of what happens after death.
Encourage use of relaxation techniques such as imagery, progressive muscle relaxation, relaxation breathing.	To reduce anxiety.
Administer anxiolytics as appropriate.	

●●● **Related NIC and NOC labels:** *NIC:* Anxiety Reduction; Coping Enhancement; Emotional Support; Spiritual Support; Reminiscence Therapy; Dying Care; Family Involvement Promotion; Grief Work Facilitation; Simple Relaxation Therapy *NOC:* Anxiety Control; Dignified Dying

Nursing Diagnosis:

Powerlessness

related to actual debility and inability to carry out normal role functions

Desired Outcome: Patient makes choices for end-of-life care.

INTERVENTIONS	RATIONALES
Reinforce use of patient's Advance Directives and advance care planning activities in guiding care.	Ensuring that patient's wishes are followed minimizes sense of powerlessness.
Remind patient and family of their continuing ability to make choices around end-of-life care.	Having control over these decisions will reduce feelings of powerlessness. Some examples include patient's right to choose whether to eat or drink, have certain care procedures performed, have or decline treatments, and actualize preferences around site of dying (e.g., home vs. institution).

●●● **Related NIC and NOC labels:** *NIC:* Decision-Making Support; Health System Guidance; Patients Rights Protection; Family Involvement Promotion *NOC:* Participation: Health Care Decisions

Nursing Diagnosis:

Spiritual Distress

related to religious, cultural, and existential beliefs about dying

Desired Outcome: Immediately following interventions, patient states that he or she has the ability to connect with spiritual/pastoral counselors to discuss issues of spirituality, existential concerns, and their meanings.

INTERVENTIONS	RATIONALES

Support patient's religious customs around end-of-life issues:
 	
  - Offer to pray with patient and family if appropriate.
 	
  - Remember that "spiritual" is not necessarily synonymous with "religious."
 	
  - Ask patient what has brought his or her life satisfaction, joy, sorrow, meaning.
 	
  - Assist family in creation of rituals (letting go, remembering, forgiving).
 	
  - Suggest planning of funeral/memorial service, music, readings, and so on.
	To provide a supportive, open environment in which patient can discuss these issues if he or she chooses.

Include priest/minister/rabbi as integral member of caregiving team.	To provide spiritual guidance and counseling.

●●● **Related NIC and NOC labels:** *NIC:* Dying Care; Spiritual Support; Forgiveness Facilitation; Reminiscence Therapy; Referral *NOC:* Dignified Dying; Spiritual Well-Being

Nursing Diagnosis:

Risk for Caregiver Role Strain

related to multiple demands on family members and resources when caring for dying loved one

Desired Outcome: Within 24 hr of this diagnosis, caregivers are assisted with providing care and are given respite.

INTERVENTIONS	RATIONALES
Identify available resources (e.g., hospice, friends, community, church members) to assist with caregiving in patient's and family members' preferred site of death.	To relieve some of the strain of caregiving.
Suggest counseling and other psychosocial support resources that assist family with maintaining integrity and avoiding conflict during strain of illness.	There may be lack of insurance funding for many activities of care (e.g., childcare, transportation, housekeeping) and other worries that caregivers may have regarding loss of time from work, loss of savings, and loss of income of ill family member.
Remind caregivers of their own health care needs. Encourage family to take breaks for meals, relaxation, and attention to nonill family members, especially young children.	To reduce stress and anxiety.

INTERVENTIONS

RATIONALES

INTERVENTIONS	RATIONALES
Offer family members unrestricted access to patient as death approaches but also encourage them to take frequent rest periods.	To provide flexibility and opportunities for rest.
If family members are unable to be present for a period of time, provide phone numbers so that they can stay in contact with staff.	To relieve stress and anxiety if they have to be away. This also may reduce guilt about not being there.

●●● **Related NIC and NOC labels:** *NIC:* Caregiver Support; Emotional Support; Respite Care; Anticipatory Guidance; Active Listening; Coping Enhancement; Grief Work Facilitation; Referral; Support System Enhancement; Family Integrity Promotion; Risk Identification *NOC:* Caregiver Emotional Health; Caregiver Physical Health; Caregiver Stressors

Nursing Diagnosis:

Anticipatory Grieving

related to impending loss of loved one

Desired Outcome: Within 24 hr of this diagnosis, family/significant others identify and express feelings appropriately and demonstrate balancing caregiving with their own physical and emotional respite needs.

INTERVENTIONS

RATIONALES

INTERVENTIONS	RATIONALES
Encourage grieving and expression of feelings by patient, family, and staff. Permit silences—do not try to say something meaningful or profound.	Anticipatory grieving is valuable. Anger is often substituted for grief.
Assist family with recalling successful past strategies for coping with grief.	Strategies that have worked in the past also may work in the present.
Respect need to use denial occasionally.	Denial is an effective coping mechanism for grief.
Give family permission to express ambivalence about impending death.	These feelings are normal, and acknowledging them may help minimize feelings of guilt about having them. For instance, "Many people in your circumstance don't want to lose their loved one, yet they wish for the suffering to be over. I wonder if you've had feelings like this?"
Offer locks of hair and other tangible mementoes to survivors.	To facilitate the grieving process.
Permit family to stay with patient after death.	To say good-bye and express grief.
Arrange bereavement follow-up for family members. For example, inform them about availability of bereavement groups, books on grieving, and available counseling resources.	To provide support to the family in their grief after the death has occurred.
Recommend judicious use of anxiolytics/sedatives for acutely grieving survivors.	To promote rest and help alleviate anxiety during their grief.
Provide phone numbers or concrete information.	To assist family in beginning process of identifying funeral plans. Participating in such tasks may help assuage grief.
Notify other health care providers (e.g., primary care provider, surgeon, ambulatory care nurses) of patient's death. Consider making a bereavement phone call or sending a sympathy card.	Condolences from health care providers are meaningful to survivors and help with grief.

●●● **Related NIC and NOC labels:** *NIC:* Coping Enhancement; Grief Work Facilitation; Dying Care; Counseling; Support System Enhancement; Visitation Facilitation *NOC:* Family Coping; Grief Resolution; Psychosocial Adjustment: Life Change

ADDITIONAL NURSING DIAGNOSES/ PROBLEMS:

9

Acute Respiratory Failure

Acute respiratory failure (ARF) is present when the lungs are unable to exchange O_2 and CO_2 adequately. Clinically, respiratory failure exists when PaO_2 is <50 mm Hg with the patient at rest and breathing room air. $PaCO_2$ ≥50 mm Hg or pH <7.35 is significant for respiratory acidosis, which is the common precursor to ARF. Four basic mechanisms are involved in the development of respiratory failure:

Alveolar hypoventilation: Occurs secondary to reduction in alveolar minute ventilation. Because differential indicators (cyanosis, somnolence) occur late in the process, the condition may go unnoticed until tissue hypoxia is severe.

Ventilation-perfusion mismatch: Considered the most common cause of hypoxemia. Normal alveolar ventilation occurs at a rate of 4 L/min, with normal pulmonary vascular blood flow occurring at a rate of 5 L/min. Normal ventilation/perfusion ratio is 0.8:1. Any disease process that interferes with either side of the equation upsets the physiologic balance and can lead to respiratory failure as a result of the reduction in arterial O_2 levels.

Diffusion disturbances: Processes that physically impair gas exchange across the alveolar-capillary membrane. Diffusion is impaired because of the increase in anatomic distance the gas must travel from alveoli to capillary and capillary to alveoli.

Right-to-left shunt: Occurs when the above processes go untreated. Large amounts of blood pass from the right side of the heart to the left and out into the general circulation without adequate ventilation; therefore blood is poorly oxygenated. Unlike the first three responses, hypoxemia secondary to right-to-left shunting does not improve with the administration of O_2 because the additional FIO_2 is not exchanged across the alveolar-capillary membrane.

HEALTH CARE SETTING

Primary care; acute care (hospitalization) resulting from complications

ASSESSMENT

Clinical indicators of ARF vary according to the underlying disease process and severity of the failure. ARF is one of the most common causes of impaired level of consciousness (LOC). Often it is misdiagnosed as heart failure, pneumonia, or cerebrovascular accident.

Early indicators: Restlessness, changes in mental status, anxiety, headache, fatigue, cool and dry skin, increased BP, tachycardia, cardiac dysrhythmias.

Intermediate indicators: Confusion, lethargy, tachypnea, hypotension caused by vasodilation, cardiac dysrhythmias.

Late indicators: Cyanosis, diaphoresis, coma, respiratory arrest.

DIAGNOSTIC TESTS

Arterial blood gas (ABG) analysis: Assesses adequacy of oxygenation and effectiveness of ventilation and is the most important diagnostic tool. Typical results are PaO_2 ≤60 mm Hg, $PaCO_2$ ≥45 mm Hg, and pH <7.35, which are consistent with severe respiratory acidosis.

Chest x-ray examination: Ascertains presence of underlying pathophysiologic condition or disease process that may be contributing to the failure.

Nursing Diagnosis:

Impaired Gas Exchange

related to inability of the lungs to exchange O_2 and CO_2 adequately

Desired Outcomes: Optimally, within 1-2 hr following intervention/treatment, patient has adequate gas exchange as evidenced by RR of 12-20 breaths/min with normal depth and pattern and absence of signs and symptoms of respiratory distress. Within 24 hr after treatment, ABGs reveal PaO_2 >60 mm Hg, $PaCO_2$ 35-45 mm Hg, and pH 7.35-7.45 (or values consistent with patient's baseline).

INTERVENTIONS	RATIONALES
Monitor for early signs and symptoms of ARF.	To enable early detection and treatment of ARF, which is one of the most common causes of impaired LOC. Early signs and symptoms include restlessness, anxiety, mental status changes, headache, fatigue, and cool and dry skin.
	Intermediate signs and symptoms of ARF include confusion and lethargy.
	Cyanosis of the lips and nail beds, diaphoresis, coma, and respiratory arrest are late indicators.
Monitor and document VS at frequent intervals.	Increased BP, tachycardia, and cardiac dysrhythmias are early indicators of ARF. Tachypnea, hypotension, and cardiac dysrhythmias are intermediate indicators of ARF.
Monitor ABG results.	To assess adequacy of oxygenation and effectiveness of ventilation. PaO_2 ≤60 mm Hg, $PaCO_2$ ≥45 mm Hg, and pH <7.35 are consistent with severe respiratory acidosis, which is the common precursor to ARF. A patient with chronic obstructive pulmonary disease (COPD) may be clinically stable with a $PaCO_2$ >45 mm Hg, and therefore determination of pH is critical with this individual. In other words, if patient's pH drops below baseline, he or she is at risk for developing ARF.
Position patient in semi-Fowler's position.	Promotes comfort and diaphragmatic descent, maximizes inhalation, and decreases work of breathing (WOB).
Deliver oxygen as prescribed.	To ensure that oxygen is within prescribed concentrations. Patients with COPD may not tolerate oxygen at a delivery >2 L/min, which can suppress the hypoxic respiratory drive.
Monitor FIO_2.	An FIO_2 of ≤0.5, along with chest physiotherapy and pharmacotherapy, often improves ABGs sufficiently to get patient out of danger.
Ensure that patient receives chest physiotherapy and coughing/deep-breathing exercises.	To mobilize secretions and promote full lung expansion, which will facilitate gas exchange.
Administer pharmacotherapy as prescribed and document effectiveness.	For example, IV aminophylline may be given to treat bronchospasms; bronchodilator therapy may be delivered via nebulizer or intermittent positive-pressure breathing (IPPB) machine to minimize CO_2 retention.

●●● **Related NIC and NOC labels:** *NIC:* Acid-Base Monitoring; Oxygen Therapy; Chest Physiotherapy; Positioning; Respiratory Monitoring; Vital Signs Monitoring; Cough Enhancement; Laboratory Data Interpretation *NOC:* Respiratory: Gas Exchange; Vital Signs Status; Tissue Perfusion: Pulmonary

Nursing Diagnosis:
Deficient Fluid Volume

related to increased insensible loss secondary to tachypnea, fever, or diaphoresis

Desired Outcome: Before hospital discharge (or within 24 hr after treatment if patient is not hospitalized), patient becomes normovolemic as evidenced by urine output ≥30 ml/hr with specific gravity 1.010–1.030, stable weight, HR and BP within patient's normal limits, central venous pressure (CVP) >2 mm Hg (5 cm H_2O), fluid intake approximating fluid output, moist mucous membranes, and normal skin turgor.

INTERVENTIONS	RATIONALES
Monitor I&O. Consider insensible losses if patient is diaphoretic and tachypneic.	To monitor trend of fluid volume.
Be alert to and report indicators of deficient fluid volume.	Indicators of deficient fluid volume include urinary output <30 ml/hr for 2 consecutive hr and urinary specific gravity >1.030.
Weigh patient daily at the same time of day, with the same clothing, and on the same scale; record weight.	Ensures consistency and accuracy of measurements.
Report weight changes of 1-1.5 kg/day.	May signal fluid volume overload/deficit.
Encourage fluid intake (at least 2.5 L/day in the unrestricted patient).	To ensure adequate hydration.
Maintain IV fluid therapy as prescribed.	To maintain fluid volume balance.
Promote oral hygiene, including lip and tongue care.	To moisten dried tissues and mucous membranes.
Provide humidity for oxygen therapy.	To decrease convective losses of moisture.

●●● **Related NIC and NOC labels:** *NIC:* Fluid Management; Fluid Monitoring; Intravenous Therapy *NOC:* Fluid Balance; Hydration

Additional Nursing Diagnoses/ Problems: (the listed disorders may be precursors to ARF)

PATIENT-FAMILY TEACHING AND DISCHARGE PLANNING

ARF is an acute condition that is symptomatically treated during the patient's hospitalization. Discharge planning and teaching should be directed at educating the patient and significant others about the underlying pathophysiology and treatment specific for that process. See sections listed above that relate specifically to the underlying pathophysiologic condition contributing to development of ARF.

Chronic Bronchitis

Chronic bronchitis is the most common respiratory disease in the United States. Airway changes that occur with this disease result from chronic airway inflammation and irritation. As the disease progresses, there is associated destruction of lung tissue used in gas exchange, resulting in inadequate ventilation. Recurrent upper respiratory infections (URIs) with *Streptococcus pneumoniae* and *Haemophilus influenzae* are common in this population secondary to the inability to clear the bronchial tree of mucus. As the disease progresses, acute exacerbations increase in severity and duration. Respiratory failure and cardiac problems can develop.

HEALTH CARE SETTING

Primary care or long-term care, with possible hospitalization resulting from complications

ASSESSMENT

Chronic indicators: Morning cough, clear and copious secretions, anorexia, cyanosis, dependent edema.

Acute indicators (exacerbation): Dyspnea, shortness of breath, orthopnea; discolored, thick, tenacious sputum.

Physical assessment: Use of accessory muscles of respiration, prolonged expiratory phase, digital clubbing, decreased thoracic expansion, barrel chest appearance, dullness over areas of consolidation, adventitious breath sounds (especially coarse rhonchi and wheezing), ankle edema, distended neck veins, bloated appearance.

DIAGNOSTIC TESTS

Chest x-ray examination: Will reveal normal anteroposterior (AP) diameter, nearly normal diaphragm position, and increased peripheral lung markings.

ABG values: Will reveal hypoxemia (PaO$_2$ <60 mm Hg) and hypercarbia (PaCO$_2$ >50-60 mm Hg) in most patients. Baseline pH may be 7.35-7.38, but during acute exacerbation, as the PaCO$_2$ increases, pH may fall below 7.35.

Oximetry: Will reveal decreased O$_2$ saturation.

Sputum culture: May reveal presence of infective organisms. Sputum specimens are best collected when the patient first wakes in the morning.

Complete blood count (CBC): Will reveal chronically elevated Hgb in the presence of chronic hypoxemia and elevated white blood cell (WBC) count in the presence of acute bacterial infection.

Pulmonary function tests: Will show reduced forced vital capacity, reduced forced expiratory volume, increased residual volume caused by trapping of air, and increased expiratory reserve volume.

Nursing Diagnosis:

Ineffective Airway Clearance

related to decreased energy, which results in ineffective cough; or *related to* presence of increased tracheobronchial secretions

Desired Outcome: Immediately following intervention, patient coughs appropriately and has effective airway clearance as evidenced by absence of adventitious breath sounds

INTERVENTIONS	RATIONALES
Auscultate breath sounds q2-4h (or as indicated by patient's condition) and after coughing.	To assess for adventitious and/or changes in breath sounds.
Teach patient the "double cough" technique.	This technique prevents small airway collapse, which can occur with forceful coughing. Steps include: - Sit upright with upper body flexed forward slightly. - Take two to three breaths and exhale passively. - Inhale again, but only to the midinspiratory point. - Exhale by coughing quickly 2-3 times.
Unless contraindicated, administer chest physiotherapy as prescribed.	To mobilize secretions.
Encourage fluid intake (≥2.5 L/day).	To decrease viscosity of sputum and promote ciliary activity, which will help mobilize secretions.

●●● **Related NIC and NOC labels:** *NIC:* Respiratory Monitoring; Chest Physiotherapy; Cough Enhancement; Fluid Monitoring *NOC:* Respiratory Status: Gas Exchange; Respiratory Status: Ventilation

Nursing Diagnosis:

Imbalanced Nutrition: Less than body requirements

related to decreased intake secondary to fatigue and anorexia

Desired Outcome: Before hospital discharge (if patient is hospitalized) or within 48 hr of interventions, patient has adequate nutrition as evidenced by stable weight, positive nitrogen (N) state on N studies, total lymphocyte count 1500-4500/mm^3, and serum albumin 3.5-5.5 g/dl.

INTERVENTIONS	RATIONALES
Monitor food and fluid intake.	Provides data to determine need for dietary consultation.
Provide diet in small, frequent meals that are nutritious.	Small meals are easier to consume in individuals who are fatigued.
Unless otherwise indicated, provide calories more from unsaturated fat sources than from carbohydrate sources.	The patient with chronic obstructive pulmonary disease (COPD) takes in less O_2 and retains CO_2. A high-fat diet generates the least amount of CO_2 for a given amount of O_2 used, whereas a diet high in carbohydrates generates the most. Foods high in fat that should be encouraged include whole milk, cream, evaporated milk, cream soups, custards, cheese, salad and cooking oils, mayonnaise, nuts, meat, poultry, and fish. High-carbohydrate sources that should be discouraged include cakes, cookies, jams, pastries, and sugar-concentrated snacks.
Discuss with patient and significant others the importance of a proper diet in treatment of chronic bronchitis.	To promote adequate nutrition and stable body weight. A knowledgeable patient is more likely to comply with the treatment plan.

●●● **Related NIC and NOC labels:** *NIC:* Nutritional Monitoring; Nutrition Therapy; Nutritional Counseling; Teaching: Prescribed Diet; Weight Management *NOC:* Nutritional Status; Nutrient Intake

ADDITIONAL NURSING DIAGNOSES/ PROBLEMS:

PATIENT-FAMILY TEACHING AND DISCHARGE PLANNING

When providing patient-family teaching, focus on sensory information, avoid giving excessive information, and initiate a visiting nurse referral for necessary follow-up teaching. Include verbal and written information about the following:

✓ Use of home O_2, including instructions for when to use it, importance of not increasing prescribed flow rate, precautions, and community resources for O_2 replacement when necessary. Request respiratory therapy consultation to assist with teaching related to O_2 therapy, if indicated.

✓ Medications, including drug name, route, purpose, dosage, schedule, precautions, drug/drug and food/drug interactions, and potential side effects. If the patient will take corticosteroids while at home, provide instructions accordingly to ensure that the patient takes the correct amount, particularly during the period in which the medication will be tapered.

✓ Signs and symptoms of heart failure that necessitate medical attention: increased dyspnea; fatigue; increased coughing; changes in the amount, color, or consistency of sputum; swelling of the ankles and legs; and sudden weight gain. Patients with COPD often have right-sided heart failure secondary to cardiac effects of the disease. For more information, see "Heart Failure," p. 195.

✓ Importance of avoiding contact with infectious individuals, especially those with respiratory infections.

✓ Recommendation that patient receive a pneumococcal vaccination and annual influenza vaccination.

✓ Review of Na^+-restricted diet and other dietary considerations as indicated. Sodium may be restricted to reduce fluid overload in the presence of cardiac complications such as heart failure. See "Heart Failure," p. 195.

✓ Importance of pacing activity level to conserve energy.

✓ Follow-up appointment with health care provider; confirm date and time of next appointment.

✓ Introduction to local chapter of American Lung Association activities and pulmonary rehabilitation programs. Physical training programs may improve ventilation and cardiac muscle function, as well as physical stamina, which may compensate for nonreversible lung disease.

✓ Phone numbers to call should questions or concerns arise about therapy or disease after discharge. Additional general information can be obtained by contacting the following organization:

American Lung Association
1740 Broadway
New York, NY 10019-4374
(212) 315-8700
www.lungusa.org

✓ For patients who smoke: elimination of smoking; refer patient to a "stop smoking" program as appropriate. The following free brochures outline ways to help patients stop smoking:

- *How to Help Your Patients Stop Using Tobacco: A National Cancer Institute Manual for the Oral Health Team*, from the Smoking and Tobacco Control Program of the National Cancer Institute; call 1-800-4-CANCER.

- *Clinical Practice Guideline: A Quick Reference Guide for Smoking Cessation Specialists*, from the Agency for Health Care Policy and Research (AHCPR); call 1-800-358-9295.

Emphysema

Pulmonary emphysema is a degenerative process characterized by enlargement of the air spaces distal to the terminal bronchioles accompanied by destruction of the alveolar walls (coalescence of the alveoli). Emphysema is a progressive disease, and affected individuals can become totally disabled because they must use all available energy for breathing. In the later stages of the disease, pulmonary hypertension develops, leading to cor pulmonale, or right-sided heart failure, a condition that produces cardiac symptoms, as well as complicating respiratory problems.

HEALTH CARE SETTING

Primary care or long-term care with possible hospitalization resulting from complications

ASSESSMENT

Chronic indicators: Nonproductive cough (unless patient also has bronchitis), dyspnea on exertion, orthopnea, shortness of breath.

Acute indicators (exacerbation): Increased dyspnea, productive cough, fever, peripheral edema, fatigue.

Physical assessment: Emaciation, increased anteroposterior (AP) chest diameter, pursed-lip breathing, hypertrophy of accessory muscles of respiration, decreased fremitus over affected lung fields, decreased thoracic excursion, hyperresonance over affected lung fields, decreased breath sounds, and prolonged expiratory phase. Digital clubbing occurs late in the disease.

DIAGNOSTIC TESTS

Chest x-ray examination: Will show hyperinflation of the lungs, increased AP diameter, lowered and flattened diaphragm, and a small cardiac silhouette. With cor pulmonale the pulmonary vasculature may appear engorged and the heart size enlarged.

Arterial blood gas (ABG) values: May reveal a slight decrease in PaO_2. As disease progresses, the PaO_2 will continue to decrease and $PaCO_2$ may increase because of hypoventilation and CO_2 retention.

Oximetry: May reveal decreased O_2 saturation.

Complete blood count (CBC): May reveal a chronically elevated red blood cell (RBC) count (polycythemia) later in the disease process as a compensatory response to chronic hypoxemia. Leukocytosis may be evident with overlying respiratory tract infection.

Pulmonary function tests: Will show an increased total lung capacity, increased residual volume, and decreased forced expiratory reserve volume. The vital capacity will be normal or slightly decreased.

Electrocardiogram (ECG): May reveal atrial and ventricular dysrhythmias. Most patients will have an atrial dysrhythmia as a result of atrial dilation and right ventricular hypertrophy caused by pulmonary hypertension.

Sputum culture: May be requested to determine presence of pulmonary infection.

Nursing Diagnosis:

Ineffective Breathing Pattern

related to decreased lung expansion secondary to chronic air flow limitations

Desired Outcome: Optimally, immediately following treatment/intervention, patient's breathing pattern improves as evidenced by reduction in or absence of dyspnea and movement toward a state of eupnea.

INTERVENTIONS	RATIONALES
Assess respiratory status q2-4h.	To be alert for indicators of respiratory distress, including restlessness, anxiety, mental status changes, shortness of breath, tachypnea, and use of accessory muscles of respiration.
Auscultate breath sounds.	To assess for and promptly report a decrease in breath sounds or an increase in adventitious breath sounds (crackles, wheezes, rhonchi), which may precede respiratory distress.
Teach pursed-lip breathing. Record patient's response to breathing technique.	Pursed-lip breathing increases intraluminal air pressure and thus internal stability to the airways and may prevent airway collapse during expiration. Steps are as follows: - Sit upright with hands on thighs or lean forward with elbows propped on over-the-bed table. - Inhale slowly through nose with mouth closed. - Form lips in an *O* shape as though whistling. - Exhale slowly through pursed lips. Exhalation should take twice as long as inhalation.
Administer bronchodilator therapy as prescribed.	To open airways by relaxing smooth muscles of the airways.
Monitor for tachycardia and dysrhythmias.	Common side effects of bronchodilator therapy.
Monitor patient's response to O_2 therapy.	High concentrations of O_2 can depress the respiratory drive in individuals with chronic CO_2 retention.
Monitor oximetry readings.	To be alert to and report O_2 saturation ≤90%.
Monitor serial ABG values.	Pao_2 likely will continue to decrease as patient's disease progresses. Patients with chronic CO_2 retention may have chronically compensated respiratory acidosis with a low-normal pH (7.35-7.38) and a $Paco_2$ >45 mm Hg.

●●● **Related NIC and NOC labels:** *NIC:* Respiratory Monitoring; Oxygen Therapy; Acid-Base Monitoring
NOC: Respiratory Status: Ventilation

Nursing Diagnosis:

Activity Intolerance

related to imbalance between oxygen supply and demand secondary to inefficient work of breathing

Desired Outcome: Patient reports decreasing dyspnea during activity or exercise and rates his or her perceived exertion (RPE) at ≤3 on a 0–10 scale.

INTERVENTIONS	RATIONALES
Maintain prescribed activity levels.	To increase patient's stamina while minimizing dyspnea. Emphysema is a progressive disease, and affected individuals can become totally disabled because they must use all available energy for breathing.
Monitor patient's respiratory response to activity. Ask patient to rate perceived exertion.	If activity intolerance is noted, patient should be instructed to stop the activity and rest. For more information, see **Activity Intolerance,** p. 67, in "Prolonged Bedrest."

Continued

INTERVENTIONS	RATIONALES
Facilitate coordination across health care providers to provide rest periods between care activities. Allow 90 min for undisturbed rest.	To decrease oxygen demand and enable adequate physiologic recovery.
Assist patient with active range-of-motion (ROM) exercises. For more information, see "Prolonged Bedrest" for **Risk for Activity Intolerance,** p. 67, and **Risk for Disuse Syndrome,** p. 69.	To help build stamina and prevent complications of decreased mobility.

●●● **Related NIC and NOC labels:** *NIC:* Activity Therapy; Energy Management; Exercise Therapy: Joint Mobility *NOC:* Endurance

Nursing Diagnosis:

Impaired Gas Exchange

related to altered oxygen supply secondary to decreased alveolar ventilation as a result of collapsed terminal airways and hyperinflated alveoli

Desired Outcomes: Optimally within 1-2 hr following treatment/intervention, patient has adequate gas exchange as evidenced by RR 12-20 breaths/min (or values consistent with patient's baseline). Before discharge from care facility, patient's ABG values are as follows: PaO_2 ≥80 mm Hg, $PaCO_2$ 35-45 mm Hg, and pH 7.35-7.45; or oximetry readings demonstrating O_2 saturation >92% or values consistent with patient's baseline.

INTERVENTIONS	RATIONALES
Observe for signs and symptoms of hypoxia.	Hypoxia (evidenced by agitation, anxiety, restlessness, changes in mental status or level of consciousness [LOC]) indicates oxygen deficiency and necessitates prompt treatment.
Recognize that cyanosis of the lips and nail beds is a late indicator of hypoxia.	Treatment is less complicated when symptoms are treated early.
Auscultate breath sounds q2-4h or more frequently as indicated by patient's condition.	To monitor for decreased or adventitious sounds (e.g., crackles, rhonchi, wheezes).
Monitor oximetry readings; report significant findings.	O_2 saturation <90% can indicate oxygenation problems and a possible need for O_2 therapy.
Monitor ABG results.	Decreasing PaO_2 and increasing $PaCO_2$ can signal respiratory compromise.
Position patient in high Fowler's position, with patient leaning forward and elbows propped on the over-the-bed table. Pad the over-the-bed table with pillows or blankets. Record patient's response to positioning.	For comfort and to promote optimal gas exchange by enabling maximal chest expansion. Leaning forward with diaphragm positioned against over-the-bed table may increase pressure of gastric contents and promote diaphragm contraction, thereby decreasing dyspnea.
Deliver and monitor O_2 and humidity as prescribed.	Patients with long-standing emphysema and CO_2 retention may not tolerate oxygen at a delivery >2 L/min, which can suppress their hypoxic respiratory drive.
	Delivering O_2 with humidity will help minimize convective losses of moisture.

●●● **Related NIC and NOC labels:** *NIC:* Acid-Base Monitoring; Laboratory Data Interpretation; Respiratory Monitoring; Positioning; Oxygen Therapy *NOC:* Respiratory Status: Gas Exchange

ADDITIONAL NURSING DIAGNOSES/ PROBLEMS:

PATIENT-FAMILY TEACHING AND DISCHARGE PLANNING

When providing patient-family teaching, focus on sensory information, avoid giving excessive information, and initiate a visiting nurse referral for necessary follow-up teaching. Include verbal and written information about the following:

✓ Use of home O_2, including instructions for when to use it, importance of not increasing prescribed flow rate, precautions, and community resources for O_2 replacement when necessary. Request respiratory therapy consultation to assist with teaching related to O_2 therapy, if indicated.

✓ Medications, including drug name, route, purpose, dosage, schedule, precautions, drug/drug and food/drug interactions, and potential side effects. If the patient will take corticosteroids while at home, provide instructions accordingly to ensure that the patient takes the correct amount, particularly during the period in which the medication will be tapered.

✓ Signs and symptoms of heart failure that necessitate medical attention: increased dyspnea; fatigue; increased coughing; changes in the amount, color, or consistency of sputum; swelling of the ankles and legs; and sudden weight gain. Patients with chronic obstructive pulmonary disease (COPD) often have right-sided heart failure secondary to cardiac effects of the disease. For more information, see "Heart Failure," p.195.

✓ Importance of avoiding contact with infectious individuals, especially those with respiratory infections.

✓ Recommendation that patient receive a pneumococcal vaccination and annual influenza vaccination.

✓ Review of Na^+-restricted diet and other dietary considerations as indicated. Sodium may be restricted to prevent fluid overload, which can occur if heart failure develops. See "Heart Failure," p. 195, for more information.

✓ Importance of pacing activity level to conserve energy.

✓ Follow-up appointment with health care provider; confirm date and time of next appointment.

✓ Introduction to local chapter of American Lung Association activities and pulmonary rehabilitation programs. Physical training programs may improve ventilation and cardiac muscle function, which may compensate for nonreversible lung disease.

✓ Phone numbers to call should questions or concerns arise about therapy or disease after discharge. Additional general information can be obtained by contacting the following organization:

American Lung Association
1740 Broadway
New York, NY 10019-4374
(212) 315-8700
www.lungusa.org

✓ For patients who smoke: elimination of smoking; refer patient to a "stop smoking" program as appropriate. The following free brochures outline ways to help patients stop smoking:

- *How to Help Your Patients Stop Using Tobacco: A National Cancer Institute Manual for the Oral Health Team,* from the Smoking and Tobacco Control Program of the National Cancer Institute; call 1-800-4-CANCER.
- *Clinical Practice Guideline: A Quick Reference Guide for Smoking Cessation Specialists,* from the Agency for Health Care Policy and Research (AHCPR); call 1-800-358-9295.

Pneumonia

Pneumonia is an acute bacterial or viral infection that causes inflammation of the lung parenchyma (alveolar spaces and interstitial tissue). As a result of the inflammation, the involved lung tissue becomes edematous and the air spaces fill with exudate (consolidation), gas exchange cannot occur, and nonoxygenated blood is shunted into the vascular system, causing hypoxemia. Bacterial pneumonias involve all or part of a lobe, whereas viral pneumonias appear diffusely throughout the lungs.

Pneumonias generally are classified into two groups: community acquired and hospital associated. A third type of pneumonia occurs in the immunocompromised individual.

- *Community acquired:* Individuals with community-acquired pneumonia generally do not require hospitalization unless an underlying medical condition, such as chronic obstructive pulmonary disease (COPD), cardiac disease, or diabetes mellitus or an immunocompromised state, complicates the illness.
- *Hospital associated (nosocomial):* This type usually occurs following aspiration of oropharyngeal flora in an individual whose resistance is altered or coughing mechanisms are impaired. Bacteria invade the lower respiratory tract via three routes: aspiration of oropharyngeal secretions (most common route), inhalation of aerosols that contain bacteria, or hematogenous spread to the lung from another site of infection (rare).
- *Pneumonia in the immunocompromised individual:* Severely immunocompromised patients are affected not only by bacteria but also by fungi *(Candida, Aspergillus),* viruses (cytomegalovirus), and protozoa *(Pneumocystis carinii).* Most commonly, *P. carinii* is seen in persons with human immunodeficiency virus (HIV) or in individuals who are immunosuppressed therapeutically following organ transplants.

HEALTH CARE SETTING

Primary care, with acute care hospitalization resulting from complications

ASSESSMENT

Findings are influenced by the patient's age, extent of disease process, underlying medical condition, and pathogen involved. Generally, any factor that alters integrity of the lower airways, thereby inhibiting ciliary activity, increases likelihood of developing pneumonia.

Signs and symptoms: Cough (productive and nonproductive), increased sputum production (rust colored, discolored, purulent, bloody, or mucoid), fever, pleuritic chest pain (more common in community-acquired bacterial pneumonias), dyspnea, chills, headache, and myalgia. Older adults may be confused or disoriented and run low-grade fevers but may present with few other signs and symptoms.

Physical assessment: Restlessness; anxiety; older adults may exhibit mental status changes, decreased skin turgor, and dry mucous membranes secondary to dehydration; presence of nasal flaring and expiratory grunt; use of accessory muscles of respiration (scalene, sternocleidomastoid, external intercostals); decreased chest expansion caused by pleuritic pain; dullness on percussion over affected (consolidated) areas; tachypnea (RR >20 breaths/min); tachycardia (HR >100 bpm); increased vocal fremitus; egophony ("e" to "a" change) over area of consolidation; decreased breath sounds; high-pitched and inspiratory crackles (rales) (increased by or heard only after coughing); low-pitched inspiratory crackles (rales) caused by airway secretions; and circumoral cyanosis (a late finding). **Note:** Findings may be normal, even with an abnormal chest x-ray.

DIAGNOSTIC TESTS

Chest x-ray examination: Confirms the presence of pneumonia (i.e., vague haziness to consolidation in the affected lung fields).

Sputum for Gram stain and culture and sensitivity tests: Sputum is obtained from the lower respiratory tract before initiation of antibiotic therapy to identify the causative organism. It can be obtained via expectoration, suctioning, transtracheal aspiration, bronchoscopy, or open-lung biopsy.

White blood cell (WBC) count: Will be increased (>11,000/mm^3) in the presence of bacterial pneumonias. Normal or low WBC count may be seen with viral or mycoplasma pneumonias.

Blood culture and sensitivity: To determine presence of bacteremia and aid in the identification of the causative organism.

Oximetry: May reveal decreased O_2 saturation.

Arterial blood gas (ABG) values: May vary, depending on the presence of underlying pulmonary or other debilitating disease, but the following is likely to occur: hypoxemia (PaO_2 <80 mm Hg) and hypocarbia ($PaCO_2$ <35 mm Hg), with a resultant respiratory alkalosis (pH >7.45), in the absence of an underlying pulmonary disease.

Serologic studies: Acute and convalescent antibody titers are drawn to diagnose viral pneumonia. A relative rise in antibody titers suggests a viral infection.

Acid-fast stains and cultures: To rule out tuberculosis.

Patients with Pneumonia

Nursing Diagnosis:

Impaired Gas Exchange

related to altered oxygen supply and alveolar-capillary membrane changes secondary to inflammatory process in the lungs

Desired Outcomes: Following intervention/treatment, patient has adequate gas exchange as evidenced by RR of 12-20 breaths/min with normal depth and pattern, absence of signs and symptoms of respiratory distress, and lung sounds clear to auscultation. At least 24 hr before hospital discharge, patient's O_2 saturation is >90% or ABGs reveal PaO_2 ≥80 mm Hg, $PaCO_2$ 35-45 mm Hg, and pH 7.35-7.45 (or values consistent with patient's baseline).

INTERVENTIONS	RATIONALES
Monitor for signs and symptoms of respiratory distress. Notify health care provider of significant findings.	Signs and symptoms of respiratory distress include restlessness, anxiety, mental status changes, shortness of breath, tachypnea, and use of accessory muscles of respiration. Cyanosis of the lips and nail beds may be a late indicator of hypoxia. Respiratory distress necessitates prompt medical intervention.
Monitor and document VS q2-4h.	A rising temperature and other changes in VS (e.g., increased HR and RR) may signal presence of infection.
Auscultate breath sounds at least q2-4h or as indicated by patient's condition.	To detect and promptly report decreased or adventitious sounds (e.g., crackles, wheezes), which can signal potential airway obstruction that would further aggravate hypoxia.
Monitor oximetry readings; report significant findings.	O_2 saturation ≤90% is a sign of a significant oxygenation problem and can indicate need for O_2 therapy.
Monitor ABG results.	Acute hypoxemia (PaO_2 <80 mm Hg) often indicates need for oxygen therapy. Hypocarbia ($PaCO_2$ <35 mm Hg), with a resultant respiratory alkalosis (pH >7.45), in the absence of an underlying pulmonary disease is consistent with pneumonia.
Position patient in semi-Fowler's position.	To provide comfort and promote diaphragmatic descent, maximize inhalation, and decrease work of breathing (WOB).
In patients with unilateral pneumonia, position on the unaffected side (i.e., "good side down") for 60-90 min at a time.	Gravity and hydrostatic pressure when patient is in this position promote perfusion and ventilation-perfusion matching.
Deliver oxygen with humidity as prescribed.	To provide oxygenation. Adding humidity decreases convective losses of moisture.

Continued

INTERVENTIONS	RATIONALES
Monitor oximetry or FIo$_2$.	To ensure that oxygen is delivered within prescribed concentrations.
Facilitate coordination across health care providers to provide rest periods between care activities. Allow 90 min for undisturbed rest.	To decrease oxygen demand in a patient whose reserves are likely limited.

●●● **Related NIC and NOC labels:** *NIC:* Oxygen Therapy; Acid-Base Monitoring; Positioning; Energy Management; Respiratory Monitoring; Vital Signs Monitoring *NOC:* Respiratory Status: Gas Exchange; Vital Signs Status

Nursing Diagnosis:

Ineffective Airway Clearance

related to presence of tracheobronchial secretions secondary to infection or related to pain and fatigue secondary to lung consolidation

Desired Outcome: Immediately following intervention, patient demonstrates effective cough as evidenced by airway free of adventitious breath sounds.

INTERVENTIONS	RATIONALES
Auscultate breath sounds q2-4h (or as indicated by patient's condition).	To determine presence of adventitious breath sounds (e.g., crackles, wheezes). If coarse crackles are present, this is a sign that patient needs to cough. Fine crackles at lung bases likely will clear with deep breathing. Wheezing is a sign of airway obstruction, which necessities prompt intervention to ensure effective gas exchange.
Inspect sputum for quantity, odor, color, and consistency; document findings.	As patient's condition worsens, sputum can become more copious and change in color from clear→white→yellow→ green, or it may show other discoloration characteristic of underlying bacterial infection (e.g., rust colored; "currant jelly").
Ensure that patient performs deep breathing with controlled coughing exercises at least q2h.	These exercises help clear airways of secretions. Controlled coughing (tightening upper abdominal muscles while coughing 2-3 times) ensures a more effective cough because it uses the diaphragmatic muscles, which increases forcefulness of the effort.
Assist patient into semi-Fowler's position.	To provide comfort and facilitate ease and effectiveness of these exercises by promoting better lung expansion (there is less lung compression by abdominal organs) and gas exchange.
Ensure that patient gets prescribed chest physiotherapy.	To promote mobilization of secretions.
Assist patient with position changes q2h. If patient is ambulatory, encourage ambulation and activity to patient's tolerance.	Movement and activity help mobilize secretions to facilitate airway clearance.
Suction as prescribed and indicated.	To clear airways.
When not contraindicated, encourage fluid intake (≥2.5 L/day).	To decrease viscosity of the sputum, which will make it easier to raise and expectorate.

Continued

INTERVENTIONS	RATIONALES
Instruct patient in use of hyperinflation device (e.g., incentive spirometer). Monitor patient's progress and document in nurse's notes.	Deep inhalation with this device expands alveoli and aids in mobilizing secretions to the airways, and coughing further mobilizes and clears the secretions. Emphasis of this therapy is on inhalation to expand the lungs maximally. Patient inhales slowly and deeply 2 × normal tidal volume and holds the breath at least 5 sec at the end of inspiration. To maintain adequate alveolar inflation, 10 such breaths/hr is recommended.
Monitor for gastric distention, headache, hypotension, and signs and symptoms of pneumothorax (shortness of breath, sharp chest pain, unilateral diminished breath sounds, dyspnea, cough).	Potential complications of hyperventilation therapy.
When appropriate, teach methods of splinting wounds or painful areas to enable cough. Administer analgesics as prescribed.	To reduce pain when coughing, which should facilitate ease with deep-breathing and coughing exercises.
Instruct patients who are unable to cough effectively in cascade cough.	A cascade cough removes secretions and improves ventilation via a succession of shorter and more forceful exhalations than are done with usual coughing exercise.
When appropriate, coordinate deep-breathing and coughing exercises with peak effectiveness of bronchodilator therapy.	To maximize potential for mobilization of secretions.

●●● **Related NIC and NOC labels:** *NIC:* Respiratory Monitoring; Chest Physiotherapy; Positioning; Airway Suctioning; Cough Enhancement; Medication Administration: Inhalation *NOC:* Respiratory Status: Gas Exchange; Respiratory Status: Ventilation

Nursing Diagnosis:

Deficient Fluid Volume

related to increased insensible loss secondary to tachypnea, fever, or diaphoresis

Desired Outcome: Before hospital discharge (or within 24 hr following intervention), patient is normovolemic as evidenced by urine output ≥30 ml/hr with specific gravity 1.010–1.030, stable weight, HR and BP within patient's normal limits, fluid intake approximating fluid output, moist mucous membranes, and normal skin turgor.

INTERVENTIONS	RATIONALES
Monitor I&O. Consider insensible losses if patient is diaphoretic and tachypneic.	To monitor trend of fluid volume.
Be alert to and report indicators of deficient fluid volume.	Indicators of deficient fluid volume include urinary output <30 ml/hr for 2 consecutive hr and urinary specific gravity >1.030.
Weigh patient daily at the same time of day, with the same clothing, and on the same scale; record weight.	Ensures consistency and accuracy of weight measurements. Weight changes of 1-1.5 kg/day can occur with fluid volume excess or deficit.
Encourage fluid intake (at least 2.5 L/day in unrestricted patient).	To ensure adequate hydration.
Maintain IV fluid therapy as prescribed.	To maintain fluid balance.

Continued

INTERVENTIONS	RATIONALES
Promote oral hygiene, including lip and tongue care.	To moisten dried tissues and mucous membranes in patients with fluid volume deficit.
Provide humidity for oxygen therapy.	To decrease convective losses of moisture.

●●● **Related NIC and NOC labels:** *NIC:* Fluid Management; Fluid Monitoring; Intravenous Therapy
NOC: Fluid Balance; Hydration

Patients at Risk for Developing Pneumonia (nosocomial pneumonia)

Nursing Diagnosis:

Risk for Infection

related to inadequate primary defenses (e.g., decreased ciliary action), invasive procedures (e.g., intubation), and/or chronic disease

Desired Outcome: Patient is free of infection as evidenced by normothermia, WBC count ≤11,000/mm^3, and sputum clear to whitish in color.

INTERVENTIONS	RATIONALES
Perform good handwashing technique before and after contact with patient (even if gloves were worn).	To prevent spread of infection by removing pathogens from hands. Hand hygiene involves using alcohol-based waterless antiseptic agent if hands are not visibly soiled or using soap and water if hands are dirty or contaminated with proteinaceous material.
Identify presurgical candidate who is at increased risk for nosocomial pneumonia.	To help ensure that at risk surgical patients remain free of infection because nosocomial pneumonia has a high morbidity and mortality rate. Factors that increase risk for nosocomial pneumonia in surgical patients include the following: older adult (>70 yr), obesity, COPD, other chronic pulmonary conditions (e.g., asthma), history of smoking, abnormal pulmonary function tests (especially decreased forced expiratory flow rate), intubation, and upper abdominal/thoracic surgery.
Provide preoperative teaching, explaining and demonstrating activities and exercises that help prevent infection/pneumonia.	Pulmonary activities that help to prevent infection/pneumonia include deep breathing, coughing, turning in bed, splinting wounds before breathing exercises, ambulation, maintaining adequate oral fluid intake, and use of hyperinflation device.
Make sure that patient verbalizes knowledge of the exercises and their rationale and returns the demonstrations appropriately.	Learning how to apply information via a return demonstration is more helpful than receiving verbal instruction alone. A knowledgeable patient is more likely to comply with therapy.
Encourage individuals who smoke to discontinue smoking.	Inhalation of toxic fumes/chemical irritants can damage cilia and lung tissue and is a factor that increases likelihood of developing pneumonia.
Refer to a community-based smoking cessation program as needed. When appropriate, discuss possibility of health care provider's prescription of transdermal nicotine patches.	To promote smoking cessation.

Continued

INTERVENTIONS	RATIONALES
Administer analgesics ½ hr before deep-breathing exercises. Support (splint) surgical wound with hands, pillows, or folded blanket placed firmly across site of incision.	To control pain, which will promote compliance with breathing exercises.
Identify patients who are at increased risk for aspiration.	Individuals with depressed level of consciousness (LOC), dysphagia, or a nasogastric (NG) or enteral tube in place are at risk for aspiration, which predisposes them to pneumonia.
Establish aspiration precautions in high-risk individuals.	Aspiration is one of the two leading causes of nosocomial pneumonia. Aspiration precautions include maintaining head of bed (HOB) at 30-degree elevation, turning patient onto side rather than back, and using continuous rather than bolus feedings when patient receives enteral alimentation.
Recognize risk factors for contamination in a patient with tracheostomy.	To minimize risk of contamination, which predisposes patient with tracheostomy to pneumonia. Risk factors include presence of underlying lung disease or other serious illness, increased colonization of oropharynx or trachea by aerobic gram-negative bacteria, greater access of bacteria to lower respiratory tract, and cross-contamination caused by manipulation of tracheostomy tube.
Use "no-touch" technique or wear sterile gloves on both hands when performing tracheostomy care until tracheostomy wound has healed or formed granulation tissue around the tube.	Loss of skin integrity or space around the tube would enable ingress of pathogens via the wound or tube.
Use sterile catheter for each suctioning procedure and sterile solutions if secretions are tenacious and catheter flushing is necessary.	This intervention and those that follow are established strategies for preventing nosocomial pneumonia.
Replace closed suction system if soiled, for mechanical failure, or per agency policy. Always replace suction system between patients.	
Always wear gloves on both hands to suction.	
Recognize the following ways in which nebulizer reservoirs can contaminate patient: introduction of nonsterile fluids or air, manipulation of nebulizer cup, or back flow of condensate from delivery tubing into reservoir or into patient when tubing is manipulated.	
Use only sterile fluids and dispense them using sterile technique.	
Replace (rather than replenish) solutions and equipment at frequent intervals.	
Change breathing circuits every week or sooner if soiled, if there is mechanical failure, or according to agency policy.	
Fill fluid reservoirs immediately before use (not far in advance).	
Discard any fluid that has condensed in tubing; do not allow it to drain back into reservoir or into patient.	
Suction prn rather than on a routine basis.	(Frequent suctioning increases risk of trauma and cross-contamination.)

●●● **Related NIC and NOC labels:** *NIC:* Infection Control; Infection Prevention; Incision Site Care; Aspiration Precautions; Environmental Management; Infection Control: Intraoperative; Artificial Airway Management; Cough Enhancement; Tube Care *NOC:* Infection Status

PATIENT-FAMILY TEACHING AND DISCHARGE PLANNING

When providing patient-family teaching, focus on sensory information, avoid giving excessive information, and initiate a visiting nurse referral for necessary follow-up teaching. Include verbal and written information about the following:

✓ Techniques that promote gas exchange and minimize stasis of secretions (e.g., deep breathing, coughing, use of hyperinflation device, increasing activity level as appropriate for patient's medical condition, percussion and postural drainage as necessary).

✓ Medications, including drug name, purpose, dosage, frequency or schedule, precautions, drug/drug and food/drug interactions, and potential side effects, particularly of antibiotics.

✓ Signs and symptoms of pneumonia and the importance of reporting them promptly to health professional should they recur. Teach patient's significant others that fatigue and changes in mental status may be the only indicator of pneumonia if patient is elderly.

✓ Importance of preventing fatigue by pacing activities and allowing frequent rest periods.

✓ Importance of avoiding exposure to individuals known to have flu and colds. Recommend that patient receive a pneumococcal vaccination and annual influenza vaccination.

✓ Minimizing factors that can cause reinfection, including overcrowded living conditions, poor nutrition, and poorly ventilated living quarters or work environment.

✓ Phone numbers to call should questions or concerns arise about therapy or disease after discharge. Additional general information can be obtained by contacting:

American Lung Association
1740 Broadway
New York, NY 10019-4374
(212) 315-8700
www.lungusa.org

✓ Information about the following free brochures that outline ways to help patients stop smoking:

- *How to Help Your Patients Stop Using Tobacco: A National Cancer Institute Manual for the Oral Health Team,* from the Smoking and Tobacco Control Program of the National Cancer Institute; call 1-800-4-CANCER.
- *Clinical Practice Guideline: A Quick Reference Guide for Smoking Cessation Specialists,* from the Agency for Health Care Policy and Research (AHCPR); call 1-800-358-9295.

Pneumothorax/ Hemothorax

Pneumothorax is an accumulation of air in the pleural space, which leads to increased intrapleural pressure. Risk factors include blunt or penetrating chest injury, chronic obstructive pulmonary disease (COPD), previous pneumothorax, and positive pressure ventilation. There are three types:

- *Spontaneous:* Also referred to as *closed pneumothorax* because the chest wall remains intact with no leak to the atmosphere. It results from the rupture of a bleb or bulla on the visceral pleural surface, usually near the apex. Generally, the cause of the rupture is unknown, although it may result from a weakness related to a respiratory infection or from an underlying pulmonary disease (e.g., COPD, tuberculosis, malignant neoplasm).
- *Traumatic:* Can be open or closed. An open pneumothorax occurs when air enters the pleural space from the atmosphere through an opening in the chest wall, such as with a gunshot wound, stab wound, or invasive medical procedure. A sucking sound may be heard over the area of penetration during inspiration, accounting for the classic wound description as a "sucking chest wound." A closed pneumothorax occurs when the visceral pleura is penetrated but the chest wall remains intact with no atmospheric leak. This usually occurs following blunt trauma that results in a fracture and dislocation of the ribs. It also may occur from the use of positive end-expiratory pressure (PEEP) or after cardiopulmonary resuscitation (CPR).
- *Tension:* Generally occurs with closed pneumothorax; also can occur with open pneumothorax when a flap of tissue acts as a one-way valve. Air enters the pleural space through the pleural tear when the individual inhales, and it continues to accumulate but cannot escape during expiration because the tissue flap closes. Tension pneumothorax is a life-threatening medical emergency.

Hemothorax is an accumulation of blood in the pleural space. Hemothorax generally results from blunt trauma to the chest wall, but it can also occur following thoracic surgery, after penetrating gunshot or stab wounds, as a result of anticoagulant therapy, after insertion of a central venous catheter, or following various thoracoabdominal organ biopsies.

HEALTH CARE SETTING

Acute care, primary care

ASSESSMENT

Clinical presentation will vary, depending on type and size of the pneumothorax or hemothorax.

Signs and symptoms:
- **Closed pneumothorax:** Shortness of breath, cough, chest tightness, chest pain
- **Open pneumothorax:** Shortness of breath, sharp chest pain
- **Tension pneumothorax:** Dyspnea, chest pain
- **Hemothorax:** Dyspnea, chest pain

Physical assessment:
- **Closed pneumothorax:** Tachypnea, decreased thoracic movement, cyanosis, subcutaneous emphysema, hyperresonance over affected area, diminished breath sounds, paradoxical movement of chest wall (may signal flail chest), change in mental status
- **Open pneumothorax:** Agitation, restlessness, tachypnea, cyanosis, presence of chest wound, hyperresonance over affected area, sucking sound on inspiration, diminished breath sounds, change in mental status
- **Tension pneumothorax:** Anxiety, tachycardia, cyanosis, jugular vein distention, tracheal deviation toward unaffected side, absent breath sounds on affected side, distant heart sounds, hypotension, change in mental status

- **Hemothorax:** Tachypnea, pallor, cyanosis, dullness over affected side, tachycardia, hypotension, diminished or absent breath sounds, change in mental status

DIAGNOSTIC TESTS

Chest x-ray examination: Will reveal the presence of air or blood in the pleural space on the affected side, size of the pneumothorax/hemothorax, and any shift in the mediastinum.

Arterial blood gas (ABG) values: Hypoxemia (PaO_2 <80 mm Hg) may be accompanied by hypercarbia ($PaCO_2$ >45 mm Hg) with resultant respiratory acidosis (pH <7.35). Arterial oxygen saturation may be decreased initially but usually returns to normal within 24 hr.

Oximetry: Will reveal decreased O_2 saturation (≤92%).

Complete blood count (CBC): May reveal decreased Hgb proportionate to the amount of blood lost in a hemothorax.

Nursing Diagnosis:

Impaired Gas Exchange

related to altered oxygen supply secondary to ventilation–perfusion mismatch

Desired Outcomes: Optimally, within 2 hr following treatment/intervention, patient exhibits adequate gas exchange and ventilatory function as evidenced by RR ≤20 breaths/min with normal depth and pattern (eupnea), no significant mental status changes, and orientation to person, place, and time. At a minimum of 24 hr before hospital discharge (or within 24 hr after intervention), patient's ABG values are as follows: PaO_2 ≥80 mm Hg and $PaCO_2$ 35-45 mm Hg (or values within patient's acceptable baseline parameters), or oximetry readings demonstrate O_2 saturation >92%.

INTERVENTIONS	RATIONALES
Monitor serial ABG results or oximetry readings for O_2 saturation. Report significant findings to health care provider.	To detect decreasing PaO_2 or O_2 saturation and increasing $PaCO_2$, which can signal impending respiratory compromise and necessitate prompt intervention.
Assess for signs of hypoxia.	Increased restlessness, anxiety, tachycardia, and changes in mental status are early indicators of hypoxia. Cyanosis may be a late sign.
Assess VS and breath sounds q2h or as indicated by patient's condition. Report significant findings.	To monitor patient's trend. Significant changes such as increased HR, increased RR, and unilateral decreased breath sounds signal a worsening or unresolved condition.
If patient has had chest tube placement or exploratory thoracotomy, assess respiratory status q15min until patient is stable. Report significant findings.	Enables prompt detection of respiratory distress for timely intervention: increased RR, diminished or absent movement of chest wall on affected side, paradoxical movement of the chest wall, increased work of breathing (WOB), use of accessory muscles of respiration, complaints of increased dyspnea, unilateral diminished breath sounds, and cyanosis.
	Chest tubes may be placed in any patients who are symptomatic to remove air or fluid from the pleural space and enable reexpansion of the lung. A thoracotomy may be indicated if patient has had ≥2 spontaneous pneumothoraces or if the current pneumothorax does not resolve within 7 days. In the presence of a hemothorax, a thoracotomy may be indicated to locate the source and control the bleeding if loss exceeds 200 ml/hr for 2 hr.
Position patient in semi-Fowler's position.	To provide comfort and enable full expansion of unaffected lung, adequate expansion of chest wall, and descent of diaphragm.

Continued

INTERVENTIONS	RATIONALES
Change patient's position q2h.	To promote drainage and lung reexpansion and facilitate alveolar perfusion.
Encourage patient to take deep breaths, providing necessary analgesia ½ hr before breathing is to take place. Teach patient how to splint thoracotomy site with arms, pillow, or folded blanket to enable adequate coughing.	Deep breathing promotes full lung expansion and decreases risk of atelectasis. Analgesia and splinting decrease discomfort during deep-breathing exercises. Coughing facilitates mobilization of tracheobronchial secretions, if present.
Deliver and monitor oxygen and humidity as indicated.	To ensure adequate oxygen levels if patient has hypoxemia, which is likely to be present if the pneumothorax/hemothorax is large. Humidity prevents convective losses of moisture.

●●● **Related NIC and NOC labels:** *NIC:* Acid-Base Management; Oxygen Therapy; Ventilation Assistance; Positioning; Respiratory Monitoring; Cough Enhancement; Vital Signs Monitoring *NOC:* Respiratory Status: Gas Exchange; Respiratory Status: Ventilation; Vital Signs Status

Nursing Diagnosis:

Ineffective Breathing Pattern

(or risk for same) *related to* decreased lung expansion secondary to malfunction of chest drainage system

Desired Outcome: Patient remains eupneic, or, immediately following intervention, patient becomes eupneic.

INTERVENTIONS	RATIONALES
Assess mental status, respiratory status, and VS at frequent intervals (q2-4h, as appropriate).	To monitor patient's status while chest drainage system is in place. The purpose of a chest drainage system is to drain air or fluid and reexpand the lung. Diminished breath sounds, along with tachycardia, restlessness, anxiety, and changes in mental status, are signs of respiratory distress that may occur as a result of chest drainage system malfunction. If these signs are present, prompt intervention is necessary to prevent further hypoxia and distress.
Tape all connections and secure chest tube to thorax with tape.	Helps ensure maintenance of closed chest drainage system.
Avoid the following: kinks in the tubing, bed and equipment compressing any component of the system, and dependent loops in the tubing.	These factors may impede removal of air and fluid from the pleural space.
Maintain fluid in underwater-seal chamber and suction chamber at appropriate levels.	The suction apparatus does not regulate the amount of suction applied to closed chest drainage system. The amount of suction is determined by the water level in the suction control chamber. Minimal bubbling in this chamber is acceptable and desirable.
Monitor bubbling in the underwater-seal chamber.	Bubbling in the underwater-seal chamber occurs on expiration and is a sign that air is leaving the pleural space.
Locate and seal any leak in the system, if possible.	Continuous bubbling in the underwater-seal chamber may be a signal that air is leaking into the drainage system.

Continued

INTERVENTIONS	RATIONALES
Monitor fluctuations in the underwater-seal chamber.	Fluctuations are characteristic of a patent chest tube. Fluctuations stop when the lung has reexpanded or there is a kink or obstruction in the chest tube.
Keep necessary emergency supplies at the bedside.	- *Petrolatum gauze pad:* to apply over insertion site if chest tube becomes dislodged. Use of this dressing provides an airtight seal to prevent recurrent pneumothorax. - *Bottle of sterile water:* submerging chest tube in a bottle of sterile water if it becomes disconnected from the underwater-seal system provides for a temporary closed chest drainage system.
Follow institution's policy about chest tube stripping. Avoid use of mechanical or handheld tube-stripping devices.	This mechanism for maintaining chest tube patency is controversial and has been associated with creating high negative pressures in the pleural space, which can damage fragile lung tissue.
Squeeze alternately hand-over-hand along the drainage tube.	This gentler method of chest tube stripping may generate sufficient pressure to move fluid along the tube and may be indicated when bloody drainage or clots are visible in the tubing.
Never clamp a chest tube without a specific directive from health care provider.	Clamping may lead to tension pneumothorax because air in the pleural space no longer can escape.

●●● **Related NIC and NOC labels:** *NIC:* Airway Management; Respiratory Monitoring; Ventilation Assistance *NOC:* Respiratory Status: Airway Patency; Respiratory Status: Ventilation

Nursing Diagnosis:

Acute Pain

related to impaired pleural integrity, inflammation, or presence of a chest tube

Desired Outcomes: Within 1 hr of intervention, patient's subjective perception of pain decreases, as documented by a pain scale. Objective indicators, such as grimacing, are absent or diminished.

INTERVENTIONS	RATIONALES
At frequent intervals, assess patient's degree of discomfort, using patient's verbal and nonverbal cues. Devise a pain scale with patient, rating pain from 0 (no pain) to 10 (worst pain).	To monitor trend of pain and determine success of subsequent pain interventions. Because of rich innervation of the pleura, chest tube placement is painful; significant analgesia is usually required.
Medicate with analgesics as prescribed, using pain scale to evaluate and document effectiveness of the medication.	To provide pain relief and determine effectiveness of the analgesia.
Encourage patient to request analgesic before pain becomes severe.	Prolonged stimulation of pain receptors results in increased sensitivity to painful stimuli and increases amount of drug required to relieve pain.
Premedicate 30 min before initiating coughing, exercising, or repositioning. Teach patient to splint affected side when coughing, moving, or repositioning.	Provides comfort during painful exercises and repositioning and facilitates compliance.

Continued

INTERVENTIONS	RATIONALES
Facilitate coordination across health care providers to provide rest periods between care activities. Allow 90 min for undisturbed rest.	Relaxation decreases oxygen demand and may decrease level of pain.
Stabilize chest tube. Tape chest tube securely to thorax.	To reduce pull or drag on latex connector tubing and prevent discomfort.
See "Pain," p. 41, for more information.	

●●● **Related NIC and NOC labels:** *NIC:* Analgesic Administration; Pain Management; Environmental Management: Comfort; Splinting *NOC:* Pain Level; Pain Control

ADDITIONAL NURSING DIAGNOSES/ PROBLEMS:

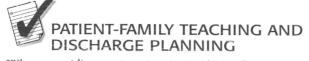

"Pain"	p. 41
"Psychosocial Support"	p. 81
"Pneumonia" for **Deficient Fluid Volume**	p. 142

PATIENT-FAMILY TEACHING AND DISCHARGE PLANNING

When providing patient-family teaching, focus on sensory information, avoid giving excessive information, and initiate a visiting nurse referral for necessary follow-up teaching. Include verbal and written information about the following:

✓ Purpose for chest tube placement and maintenance.

✓ Potential for recurrence of spontaneous pneumothorax. Average time between occurrences is 2-3 yr. Explain the importance of seeking medical care immediately if symptoms recur.

✓ Medications, including drug name, purpose, dosage, schedule, precautions, drug/drug and food/drug interactions, and potential side effects.

Pulmonary Embolus

The most common pulmonary perfusion abnormality is a pulmonary embolus (PE). It is caused by the passage of a foreign substance (blood clot, fat, air, or amniotic fluid) into the pulmonary artery or its branches, with resulting obstruction of the blood supply to lung tissue and subsequent collapse. The most common source is a dislodged blood clot from the systemic circulation, typically the deep veins of the legs or pelvis. Thrombus formation is the result of the following factors: blood stasis, alterations in clotting factors, and injury to vessel walls.

HEALTH CARE SETTING

Acute care

ASSESSMENT

Signs and symptoms often are nonspecific and variable, depending on the extent of the obstruction and whether the patient has infarction as a result of the obstruction.

Pulmonary embolus: Sudden onset of dyspnea and sharp chest pain, restlessness, anxiety, nonproductive cough or hemoptysis, palpitations, nausea, and syncope. With a large embolism, oppressive substernal chest discomfort will be present.

Pulmonary infarction: Fever, pleuritic chest pain, and hemoptysis.

Physical assessment: Tachypnea, tachycardia, hypotension, crackles (rales), decreased chest wall excursion secondary to splinting, S_3 and S_4 gallop rhythms, transient pleural friction rub, jugular venous distention, diaphoresis, edema, and cyanosis. Temperature may be elevated if infarction has occurred.

History and risk factors:
- *Prolonged immobility:* Especially significant when it coexists with surgical or nonsurgical trauma, carcinoma, or cardiopulmonary disease. Risk increases as duration of immobility increases.

- *Cardiac disorders:* Atrial fibrillation, heart failure, myocardial infarction, rheumatic heart disease.
- *Surgical intervention:* Risk increases in postoperative period, especially for patients with pelvic, thoracic, and abdominal surgery and for those with exten-sive burns or musculoskeletal injuries of the hip or knee.
- *Pregnancy:* Especially during the postpartum period.
- *Chronic pulmonary disease*
- *Trauma:* Especially fractures of the lower extremities and burns. The degree of risk is related to the severity, site, and extent of trauma.
- *Carcinoma:* Particularly neoplasms involving the breast, lung, pancreas, and genitourinary and alimentary tracts.
- *Obesity:* A 20% increase in ideal body weight is associated with an increased incidence of PE.
- *Varicose veins or prior thromboembolic disease*
- *Age:* Risk of thromboembolism is greatest for patients between 55 and 65 years of age.

Specific findings for fat embolus: Typically, patient is asymptomatic for 12-24 hr following embolization; this period ends with sudden cardiopulmonary and neurologic deterioration: apprehension, restlessness, mental status changes, confusion, delirium, coma, and dyspnea.

Physical assessment for fat embolus: Tachypnea, tachycardia, and hypertension; fever; petechiae, especially of the conjunctivae, neck, upper torso, axillae, and proximal arms; inspiratory crowing; pulmonary edema; profuse tracheobronchial secretions; fat globules in the sputum; and expiratory wheezes.

History and risk factors for fat embolus:
- Multiple long bone fractures: especially fractures of the femur and pelvis
- Trauma to adipose tissue or liver
- Burns
- Osteomyelitis
- Sickle cell crisis

DIAGNOSTIC TESTS

General findings for pulmonary emboli

Arterial blood gas (ABG) values: Hypoxemia (PaO_2 <80 mm Hg), hypocarbia ($PaCO_2$ <35 mm Hg), and respiratory alkalosis (pH >7.45) usually are present. A normal PaO_2 does not rule out the presence of pulmonary emboli.

Chest x-ray examination: Initially, the chest x-ray is normal or an elevated hemidiaphragm may be present. After 24 hr, x-ray examination may reveal small infiltrates secondary to atelectasis that result from the decrease in surfactant. If pulmonary infarction is present, infiltrates and pleural effusions may be seen within 12-36 hr.

Electrocardiogram (ECG): If PEs are extensive, signs of acute pulmonary hypertension may be present: right-shift QRS axes, tall and peaked P waves, ST-segment changes, and T-wave inversion in leads V1-V4.

Pulmonary ventilation-perfusion scan: Used to detect abnormalities of ventilation or perfusion in the pulmonary system. Radiopaque agents are inhaled and injected peripherally. Images of both agents' distribution throughout the lung are scanned. If the scan shows a mismatch of ventilation and perfusion (i.e., a pattern of normal ventilation with decreased perfusion), vascular obstruction is suggested.

Pulmonary angiography: The definitive study for PE. It is an invasive procedure that involves right-sided heart catheterization and injection of dye into the pulmonary artery (PA) to visualize pulmonary vessels. An abrupt vessel "cutoff" may be seen at the site of embolization. Usually, filling defects are seen. More specific findings are abnormal blood vessel diameters (i.e., obstruction of right PA would cause dilation of left PA) and shapes (i.e., the affected blood vessel may taper to a sharp point and disappear).

Findings specific for fat emboli

ABG values: Should be drawn on patients at risk for fat embolus for the first 48 hr following injury because early hypoxemia indicative of fat embolus is apparent only with laboratory assessment. Hypoxemia (PaO_2 <80 mm Hg) and hypercarbia ($PaCO_2$ >45 mm Hg) will be present with respiratory acidosis (pH <7.35).

Chest x-ray examination: A pattern similar to adult respiratory distress syndrome (ARDS) is seen: diffuse, extensive bilateral interstitial and alveolar infiltrates.

Complete blood count (CBC): May reveal decreased Hgb and Hct secondary to hemorrhage into the lung. In addition, thrombocytopenia ($\leq150,000/mm^3$) is indicative of fat embolism.

Serum lipase: Will rise with fat embolism.

Urinalysis: May reveal fat globules following fat embolus.

Nursing Diagnosis:

Impaired Gas Exchange

related to altered oxygen supply secondary to ventilation-perfusion mismatch

Desired Outcomes: Within 2-4 hr following intervention/treatment, patient exhibits adequate gas exchange and ventilatory function as evidenced by RR 12-20 breaths/min with normal pattern and depth (eupnea), no significant changes in mental status, and orientation to person, place, and time. At a minimum of 24 hr before hospital discharge, patient has O_2 saturation >92% or PaO_2 $\geq$80 mm Hg, $PaCO_2$ 35-45 mm Hg, and pH 7.35-7.45 (or values consistent with patient's acceptable baseline parameters).

INTERVENTIONS	RATIONALES
Monitor patient for RR increased from baseline, increasing dyspnea, anxiety, sharp chest pain, restlessness, confusion, and cyanosis.	Signs and symptoms of increasing respiratory distress and indicators of PE.
As indicated, monitor oximetry readings; report O_2 saturation $\leq$92%.	May indicate need for O_2 therapy. Hypoxia is common with PE, although its absence does not mean that patient does not have a PE.
Elevate HOB 30 degrees.	For comfort and optimal gas exchange by preventing abdominal contents from inhibiting lung expansion.
When positioning patient in lateral position, ensure that area of the lung affected by the embolus is not dependent.	Turning patient so that affected area of the lung is dependent may cause oxygen desaturation, especially in the presence of low cardiac output or decreased Hgb levels.

Continued

INTERVENTIONS	RATIONALES
Avoid positioning patient with knees bent. Instruct patient not to cross legs when lying in bed or sitting in a chair.	These positions impede venous return from the legs and can increase risk of PE.
Limit or pace patient's activities and procedures.	Decreases metabolic demands for oxygen.
Ensure that patient performs deep-breathing and coughing exercises 3-5 times q2h.	To mobilize secretions and improve ventilation.
Ensure delivery of prescribed concentrations and humidity of oxygen.	To maintain a PaO_2 >60 mm Hg and optimally ≥80 mm Hg. Humidifying the oxygen minimizes convective losses.
Monitor serial ABG values. Report significant findings.	To assess response to treatment. A poor response to treatment or worsening ABG values necessitates prompt reporting for timely evaluation and further treatment.

●●● **Related NIC and NOC labels:** *NIC:* Oxygen Therapy; Respiratory Monitoring; Acid-Base Monitoring; Positioning; Cough Enhancement; Embolus Care: Pulmonary; Energy Management *NOC:* Tissue Perfusion: Pulmonary; Respiratory Status: Ventilation; Respiratory Status: Gas Exchange

Nursing Diagnosis:

Ineffective Protection

related to risk of prolonged bleeding or hemorrhage secondary to anticoagulation therapy

Desired Outcome: Patient is free of frank or occult bleeding; body secretions/excretions test negative for blood.

INTERVENTIONS	RATIONALES
Monitor VS q2-4h, depending on patient's status.	Hypotension, tachycardia, and tachypnea are signs of bleeding/hemorrhage, which can occur with anticoagulant therapy
At least once each shift check stool, urine, emesis, and nasogastric (NG) drainage for blood via agency-approved protocols.	To determine if blood is present in these body fluids.
At least once each shift inspect wounds, oral mucous membranes, any entry site of an invasive procedure, and nares.	To assess for evidence of bleeding.
At least once each shift inspect torso and extremities for petechiae or ecchymoses.	Petechiae and ecchymoses are signs of bleeding within the tissues.
Do not give an IM injection unless it is unavoidable. If parenteral medications are mandatory, attempt to administer using a smaller-gauge needle.	To prevent bleeding and hematoma formation caused by larger puncture wounds.
Apply pressure to all venipuncture or arterial puncture sites until bleeding stops.	To ensure that all bleeding stops completely, it is necessary to apply pressure for a longer than usual amount of time.
Ensure easy access to antidotes for prescribed treatment.	*Protamine sulfate:* 1 mg counteracts 100 U heparin. Usual initial dose is 50 mg. Fatal hemorrhage occurs in 1%-2% of patients undergoing heparin therapy. *Vitamin K* (*vitamin K$_1$* [Mephyton or phytonadione] or K$_3$ [menadione]): 20 mg given SC counteracts effects of oral anticoagulants.

Continued

INTERVENTIONS	RATIONALES
	Aminocaproic acid (e.g., Amicar): administered via slow IV infusion of 5 g. Reverses fibrinolytic condition related to thrombolytic therapy.
If patient is receiving heparin therapy, monitor serial partial thromboplastin time (PTT) or International Normalized Ratio (INR).	To ensure that it is within desired range: 1.5-2.5 × control for PTT or 2.0-3.0 for INR. Values outside these ranges should be reported for timely intervention.
If patient is receiving warfarin (Coumadin) therapy, monitor serial prothrombin time (PT).	To ensure that it is within desired range: 1.25-1.5 × control or an INR value of 2.0-3.0. Values outside these ranges should be reported for timely intervention.
Establish compatibility of all drugs before administering them.	To prevent negative interactions with anticoagulants or thrombolytic therapy.
	The following agents decrease the effect of heparin therapy: digitalis, tetracycline, nicotine, and antihistamines. Consult pharmacist about compatibility before infusing other IV drugs through heparin IV line.
	Numerous drugs result in a decrease or increase in response to treatment with warfarin. Consult pharmacist to obtain specific information about patient's medication profile.
	Although no specific drug interactions are currently known for thrombolytic therapy (e.g., streptokinase, urokinase), new drugs are always coming on the market, and therefore it is good practice to consult a pharmacist before infusing any medication through the same IV line.
Avoid use of *any* drug that contains aspirin and nonsteroidal antiinflammatory drugs (NSAIDs), such as ibuprofen.	Aspirin and NSAIDs are platelet aggregation inhibitors and can prolong episodes of bleeding.
Discuss with patient and significant others the effects of anticoagulant therapy and importance of reporting signs of bleeding promptly.	Hematuria, melena, frank bleeding from the mouth, epistaxis, hemoptysis, and excessive vaginal bleeding (menometrorrhagia) are potential effects of anticoagulant therapy and necessitate timely intervention to prevent further blood loss.
Teach necessity of using sponge-tipped applicators and mouthwash for oral care.	To minimize risk of gum bleeding.
Instruct patient to shave with an electric rather than a straight or safety razor.	To avoid cuts, which could result in severe bleeding.
If patient is restless and combative, pad the side rails, restrain as necessary, and use extreme care when moving patient.	To prevent falls and avoid bumping extremities into side rails, which could result in severe bleeding.

●●● **Related NIC and NOC labels:** *NIC:* Bleeding Precautions; Hemorrhage Control *NOC:* Coagulation Status

Nursing Diagnosis:

Deficient Knowledge:

Oral anticoagulant therapy, potential side effects, and foods and medications to avoid during therapy

Desired Outcome: Before hospital discharge, patient verbalizes accurate knowledge about the prescribed anticoagulant drug, the potential side effects, and foods and medications to avoid while receiving oral anticoagulant therapy.

INTERVENTIONS	RATIONALES
Determine patient's knowledge of oral anticoagulant therapy. As appropriate, discuss drug name, purpose, dose, schedule, precautions, food/drug and drug/drug interactions, and side effects.	To develop an individualized teaching plan that will ensure patient has sufficient knowledge of prescribed drug therapy. Knowledgeable patients are more likely to be compliant with therapy.
Teach potential side effects/complications of anticoagulant therapy: easy bruising, prolonged bleeding from cuts, spontaneous nosebleeds, bleeding gums, black and tarry or bloody stools, vaginal bleeding, and blood in urine and sputum.	Increases patient's awareness of side effects and complications to report to health care provider for timely intervention.
Discuss importance of laboratory testing and follow-up visits with health care provider.	Laboratory testing helps ensure that patient's blood clotting time stays within therapeutic range. To promote safety, patient needs close management by health care provider while undergoing anticoagulant therapy.
Explain importance of informing all health care providers (e.g., dentists, physicians) that patient is taking an anticoagulant. Suggest patient wear a Medic-Alert tag or other method of informing health care providers about the anticoagulant therapy.	To ensure that patient is not given drugs or therapies that will have adverse effects on anticoagulant therapy, causing greater risk for hemorrhaging or clotting.
Teach patient to avoid foods high in vitamin K.	Foods high in vitamin K (e.g., fish, bananas, dark green vegetables, tomatoes, cauliflower) interfere with anticoagulation.
Caution patient that a soft-bristled, rather than hard-bristled, toothbrush and an electric, rather than a straight or safety, razor should be used during anticoagulant therapy.	To minimize risk of injury that could cause severe bleeding.
Instruct patient to consult health care provider before taking over-the-counter (OTC) or prescribed drugs that were used before initiating anticoagulants.	Aspirin, cimetidine, and trimethaphan are among the many drugs that enhance the response to warfarin. Drugs that decrease the response include antacids, diuretics, oral contraceptives, and barbiturates, among others.

●●● **Related NIC and NOC labels:** *NIC:* Teaching: Prescribed Medication; Medication Management
NOC: Knowledge: Medication

ADDITIONAL NURSING DIAGNOSES/ PROBLEMS:

"Perioperative Care"	p. 47
"Prolonged Bedrest"	p. 67
"Venous Thrombosis/Thrombophlebitis"	p. 217

PATIENT-FAMILY TEACHING AND DISCHARGE PLANNING

When providing patient-family teaching, focus on sensory information, avoid giving excessive information, and initiate a visiting nurse referral if indicated for necessary follow-up teaching. Include verbal and written information about the following:

✓ Risk factors related to the development of thrombi and embolization and preventive measures to reduce the risk.

✓ Signs and symptoms of *thrombophlebitis:* swelling of the calf; tenderness or warmth in the involved area; possible presence of pain in affected calf when ankle is dorsiflexed; slight fever; and distention of distal veins, coolness, edema, and pale color in the distal affected leg.

✓ Signs and symptoms of *pulmonary embolus:* sudden onset of dyspnea and anxiety, nonproductive cough or hemoptysis, palpitations, nausea, and syncope.

✓ Rationale and application procedure for antiembolism hose. These hose prevent venous stasis, a risk factor for PE, by promoting venous return. Explain that patient should put them on in the morning before getting out of bed and after elevating the legs.

✓ Importance of preventing impairment of venous return from lower extremities by avoiding prolonged sitting, crossing legs, and constrictive clothing.

✓ Prescribed medications, including drug name, purpose, dosage, schedule, precautions, drug/drug and food/drug interactions, and potential side effects. Remind patient of necessity for continued laboratory monitoring during anticoagulant therapy.

Note: Rehabilitation and family teaching concepts for fat emboli are nonspecific.

15

Pulmonary Tuberculosis

Tuberculosis (TB) is a highly infectious disease spread by contact with respiratory droplets containing mycobacteria, generally the *Mycobacterium tuberculosis* bacillus in humans. The most common mode of transmission is inhalation of bacilli in airborne mucus droplets from sputum of persons with active disease. Less frequently, transmission may result from ingestion or skin penetration. People who are immunocompromised are at a much greater risk for development of TB disease, especially those with HIV disease. Although the majority of TB cases are pulmonary, TB can occur in almost any part of the body or as disseminated disease.

HEALTH CARE SETTING

Primary care or long-term care, with possible hospitalization (acute care) resulting from complications

ASSESSMENT

Note: Symptomatic patients who may have TB must wear a regular surgical mask and cover all coughs with a tissue. It is important to mask and isolate suspect patients as quickly as possible to minimize the risk of transmission to other patients and hospital staff. Also, close contacts of the patient require identification so that they can undergo evaluation for the presence of infection.

Signs and symptoms: Cough, hemoptysis, afternoon temperature elevation, night sweats, anorexia, weight loss, chest pain, lethargy, and dyspnea.

DIAGNOSTIC TESTS

Sputum culture: Three sputum cultures are obtained on separate days and sent for smear and culture to ascertain presence of *M. tuberculosis;* will not be positive during latency period.

Acid-fast stain: Detection of acid-fast bacilli (AFB) in stained smears examined under a microscope usually provides the first bacteriologic evidence of TB. Smear results should be available within 24 hr of specimen collection. AFB in the smear may be mycobacteria other than *M. tuberculosis;* many patients can have TB and have a negative smear. Specimens may be collected by tracheal washing, thoracentesis of pleural fluid, and lung biopsy.

Chest x-ray examination: Involvement is most characteristically evident in the apex and posterior segments of the upper lobes. Although not diagnostically definitive, the film will reveal calcification at original site, enlargement of hilar lymph nodes, parenchymal infiltrate, pleural effusion, and cavitation. Patients with HIV infection may have atypical radiographic presentation of TB. Any abnormality in an AIDS patient's chest x-ray should be considered possible TB until ruled out.

Intradermal injection of antigen: Purified protein derivative (PPD). The test is considered positive when an area of induration >10 mm is present within 48-72 hr after injection. High-risk categories such as HIV infected and recently exposed are considered positive with only 5-mm induration. Those who are immunocompromised and some patients with active TB may have a negative PPD test, even in the presence of active TB disease. A positive test indicates past infection and presence of antibodies; it is not definitive of active disease.

Gastric washings: May reveal presence of tubercle bacilli secondary to swallowed sputum.

Nursing Diagnosis:

Deficient Knowledge:

The spread of TB and the procedure for Airborne Infection Isolation

Desired Outcome: Immediately following instruction, patient and significant others verbalize how
  TB is spread and the measures necessary to prevent the spread.

INTERVENTIONS	RATIONALES
Teach patient about TB and the mechanism by which it is spread (respiratory droplet aerosol). Explain Airborne Infection Isolation to patient and significant others. Post a notice of isolation/airborne precautions on patient's room door.	A well-informed patient is more likely to comply with precautions against spreading the disease.
	Until antimicrobial therapy is successful as indicated by AFB smears, AFB isolation (or "airborne precautions" in the nomenclature of Standard Precautions) requires a private room with special ventilation that dilutes and removes airborne contaminants and controls the direction of airflow. The negative pressure is monitored continuously or checked and recorded daily while patient is isolated in this room. Patient should wear a regular surgical mask if it is necessary to leave the room.
Remind staff and visitors of need to keep door to patient's room closed.	To enable effective function of the ventilation system.
Explain to staff and visitors the importance of wearing high-efficiency masks, including their proper fit and use. Provide masks at doorway or other convenient place.	N-95 respirators, designed to provide a tight face seal and filter particles in the 1- to 5-µm range, are worn by all individuals entering patient's room to reduce possibility of infection.
Teach patient procedure to follow when coughing or sneezing.	To reduce possibility of spreading infection, patient should cover mouth and nose with tissue when sneezing or coughing and dispose of used tissue in container suitable for biohazardous waste disposal.
For more information, see Appendix for "Infection Prevention and Control," p. 831.	

●●● **Related NIC and NOC labels:** *NIC:* Infection Protection; Infection Control; Teaching: Disease
Process *NOC:* Knowledge: Disease Process; Knowledge: Infection Control

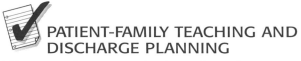 PATIENT-FAMILY TEACHING AND DISCHARGE PLANNING

When providing patient-family teaching, focus on sensory information, avoid giving excessive information, and initiate a visiting nurse referral if indicated for necessary follow-up teaching. Include verbal and written information about the following:

✓ Importance of good handwashing technique.

✓ Antituberculosis medications, including drug name, purpose, dosage, schedule, precautions, drug/drug and food/drug interactions, and potential side effects. Remind patient that medications are to be taken without interruption for the pre-

scribed period. Remind patient of the need for continued laboratory monitoring for complications of pharmacotherapy.

✓ Importance of periodic reculturing of sputum.

✓ Phone numbers to call should questions or concerns arise about therapy or disease after discharge. Additional general information can be obtained by contacting:

American Lung Association
1740 Broadway
New York, NY 10019-4374
(212) 315-8700
www.lungusa.org

Aneurysms: Abdominal, Thoracic, and Femoral

An aneurysm is a local dilation of a blood vessel. More precisely, it is a 50% increase in diameter of any vessel. The most likely cause of aneurysm is hereditary lack of elastin, although vessel wall trauma, congenital defect, infection, and atherosclerosis may be other causes. Loss of vessel wall elasticity and atherosclerotic deposits cause the vessel to weaken, resulting in gradual dilation. Acute hypertension can weaken the vessel wall further with the shearing force of the increased systolic blood pressure. Unless this condition is recognized and surgically treated, rupture and exsanguination can occur. Although aneurysms can develop in any vessel, peripheral vessel aneurysms are most commonly found in the infrarenal aorta. Until the aneurysm reaches sufficient size to press on adjacent organs, the individual may be asymptomatic. Complications include rupture and bleeding, exsanguination, and embolization.

- *Fusiform aneurysm:* The weakened arterial wall allows dilation around the entire circumference of the vessel.
- *Saccular aneurysms:* An isolated portion of the arterial wall weakens, and a balloonlike deficit is created.
- *Dissecting aneurysms:* These occur in vessels that have atherosclerotic lesions and develop intimal tears, allowing bleeding into the layers of the vessel, which causes false lumens to form that can obstruct or limit blood flow in the true lumen of the vessel.

HEALTH CARE SETTING

Chronic aneurysms in which surgery is not imminent may be followed in primary care. When there is rupture or dissection, preoperative and immediate postoperative care may be done in intensive care, followed by a step-down unit for postoperative care. Some patients may require home care assistance after they are discharged.

ASSESSMENT

Chronic indicators:

- *Abdominal aneurysm:* Patient describes sensation of heartbeat in the abdomen. Chronic abdominal pain in the middle or lower abdomen also may be present. This form occurs more frequently in men and represents approximately 80% of all aneurysms.
- *Thoracic aneurysm:* Patient may be asymptomatic for years. Pressure from the aneurysm on adjacent structures can result in dull pain in the upper back, dyspnea, cough, dysphagia, and hoarseness.
- *Femoral aneurysm:* Signs of decreased distal arterial blood flow occur. See the indicators discussed under "Atherosclerotic Arterial Occlusive Disease."

Acute indicators (rupture or dissection): Sudden onset of severe pain often described as tearing or ripping, pallor, diaphoresis, and sudden loss of consciousness.

Pain with aneurysm at ascending aorta: Nonradiating, central chest pain.

Pain with aneurysm at distal aorta: Radiation to back, abdomen, and legs.

Physical assessment: Decreased BP and peripheral pulses, tachycardia, cyanosis, and cool, clammy skin. Patient may have pulsating abdominal mass or systolic bruit over the abdomen (abdominal aneurysm) or a diastolic murmur (thoracic aneurysm).

DIAGNOSTIC TESTS

Chest x-ray examination: May reveal outline of an aneurysm, especially if there is calcification.

Aortography: Uses contrast dye to locate the lesion and identify its size, as well as the condition of the proximal and distal vessels.

Ultrasound: May assist in diagnosis when x-ray and physical examination are inconclusive. The sound waves may help determine the size, shape, and location of the aneurysm.

Digital subtraction angiography (DSA): Confirms diagnosis via computed tomography (CT), which visualizes the arteries radiographically.

Electrocardiogram (ECG): May help differentiate the pain of thoracic aneurysm from that of myocardial infarction (MI).

Transesophageal echocardiography: Provides clearer ultrasonic images of the heart by avoiding interposition of subcutaneous tissues, bony thorax, and lungs. A high-frequency transducer on an endoscope is placed in the esophagus behind the heart or advanced to the stomach to allow an inferior view of the heart to identify any associated aneurysms.

CT scan: Determines site of the intimal tear and size of the aneurysm.

Arteriography: Important before surgery to identify proximal and distal blood vessels.

Nursing Diagnosis:

Ineffective Peripheral or Renal Tissue Perfusion

(or risk of same) *related to* interrupted arterial flow secondary to postoperative embolization, occlusion of graft, or bleeding from rupture of surgical site

Desired Outcome: Patient maintains adequate peripheral and renal perfusion as evidenced by peripheral pulse amplitude >2+ on a 0-4+ scale (or N on an ADWNB scale); brisk capillary refill (<2 sec); baseline extremity sensation, motor function, color, and temperature; and urinary output ≥30 ml/hr.

INTERVENTIONS	RATIONALES
Assess peripheral pulses at least hourly and compare them bilaterally.	To establish a baseline and ongoing assessment of peripheral perfusion trend in patient who has had surgical resection of an aneurysm.
Report decreases in amplitude or absence of a pulse.	Pulse amplitude ≤2+ (or other than "N") could signal embolization. **Note:** Some health care centers use A (absent), D (requires Doppler), W (weak), N (normal), and B (bounding) to describe peripheral pulses.
Assess urine output q1-2h after surgery.	To assess renal perfusion. Output <30 ml/hr may signal impaired renal perfusion resulting from surgical procedure, embolization, or bleeding.
Assess peripheral sensation with VS, especially two-point discrimination and paresthesias; compare bilaterally. Instruct patient to report impaired sensation promptly to staff members. Report significant findings to health care provider.	Impaired sensation could signal embolization or bleeding, and it must be reported promptly for timely intervention.
Report to health care provider any changes in color, capillary refill, temperature, and motor function of the extremities.	These are assessments of peripheral perfusion; changes from baseline (e.g., capillary refill ≥3 sec, coolness, pallor or mottling, and decreased motor function) may signal embolization or bleeding. Arterial obstruction, if present, must be treated emergently to prevent loss of the extremity.
Maintain patient on bedrest until otherwise directed.	To maintain integrity of graft and minimize risk of postoperative embolization.
Keep patient flat.	To maintain graft patency and ensure healing with decreased risk of embolization. Flexing a joint near the graft could cut off blood supply to the graft.

Continued

INTERVENTIONS	RATIONALES
If patient has a lumbar drain for a thoracoabdominal aneurysm repair, assess cerebrospinal fluid (CSF)/spinal pressure. Maintain and drain the device per directive of health care provider.	An increase in spinal fluid pressure could compress the spinal cord and nerves.

●●● **Related NIC and NOC labels:** *NIC:* Circulatory Care: Arterial Insufficiency; Embolus Care: Peripheral; Positioning; *NOC:* Tissue Perfusion: Peripheral; Circulation Status

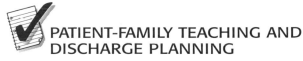

PATIENT-FAMILY TEACHING AND DISCHARGE PLANNING

When providing patient-family teaching, focus on sensory information, avoid giving excessive information, and initiate a visiting nurse referral for necessary follow-up teaching. Include verbal and written information about the following:

✓ Importance of regular medical follow-up to ensure graft patency and prompt identification of the development of a new aneurysm.

✓ Prevention of recurrence of aneurysm by avoiding factors that accelerate atherosclerosis, such as cigarette smoking, obesity, and hypertension.

✓ Necessity of a regularly scheduled exercise program that alternates exercise with rest.

✓ Indicators of wound infection and thrombus or embolus formation and the need to report them promptly to health care provider should they occur.

✓ Medications, including drug name, purpose, dosage, schedule, precautions, drug/drug and food/drug interactions, and potential side effects.

✓ Phone number of nurse available to discuss concerns and questions or clarify unclear instructions.

✓ Importance of follow-up visits with health care provider; confirm date and time of next appointment.

✓ Potential for aneurysm rupture if surgery is not immediately planned.

✓ Symptoms of rupture, including sudden onset of severe pain, often described as tearing or ripping; pallor; diaphoresis; and sudden loss of consciousness.

✓ Importance of seeking immediate medical attention should any signs and symptoms of rupture occur.

✓ Need for home blood pressure measurement.

✓ Numbers of emergency services in the area.

✓ Potential need for ultrasound for other family members to rule out aneurysm.

Atherosclerotic Arterial Occlusive Disease

Arteriosclerosis is a normal aging process resulting in changes in the arteries, including thickening of the walls, loss of elasticity, increase in calcium deposits, and, usually, an increase in external diameter and a decrease in internal diameter. In contrast, *atherosclerosis* refers to a pathologic process in which there is a proliferation of smooth muscle cells and an accumulation of lipids in the intima of the large and middle caliber arteries. Although the two processes differ, they usually occur simultaneously.

The process of atherosclerotic disease results in narrowing of the arterial lumen, which limits blood flow. Thrombosis or aneurysm can occur, depending on the reaction of the tissue that is supplied by the atherosclerotic vessels. Arterial occlusion and insufficiency are usually found in the lower extremities in patients older than 50 yr.

HEALTH CARE SETTING

Acute care or primary care

ASSESSMENT

Signs and symptoms: Severe, cramping pain (called *intermittent claudication*) with exercise and relieved by rest. It is indicative of ischemia secondary to decreased blood flow. The patient also may have delayed healing, collapsed veins, decreased sensory or motor function, leg ulcers, gangrene, or dependent rubor.

Physical assessment: Decreased pulse amplitude, decreased hair distribution, bluish discoloration of the extremities, and areas of decreased circulation. The skin may appear shiny and the nails thickened. Audible bruits may be assessed with a stethoscope over partially occluded vessels. Capillary filling will be ≥2 sec (with normal circulation, capillary filling occurs in <2 sec), and amplitude of peripheral pulses will be decreased or only detected by Doppler examination.

Risk factors: Hypertension, cigarette smoking, diabetes mellitus, family history of atherosclerotic disease, and hyperlipoproteinemia. Use of β-blocker drugs can exacerbate patient's symptoms.

DIAGNOSTIC TESTS

Angiography of peripheral vasculature: Locates obstruction and reveals extent of vascular lesions. This invasive study usually is done only if surgery is planned.

Duplex imaging: Uses ultrasound to assess arteries for plaque formation and measurement of flow and pressure.

Doppler flow studies: Use a transducer that emits sound waves through a probe to determine the amount of blood flow in arteries in which palpable pulses are difficult to obtain.

Digital subtraction angiography (DSA): Uses computed tomography (CT) to visualize arteries radiologically and determine presence and extent of occlusion.

Exercise testing: Determines the amount of exercise that precipitates ischemia and claudication.

Oscillometry: Uses a BP cuff connected to a manometer to locate occlusive sites, as evidenced by decreased pressure readings.

Ankle-brachial index (ABI): Determines the degree of arterial occlusion and subsequent ischemia. Blood pressure is determined at the ankle (using either posterior tibial or dorsalis pedis pulses) and at the brachial artery. The pressure obtained at the ankle is divided by that at the brachial artery. Normally the ABI is >1.0; resting pain occurs with an ABI ≤0.3.

See "Coronary Heart Disease," p. 179, for a discussion of additional markers for assessing cardiac and vascular disease.

Nursing Diagnosis:

Impaired Tissue Integrity: Lower extremities

(or risk of same) *related to* altered arterial circulation secondary to atherosclerotic process

Desired Outcome: Patient's lower extremity tissue remains intact.

INTERVENTIONS	RATIONALES
Assess leg(s) for ulcerations and/or impaired healing of minor trauma. Report significant findings.	A decrease in circulation significantly decreases oxygen delivery to the tissues and subsequently impairs healing of even the most minor break in the skin. A baseline assessment will enable subsequent comparison for improving or worsening condition. Prompt assessment of a worsening condition enables timely intervention.
Teach patient rationale for elevating head of bed (HOB). Explain that this can be accomplished at home by raising HOB on 6-inch blocks.	To increase circulation to lower extremities (LE), which optimally will improve integrity of patient's tissue.
Stress importance of walking and range-of-motion (ROM) exercises for hip, knee, and ankle.	These exercises increase circulation and promote collateral circulation.
Discuss an exercise program with health care provider and describe routine to patient.	Knowledge promotes compliance with the medical regimen, which provides a means for pain relief. Often this includes walking to patient's tolerance (without pain).
	Note: Bedrest without exercise may be prescribed in acute, severe cases to decrease oxygen demand to the tissues, which optimally will decrease pain.
If prescribed, teach Buerger-Allen exercises.	Buerger-Allen exercises increase circulation to the LE and are performed as follows:
	- Patient lies flat in bed with legs elevated above level of heart for 2-3 min.
	- Patient sits on edge of bed for 2-3 min with legs relaxed and dependent.
	- In same position, patient flexes, extends, inverts, and everts feet, holding each position for 30 sec.
	- Patient lies flat with legs at heart level and covered with a warm blanket for approximately 5 min.
Teach patient to assess peripheral pulses, warmth, and color of LE and to remain alert to signs of infection. Teach patient to assess LE for ulcers and cuts and to see health care provider if they do not heal in 2 wk.	Monitoring status of LE keeps patient and health care provider informed of changes in circulatory status, as well as infection.
If patient smokes, provide smoking cessation literature.	Smoking causes vasoconstriction of the arteries, thereby decreasing blood flow to the smaller arterioles of the extremities.
Discuss importance of keeping warm by wearing socks when walking or in bed.	Decreased circulation because of vasoconstriction results in cooler blood to the LE and hence hypothermia. Keeping warm promotes vasodilation and blood supply.

Continued

INTERVENTIONS	RATIONALES
Caution patient about using heating pads.	Heating pads increase metabolism and may promote ischemia if circulation is limited. Also, patient's sensitivity to temperature often is decreased, and burns can result.
Caution patient to cover all exposed areas when going outside in cooler weather.	To prevent hypothermia, to which patient with decreased circulation may be prone.
Teach patient to maintain moderate room temperatures and avoid temperature extremes.	To promote consistent arterial flow and decrease incidents of spasm.
If prescribed, administer pentoxyphylline (Trental).	To increase flexibility of erythrocytes, prevent aggregation of red blood cells (RBCs) and platelets, and decrease blood viscosity, which optimally will increase circulation at the capillary level.

●●● **Related NIC and NOC labels:** *NIC:* Circulatory Care: Arterial Insufficiency; Circulatory Precautions; Medication Administration; *NOC:* Tissue Integrity: Skin & Mucous Membranes; Wound Healing: Secondary Intention

Nursing Diagnosis:

Chronic Pain

related to atherosclerotic obstructions and ischemia

Desired Outcomes: By the time of discharge from health care setting (or within 24 hr of intervention), patient's subjective perception of chronic pain decreases as documented by a pain scale. Objective indicators, such as grimacing, are absent.

INTERVENTIONS	RATIONALES
Assess for presence of pain, using a pain scale from 0 (no pain) to 10 (worst pain).	To determine degree and trend of pain.
Administer pain medications as prescribed.	To reduce pain. Usually mild analgesics are given.
Document pain relief achieved using pain scale.	To determine effectiveness of the medication.
Teach patient to rest and stop exercising before claudication occurs.	Intermittent claudication is severe, cramping pain that occurs as a result of ischemia after extended periods of exercise and is relieved by rest.
Because the pain may be chronic and continuous, explore alternate methods of pain relief, such as visualization, guided imagery, biofeedback, meditation, and relaxation exercises or tapes.	To augment pain relief from analgesics and decrease discomfort using nonpharmacologic methods, which do not have side effects.
Institute measures such as Buerger-Allen exercises (see **Impaired Tissue Integrity,** p. 166) and walking.	To increase circulation to ischemic extremities, which optimally will increase patient's comfort level.
Advise about possibility of "rest" pain.	Occurs at night when patient is recumbent and decreases when legs are in a dependent position with gravity assisting in delivery of blood and oxygen to the LE.

●●● **Related NIC and NOC labels:** *NIC:* Pain Management; Analgesic Administration; Simple Relaxation Therapy; Biofeedback; Exercise Therapy: Ambulation; Exercise Promotion: Stretching; Simple Guided Imagery *NOC:* Pain Control; Pain: Disruptive Effects

Nursing Diagnosis:

Deficient Knowledge:

Potential for infection and impaired tissue integrity caused by decreased arterial circulation

Desired Outcome: Immediately following teaching, patient verbalizes accurate knowledge about the potential for infection and impaired tissue integrity, as well as measures to prevent these problems.

INTERVENTIONS	RATIONALES
Teach how to assess for signs of infection or problems with skin integrity and to report significant findings to health care provider.	Facilitates understanding of symptoms that occur with infection or impaired skin integrity and knowledge of symptoms that should be reported for timely intervention.
Caution about increased potential for easily traumatizing the skin (e.g., from bumping LE).	Decreased circulation in the LE diminishes the healing process after tissue trauma.
Instruct patient to inspect both feet each day for any open wounds or bruises. If necessary, suggest that patient use a long-handled mirror to see bottoms of the feet. Advise patient to report any open areas to health care provider.	Open wounds can lead to infection and should be reported promptly for timely intervention.
Stress importance of wearing shoes or slippers that fit properly.	Improper fit can lead to traumatized tissue.
Instruct patient to cut toenails straight across or to have them cut by a podiatrist.	To prevent ingrown toenails, which can lead to infection.
Encourage patient to keep feet clean and dry, using mild soap and warm water for cleansing, and to apply a mild lotion.	To promote hygiene and prevent dryness, which could result in skin breakdown that can lead to infection.
Advise patient not to scratch or rub the skin on the feet.	This can result in abrasions that easily can become infected.
Suggest that patient keep feet warm with loose-fitting socks and warm soaks.	Decreased circulation leaves patient vulnerable to hypothermia. Keeping warm promotes vasodilation and increased blood supply to the area.
Caution patient to check temperature of warm soaks and bath water carefully.	To protect skin from burns in a patient whose temperature sensitivity is decreased.
Discuss endarterectomy, bypass vascular grafting, and angioplasty as indicated.	These are possible surgical corrections.

●●● **Related NIC and NOC labels:** *NIC:* Infection Protection; Teaching: Disease Process *NOC:* Knowledge: Infection Control

Nursing Diagnosis:

Ineffective Peripheral Tissue Perfusion

(or risk of same) *related to* interrupted arterial flow with postsurgical graft occlusion

Desired Outcome: Patient has adequate peripheral perfusion as evidenced by peripheral pulse amplitude >2+ on a 0-4+ scale (or "N" on an ADWNB scale), BP within 20 mm Hg of baseline BP, and absence of the six *P*s (see below) in the involved extremities.

INTERVENTIONS	RATIONALES
Assess peripheral pulses and involved extremity for the six *P*s: pain, pallor, pulselessness, paresthesia, polar (coolness), and paralysis. Report significant findings.	Sensory changes (i.e., pain, loss of two-point discrimination, and paresthesias) usually precede other symptoms of ischemia. Such findings should be reported promptly for timely intervention. **Note:** Some health care settings document pulses as A (absent), D (requires Doppler), W (weak), N (normal), or B (bounding).
Monitor BP. Report to health care provider any significant increase or decrease (>15-20 mm Hg, or as directed).	BP is another indicator of peripheral perfusion pressure. An increase in BP may interrupt the surgical site; decreased BP may cause graft occlusion.
If necessary, use Doppler ultrasonic probe to check pulses, holding probe to the skin at a 45-degree angle to blood vessel. Record presence or absence of pulsations, as well as rate, character, frequency, and intensity of the sounds.	Doppler probes are able to evaluate amount of blood flow in arteries in which pulses are difficult to palpate. In the presence of normal blood flow, wavelike, whooshing sounds will be heard.
Use a foot cradle to keep sheets and blankets off legs and feet.	Keeps sources of irritation away from sensitive LE.
For the first 48-72 hr after surgery (or as directed), prevent acute joint flexion in the presence of a graft.	Flexing the joint can impede blood flow.

●●● **Related NIC and NOC labels:** *NIC:* Circulatory Care: Arterial Insufficiency; Positioning *NOC:* Tissue Perfusion: Peripheral

Nursing Diagnosis:

Ineffective Renal Tissue Perfusion

related to interrupted blood flow during surgery and potential embolization after surgery

Desired Outcome: Within 1 hr after surgery, patient has adequate renal perfusion as evidenced by urinary output ≥30 ml/hr.

INTERVENTIONS	RATIONALES
Monitor I&O. Report output <30 ml/hr.	Decreased urinary output is a sign of decreased renal perfusion. During many vascular surgical procedures, the aorta is clamped temporarily to facilitate endarterectomy and grafting. Although all body systems are affected to a degree, the renal system is especially sensitive to the lack of blood flow.
Monitor results of renal function tests.	To determine increases in serum creatinine (>1.5 mg/dl) and blood urea nitrogen (BUN) (>20 mg/dl), which can occur with decreasing renal function.
Monitor for distended neck veins, crackles (rales), peripheral edema.	These are signs of fluid retention.
In the absence of acute cardiac or renal failure, encourage adequate fluid intake (2-3 L/day).	To help maintain adequate renal blood flow and promote fluid balance.

●●● **Related NIC and NOC labels:** *NIC:* Laboratory Data Interpretation; Fluid Monitoring *NOC:* Tissue Perfusion: Abdominal Organs

ADDITIONAL NURSING DIAGNOSES/ PROBLEMS:

"Perioperative Care"   p. 47

PATIENT-FAMILY TEACHING AND DISCHARGE PLANNING

When providing patient-family teaching, focus on sensory information, avoid giving excessive information, and initiate a visiting nurse referral for necessary follow-up teaching. Include verbal and written information about the following:

✔ Referral to smoking cessation program in your area if appropriate. The following free brochures outline ways to help patients stop smoking:

- *How to Help Your Patients Stop Using Tobacco: A National Cancer Institute Manual for the Oral Health Team,* from the Smoking and Tobacco Control Program of the National Cancer Institute; call 1-800-4-CANCER.

- *Clinical Practice Guideline: A Quick Reference Guide for Smoking Cessation Specialists,* from the Agency for Health Care Policy and Research (AHCPR); call 1-800-358-9295.

✔ Importance of avoiding factors and activities that cause vasoconstriction (e.g., tight clothing, smoking, cold exposure).

✔ Exercise program as prescribed by health care provider; importance of rest periods if claudication occurs.

✔ Skin and foot care.

✔ Measures that optimize arterial blood flow, such as keeping warm and raising HOB on blocks to promote circulation to the lower extremities.

✔ Medications, including drug name, purpose, dosage, schedule, precautions, drug/drug and food/drug interactions, and potential side effects.

Cardiac and Noncardiac Shock (Circulatory Failure)

A shock state exists when tissue perfusion decreases to the point of cellular metabolic dysfunction. Shock is classified according to the causative event. *Hematogenic (hemorrhagic or hypovolemic)* shock occurs when blood volume is insufficient to meet metabolic needs of the tissues, as with severe hemorrhage. *Cardiogenic shock* occurs when cardiac failure results in decreased tissue perfusion, as in myocardial infarction (MI). *Distributive shock conditions* are characterized by displacement of a significant amount of vascular volume. The three types of distributive shock are:

- **Neurogenic shock:** Results from a neurologic event (e.g., head injury) that causes massive vasodilation and decreased perfusion pressures.
- **Anaphylactic shock:** Caused by a severe systemic response to an allergen (foreign protein), resulting in massive vasodilation, increased capillary permeability, decreased perfusion, decreased venous return, and subsequent decreased cardiac output.
- **Septic shock:** Occurs when bacterial toxins cause an overwhelming systemic infection.

Regardless of the cause, shock results in cellular hypoxia secondary to decreased perfusion and ultimately in cellular, tissue, and organ dysfunction. A prolonged shock state can result in death, so early recognition and intervention are essential.

HEALTH CARE SETTING

Critical care unit (e.g., cardiogenic shock in coronary care unit, distributive shock in medical intensive care unit [ICU])

ASSESSMENT

Early signs and symptoms: Cool, pale, and clammy skin; decreased pulse strength; dry and pale mucous membranes; restlessness; hyperventilation; anxiety; nausea; thirst; weakness.

Physical assessment: Rapid HR, decreased pulse pressure, decreased systolic BP, and increased diastolic BP secondary to catecholamine (sympathetic nervous system [SNS]) response.

Late signs and symptoms: Decreased urinary output, hypothermia, drowsiness, diaphoresis, confusion, and lethargy, all of which can progress to a comatose state.

Physical assessment: Irregular HR; continually decreasing BP, usually with systolic pressure palpable at 60 mm Hg or less; rapid and possibly irregular RR.

DIAGNOSTIC TESTS

Diagnosis is usually based on presenting symptoms and clinical signs. Patients in critical care will most likely have pulmonary artery (PA) catheters placed into the right side of the heart. Measurement of volume levels, cardiac output, and pressures inside the chambers helps diagnose fluid levels and heart performance. SvO_2 monitoring also is possible via PA catheters. It enables measurement of mixed venous oxygen saturation and is especially useful in septic shock patients, for whom measurement of SvO_2, along with cellular consumption, enables close monitoring of trend and facilitates treatment.

Arterial blood gas (ABG) values: Will reveal metabolic acidosis (bicarbonate [HCO_3^-] <22 mEq/L and pH <7.40) caused by anaerobic metabolism.

Serial measurement of urinary output: Less than 30 ml/hr indicates decreased perfusion and decreased renal function.

Blood urea nitrogen (BUN) and creatinine: Increase with decreased renal perfusion (a late finding).

Blood glucose: Hyperglycemia may be present because of epinephrine-induced glycogenolysis.

For septic shock:

Serum electrolyte levels: Identify renal complications and metabolic dysfunctions as evidenced by hyperkalemia and hypernatremia.

Blood culture: To identify the causative organism.

White blood cell (WBC) count and erythrocyte sedimentation rate (ESR): Elevated in the presence of infection.

For hematogenic shock:

Complete blood count (CBC): Hct and Hgb will be decreased because of decreased blood volume.

For anaphylactic shock:

WBC count: Will reveal increased eosinophils, a type of granulocyte that appears in the presence of allergic reaction.

Nursing Diagnosis:

Ineffective Peripheral, Cardiopulmonary, Cerebral, and Renal Tissue Perfusion

related to decreased circulating blood volume

Desired Outcome: Within 1 hr of intervention/treatment, patient has adequate perfusion as evidenced by peripheral pulse amplitude >2+ on a 0-4+ scale; brisk capillary refill (<2 sec); BP within patient's normal range; central venous pressure (CVP) ≥5 cm H_2O; HR regular and ≤100 bpm; no significant change in mental status; orientation to person, place, and time; and urine output ≥30 ml/hr.

INTERVENTIONS	RATIONALES
Assess and document peripheral perfusion status.	Decreased peripheral perfusion is an early sign of decreased cardiac output and shock.
	Coolness and pallor of the extremities, decreased amplitude of pulses, and delayed capillary refill are significant findings for decreased cardiac output and all shock types.
Monitor BP at frequent intervals; assess for altered mentation, dizziness, and decreased urinary output.	Decreased systolic BP and increased diastolic BP (narrowing pulse pressure) are signs that the body is attempting to compensate for a decrease in cardiac output or lack of volume and are early signs of shock.
	BP >20 mm Hg below patient's normal range, along with dizziness, altered mentation, and decreased urinary output, indicates hypotension and decreased cardiac output.
If hypotension is present, place patient in a supine position.	To promote venous return. **Caution:** BP must be ≥80/60 mm Hg because this level ensures adequate coronary and renal artery perfusion.
Caution: Avoid Trendelenburg position.	This position can flood the baroreceptors and subsequently knock out the compensatory mechanism for hypotension.
Monitor CVP (if line is inserted).	To determine adequacy of venous return and blood volume. A range of 5-10 cm H_2O usually is considered adequate. Values near zero can indicate hypovolemia, especially when associated with decreased urinary output, vasoconstriction, and increased HR, which are found with hypovolemia. Increased CVP may signal cardiogenic shock.
Observe for restlessness, confusion, mental status changes, and decreased level of consciousness (LOC).	Indicators of decreased cerebral perfusion.

Continued

INTERVENTIONS	RATIONALES
If positive indicators are present, raise side rails and place bed in its lowest position. Observe patient frequently and reorient as indicated.	To protect patient from injury.
Monitor for chest pain and an irregular HR.	Indicators of decreased coronary artery perfusion.
Monitor urinary output hourly. Notify health care provider if it is <30 ml/hr in the presence of adequate intake.	Decreased urinary output is a sign of decreased cardiac output and renal perfusion.
Check weight daily for evidence of gain.	Weight gain may be a signal of fluid retention, which can occur with decreased renal perfusion.
Monitor laboratory results for BUN and creatinine values. Report increases.	Elevated BUN (>20 mg/dl) and creatinine (>1.5 mg/dl) levels signal decreased renal perfusion.
Monitor serum electrolyte values for evidence of imbalances, particularly of Na^+ and K^+.	Hypernatremia (Na^+ >147 mEq/L) and hyperkalemia (K^+ >5 mEq/L) may be signs of renal and metabolic complications in shock.
Monitor patient for muscle weakness, hyporeflexia, and irregular HR.	Signs of hyperkalemia.
Also monitor for fluid retention and edema.	Hypernatremia can contribute to these problems.
Administer fluids as prescribed.	To increase vascular volume. The type and amount of fluid will depend on the type of shock and patient's clinical situation.
	Cardiogenic shock: Fluids are probably limited to prevent overload (the heart is not able to handle the volume already in the intravascular space), yet dehydration must be avoided. Decreasing preload (fluids) may be the treatment of choice to take the workload off the heart.
	Hypovolemic shock: The amount lost is replaced. Ringer's solution, as much as 1000 ml/hr, may be administered if volume loss is severe. Ringer's lactate replaces circulating volume and electrolytes. Blood replacement, if Hgb is low, will increase oxygen carrying capacity and therefore delivery to the tissues. Colloid infusion may be necessary when blood is not needed. Colloids such as albumin replace circulating proteins. Proteins hold on to intravascular volume better than crystalloids (Ringer's).
	Septic shock: Ringer's solution, plasma, and blood are administered. Ringer's lactate replaces circulating volume and electrolytes. Blood replacement, if Hgb is low, will increase oxygen carrying capacity and therefore delivery to the tissues. Colloid infusion may be necessary when blood is not needed. Colloids such as albumin replace circulating proteins. Proteins hold on to intravascular volume better than crystalloids (Ringer's).

●●● **Related NIC and NOC labels:** *NIC:* Circulatory Precautions: Shock Management: Cardiac; Fluid Management; Vital Signs Monitoring; Blood Products Administration; Fluid Monitoring; Shock Prevention; Hypovolemia Management; Fluid Resuscitation; Laboratory Data Interpretation; Intravenous Therapy; Electrolyte Management; Neurologic Monitoring; Positioning *NOC:* Tissue Perfusion: Abdominal Organs; Tissue Perfusion: Peripheral; Electrolyte & Acid-Base Balance; Circulation Status; Tissue Perfusion: Cerebral; Tissue Perfusion: Cardiac; Tissue Perfusion: Pulmonary

Nursing Diagnosis:

Impaired Gas Exchange

related to pulmonary congestion from left-sided heart failure or altered utilization of O_2 at the capillary bed from a decrease in delivery

Desired Outcome: Within 1 hr of intervention, patient has adequate gas exchange as evidenced by O_2 saturation >92%; partial pressure of dissolved oxygen in arterial blood (PaO_2) ≥80 mm Hg; partial pressure of dissolved carbon dioxide in arterial blood ($PaCO_2$) ≤45 mm Hg; pH ≥7.35; presence of eupnea; and orientation to person, place, and time.

INTERVENTIONS	RATIONALES
Monitor ABG results. Report significant findings.	A diagnostic tool to assess acid-base balance and oxygenation status. Significant findings in shock include decreased PaO_2 (indicates presence of hypoxemia), increased $PaCO_2$ (indicates presence of hypercarbia), or decreased pH and increased $PaCO_2$ (indicates presence of acidosis). These values may signal respiratory failure or distress.
Monitor oximetry readings. Report significant findings.	Readings ≤92% are indicators of significantly decreased oxygenation and signal the need to increase or implement supplemental oxygen or other respiratory intervention.
Monitor respirations q30min; note and report presence of tachypnea or dyspnea.	Fast or labored breaths may signal respiratory distress and possibly respiratory failure and the need for supplemental oxygen or other respiratory intervention. Tachypnea or dyspnea also may be a sign of pain, anxiety, or infection.
Be alert to mental status changes, restlessness, irritability, and confusion.	Indicators of hypoxia.
Teach patient to breathe slowly and deeply in through the nose and out through the mouth.	Slows the respiratory cycle for better alveolar gas exchange.
Ensure that patient has a patent airway; suction secretions as needed.	To promote movement of air.
Administer O_2 as prescribed.	To increase oxygen supply.
Deliver O_2 with humidity.	To help prevent its convective drying effects on oral and nasal mucosa.

●●● **Related NIC and NOC labels:** *NIC:* Acid-Base Monitoring; Acid-Base Management; Laboratory Data Interpretation; Respiratory Monitoring; Oxygen Therapy; Airway Suctioning *NOC:* Tissue Perfusion: Pulmonary; Respiratory Status: Ventilation; Respiratory Status: Gas Exchange

ADDITIONAL NURSING DIAGNOSES/ PROBLEMS:

"Psychosocial Support"	p. 81
"Psychosocial Support for the Patient's Family and Significant Others"	p. 95

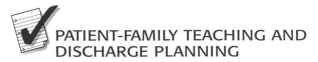

PATIENT-FAMILY TEACHING AND DISCHARGE PLANNING

For interventions, see discussion of patient's primary diagnosis.

Cardiac Surgery

Surgical intervention continues to be a mainstay in the treatment of acquired and congenital heart disease.

Coronary artery bypass grafting (CABG) is a technique used to treat blocked coronary arteries; a portion of the saphenous vein, internal mammary artery, gastroepiploic artery, or radial artery is excised and anastomosed from the aorta to below the blocked artery, thereby revascularizing the affected myocardium.

Valve replacement, another type of cardiac surgery, is performed for patients with valvular stenosis or valvular incompetence of the mitral, tricuspid, pulmonary, or aortic valve.

Other cardiac surgery is also performed to correct heart defects that are either acquired or congenital, such as ventricular aneurysm, ventricular or atrial septal defects, transposition of the great vessels, and tetralogy of Fallot.

Heart transplantation has become an accepted treatment modality for some patients diagnosed with end-stage cardiomyopathy. The availability of acceptable donor organs remains a problem. Immunosuppressive treatment to prevent organ rejection after heart transplantation is similar to that of patients who receive a renal transplant. See "Care of the Renal Transplant Recipient," p. 261.

Combined heart-lung transplantation is used for patients with end-stage disease affecting both organs.

HEALTH CARE SETTING

Under normal circumstances, patients are admitted to the hospital the day of surgery. After surgery, most patients are in an intensive care unit (ICU) for 24 hr and then transferred to a step-down unit for 3-5 days, although heart transplant patients have a longer stay.

Nursing Diagnosis:

Deficient Knowledge:

Diagnosis, surgical procedure, preoperative routine, and postoperative course

Desired Outcome: Before surgery, patient verbalizes accurate knowledge about the diagnosis, surgical procedure, and preoperative and postoperative regimens.

INTERVENTIONS	RATIONALES
Assess patient's level of knowledge about the diagnosis and surgical procedure and provide information as necessary. Encourage questions and allow time for verbalization of concerns and fears.	Some patients may be knowledgeable and others may not be. Some find detailed explanations helpful; others prefer very brief and simple explanations. The amount of information given should depend on the patient, enabling an individualized teaching plan.
If appropriate for patient, provide orientation to the ICU and equipment that will be used postoperatively.	To reduce anxiety and facilitate understanding of the equipment.

Continued

INTERVENTIONS	RATIONALES
Provide instructions and purpose for deep breathing and coughing.	Deep breathing and coughing are essential postoperative techniques that reinflate the lungs after heart-lung bypass and help prevent atelectasis and pneumonia.
Reassure patient that postoperative discomfort will be relieved with medication.	To reduce anxiety about postoperative pain. **Note:** Pain after a midline sternotomy (the usual incision with cardiac surgery) usually is less than that with the thoracotomy approach because the somatic nerves are not divided by the surgical incision in the former.
Advise patient that in the immediate postoperative period, speaking will be limited.	An endotracheal tube that will assist with breathing will prevent speech. Other means of communicating (e.g., nodding, writing) will be necessary. This knowledge will prepare patient for use of alternative means of communicating in the postoperative period.
For more details, see this nursing diagnosis in "Perioperative Care," p. 47.	

●●● **Related NIC and NOC labels:** *NIC:* Preparatory Sensory Information; Teaching: Procedure/Treatment; Anxiety Reduction; Learning Facilitation; Teaching: Disease Process *NOC:* Knowledge: Treatment Procedures

Nursing Diagnosis:

Activity Intolerance

related to generalized weakness and bedrest secondary to cardiac surgery

Desired Outcome: By a minimum of 24 hr before discharge from care facility, patient rates perceived exertion at ≤3 on a 0-10 scale and exhibits cardiac tolerance to activity after cardiac surgery as evidenced by HR ≤110 bpm, systolic BP within 20 mm Hg of resting systolic BP, and RR ≤20 breaths/min with normal depth and pattern (eupnea).

INTERVENTIONS	RATIONALES
Ask patient to rate perceived exertion (RPE) during activity. Monitor for evidence of activity intolerance. For details, see **Risk for Activity Intolerance** in "Prolonged Bedrest," p. 67. Notify health care provider of significant findings.	An RPE >3, along with cool and diaphoretic skin, is a signal to stop the activity and notify health care provider.
Monitor VS at frequent intervals, especially during range-of-motion (ROM) exercises and other in-bed activities. Notify health care provider of significant findings.	Hypotension, tachycardia, crackles (rales), tachypnea, and decreased amplitude of peripheral pulses are indicators of cardiac failure and should be reported promptly for timely intervention. Be especially alert to a decrease >20 mm Hg of resting systolic BP inasmuch as a mean BP of 50 mm Hg is required for adequate brain perfusion.
Facilitate coordination of health care providers to allow rest periods between care activities. Ensure 90 min for undisturbed rest.	To decrease cardiac workload. An increased cardiac workload is likely if too many activities are performed without concomitant rest.
As prescribed, administer medications, such as β-blockers.	These medications decrease myocardial O_2 consumption and may enable increased cardiac tolerance to activity.
Assist with exercises, depending on tolerance and prescribed activity limitations.	To decrease cardiac workload and promote exercise tolerance.

Continued

INTERVENTIONS	RATIONALES
As prescribed, initiate physical therapy.	To increase activity tolerance and provide instructions for home exercise program.
See **Risk for Activity Intolerance**, p. 67, and **Risk for Disuse Syndrome**, p. 69, for a discussion of in-bed exercises.	

●●● **Related NIC and NOC labels:** *NIC:* Energy Management; Exercise Promotion; Cardiac Care: Rehabilitative; Medication Management *NOC:* Energy Conservation; Activity Tolerance

Nursing Diagnosis:

Imbalanced Nutrition: More than body requirements

of calories, sodium, or fats

Desired Outcome: Within the 24-hr period before hospital discharge, patient demonstrates accurate knowledge of the dietary regimen by planning a 3-day menu that includes and excludes appropriate foods.

INTERVENTIONS	RATIONALES
If patient is over ideal body weight, explain necessity of a low-calorie diet.	Being overweight is a risk factor for cardiac disease.
Explain how to decrease dietary intake of saturated (animal) fats and increase intake of polyunsaturated (vegetable oil) fats.	Knowledge of acceptable fats promotes compliance with dietary plan.
Teach patient to limit dietary intake of cholesterol to <300 mg/day. Encourage use of food labels to determine cholesterol content of foods.	A high serum lipid level is a risk factor for cardiac disease.
Teach patient to limit dietary intake of refined/processed sugar.	Sugar is a short-acting energy source that can result in hunger, followed by eating more foods that are stored as fat.
Teach patient to limit dietary intake of sodium chloride (NaCl) to <4 g/day (mild restriction). Encourage use of food labels to determine Na⁺ content of foods.	Limiting sodium helps control fluid retention and hypertension, which would otherwise increase cardiac workload and myocardial O_2 demand.
Instruct patient and significant other in use of "Nutrition Facts" (federally mandated public information on all food product labels) to determine amount of calories, total fat, saturated fat, cholesterol, and sodium in foods.	To increase knowledge for making better food choices and promoting compliance with dietary plan. Patient should be especially aware of the serving size listed for respective nutrients; that is, a serving size listed as 4 oz on a package containing 12 oz would mean patient would get 3 times the amount of each ingredient if the patient eats the entire contents of the container!
Encourage intake of a healthy, balanced diet.	A healthy, balanced diet incorporates fresh fruits, natural (unrefined or unprocessed) carbohydrates, fish, poultry, legumes, fresh vegetables, and grains.
Ask patient to prepare a 3-day menu that includes and excludes appropriate foods.	A return demonstration is a proven way of enhancing knowledge, which optimally will promote compliance.

●●● **Related NIC and NOC labels:** *NIC:* Weight Reduction Assistance; Nutritional Counseling; Teaching: Prescribed Diet; Referral *NOC:* Weight Control; Nutritional Status: Nutrient Intake

ADDITIONAL NURSING DIAGNOSES/ PROBLEMS:

PATIENT-FAMILY TEACHING AND DISCHARGE PLANNING

When providing patient-family teaching, focus on sensory information, avoid giving excessive information, and initiate a visiting nurse referral for necessary follow-up teaching. Include written information with verbal reinforcement and time for questions about the following:

✓ Medications, including drug name, dosage, schedule, purpose, precautions, drug/drug and food/drug interactions, and potential side effects.

✓ Untoward symptoms requiring medical attention for patients taking warfarin (Coumadin), such as bleeding from the nose (epistaxis) or gums, hemoptysis, hematemesis, hematuria, melena, hematochezia, menometrorrhagia, and excessive bruising. In addition, stress the following: take warfarin at the same time every day; notify health care provider if *any* signs of bleeding occur; keep appointments for physical therapy checks; avoid over-the-counter (OTC) and herbal medications unless approved by health care provider; carry a Medic-Alert bracelet or card; avoid constrictive or restrictive clothing; use soft-bristled toothbrush and electric razor; maintain vitamins and foods high in vitamin K at a constant intake. Too much intake can reverse the Coumadin effect and therefore bleeding. Change or too little intake can cause more clotting and need for more Coumadin.

✓ Maintenance of low-Na^+, low-fat, and low-cholesterol diet. Encourage patients to use food labels to determine sodium, fat, and cholesterol content of foods.

✓ Importance of pacing activities at home and allowing frequent rest periods.

✓ Technique for assessing radial pulse, temperature, and weight, if these indicators require monitoring at home, and reporting significant changes to health care provider.

✓ Introduction to local American Heart Association activities. Either provide the address or phone number for the local chapter or encourage the patient to write for information to the following address:

American Heart Association
7320 Greenville Avenue
Dallas, TX 75231
(800) 242-8721
www.americanheart.org

✓ For patients awaiting heart transplantation, provide the following information, as appropriate:

The United Network for Organ Sharing
UNOS Communication Department
P.O. Box 13770
Richmond, VA 23225
(804) 330-8561 or (800) 243-6667 (voice mail)
www.unos.org

✓ Phone number of nurse available to discuss concerns and questions or clarify unclear instructions.

✓ Importance of follow-up visits with health care provider; confirm date and time of next appointment.

✓ Signs and symptoms that necessitate immediate medical attention: edema, chest pain, dyspnea, shortness of breath, weight gain, and decrease in exercise tolerance.

✓ Activity restrictions (e.g., no heavy lifting, pushing, or pulling anything heavier than 5 lb with the upper extremities for at least 6 wk); prescribed exercise program; and resumption of sexual activity, work, and driving a car, as directed. Instruct patient to avoid prolonged sitting, which in a cardiac surgery patient can cause deep vein thrombosis (DVT).

✓ Care of incision site; importance of assessing for signs of infection, such as drainage, swelling, fever, persistent redness, and local warmth and tenderness.

✓ Referral to a cardiac rehabilitation program.

✓ Discussion of patient's home environment and potential need for changes or adaptations (e.g., too many steps to climb, activities of daily living [ADL] that are too strenuous).

Coronary Heart Disease

The coronary arteries are the vessels that supply the myocardial muscle with O_2 and the nutrients necessary for optimal function. Atherosclerotic lesions within these arteries are a major cause of obstruction and subsequent ischemia, which ultimately can lead to myocardial infarction (MI). Other mechanisms include spasm, platelet aggregation, and thrombus formation. The most common symptom of coronary heart disease (CHD) is angina, a result of decreasing blood flow and decreased O_2 supply through narrowed or obstructed arteries (ischemia). This often occurs during exercise, but it may occur at rest or during a condition of decreased perfusion, such as an episode of hypotension. Often, CHD is diagnosed only after the patient is seen for angina or MI. It is important to note that symptoms do not appear until approximately 75% of the artery is occluded. CHD is the number one killer of both men and women in the United States. After 65 years of age, death from CHD occurs slightly (11%) more frequently in women than in men.

HEALTH CARE SETTING

Primary care, acute care, coronary care unit

ASSESSMENT

Chronic indicators: Stable or progressively worsening angina that occurs when myocardial demand for O_2 is more than the supply, such as during exercise. The pain usually is described as pressure or a crushing or burning substernal pain that radiates down one or both arms. It can be felt also in the neck, cheeks, and teeth. Usually it is relieved by discontinuation of exercise or administration of nitroglycerin (NTG).

Acute indicators: CHD is considered unstable (acute) when angina becomes more frequent and is unrelieved by NTG and rest, when it occurs during sleep or rest, or when it occurs with progressively lower levels of exercise.

Risk factors: Family history, increasing age, male gender, smoking, low high-density lipoprotein (HDL), high serum lipid levels, increased homocysteine level, diabetes mellitus, hypertension, obesity, glucose intolerance, hyperinsulinemia in the absence of diabetes mellitus, and sedentary and stressful lifestyle. Some patients may not demonstrate any of these risk factors.

DIAGNOSTIC TESTS

Electrocardiogram (ECG): Usually normal unless MI has occurred or the individual is experiencing angina at the time of the test. If ECG is performed during angina, characteristic changes include ST-segment depression in leads over the area of ischemia.

Serum enzymes: To rule out acute MI. See "Myocardial Infarction," p. 203.

Chest x-ray examination: Usually normal unless heart failure is present.

Stress tests:

- *Exercise treadmill test:* To determine amount of exercise-induced ischemia, hemodynamic response, and ECG changes with exercise. Significant findings include 1 mm or more ST-segment depression or elevation, dysrhythmia, or sudden decrease in BP.
- *Stress echocardiogram:* Combination of stress exercise test and echocardiogram. A stress-induced imbalance in myocardial supply/demand ratio will produce myocardial ischemia and regional wall motion abnormality.
- *Dobutamine stress echocardiogram:* Dobutamine is used as a stress agent in combination with an echocardiogram for patients who cannot exercise. Dobutamine causes myocardial contractility, simulating a working heart. It may cause ischemia in patients with CHD, resulting in a wall motion abnormality.

Cardiac nuclear imaging modalities:

Myocardial perfusion imaging:

▪ Detection of CHD by differential blood flow through the left ventricular myocardium. Normal blood flow and normal tracer uptake are seen with normal coronary arteries; diminished flow and diminished tracer uptake are found with coronary stenosis. A perfusion abnormality will be present in an area of MI.

▪ Radiopharmaceutical agents used are thallium-201 and technetium-99m sestamibi. Adenosine and dipyridamole are pharmacologic stress agents used in combination with a radiopharmaceutical agent if the patient is unable to exercise or fails to reach 85% of age-predicted maximum HR.

▪ Single photon emission computed tomography (SPECT): Used to develop three-dimensional views of cardiac processes and cellular level metabolism by viewing the heart from several different angles and using tomography methods to reconstruct the image. SPECT enables clearer resolution of myocardial ischemia and better quantification of cardiac damage.

Technetium-99m pyrophosphate: Taken up by infarcted myocardial tissue. MI will show up as a "hot spot" on the scan.

Radionuclide angiography: Used to evaluate left and right ventricular ejection fraction, left ventricular volume, and regional wall motion. The first pass technique is a fast acquisition of myocardial images. The gated pool ejection or multiple-gated acquisition (MUGA) scan permits calculation of the amount of blood ejected with ventricular contraction and is used for risk stratification of patients after MI or heart failure.

Ambulatory monitoring: A 24-hr ECG monitoring that can show activity-induced ST-segment changes or ischemia-induced dysrhythmias.

Coronary arteriography via cardiac catheterization: Provides the ultimate diagnosis of CHD. Arterial lesions (plaque)

are located, and the amount of occlusion is determined. At this time, feasibility for coronary artery bypass grafting (CABG) or angioplasty is determined. For details about these procedures, see "Cardiac Surgery," p. 175.

Intravascular ultrasound (IVUS): To assess degree of atherosclerosis during coronary angiogram. A flexible catheter with a miniature transducer at the tip is threaded from an arteriotomy (commonly femoral) retrograde to the coronary arteries to provide information on the interior of the coronary arteries. Ultrasound is used to create a cross-sectional image of the three layers of the arterial wall and its lumen.

Additional markers for assessing cardiovascular disease: Blood markers that look promising for diagnosing and identifying patients at risk for CHD and vascular/arterial disease include the following:

• *Lipoprotein(a):* A promising marker for detecting premature CHD. Lipoprotein(a), a particle very similar to LDL, may interfere with endothelium-dependent vasodilation. A level >30 mg/dl is associated with a greater risk of MI.

• *Homocysteine:* An elevated level may aggravate atherosclerosis by interfering with endothelium-dependent vasodilation. It also may adversely affect the coagulation cascade by increasing platelet adhesiveness and aggregation of clotting factors. Mild elevation is 10-15 µmol/L; moderate elevation is 16-30 µmol/L; moderate–severe level is 31-100 µmol/L; and severe level is ≥100 µmol/L.

• *High sensitive C-reactive protein (Hs-CRP):* Plasma concentrations of this glycoprotein increase during an inflammatory response. It has been shown to have predictive value for stroke, first myocardial infarction, and peripheral vascular disease. Aspirin, acting as an anti-inflammatory agent, significantly reduces the risk of myocardial infarction. Patients with higher Hs-CRP levels taking aspirin benefit the most. At a level >2.1 mg/L the patient is at great risk.

Nursing Diagnosis:

Acute Pain (Angina)

related to decreased oxygen supply to the myocardium

Desired Outcomes: Within 30 min of onset of pain, patient's subjective perception of angina decreases, as documented by a pain scale. Objective indicators, such as grimacing and diaphoresis, are absent.

INTERVENTIONS	RATIONALES
Assess location, character, and severity of pain. Record severity on a subjective 0 (no pain) to 10 (worst pain) scale. Also record number of NTG tablets needed to relieve each episode, the factor or event that precipitated pain, and alleviating factors. Document angina relief obtained, using pain scale.	To monitor degree, character, precipitator, and trend of pain and document amount of relief obtained, including number of NTG tablets to alleviate it.

Continued

INTERVENTIONS	RATIONALES
Keep sublingual NTG within reach of patient and explain that it is to be taken as soon as angina begins, repeating q5min ×3 if necessary. As prescribed, administer long-acting and/or topical nitrates.	To increase microcirculation, perfusion to the myocardium, and venous dilation. Venous dilation causes pooling of blood in the periphery so that less blood comes back to the right side of the heart. This decrease in return to the right side of the heart lowers O_2 demand.
Stay with patient and provide reassurance during periods of angina. If indicated, request that visitors leave the room.	To reduce anxiety, which might otherwise worsen the angina.
Monitor HR and BP during episodes of chest pain.	To detect irregularities in HR and changes in systolic BP >20 mm Hg from baseline. Increases in both HR and BP signal increased myocardial O_2 demands.
Monitor for presence of headache and hypotension after administering NTG.	Side effects of NTG.
Keep patient recumbent during angina and NTG administration.	To minimize potential for headache/hypotension by enabling better blood return to the heart and head.
Administer O_2 as prescribed.	To increase O_2 supply to the myocardium.
Deliver O_2 with humidity.	To help prevent oxygen's convective drying effects on oral and nasal mucosa.
Emphasize importance of immediately reporting angina to health care team.	Early treatment decreases morbidity and mortality.
Instruct patient to avoid activities and factors known to cause stress.	Stress may precipitate angina.
Discuss value of relaxation techniques, including tapes, soothing music, biofeedback, meditation, or yoga. See **Health-Seeking Behaviors**, p. 183.	To reduce stress and anxiety, which may otherwise precipitate angina.
Administer angiotensin-converting enzyme (ACE) inhibitor as prescribed.	ACE inhibitors block conversion of angiotension I to angiotensin II, which is a potent vasoconstrictor. Subsequently, an ACE inhibitor causes vasodilation of the arterial system, decreasing afterload beyond the aortic valve. Therefore the heart will not have to work as hard during systole against a less vasoconstricted aorta.
Administer β-blockers as prescribed.	These drugs block beta stimulation to the sinoatrial (S-A) node and myocardium. Heart rate and contractility are decreased, subsequently decreasing workload of the heart.
Administer calcium channel blockers as prescribed.	To decrease coronary artery vasospasm, a potential cause of ischemia and subsequent angina.

●●● **Related NIC and NOC labels:** *NIC:* Medication Management; Pain Management; Biofeedback; Emotional Support; Meditation Facilitation; Presence; Simple Relaxation Therapy; Anxiety Reduction; Music Therapy; Oxygen Therapy; Progressive Muscle Relaxation *NOC:* Comfort Level; Pain Control

Nursing Diagnosis:

Activity Intolerance

related to generalized weakness and imbalance between oxygen supply and demand secondary to tissue ischemia (MI)

Desired Outcome: During activity, patient rates perceived exertion at ≤3 on a 0-10 scale and exhibits cardiac tolerance to activity as evidenced by RR ≤20 breaths/min, HR ≤120 bpm (or within 20 bpm of resting HR), systolic BP within 20 mm Hg of patient's resting systolic BP, and absence of chest pain and new dysrhythmias.

INTERVENTIONS	RATIONALES
Observe for and report increasing frequency of angina, angina that occurs at rest, angina that is unrelieved by NTG, or decreased exercise tolerance without angina.	To detect evidence of imbalance between oxygen supply and demand and hence potential activity intolerance.
Assess patient's response to activity.	Chest pain, increase in HR (>20 bpm), change in systolic BP (>20 mm Hg over or under resting BP), excessive fatigue, and shortness of breath are signs of activity intolerance.
Ask patient to rate perceived exertion (RPE).	RPE >3 is a signal to stop the activity.
Assist patient with recognizing and limiting activities that increase oxygen demand such as exercise and anxiety.	To help patient control factors that increase ischemia.
Administer O_2 as prescribed for angina episodes.	To increase oxygen supply to the myocardium.
Deliver O_2 with humidity.	To help prevent oxygen's convective drying effects on oral and nasal mucosa.
Have patient perform ROM exercises, depending on tolerance and prescribed activity limitations.	Cardiac intolerance to activity can be further aggravated by prolonged bedrest.
Consult health care provider about cardiac rehabilitation or in-bed exercises and activities that can be performed by patient as the condition improves.	Enables progressive pacing of patient toward his or her activity potential.
For more detail, see "Prolonged Bedrest" for **Risk for Activity Intolerance,** p. 67, and **Risk for Disuse Syndrome,** p. 69.	

●●● **Related NIC and NOC labels:** *NIC:* Energy Management; Exercise Promotion; Cardiac Care: Rehabilitative; Teaching: Prescribed Activity/Exercise; Oxygen Therapy *NOC:* Activity Tolerance; Energy Conservation

Nursing Diagnosis:

Imbalanced Nutrition: More than body requirements

of calories, sodium, or fats

Desired Outcome: Within the 24-hr period before hospital discharge (or immediately following teaching intervention if patient is not hospitalized), patient demonstrates accurate knowledge of the dietary regimen by planning a 3-day menu that includes and excludes appropriate foods.

INTERVENTIONS	RATIONALES
If patient is over ideal body weight, explain that a low-calorie diet is necessary.	Being overweight is a risk factor for CHD and puts more workload on the heart.
Show patient how to decrease dietary intake of saturated (animal) fats and increase intake of polyunsaturated (vegetable oil) fats.	Reducing dietary saturated fat is effective in lowering risk of heart and blood vessel disease in many individuals.
Teach patient to limit dietary intake of cholesterol to <300 mg/day. Encourage use of food labels to determine cholesterol content of foods.	Reducing cholesterol intake is effective in lowering risk of heart and blood vessel disease in many individuals.
Teach patient to limit dietary intake of refined/processed sugar.	Refined sugars are empty calories that can convert to fat stores.
Teach patient to limit dietary intake of sodium chloride (NaCl) to <4 g/day (mild restriction). Encourage use of food labels to determine Na^+ content of foods.	Increased sodium intake can lead to water retention by the kidneys. This increased fluid/vascular volume puts more work on the heart.

Continued

INTERVENTIONS	RATIONALES
Instruct patient and significant other in use of "Nutrition Facts" (federally mandated public information on all food product labels).	Teaches actual amount of calories, total fat, saturated fat, cholesterol, and sodium in foods and assists in making better food choices. Patient should be especially aware of the serving size listed for respective nutrients; that is, a serving size listed as 4 oz on a package containing 12 oz would mean that patient would get 3 times the amount of each ingredient if the patient eats the entire contents of the container!
Encourage intake of fresh fruits, natural (unrefined or unprocessed) carbohydrates, fish, poultry, legumes, fresh vegetables, and grains.	To ensure a healthy, balanced diet.
Ask patient to use this new knowledge to plan a 3-day menu that includes and excludes appropriate foods.	Applying learned knowledge by return demonstration is a proven way of maintaining knowledge, which optimally also will promote compliance.

●●● **Related NIC and NOC labels:** *NIC:* Weight Reduction Assistance; Nutrition Management; Nutritional Counseling; Teaching: Prescribed Diet; Referral *NOC:* Weight Control; Nutritional Status: Nutrient Intake

Nursing Diagnosis:

Health-Seeking Behaviors:

Relaxation technique effective for stress reduction

Desired Outcome: Patient reports subjective relief of stress after using relaxation technique.

INTERVENTIONS	RATIONALES
Discuss importance of relaxation.	Relaxation helps to decrease nervous system tone (sympathetic), energy requirements, and O_2 consumption. A knowledgeable individual is more likely to comply with this and other techniques that promote relaxation.

Speaking slowly and softly, give patient the following guidelines:
 	
  - Find a comfortable position. Close your eyes.
 	
  - Begin by concentrating on your feet and toes; tighten the muscles in your feet and toes and hold this tightness for a count of three. Now slowly relax your feet and toes. Feel or imagine the tension flowing out of your feet and toes. Now concentrate on your lower legs. Tense the muscles of your lower legs for a count of three. Now slowly release this tightness and feel the tension drain from your lower legs. Continue with this purposeful tightening and relaxation with each successive major body part, moving up the body, until finally you reach your facial muscles. When you reach your face, tighten the muscles of your face for a count of three. When you go to relax the muscles in your face, take a deep breath and exhale. As you breathe out, imagine that you are blowing all the tension of your body out and away from you, leaving you totally relaxed and calm.
	To promote relaxation and decrease energy requirements. Many techniques use breathing, concentration, or imagery. This technique can be used easily by anyone.

Continued

INTERVENTIONS	RATIONALES
- Now breathe through your nose. Concentrate on feeling the air move in and out. As you exhale, say the word *one* silently to yourself. Again continue feeling the air move in and out of your lungs. Continue for approximately 20 min. - Try to clear your mind of worries; be passive. Let relaxation occur. If distractions appear, gently push them away. Continue breathing through your nose, repeating *one* silently. - After approximately 20 min, slowly begin to allow yourself to become aware of your surroundings. Keep your eyes closed for a few moments. - Open your eyes.	
Encourage patient to practice this technique 2-3 times/day or whenever feeling stressed or tense.	Although this technique may feel strange at first, it becomes easier and more effective with each practice.
Suggest that patient play baroque or new-age music during relaxation exercise.	Baroque or new age music, played softly, helps many individuals achieve an even greater state of relaxation.

●●● **Related NIC and NOC labels:** *NIC:* Health Education *NOC:* Health Promoting Behavior

Nursing Diagnosis:

Deficient Knowledge:

Purpose, precautions, and side effects of nitrates

Desired Outcome: Within the 24-hr period before hospital discharge (or immediately following instruction if patient is not hospitalized), patient verbalizes accurate understanding of the purpose, precautions, and side effects of the prescribed nitrates.

INTERVENTIONS	RATIONALES
Teach patient the purpose of the prescribed nitrates (e.g., NTG).	These drugs are given during angina to increase microcirculation, venous dilation, and blood to the myocardium, which should decrease angina. A patient who is knowledgeable about the purpose of this drug will be more likely to comply with the therapy.
Instruct patient to report to health care provider or staff the presence of a headache.	The vasodilation effect of NTG can result in transient headaches, in which case the health care provider may alter the dose.
Teach patient to assume a recumbent position if a headache occurs.	May reduce pain by enabling better blood return to the heart and head.
Instruct patient to rise slowly from a sitting or lying position and to remain by the chair or bed for 1 min after standing.	Vasodilation from nitrates may also decrease BP, which can result in orthostatic hypotension.

●●● **Related NIC and NOC labels:** *NIC:* Teaching: Prescribed Medication *NOC:* Knowledge: Medication

Nursing Diagnosis:

Deficient Knowledge:

Purpose, precautions, and side effects of β-blockers

Desired Outcome: Within the 24-hr period before hospital discharge (or immediately following instruction if patient is not hospitalized), patient verbalizes accurate understanding of the purpose, precautions, and side effects of β-blockers.

INTERVENTIONS	RATIONALES
Teach patient the purpose of β-blockers if prescribed.	These drugs block beta stimulation to the S-A node and myocardium. The heart rate and contractility are decreased, subsequently decreasing the workload of the heart. A patient who is knowledgeable about the purpose of this drug will be more likely to comply with the therapy.
Instruct patient to be alert to depression, fatigue, dizziness, erythematous rash, respiratory distress, and sexual dysfunction.	Can occur as side effects of β-blockers and should be reported to staff or health care provider, who may alter the dose or frequency.
Teach patient how to assess for weight gain and edema and importance of reporting signs and symptoms promptly if they occur.	Weight gain and peripheral and sacral edema can occur as side effects of β-blockers and should be reported promptly for timely intervention.
Explain that BP and HR are assessed before administration of β-blockers.	These drugs can cause hypotension and excessive slowing of the heart.
Caution patient not to omit or abruptly stop taking β-blockers.	May result in rebound tachycardia causing angina or MI.

●●● **Related NIC and NOC labels:** *NIC:* Teaching: Prescribed Medication *NOC:* Knowledge: Medication

Nursing Diagnosis:

Deficient Knowledge:

Disease process and lifestyle implications of CHD

Desired Outcome: Within the 24-hr period before hospital discharge (or following instruction if patient is not hospitalized), patient verbalizes accurate knowledge about the disease process of CHD and the concomitant lifestyle implications.

INTERVENTIONS	RATIONALES
Teach patient about CHD, including pathophysiologic processes of cardiac ischemia, angina, and infarction.	To increase patient's knowledge of health status, which optimally will increase compliance with the treatment regimen.
Assist with identifying risk factors for CHD.	Risk factor identification optimally will result in risk factor modification, including: - Diet low in cholesterol and saturated fat - Smoking cessation - Regular activity/exercise programs

Continued

INTERVENTIONS	**RATIONALES**
Discuss symptoms that necessitate medical attention.	Progression to unstable angina, loss of consciousness, decreased exercise tolerance, angina that is unrelieved by NTG, increasing frequency of angina, and need to increase number of NTG tablets to relieve angina are symptoms that necessitate medical attention to prevent MI.
Discuss guidelines for sexual activity, if indicated.	Resting before intercourse, finding a comfortable position, taking prophylactic NTG, and postponing intercourse for 1-1½ hr after a heavy meal are valid guidelines that help minimize oxygen demand on the heart.
Discuss medical procedures, such as cardiac catheterization, and surgical procedures, such as percutaneous transluminal coronary angioplasty (PTCA), directional coronary atherectomy, and CABG, as appropriate.	Coronary arteriography via cardiac catheterization provides the ultimate diagnosis of CHD. Arterial lesions (plaque) are located, and the amount of occlusion and feasibility for cardiac surgery are determined.
	PTCA improves coronary blood flow by using a balloon inflation catheter to rupture plaque and dilate the artery. A mesh stent is placed to keep the artery open. It is a common alternative to bypass surgery for individuals with discrete lesions.
	Directional coronary atherectomy uses a special catheter that contains a balloon (for stabilization of the catheter), a cutting device that "shaves" the lesion, and a nose cone in which the shaved lesions are placed to remove atherosclerotic deposits in the coronary arteries.
	See "Cardiac Surgery," p. 175, for a discussion of CABG.

●●● **Related NIC and NOC labels:** *NIC:* Teaching: Disease Process; Discharge Planning; Teaching: Prescribed Diet; Teaching: Prescribed Activity/Exercise; Teaching: Procedure/Treatment *NOC:* Knowledge: Disease Process; Knowledge: Illness Care; Knowledge: Treatment/Procedures; Knowledge: Treatment Regimen

PATIENT-FAMILY TEACHING AND DISCHARGE PLANNING

When providing patient-family teaching, focus on sensory information, avoid giving excessive information, and initiate a visiting nurse referral for necessary follow-up teaching. Include verbal and written information about the following:

✓ Medications, including drug name, dosage, purpose, schedule, precautions, drug/drug and food/drug interactions, and potential side effects. Discuss the potential for headache and dizziness after NTG administration. Caution patient about using NTG more frequently than prescribed and notifying health care provider if three tablets do not relieve angina.

✓ If patient will begin taking statin drug (e.g., atorvastatin [Lipitor]) either during hospitalization or after hospital discharge, explain its purpose: The statin drugs are believed to slow the progression of CHD and stabilize the plaque. They may aid in decreasing the inflammatory response, which is a theory currently recognized as the response mechanism in a diseased coronary artery.

✓ If antiplatelet therapy (e.g., aspirin, clopidrogel [Plavix]) has been prescribed, the importance of notifying other health

care providers and recognizing the signs of bleeding. See this section in "Myocardial Infarction," p. 209, for detail.

✓ Importance of reducing or eliminating intake of caffeine, which causes vasoconstriction and increases HR.

✓ Dietary changes: low saturated fat, low Na⁺, low cholesterol, and need for weight loss if appropriate. Encourage use of food labels to determine caloric, cholesterol, fat, and Na⁺ content of foods.

✓ Pulse monitoring: how to self-measure pulse, including parameters for target heart rates and limits.

✓ Prescribed exercise program and importance of maintaining a regular exercise schedule. Remind patient of the need to measure pulse, stop if pain occurs, and stay within prescribed exercise limits. Caution patient not to exercise during extremes of weather (hot or cold), which can place an additional strain on the heart.

✓ Indicators that necessitate medical attention: progression to unstable angina, loss of consciousness, decreased exercise tolerance, unrelieved pain, angina that is unrelieved by NTG, increasing frequency of angina, and need to increase number of NTG tablets to relieve angina. Stress importance of seeking aid of emergency medical services (EMS) and not driving self to emergency center if these indicators occur.

✓ Elimination of smoking; refer patient to a "stop smoking" program as appropriate. The following free brochures outline ways to help patients stop smoking:

- *How to Help Your Patients Stop Using Tobacco: A National Cancer Institute Manual for the Oral Health Team,* from the Smoking and Tobacco Control Program of the National Cancer Institute; call 1-800-4-CANCER.
- *Clinical Practice Guideline: A Quick Reference Guide for Smoking Cessation Specialists,* from the Agency for Health Care Policy and Research (AHCPR); call 1-800-358-9295.

✓ Importance of involvement and support of significant others in patient's lifestyle changes.

✓ Importance of getting BP checked at regular intervals (at least monthly if the patient is hypertensive). Suggest purchase of BP cuff for home use.

✓ Importance of avoiding strenuous activity for at least 1 hr after meals to avoid excessive O_2 demands.

✓ Importance of reporting to health care provider any change in the pattern or frequency of angina.

✓ Sexual activity guidelines:

- Rest is beneficial before sexual activity.
- Medications such as NTG may be taken prophylactically if pain occurs with activity.
- Postpone sexual activity for 1-1½ hr after a meal.

✓ Phone numbers to call should questions or concerns arise about therapy or this condition after discharge. Additional general information can be obtained by contacting the following organization:

National Center for Cardiac Information
8180 Greensboro Drive #1070
McLean, VA 22102
(703) 356-6568

✓ Availability of community and medical support, such as American Heart Association. Either provide the address or phone number for the local chapter or encourage the patient to write for information to the following address:

American Heart Association
7320 Greenville Avenue
Dallas, TX 75231
(800) 242-8721
www.americanheart.org

Dysrhythmias and Conduction Disturbances

D ysrhythmias are abnormal rhythms of the heart's electrical system. They can originate in any part of the conduction system, such as the sinus node, atrium, atrioventricular (A-V) node, His-Purkinje system, bundle branches, and ventricular tissue. Although a variety of diseases may cause dysrhythmias, the most common are coronary heart disease (CHD) and myocardial infarction (MI). Other causes include electrolyte imbalance, changes in oxygenation, and drug toxicity. Cardiac dysrhythmias may result from the following mechanisms

Disturbances in automaticity: May involve an increase or decrease in automaticity in the sinus node (i.e., sinus tachycardia or sinus bradycardia). Premature beats may arise via this mechanism from the atria, junction, or ventricles. Abnormal rhythms, such as atrial or ventricular tachycardia, also may occur.

Disturbances in conductivity: Conduction may be too rapid, as in conditions caused by an accessory pathway (e.g., Wolff-Parkinson-White syndrome), or too slow (e.g., A-V block). Reentry is a situation in which a stimulus reexcites a conduction pathway through which it already has passed. Once started, this impulse may circulate repeatedly. For reentry to occur, there must be two different pathways for conduction: one with slowed conduction and one with unidirectional block.

Combinations of altered automaticity and conductivity: Observed when several dysrhythmias are noted (e.g., first-degree A-V block, or a disturbance in conductivity; and premature atrial contractions, or a disturbance in automaticity).

HEALTH CARE SETTING

Primary care with possible hospitalization in coronary care unit (CCU) resulting from complications

ASSESSMENT

Signs and symptoms: Can vary on a continuum from absence of symptoms to complete cardiopulmonary collapse. General indicators include alterations in level of consciousness (LOC), vertigo, syncope, seizures, weakness, fatigue, activity intolerance, shortness of breath, dyspnea on exertion, chest pain, palpitations, sensation of "skipped beats," anxiety, and restlessness.

Physical assessment: Increases or decreases in HR, BP, and RR; dusky color or pallor; crackles (rales); cool skin; decreased urine output; and paradoxical pulse and abnormal heart sounds (e.g., paradoxical splitting of S_1 and S_2).

Electrocardiogram (ECG): Some findings seen with various dysrhythmias include abnormalities in rate such as sinus bradycardia or sinus tachycardia, irregular rhythm such as atrial fibrillation, extra beats such as premature atrial contractions (PACs) and premature junctional contractions (PJCs), wide and bizarre-looking beats such as premature ventricular contractions (PVCs) and ventricular tachycardia (VT), a fibrillating baseline such as ventricular fibrillation (VF), and a straight line as with asystole.

History and risk factors: CHD, recent MI, electrolyte disturbances, and drug toxicity.

DIAGNOSTIC TESTS

12-lead ECG: To detect dysrhythmias and identify possible cause.

Serum electrolyte levels: To identify electrolyte abnormalities, which can precipitate dysrhythmias. The most common are hyperkalemia, hypokalemia, and hypomagnesemia.

Drug levels: To identify toxicities (e.g., of digoxin, quinidine, procainamide, aminophylline) that can precipitate dysrhythmias.

Ambulatory monitoring (e.g., Holter monitor or cardiac event recorder): To identify subtle dysrhythmias and associate abnormal rhythms by means of the patient's symptoms.

Electrophysiologic study: Invasive test in which two to three catheters are placed into the heart, giving the heart a pacing stimulus at varying sites and of varying voltages. The test determines origin of dysrhythmia, inducibility, and effectiveness of drug therapy or ablation procedure in dysrhythmia suppression.

Exercise stress testing: Used in conjunction with Holter monitoring to detect advanced grades of PVCs (those caused by ischemia) and to guide therapy. During the test, ECG and BP readings are taken while the patient walks on a treadmill or pedals a stationary bicycle; response to a constant or increasing workload is observed. The test continues until the patient reaches target heart rate or symptoms such as chest pain, severe fatigue, dysrhythmias, or abnormal BP occur.

Oximetry or arterial blood gas (ABG) values: To document trend of hypoxemia.

Nursing Diagnosis:

Decreased Cardiac Output

related to altered rate, rhythm, or conduction or negative inotropic changes secondary to cardiac disease

Desired Outcome: Within 1 hr of treatment/intervention, patient has adequate cardiac output as evidenced by BP ≥90/60 mm Hg, HR 60-100 bpm, and normal sinus rhythm on ECG.

INTERVENTIONS	RATIONALES
Monitor patient's heart rhythm continuously.	To determine whether dysrhythmias occur or increase in occurrence.
In the presence of dysrhythmias, assess for signs of decreased cardiac output; document findings. Report significant findings to health care provider.	Signs of decreased cardiac output include decreased BP and symptoms such as unrelieved and prolonged palpitations, chest pain, shortness of breath, rapid pulse (>150 bpm), dizziness, sensation of skipped beat, palpitations, and syncope.
	Decreased cardiac output should be reported promptly for timely intervention. Patient likely will be transferred to CCU for specialized and intensive care and monitoring.
Document dysrhythmias with rhythm strip. Use a 12-lead ECG as necessary.	To identify dysrhythmias and their general trend.
Monitor patient's laboratory data, particularly electrolyte and digoxin levels.	Serum K⁺ levels <3.5 mEq/L or >5 mEq/L can cause dysrhythmias. Digoxin level affects heart rate.
Administer antidysrhythmic agent as prescribed; note patient's response to therapy based on action of the following classifications:	
Class IA: quinidine, procainamide, disopyramide	Decreases depolarization moderately and prolongs repolarization.
Class IB: phenytoin, mexiletine, tocainide	Decreases depolarization and shortens repolarization.
Class IC: encainide, flecainide, propafenone	Significantly decreases depolarization with minimal effect on repolarization.
Class II: β-blockers; propranolol, metoprolol, atenolol, acebutolol	Slows sinus automatically, slows conduction via A-V node, controls ventricular response to supraventricular tachycardias, and shortens the action potential of Purkinje fibers.

Continued

INTERVENTIONS	RATIONALES
Class III: bretylium, amiodarone, sotalol	Increases the action potential and refractory period of Purkinje fibers, increases ventricular fibrillation threshold, restores injured myocardial cell electrophysiology toward normal, and suppresses reentrant dysrhythmias.
Class IV: calcium channel blocker; verapamil, diltiazem, nifedipine	Depresses automaticity in the S-A and A-V nodes, blocks the slow calcium current in the A-V junctional tissue, reduces conduction via the A-V node, and is useful in treating tachydysrhythmias because of A-V junction reentry. This class of drugs also vasodilates.
Provide O_2 as prescribed.	O_2 may be beneficial if dysrhythmias are related to ischemia.
Deliver O_2 with humidity.	To help prevent oxygen's convective drying effects on oral and nasal mucosa.
Maintain a quiet environment and administer pain medications promptly.	Both stress and pain can increase sympathetic tone and cause dysrhythmias.
If life-threatening dysrhythmias occur, initiate emergency procedures and cardiopulmonary resuscitation (CPR; as indicated by advanced cardiac life support [ACLS] protocol). Treat dysrhythmias as prescribed.	To provide circulation to vital organs and restore heart to normal or viable rhythm.
When dysrhythmias occur, stay with patient; provide support and reassurance while performing assessments and administering treatment.	To reduce stress and provide comfort, which optimally will decrease dysrhythmias.

●●● **Related NIC and NOC labels:** *NIC:* Dysrhythmia Management; Cardiac Care: Acute; Electrolyte Monitoring; Vital Signs Monitoring; Medication Administration; Emergency Care *NOC:* Cardiac Pump Effectiveness; Vital Signs Status

Nursing Diagnosis:

Deficient Knowledge:

Mechanism by which dysrhythmias occur and lifestyle implications

Desired Outcome: Within the 24-hr period before hospital discharge (or immediately after teaching if patient is not hospitalized), patient and significant other verbalize accurate knowledge about causes of dysrhythmias and implications for patient's lifestyle modifications.

INTERVENTIONS	RATIONALES
Discuss causal mechanisms for dysrhythmias, including resulting symptoms. Use a heart model or diagrams as necessary.	To increase patient's knowledge about health status. Visual aids augment understanding of verbal information. A knowledgeable patient is more likely to comply with the treatment.
Teach signs and symptoms of dysrhythmias that necessitate medical attention.	Indicators such as unrelieved and prolonged palpitations, chest pain, shortness of breath, rapid pulse (>150 bpm), dizziness, and syncope are serious and should be reported promptly for timely intervention.

Continued

INTERVENTIONS	RATIONALES
Teach patient and significant other how to check pulse rate for a full minute.	Checking pulse for a full minute ensures a better average of the rate and rhythm than if it were measured for 15 seconds and multiplied by 4.
Teach patient and significant other about medications that will be taken after hospital discharge, including drug name, purpose, dosage, schedule, precautions, drug/drug and food/drug interactions, and potential side effects.	The more knowledgeable the patient is, the more likely he or she is to comply with therapy and report side effects and complications promptly for timely intervention.
Stress that patient will be taking long-term antidysrhythmic therapy and that it could be life-threatening to stop or skip these medications without health care provider's approval.	Stopping treatment may decrease blood levels effective for dysrhythmia suppression.
Advise patient and significant other about the availability of support groups and counseling; provide appropriate community referrals. Explain that anxiety and fear, along with periodic feelings of denial, depression, anger, and confusion, are normal following this experience.	Patients who survive sudden cardiac arrest may experience nightmares or other sleep disturbances at home.
Stress importance of leading a normal and productive life.	This may seem difficult for a patient who fears breakthrough of life-threatening dysrhythmias and alters his or her life accordingly.
If patient is going on vacation, advise taking along sufficient medication and investigating health care facilities in the area.	Being informed of local medical facilities may help reduce stress.
Advise patient and significant other to take CPR classes; provide addresses of community programs.	To learn emergency life-saving procedure in the event that it becomes necessary.
Explain dietary restrictions that individuals with recurrent dysrhythmias should follow. Discuss need for reduced intake of products containing caffeine, including coffee, tea, chocolate, and colas. Because of the overlap between dysrhythmias and CHD, provide instruction for a general low-cholesterol diet. Encourage patients to use food labels to determine cholesterol content of foods.	Caffeine is a stimulant that can cause abnormal heart rhythms. Patients with CHD require a low-cholesterol diet to decrease hyperlipidemia.
As indicated, teach patient relaxation techniques. See **Health-Seeking Behaviors:** Relaxation technique effective for stress reduction, p. 183.	To reduce stress and enable patient to decrease sympathetic tone.

If patient has had an implantable cardioverter-defibrillator (ICD) inserted, teach the following:

INTERVENTIONS	RATIONALES
The ICD is programmed to deliver the electrical stimulus at a predetermined rate and/or after assessing morphology of the ECG. First- and second-generation ICDs provide for only cardioversion or defibrillation; third-generation ICDs also provide overdrive pacing and backup ventricular pacing.	ICD is recommended for patients who have survived an episode of sudden cardiac death (cardiac arrest), patients with CHD who have had a cardiac arrest, and those in whom conventional antidysrhythmic therapy has failed.
The pulse generator, which is powered by lithium batteries, is surgically inserted (in the operating room [OR] or catheterization laboratory) into a "pocket" formed in the pectoral area. Leads are tunneled beneath the skin from the pocket to the subclavian vein through which they are advanced to the right ventricle.	
Postoperative complications include atelectasis, pneumonia, seroma at the generator "pocket," pneumothorax, and thrombosis. Lead migration and lead fracture are the two most common structural problems. Interference from unipolar pacemakers and "myopotentials" (electrical interference) are common mechanical complications.	Patient should be informed of these complications and structural problems to report them promptly for timely intervention.

Continued

INTERVENTIONS	RATIONALES
ICDs may need to be deactivated during surgical procedures, use of electrocautery, and magnetic resonance imaging (MRI).	Some procedures interfere with and may change programming of the device. In addition, the ICD may "see" these procedures as a dysrhythmia and shock the patient.
Patient should keep a pocket card on hand with all relevant ICD data on it.	Ensures that medical information is available at all times should a medical event occur.
Explain importance of follow-up care; confirm date and time of next appointment if known.	Ensures proper functioning of device. Outpatient Holter monitoring also may be performed periodically.
If patient has had radio frequency (RF) ablation, teach the following:	
This is a procedure in which the catheter is placed in the heart via cardiac catheterization. RF waves are applied to the area in which the dysrhythmia originates, causing controlled, localized necrosis of the area.	This procedure is used for conduction disturbances such as Wolff-Parkinson-White syndrome and some forms of A-V block.

●●● **Related NIC and NOC labels:** *NIC:* Teaching: Disease Process; Teaching: Individual; Discharge Planning; Teaching: Prescribed Medication; Teaching: Procedure/Treatment; Teaching: Psychomotor Skills *NOC:* Knowledge: Disease Process; Knowledge: Illness Care; Knowledge: Treatment Procedures; Knowledge: Medication; Knowledge: Diet; Knowledge: Prescribed Activity

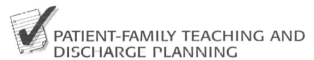

PATIENT-FAMILY TEACHING AND DISCHARGE PLANNING

See **Deficient Knowledge,** earlier, as well as patient's primary diagnosis.

Heart Failure

Heart (cardiac) failure is not a disease in and of itself, it is the end product of a variety of insults to the heart that result in its failure as a pump. Heart failure is the state in which the heart is unable to pump blood at a rate sufficient to meet metabolic requirements of the tissues. With systolic dysfunction, there is abnormal contraction of the pumping chambers of the heart; whereas with diastolic dysfunction the pumping chamber may contract normally, but it is stiff and does not relax properly. Heart failure can occur as a result of myocardial or cardiac muscle damage, such as after large infarcts, or when an adequate cardiac muscle is stressed or forced to work harder over a period of time. When the heart is unable to pump sufficient blood to meet metabolic demands, it relies on three main compensatory mechanisms.

- **Increasing cardiac fluid** to increase fiber length and subsequent force of contraction (Frank-Starling law).
- **Increasing catecholamine discharge** (epinephrine and norepinephrine) to increase contractility.
- **Myocardial hypertrophy** to increase the mass of working contractile tissue. The hypertrophy will be either right sided, left sided, or both, depending on the cause of failure.

HEALTH CARE SETTING

Primary care with possible hospitalization resulting from complications

ASSESSMENT

Signs and symptoms: Orthopnea, nocturnal dyspnea, dyspnea on exertion (DOE), fatigue, chest pain, dizziness, weakness, nocturia, cardiac cachexia (malnutrition/wasting), and confusion, which can occur late in the disease. In addition, decreased right ventricular output can cause increased central venous pressure (CVP), distended neck veins, and peripheral edema; decreased left ventricular output can cause dyspnea and shortness of breath, as well as other indicators of pulmonary edema.

Physical assessment: Decreased BP, dysrhythmias, tachycardia, tachypnea, increased venous pulsations and pressure, crackles (rales), pitting edema, ascites, galloping heart sounds, and pulsus alternans (alternating strong and weak heartbeats). Cardiac monitor would show ventricular ectopy and possibly ventricular tachycardia. Hepatomegaly may occur in the presence of right-sided or left-sided heart failure.

History of: Sleeping on extra pillows to enhance respirations, decreased exercise tolerance, increasing shortness of breath, coronary heart disease (CHD), and risk factors for CHD, including family history, increasing age, male gender, smoking, low high-density lipoprotein (HDL), high serum lipid levels, increased homocysteine level, diabetes mellitus, hypertension, obesity, glucose intolerance, and sedentary and stressful lifestyle.

DIAGNOSTIC TESTS

Chest x-ray examination: Will show cardiomegaly and engorged pulmonary vasculature.

Serum electrolytes: May reveal hyponatremia (dilutional); hyperkalemia if glomerular filtration is decreased; or hypokalemia, which can result from some diuretics.

Serum enzymes: May reveal an elevated aspartate aminotransferase (AST) level with hepatic congestion and decreased liver function.

Serum bilirubin: May reveal hyperbilirubinemia in the presence of liver dysfunction following hepatomegaly with right-sided heart failure.

Complete blood count (CBC): May reveal decreased Hgb and Hct levels in the presence of anemia.

B-type natriuretic peptide (BNP): BNP is a hormone secreted from the heart's ventricles in response to increased pressure and volume in the organ. BNP helps relieve this stress by promoting release of fluid and sodium from the body. BNP levels may be elevated in the blood of people with heart failure.

Serum albumin: Albumin levels may be helpful in determining a patient's nutritional status, as well as effective circulating proteins in the vascular space. Lower protein levels in the blood are associated with an increased risk of third spacing of fluids.

Invasive hemodynamic monitoring: Patients in critical care most likely will have pulmonary artery (PA) catheters placed into the right side of the heart. Measurement of volume levels, cardiac output, and pressures inside the chambers helps diagnose fluid levels and heart performance.

Ejection fraction (EF): Provides an indirect measure of the effectiveness of the heart as a pump. EF is the fraction (pro-portion) of the blood ejected from the left ventricle during systole. This may be determined via cardiac catheterization or echocardiogram.

Noninvasive testing: Impedance cardiography is a non-invasive technique that follows the trend of fluid and cardiac performance via strategic placement of electrodes. Parameters include cardiac output/index and thoracic fluid content.

Nursing Diagnosis:

Excess Fluid Volume

related to presence of compensatory regulatory mechanisms secondary to decreased cardiac output

Desired Outcome: Within the 24-hr period after treatment or before hospital discharge, patient becomes normovolemic as evidenced by urinary output $\geq$30 ml/hr, balanced I&O, stable weight (or weight loss attributable to fluid loss), edema $\leq$1+ on a 0-4+ scale, HR $\leq$100 bpm, and absence of crackles (rales) and S_3 heart sound.

INTERVENTIONS	RATIONALES
Auscultate lung fields at least q8h; report presence of crackles.	Crackles occur with fluid volume excess and left-sided heart failure.
Monitor and document I&O at least q8h. Report imbalances, including urinary output <30 ml/hr.	Decreased urinary output can occur with decreased cardiac output, which can cause decreasing renal blood flow.
Monitor weight daily and report unusual gains. Be alert to presence of pitting edema.	Weight gain and pitting edema occur with excess fluid retention and heart failure.
	Their presence is a key determinate of whether a patient should be readmitted to the hospital or treated on an outpatient basis. If diligent assessment is maintained, rehospitalization can be decreased tremendously.
	To assess for pitting edema, apply firm pressure to the edematous area with a finger. If indentation remains after the finger has been removed, pitting edema is present.
Auscultate heart sounds; be alert to S_3 gallop.	S_3 gallop is an early sign of left-sided heart failure and is a defining characteristic of excess fluid volume.
Administer diuretics as prescribed.	To promote normovolemia by controlling fluid accumulation and reducing blood volume.
Observe for hypotension, decreased CVP (<5 cm H_2O [if available]), and tachycardia.	These indicators of decreased effective circulating volume can occur because of the disease process (fluids shift from the vascular space into the interstitial space [third spacing] caused by high fluid volume and decreased proteins) and diuretics, which remove much of the remaining fluid in the vascular space.
Monitor potassium (K^+) levels and notify health care provider of levels <3.5 mEq/L.	Potassium loss can occur with use of some diuretics, such as furosemide.
If appropriate, teach importance of decreasing intake of Na^+ (or table salt).	Hypernatremia can promote excess fluid retention.

Continued

INTERVENTIONS	RATIONALES
Administer nesiritide (Natrecor) IV infusion if it is prescribed.	Natrecor belongs to a new class of drugs called human B-type natriuretic peptides (hBNP) and is made by genetically recombining the hBNP naturally found in the body. This medication helps to improve breathing by decreasing shortness of breath and helps to decrease vascular volume by increasing urinary output.
If fluids are limited, help relieve thirst by offering ice chips or popsicles. Record amount of intake on I&O record.	To provide minimal amounts of fluid while helping to relieve thirst. **Note:** Some care centers recommend small amounts of room-temperature water instead because it appears to relieve thirst better.
As prescribed, administer blood products or albumin.	Blood products and albumin are colloids/protein that play a part in intravascular volume homeostasis. Protein levels must be maintained in order for patient to retain water in the vascular space. Water moves to areas of higher concentration of solutes and pressure. If proteins are decreased in the vascular space, water moves to the interstitial space (third spacing). In addition, patients in a chronic sick state may have depleted levels of protein because of decreased oral protein intake.

●●● **Related NIC and NOC labels:** *NIC:* Fluid/Electrolyte Management; Fluid Monitoring; Hypervolemia Management; Laboratory Data Interpretation; Nutrition Management; Vital Signs Monitoring; Cardiac Care: Acute; Respiratory Monitoring *NOC:* Fluid Balance; Electrolyte & Acid-Base Balance

Nursing Diagnosis:

Deficient Knowledge:

Purpose, precautions, and side effects of diuretic therapy

Desired Outcome: Within the 24-hr period before hospital discharge (or immediately after teaching if patient is not hospitalized), patient verbalizes accurate knowledge of the purpose, precautions, and side effects of diuretic therapy.

INTERVENTIONS	RATIONALES
Teach patient the purpose of the prescribed diuretic.	These drugs control fluid accumulation and reduce blood volume. A patient who is knowledgeable about purpose of the drug will be more likely to comply with the therapy.
Depending on type of diuretic used, teach patient to report signs and symptoms of the following:	A knowledgeable patient will know how to monitor for and report symptoms that necessitate medical attention.
- *Hypokalemia:* anorexia, irregular pulse, nausea, apathy, and muscle cramps.	Use of furosemide, a potassium-wasting diuretic, can cause these symptoms.
- *Hyperkalemia:* muscle weakness, hyporeflexia, and irregular HR (ventricular ectopy if on cardiac monitoring), which can occur with K^+-sparing diuretics.	Use of amiloride, a K^+-sparing diuretic, can cause these symptoms.
- *Hyponatremia:* fatigue, weakness, and edema.	Use of bumetanide, a diuretic that promotes excretion of NaCl, may cause these symptoms.

Continued

INTERVENTIONS	RATIONALES
For patients on long-term diuretic therapy, explain importance of follow-up monitoring of blood levels of Na⁺ and K⁺.	Although the most common electrolyte problem with diuretic use is hypokalemia, the potential for hyperkalemia and electrolyte imbalance of sodium continues with long-term therapy.
For patients receiving K⁺-wasting diuretics (e.g., furosemide), teach need to consume high-potassium foods.	Foods high in potassium content, such as apricots, bananas, oranges, and raisins, will help replenish potassium lost via diuretics.
As appropriate, instruct patient to use care when rising from a sitting or recumbent position.	To prevent injury from orthostatic hypotension, which can occur with diuretic use because of diuresis.

●●● **Related NIC and NOC labels:** *NIC:* Teaching: Prescribed Medication *NOC:* Knowledge: Medication

Nursing Diagnosis:

Deficient Knowledge:

Purpose, precautions, and side effects of digitalis therapy

Desired Outcome: Within the 24-hr period before hospital discharge (or immediately following teaching for a patient who is not hospitalized), patient verbalizes accurate understanding of the purpose, precautions, and side effects of digitalis therapy.

INTERVENTIONS	RATIONALES
Teach patient the purpose of digitalis therapy.	Digitalis slows conduction through the atrioventricular (A-V) node and increases strength of contractility. Although not a first-line drug as originally believed for heart failure patients, it is used for dysrhythmia management when atrial fibrillation coexists. A patient who is knowledgeable about the purpose of digitalis will be more likely to comply with the therapy.
Teach technique and importance of assessing HR before taking digitalis.	Although patient should obtain HR parameters from health care provider, digitalis is usually withheld when HR is <60 bpm (unless patient's usual HR before digitalis administration is <60 bpm).
Also instruct patient to hold dose if there is a ≥20 bpm change from his or her normal rate.	May signal that patient is receiving too much medication and should be reported to health care provider.
Teach patient to notify health care provider if he or she has omitted a dose because of a slow or significantly changed HR.	Dose adjustment may be necessary if a slowing of the HR persists.
Explain that serum K⁺ levels are monitored routinely.	Low K⁺ levels can potentiate digitalis toxicity.
Explain that apical HR and peripheral pulses are assessed by health care provider for irregularity.	Irregularity may signal presence of dysrhythmias (i.e., heart block), which is associated with digitalis toxicity.
Teach patient to be alert to nausea, vomiting, anorexia, headache, diarrhea, blurred vision, yellow-haze vision, and mental confusion. Explain importance of reporting signs and symptoms promptly to health care provider or staff if they occur.	These are indicators of digitalis toxicity and necessitate prompt medical attention.
For more information see **Decreased Cardiac Output,** p. 200.	

●●● **Related NIC and NOC labels:** *NIC:* Teaching: Prescribed Medication *NOC:* Knowledge: Medication

Nursing Diagnosis:

Deficient Knowledge:

Purpose, precautions, and side effects of vasodilators

Desired Outcome: Within the 24-hr period before hospital discharge (or immediately after teaching if patient is not hospitalized), patient verbalizes accurate understanding of the purpose, precautions, and side effects of vasodilators.

INTERVENTIONS	RATIONALES
Teach patient the purpose of vasodilator therapy.	Vasodilators such as sodium nitroprusside, nitroglycerin, angiotensin-converting enzyme (ACE) inhibitors, α-blockers, and angiotensin II receptor blockers, decrease afterload by dilating the arteries to decrease workload of the left ventricle. Nitroglycerin is a vasodilator that also decreases preload by reducing blood flow to the right side of the heart, which reduces right-sided workload. A patient who is knowledgeable about the purpose of vasodilators is more likely to comply with the therapy.
Explain that a headache can occur after administration of a vasodilator.	Headache may occur because of dilation of the cranial vessels or from orthostatic hypotension.
Suggest that if this occurs patient should lie down.	A supine position may help alleviate the pain by increasing blood flow to the heart and head, although increasing blood flow to the head may worsen the headache. Pain medication and decreasing dosage of the drug may be necessary
Teach importance of assessment for weight gain and signs of peripheral or sacral edema.	A possible side effect of vasodilator therapy is a decrease in venous return to the right side of the heart with subsequent accumulation in the periphery
For patients on long-term ACE inhibitor therapy, explain importance of follow-up monitoring of blood levels of serum creatinine	ACE inhibitors may cause kidney damage, resulting in decreased creatinine clearance. If this occurs, patient may need to be taken off the drug.
Instruct patients taking ACE inhibitors to notify health care provider if a cough develops.	Cough is a common and expected side effect of ACE inhibitors. If the cough becomes severe, the health care provider may consider replacement with an angiotensin receptor blocker (ARB). Examples of ARBs include (losartan (Cozaar), valsartan (Diovan), irbesartan (Avapro), and candesartan (Atacand).
Teach importance of using care when rising from a sitting or recumbent position.	To prevent injury from orthostatic hypotension, a potential side effect of ACE inhibitors.
Teach technique and importance of assessing BP before taking medication.	Vasodilators can cause an excessive reduction in BP; therefore patient should be taught BP monitoring technique and importance of BP assessment before taking each dose. It is possible to purchase automatic BP machines from local pharmacies. If necessary, reimbursement or funding information can be obtained from a social worker.
Explain that patient should obtain BP parameters from health care provider.	Although patient will need to obtain actual parameters from health care provider, the drug is usually withheld when BP is <90/60 mm Hg.
Teach patient to notify health care provider if he or she has omitted a dose because of a low or significantly changed BP.	It may be necessary to lower the dose or change the drug.

●●● **Related NIC and NOC labels:** *NIC:* Teaching: Prescribed Medication *NOC:* Knowledge: Medication

Nursing Diagnosis:

Deficient Knowledge:

Purpose, precautions, and side effects of β-blockers

Desired Outcome: Within the 24-hr period before hospital discharge (or immediately following teaching if patient is not hospitalized), patient verbalizes accurate understanding of the purpose, precautions, and side effects of β-blockers.

INTERVENTIONS	RATIONALES
Teach patient the purpose of β-blocker therapy	These drugs decrease HR and myocardial irritability, thereby decreasing myocardial workload. A patient knowledgeable about the purpose of the β-blocker will be more likely to comply with the therapy.
Teach patient possible side effects of β-blockers.	Possible side effects of β-blockers include depression, fatigue, dizziness, erythematous rash, respiratory distress, and sexual dysfunction.
Explain importance of notifying health care provider promptly if these side effects occur.	Health care provider may lower the dose or frequency if these symptoms occur.
Explain that BP and HR are assessed before administration of β-blockers.	These drugs can cause hypotension and excessive slowing of the heart; values outside prescribed parameters may necessitate dose modification by health care provider.
Caution patient not to omit or abruptly stop taking β-blockers.	May result in rebound tachycardia causing angina or myocardial infarction (MI).

●●● **Related NIC and NOC labels:** *NIC:* Teaching: Prescribed Medication *NOC:* Knowledge: Medication

Nursing Diagnosis:

Decreased Cardiac Output

related to negative inotropic changes (decreased cardiac contractility) secondary to compensatory regulatory mechanisms and loss of myocardial muscle function

Desired Outcomes: Patient has adequate cardiac output within 1 hr of treatment/intervention as evidenced by systolic BP ≥90 mm Hg, HR ≤100 bpm, urinary output ≥30 ml/hr, RR 12-20 breaths/min with normal depth and pattern (eupnea), O_2 saturation >92%, absence of crackles (rales) and S_3 heart sound, edema ≤1+ on a 0-4+ scale, and orientation to person, place, and time. Peripheral pulse amplitude is >2+ on a 0-4+ scale.

INTERVENTIONS	RATIONALES
Assess for and document restlessness and/or change in mental status or level of consciousness (LOC), extra heart sounds (e.g., S_3), decreased peripheral pulse amplitude, systolic BP <90 mm Hg, HR >100 bpm, and O_2 saturation (via oximetry readings) ≤92%.	These signs and symptoms signal decreased cardiac output. Cardiac output declines as heart failure progresses.
Monitor for and report dyspnea, crackles, and shortness of breath.	Indicators of fluid accumulation in the lungs and may be a direct indicator of left ventricular failure and decreased cardiac output.

Continued

INTERVENTIONS	RATIONALES
Administer O₂ as prescribed, usually 2-4 L/min per nasal cannula.	To increase oxygen delivery to the myocardium and improve prognosis. Hypoxia adds stress to the compromised myocardium.
Deliver O₂ with humidity.	To help prevent convective drying effect of oxygen on oral and nasal mucosa.
Raise head of bed (HOB) 30 degrees or place patient in position of comfort.	To decrease work of breathing and reduce cardiac workload.
Be alert to and report decreasing urine output (particularly <30 ml/hr) and increasing specific gravity (>1.030).	Can occur as a result of decreased cardiac contractility causing decreased renal perfusion and fluid retention.
Assess for peripheral (sacral, pedal) edema.	Can occur with right-sided MI/heart failure.
Be aware that dysrhythmia management may be necessary under guidance of an electrophysiologist/cardiologist.	Dysrhythmias have become a major factor in quality-of-life issues and rehospitalization in patients with heart failure. Many of those patients require an implantable cardioverter-defibrillator (ICD) because of repeated life-threatening episodes of ventricular tachycardia from an irritable myocardium. Patients with ventricular asynchrony, as seen in bundle branch blocks, may benefit from a biventricular pacer. Pacing each ventricle in synchrony may result in a better cardiac output.
Administer milrinone (Primacor), dobutamine, ACE inhibitors, and vasodilators as prescribed.	These medications increase cardiac contractility and decrease resistance in the arterial system to promote cardiac output.
If the patient is unstable, prepare patient for possible transfer to coronary care unit (CCU).	For close monitoring.

ADDITIONAL NURSING DIAGNOSES/ PROBLEMS:

PATIENT-FAMILY TEACHING AND DISCHARGE PLANNING

When providing patient-family teaching, focus on sensory information, avoid giving excessive information, and initiate a visiting nurse referral for necessary follow-up teaching. Include verbal and written information about the following:

✓ Medications, including drug name, purpose, dosage, schedule, precautions, drug/drug and food/drug interactions, and potential side effects. Stress importance of taking medications regularly and not stopping them without health care provider consultation. Teach patient and significant other how to measure HR for digitalis therapy and/or BP for ACE inhibitor and β-blocker therapy.

✓ Diet: Advise patient that Na⁺ restriction may be lessened as cardiac function improves. Assist with diet planning or refer to a nutrition specialist if major dietary changes are necessary. Encourage patients to use food labels to determine Na⁺ content of foods.

✓ Signs and symptoms that necessitate medical attention: irregular pulse, bradycardia, unusual shortness of breath, increased orthopnea, decreased exercise tolerance, and unusual or steady weight gain.

✓ Importance of quitting smoking, which causes vasoconstriction and increases cardiac workload. Refer patient to a "stop smoking" program as appropriate. The following free brochures outline ways to help patients stop smoking:

- *How to Help Your Patients Stop Using Tobacco: A National Cancer Institute Manual for the Oral Health Team,* from the Smoking and Tobacco Control Program of the National Cancer Institute; call 1-800-4-CANCER.
- *Clinical Practice Guideline: A Quick Reference Guide for Smoking Cessation Specialists,* from the Agency for Health Care Policy and Research (AHCPR); call 1-800-358-9295.

✓ Importance of limiting exertional activities at home (e.g., minimize bending and lifting and avoid stair climbing).

However, stress importance of a progressive increase in activity to prevent problems of deconditioning.

✓Dysrhythmia management as indicated. Many of these patients may need an ICD. See discussion under **Decreased Cardiac Output,** earlier. Also see "Dysrhythmias and Conduction Disturbances," p. 189.

✓Emergency phone numbers to call if needed.

✓Importance of follow-up care; confirm date and time of next medical appointment.

Myocardial Infarction

Ischemic heart disease accounts for approximately one third of all deaths in the United States, and of patients with ischemic heart disease, half die because of myocardial infarction (MI). Most MIs are caused by critical narrowing of the coronary arteries as a result of atherosclerosis followed by thrombus formation or coronary artery spasm. When ischemia is prolonged and unrelieved, irreversible damage (infarction) occurs. MI can occur in various areas of the heart, depending on location of the coronary artery occlusion and distribution of blood supply.

HEALTH CARE SETTING

Acute care, coronary care unit (CCU), emergency care, cardiac rehabilitation unit

ASSESSMENT

Signs and symptoms: Chest pain, substernal pressure and burning, pain that radiates to the jaw, shoulder, or arm. Weakness, diaphoresis, nausea, vomiting, and acute anxiety also can occur. HR can be abnormally slow (bradycardia) or rapid (tachycardia). Nontraditional indicators include vague feelings of not feeling well or flulike symptoms. Some individuals have no symptoms at all.

Physical assessment: Possible minor hypotension, increasing RR, and crackles (rales) if ventricular failure occurs. Temperature elevations to 39.4° C (104° F) can occur secondary to the inflammatory process. Intensity of S_1 and S_2 heart sounds may be decreased, and pulmonary congestion will occur if papillary muscle rupture has occurred. S_3 and S_4 sounds may be present if heart failure has occurred.

History of: Sudden onset of intense chest pain that is unrelieved by stopping activity or taking nitroglycerin (NTG), positive family history, cigarette smoking, hypercholesterolemia, hypertension, obesity, diabetes mellitus, and stressful or sedentary lifestyle.

DIAGNOSTIC TESTS

Serum enzymes: Will reveal myocardial muscle damage. Myocardial necrosis is associated with a release of enzymes,

myoglobin, and contractile proteins. Troponin T and troponin I are diagnostic cardiac markers that increase 3 hr after injury and are preferred because they remain elevated for 10-14 days. Serial examination (q6h × 3) of the CPK-MB isoenzyme is useful to quantify the amount of MI and to time the onset of infarction.

Serial electrocardiograms (ECGs): For comparison with the baseline. Lead changes, including ST-segment elevation, T-wave inversion, and formation of Q waves, identify the area of infarct.

Chest x-ray examination: May reveal cardiomegaly and signs of left ventricular failure.

Stress tests: See "Coronary Heart Disease," p. 179, for discussion of ischemia and myocardial viability assessment after MI.

Radionuclide studies: Noninvasive diagnostic testing to determine functioning of the cardiac muscle. They are used to localize area of infarct and determine level of contractility. See discussion in "Coronary Heart Disease," p. 179.

Echocardiography: Detects abnormalities in the valves and ventricular wall motion, which usually correspond to the ECG site of infarction.

Transesophageal echocardiography (TEE): Provides clearer ultrasonic images of the heart by avoiding interposition of subcutaneous tissues, bony thorax, and lungs. A high-frequency transducer on an endoscope is placed in the esophagus behind the heart or advanced to the stomach to allow an inferior view of the heart.

Hemodynamic monitoring in the CCU: Measures cardiac output and pulmonary artery pressures, which may reflect significant myocardial injury and dysfunction.

Angiocardiography: Determines areas of stenosis or occlusion and suitability for coronary artery bypass grafting (CABG) or percutaneous transluminal coronary angioplasty (PTCA). This test remains the gold standard for assessing cardiac perfusion.

Arterial blood gas (ABG) analysis: May reveal hypoxemia (decreased partial pressure of dissolved oxygen in arterial blood

[PaO_2]) and hyperventilation (decreased partial pressure of dissolved carbon dioxide in arterial blood [$PaCO_2$]).

Complete blood count (CBC): May reveal leukocytosis secondary to the inflammatory process.

See "Coronary Heart Disease," p. 179, for a discussion of additional markers for assessing cardiac and vascular disease.

Nursing Diagnosis:

Acute Pain

related to ischemia and infarction of myocardial tissue

Desired Outcomes: Patient's subjective perception of pain decreases within 30 min of onset as documented by a pain scale. Objective indicators, such as grimacing and diaphoresis, are absent. Within 1 hr of interventions, VS return to baseline and ECG changes resolve.

INTERVENTIONS	RATIONALES
Along with VS, assess location, character, duration, and intensity of pain. Use a pain scale, rating pain from 0 (no pain) to 10 (worst pain patient has ever experienced).	To quantify character, location, duration, and intensity of discomfort. The pain scale enables comparison to baseline to quantify degree of relief obtained.
Also use the PQRST mnemonic.	The PQRST mnemonic facilitates detailed information about the chest pain and its cause, and some components may help differentiate cardiac causes from noncardiac causes.
	- **P** = Provoked/palliative: Was the pain provoked by activity, or what preceded the pain? For example, cardiac causes may include exercising and yard work. An example of a noncardiac cause may be a sports injury involving a blow to the right chest that results in a collapsed lung.
	- **Q** = Quality: Patient describes characteristics of the pain (e.g., burning, crushing, stabbing).
	- **R** = Region/radiation: Where did the pain start; does the pain radiate anywhere (e.g., jaw, arm, shoulder)?
	- **S** = Severity: Pain is rated on a scale of 0-10 (0 being no pain and 10 being most painful).
	- **T** = Timing: Description of duration of the pain and time of day symptoms began.
Assess for discomfort symptoms associated with MI.	Nausea, vomiting, dyspnea, orthopnea, diaphoresis, weakness, fatigue, anxiety, and apprehension also may be present in acute MI.
Obtain ECG strip and/or 12-lead ECG.	To assess cardiac rhythm for ST-segment changes along with the pain and possibly determine whether patient is experiencing acute MI or angina/myocardial ischemia. ST-segment elevation is usually consistent with acute MI, although ST-segment depression may signal reciprocal changes opposite the area of injury. ST-segment depression and T-wave inversion are seen with ischemia.
Assess and document BP and HR with episodes of pain.	BP and HR may increase because of sympathetic stimulation that occurs with pain, or the body's response to a decrease in BP and HR may stimulate the sympathetic nervous system, causing catecholamine release to increase these values.
	A decrease in BP and HR may occur as a result of parasympathetic stimulation common in inferior and septal MIs.

Continued

INTERVENTIONS	RATIONALES
Assess for nausea.	May signal ischemia when inferior or right side of heart is involved.
Administer prescribed pain medications (usually morphine sulfate) and document quality of relief obtained, using pain scale.	Morphine is an opiate analgesic and vasodilator. Not only does it reduce pain, but its secondary dilatory effects can reduce myocardial ischemia as well.
Administer NTG as prescribed.	NTG is a vasodilator that decreases myocardial ischemia to promote pain relief.
Time the interval from administration to expressed relief using the pain scale.	To assess effectiveness of pain medication.
Provide reassurance during episodes of pain; stay with patient if possible.	To reduce anxiety, which might otherwise increase the pain.
Observe for and report hypotension, slowed RR, and decreased level of consciousness (LOC).	Possible side effects of pain medications.
Administer O_2 as prescribed, usually 2-4 L/min per nasal cannula.	To increase oxygen supply to the myocardium, which likely will reduce or eliminate discomfort. Hypoxia adds stress to the compromised myocardium.
Deliver O_2 with humidity.	To help prevent oxygen's convective drying effects on oral and nasal mucosa.
Elevate head of bed (HOB) 30 degrees or in position of comfort.	Elevating HOB enables better expansion of the lungs to promote ventilation and gas exchange. The resulting decreased work of breathing (WOB) promotes comfort.
If appropriate, prepare patient for transport to CCU or cardiac catheterization laboratory.	For close monitoring or emergency intervention.

●●● **Related NIC and NOC labels:** *NIC:* Pain Management; Medication Administration; Positioning; Presence; Anxiety Reduction; Oxygen Therapy *NOC:* Comfort Level

Nursing Diagnosis:

Decreased Cardiac Output

related to negative inotropic changes (decreased cardiac contractility) secondary to ischemia and infarction

Desired Outcomes: Patient has adequate cardiac output within 1 hr of treatment/intervention as evidenced by systolic BP ≥90 mm Hg; HR ≤100 bpm; urinary output ≥30 ml/hr; RR 12-20 breaths/min with normal depth and pattern (eupnea); O_2 saturation >92%; absence of crackles (rales); edema ≤1+ on a 0-4+ scale; orientation to person, place, and time; and peripheral pulse amplitude >2+ on a 0-4+ scale. If hemodynamic monitoring is used, the following values are present within 24 hr of this diagnosis: measured cardiac output (CO) 4-7 L/min, right atrial pressure (RAP) 4-6 mm Hg, pulmonary artery pressure (PAP) 20-30/8-15 mm Hg, and pulmonary artery wedge pressure (PAWP) 6-12 mm Hg.

INTERVENTIONS	RATIONALES
Assess for and document the following: restlessness and/or change in mental status or LOC, extra heart sounds (e.g., S_3), decreased peripheral pulse amplitude, systolic BP <90 mm Hg, HR >100 bpm, and O_2 saturation (via oximetry readings) ≤92%.	Indicators of decreased cardiac output.

Continued

INTERVENTIONS	RATIONALES
Observe for and report dyspnea, crackles, and shortness of breath.	Indicators of fluid accumulation in the lungs and may be a direct indicator of left ventricular failure and decreased cardiac output.
If a pulmonary artery line is present, record hemodynamic readings q1-2h and prn.	To monitor for PAWP >18 mm Hg (a sign of vascular volume overload), CO <4 L/min, and cardiac index (CI) <2.5 L/min/m², which are signals of decreasing cardiac function. CI is obtained by dividing measured CO by body surface area.
Administer O₂ as prescribed, usually 2-4 L/min per nasal cannula.	To increase oxygen supply to the myocardium. Hypoxia adds stress to the compromised myocardium.
Deliver O₂ with humidity.	To help prevent convective drying effect of oxygen on oral and nasal mucosa.
Raise HOB 30 degrees or place patient in position of comfort.	To reduce cardiac workload and WOB by enabling better lung expansion to promote ventilation and gas exchange.
Be alert to and report decreasing urine output (particularly <30 ml/hr) and increasing specific gravity (>1.030).	Can occur as a result of decreased cardiac contractility, which leads to decreased renal perfusion and fluid retention.
Assess for peripheral (sacral, pedal) edema.	Can occur with right-sided MI/heart failure.
Maintain IV infusion as prescribed.	To ensure access for emergency/IV medications and fluids.
Administer and titrate medications as prescribed.	Inotropic agents (e.g., dobutamine, milrinone) increase strength of contractions to help keep CO >4 L and promote adequate perfusion to the body. Use of these agents usually necessitates transfer of patient to CCU to monitor vasoactive effects.
	Vasodilators (e.g., sodium nitroprusside and nitroglycerine) decrease cardiac workload by decreasing sympathetic nervous system vasoconstriction. When used with IV inotropes, the combination results in increased contractility (inotrope) and decreased afterload (vasodilator). Usually patient is transferred to CCU when vasodilator is given IV. IV vasodilators are fast acting and must be monitored closely, necessitating frequent checks of VS, which is not feasible on a medical floor.
	β-Blockers block beta stimulation to the sinoatrial (S-A) node and myocardium. Heart rate and contractility are decreased, subsequently decreasing workload of the heart.
If patient is on a medical floor and his or her condition deteriorates, prepare for possible transfer to CCU.	For closer monitoring, which may include a pulmonary artery catheter for monitoring heart function and an arterial line for continuous BP monitoring and frequent blood drawing.

●●● **Related NIC and NOC labels:** *NIC:* Cardiac Care: Acute; Fluid Management; Vital Signs Monitoring; Emergency Care *NOC:* Cardiac Pump Effectiveness; Tissue Perfusion: Abdominal Organs; Tissue Perfusion: Peripheral; Vital Signs Status

Nursing Diagnosis:

Activity Intolerance

related to imbalance between oxygen supply and demand secondary to decreased strength of cardiac contraction and decreased cardiac output

Desired Outcome: During exercise/activity, patient rates perceived exertion (RPE) at ≤3 on a 0-10 scale and exhibits cardiac tolerance to activity as evidenced by systolic BP within 20 mm Hg of resting systolic BP, RR ≤20 breaths/min, and HR ≤120 bpm (or ≤20 bpm over resting HR).

INTERVENTIONS	RATIONALES
Ask patient to rate perceived exertion before, during, and after activity and monitor for evidence of activity intolerance. For details, see **Risk for Activity Intolerance** in "Prolonged Bedrest," p. 67. Notify health care provider of significant findings.	The patient should not experience RPE >3. If this happens, reduce the intensity and increase the frequency of the activity until RPE ≤3 is achieved.
Observe for and report decreasing BP, pale and cold extremities, oliguria, decreased peripheral pulses, and increased HR.	These are signs of decreased cardiac output or cardiac failure. HR >20 bpm from baseline may increase O_2 demands of the heart. Set HR parameters on cardiac monitor accordingly.
Administer O_2 and medications as prescribed.	To increase oxygen supply. Activity increases O_2 utilization, and hypoxia adds stress to the compromised myocardium.
Deliver O_2 with humidity.	To help prevent convective drying effect of oxygen on oral and nasal mucosa.
During acute periods of decreased cardiac output and as prescribed, keep personal articles within reach, provide a calm and quiet atmosphere, and limit visitors.	To support patient in maintaining bedrest, thereby ensuring periods of undisturbed rest, which will decrease oxygen consumption.
Assist patient to commode when bathroom privileges are allowed.	Patient may be weak and require assistance to prevent falling.
Assist patient with passive or assistive range-of-motion (ROM) exercises, as determined by activity tolerance and activity limitations. Consult health care provider about type and amount of in-bed exercises that patient can perform as his or her condition improves.	To prevent joint and muscle problems caused by prolonged bedrest.
Also discuss with health care provider patient's participation in an exercise program after hospital discharge.	Cardiac rehabilitation is a must for all patients who have had MI. It is a closely monitored program that teaches patients about risk factor reduction to prevent another MI and how to have a better quality of life after an MI.
As appropriate, teach patient self-measurement of HR for gauging exercise tolerance.	A HR that is too high increases myocardial O_2 demand; a HR that is too low may cause more ischemia. Patient should use exertion scale and pain scale to gauge exercise tolerance and ensure that HR is <20 bpm above baseline or as prescribed by health care provider.
Facilitate coordination of health care providers. Ensure 90 min for undisturbed rest.	To provide rest periods between care activities to decrease cardiac workload.
For further interventions, see "Prolonged Bedrest," **Risk for Activity Intolerance,** p. 67, and **Risk for Disuse Syndrome,** p. 69.	

●●● **Related NIC and NOC labels:** *NIC:* Energy Management; Cardiac Care: Rehabilitative; Environmental Management; Exercise Therapy: Joint Mobility; Self-Care Assistance; *NOC:* Activity Tolerance; Energy Conservation; Self-Care: Activities of Daily Living

Nursing Diagnosis:

Impaired Gas Exchange

related to alveolar–capillary membrane changes secondary to fluid accumulation in the lungs

Desired Outcomes: Patient has adequate gas exchange within 30 min of treatment/intervention as evidenced by a state of eupnea. For at least the 24-hr period before hospital discharge, patient's PaO_2 is ≥80 mm Hg, $PaCO_2$ is 35–45 mm Hg, and O_2 saturation is >92%.

INTERVENTIONS	RATIONALES
Assess ABG levels.	To monitor for hypoxemia (decreased PaO_2) and hyperventilation (decreased $PaCO_2$), which are findings consistent with MI.
Monitor O_2 saturation via oximetry; report O_2 saturation ≤92% to health care provider.	Indicates decreased oxygenation and signals need to increase or implement supplemental oxygen or other respiratory intervention.
Auscultate lung fields for presence of crackles.	Can occur with fluid accumulation in the lungs, which makes gas exchange more difficult.
Monitor for changes in respiratory pattern (increased dyspnea or decreased RR); report immediately if they occur.	Can occur with an extension of the infarction and decreased CO, causing more fluid backup into the lungs. This necessitates immediate intervention. For example, patient may need oxygen or vasodilator or other medication intervention. Other patients may require invasive interventions, such as angioplasty or CABG surgery.
Monitor BP. In the absence of marked hypotension, place patient in semi-Fowler's position (HOB up 30-45 degrees) or to patient's level of comfort.	To ease dyspnea by decreasing WOB and cardiac workload. In the presence of hypotension, patient should lie as flat as comfortable to facilitate blood flow back to the heart and brain.
Administer O_2 as prescribed.	To increase oxygen supply. Hypoxia adds stress to the compromised myocardium.
Deliver O_2 with humidity.	To help prevent oxygen's drying effects on oral and nasal mucosa.
Administer prescribed analgesics (usually morphine sulfate).	To decrease cardiac workload by vasodilation and ease respiratory effort.

●●● **Related NIC and NOC labels:** *NIC:* Oxygen Therapy; Acid-Base Management; Respiratory Monitoring; Vital Signs Monitoring; Laboratory Data Interpretation; Positioning; Oxygen Therapy *NOC:* Respiratory Status: Gas Exchange; Electrolyte & Acid-Base Balance; Vital Signs Status

ADDITIONAL NURSING DIAGNOSES/ PROBLEMS:

PATIENT-FAMILY TEACHING AND DISCHARGE PLANNING

When providing patient–family teaching, focus on sensory information, avoid giving excessive information, and initiate a visiting nurse referral for necessary follow-up teaching. Include verbal and written information about the following:

✓ Process of MI and extent of patient's injury.

✓ Indicators that necessitate immediate medical attention: unrelieved pain, decreased activity tolerance, sudden onset of shortness of breath, weight gain, nausea, irregular pulse.

✓ Medications, including drug name, purpose, dosage, schedule, precautions, drug/drug and food/drug interactions, and potential side effects. Provide instructions for taking prophylactic NTG before activities, such as sexual activity. It is important to take all medications as prescribed. Cessation of acetylsalicylic acid (ASA) or antiplatelet drugs could cause formation of blood clots in the diseased coronary artery.

✓ If patient will begin taking statin drug (e.g., atorvastatin [Lipitor]) either during hospitalization or after hospital discharge, explain its purpose: The statin drugs are believed to slow the progression of coronary heart disease and stabilize the plaque. They may aid in decreasing the inflammatory response, which is a theory currently recognized as the response mechanism in a diseased coronary artery.

✓ Recommendation for use of folate and vitamins B_{12} and B_6, which along with low homocysteine levels, is associated with better patient outcomes.

✓ When making appointments with other health care providers and dentists, the necessity of explaining that an antiplatelet drug is being taken.

✓Indicators of bleeding as a result of taking an antiplatelet drug that necessitate immediate medical attention: hematuria, hematemesis, menometrorrhagia, hematochezia, melena, epistaxis, bleeding gums, ecchymosis, hemoptysis, dizziness, and weakness.

✓Importance of avoiding over-the-counter (OTC) medications (e.g., aspirin, ibuprofen, which prolong coagulation time) without consulting health care provider or nurse.

✓As indicated, information about angioplasty with stent or CABG surgery.

✓Exercise program specific to patient's condition. Issue guidelines for walking. Caution patient to start slowly, walk 3-5 times/wk, warm up and cool down with stretching exercises, notify health care provider of any change in exercise tolerance, avoid overexertion, and stop when tired.

✓Importance of avoiding overexertion and getting rest when tired.

✓Resumption of sexual activity as directed, usually after 2-4 wk, but this varies with each patient.

✓Diet regimen as prescribed. Provide information regarding low-cholesterol, low-fat, and low-Na^+ diets. Encourage patients to use food labels to determine cholesterol, fat, and Na^+ content of foods.

✓Cessation of smoking. Refer patient to a "stop smoking" program as appropriate. The following free brochures outline ways to help patients stop smoking:
- *How to Help Your Patients Stop Using Tobacco: A National Cancer Institute Manual for the Oral Health Team,* from the Smoking and Tobacco Control Program of the National Cancer Institute; call 1-800-4-CANCER.
- *Clinical Practice Guideline: A Quick Reference Guide for Smoking Cessation Specialists,* from the Agency for Health Care Policy and Research (AHCPR); call 1-800-358-9295.

✓Phone number and address of local American Heart Association branch, local heart rehabilitation programs, family health care provider, and primary nurse. Either provide address or phone number for local chapter or encourage patient to write for information to the following address:

American Heart Association
7320 Greenville Avenue
Dallas, TX 75231
(800) 242-8721
www.americanheart.org

✓Additional general information can be obtained by contacting the following organization:

National Center for Cardiac Information
8180 Greensboro Drive #1070
McLean, VA 22102
(703) 356-6568
www.cardiacinfo.org

✓Referral to stress management programs if appropriate.

Pulmonary Hypertension

As blood passes through the pulmonary vasculature, it exchanges CO_2 and particulate matter for O_2. Normally the pulmonary vascular bed offers little resistance to blood flow, but when resistance occurs, pulmonary hypertension results. Pulmonary hypertension can be primary (rare), which has a poor prognosis and affects primarily young and middle-age women, or it can be secondary (most common), which often responds to therapy and is found in a variety of medical conditions. The cause of primary pulmonary hypertension is unknown. Possible causes of secondary pulmonary hypertension include increased pulmonary blood flow from a ventricular or atrial shunt, left ventricular failure, chronic hypoxia related to chronic obstructive pulmonary disease (COPD) pulmonary embolus, pulmonary stenosis, or any physiologic occurrence that increases pulmonary vascular resistance or constriction of the vessels in the pulmonary tree.

HEALTH CARE SETTING

Primary care with possible hospitalization in medical-surgical unit resulting from complications or in a special center for heart-lung transplantation

ASSESSMENT

Acute indicators: Exertional dyspnea, syncope, and precordial chest pain, all of which result from low cardiac output or hypoxia. Cough and palpitations also can occur.

Chronic indicators: Signs of right or left ventricular failure:

- **Right ventricular failure:** Peripheral edema, increased venous pressure and pulsations, liver engorgement, distended neck veins.
- **Left ventricular failure:** Dyspnea; shortness of breath, particularly on exertion; decreased BP; oliguria; orthopnea; anorexia.

Physical assessment: Cyanosis from decreased cardiac output and subsequent systemic vasoconstriction, possible systolic murmur caused by tricuspid regurgitation or pulmonary stenosis, diastolic murmur caused by pulmonary valvular incompetence, and accentuated S_2 heart sound.

DIAGNOSTIC TESTS

Chest x-ray examination: Will show enlargement of the pulmonary artery and right atrium and ventricle. Pulmonary vasculature may appear engorged.

Echocardiography: Often valuable for showing increased right ventricular dimension, thickened right ventricular wall, and possible tricuspid or pulmonary valve dysfunction.

Radionuclide imaging: For example, equilibrium-gated blood pool imaging and thallium imaging to assess function of the right ventricle.

Right heart catheterization: Necessary to confirm pulmonary hypertension. Pulmonary vascular resistance will be very high, and pulmonary artery and right ventricular pressures can approach or equal systemic arterial pressures.

Pulmonary perfusion scintigraphy (perfusion scan): A noninvasive way to assess pulmonary blood flow. This study involves IV injection of serum albumin tagged with trace amounts of a radioisotope, most often technetium. The particles pass through the circulation and lodge in the pulmonary vascular bed. Subsequent scanning reveals concentrations of particles in areas of adequate pulmonary blood flow.

Electrocardiogram (ECG): Will show evidence of right atrial enlargement and right ventricular enlargement (evidenced by right axis deviation and tall, peaked P waves) secondary to the increased pressure needed to force blood through the hypertensive pulmonary vascular bed.

Pulmonary function test: Results are usually normal, although some individuals will have increased residual volume, reduced maximum voluntary ventilation, and decreased vital capacity.

Arterial blood gas (ABG) analysis: May show low partial pressure of dissolved carbon dioxide in arterial blood ($PaCO_2$) and high pH, which occur with hyperventilation, or increased $PaCO_2$ with decreased gas exchange.

Pulse oximetry: May show decreased O_2 saturation (e.g., ≤92%).

Complete blood count (CBC): Polycythemia can occur in the presence of chronic hypoxemia as a result of compensation.

Liver function tests: May be abnormal if venous congestion is significant. Examples include increased aspartate aminotransferase (AST) or alanine aminotransferase (ALT) and bilirubin.

Open lung biopsy: May be done to establish the type of disorder causing the hypertension.

Nursing Diagnosis:

Impaired Gas Exchange

related to altered blood flow secondary to pulmonary capillary constriction

Desired Outcome: Patient has improved gas exchange by at least 24 hr after intervention or before hospital discharge, as evidenced by O_2 saturation >92% (≥90% for patients with COPD) and partial pressure of dissolved oxygen in arterial blood (PaO_2) ≥80 mm Hg.

INTERVENTIONS	RATIONALES
Monitor and document oximetry levels; report O_2 saturation ≤92% to health care provider.	To detect low O_2 saturation (≤92%), which may signal need for oxygen supplementation.
Monitor ABG results. Report significant findings to health care provider.	To detect signs of hypoventilation (decreased PaO_2, increased $PaCO_2$, and decreased pH), which can signal respiratory failure, or hyperventilation (low $PaCO_2$ and high pH), which can occur with anxiety or respiratory distress. Hypoxemia is the key gas deficit seen with pulmonary vascular vasoconstriction. Blood flow through the lungs is impaired, making it difficult to exchange O_2 for CO_2. O_2 becomes low (hypoxemia) and CO_2 becomes high (hypercarbia). Hypercarbia causes a change in pH to the acid side. Although initially respiratory in origin, hypoxemia eventually results in metabolic acidosis because of lactic acid production. Values outside of normal or acceptable range should be reported for timely intervention.
Auscultate lung fields q4-8h, or more frequently as indicated.	To detect and report presence of adventitious sounds (especially crackles), which can occur with fluid extravasation.
Assess respiratory rate, pattern, and depth; chest excursion; and use of accessory muscles of respiration q4h.	Increased respiratory rate, abdominal breathing, use of accessory muscles, and nasal flaring are signals of hypoxia and respiratory distress.
Observe for and document presence of cyanosis or skin color change.	Can be a late sign of hypoxia and decreased perfusion.
Monitor mental status and report changes in mental acuity or level of consciousness (LOC).	Mental status changes and decreased LOC occur with hypoxemia and hypercarbia.
Help patient into Fowler's position (head of bed [HOB] up 90 degrees), if possible.	To reduce work of breathing (WOB) and maximize chest excursion.
Teach patient to take slow, deep breaths.	To promote gas exchange, as well as help patient relax.
Administer prescribed low-flow O_2 as indicated.	To increase supply of oxygen.
Deliver O_2 with humidity.	To help prevent oxygen's convective drying effects on oral and nasal mucosa.

●●● **Related NIC and NOC labels:** *NIC:* Oxygen Therapy; Positioning; Respiratory Monitoring; Laboratory Data Interpretation; Acid-Base Management *NOC:* Respiratory Status: Gas Exchange

Nursing Diagnosis:

Activity Intolerance

related to generalized weakness and imbalance between oxygen supply and demand secondary to right and left ventricular failure

Desired Outcome:

By at least 24 hr after intervention or before hospital discharge, patient rates perceived exertion (RPE) at ≤3 on a 0-10 scale and exhibits cardiac tolerance to activity as evidenced by RR ≤20 breaths/min, HR ≤20 bpm over resting HR, and systolic BP within 20 mm Hg of resting range.

INTERVENTIONS	RATIONALES
Ask patient to rate perceived exertion during activity and monitor for evidence of activity intolerance. For details, see **Risk for Activity Intolerance** in "Prolonged Bedrest," p. 67. Notify health care provider of significant findings.	To determine if activity intolerance is present (RPE >3).
Perform a baseline assessment of patient's VS. Observe for and document any changes in VS during or immediately after activity.	RR >20 breaths/min and HR >20 bpm over resting HR are signals of activity intolerance.
Measure and document I&O and weight, reporting any steady gains or losses. Be alert to peripheral edema, both pedal and sacral; ascites; distended neck veins; and increased central venous pressure (CVP) (>12 cm H_2O).	These are signs and symptoms of right-sided heart failure. Over time, pulmonary hypertension will have a profound effect on the function of the right side of the heart. Tracking these changes can help gauge severity.
Also monitor for dyspnea, shortness of breath, crackles, and decreased O_2 saturation (≤92%) as determined by oximetry.	These are signs of left ventricular failure. Left ventricular failure can cause pulmonary hypertension, which is more common than pulmonary hypertension causing left ventricular failure.
Administer diuretics, vasodilators, and calcium channel blockers as prescribed.	Diuretics are given if an increase in volume is compromising right-sided or left-sided workload of the heart. Vasodilators and calcium antagonists are given to decrease pulmonary artery pressure via vasodilation.
Facilitate coordination of health care providers to allow rest periods between care activities. Allow 90 min for undisturbed rest.	To decrease oxygen demand.
If necessary, limit visitors.	To facilitate adequate rest, which will help decrease oxygen demand.
Keep frequently used items within patient's reach.	To decrease exertion as much as possible.
Assist with maintaining prescribed activity level and progress as tolerated. If activity intolerance is observed, stop the activity and have patient rest.	To increase patient's activity tolerance while preventing overexertion.
Assist with range-of-motion (ROM) exercises at frequent intervals. Plan progressive ambulation and exercise based on patient's tolerance and prescribed activity restrictions.	To help prevent complications caused by immobility while avoiding overexertion.

●●● **Related NIC and NOC labels:** *NIC:* Energy Management; Medication Management; Visitation Facilitation; Exercise Promotion; Environmental Management *NOC:* Activity Tolerance; Energy Conservation; Endurance

Nursing Diagnosis:

Deficient Knowledge:

Disease process and treatment

Desired Outcome: Immediately following teaching or within 24 hr before hospital discharge, patient and significant other verbalize accurate knowledge of the disease, its treatment, and measures that promote wellness.

INTERVENTIONS	RATIONALES
Assess patient's level of knowledge of the disease process and its treatment.	To enable development of an individualized teaching plan. A knowledgeable patient is more likely to comply with treatment.
Discuss purposes of the medications:	
Vasodilators	To ease workload of the heart.
Calcium antagonists	To "relax" the heart.
Diuretics	Prevent fluid accumulation. They are indicated if right-sided or left-sided heart failure is present.
Anticoagulant (warfarin sodium)	Promotes improved long-term survival if pulmonary emboli are the source of the pulmonary vascular resistance.
Provide emotional support to patient adapting to the concept of having a chronic disease.	Reinforces need to comply with lifetime therapy while also expressing empathy.
If the cause of pulmonary hypertension is known, reinforce explanations of the disease process and treatment.	A knowledgeable patient is more likely to comply with the treatment regimen.
Discuss lifestyle changes that may be required.	To prevent future complications and facilitate self-control of the disease process.
Explain value of relaxation techniques, including tapes, soothing music, meditation, and biofeedback.	Relaxation helps decrease nervous system tone (sympathetic), energy requirements, and O_2 consumption.
If patient smokes, encourage smoking cessation. Provide materials that explain benefits of quitting smoking, such as pamphlets prepared by American Heart Association. Provide phone number for local smoking cessation programs.	Smoking increases workload of the heart by causing vasoconstriction. Either provide address or phone number for the local chapter or encourage patient to write for information to the following address: American Heart Association 7320 Greenville Avenue Dallas, TX 75231 (800) 242-8721 www.americanheart.org
Confer with health care provider about type of exercise program that will benefit patient; provide patient teaching as indicated.	Exercise is good for vascular tone. However, increasing circulation as it relates to pulmonary hypertension will be determined by health care provider and physical therapist.

●●● **Related NIC and NOC labels:** *NIC:* Teaching: Disease Process; Discharge Planning; Teaching: Prescribed Medication *NOC:* Knowledge: Disease Process; Knowledge: Medication; Knowledge: Illness Care

ADDITIONAL NURSING DIAGNOSES/ PROBLEMS:

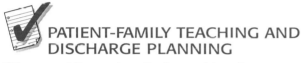

PATIENT-FAMILY TEACHING AND DISCHARGE PLANNING

When providing patient-family teaching, focus on sensory information, avoid giving too much information, and initiate a visiting nurse referral for necessary follow-up teaching. Include verbal and written information about the following:

✓ Indicators that necessitate medical attention: decreased exercise tolerance, increasing shortness of breath or dyspnea, swelling of ankles and legs, steady weight gain.

✓ Medications, including drug name, purpose, dosage, schedule, precautions, drug/drug and food/drug interactions, and potential side effects.

✓ Cessation of smoking; refer patient to a "stop smoking" program as appropriate. The following free brochures outline ways to help patients stop smoking:

- *How to Help Your Patients Stop Using Tobacco: A National Cancer Institute Manual for the Oral Health Team,* from the Smoking and Tobacco Control Program of the National Cancer Institute; call 1-800-4-CANCER.
- *Clinical Practice Guideline: A Quick Reference Guide for Smoking Cessation Specialists,* from the Agency for Health Care Policy and Research (AHCPR); call 1-800-358-9295.

✓ For additional information see **Deficient Knowledge,** p. 214.

Venous Thrombosis/ Thrombophlebitis

Although venous thrombosis and thrombophlebitis are different disorders, clinically the terms are used interchangeably to refer to the development of a venous thrombus or thrombi, with associated inflammation. Disturbances in the venous system can have a variety of causes and precipitating factors, including stasis of blood, hemoconcentration, venous trauma, inflammation, or hypercoagulable states. Venous stasis can occur with heart failure, shock states, immobility from prolonged bedrest, structural disorders of the veins, immobility on the operating room table, or abdominal, pelvic, or orthopedic operative procedures. Venous thrombosis and thrombophlebitis most often occur in the lower extremities, and the most serious complication is embolization.

HEALTH CARE SETTING

Primary care with hospitalization resulting from complications

ASSESSMENT

Signs and symptoms: Assessments may be divided into those in the area of the thrombus (associated with inflammation) and those distal to the clot (associated with venous congestion). Over the site of thrombus the assessments include pain, tenderness, erythema, local warmth, and increased limb circumference. A knot or bump occasionally can be felt on palpation. Distal to the area of thrombus the extremity will be cool, pale or cyanotic, and edematous and display prominent superficial veins. Additional findings include unilateral leg swelling, fever, and tachycardia. Sometimes the condition is clinically "silent," and the presenting sign is a pulmonary embolus (PE). See "Pulmonary Embolus," p. 153.

Risk factors: Prolonged bedrest and immobility, leg trauma, recent surgery, use of oral contraceptives, obesity, varicose veins.

DIAGNOSTIC TESTS

Contrast phlebography (venography): A contrast dye is injected into the venous system that is to be studied, allowing visualization of the veins by showing filling or absence of filling.

Doppler ultrasound: Identifies changes in blood flow secondary to presence of a thrombus.

Duplex imaging: Use of ultrasound to assess veins for flow and pressure.

α-Fibrinogen injection test: Useful screening device for early detection of thrombosis because the isotope identifies clots that are forming.

Impedance plethysmography: Estimates blood flow using measures of resistance and normal changes that occur during pulsatile blood flow.

Elevated erythrocyte sedimentation rate (ESR): Normal ESR (Westergren method) is 0-15 mm/hr in males younger than 50 yr and 0-20 mm/hr in males older than 50 yr; it is 0-20 mm/hr in females younger than 50 yr and 0-30 mm/hr in females older than 50 yr.

Nursing Diagnosis:

Ineffective Peripheral and Cardiopulmonary Tissue Perfusion

(or risk of same) *related to* interrupted blood flow secondary to embolization from thrombus formation

Desired Outcome: Optimally patient maintains adequate peripheral and cardiopulmonary perfusion as evidenced by normal extremity color, temperature, and sensation; RR 12–20 breaths/min with normal depth and pattern (eupnea); HR ≤100 bpm; BP within 20 mm Hg of baseline BP; O_2 saturation >92%; and normal breath sounds.

INTERVENTIONS	RATIONALES
Be alert to and promptly report pain, erythema, increased limb girth, local warmth, distal pale skin, edema, and venous dilation. If indicators appear, maintain patient on bedrest and notify health care provider promptly.	Early indicators of peripheral thrombus formation, which necessitate prompt medical attention to prevent embolization.
Monitor for and immediately report sudden onset of chest pain, dyspnea, tachypnea, tachycardia, hypotension, hemoptysis, shallow respirations, crackles (rales), O_2 saturation ≤92%, decreased breath sounds, and diaphoresis.	Signs of PE, a life-threatening situation. Should they occur, prompt medical attention is crucial.
Administer anticoagulants as prescribed. Ensure correct dosing of heparin infusion.	To prevent further development of deep vein thrombosis (DVT). Heparin is used during the acute phase, and long-term warfarin therapy is used after the acute phase. Low-molecular-weight heparin is administered SC, enabling outpatient management of DVT. Correct dosing is essential to avoid bleeding while preventing clot formation. **Note:** Some surgeons implant a filter in the vena cava to collect clots for patients with a history of embolization.
Keep patient on bedrest, provide gentle range-of-motion (ROM) exercises, and apply support hose, sequential compression devices, or pneumatic foot compression devices as prescribed.	To decrease lower extremity edema and minimize risk of or prevent further DVT.
Caution: In the presence of DVT/clot, avoid these interventions.	To prevent embolization.
If patient is on long-term warfarin therapy, explain importance of frequent prothrombin time (PT) checks.	To ensure maintenance of therapeutic anticoagulation level.

●●● **Related NIC and NOC labels:** *NIC:* Bleeding Precautions; Embolus Care: Peripheral; Embolus Care: Pulmonary; Embolus Precautions; Medication Administration *NOC:* Circulation Status; Tissue Perfusion: Pulmonary; Tissue Perfusion: Peripheral

Nursing Diagnosis:

Acute Pain

related to inflammatory process caused by thrombus formation

Desired Outcomes: Within 1 hr of intervention, patient's subjective perception of pain decreases, as documented by a pain scale. Objective indicators, such as grimacing, are absent.

INTERVENTIONS	RATIONALES
Monitor patient for presence of pain. Document degree of pain, using a pain scale from 0 (no pain) to 10 (worst pain).	To evaluate trend of pain, determine most effective analgesic, relieve pain, and enable more accurate assessment of degree of pain relief obtained.
Administer analgesics, usually acetaminophen, as prescribed, and document relief obtained using pain scale.	

Continued

INTERVENTIONS	RATIONALES
Ensure that patient maintains bedrest during acute phase.	To minimize painful engorgement and potential for embolization. The efficacy of this treatment continues to be debated.
If prescribed, apply warm, moist packs. Be sure that packs are warm (but not extremely so) and not allowed to cool. If appropriate, use a Kock-Mason dressing (warm towel covered by plastic wrap and a K-pad).	Continuous moist heat reduces discomfort and pain by promoting vasodilation and blood supply.
Keep legs elevated above heart level (but not >45 degrees).	To promote venous return and reduce engorgement. A greater angle could result in cutting off circulation at the pelvic area, increasing risk for thrombus formation.

●●● **Related NIC and NOC labels:** *NIC:* Pain Management; Analgesic Administration; Positioning; Heat Application *NOC:* Comfort Level; Pain Control

Nursing Diagnosis:

Ineffective Peripheral Tissue Perfusion

(or risk of same) *related to* interrupted venous flow secondary to venous engorgement or edema

Desired Outcome: Within the 24-hr period following interventions, patient has adequate peripheral perfusion as evidenced by absence of discomfort and normal extremity temperature, color, sensation, and motor function.

INTERVENTIONS	RATIONALES
Assess for signs of inadequate peripheral perfusion.	Pain; cool skin temperature, pallor, decreased motor or sensory function; and venous engorgement (prominence) in lower extremities are signs of inadequate peripheral perfusion.
Elevate patient's legs above heart level (but not >45 degrees).	To promote venous drainage. Elevating legs greater than 45 degrees could decrease circulation at the pelvic area, increasing risk of thrombus formation.
As prescribed for patients without evidence of thrombus formation, apply antiembolic hose.	Antiembolic hose compress superficial veins to prevent their distention and promote flow of blood back to the heart, thereby promoting comfort and decreasing risk of DVT.
Remove stockings for approximately 15 min q8h.	Enables skin inspection for evidence of irritation and decreased circulation.
Apply sequential compression devices or pneumatic foot compression devices as prescribed.	These devices increase blood flow in the deep and superficial veins to prevent DVT and are often indicated for patients who are mostly immobile.
Remove these devices for 15 min q8h and inspect underlying skin for irritation.	Enables skin inspection for evidence of irritation and decreased circulation.
Encourage patient to perform ankle circling and active or assisted ROM exercises of the lower extremities. Perform passive ROM exercises if patient cannot.	To prevent venous stasis, which is a known cause of venous disorders.
Caution: If there are any signs of acute thrombus formation, such as calf hardness or tenderness, exercises are contraindicated. Notify health care provider.	Increases risk of embolization.

Continued

INTERVENTIONS	RATIONALES
Encourage deep breathing.	Deep breathing creates increased negative pressure in the lungs and thorax, which aids in emptying the large veins.
Assess peripheral pulses regularly.	To confirm presence of good arterial flow. Arterial circulation usually will not be impaired unless there is arterial disease or severe edema compressing arterial flow.

●●● **Related NIC and NOC labels:** *NIC:* Circulatory Care: Venous Insufficiency; Circulatory Precautions; Positioning; Pneumatic Tourniquet Precautions *NOC:* Tissue Perfusion: Peripheral

Nursing Diagnosis:

Deficient Knowledge:

Disease process with venous thrombosis/thrombophlebitis and the necessary at-home treatment/management measures

Desired Outcome: Immediately following instruction (or within the 24-hr period before hospital discharge), patient verbalizes accurate knowledge of the disease process and treatment/management measures that are to occur at home.

INTERVENTIONS	RATIONALES
Discuss process of venous thrombosis/thrombophlebitis and ways to prevent thrombosis and discomfort.	Educates patient about how to prevent thrombosis and discomfort. Avoiding restrictive clothing, avoiding prolonged periods of standing, and elevating legs above heart level when sitting promote venous return and help prevent DVT while promoting comfort. In addition, regular walking and active ankle and leg ROM exercises promote venous return, strengthen leg muscles, and facilitate development of collateral vessels.
Teach signs of venous stasis ulcers and importance of reporting them to health care provider.	Such indicators as redness, swelling, and skin breakdown are signals of venous stasis ulcers, and they require medical attention before they lead to complications such as infection or even gangrene.
Stress importance of avoiding trauma to extremities and keeping skin clean and dry.	Avoiding trauma decreases risk of skin breakdown; clean and dry skin helps prevent infection that could develop in broken skin.
Instruct patient to inspect both feet each day. If necessary, suggest use of a long-handled mirror to see bottoms of the feet. Teach patient to report problems to health care provider.	To detect bruises or open wounds inasmuch as tissues of the lower extremities are especially affected by decreased perfusion and prone to injury. In addition, patients on anticoagulant therapy are at risk for bruising and bleeding. This can result in open wounds, which can lead to infection and even gangrene. Patient needs to report problems promptly for timely intervention.
Discuss prescribed exercise program.	Walking and other exercise involving the lower extremities prevent venous stasis, strengthen lower leg muscles, and help develop collateral vessels, where circulation may be routed.
Teach patient how to wear antiembolic hose if prescribed.	Decreasing venous distention with these hose optimally will increase blood flow back to the heart.

Continued

INTERVENTIONS	RATIONALES
Ensure that the hose fit properly without wrinkling.	For example, some hose are worn snug over the feet and progressively less snug as they reach the knee or thigh. Such hose facilitate movement of blood forward and up, increasing blood return to the heart.

●●● **Related NIC and NOC labels:** *NIC:* Teaching: Disease Process; Discharge Planning; Teaching: Prescribed Activity/Exercise; Teaching: Psychomotor Skill *NOC:* Knowledge: Disease Process; Knowledge: Illness Care; Knowledge: Prescribed Activity

ADDITIONAL NURSING DIAGNOSES/ PROBLEMS:

"Pulmonary Embolus" for **Ineffective**   p. 155
Protection related to prolonged bleeding
or hemorrhage secondary to
anticoagulation therapy

PATIENT-FAMILY TEACHING AND DISCHARGE PLANNING

When providing patient-family teaching, focus on sensory information, avoid giving excessive information, and initiate a visiting nurse referral for necessary follow-up teaching. Include verbal and written information about the following:

✓ See **Deficient Knowledge,** earlier, for topics to discuss (both verbally and through written information) with the patient and significant other.

✓ If patient is discharged from hospital on warfarin therapy, provide information about the following:

- As directed, see health care provider for scheduled PT checks.

- Take warfarin (Coumadin) at same time each day; do not skip days unless directed to by health care provider.
- Wear a Medic-Alert bracelet.
- Avoid alcohol consumption and changes in diet. Maintain vitamins and foods with vitamin K at a constant intake. Too much intake can reverse the Coumadin effect and therefore bleeding. Change or too little intake can cause more clotting and the need for more Coumadin.
- When making appointments with other health care providers and dentists, inform them that warfarin is being taken.
- Be alert to indicators that necessitate immediate medical attention: hematuria, hematemesis, menometrorrhagia, hematochezia, melena, epistaxis, bleeding gums, ecchymosis, hemoptysis, dizziness, and weakness.
- Avoid taking over-the-counter (OTC) medications (e.g., aspirin, ibuprofen, which also prolongs coagulation time) without consulting health care provider or nurse.

Acute Renal Failure

Acute renal failure (ARF) is a sudden loss of renal function, which may or may not be accompanied by oliguria. Although the alteration in renal function usually is reversible, ARF may be associated with a mortality of 40%-80%. Mortality varies greatly with the cause of ARF, the patient's age, and comorbid conditions.

The causes of ARF are classified according to development as prerenal, intrinsic, and postrenal:

- *Prerenal failure:* A decrease in renal function secondary to decreased renal perfusion but without renal parenchymal damage. Causes of prerenal failure include fluid volume deficit, vasodilation (e.g., shock), renovascular obstruction, and decreased cardiac function.
- *Intrinsic renal failure:* The most common cause of intrinsic renal failure, or renal failure that develops secondary to renal parenchymal damage, is acute tubular necrosis (ATN). Although typically associated with prolonged ischemia (prerenal failure) or exposure to nephrotoxins (aminoglycoside antibiotics, nonsteroidal antiinflammatory drugs [NSAIDs], heavy metals, myoglobin, organic solvents, radiographic contrast media), ATN also can occur after transfusion reactions, septic abortions, or crushing injuries.
- *Postrenal failure:* A reduction in urine output because of obstruction to urine flow. Conditions causing postrenal failure can include neurogenic bladder, tumors, and urethral strictures. Early detection of prerenal and postrenal failure is essential because, if prolonged, they can lead to parenchymal damage.

HEALTH CARE SETTING

Acute medical-surgical care unit

ASSESSMENT

Electrolyte disturbance: Muscle weakness and dysrhythmias.
Excess fluid volume: Oliguria, pitting edema, hypertension, pulmonary edema.

Metabolic acidosis: Kussmaul respirations (hyperventilation), lethargy, headache.
Uremia (retention of metabolic wastes): Altered mental state, anorexia, nausea, diarrhea, pale and sallow skin, purpura, decreased resistance to infection, anemia, fatigue. **Note:** Uremia adversely affects all body systems.
Physical assessment: Pallor, edema (peripheral, periorbital, sacral), crackles (rales), and elevated BP in patient who has fluid overload.
History of: Exposure to nephrotoxic substances, traumatic or crush injury, recent blood transfusion, prolonged hypotensive episodes or decreased renal perfusion, sepsis, exposure to radiolucent contrast media, or prostatic hypertrophy.

DIAGNOSTIC TESTS

Blood urea nitrogen (BUN) and serum creatinine: To assess the progression and management of ARF. Both BUN and creatinine will increase as renal function and renal excretion decrease.
Serum bicarbonate: To assess for metabolic acidosis in the absence of arterial blood gas (ABG) results. Low levels of serum bicarbonate indicate metabolic acidosis.
Creatinine clearance: Measures the ability of the kidney to clear the blood of creatinine. **Note:** Failure to collect all urine during the period of study can invalidate the test.
Urinalysis: Can provide information about the cause and location of renal disease as reflected by abnormal urinary sediment (renal tubular cell casts and renal tubular cells).
Urinary osmolarity and urinary Na^+ levels: To rule out renal perfusion problems (prerenal). In ATN the kidney loses the ability to adjust urine concentration and conserve Na^+, producing a urine sodium level >40 mEq/L (in prerenal azotemia the urine sodium is <20 mEq/L).
Note: All urine samples should be sent to the laboratory immediately after collection or refrigerated if this is not possible. Urine left at room temperature has greater potential for bacterial growth, turbidity, and alkalinity, any of which can distort the reading.

Renal ultrasound: Provides information about renal anatomy and pelvic structures, evaluates renal masses, and detects obstruction and hydronephrosis.

Renal scan: Provides information about the perfusion and function of the kidneys.

Computed tomography (CT) scan: Identifies dilation of renal calices in obstructive processes.

Retrograde urography: Assesses for postrenal causes, that is, obstruction.

Nursing Diagnosis:

Excess Fluid Volume

related to compromised regulatory mechanisms secondary to renal dysfunction: *Oliguric phase*

Desired Outcome: Patient adheres to prescribed fluid restrictions and begins move toward normovolemia within 24 hr of this diagnosis as evidenced by decreasing or stable weight, normal breath sounds, edema ≤1+ on a 0-4+ scale, central venous pressure (CVP) ≤12 cm H_2O, and BP and HR within patient's normal range.

INTERVENTIONS	RATIONALES
Closely monitor and document I&O. Review results of acid-base, serum bicarbonate, and electrolyte studies if they have been requested.	To detect trend of fluid volume, particularly decreasing urinary output when compared to intake. Patients with ARF may/may not develop oliguria. Urine volume does not necessarily reflect renal function in patients with ARF. For example, in postrenal failure, large volumes of urine may be associated with relief of obstruction. In ARF the kidneys lose their ability to maintain biochemical homeostasis. This causes retention of metabolic wastes and dramatic alterations in fluid, electrolyte, and acid-base balance. For details about likely electrolyte imbalances and metabolic acidosis, see **Ineffective Protection,** p. 226.
Monitor weight daily.	The patient should lose 0.5 kg/day if not eating; a sudden weight gain suggests excessive fluid volume.
Weigh patient at the same time each day, using the same scale and with patient wearing the same amount of clothing.	To ensure that weight measurements are performed under the same conditions with each assessment, thereby facilitating more precise measurements.
Assess for and document degree of edema, hypertension, crackles, tachycardia, distended neck veins, shortness of breath, and increased CVP.	These are indicators of fluid volume excess. In ARF, dependent edema likely will be detected in the legs or feet of patients who are ambulatory, whereas the sacral area will be edematous in those who are on bedrest. Periorbital edema may also result from excessive fluid overload. Jugular veins are likely to be distended with head of bed (HOB) elevated 45 degrees owing to increased intravascular volume if patient has excessive fluid volume. Crackles and shortness of breath can occur as a result of pulmonary fluid volume overload. Low serum albumin decreases colloid osmotic pressure, allowing fluid to leak into the extravascular space. Low serum albumin also may contribute to generalized edema and pulmonary edema.
	Hypertension, tachycardia, and increased CVP may result from sodium and fluid retention. Decreased renal perfusion also may activate the renin-angiotensin system, exacerbating these symptoms.
Monitor results of BUN, serum creatinine, and creatinine clearance tests.	Although both BUN and creatinine will increase as renal function and renal excretion decrease, creatinine is a better indicator of renal function because it is not affected by diet,

Continued

INTERVENTIONS	RATIONALES
	hydration, or tissue catabolism. Creatinine clearance measures the ability of the kidney to clear the blood of creatinine and approximates the glomerular filtration rate. It will decrease as renal function decreases. **Note:** Creatinine clearance is normally decreased in older persons.
Administer medications that promote diuresis as prescribed.	Control of fluid overload in ARF may include use of large doses of furosemide in nonoliguric patients to induce diuresis.
Carefully adhere to prescribed fluid restriction.	To help patient return to normovolemia. Fluids usually are restricted on the basis of "replace losses + 400 ml/24 hr." Insensible fluid losses are only partially replaced to offset water formed during the metabolism of proteins, carbohydrates, and fats.
Provide oral hygiene at frequent intervals and offer fluids in the form of ice chips or popsicles. Hard candies also may be given. Spread allotted fluids evenly over a 24-hr period and record amount given. Remind patient and significant others about need for fluid restriction.	To minimize thirst during fluid restriction. **Note:** Patients nourished via total parenteral nutrition (TPN) are at increased risk for fluid overload because of the necessary fluid volume involved and its hypertonicity.
Arrange for or administer renal dialysis as prescribed. For more information, see "Hemodialysis," p. 251, or "Peritoneal Dialysis," p. 257, as indicated.	Hemodialysis treatments remove excess fluid through the process of ultrafiltration (removal of fluids using pressure). Peritoneal dialysis removes fluid via osmotic pressures across the peritoneal membrane. The present trend is to use dialysis early in ARF. It is done q1-3days (but may be done continuously in critical care). Prophylactic use of dialysis has reduced the incidence of complications and rate of death in patients with ARF.

●●● **Related NIC and NOC labels:** *NIC:* Fluid Management; Fluid Monitoring; Fluid & Electrolyte Management; Hypervolemia Management *NOC:* Fluid Balance; Electrolyte & Acid/Base Balance

Nursing Diagnosis:

Risk for Deficient Fluid Volume

related to active loss secondary to excessive urinary output: *Diuretic phase*

Desired Outcome: Patient becomes normovolemic without first becoming fluid volume deficient as evidenced by stable weight, balanced I&O, good skin turgor, CVP $\geq$5 cm H_2O, and BP and HR within patient's normal range.

INTERVENTIONS	RATIONALES
Closely monitor and document I&O.	To detect trend of fluid volume. Following relief of the obstruction in patients with postrenal failure, postobstructive diuresis may occur if the kidney is unable to concentrate the urine. Consequently, large volumes of solute and fluid may be lost (8-20 L/day of urinary losses), resulting in volume depletion.
Monitor weight daily.	A weight loss $\geq$0.5 kg/day may reflect excessive volume loss.
Weigh patient at the same time each day, using the same scale and with patient wearing the same amount of clothing.	To ensure that weight measurements are performed under the same conditions, thereby facilitating precise measurements.

Continued

INTERVENTIONS	RATIONALES
Monitor for complaints of light-headedness, poor skin turgor, hypotension, postural hypotension, tachycardia, and decreased CVP.	Indicators of volume depletion that may result from loss of intravascular volume caused by urinary fluid losses.
As prescribed, encourage fluids in dehydrated patient or replace fluids and electrolytes intravenously as prescribed.	To promote rehydration and prevent life-threatening electrolyte abnormalities caused by the large-volume urinary and solute losses.
Report significant findings as mentioned above to health care provider.	To ensure timely intervention. Although renal function usually can be reversed, there is a mortality rate of 40%-80% associated with ARF, depending on cause and patient's age and comorbid conditions.

●●● **Related NIC and NOC labels:** *NIC:* Fluid Management; Fluid Monitoring; Hypovolemia Management *NOC:* Fluid Balance; Hydration

Nursing Diagnosis:

Imbalanced Nutrition: Less than body requirements

related to nausea, vomiting, anorexia, and dietary restrictions

Desired Outcome: Within 2 days of admission, patient has stable weight and demonstrates optimal intake of food within restrictions, as indicated.

INTERVENTIONS	RATIONALES
Alert health care providers to symptoms of gastric dysfunction and monitor BUN levels.	The presence of nausea, vomiting, and anorexia may signal increased uremia. BUN levels >80-100 mg/dl usually require dialytic therapy.
Provide frequent, small meals in a pleasant atmosphere, especially controlling unpleasant odors.	Smaller, more frequent meals are usually better tolerated than larger meals.
Administer prescribed antiemetics as necessary. Instruct patient to request medication before discomfort becomes severe.	Antiemetics (e.g., hydroxyzine, ondansetron, prochlorperazine, and promethazine) are given to reduce nausea.
Coordinate meal planning and dietary teaching with patient, significant others, and renal dietitian. Provide fact sheets that list foods to restrict.	Dietary restriction may include reduced protein, Na$^+$, K$^+$, phosphorus, and fluid intake. Protein is limited to minimize retention of nitrogenous wastes. Sodium is limited to prevent thirst and fluid retention. Potassium and phosphorus are limited because of the kidney's decreased ability to excrete them.
Demonstrate with sample menus examples of how dietary restrictions may be incorporated into daily meals.	Sample menus show patient how to apply this new knowledge.

●●● **Related NIC and NOC labels:** *NIC:* Nutrition Management; Nutrition Monitoring; Weight Gain Assistance *NOC:* Nutritional Status: Food Intake

Nursing Diagnosis:

Ineffective Protection

related to neurosensory, musculoskeletal, and cardiac changes secondary to uremia, electrolyte imbalance, and metabolic acidosis

Desired Outcomes: After treatment, patient verbalizes orientation to person, place, and time and is free of injury caused by neurosensory, musculoskeletal, or cardiac disturbances. Within the 24-hr period before hospital discharge, patient verbalizes the signs and symptoms of electrolyte imbalance and metabolic acidosis and the importance of reporting them promptly should they occur.

INTERVENTIONS	RATIONALES
Assess for and teach patient indicators of electrolyte disturbances, uremia, and metabolic acidosis, which can occur in ARF.	In ARF, the kidneys lose the ability to maintain biochemical homeostasis, causing retention of metabolic wastes and dramatic alterations in fluid, electrolyte, and acid-base balance. The following may occur: - *Hypokalemia:* Muscle weakness, lethargy, dysrhythmias, abdominal distention, and nausea and vomiting (secondary to ileus). It may occur during the diuretic phase because of urinary potassium losses. - *Hyperkalemia:* Muscle cramps, dysrhythmias, muscle weakness, and peaked T waves on ECG. Hyperkalemia is a common and potentially fatal complication of ARF during the oliguric phase. It may occur if the kidney is unable to excrete potassium ions into the urine. **Caution:** A normal serum K^+ level is necessary for normal cardiac function. - *Hypocalcemia:* Neuromuscular irritability, for example, positive Trousseau's sign (carpopedal spasm) and Chvostek's sign (facial muscle spasm), and paresthesias. Hypocalcemia may occur because of increased serum phosphate (there is a reciprocal relationship between calcium and phosphorus—as one rises, the other decreases). - *Hyperphosphatemia:* Although usually asymptomatic, may cause bone or joint pain, painful/itchy skin lesions. Serum phosphorus may increase because of a decreased ability of the kidneys to excrete this ion. - *Uremia:* Anorexia, nausea, metallic taste in the mouth, irritability, confusion, lethargy, restlessness, and itching. Uremic symptoms result from increased BUN as the kidney loses its ability to excrete nitrogenous wastes. - *Metabolic acidosis:* Rapid, deep respirations; confusion. A buildup of hydrogen ions occurs in the serum because of the kidneys' inability to buffer and secrete this ion.
Avoid giving patient foods high in K^+.	To help patient's potassium levels return to more normal levels. Salt substitutes also contain K^+ and should be avoided along with apricots, avocados, bananas, cantaloupe, carrots, cauliflower, chocolate, dried beans and peas, dried fruit, mushrooms, nuts, oranges, peanuts, potatoes, prune juice, pumpkins, spinach, sweet potatoes, Swiss chard, tomatoes, and watermelon.
Maintain adequate nutritional intake (especially calories).	If caloric intake is inadequate, body protein will be used for energy, resulting in increased end products of protein metabolism (i.e., nitrogenous wastes). A high-carbohydrate diet helps to minimize tissue catabolism and production of nitrogenous wastes.
Prevent infections.	To minimize tissue catabolism by controlling fevers.

Continued

INTERVENTIONS	RATIONALES
Avoid or use cautiously NSAIDs, angiotensin-converting enzyme (ACE) inhibitors, and K$^+$-sparing diuretics.	These medications may cause an increase in serum K$^+$ and should be avoided or used with caution. **Note:** Soon after renal disease is initially diagnosed, ACE inhibitors may be prescribed for their renal protective effects. However, after chronic renal failure has developed, ACE inhibitors may be contraindicated because of the risk of hyperkalemia and their potential to increase rate of progression to end-stage renal disease (ESRD).
Prepare patient for possibility of altered taste and smell.	May occur with uremia.
Avoid use of magnesium-containing medications.	Patients with renal failure are at risk for increased magnesium levels because of decreased urinary excretion of dietary magnesium. Patients using magnesium-containing antacids such as Maalox typically are switched to aluminum hydroxide preparations such as AlternaGEL or Amphojel. Milk of Magnesia should be substituted with another, nonmagnesium-containing, laxative such as casanthranol.
Administer aluminum hydroxide or calcium antacids as prescribed.	To control hyperphosphatemia. **Note:** Aluminum-containing phosphate binders should not be used long term because they have the potential to cause bone damage.
Administer other medications as prescribed:	
- Diuretics	Used in nonoliguric ARF for fluid removal. For example, furosemide (Lasix) (100-200 mg) or mannitol (12.5 g) may be given early in ARF to limit or prevent development of oliguria.
- Antihypertensives	To control BP in the presence of underlying illness, fluid overload, sodium retention, or stimulation of the renin-angiotensin system in patients with renal ischemia.
- Cation exchange resins (Kayexalate).	To control hyperkalemia. Kayexalate is most effectively administered orally, but it may be administered as an enema. The resin acts in the intestinal tract via exchange of sodium ions (from the Kayexalate) for potassium ions. Kayexalate is usually administered with sorbitol to prevent constipation and fecal impaction. **Note:** Severe hyperkalemia may be treated also with *IV sodium bicarbonate,* which shifts K$^+$ into the cells temporarily, or *glucose and insulin.* Insulin also helps move K$^+$ into the cells, and glucose helps prevent dangerous hypoglycemia, which could result from the insulin. *IV calcium* is given to reverse the cardiac effects of life-threatening hyperkalemia.
- Calcium or vitamin D supplements	For patients with hypocalcemia.
- Sodium bicarbonate	To treat metabolic acidosis when serum bicarbonate level is <15 mmol/L. It is used cautiously in patients with hypocalcemia, edema, or sodium retention. Rapidly rising serum PH may result in muscle spasms in patients with hypocalcemia.
- Vitamins B and C	To replace losses if patient is on dialysis.
Assure patient and significant other that irritability, restlessness, and altered thinking are temporary. Facilitate orientation through calendars, radios, familiar objects, and frequent reorientation.	Reassurance may help allay added anxiety. To orient patient to place and time.

Continued

INTERVENTIONS

RATIONALES

INTERVENTIONS	RATIONALES
Ensure safety measures (e.g., padded side rails, airway) for patients who are confused or severely hypocalcemic. For patients who exhibit signs of hyperkalemia, have emergency supplies (e.g., manual resuscitator bag, crash cart, and emergency drug tray) available.	For patient's protection until electrolyte disturbance is reversed.

●●● **Related NIC and NOC labels:** *NIC:* Cerebral Profusion Promotion; Neurologic Monitoring
NOC: Neurologic Status: Consciousness

Nursing Diagnosis:

Risk for Infection

related to presence of uremia

Desired Outcome: Patient is free of infection as evidenced by normothermia, white blood cell
(WBC) count $\leq 11,000/mm^3$, urine that is clear and of normal odor, normal breath sounds,
eupnea, and absence of erythema, warmth, tenderness, swelling, and drainage at the catheter or
intravenous access sites.
Note: One of the primary causes of death in ARF is sepsis.

INTERVENTIONS

RATIONALES

INTERVENTIONS	RATIONALES
Monitor temperature and secretions for indicators of infection.	Even minor increases in temperature can be significant because uremia masks the febrile response and inhibits the body's ability to fight infection.
Use meticulous sterile technique when changing dressings or manipulating venous catheters, IV lines, or indwelling catheters.	To prevent infection via spread of pathogens.
Avoid long-term use of indwelling urinary catheters. Whenever possible, use intermittent catheterization instead.	Indwelling urinary catheters are a common source of infection.
Provide oral hygiene and skin care at frequent intervals.	Intact skin and oral mucous membranes are barriers to infection.
Use emollients and gentle soap.	To avoid drying and cracking of skin, which could lead to breakdown and infection.
Rinse off all soap when bathing patient.	Soap residue may further irritate skin and affects its integrity.
For more information, see Appendix for "Infection Prevention and Control," p. 831.	

●●● **Related NIC and NOC labels:** *NIC:* Infection Control; Infection Prevention *NOC:* Infection Status;
Immune Status

ADDITIONAL NURSING DIAGNOSES/ PROBLEMS:

✔ PATIENT-FAMILY TEACHING AND DISCHARGE PLANNING

When providing patient-family teaching, focus on sensory information, avoid giving excessive information, and initiate a visiting nurse referral for necessary follow-up teaching. Include verbal and written information about the following:

✔Medications, including drug name, purpose, dosage, schedule, drug/drug and food/drug interactions, precautions, and potential side effects.

✔Diet: Include fact sheets that list foods to restrict. Provide sample menus with examples of how dietary restrictions may be incorporated into daily meals.

✔Care and observation of dialysis access if patient is being discharged with one (see "Hemodialysis," p. 251, or "Peritoneal Dialysis," p. 257).

✔Importance of continued medical follow-up of renal function.

✔Signs and symptoms of potential complications. These should include indicators of infection (see **Risk for Infection,** p. 229); electrolyte imbalance (see **Ineffective Protection,** p. 226); **Excess Fluid Volume,** p. 224; and bleeding (especially from the gastrointestinal [GI] tract for patients who are uremic).

✔Phone numbers to call should questions or concerns arise about therapy or disease after discharge. Additional general information can be obtained by contacting:

National Kidney and Urologic Diseases Information
   Clearinghouse
3 Information Way
Bethesda, MD 20892-3580
(301) 654-4415
Fax: (301) 907-8906
www.niddk.nih.gov/health/kidney/nkudic.htm

National Kidney Foundation
30 E. 33rd Street, Suite 1100
New York, NY 10016
(800) 622-9010
Fax: (212) 689-9261
www.kidney.org

In addition

✔If patient requires dialysis after discharge, coordinate discharge planning with dialysis unit staff.

Benign Prostatic Hypertrophy

The prostate is an encapsulated gland that surrounds the male urethra below the bladder neck and produces a thin, milky fluid during ejaculation. As a man ages, the prostate gland grows larger. Although the exact cause of the enlargement is unknown, one theory is that hormonal changes affect the estrogen/androgen balance. This noncancerous enlargement is common in men older than 50 yr, and as many as 80% of men older than 65 yr are believed to have symptoms of prostatic enlargement. Treatment is given when symptoms of bladder outlet obstruction appear.

HEALTH CARE SETTING

Primary care; outpatient acute (surgical) care

ASSESSMENT

Chronic indicators: Urinary frequency, hesitancy, urgency, retention, and dribbling or postvoid dribbling; slow urinary stream; nocturia (several times each night); hematuria. Scores on American Urological Association (AUA) questionnaire are 0-7 (mild), 8-19 (moderate), and 20-35 (severe).

Acute indicators/bladder outlet obstruction: Anuria, nausea, vomiting, severe suprapubic pain, severe and constant urgency, flank pain during micturition.

Physical assessment: Bladder distention, kettle drum sound with percussion over the distended bladder. Rectal examination reveals a smooth, firm, symmetric, and elastic enlargement of the prostate.

DIAGNOSTIC TESTS

Urinalysis: Checks for the presence of white blood cells (WBCs), leukocyte esterase, WBC casts, bacteria, and microscopic hematuria.

Urine culture and sensitivity: Verifies presence of an infecting organism, identifies the type of organism, and determines the organism's antibiotic sensitivities. **Note:** All urine specimens should be sent to the laboratory immediately after they are obtained, or they should be refrigerated if this is not possible (specimens for urine culture should not be refrigerated). Urine left at room temperature has a greater potential for bacterial growth, turbidity, and alkaline pH, any of which can distort the test results.

Hct and Hgb: Decreased values may signal mild anemia from local bleeding.

Blood urea nitrogen (BUN) and creatinine: To evaluate renal and urinary function. **Note:** BUN can be affected by the patient's hydration status, and the results must be evaluated accordingly. fluid volume excess reduces BUN levels, whereas fluid volume deficit will increase them. Serum creatinine may not be a reliable indicator of renal function in the older adult because of decreased muscle mass and decreased glomerular filtration rate; results of this test must be evaluated along with those of urine creatinine clearance, other renal function studies, and the patient's age.

Prostate-specific antigen (PSA): Elevated above normal (0-4 ng/ml; normal range may increase with age) correlates well with positive digital examination findings. This glycoprotein is produced only by the prostate and reflects prostate size.

Cystoscopy: To visualize the prostate gland, estimate its size, and ascertain the presence of any damage to the bladder wall secondary to an enlarged prostate. **Note:** Because patients undergoing cystoscopy are susceptible to septic shock, this procedure is contraindicated in patients with acute urinary tract infection (UTI) because of the possible danger of hematogenic spread of gram-negative bacteria.

Transrectal ultrasound (TRUS): Assesses the size and shape of the prostate via a probe inserted into the rectum.

Maximal urinary flow rate (MUFR): MUFR <15 ml/sec indicates significant obstruction to flow.

Postvoid residual (PVR) volume: A normal volume is <12 ml; higher volumes signal obstructive process.

Nursing Diagnosis:

Risk for Deficient Fluid Volume

related to postsurgical bleeding/hemorrhage

Desired Outcomes: Patient remains normovolemic as evidenced by balanced I&O, HR ≤100 bpm (or within patient's normal range), BP ≥90/60 mm Hg (or within patient's normal range), RR ≤20 breaths/min, and skin that is warm, dry, and of normal color. Following instruction, patient relates actions that may result in hemorrhage of the prostatic capsule and participates in interventions to prevent them.

INTERVENTIONS	RATIONALES
On patient's return from recovery room, monitor VS as patient's condition warrants or per agency protocol.	To evaluate trend of patient's recovery. Increasing pulse, decreasing BP, diaphoresis, pallor, and increasing respirations can occur with hemorrhage and impending shock.
Monitor and document I&O q8h. Subtract amount of fluid used with continuous bladder irrigation (CBI) from total output.	To evaluate trend of patient's hydration status and assess for postsurgical bleeding.
Monitor catheter drainage closely for first 24 hr.	To assess for color and consistency. Drainage should lighten to pink or blood tinged within 24 hr after surgery. Dark red drainage that does not lighten to reddish pink or drainage that remains thick in consistency after irrigation can signal bleeding within the operative site.
Be alert to bright red, thick drainage at any time.	Can occur with arterial bleeding within the operative site.
Do not measure temperature rectally or insert tubes or enemas into rectum. Instruct patient not to strain with bowel movements or sit for long periods.	Any of these actions can result in pressure on the prostatic capsule and may lead to hemorrhage.
Obtain prescription for and provide stool softeners or cathartics as necessary. Encourage a diet high in fiber and increase fluid intake.	To aid in producing soft stool and preventing straining.
Maintain traction on indwelling catheter for 4-8 hr after surgery or as directed.	The surgeon may establish traction on indwelling urethral catheter in the operating room to help prevent bleeding.
Monitor patient for signs of disseminated intravascular coagulation (DIC). Report significant findings promptly if they occur. For more information, see "Disseminated Intravascular Coagulation," p. 515.	DIC can result from release of large amounts of tissue thromboplastins during a transurethral prostatectomy (TURP). Indicators of DIC include active bleeding (dark red) without clots and unusual oozing from all puncture sites.

●●● **Related NIC and NOC labels:** *NIC:* Bleeding Precautions; Fluid Monitoring; Vital Signs Monitoring; Hemorrhage Control *NOC:* Fluid Balance

Nursing Diagnosis:

Risk for Infection (Septic shock)

related to invasive procedure (cystoscopy or TURP) resulting in introduction of gram-negative bacteria leading to septic shock

Desired Outcome: Patient is free of gram-negative infection as evidenced by normothermia; urinary output ≥30 ml/hr; RR 12-20 breaths/min; HR and BP within patient's normal range;no mental status changes; and orientation to person, place, and time (within patient's normal range).

INTERVENTIONS	RATIONALES
Monitor VS and mentation status at frequent intervals for indicators of the early (warm) stage of septic shock.	Mental status changes such as inappropriate behavior, personality changes, restlessness, increasing lethargy, and disorientation may signal hypoxia caused by decreased cerebral perfusion during the early stage of septic shock.
During first 24 hr after surgery, be alert to temperatures of 38.3°-40° C (101°-104° F) and to moderately increased RR and HR and decreased BP.	These findings can occur in presence of infection and are caused by increased metabolic activity and release of pyrogens.
Be especially alert to classic circulatory signs of collapse.	Classic circulatory signs of collapse occur in the late (cold) stage of septic shock and include profoundly decreased BP (because of decreased stroke volume), greatly increased and weakened HR (compensatory mechanism to maintain cardiac output), and decreased RR (because of respiratory center depression).
Monitor patient's skin for flushing and warmth.	These are early signs of septic shock and are caused by vasodilation.
Be especially alert to skin that becomes clammy, cool, and pale.	Clammy, cool, and pale skin occurs because of the sustained vasoconstriction that happens during the cold stage of septic shock.
Monitor urinary output for decrease.	A decrease in urinary output can signal development of shock.
Notify health care provider promptly if septic shock is suspected. Prepare for the following if septic shock is confirmed: IV infusion (e.g., lactated Ringer's or normal saline); oxygen administration, specimens for WBC, arterial blood gas (ABG), and electrolyte values; and administration of antibiotics.	Accurate assessment and prompt treatment of patient in the early (warm) stage of septic shock greatly improve the prognosis.
Teach indicators of infection and early septic shock to patient and stress importance of notifying staff promptly if they occur after cystoscopy or TURP.	Same as above.
For more information, see Appendix for "Infection Prevention and Control," p. 831.	

●●● **Related NIC and NOC labels:** *NIC:* Infection Control: Intraoperative; Vital Signs Monitoring
NOC: Infection Status

Nursing Diagnosis:

Excess Fluid Volume

(or risk for same) *related to* absorption of irrigating fluid during surgery (TURP syndrome)

Desired Outcomes: Optimally within 24 hr following surgery, patient is normovolemic as evidenced by balanced I&O (after subtraction of irrigant from total output); orientation to person, place, and time with no significant changes in mental status; BP and HR within patient's normal range; absence of dysrhythmias; and electrolyte values within normal range. Urinary output is ≥30 ml/hr.

INTERVENTIONS	RATIONALES
Monitor and record VS.	To assess hydration status along with corresponding electrolyte status. Sudden increases in BP with corresponding decrease in HR can occur with fluid volume excess. Dysrhythmias, including irregular HR and skipped beats, can signal electrolyte imbalance.
Monitor and record I&O. To determine true amount of urinary output, subtract amount of irrigant (CBI) from total output. Report discrepancies.	Large amounts of fluid, commonly plain sterile water, are used to irrigate the bladder during operative cystoscopy to remove blood and tissue, thereby enabling visualization of the surgical field. Over time, this fluid may be absorbed through the bladder wall into the systemic circulation.
Monitor patient's mental and motor status. Assess for presence of muscle twitching, seizures, and changes in mentation.	These are signs of water intoxication and electrolyte imbalance, which can occur within 24 hr after surgery because of the high volumes of fluid used in irrigation.
Monitor electrolyte values, in particular Na^+, for evidence of hyponatremia.	Normal range for Na^+ is 137-147 mEq/L. Values less than that signal hyponatremia, which can occur with absorption of the extra fluids and its dilutional effect.
Promptly report indications of fluid overload and electrolyte imbalance to health care provider.	To ensure prompt treatment, which may include diuretics.

●●● **Related NIC and NOC labels:** *NIC:* Fluid Management; Fluid Monitoring; Fluid/Electrolyte Management; Electrolyte Management: Hyponatremia; Laboratory Data Interpretation; Vital Sign Monitoring; Neurologic Monitoring *NOC:* Electrolyte & Acid/Base Balance; Fluid Balance

Nursing Diagnosis:

Acute Pain

related to bladder spasms

Desired Outcomes: Within 1 hr of intervention, patient's subjective perception of pain decreases, as documented by a pain scale. Objective indicators, such as grimacing, are absent or diminished.

INTERVENTIONS	RATIONALES
Assess and document quality, location, and duration of pain. Devise a pain scale with patient, rating pain from 0 (no pain) to 10 (worst pain).	To establish a baseline, monitor trend of pain, and determine subsequent response to medication.
Medicate patient with prescribed analgesics, narcotics, and antispasmodics as appropriate; evaluate and document patient's response, using the pain scale.	To relieve pain and spasms.
For patients in whom the retropubic approach was used, avoid use of suppositories.	Suppositories (e.g., belladonna and opium [B&O] suppositories) are contraindicated because of the potential for disrupting the incision, which is close to the rectum. Oral anticholinergics, such as oxybutynin, are used instead.
Instruct patient to request analgesic before pain becomes severe.	Prolonged stimulation of the pain receptors results in increased sensitivity to painful stimuli and will increase amount of drug required to relieve pain.
Provide warm blankets or heating pad to affected area.	To increase regional circulation and relax tense muscles.
Monitor for leakage around catheter.	Can signal presence of bladder spasms.

Continued

INTERVENTIONS	RATIONALES
If patient has spasms, assure him that they are normal.	Spasms can occur from irritation of the bladder mucosa by the catheter balloon or from a clot that results in backup of urine into the bladder with concomitant irritation of the mucosa.
Encourage fluid intake.	Adequate hydration helps prevent spasms.
If health care provider has prescribed catheter irrigation for removal of clots, follow instructions carefully.	To prevent discomfort and injury to patient.
Monitor for presence of clots in the tubing. If clots inhibit flow of urine, irrigate catheter by hand according to agency or health care provider's directive.	If output is less than or equals amount of irrigant or patient complains that his bladder is full, the catheter may be clogged with clots. If clots are present for patient with CBI, the rate of bladder irrigation should be adjusted to maintain light red urine (with clots). Optimally, total output should be greater than the amount of irrigant instilled.

●●● **Related NIC and NOC labels:** *NIC:* Medication Management; Pain Management; Heat/Cold Application *NOC:* Pain Control; Comfort Level

Nursing Diagnosis:

Risk for Impaired Skin Integrity

related to presence of wound drainage from suprapubic or retropubic prostatectomy

Desired Outcome: Patient's skin remains nonerythemic and intact.

INTERVENTIONS	RATIONALES
Monitor incisional dressings frequently during first 24 hr and change or reinforce as needed.	If incision has been made into the bladder, irritation can result from prolonged contact of urine with the skin.
Use Montgomery straps or gauze net (Surginet) rather than tape to secure the dressing.	To ensure dressing is secure without the damage that tape can cause to the skin.
If drainage is copious after drain removal, apply wound drainage or ostomy pouch with skin barrier over the incision.	To provide a barrier between the skin and drainage.
Use pouch with an antireflux valve.	To prevent contamination from reflux.

●●● **Related NIC and NOC labels:** *NIC:* Incision Site Care; Wound Care: Drainage *NOC:* Wound Healing: Primary Intention; Tissue Integrity: Skin

Nursing Diagnosis:

Sexual Dysfunction

related to fear of impotence caused by lack of knowledge about postsurgical sexual function

Desired Outcome: Within the 24-hr period following intervention/patient teaching, patient discusses concerns about sexuality and relates accurate understanding about his sexual function.

INTERVENTIONS	RATIONALES
Assess patient's level of readiness to discuss sexual function; provide opportunities for patient to discuss fears and anxieties.	Ensures appropriate time to provide patient teaching and enables nurse to determine patient's specific fears and anxieties.
Assure patient who has had a simple prostatectomy that ability to attain and maintain an erection is unaltered.	Retrograde ejaculation (backward flow of seminal fluid into the bladder, which is eliminated with next urination) or "dry" ejaculation will occur in most patients, but this probably will end after a few months. However, it will not affect ability to achieve orgasm.
Encourage communication between patient and his significant other.	Communication likely will diminish anxiety.
Be aware of your own feelings about sexuality.	If you are uncomfortable discussing sexuality, request that another staff member take responsibility for discussing concerns with patient.
As indicated, encourage continuation of counseling after hospital discharge.	Conferring with health care provider and social services will help identify appropriate referrals.

●●● **Related NIC and NOC labels:** *NIC:* Sexual Counseling; Teaching *NOC:* Sexual Functioning

Nursing Diagnosis:

Perceived Constipation

(or risk for same) *related to* postsurgical discomfort or fear of exerting excess pressure on prostatic capsule

Desired Outcome: By the third to fourth postoperative day, patient relates the presence of a bowel pattern that is normal for him with minimal pain or straining.

INTERVENTIONS	RATIONALES
Document presence or absence and quality of bowel sounds in all four abdominal quadrants and question patient about his urge to have a bowel movement.	A patient whose bowel sounds have not yet returned but who states that he needs to have a bowel movement during the first 24 hr after surgery may have clots in the bladder that are creating pressure on the rectum. Assess for the presence of clots (see **Acute Pain,** earlier) and irrigate the catheter as indicated.
Gather baseline information on patient's normal bowel pattern and document findings.	Each patient has a bowel pattern that is normal for him.
Unless contraindicated, encourage patient to drink 2-3 L of fluid/day on the day after surgery.	Adequate hydration helps ensure a softer stool with less tendency to strain.
Consult health care provider and dietitian about need for increased fiber in patient's diet.	Adding bulk to stools will minimize risk of damaging the prostatic capsule by straining.
Teach patient to avoid straining when defecating.	Prevents excess pressure on the prostatic capsule.
Encourage patient to ambulate and be as active as possible.	Increased activity helps promote bowel movements by increasing peristalsis.
Consult health care provider about use of stool softeners for patient during postoperative period.	Soft stool will be less painful to evacuate following surgery and will cause less straining.
See "Prolonged Bedrest" for **Constipation,** p. 62, for more information.	

●●● **Related NIC and NOC labels:** *NIC:* Bowel Management; Fluid Management; Pain Management; Nutrition Management; Exercise Promotion; Medication Administration *NOC:* Bowel Elimination; Hydration; Symptom Control

Nursing Diagnosis:

Urge Urinary Incontinence

(or risk for same) *related to* urethral irritation after removal of urethral catheter

Desired Outcome: Patient reports increasing periods of time between voidings by the second postoperative day and regains normal pattern of voiding within 4-6 wk after surgery.

INTERVENTIONS	RATIONALES
Before removing urethral catheter, explain to patient that he may void in small amounts for first 12 hr after catheter removal. Note and document time and amount of each voiding.	Irritation from the catheter may cause patient to void in small amounts. Initially patient may void q15-30min, but the interval between voidings should increase toward a more normal pattern.
Instruct patient to save urine in a urinal for first 24 hr after surgery. Inspect each voiding for color and consistency.	First urine specimens can be dark red from passage of old blood. Each successive specimen should be lighter in color.
Encourage patient to drink 2.5-3 L/day if it is not contraindicated.	Low intake leads to highly concentrated urine, which irritates the bladder and can lead to incontinence.
Before hospital discharge, inform patient that dribbling may occur for first 4-6 wk after surgery.	Dribbling occurs because of disturbance of the bladder neck and urethra during prostate removal. As muscles strengthen and healing occurs (the urethra reaches normal size and function), dribbling stops.
Teach patient Kegel exercises (see p. 240).	To improve sphincter control.

●●● **Related NIC and NOC labels:** *NIC.* Urinary Elimination Management; Fluid Management; Pelvic Muscle Exercise; Teaching: Procedure/Treatment *NOC:* Urinary Continence; Urinary Elimination

Nursing Diagnosis:

Acute Confusion

(or risk for same) *related to* fluid volume deficit secondary to postsurgical bleeding/hemorrhage; fluid volume excess secondary to absorption of irrigating fluid during surgery; or cerebral hypoxia secondary to infectious process or sepsis

Desired Outcomes: Patient's mental status returns to normal for patient within 3 days of treatment. Patient exhibits no evidence of injury as a result of altered mental status.

INTERVENTIONS	RATIONALES
Assess patient's baseline level of consciousness (LOC) and mental status on admission. Document patient's response.	Asking patient to perform a three-step task (i.e., "Raise your right hand, place it on your left shoulder, and then place the right hand by your side.") is an effective way to evaluate baseline mental status because patient may be admitted with chronic confusion. Short-term memory can be tested by showing patient how to use call light, having patient return the demonstration, and then waiting 5 min before having patient demonstrate use of call light again. Inability to remember beyond 5 min indicates poor short-term memory. Patient's baseline status can then be compared with postsurgical status for evaluation, which will help determine presence of acute confusion.

Continued

INTERVENTIONS	RATIONALES
Obtain description of prehospital functional and mental status from sources familiar with patient (e.g., patient's family, friends, personnel at nursing home or residential care facility).	This ensures that patient's current/postsurgical status is compared with his normal status.
Identify cause of acute confusion.	The cause may be reversible.
- Assess oximetry or request ABG values.	To determine oxygenation levels. Low levels of oxygen can contribute to diminished mental status.
- Check serum or fingerstick glucose.	To determine glucose levels. Hypoglycemia can affect mental status.
- Request current serum electrolytes and complete blood count (CBC).	To ascertain imbalances and/or presence of elevated WBC count as a determinant of infection, either of which can affect mental status.
- Assess hydration status by reviewing I&O records after surgery. Note any imbalances either way; output should match intake.	Both excess and deficient fluid volumes can affect mental status.
- Assess legs for presence of dependent edema.	Can signal overhydration with poor venous return.
- Assess cardiac and lung status for presence of abnormal heart sounds or rhythms and presence of crackles (rales) in lung bases.	Can indicate fluid excess.
- Assess mouth for furrowed tongue and dry mucous membranes.	Signals of fluid volume deficit.
For oximetry readings ≤92%, anticipate initiation of oxygen therapy to increase oxygenation.	Patients usually require supplementary oxygen at these levels. Decreased levels of oxygen can adversely affect mental status.
As appropriate, anticipate initiation of antibiotics in the presence of sepsis; diuretics to increase diuresis; or increased fluid intake by mouth or IV to rehydrate patient.	Interventions that may help reverse acute confusion.
As appropriate, have patient wear glasses and hearing aid or keep them close to the bedside and within patient's easy reach.	Disturbed sensory perception can contribute to confusion.
Keep patient's urinal and other frequently used items within easy reach.	If patient has a short-term memory problem, he cannot be expected to use call light.
As indicated by mental status, check on patient frequently or every time you pass by the room.	Helps ensure patient's safety.
If indicated, place patient close to nurse's station if possible and in a nonstimulating environment.	Provides a safer and less confusing environment for patient.
Provide music but avoid use of TV.	Individuals who are acutely confused regarding place and time often think action on TV is happening in the room.
Attempt to reorient patient to surroundings as needed. Keep clock and calendar at the bedside and remind patient verbally of date and place.	To help reduce confusion.
Encourage patient or significant other to bring items familiar to patient. These items can be simple and include blankets, bedspreads, and pictures of family or pets.	To provide a foundation for orientation.
Avoid arguing with patients who are confused.	Arguing with confused patients likely will increase their belligerence. If patient becomes belligerent, angry, or argumentative while you are attempting to reorient him, stop this approach. Do not argue with patient or patient's interpretation of the environment. State "I can understand why you may (hear, think, see) that."

Continued

INTERVENTIONS	RATIONALES
If patient displays hostile behavior or misperceives your role (e.g., nurse becomes thief, jailer), leave the room. Return in 15 min. Introduce yourself to patient as though you have never met. Begin dialogue anew.	Patients who are acutely confused have poor short-term memory and may not remember previous encounter or that you were involved in that encounter.
Use distraction techniques if necessary.	Distraction is an effective technique with individuals who are confused. If patient attempts to leave the hospital, walk with him and ask him to tell you about his destination (e.g., "That sounds like a wonderful place! Tell me about it."). Keep tone pleasant and conversational. Continue walking with patient away from exits and doors around the unit. After a few minutes, attempt to guide patient back to his room.
If patient has permanent or severe cognitive impairment, check on him frequently and reorient to baseline mental status as indicated; however, do not argue with patient about his perception of reality.	Arguing can cause a cognitively impaired person to become aggressive and combative. Patients with severe cognitive impairments (e.g., Alzheimer disease, dementia) also can experience acute confusional states (i.e., delirium) and can be returned to their baseline mental state.

●●● **Related NIC and NOC labels:** *NIC:* Delirium Management; Delusion Management; Reality Orientation; Cognitive Stimulation; Cerebral Perfusion Management; Environmental Management: Safety; Fall Prevention; Neurologic Monitoring; Hypoglycemia Management; Distraction; Fluid/Electrolyte Management; Calming Technique *NOC:* Cognitive Orientation; Distorted Thought Control; Information Processing; Safety Behavior: Personal

Nursing Diagnosis:

Stress Urinary Incontinence

(or risk for same) *related to* temporary loss of muscle tone in the urethral sphincter after radical prostatectomy

Desired Outcome: Within the 24-hr period before hospital discharge, patient relates understanding of the cause of the temporary incontinence and the regimen that must be observed to promote bladder control.

INTERVENTIONS	RATIONALES
Explain to patient that there is a potential for urinary incontinence after prostatectomy but that it should resolve within 6 mo. Describe reason for the incontinence, using aids such as anatomic illustrations.	A knowledgeable patient likely will comply with the therapeutic regimen. Understanding that incontinence is a possibility but that it usually resolves should be encouraging.
Encourage patient to maintain adequate fluid intake of at least 2-3 L/day (unless contraindicated by an underlying cardiac dysfunction or other disorder).	Dilute urine is less irritating to the prostatic fossa and less likely to result in incontinence.
Instruct patient to avoid caffeine-containing drinks.	These fluids irritate the bladder and have a mild diuretic effect, making bladder control even more difficult.
Establish a bladder routine with patient before hospital discharge.	The goal of bladder training is to reduce the number of small voidings and thereby return patient to a more normal bladder function.
	- The amount of time between voidings is determined to estimate how long the patient can hold his urine.

Continued

INTERVENTIONS	RATIONALES
	- Patient schedules times for emptying his bladder and has a copy of the written schedule. An example initially would be q1-2h when awake and q4h at night. Then if this is successful, the patient lengthens the intervals between voidings.
Teach patient Kegel exercises. See **Deficient Knowledge:** Pelvic muscle (Kegel) exercise program, below.	To promote sphincter control, thereby decreasing incontinence episodes.
Remind patient to discuss any incontinence problems with health care provider during follow-up examinations.	To ensure that his needs are addressed and treated.

●●● **Related NIC and NOC labels:** *NIC:* Pelvic Muscle Exercise; Bladder Training; Teaching: Individual *NOC:* Urinary Continence; Urinary Elimination

Nursing Diagnosis:

Deficient Knowledge:

Pelvic muscle (Kegel) exercise program to strengthen perineal muscles (effective for individuals with mild to moderate stress incontinence)

Desired Outcome: Within the 24-hr period following teaching, patient verbalizes and demonstrates accurate knowledge about the pelvic muscle (Kegel) exercise program.

INTERVENTIONS	RATIONALES
Explain purpose of Kegel exercises.	Kegel exercises strengthen pelvic area muscles, which will help regain bladder control.
Assist patient with identifying correct muscle group.	A common error when attempting to perform these exercises is contracting the buttocks, quadriceps, and abdominal muscles.
	- Patient attempts to shut off urinary flow after beginning urination, holds for a few seconds, and then starts the stream again. This strengthens the proximal muscle. If this can be accomplished, the correct muscle is being exercised.
	- Patient contracts the muscle around the anus as though to stop a bowel movement. This strengthens the distal muscle.
	- Patient repeats these exercises 10-20 times, qid. These exercises must be done frequently throughout the day and for 2-9 mo before benefits may be obtained.

●●● **Related NIC and NOC labels:** *NIC:* Teaching: Prescribed Exercise *NOC:* Knowledge: Prescribed Activity (Exercise)

ADDITIONAL NURSING DIAGNOSES/ PROBLEMS:

Perioperative Care   p. 47

PATIENT-FAMILY TEACHING AND DISCHARGE PLANNING

When providing patient-family teaching, focus on sensory information, avoid giving excessive information, and initiate a visiting nurse referral for necessary follow-up teaching. Include verbal and written information about the following:

✓ Medications, including drug name, purpose, dosage, schedule, precautions, drug/drug and food/drug interactions, and potential side effects.

✓ Necessity of reporting the following indicators of UTI to health care provider: chills; fever; hematuria; flank, costovertebral angle (CVA), suprapubic, low back, buttock, or scrotal pain; cloudy and foul-smelling urine; frequency; urgency; dysuria; and increasing or recurring incontinence.

✓ Care of incision, if appropriate, including cleansing, dressing changes, and bathing. Advise patient to be aware of indicators of infection: persistent redness, increasing pain, edema, increased warmth along incision, or purulent or increased drainage.

✓ Care of catheters or drains if patient is discharged with them.

✓ Daily fluid requirement of at least 2-3 L/day in non-restricted patients.

✓ Importance of increasing fluids and dietary fiber or taking stool softeners to soften stools. This will minimize risk of damage to the prostatic capsule by preventing straining with bowel movements. Caution patient to avoid using suppositories or enemas for treatment of constipation.

✓ Use of a sofa, reclining chair, or footstool to promote venous drainage from legs and to distribute weight on perineum, not the rectum.

✓ Avoiding the following activities for the period of time prescribed by health care provider: sitting for long periods, heavy lifting (>10 lb), and sexual intercourse.

✓ Kegel exercises to help regain urinary sphincter control for postoperative dribbling.

✓ As appropriate, refer patients to U.S. Agency for Health Care Policy and Research (AHCPR) publication, "Treating your Enlarged Prostate," available by calling the AHCPR Publications Clearinghouse at (800) 358-9295.

✓ For patients experiencing impotence, provide the following information, as appropriate:

Impotents Anonymous (IA)
119 South Ruth Street
Maryville, TN 37803-5746
(615) 983-6092

Chronic Renal Failure

Chronic renal failure (CRF), also known as chronic kidney disease, is a progressive, irreversible loss of kidney function that develops over days to years. Eventually it can progress to end-stage renal disease (ESRD), at which time renal replacement therapy (dialysis or transplantation) is required to sustain life. Before ESRD the individual with CRF can lead a relatively normal life managed by diet and medications. The length of this period varies, depending on the cause of renal disease and the patient's level of renal function at the time of diagnosis.

Of the many causes of CRF, some of the most common are glomerulonephritis (GN), diabetes mellitus, hypertension, and polycystic kidney disease. Regardless of the cause, the clinical presentation of CRF, particularly as the individual approaches ESRD, is similar. Retention of metabolic end products and accompanying fluid and electrolyte imbalances adversely affect all body systems. Alterations in neuromuscular, cardiovascular, and gastrointestinal (GI) function are common. Renal osteodystrophy and anemia are early and frequent complications. The collective manifestations of CRF are termed *uremia.*

HEALTH CARE SETTING

Primary care with possible hospitalization resulting from complications or during ESRD

ASSESSMENT

Fluid volume abnormalities: Crackles (rales), hypertension, edema, oliguria, anuria.

Anemia: Fatigue, shortness of breath on exertion, lethargy, angina (if anemia is severe).

Electrolyte disturbances: Muscle weakness, dysrhythmias, neuromuscular irritability, tetany. With *hyperphosphatemia,* the patient may have bone/joint pain, pruritus, and skin rashes.

Uremia—retention of metabolic wastes: Weakness, malaise, anorexia, dry and discolored skin, peripheral neuropathy, irritability, clouded thinking, ammonia odor to breath, metallic taste in mouth, nausea, vomiting. **Note:** Uremia adversely affects all body systems.

Metabolic acidosis: Deep respirations, lethargy, headache.

Potential Acute Complications

Heart failure: Crackles (rales), dyspnea, orthopnea.

Pericarditis: Chest pain, shortness of breath.

Cardiac tamponade: Hypotension, distant heart sounds, pulsus paradoxus (exaggerated inspiratory drop in systolic BP).

Physical assessment: Pallor, dry and discolored skin, edema (peripheral, periorbital, sacral). With fluid overload, crackles and elevated BP may be present.

History of: GN, diabetes mellitus, polycystic kidney disease, hypertension, systemic lupus erythematosus, chronic pyelonephritis, and analgesic abuse, especially the combination of phenacetin and aspirin.

DIAGNOSTIC TESTS

Blood urea nitrogen (BUN) and serum creatinine: Both will be elevated. **Note:** Nonrenal problems, such as dehydration or GI bleeding, also can cause the BUN to increase, but there will not be a corresponding increase in creatinine.

Serum Hgb and Hct: Measures of anemia. In progressive renal insufficiency, as creatinine clearance declines, the kidney loses its ability to produce sufficient levels of erythropoietin. Declining erythropoietin levels result in decreased red blood cell production, which, in turn, leads to decreased Hgb and Hct and hence anemia.

Creatinine clearance: Measures the ability of the kidneys to clear the blood of creatinine and approximates the glomerular filtration rate (GFR). Creatinine clearance will decrease as renal function decreases. Dialysis is usually begun when the GFR is 12 ml/min when the patient is symptomatic or when the GFR is <6 ml/min. Creatinine clearance normally is decreased in older adults. **Note:** Failure to collect all urine specimens during the period of study will invalidate the test.

X-ray examinations of the kidneys, ureters, and bladder (KUB): Documents the presence of two kidneys, changes in size or shape, and some forms of obstruction. Intravenous pyelogram (IVP), renal ultrasound, renal biopsy, renal scan (using radionuclides), and computed tomography (CT).

IVP, renal ultrasound, renal biopsy, renal scan (using radionuclides), and CT scan: Additional tests for determining the cause of renal insufficiency. Once the patient has reached ESRD, these tests are not performed.

Serum chemistries, chest and hand x-rays, and nerve conduction velocity test: To assess for development and progression of uremia and its complications.

Nursing Diagnosis:
Activity Intolerance

related to generalized weakness secondary to anemia and uremia

Desired Outcome: Following treatment, patient rates perceived exertion at ≤3 on a 0-10 scale and exhibits improving endurance to activity as evidenced by HR ≤20 bpm over resting HR, systolic BP ≤20 mm Hg over or under resting systolic pressure, and RR ≤20 breaths/min with normal depth and pattern (eupnea). **Note:** Anemia is better tolerated in the uremic patient than in the nonuremic patient.

INTERVENTIONS	RATIONALES
Monitor patient during activity and ask patient to rate perceived exertion (RPE, see **Risk for Activity Intolerance,** p. 67, in "Prolonged Bedrest," for details).	To assess degree of activity intolerance. Optimally RPE should be at ≤3 on a 0-10 scale.
Administer parenteral or oral iron as prescribed.	Anemia is an early and frequent complication of CRF. Anemia results primarily from decreased erythropoietin production in the failing kidney. Uremia and iron deficiency (related to decreased dietary intake) also contribute to anemia in CRF. Current practice guidelines recommend that iron be replaced before starting epoetin alfa (Epogen). Adequate iron stores may be sufficient to correct iron deficiency anemia. Iron stores are required to maximize effectiveness of epoetin alfa. **Caution:** Anaphylaxis is a potential complication of ferrous iron administration.
Do not administer ferrous sulfate at same time as antacids.	To maximize absorption of ferrous sulfate, antacids or calcium carbonate medications are given at least 1 hr before or after ferrous sulfate.
Administer epoetin alfa SC or IV as prescribed to treat anemia.	Current clinical practice guidelines recommend that epoetin alfa be started when Hgb decreases to below 10 g/dl. Target Hgb for patients receiving epoetin alfa is 11.5 g/dl (or a range of 11-12 g/dl). Epoetin alfa may be contraindicated in patients with uncontrolled hypertension or sensitivity to human albumin.
Gently mix container.	Shaking may denature the glycoprotein.
Monitor for and report promptly increased hypertension, dyspnea, chest pain, seizures, severe headache, calf pain, erythema, and swelling.	These are potential untoward effects of epoetin alfa therapy. Dose adjustment or discontinuation may be necessary. Patients with uncontrolled hypertension should not be started on Epogen therapy until their hypertension is controlled. Blood pressure must be closely monitored in all patients during initiation of therapy. Hypertension may occur as a side effect of Epogen therapy during the period

Continued

INTERVENTIONS	RATIONALES
	in which Hct levels are rapidly rising, even in nonhypertensive patients. Headaches may accompany the rise in blood pressure. Epogen has also been associated with increased thrombotic events in some studies. Patients should be monitored for evidence of thrombotic events (i.e., symptoms of myocardial infarction [MI], deep vein thrombosis [DVT], cerebrovascular accident [CVA], transient ischemic attack [TIA], or clotting of the vascular access in hemodialysis patients), and those symptoms should be reported immediately to the health care provider. Epogen should be used with caution in patients with a known seizure history. There is an increased risk of seizures in CRF patients within the first 3 mo of Epogen therapy.
For patients with dietary restrictions or who are on dialysis, administer multivitamins and folic acid.	Water-soluble vitamins are lost during dialysis. Folic acid deficiency may contribute to anemia.
Notify health care provider of increased weakness, fatigue, dyspnea, chest pain, or further decreases in Hct.	To monitor for and enable rapid treatment of anemia and dose adjustments of epoetin alfa.
In addition:	
• Coordinate laboratory studies.	To minimize blood drawing.
• Observe for and report evidence of occult blood and blood loss.	Blood loss can cause anemia.
• Assist with identifying activities that Increase fatigue and adjusting those activities accordingly.	To minimize fatigue while attempting to promote tolerance to activity.
• Assist with activities of daily living (ADL) while encouraging maximum independence to tolerance. Establish realistic, progressive exercises and activity goals that are designed to increase endurance. Ensure that they are within patient's prescribed limitations. Examples are found in **Risk for Activity Intolerance,** p. 67, and **Risk for Disuse Syndrome,** p. 69, in "Prolonged Bedrest."	Same as above.
Administer packed red blood cells as prescribed.	To treat severe or symptomatic anemia.

●●● **Related NIC and NOC labels:** *NIC:* Energy Management; Nutrition Management: Medication Management *NOC:* Activity Tolerance; Endurance; Energy Conservation; Self-Care: Activities of Daily Living (ADL)

Nursing Diagnosis:

Impaired Skin Integrity

related to pruritus and dry skin secondary to uremia and edema

Desired Outcome: Patient's skin remains intact and free of erythema and abrasions.

INTERVENTIONS	RATIONALES
Monitor for presence/degree of pruritus.	Pruritus is common in patients with uremia and occurs when accumulating nitrogenous wastes begin to be excreted through the skin, causing frequent and intense itching with scratching. Pruritus also may result from prolonged hyperphosphatemia.

Continued

INTERVENTIONS	RATIONALES
Encourage use of phosphate binders and reduction of dietary phosphorus if elevated phosphorus level is a problem. Give phosphate binders with meals for maximum effect.	Pruritus often decreases with a reduction in BUN and improved phosphorus control. Phosphate binders are medications that, when taken with food, bind dietary phosphorous and prevent GI absorption. Calcium carbonate, sevelamer hydrochloride (Renagel), aluminum hydroxide, and calcium acetate are common phosphate binders.
If necessary, administer antihistamines as prescribed.	To help control itching.
Keep patient's fingernails short.	If patient is unable to control scratching, short fingernails will cause less damage.
Instruct patient to monitor scratches for evidence of infection and seek early medical attention should signs and symptoms of infection appear.	Uremia retards wound healing; nonintact skin can lead to infection.
Encourage use of skin emollients. Teach patients to avoid harsh soaps and excessive bathing and to bathe every other day and use bath oils as needed if dry skin is a problem.	To reduce dry, scaly skin. Uremic skin is often dry and scaly because of reduction in oil gland activity.
Advise patient and significant others that bruising can occur easily.	Patients with uremia are at increased risk for bruising because of clotting abnormalities and capillary fragility.
Provide scheduled skin care and position changes for individuals with edema.	To decrease risk of skin/tissue damage resulting from decreased perfusion and increased pressure.

●●● **Related NIC and NOC labels:** *NIC:* Skin Care: Topical Treatments; Positioning; Medication Management; Nutrition Management *NOC:* Tissue Integrity: Skin & Mucous Membranes

Nursing Diagnosis:

Deficient Knowledge:

Need for frequent BP checks and adherence to antihypertensive therapy and potential for change in insulin requirements for individuals who have diabetes

Desired Outcomes: Within the 24-hr period before hospital discharge (or immediately following teaching if patient is not hospitalized), patient verbalizes accurate knowledge about the importance of frequent BP checks and adherence to antihypertensive therapy. The patient with diabetes mellitus (DM) verbalizes understanding about the potential for change in insulin requirements.

INTERVENTIONS	RATIONALES
Teach importance of getting BP checked at frequent intervals and adhering to prescribed antihypertensive therapy.	Patients with CRF may experience hypertension because of fluid overload, excess renin secretion, or arteriosclerotic disease. Control of hypertension may slow progression of chronic renal insufficiency.
Teach patient to take antihypertensive medications as prescribed.	To help keep BP within optimal levels.
Teach patients with DM that insulin requirements often decrease as renal function decreases.	Anorexia or nausea/vomiting, which occur with uremia, may decrease dietary consumption and thereby decrease insulin requirements.
Instruct these patients to be alert to weakness, blurred vision, headache, diaphoresis, and shaking.	Indicators of hypoglycemia, which can occur as insulin requirements decrease.

●●● **Related NIC and NOC labels:** *NIC:* Teaching: Prescribed Medications; Teaching: Procedure *NOC:* Knowledge: Treatment Procedure; Knowledge: Medication

Nursing Diagnosis:

Deficient Knowledge:

Dietary restrictions and prescribed therapies used to treat systemic complications of ESRD

Desired Outcome: Immediately following teaching, patient verbalizes accurate knowledge about the importance of dietary restrictions and adherence to prescribed therapies in the treatment of ESRD.

INTERVENTIONS	RATIONALES
Teach patient how to manage nutrition.	A knowledgeable patient is more likely to follow the dietary regimen.
Explain importance of restricting protein and phosphorus initially.	To slow progression of CRF and prevent early development of renal osteodystrophy. Protein restriction decreases production of nitrogenous wastes. Prolonged or overrestriction of protein may lead to malnutrition. Referral to a renal dietitian is recommended for calculation of each patient's optimal protein requirement.
	As kidney function declines, the kidney loses its ability to excrete phosphate. High levels of serum phosphate contribute to development of renal osteodystrophy and secondary hyperparathyroidism. Foods high in phosphorus content include meats (especially organ meats), fish, poultry, milk and milk products, whole grains, seeds, nuts, eggs and egg products, and dried beans and peas.
Explain how to increase carbohydrates for patients on protein-restricted diets.	To ensure adequate caloric intake to prevent tissue catabolism (contributing to the buildup of nitrogenous wastes).
As patient approaches ESRD, explain necessity of limiting Na^+ intake.	To reduce thirst and fluid retention. Foods high in sodium content include bouillon, celery, cheeses, dried fruits, frozen or canned foods, packaged foods, monosodium glutamate (MSG), mustard, olives, pickles, preserved meats, salad dressings and prepared sauces, sauerkraut, snack foods, soups, and soy sauce.
Teach how to limit K^+ intake.	The kidneys have decreased ability to excrete this ion in CRF. Foods high in potassium content include apricots, artichokes, avocados, bananas, cantaloupe, carrots, cauliflower, chocolate, dried beans and peas, dried fruit, mushrooms, nuts, oranges, peanuts, potatoes, prune juice, pumpkin, spinach, sweet potatoes, Swiss chard, tomatoes, and watermelon. Salt substitutes also contain potassium.
For patients on protein-restricted diets, explain how to restrict protein intake to protein sources primarily of high biologic value.	Protein may be restricted to limit production of nitrogenous wastes. Foods that contain the essential amino acids (the amino acids that the body needs) are called high biologic value proteins. High biologic value proteins include dairy foods, eggs, meat, poultry, and fish. Other protein sources contain nonessential amino acids (amino acids the body can produce from the essential amino acids). Nonessential amino acids increase the kidneys' workload as they are excreted as wastes. The goal of protein-restricted diets is to balance the increased workload on the kidneys (in terms of nitrogenous waste production) and the potential for malnutrition.
Recommend a referral to a renal dietitian to ensure adequate protein intake.	Overrestriction of protein may lead to malnutrition.

Continued

INTERVENTIONS	RATIONALES
Teach importance of taking sevelamer hydrochloride (Renagel), aluminum hydroxide, calcium carbonate, or calcium acetate with meals as prescribed.	These calcium binders assist in the control of hyperphosphatemia by binding dietary phosphorus. The bound phosphate is excreted in the stool.
Teach importance of taking vitamin D preparations as prescribed.	To prevent renal osteodystrophy and secondary hyperparathyroidism. As kidney function declines, the kidney is unable to produce an adequate supply of vitamin D. Hypocalcemia and hyperphosphatemia stimulate the parathyroid gland. Without an adequate supply of vitamin D, the body is unable to regulate the parathyroid gland, and secondary hyperparathyroidism occurs as a result.
Advise patient of the need for frequent laboratory monitoring of serum phosphorus, serum calcium, and parathyroid hormone.	Hypercalcemia may result from administration of calcium-based phosphate binders and vitamin D analogs. Increased serum phosphate levels may indicate the need for increased dietary phosphorus restrictions or the need to increase dose of phosphate binders, or they may occur as a result of vitamin D analog administration. Oversuppression of the parathyroid gland may occur as a result of administration of vitamin D analogs.

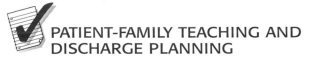

PATIENT-FAMILY TEACHING AND DISCHARGE PLANNING

When providing patient-family teaching, focus on sensory information, avoid giving excessive information, and initiate a visiting nurse referral for necessary follow-up teaching. Include verbal and written information about the following:

✓ Medications, including drug name, purpose, dosage, schedule, drug/drug and food/drug interactions, precautions, and potential side effects.

✓ For patients not on dialysis but requiring epoetin alfa, teach patient and/or significant other about preparation of the medication and SC injections. Demonstrate how to mix the container gently (shaking may denature the glycoprotein); use only one dose per vial (do not reenter used vials; discard unused portions). Instruct patient and/or significant other to store epoetin alfa in refrigerator but not to allow it to freeze. Teach importance of monitoring for and rapidly reporting to health care provider any of the following possible side effects: dyspnea, chest pain, seizures, severe headache, increased BP, and calf swelling, tenderness, or redness.

✓ Diet, including fact sheet listing foods that are to be restricted or limited. Inform patient that diet and fluid restrictions may be altered as renal function decreases. Provide sample menus and have patient demonstrate understanding by preparing 3-day menus that incorporate dietary restrictions.

✓ Care and observation of dialysis access if patient has one (see "Hemodialysis," p. 251, and "Peritoneal Dialysis," p. 257).

✓ Signs and symptoms that necessitate medical attention. These include symptoms of electrolyte imbalances: irregular pulse, muscle cramping, muscle weakness, tetany; symptoms of infection: fever; symptoms of declining renal function and retained fluid: unusual shortness of breath or edema, sudden change in urine output, and irregular pulse.

✓ Need for continued medical follow-up; confirm date and time of next health care provider appointment.

✓ Importance of avoiding infections and seeking treatment promptly should one develop. Teach indicators of frequently encountered infections, including upper respiratory infection (URI), urinary tract infection (UTI), impetigo, and otitis media.

✓ Phone numbers to call should questions or concerns arise about therapy or disease after discharge. Additional general information can be obtained by contacting:

National Institute of Diabetes and Digestive and
   Kidney Diseases
31 Center Drive
Bethesda, MD 20892-2560
www.niddk.nih.gov

National Kidney and Urologic Diseases Information
   Clearinghouse
3 Information Way
Bethesda, MD 20892-3580
(301) 654-4415
Fax: (301) 907-8906
www.niddk.nih.gov/health/kidney/nkudic.htm

National Kidney Foundation
30 E. 33rd Street, Suite 1100
New York, NY 10016
(800) 622-9010
Fax: (212) 689-9261
www.kidney.org

✓ For patient with or approaching ESRD, data concerning various treatment options and support groups. The local chapter of the National Kidney Foundation can be helpful in identifying support groups and organizations in the area. Patient and significant others should meet with renal dietitian and social worker before discharge.

✓ Coordination of discharge planning and teaching with dialysis unit or facility. If possible, have patient visit dialysis unit before discharge.

✓ For the individual with ESRD, importance of coordinating all medical care through nephrologist and importance of alerting all medical and dental personnel to ESRD status, because of increased risk of infection and need to adjust medication dosages. In addition, dentists may want to premedicate ESRD patients with antibiotics before dental work and avoid scheduling dental work on the day of dialysis because of heparinization that is used with dialytic therapy.

29

Hemodialysis

Care of patients undergoing dialysis can be complex, and the actual dialysis (especially hemodialysis) is generally performed by nurses with specialized education and guided experience. This section does not focus on the specific care of patients during dialysis but rather provides essential background data, especially the special issues related to patients who are undergoing hemodialysis.

During hemodialysis, blood is removed via a special vascular access, heparinized, pumped through an artificial kidney (dialyzer), and then returned to the patient's circulation. Hemodialysis is a temporary, acute procedure performed as needed, or it is performed long term 2-4 times/wk for 3-5 hr each treatment.

Hemodialysis may be indicated for patients with acute renal failure or acute episodes of renal insufficiency that cannot be managed by diet, medications, and fluid restriction; end-stage renal disease (ESRD); drug overdose; hyperkalemia; fluid overload; and metabolic acidosis.

HEALTH CARE SETTING

Dialysis center, with possible hospitalization in acute care setting during initiation of therapy

COMPONENTS OF HEMODIALYSIS

Artificial kidney (dialyzer): Composed of a blood compartment and dialysate compartment, separated by a semipermeable membrane that allows the diffusion of solutes and the filtration of water. Protein and bacteria do not cross the artificial membrane.

Dialysate: An electrolyte solution similar in composition to normal plasma. Each of the constituents may be varied according to patient need. The most commonly altered components are K^+ and bicarbonate. Glucose may be added to prevent sudden drops in serum osmolality and serum glucose during dialysis.

Vascular access: Necessary to provide a blood flow rate of 200-500 ml/min for an effective dialysis. Vascular access sites may include an arteriovenous fistula, arteriovenous graft, arteriovenous shunt (less commonly used), and subclavian or femoral vein catheterization.

Nursing Diagnosis:
Risk for Imbalanced Fluid Volume

related to excessive fluid removal during dialysis or bleeding caused by heparinization; *or related to* compromised regulatory mechanism resulting in fluid retention secondary to renal failure

Desired Outcomes: Postdialysis patient is normovolemic as evidenced by stable weight, RR 12-20 breaths/min with normal depth and pattern (eupnea), central venous pressure (CVP) 5-12 cm H_2O, HR and BP within patient's normal range, and absence of abnormal breath sounds and abnormal bleeding. Immediately after instruction, patient relates the signs and symptoms of fluid volume excess and deficit.

INTERVENTIONS	RATIONALES
Monitor I&O and daily weight. Weigh patient at same time each day, using same scale and with patient wearing same amount of clothing (or with same items on bed if using a bed scale).	Intake greater than output and steady weight gain indicate retained fluid. In addition, patient's weight is an important guideline for determining quantity of fluid that needs to be removed during dialysis. Consistency in weighing patient is important to ensure a measurement that is as precise as possible.
Monitor for and report edema, hypertension, crackles (rales), tachycardia, distended neck veins, shortness of breath, and increased CVP. Teach relevant symptoms to patient.	Indicators of fluid volume excess. Dependent edema likely will be detected in the legs or feet of patients who are ambulatory, whereas the sacral area will be edematous in those who are on bedrest. Periorbital edema also may result from excessive fluid overload. Jugular veins are likely to be distended with head of bed (HOB) elevated 45 degrees owing to increased intravascular volume if patient has excessive fluid volume. Crackles and shortness of breath can occur as a result of fluid volume overload. Low serum albumin decreases colloid osmotic pressure, allowing fluid to leak into the extravascular space. Low serum albumin also may contribute to generalized edema and pulmonary edema. Hypertension, tachycardia, and increased CVP may result from sodium and fluid retention.
Clarify antihypertensive medication prescriptions with health care provider.	Antihypertensive medications usually are held before and during dialysis to help prevent hypotension during dialysis.
After dialysis, monitor for and report hypotension, decreased CVP, tachycardia, and complaints of dizziness or light-headedness.	Indicators of fluid volume deficit, which may result from rapid or excessive fluid losses during dialysis. It should be noted that patients with uremia may not develop compensatory tachycardia owing to autonomic neuropathy, which can occur in uremia.
Describe signs and symptoms to patient.	If these signs and symptoms occur, patient will be able to report them promptly to staff or health care provider for timely intervention.
Monitor for postdialysis bleeding (needle sites, incisions). Alert patient to potential for bleeding from these areas.	Can occur because of use of heparin during dialysis.
Do not give IM injection for at least 1 hr after dialysis.	To prevent hematoma formation.
Test all stools for presence of blood. Report significant findings.	Gastrointestinal (GI) bleeding is common in patients with renal failure, especially after heparinization.

●●● **Related NIC and NOC labels:** *NIC:* Fluid Monitoring; Hemodialysis Therapy; Bleeding Precautions
NOC: Fluid Balance; Hydration

Nursing Diagnosis:

Risk for Deficient Fluid Volume

related to bleeding/hemorrhage that can occur with vascular access puncture or disconnection

Nursing Diagnosis:

Risk for Ineffective Peripheral Tissue Perfusion

related to interrupted blood flow that can occur with clotting in the vascular access; *and*

Nursing Diagnosis:

Risk for Infection

related to invasive procedure (creation of the vascular access for hemodialysis)

Desired Outcomes: Patient's vascular access remains intact and connected, and patient remains normovolemic (see description in preceding nursing diagnosis). Patient has adequate tissue perfusion as evidenced by normal skin temperature and color and brisk capillary refill (<2 sec) distal to the vascular access. Patient's access is patent as evidenced by presence of bright red blood within shunt tubing or presence of thrill with palpation and bruit with auscultation of fistula or graft. Patient is free of infection as evidenced by normothermia and absence of erythema, local warmth, exudate, swelling, and tenderness at the access site.

INTERVENTIONS	RATIONALES
After surgical creation of the vascular access, auscultate for bruit and palpate for thrill.	To ensure that patient's vascular access is patent. A bruit is a hissing sound that is made when blood moves through the access. A thrill is a vibration felt when placing hand over the access, denoting blood flow.
Report complaints of severe or unrelieved pain, numbness, and tingling of the area of vascular access or extremity distal to the access. Notify health care provider if extremity distal to the vascular access becomes cool or swollen, has decreased capillary refill, or is discolored.	Can signal impaired tissue perfusion caused by occlusion of the vascular access.
Elevate extremity that has the vascular access.	Postoperative swelling along graft or fistula or area around the shunt is expected.
Follow the three principles of nursing care common to all types of vascular access: (1) prevent bleeding, (2) prevent clotting, and (3) prevent infection. Explain monitoring and care procedures to patient. Vascular accesses include the following:	The vascular access is the patient's lifeline, and it must be monitored closely and handled with care. A knowledgeable patient is likely to comply with these principles as well.
Subclavian or femoral lines:	External, temporary catheters inserted into a large vein.
1. Anchor catheter securely. Tape all connections. Keep clamps at bedside in case line becomes disconnected. If the line is removed or accidently pulled out, apply firm pressure to site for at least 10 min.	These actions prevent bleeding.
Caution: An air embolus can occur if a subclavian line accidently becomes pulled out or disconnected.	
- If air embolus occurs, immediately clamp the line.	To help prevent air from blocking the pulmonary artery.
- Turn patient onto a left-side-lying position; lower HOB into Trendelenburg position.	To increase intrathoracic pressure. This will decrease the flow of inspiratory air into the vein and keep air away from the pulmonary valve.
- Administer 100% oxygen by mask and obtain VS. Notify health care provider stat!	To provide cardiorespiratory support.
2. Prime the line with heparin or by constant infusion with a heparinized solution. Follow protocol or obtain specific directions from health care provider. Attach a label to all lines that are primed with heparin to alert other personnel.	This measure keeps the line patent by preventing clotting.
3. Monitor for and report presence of erythema, local warmth, exudate, swelling, and tenderness at exit site. Report and culture any drainage.	These measures assess for infection.

Continued

INTERVENTIONS	RATIONALES
Perform sterile dressing changes according to agency protocol.	This measure helps prevent infection.
Avoid use of these lines for instillation of IV medications or blood letting.	These procedures increase risk of line infection.
Fistula, graft, or shunt	*Fistula or graft:* Internal, permanent connection between an artery and a vein, or the insertion of an internal graft that is joined to an artery and vein. Grafts can be straight or U shaped. *Shunts* are similar to a fistula or graft in that they are plastic tubes used to connect an artery and vein. However, they exit the skin and can be disconnected to allow connection to dialysis. Shunts are usually temporary. Shunts, grafts, or fistulas are located in the arm or thigh.
1. Inspect needle puncture sites. - If bleeding occurs, apply just enough pressure over the site to stop it. - Release the pressure and check for bleeding q5-10min. - Check shunt connections postdialysis.	These measures assess for and intervene in the presence of bleeding. To ensure that connections are securely sealed to prevent embolus and loss of blood.
If a shunt becomes disconnected, clamp the ends and follow hospital protocol for cleansing connections before reconnection.	To prevent infection while preventing an air embolus and loss of blood.
2. Do not take BP, start IV, or draw blood in arm with shunt, graft, or fistula. Teach patient to avoid tight clothing, jewelry, name bands, or restraint on affected extremity.	These procedures or wearing these articles could cause blood to clot in the vascular access.
Palpate for thrill and auscultate for bruit at least every shift and after hypotensive episodes. Notify health care provider *stat* if bruit or thrill has changed significantly or is absent.	To ensure that vascular access is patent.
3. Observe for and report presence of erythema, local warmth, swelling, exudate, and unusual tenderness at graft, fistula, or shunt site. Culture and report any drainage.	These measures assess for infection.

●●● **Related NIC and NOC labels:** *NIC:* Circulatory Care Neurologic Monitoring; Positioning; Specimen Management; Incision Site Care; Infection Protection; Bleeding Precautions *NOC:* Sensory Function: Cutaneous; Tissue Integrity: Skin and Mucous Membranes; Infection Status; Wound Healing: Primary Intention; Fluid Balance

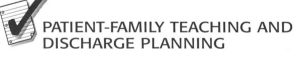

PATIENT-FAMILY TEACHING AND DISCHARGE PLANNING

When providing patient-family teaching, focus on sensory information, avoid giving excessive information, and initiate a visiting nurse referral if indicated for follow-up teaching. Include verbal and written information about the following:

✓ Medications, including drug name, purpose, dosage, schedule, drug/drug and food/drug interactions, precautions, and potential side effects.

✓ Diet: Include fact sheets that list foods to limit or restrict. Review fluid restrictions. Provide sample menus with examples of how dietary restrictions may be incorporated into daily meals. Have patient demonstrate understanding of dietary restrictions by preparing 3-day menus.

✓ Care of fistula or graft to prevent/detect bleeding, clotting, and infection.

✓ Importance of continued medical follow-up; confirm date and time of next health care provider and hemodialysis appointments.

✓ Signs and symptoms that necessitate medical attention: increased weight gain, unusual shortness of breath, edema, dizziness or fainting, fever, increased hypertension, redness around access site, decrease in bruit or thrill (fistulas, graft), prolonged bleeding from fistula or graft, discoloration or coldness distal to fistula or graft, accidental pulling on subclavian line.

✓ Phone numbers to call should questions or concerns arise about therapy or disease after discharge. Additional general information can be obtained by contacting:

National Kidney and Urologic Diseases Information
  Clearinghouse
3 Information Way
Bethesda, MD 20892-3580
(301) 654-4415
Fax: (301) 907-8906
www.niddk.nih.gov/health/kidney/nkudic.htm

National Kidney Foundation
30 E. 33rd Street, Suite 1100
New York, NY 10016
(800) 622-9010
Fax: (212) 689-9261
www.kidney.org

Peritoneal Dialysis

This section does not focus on the specific care of patients during dialysis but rather provides essential background data for nursing care of patients who are undergoing peritoneal dialysis.

Peritoneal dialysis (PD) uses the peritoneum as the dialysis membrane. Dialysate is instilled into the peritoneal cavity via a catheter surgically placed in the abdominal wall. Once the dialysate is within the abdominal cavity, movement of solutes and fluid occurs between the patient's capillary blood and the dialysate. At set intervals the peritoneal cavity is drained, and new dialysate is instilled.

PD may be indicated for patients with acute renal failure or acute episodes of renal insufficiency that cannot be managed by diet, medications, and fluid restriction. Indicators for use of PD in acute respiratory failure (ARF) include uremia, electrolyte imbalances, fluid overload, hemodynamic instability, and contraindications for hemodialysis. PD is also indicated for patients with end-stage renal disease (ESRD) and may be the preferred modality in ESRD patients with poor vasculature, heart failure, severe heart disease, or cardiomyopathy.

COMPONENTS OF DIALYSIS

- **Catheter:** Silastic tube that is either implanted using general anesthesia as a surgical procedure for patients who will have long-term treatment or inserted using local anesthesic at the bedside for short-term dialysis.
- **Dialysate:** Sterile electrolyte solution similar in composition to normal plasma. The electrolyte composition of the dialysate can be adjusted according to individual need. The most commonly adjusted electrolyte is K^+. Glucose is added to the dialysate in varying concentrations to remove excess body fluid via osmosis. **Note:** Some glucose crosses the peritoneal membrane and enters the patient's blood. Patients with diabetes mellitus may require additional insulin. Observe for and report indicators of hyperglycemia

(e.g., complaints of thirst, changes in sensorium). Insulin and other medications, such as heparin and potassium xylocaine, may be added directly to the dialysate by dialysis nurses.

TYPES OF DIALYSIS

Intermittent peritoneal dialysis (IPD): The patient receives dialysis for periods of 8-10 hr, 4-5 times/wk. A predetermined amount of dialysate (usually 2 L) is instilled for a set length of time (usually 20-30 min). It is then allowed to drain by gravity, and the process is repeated. IPD can be performed manually with individual bags or mechanically using a proportioning machine or cycler. The patient is restricted to a chair or bed. PD can be performed also as an acute, temporary procedure. Continuous hourly exchanges are performed for 48-72 hr. The patient is restricted to bed.

Continuous ambulatory peritoneal dialysis (CAPD): Using sterile technique, the patient attaches a new bag of dialysate to the peritoneal catheter, allows the dialysate to drain out, and then allows new dialysate to drain in. The patient then clamps the catheter and places a new cap on the tubing using sterile technique. This process is repeated q4-6hr (8 hr at night), 7 days/wk. CAPD is used primarily for ESRD.

Continuous cycling peritoneal dialysis (CCPD): This is a combination of IPD and CAPD. A cycler performs dialysate exchanges at night. In the morning the final exchange is instilled and left in the peritoneal cavity for the entire day. At the end of the day, the fourth exchange is allowed to drain out, and the process is repeated. The patient is ambulatory by day and restricted to bed at night. CCPD is commonly done every night.

HEALTH CARE SETTING

For IPD: Dialysis center; acute care if patient has complications
For CAPD and CCPD: Home setting; acute care if patient has complications

Nursing Diagnosis:

Risk for Infection

related to invasive procedure (direct access of the catheter to the peritoneum)

Desired Outcomes: Patient is free of infection as evidenced by normothermia and absence of the following: abdominal pain, cloudy outflow, nausea, malaise, erythema, edema, and increased local warmth, drainage, and tenderness at the exit site. Before discharge from dialysis center or following outpatient instruction, patient verbalizes signs and symptoms of infection and the need for sterile technique for bag, tubing, and dressing changes.

INTERVENTIONS	RATIONALES
Monitor for and report indications of peritonitis. Teach these indicators to patient.	The most common complication of PD is peritonitis. Indicators include fever, abdominal pain, distention, abdominal wall rigidity, rebound tenderness, cloudy outflow, nausea, and malaise.
Use sterile technique and teach patient that it is essential that sterile technique be used when connecting and disconnecting catheter from dialysis system.	To minimize risk of peritonitis and other infections.
Maintain sterile technique when adding medications to dialysate.	The dialysate must remain sterile because it is instilled directly into the body.
Follow agency policy for care of catheter exit site.	Exit site infections may lead to development of peritonitis.
Observe for and report erythema, local warmth, edema, drainage, or tenderness at exit site. Culture any exudate and report results to health care provider. Teach these indicators to patient.	Signs of infection at the exit site.
Report to health care provider if dialysate leaks around catheter exit site. Teach patient to do the same.	This can indicate an obstruction or need for another purse-string suture around catheter site. Leakage around the exit site has been associated with an increased risk of tunnel infections, exit site infections, and peritonitis. Organisms may track through the subcutaneous tissue into the peritoneum, causing infection.

●●● **Related NIC and NOC labels:** *NIC:* Infection Protection; Incision Site Care; Specimen Management
NOC: Infection Status

Nursing Diagnosis:

Risk for Imbalanced Fluid Volume

related to excess fluid volume secondary to inadequacy of exchanges; or *related to* deficient fluid volume secondary to hypertonicity of the dialysate

Desired Outcomes: Postdialysis the patient is normovolemic as evidenced by balanced I&O, stable weight, absence of peripheral and periorbital edema, good skin turgor, central venous pressure (CVP) 5-12 cm H_2O, RR 12-20 breaths/min with normal depth and pattern (eupnea), and BP and HR within patient's normal range. The volume of dialysate outflow equals or exceeds inflow.

INTERVENTIONS	RATIONALES
Monitor for and report indicators of fluid overload, such as edema, hypertension, dyspnea, tachycardia, distended neck veins, or increased CVP. Also be alert to incomplete dialysate returns.	Fluid retention can occur because of catheter complications that prevent adequate outflow, a severely scarred peritoneum that prevents adequate exchange, or inadequate dialysis prescriptions. Accurate measurement and recording of outflow are critical to detect these problems promptly.
Monitor for the following and intervene as indicated: - *Full colon:* Use stool softeners, high-fiber diet, laxatives, or enemas if necessary. - *Catheter occlusion by fibrin* (usually occurs soon after insertion): Obtain prescription to irrigate with heparinized saline. - *Catheter obstruction by omentum:* Turn patient from side to side, elevate head of bed (HOB) or foot of bed, or apply firm pressure to the abdomen. Notify health care provider for unresolved outflow problems.	These factors are potential causes of outflow problems, and they necessitate intervention to reverse the problem.
Monitor I&O and weight daily. Weigh patient at the same time each day, using the same scale and with patient wearing the same amount of clothing (or with same items on the bed if using a bed scale).	Patient's weight is one of the key indicators in choosing dialysis solutions. For example, a steady weight gain indicates fluid retention and may indicate a need for increased dialysis. Weighing patient under the same conditions helps ensure accurate measurement of fluid status.
If respiratory distress occurs, elevate HOB, drain the dialysate, and notify dialysis nurse and/or health care provider.	Respiratory distress can occur because of compression of the diaphragm by the dialysate, especially when patient is supine. Raising HOB may help alleviate this problem because the diaphragm will be less compressed by the dialysis solution. Should respiratory distress continue, the dialysis nurse should be notified because drainage of the solution may alleviate diaphragmatic pressure.
Monitor for gross bloody outflow.	Bloody outflow may appear with initial exchanges as a sign of peritonitis (see earlier nursing diagnosis).
Report it to health care provider if patient also exhibits other signs of peritonitis.	Because bloody outflow can also appear as a result of menstruation, the nurse should ask female patient if she is menstruating during assessment for signs and symptoms of peritonitis.
Assess for and report indicators of volume depletion.	Volume depletion (e.g., poor skin turgor, hypotension, tachycardia, and decreased CVP) can occur with excessive use of hypertonic dialysate and should be reported promptly for timely intervention.

●●● **Related NIC and NOC labels:** *NIC:* Fluid Monitoring; Vital Signs Monitoring; Peritoneal Dialysis Therapy *NOC:* Fluid Balance

Nursing Diagnosis:

Imbalanced Nutrition: Less than body requirements

related to protein loss in the dialysate

Desired Outcomes: At a minimum of 24 hr before hospital discharge or within 2-3 days following intervention/instruction for patient who is not hospitalized, patient exhibits adequate nutrition as evidenced by stable weight and serum albumin 3.5-5.5 g/dl. Following patient teaching, patient's protein intake is 1.2-1.5 g/kg body weight/day.

INTERVENTIONS	RATIONALES
Ensure adequate dietary intake of protein: 1.2-1.5 g/kg body weight/day.	Protein crosses the peritoneum, and a significant amount is lost in the dialysate. An increased intake of protein is necessary to prevent excessive tissue catabolism. Protein loss increases with peritonitis.
Ensure that a dietary evaluation and teaching program are initiated when patient changes from one type of dialysis to the other. Refer patient to a renal dietitian if one is available.	Sodium and potassium restrictions typically are less for a patient receiving peritoneal dialysis than for one on hemodialysis. This is due, in part, to the fact that dialysis is provided continuously to peritoneal dialysis patients versus only 3 times/wk for those receiving hemodialysis.
Provide list of restricted and encouraged foods (based on input of dietitian) with menus that illustrate their integration into the daily diet. Have patient plan a 3-day menu that incorporates appropriate foods and restrictions.	To ensure understanding of dietary restrictions. Asking patient to apply newly learned information via menu planning is a valid way of teaching and evaluating patient's understanding.

●●● **Related NIC and NOC labels:** *NIC:* Nutrition Monitoring; Nutrition Management; Teaching: Prescribed Diet *NOC:* Nutritional Status: Nutrient Intake

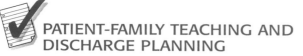

PATIENT-FAMILY TEACHING AND DISCHARGE PLANNING

When providing patient-family teaching, focus on sensory information, avoid giving excessive information, and initiate a visiting nurse referral if indicated for follow-up teaching. Include verbal and written information about the following:

✓ Medications, including drug name, purpose, dosage, schedule, drug/drug and food/drug interactions, precautions, and potential side effects.

✓ Diet: Include fact sheets that list foods to limit or restrict. Review fluid restrictions. Provide sample menus with examples of how dietary restrictions may be incorporated into daily meals. Have patient demonstrate understanding of dietary restrictions by preparing 3-day menus.

✓ Care and observation of exit site as per agency protocol.

✓ Importance of continued medical follow-up; confirm date and time of next health care provider appointment.

✓ Signs and symptoms that necessitate medical attention. For example, symptoms that may indicate need for alteration in dialysis prescription: increased weight gain, unusual short-ness of breath, edema, dizziness or fainting; symptoms that may indicate infection: fever, abdominal pain, redness or discharge from exit site, cloudy or decreased outflow, or nausea.

✓ Phone numbers to call should questions or concerns arise about therapy or disease after discharge. Additional general information can be obtained by contacting:

National Kidney and Urologic Diseases Information Clearinghouse
3 Information Way
Bethesda, MD 20892-3580
(301) 654-4415
Fax: (301) 907-8906
www.niddk.nih.gov/health/kidney/nkudic.htm

National Kidney Foundation
30 E. 33rd Street, Suite 1100
New York, NY 10016
(800) 622-9010
Fax: (212) 689-9261
www.kidney.org

Care of the Renal Transplant Recipient

Annually over 14,000 patients with end-stage renal disease (ESRD) receive a renal transplant. A small but increasing number of patients with ESRD and diabetes receive a combined kidney-pancreas transplant. Although patients receive transplants at major medical centers and are cared for postoperatively in specialized units, they may be admitted to any hospital for treatment of a rejection episode, medication complication, or unrelated illness. The majority of the transplanted kidneys come from cadavers, although living family members or friends also might donate. The organs for combined kidney-pancreas transplants come from a single cadaveric donor. Unless the graft is donated from an identical twin, transplant success depends on the suppression of graft rejection. This is accomplished by carefully matching donors to recipients through tissue typing before transplantation and immunosuppression after transplantation. Rejection is the major complication of renal transplant. Long-term complications occur secondary to the use of immunosuppressive agents and include infection, hypertension, cardiovascular disease, chronic liver disease, bone demineralization, cataracts, gastrointestinal (GI) hemorrhage, and cancer.

The transplant experience usually is a planned, elective surgery. There are strict criteria for being accepted into the program and many contraindications for the surgery. An extensive preoperative evaluation includes assessment of physical, cognitive, emotional, and financial readiness for this life change.

HEALTH CARE SETTING

Transplant center; acute care surgical unit or critical care unit for complications or rejection

IMMUNOSUPPRESSION

Suppression of the patient's immune system and prevention of rejection are vital for the patient's acceptance of the transplanted kidney. Currently used immunosuppressive drugs provide a nonpermanent form of tolerance. Immunosuppression is necessary for the life of the graft. Despite advances in understanding immunology, these medications put the transplant patient at increased risk for infection and development of malignancy in the long term.

REJECTION

Although significant improvements in graft survival have been made in the past decade, graft rejection is a major reason for graft loss in kidney transplantation. The four types of rejection include the following:

- **Hyperacute:** Occurs within minutes to hours after transplant owing to cytotoxic antibodies against donor-specific antigens. This type occurs rarely.
- **Accelerated:** Occurs 2-6 days after transplant because of prior sensitization of antigens similar to those of the donor to newly developed donor-specific antibodies. This is more common in patients who have undergone previous transplantation and is usually resistant to antibody therapy.
- **Acute:** There are two types of rejection that are considered acute—acute cellular rejection and acute vascular rejection. The most common form of acute cellular rejection occurs 1 wk to 4 mo after surgery and has the potential for reversibility. Patients are usually treated with increased immunosuppression. Vascular rejection occurs on a humoral level and is not as amenable to drug therapy. Vascular rejection is generally caused by hemodynamic compromise to the graft.
- **Chronic:** Occurs months to years after transplant. It is irreversible and managed conservatively with diet and antihypertensives until dialysis is required. Chronic rejection is a slow process that generally manifests as hypertension, proteinuria, and a decline in kidney func-

tion leading to renal failure. Diagnosis is made by clinical symptoms and kidney biopsy.

Indicators of rejection: Oliguria, tenderness over graft site (located in iliac fossa), sudden weight gain (2-3 lb/day), fever, malaise, hypertension, and increased blood urea nitrogen (BUN) and serum creatinine. In addition, hyperglycemia will develop with combined kidney-pancreas transplants.

Nursing Diagnosis:

Deficient Knowledge:

Immunosuppressive maintenance medication management

Desired Outcome: Immediately following teaching and on an ongoing basis, patient verbalizes accurate understanding of the prescribed immunosuppressive maintenance medications, including purpose and potential side effects.

INTERVENTIONS	RATIONALES
Teach patient and family the importance of taking the prescribed medications, their purpose and side effects, and the appropriate procedures for taking them.	Medications prevent rejection of the transplanted kidney; a knowledgeable patient is more likely to comply with this critically important element of therapy. Preoperative medication instruction begins early, and every member of the transplant team discusses side effects of these medications. Posttransplant follow-up generally occurs twice per week during the first month, once per week for the next month, and then once every other week until once per month for the rest of the patient's life.
	Immunosuppressive maintenance medication management ("triple therapy") typically includes a combination of the following drug families: antiinterleukins/calcineurin inhibitor, antiproliferative antimetabolite agents, and antiinflammatory agents. Each of these agents works on a different and separate level of the complex immunosuppressant cascade. The goal of these drugs is prevention of patient's immune system from attacking the newly transplanted kidney.
1. Antiinterleukin agents	
Cyclosporine (Sandimmune, Neoral, Gengraf)	Suppresses immune response by inhibiting the first phase of T-cell activation. Initial posttransplant dosages are 15 mg/kg/day, which are slowly tapered to a maintenance level of 5-10 mg/kg/day. Route is either PO or IV.
Teach patient the following:	
- Importance of keeping regularly scheduled appointments with health care provider and for laboratory work.	Serum levels should be closely monitored to ensure optimum effect while avoiding adverse side effects.
- Be alert to and report immediately: headaches, confusion, tremors, hypertension, and irregular heartbeat.	Adverse drug side effects. Hirsutism, gum hyperplasia/bleeding, diarrhea, leg cramps, and loss of appetite also may occur but are less urgent. Hirsutism, for example, can be managed with electrolysis, bleaching, creams, or waxing.
- Although this drug is most commonly prescribed in capsule form, if a liquid form is required, follow label directions precisely.	Taking this medication as prescribed decreases risk of drug/food interactions, as well as reaction of the drug with the container in which it is mixed. Most pharmacists counsel that cyclosporine should not be mixed in a plastic or foam container because the drug adheres to the sides of the container. Taking the medication at the same time each day enables better absorption and increased efficacy.

Continued

INTERVENTIONS	**RATIONALES**
- Do not use grapefruit juice or products containing grapefruit juice, such as Fresca.	Grapefruit juice is a cytochrome P450 inhibitor that could interact with cyclosporine, causing increased drug levels.
- Discuss oral problems with dentist. Use soft toothbrush. Inspect mouth daily and report sores that develop to transplant health care provider.	Gingival hyperplasia and oral bleeding can occur. Immunosuppressive medications put patients at risk for oral lesions or thrush or other opportunistic oral infections.
- As indicated, ensure effective contraception.	In animal trials, this drug has interfered with normal prenatal development.
Tacrolimus (FK506, Prograf): **Note:** This drug is used in place of cyclosporine.	Inhibits T-cell activity to suppress the inflammatory response, thereby aiding in rejection prevention. Dosage is 0.15-0.3 mg/kg/day; oral administration is preferred.
Teach patient to be alert to and report tremor, headache, insomnia, constipation, diarrhea, and vomiting.	Side effects.
Teach importance of scheduled assessments of laboratory values.	Renal or liver dysfunction, hyperkalemia, and increased glucose levels can occur.
Sirolimus (Rapamune)	Inhibits T cell from recognizing interleukin-2 (IL-2) of the immune response. It is for oral use only and is available in liquid and tablet forms. It is given 4 hr after cyclosporine. Azathioprine is discontinued before initiating sirolimus.
Teach patient the following:	
- If liquid form is prescribed, mix only with water or orange juice.	Sirolimus is metabolized by the CYP3A4 enzyme system in the gut and liver. Other liquids may act as inducers or inhibitors.
- Avoid meals that are high in fat content when taking the drug.	Fat alters bioavailability of the drug
- Effective contraception must be used.	In animal trials, this drug has interfered with normal prenatal development.
- Be alert to and report edema, weight gain, tremor, insomnia, arthralgia, nausea, vomiting, diarrhea, acne, and rash.	Side effects.
- Be sure to follow through with scheduled laboratory assessments.	Increased serum creatinine, hypertension, anemia, hyperkalemia, hyperlipidemia, and hyperphosphatemia can occur when taking this drug.
Diltiazem (Cardizem CD)	This is not an antiinterleukin agent but rather an adjunct drug used to potentiate effects of cyclosporine, tacrolimus, or sirolimus. In addition to potentiating the effects of these drugs, it also may decrease hypertension by dilating afferent arterioles in the kidney.
Teach patient to be alert to and report dizziness, edema, headache, slowed heart rate, or weakness. Nausea and constipation also can occur, as can dysuria and rash.	Side effects.
2. Antiproliferative agents	
Azathioprine (Imuran)	Alters immune response in renal transplant recipients and prevents acute rejection by inhibiting T-cell replication and B-cell immune responses. Maintenance usually is accomplished with 1 mg/kg or less daily.
Teach patient the following:	
- Importance of keeping regularly scheduled appointments with health care provider and for laboratory work.	Dosage is adjusted based on white blood cell (WBC) count.

Continued

INTERVENTIONS	**RATIONALES**
- Be alert to and report changes in size and shape of moles. Avoid prolonged sun exposure; use at least SPF 20 sunscreen.	Risk of skin cancer is 3-5 × greater with this drug than with other immunosuppressive agents.
- Take drug with food.	Nausea, vomiting, and diarrhea can occur. Taking with food helps decrease gastric irritation. Patient should contact transplant nurse if symptoms persist.
- Avoid contact with persons with colds/flu and other common illnesses. Maintain good hygiene by bathing daily and shampooing regularly. Ensure good oral hygiene.	Measures to manage increased susceptibility to infection, a side effect of azathioprine.
- Gently brush teeth with soft-bristled toothbrush after each meal. Wait at least 3 mo after transplant before having dental procedures.	Mouth sores are a side effect of this drug.
- Explain that although hair will thin on this drug, patient will not go bald.	Knowledge that hair will grow back is likely to be reassuring.
- Notify health care provider if bruising occurs or blood appears in stool or urine.	There is an increased tendency to bleed when taking this drug because the platelet count is reduced.
Mycophenolate (CellCept)	Suppresses immune-mediated inflammatory response in renal transplant patients. It prevents acute rejection by inhibiting T and B lymphocytes. It is given in combination with other drugs to prevent rejection.
Teach patient the following:	
Be alert to and report nausea, vomiting, and diarrhea.	Drug side effects.
Take only on empty stomach.	Improves drug absorption.
Do cut tablets, open capsules, or handle medication inside tablets or capsules. Ensure that effective contraception is used.	In animal trials, this drug has been found to be teratogenic (interfering with prenatal development).
3. Antiinflammatory agent	
Prednisone	Suppresses/prevents cell-mediated immune response. Initial maintenance dosages vary but usually are 0.5 mg/kg/day. Gradually the maintenance dose may be reduced to 10 mg/day and then tapered off completely around 3 mo posttransplant.
Teach patient the following:	
Be alert to and report the following: signs of infection, hypertension, bruising, muscle wasting, bone pain, cataracts, acne, mood and behavior changes, increased appetite, weight gain, night sweats, and cushingoid changes.	Side effects of this drug. They should be reported to transplant team because medications can be substituted and side effects decreased. Support is available.
If bothersome side effects occur:	
- Practice good skin hygiene; if acne develops, request medicated soap or cream from health care provider.	To treat acne.
- Avoid turtlenecks; wear makeup if appropriate.	To minimize appearance of moonface.
- Try to control caloric intake.	Appetite will be increased. It is easier to keep weight off than it is to try to lose it later.
- Become involved in an exercise program.	Muscle wasting is a side effect of this drug.
- Inform family and friends that you may be susceptible to mood swings.	Individuals who are informed of this side effect likely will be more supportive during those periods.
- Take the drug with food.	Decreases stomach irritation.

Continued

INTERVENTIONS	RATIONALES
- Individuals with diabetes will need to adjust insulin dosages.	Prednisone increases blood sugar, which will necessitate more insulin. As prednisone dose is decreased, need for insulin will decrease.
- Avoid contact with persons with colds/flu and other common illnesses. Maintain good hygiene by bathing daily and shampooing regularly. Ensure good oral hygiene.	Measures to manage increased susceptibility to infection.
Wear a Medic-Alert bracelet.	To alert other medical professionals that this drug is being used.

●●● **Related NIC and NOC labels:** *NIC:* Teaching: Prescribed Medication *NOC:* Knowledge: Medication

Nursing Diagnosis:

Deficient Knowledge:

Medication regimen for acute rejection episode

Desired Outcome: Immediately following teaching, patient verbalizes accurate understanding of the medications used during an acute rejection episode, if it occurs, including purpose and potential side effects.

INTERVENTIONS	RATIONALES
See first intervention in previous nursing diagnosis.	
Antilymphocyte globulin (ALG)	Decreases T cells, which helps prevent rejection. It is given IV in doses of 10-30 mg/kg/day.
Teach patient the following:	
- Be alert to chills, fever, rash, joint pain, and anaphylaxis.	These are the immediate side effects of this drug.
- Be aware of the potential for malignancy and increased risk of infection.	Potential adverse effects.
Monoclonal antibody (Orthocione OKT3)	Blocks T-cell function to help reverse renal rejection. It is given IV bolus in <1 min. Recommended therapy is to precede dosage with methylprednisolone 1 mg/kg IV and follow 30 min after the dosage with 100 mg of hydrocortisone.
Teach patient the following:	
- Be alert to fever, chills, tremor, headache, vomiting, nausea, dyspnea, and bronchospasm.	Immediate side effects.
- Be aware of increased risk of infection and potential for malignancy.	Potential adverse effects.
- Patients receiving initial doses require close monitoring because of the high incidence of side effects.	Respiratory side effects, especially pulmonary edema, are more likely to occur if patient has excess fluid volume. Ideally patients should be within 3% of their "dry weight" while taking this drug.
Prednisone	During acute rejection, dosage may be increased to 2-3 mg/kg/day followed with gradually tapering the dose. See discussion in the previous nursing diagnosis.
Sirolimus	See discussion in previous nursing diagnosis.

●●● **Related NIC and NOC labels:** *NIC:* Teaching: Prescribed Medication *NOC:* Knowledge: Medication

Nursing Diagnosis:

Ineffective Tissue Perfusion: Renal

(or risk for same) *related to* decreased cellular exchange secondary to rejection of kidney and renal failure; or *related to* complications of surgery such as ureteral obstruction or thrombosis of graft

Desired Outcome: Optimally within 24 hr after interventions, patient attains hemodynamic stability and has stable I&O with urinary output >100 ml/hr, stable weight, clear breath sounds, and no evidence of edema.

INTERVENTIONS	RATIONALES
Initially during the postoperative period, monitor I&O q30min-1h per institution transplant protocol until output exceeds 30 ml/hr.	Urine output is generally a good indicator of tissue perfusion in a healthy kidney. Decreased or absent urinary output compared to input may indicate poor renal perfusion, impaired glomerular filtration, and/or acute rejection.
Monitor hemodynamic status by assessing central venous pressure (CVP) readings and BP and pulse q2-4h on first postoperative day and q4-12h thereafter as patient's condition warrants.	Increases from baseline may indicate fluid overload caused by lack of kidney function.
	The goal is for BP and pulse to be within 20% of patient's baseline readings and BP to be <200/110 mm Hg. CVP measurements can detect disorders before changes in VS develop. Although normal CVP levels are between 3-15 mm Hg, CVP >10 mm Hg should be reported to transplant team inasmuch as it may signal a trend.
Assess breath sounds q4-8h, adjusting frequency as patient's condition warrants.	Adventitious breath sounds are indicators of fluid volume excess and the kidney's inability to regulate this excess. This can lead to heart failure.
Document urine color and characteristics. Report any changes.	In a healthy kidney, darkening of the urine may indicate dehydration.
Weigh patient daily before breakfast using the same scale and with patient wearing same amount of clothing.	Weight is an important indicator of fluid status. Weight gain in the early postoperative period (first 48-72 hr) suggests fluid volume excess owing to IV fluids during surgery. Weight gain later in the postoperative period (with no IV fluids) may be a result of excessive intake of calories and increasing fat stores, side effects from antirejection medication, or declining function of the kidney with resultant inability to regulate body fluids. Weight loss (compared with preoperative weight) is expected in the immediate postoperative period as a normal physiologic response.
Assess face, hands, shins, feet, and lumbosacral area for edema.	Edema occurs primarily in dependent areas of the body (e.g., hands, feet, and lumbosacral area).
Check for presence of pitting by making a thumbprint in the shin, foot, or sacral area.	An indentation or pit that remains signals pitting edema. An individual can gain up to 10 lb (4.5 kg) before pitting edema is present. Periorbital edema may be an early sign of this fluid shift because these fragile tissues are distended by even minimal fluid accumulation. Dependent edema may indicate rejection of the kidney or toxicity from cyclosporine or tacrolimus.
Measure lower extremity diameters with a millimeter measuring tape. Report increases based on parameters given by transplant team.	Measurements provide objective data for assessment of increasing edema.

Continued

INTERVENTIONS	RATIONALES
Monitor urine specific gravity, serum electrolytes (sodium and potassium), BUN, and creatinine levels.	Hyponatremia may result from fluid overload (dilutional) or inability of the kidney to conserve sodium. Hypernatremia indicates a deficit of body water. Lack of renal excretion and/or retention of potassium by the kidney in order to excrete excess H^+ (to correct acidosis) leads to hyperkalemia. Urine specific gravity measures the kidney's ability to concentrate urine. In renal failure the specific gravity is usually ≤1.010, indicating loss of ability to concentrate the urine. Rising BUN and creatinine are measures of renal dysfunction/failure. Creatinine is the most effective indicator because it is not influenced by hydration, diet, or tissue catabolism.
As indicated, provide a dietary consultation for renal diet and teaching.	Consultation with a dietitian or nutritional support team will help determine patient's caloric and nutrient needs within prescribed restrictions. A low-protein diet may be indicated because of ketoacid formation during digestion, which places greater demands on the kidney. If patient is in acute renal failure, restrictions of potassium, sodium, and phosphorus may be needed to decrease further renal damage.
Assess for indicators of graft rejection. (See signs and symptoms of rejection in introductory data.)	
Early phase: Monitor urinary elimination by assessing patency of indwelling catheter and urinary output qh during the first 24hr, then q2-4h as patient's condition warrants. Notify health care provider if urinary catheter is not draining or if urinary output is <100 ml/hr.	If decreased urinary output occurs in the early phase (first 18 hr), it may be the result of acute tubular necrosis (ATN) or mechanical obstruction (i.e., catheter obstruction, ureteral obstruction, surgical stitch, or thrombosis). Ischemia resulting from obstruction can damage nephrons, ultimately decreasing tissue perfusion.
If indicated, irrigate catheter using 30 ml normal saline and a catheter-tip syringe.	A measure to help assess for cause of these symptoms. Patient's catheter may be obstructed or a larger catheter may be needed.
If ATN is suspected, restrict fluids to 1500 ml/24 hr. It may be necessary to restrict potassium and phosphate as well.	In ATN, necrosis and sloughing of the epithelium and blockage of the tubules occur. Intimal arteritis with necrosis and hemorrhage may occur in severe cases of acute rejection. Because of this, renal perfusion and ability of the kidney to excrete excess fluid, potassium, and phosphate are diminished.
As indicated, prepare patient for a renal duplex ultrasound to rule out thrombosis or hydronephrosis.	Thrombosis and hydronephrosis of the graft are potential causes of decreased renal perfusion leading to decreased urinary output. Noninvasive studies demonstrating good flow, vessel patency, and absence of hydronephrosis will confirm the graft is fundamentally sound.
If thrombosis or hydronephrosis is diagnosed, prepare patient for emergency surgery.	A thrombus can be removed from the vessels of the graft, and a ureteral stent or nephrostomy tube may be placed to relieve obstruction and hydronephrosis. Dialysis can be continued postoperatively until the transplanted kidney recovers.
Late phase: Assess VS for changes in BP (±20% from baseline), increased body temperature, and increased pulse. Assess breath sounds for crackles or other adventitious sounds indicative of excessive fluid volume as a result of decreased renal perfusion.	If such problems occur during the late phase (>24 hr after transplant through hospital discharge), they may be the result of rejection, thrombosis, nephrotoxicity (side effect of cyclosporine), ureteral obstruction resulting in hydronephrosis, bladder dysfunction, or infection.
Assess patency of indwelling catheter (as discussed under "early phase") or check postvoid residual as indicated. Obtain a urinalysis and culture as appropriate.	If the bladder is retaining urine and an indwelling catheter is present, it is usually removed, and clean intermittent catheterization is used instead to decrease risk of urinary infection.

Continued

INTERVENTIONS	RATIONALES
Prepare patient for tests such as a renal duplex ultrasound or renal biopsy by explaining procedure, rationale, and sensations to expect.	A renal duplex ultrasound is a noninvasive procedure in which ultrasound waves transmit through tissues of the kidney to reveal whether ureteral obstruction, hydronephrosis, or perinephric fluid collection is present. If obstruction is present, the patient usually returns to the operating room where a ureteral stent or nephrostomy tube is placed to relieve hydronephrosis, or a thrombectomy is performed to promote renal blood flow.
	A renal biopsy is invasive in that a small area of skin is prepared with a local anesthetic, and an open-bore needle is inserted into the kidney to remove a tissue sample. The patient may feel pressure, but if skin is anesthetized well, pain should not occur. A renal biopsy will confirm a late rejection episode and may help determine cause. Dialysis can be reinitiated until the transplanted kidney recovers.
If rejection is confirmed, administer high-dose corticosteroids or drugs such as OKT3 as prescribed.	When the cause of rejection is cellularly mediated and involves T lymphocytes and various lymphokines (seen in the tissue biopsy), then high-dose corticosteroids or antilymphocyte preparations such as OKT3 may be used to halt the rejection process.
If nephrotoxicity is confirmed, anticipate altered dosages of patient's medications.	Medication doses will be changed accordingly to decrease stress on the kidney.

●●● **Related NIC and NOC labels:** *NIC:* Bedside Laboratory Testing; Electrolyte Monitoring; Laboratory Data Interpretation; Vital Signs Monitoring; Invasive Hemodynamic Monitoring; Shock Management
NOC: Fluid Balance; Urinary Elimination

Nursing Diagnosis:
Risk for Infection

related to invasive procedures, exposure to infected individuals, and immunosuppression

Desired Outcomes: Patient is free of infection as evidenced by normothermia, HR ≤100 bpm (or within patient's normal range), RR 12-20 breaths/min with normal depth and pattern, and absence of erythema, edema, increased local warmth, tenderness, or purulent drainage at wounds or catheter exit sites. Patient is free of signs and symptoms of oral, esophageal, respiratory, GI, genitourinary, and cutaneous infections. Patient verbalizes indicators of infection and the importance of reporting them promptly to health care provider or staff.

INTERVENTIONS	RATIONALES
When caring for patient, increase your sensitivity to *any* indicator of infection as a cue to increase depth and frequency of assessments for infection.	These patients are taking large doses of immunosuppressive agents, and their immune response and thus response to infectious agents will be muted. Infections therefore are potentially life threatening in an individual who is immunosuppressed.
Be especially sensitive to low-grade temperature elevation, fever, and unexplained tachycardia.	Indicators that might signal infection in a transplant recipient.

Continued

INTERVENTIONS	RATIONALES
Instruct patient to be alert to signs and symptoms of commonly encountered infections and importance of reporting them promptly.	These include *urinary tract infection* (UTI)—cloudy and malodorous urine; dysuria, frequency, and urgency; pain in the suprapubic area, buttock, thighs, labia, or scrotum; *upper respiratory tract infection* (URI)—productive cough, malodorous, purulent, colored, and copious secretions, chest pain or heaviness; *pharyngitis*—painful swallowing; *otitis media*—malaise, earache; *impetigo*—inflamed or draining areas on the skin.
	Prompt reporting of these indicators is essential because infections can be life threatening in a patient undergoing immunosuppression.
Monitor for symptoms of cytomegalovirus (CMV) and other infections, including fever, malaise, fatigue, and muscle aches. Teach patient importance of avoiding exposure to individuals known to have infections.	CMV is a common infectious agent among these patients. Other infectious complications include *Legionella pneumophila;* cutaneous herpes simplex (shingles); varicella zoster (chickenpox); Epstein-Barr virus (EBV); oral, esophageal, deep fungal, or mycotic pseudoaneurysm caused by *candida;* and *Pneumocystis carinii.*
Teach patient importance of good handwashing.	Washing hands consistently is a proven method of removing pathogens from the skin that could otherwise cause infection and is especially important in patients whose immune systems are compromised.
Administer prophylactic antibiotics as prescribed.	Some health care providers encourage antibiotics for any minor invasive procedures, including dental cleaning. Prophylactic antibiotics reduce infection risk, which can occur in even minor procedures.
Use sterile technique with all invasive procedures and dressing changes.	To reduce possibility of infection, which is increased with invasive procedures into the body and involving nonintact skin.
If patient is a smoker, be aggressive in advising smoking cessation. Recommend an approach such as a nicotine patch or gum and ask patient to set a date for cessation. Refer patient to a smoking cessation program. If patient lapses, encourage him or her to keep trying.	Smoking increases susceptibility to respiratory infection because it damages protective mechanisms such as cilia in the lungs. Smoking also causes detrimental changes to blood pressure, HR, cholesterol levels, and clotting factors.
For more information, see Appendix for "Infection Prevention and Control," p. 831.	

●●● **Related NIC and NOC labels:** *NIC:* Infection Control; Communicable Disease Management; Vital Signs Monitoring; Health Education *NOC:* Infection Status; Immune Status

Nursing Diagnosis:

Deficient Knowledge:

Signs and symptoms of rejection, side effects of immunosuppressive agents, transplantation complications, and importance of protecting the existing hemodialysis vascular access

Desired Outcome: Immediately following teaching and on an ongoing basis, patient verbalizes accurate knowledge of the signs and symptoms of rejection, the side effects of immunosuppressive therapy, complications of transplantation, and the importance of protecting the hemodialysis vascular access.

INTERVENTIONS	RATIONALES
Explain importance of keeping laboratory appointments for monitoring BUN and serum creatinine values.	These tests evaluate kidney status: as renal function decreases, BUN and creatinine values will increase.
Explain that serial monitoring of drug levels is essential as well.	These levels guide therapeutic drug regimen and treatment plan.
Teach patient signs and symptoms of rejection and importance of reporting these indicators promptly:	Signs and symptoms of rejection necessitate prompt intervention to save the kidney. These include oliguria, tenderness over transplanted kidney (located in iliac fossa), sudden weight gain (>5 lb in 2 days), fever, malaise, hypertension, and increased BUN (>20 mg/dl) and serum creatinine (>1.5 mg/dl). In addition, patient may have body aches, swelling in legs or hands, and temperature >100° F.
Provide patient with a notebook in which to record daily VS and weight measurements. Instruct patient to weigh self at the same time each day, using the same scale and wearing the same amount of clothing. Remind patient to bring the notebook to all outpatient visits and to report abnormal values promptly should they occur.	To monitor trend of VS and weight measurements. Using same standards daily ensures accuracy with weight measurements.
Alert patient to signs and symptoms of GI bleeding and importance of reporting these symptoms promptly should they occur.	GI bleeding is a potential side effect of immunosuppressive agents and can be life threatening if it is excessive. Prompt reporting of the onset of these symptoms (e.g., tarry stools, "coffee-ground" emesis, orthostatic changes, dizziness, tachycardia, increasing fatigue and weakness) enables health care provider to adjust medications or add medications such as antacids and H$_2$-receptor blockers to treat cause of the bleeding.
Teach patient and/or significant others how to measure BP and provide guidelines for values that would necessitate notification of health care provider or staff member.	In a patient who has undergone renal transplantation, hypertension may develop for a variety of reasons, including cyclosporine or steroid use, rejection, or renal artery stenosis. In addition, patient may have had hypertension before the transplant. A value that would necessitate notification of the health care provider is BP 20% above or below patient's "normal" BP. This value and parameters for calling health care provider are generally agreed on before patient leaves the hospital.
If patient has a fistula, shunt, or graft (hemodialysis vascular access), explain that it must be handled with care. See "Hemodialysis," pp. 252-254, for more information.	Patient will need the fistula, shunt, or graft if a return to dialysis is indicated, and therefore it must be handled carefully. Taking BPs, drawing blood, and starting IVs are contraindicated in the arm with the vascular access, and therefore patient should warn others about these contraindications.
Stress need for continued medical evaluation of the transplant.	To ensure that kidney is working properly and patient is not undergoing rejection.

●●● **Related NIC and NOC labels:** *NIC:* Teaching: Prescribed Medications; Teaching: Individual
NOC: Knowledge: Treatment Regimen

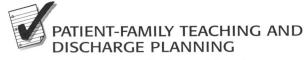

PATIENT-FAMILY TEACHING AND DISCHARGE PLANNING

When providing patient-family teaching, focus on sensory information, avoid giving excessive information, and make appropriate referrals (e.g., visiting or home health nurse, community health resources) for follow-up teaching. Include verbal and written information about the following:

✔ Medications, including name, dosage, purpose, schedule, precautions, drug/drug and food/drug interactions, and potential side effects. Provide guidelines for how to cope with medication side effects.

✓ Measures for preventing infection, including incision care. Stress to patient that infections can be life threatening because of immunosuppression.

✓ Prescribed diet and activity level progression.

✓ Community resources for emotional and financial support.

✓ Importance of follow-up care to ensure long-term viability of transplanted kidney.

✓ Phone numbers to call should problems or questions arise after discharge from care facility.

✓ Internet resources:

United Network for Organ Sharing
www.unos.org

National Kidney Disease Education Program
www.nkdep.nih.gov/

National Kidney Foundation
www.kidney.org

International Transplant Nurses Society
www.transweb.org/itns

Transplant Recipients International Organization (TRIO)
www.primenet.com/ntrio

✓ Also see discussions in **Deficient Knowledge:** Signs and symptoms of rejection, side effects of immunosuppressive agents, transplantation complications, and importance of protecting the existing hemodialysis vascular access, earlier.

Ureteral Calculi

Ureteral calculi (stones) are the third most common urologic condition after urinary tract infections (UTIs) and pathologic conditions of the prostate. Although the cause of stones is unknown in 50% of reported cases, it is believed that they originate in the kidney and are passed through the kidney into the ureter. About 90% of all stones pass from the ureter into the bladder and out of the urinary system spontaneously.

HEALTH CARE SETTING

Primary care; may require hospitalization for complications or surgery

ASSESSMENT

Signs and symptoms: Pain that is sharp, sudden, and intense or dull and aching; located in the flank area; and frequently radiating toward the groin. Pain may be intermittent (colic) as the stone moves along the ureter and may subside when it enters the bladder. Nausea, vomiting, diarrhea, abdominal pain, and paralytic ileus may occur. Patient may experience urgency and frequency, void in small amounts, and have hematuria. Fever may indicate an infected stone or secondary UTI.

Physical assessment: Hypertension, pallor, diaphoresis, tachycardia, and tachypnea may be noted. Costovertebral angle (CVA) tenderness and guarding may be present. Bowel sounds may be absent secondary to ileus, and the abdomen may be distended and tympanic. The patient will be restless and unable to find a position of comfort.

History of: Sedentary lifestyle; residence in geographic area in which water supply is high in stone-forming minerals; vitamin A deficiency; vitamin D excess; hereditary cystinuria; treatment with acetazolamide, which is given for glaucoma; inflammatory bowel disease; recurrent UTIs; prolonged periods of immobilization; gout or prophylactic therapy with allopurinol; decreased fluid intake; hyperparathyroidism; Paget's disease; sarcoidosis; and familial history of calculi or renal disease such as renal tubular acidosis.

DIAGNOSTIC TESTS

Serum tests: To assess calcium levels >5.3 mEq/L, phosphorus levels >2.6 mEq/L, and uric acid levels >7.5 mg/dl, which have been implicated in the formation of stones.

BUN and creatinine tests: To evaluate renal-urinary function. Abnormalities are reflected by high blood urea nitrogen (BUN) and serum creatinine levels and low urine creatinine levels. **Note:** BUN levels are affected by fluid volume excess and deficit. Volume excess will reduce BUN levels, whereas volume deficit will increase levels. For the older adult, serum creatinine level may not be a reliable measure of renal function because of reduced muscle mass and a decreased glomerular filtration rate. These tests must be evaluated based on an adjustment for the patient's age and hydration status and in comparison with other renal urinary tests.

Urinalysis: To provide baseline data on the functioning of the urinary system, detect metabolic disease, and assess for the presence of UTI. A cloudy or hazy appearance, foul odor, pH >8.0, and the presence of red blood cells (RBCs), leukocyte esterase, white blood cells (WBCs), and WBC casts signal UTI. A pH <5 is associated with uric acid calculi, whereas a pH ≥7.5 may signal presence of urea-splitting organisms (responsible for magnesium-ammonium-phosphate or struvite calculi).

Urine culture: To determine type of bacteria present in the genitourinary tract. To avoid contamination, a midstream specimen should be collected.

24-hr urine collection: To test for high levels of uric acid, cystine, oxalate, calcium, phosphorus, or creatinine.

Note: All urine samples should be sent to the laboratory immediately after they are obtained or refrigerated if this is not possible (specimens for culture are *not* refrigerated). Urine left at room temperature has greater potential for bacterial growth, turbidity, and alkaline pH, any of which can distort the reading.

Kidney, ureter, bladder (KUB) x-ray: To outline gross structural changes in the kidneys and urinary system. Typically, calcified calculi are seen (90% of urinary calculi are radiopaque, i.e., calcium or cystine). Serial radiography monitors progressive movement of the stone. Plain x-rays of the skeletal system may reveal Paget's disease, sarcoidosis, or changes associated with prolonged immobilization.

Excretory urogram/intravenous pyelogram (IVP): Used to visualize the kidneys, renal pelvis, ureters, and bladder. This test also outlines nonradiopaque stones within the ureters; nonradiopaque stones (such as uric acid calculi) are seen as radiolucent defects in the contrast media.

Renal ultrasound: To identify ureteral dilation and presence of stones in the ureters.

Computed tomography (CT) scan with or without injection of contrast medium: To distinguish cysts, tumors, calculi, and other masses and determine presence of ureteral dilation and bladder distention.

Nursing Diagnosis:

Acute Pain

related to presence of the calculus or the surgical procedure to remove it

Desired Outcomes: Patient's subjective perception of pain decreases within 1 hr of intervention, as documented by a pain scale. Objective indicators, such as grimacing, are absent or diminished.

INTERVENTIONS	RATIONALES
Assess and document quality, location, intensity, and duration of pain. Devise a pain scale with patient that ranges from 0 (no pain) to 10 (worst pain).	To determine intensity and trend of pain and subsequent relief obtained.
Notify health care provider of sudden and/or severe pain.	A sign that a stone is passing through the ureter.
Notify health care provider of a sudden cessation of pain. Strain all urine for solid matter and send it to the laboratory for analysis.	Can signal passage of the stone.
Medicate patient with prescribed analgesics, narcotics, and antispasmodics. Evaluate and document response based on the pain scale. Provide warm blankets, heating pad to affected area, or warm baths.	To relieve pain and ureteral spasms. **Note:** Morphine increases ureteral peristalsis, which aids in stone passage, but ureteral peristalsis can increase pain.
Encourage patient to request medication before discomfort becomes severe.	Pain is easier to manage when it is treated before it gets too severe because prolonged stimulation of pain receptors increases sensitivity to painful stimuli and increases amount of drug required to relieve pain.
Administer antiemetics (e.g., hydroxyzine, ondansetron, prochlorperazine, promethazine) as prescribed.	To promote comfort from nausea and vomiting.
Provide dissolution agent as instructed.	Dissolution agents such as orange juice alkalinize urine and work to shrink stones so that they can pass through the ureter.
Provide back rubs.	Back rubs are especially helpful for postoperative patients who were in the lithotomy position during surgery.
See "Pain," p. 41, for other interventions.	

●●● **Related NIC and NOC labels:** *NIC:* Medication Management; Pain Management; Simple Massage; Heat Application *NOC:* Comfort Level; Pain Control; Pain Level

Nursing Diagnosis:

Impaired Urinary Elimination (Dysuria, Urgency, Frequency)

related to obstruction caused by ureteral calculus

Desired Outcomes: Patient relates the return of a normal voiding pattern within 2 days. Patient demonstrates ability to record I&O and strain urine for stones.

INTERVENTIONS	RATIONALES
Determine and document patient's normal voiding pattern.	To establish a baseline for subsequent assessment.
Monitor and document quality and color of the urine.	Optimally, urine is straw colored and clear and has a characteristic odor. Dark urine is often indicative of dehydration, and blood-tinged urine can result from rupture of ureteral capillaries as the calculus passes through the ureter.
In patients for whom fluids are not restricted, encourage fluid intake of at least 2 L/day.	To help flush calculus through the ureter into the bladder and out through the system
Record accurate I&O; teach patient how to record I&O.	Output that is less than input could signal an obstruction. Patient should participate in I&O documentation to ensure that all output and intake is being recorded.
Strain all urine for evidence of solid matter; teach patient the procedure.	To detect passage of stones.
Send any solid matter to the laboratory for analysis.	To test for high levels of uric acid, cystine, oxalate, calcium, or phosphorus, which would signal presence and type of stones.

●●● **Related NIC and NOC labels:** *NIC:* Fluid Management; Urinary Elimination Management
NOC: Urinary Continence; Urinary Elimination

Nursing Diagnosis:

Impaired Urinary Elimination

related to obstruction or positional problems of the ureteral catheter

Desired Outcome: Following intervention, patient has output from the ureteral catheter and is free of spasms or flank pain after ureteral catheter has been removed.

INTERVENTIONS	RATIONALES
If patient has more than one ureteral catheter, label one *right* and the other *left*; keep all drainage records separate.	Occasionally, patients return from surgery with ureteral catheters. Ureteral catheters, also known as stents, are positioned postoperatively to enable healing and promote ureteral patency in the presence of edema. If patient has two ureteral catheters, separate output records are used to identify how each ureter is functioning.
Monitor output from ureteral catheter.	Amount will vary with each patient and will depend on catheter dimension.
If drainage is scanty or absent, milk catheter and tubing gently. If this fails, notify health care provider.	To try to dislodge the obstruction.
Caution: Never irrigate catheter without specific health care provider instructions to do so. If irrigation is prescribed, use gentle pressure and sterile technique.	There is potential for ureteral damage during irrigation caused by overdistention and/or introduction of pathogens.
Always aspirate with sterile syringe before instillation. Use another sterile syringe to insert amounts no greater than 3 ml per instillation.	To prevent infection and ureteral damage caused by overdistention.
Explain to patient that semi-Fowler's and side-lying positions are acceptable, but Fowler's position should be avoided.	Typically, patient will require bedrest if ureteral catheter is indwelling. Sutures are seldom used, and gravity resulting from Fowler's position could cause catheter to move into the bladder.

Continued

INTERVENTIONS	RATIONALES
Monitor urethral catheter as well.	Ureteral catheters are often attached to the urethral catheter after placement in the ureters to stabilize the ureteral catheters.
	The urethral catheter should be monitored to detect movement and to ensure that it is securely attached to patient.
After ureteral catheters have been removed (usually simultaneously with urethral catheter), monitor for and report flank pain, CVA tenderness, nausea, and vomiting.	Indicators of ureteral obstruction, which necessitates prompt intervention.

●●● **Related NIC and NOC labels:** *NIC:* Tube Care: Urinary *NOC:* Urinary Elimination

Nursing Diagnosis:

Risk for Impaired Skin Integrity

related to wound drainage after ureterolithotomy or procedures entering the ureter

Desired Outcome: Patient's skin surrounding the wound site remains nonerythemic and intact.

INTERVENTIONS	RATIONALES
Monitor incisional dressings frequently during first 24 hr and change or reinforce as needed. Note and document odor, consistency, and color of drainage.	Immediately after surgery, drainage may be red. Flank approaches to the ureter require muscle-splitting incisions and result in significant postoperative oozing of blood. Because drainage will also include urine leaking from the entered ureter, excoriation can result from prolonged contact of urine with the skin.
Use Montgomery straps or net wraps (e.g., Surginet) rather than tape to secure dressing.	To facilitate frequent dressing changes without harming the skin with tape removal.
If drainage is copious after drain removal, apply wound drainage or ostomy pouch with a skin barrier over the incision.	To prevent contact of wound drainage with the skin.
Use a pouch with an antireflux valve.	To prevent contamination from reflux.

●●● **Related NIC and NOC labels:** *NIC:* Skin Surveillance; Skin Care: Topical Treatments; Wound Care; Incision Site Care *NOC:* Tissue Integrity: Skin and Mucous Membranes; Wound Healing: Primary Intention

Nursing Diagnosis:

Deficient Knowledge:

Dietary regimen and prophylactic pharmacotherapy and their relationship to calculus formation or prevention

Desired Outcomes: Immediately following teaching, patient verbalizes accurate knowledge about foods and liquids to limit to prevent stone formation and within 24 hr demonstrates this knowledge by planning a 3-day menu that excludes or limits these foods. Immediately following teaching, patient verbalizes accurate understanding of medications used to prevent stone formation.

INTERVENTIONS	RATIONALES
Assess patient's knowledge about diet and its relationship to stone formation.	To determine patient's baseline knowledge, which will enable formulation of an individualized teaching plan.
Advise patient to maintain a urine output of 3 L/day.	Increasing urine output reduces saturation of stone-forming solutes.
Teach patient to maintain adequate hydration of at least 3 L/day.	Good hydration after meals and exercise is important because patient's solute load is highest at these times.
Caution: Persons with cardiac, liver, or renal disease require special fluid intake instructions from their health care provider.	These patients likely will need some degree of fluid restriction to prevent fluid overload.
Teach technique for measuring urine specific gravity via a hydrometer.	To follow trend of specific gravity. To minimize stone formation, specific gravity should remain <1.010.
As appropriate, provide the following information:	
For uric acid stones:	
- Limit intake of lean meat, legumes, whole grains; limit protein intake to 1 g/kg/day.	These foods are high in purine, which can lead to formation of uric acid stones.
- Allopurinol or sodium bicarbonate may be given prophylactically.	Allopurinol may be given to reduce uric acid production. Sodium bicarbonate may be given to alkalinize the urine, keeping the pH at ≥6.5 and thus preventing acid stone formation.
For calcium stones:	
- Limit intake of milk, cheese, green leafy vegetables, and yogurt. Also limit intake of sodium, refined carbohydrates, and animal proteins.	These foods are high in calcium. A low-Na^+ diet helps reduce intestinal absorption of calcium. Refined carbohydrates and animal proteins cause hypercalciuria.
- Encourage patient to eat foods high in natural fiber content (e.g., bran, prunes, apples)	Foods high in natural fiber provide phytic acid, which binds with dietary calcium.
- Explain that sodium cellulose phosphate, 5 g, may be given tid before each meal. It should be used with caution in postmenopausal women at risk for osteoporosis.	Sodium cellulose phosphate, when used with a calcium-restricted diet, reduces risk of stone formation by binding with intestinal calcium and thus increasing calcium excretion.
- Explain that orthophosphates (potassium acid phosphate and disodium and dipotassium phosphates) or thiazides also may be given for calcium stones.	To decrease urinary excretion of citrate and pyrophosphate and thus inhibit stone formation.
For oxalate stones:	
- Limit intake of chocolate, caffeine-containing drinks (including instant and decaffeinated coffees), beets, spinach, and peanuts.	These foods are high in oxalate.
- Explain that cholestyramine, 4 g qid, may be prescribed.	Cholestyramine binds with oxalate enterally.
- Caution that vitamin C supplements should be avoided.	As much as half of these supplements is converted to oxalic acid.
For cystine stones:	
- Explain that sodium bicarbonate or sodium-potassium citrate solution may be prescribed.	To increase urinary pH (≥7.5). Cystine stones need a lower pH in order to form.
- Explain that penicillamine or tiopronin may be given.	To lower cystine levels in the urine.
Ask patient to plan a 3-day menu that includes or excludes appropriate foods.	To determine patient's level of understanding of the prescribed diet and areas in which teaching should be reinforced. This effort by patient also will reinforce learning.

●●● **Related NIC and NOC labels:** *NIC:* Teaching; Prescribed Diet; Teaching: Prescribed Medications
NOC: Knowledge: Diet; Knowledge: Medications

ADDITIONAL NURSING DIAGNOSES/ PROBLEMS:

"Perioperative Care"   p. 47

PATIENT-FAMILY TEACHING AND DISCHARGE PLANNING

When providing patient-family teaching, focus on sensory information, avoid giving excessive information, and initiate a visiting nurse referral for necessary follow-up teaching. Include verbal and written information about the following:

✓ Medications, including drug name, purpose, dosage, schedule, drug/drug and food/drug interactions, precautions, and potential side effects.

✓ Indicators of UTI that necessitate medical attention: chills; fever; hematuria; flank, CVA, suprapubic, low back, buttock, scrotal, or labial pain; cloudy and foul-smelling urine; frequency; urgency; dysuria; and increasing or recurring incontinence.

✓ Care of incision, including cleansing and dressing. Teach patient signs and symptoms of local infection, including redness, swelling, local warmth, tenderness, and purulent drainage.

✓ Care of drains or catheters if patient is discharged with them.

✓ Importance of daily fluid intake of at least 2-3 L/day in nonrestricted patients.

✓ Dietary changes as specified by health care provider. Include fact sheets that list foods to restrict or add to the diet. Provide sample menus with examples of how dietary restrictions and requirements may be incorporated into daily meals.

✓ Activity restrictions as directed for patient who has had surgery: avoid lifting heavy objects (>10 lb) for the first 6 wk, be alert to fatigue, get maximum rest, and increase activities gradually to tolerance.

✓ Use of nitrazine paper to assess pH of urine. Desired pH will be determined by type of stone formation to which the patient is prone. Instructions for use are on nitrazine container.

✓ Importance of walking or other exercise to decrease risk of stone formation.

Urinary Diversions

When the bladder must be bypassed or is removed, a urinary diversion is created. Urinary diversions most commonly are created for individuals with bladder cancer. However, malignancies of the prostate, urethra, vagina, uterus, or cervix may require creation of a urinary diversion if anterior, posterior, or total pelvic exenteration must be done. Individuals with severe, nonmalignant urinary problems, such as radiation damage to the bladder, vesicovaginal fistula, urethrovaginal fistula, neurogenic bladder, radiation or interstitial cystitis, or urinary incontinence that cannot be managed conservatively, also are candidates for urinary diversion. A radical cystectomy may or may not accompany placement of a urinary diversion. Although most urinary diversions are permanent, some act as a temporary bypass of urine, and undiversion (reversal) can be performed if the patient's condition changes.

Intestinal (ileal) conduit: Any segment of bowel may be used to create a passageway for urine, but the ileal conduit is most commonly used. A 15-20 cm section of the ileum is resected from the intestine to form a passageway for the urine. The proximal end is closed, and the distal end is brought out through the abdomen, forming a stoma. The ureters are resected from the bladder and anastomosed to the ileal segment. The intestine is reanastomosed, and therefore bowel function is unaffected. Occasionally jejunum is used for the conduit. However, jejunal-conduit syndrome (hyperkalemia, hyponatremia, hypochloremia) frequently occurs.

Cutaneous ureterostomy: The ureters are resected from the bladder and brought out through the surface of the abdomen, either separately or with one attached to the other inside the body, resulting in only one abdominal stoma. Stenosis and ascending urinary tract infections (UTIs) are a common problem with this diversion.

Continent urinary diversion: There are several different continent procedures, but the two that are most commonly performed are the Indiana reservoir and the Kock continent urostomy. All continent urinary diversions are constructed with the following three components: a reservoir or reconstructed bladder, a continence mechanism, and an antireflux mechanism. The antireflux mechanism is established via use of the ileocecal valve, which acts as a one-way valve keeping urine in the reservoir until a catheter is passed through the skin-level stoma. The presence of a tapered ileal segment further strengthens the continence mechanism by creating increased resistance to urine outflow pressures. The ureters are attached at an angle to the wall of the cecum, preventing reflux of urine to the kidneys.

Orthotopic urinary diversion: Creates a pseudobladder from the ileum to which the urethra is attached to reestablish lower urinary tract function. Because this procedure requires an intact and functional external urethral sphincter, it is possible more frequently in males.

HEALTH CARE SETTING

Surgical unit; primary care

Nursing Diagnosis:

Anxiety

related to threat to self-concept, interaction patterns, or health status secondary to urinary diversion surgery

Desired Outcome: Within the 24-hr period before surgery, patient communicates fears and concerns, relates the attainment of increased psychologic and physical comfort, and exhibits effective coping mechanisms.

INTERVENTIONS	RATIONALES
Assess patient's perceptions of impending surgery and resulting body function changes. Listen actively.	Provides an opportunity for patient to express fears and anxieties and for nurse to evaluate the response. For example, "You seem very concerned about next week's surgery." Anger, denial, withdrawal, and demanding behaviors may be coping responses.
Acknowledge patient's anxieties and concerns.	Helps focus attention on anxieties and concerns so that they can be dealt with.
Provide brief, basic information regarding physiology of the procedure and equipment that will be used after surgery, including tubes and drains.	Knowledge is one of the best means of decreasing anxiety.
Show patient pouches that will be used after surgery. Assure patient that the pouch usually cannot be seen through clothing and that it is odor resistant.	Patient may worry that others will be able to see and smell the pouch.
For patient about to undergo a continent urostomy, explain that a pouching system may be needed for a short time after surgery. Explain that teaching about accessing the continent urostomy will be done before hospital discharge.	Decreases anxiety and reassures patient that he or she will be taught necessary skills before going home.
Discuss activities of daily living (ADL) with patient.	This information decreases anxiety that such ADL as showers, baths, and swimming can continue and that diet is not affected after the early postoperative period.
As appropriate, ask patient what information has been relayed by surgeon about sexual implications of the surgery.	Patient may be very anxious about sexual implications of this surgery but afraid to ask. Asking this question will help establish an open relationship between patient and primary nurse and inform nurse if patient has understood information given by the surgeon. For example, some males undergoing radical cystectomy with urinary diversion may become impotent, but recent surgical advances have enabled preservation of potency for others.
Arrange for a visit by the enterostomal therapy (ET) nurse during the preoperative period. Collaborate with surgeon, ET nurse, and patient to identify and mark the most appropriate site for the stoma.	Showing patient the actual spot for placement may help alleviate anxiety by reinforcing that impact on lifestyle and body image will be minimal.

●●● **Related NIC and NOC labels:** *NIC:* Anxiety reduction; Active Listening; Emotional Support; Teaching: Preoperative; Preparatory Sensory Information *NOC:* Anxiety Control; Coping

Nursing Diagnosis:

Ineffective Protection

related to neurosensory, musculoskeletal, and cardiac changes secondary to hyperchloremic metabolic acidosis with hypokalemia

Desired Outcome: Patient verbalizes orientation to person, place, and time (within patient's normal range) and remains free of injury caused by neurosensory, musculoskeletal, and cardiac changes.

INTERVENTIONS	RATIONALES
For patients with ileal conduits, assess for nausea and changes in level of consciousness (LOC; ranging from sleepiness to combativeness), muscle tone (ranging from convulsions to flaccidity), and irregular HR.	These are indicators of hypokalemia and metabolic acidosis. They can occur secondary to reabsorption of Na^+ and Cl^- from the urine in the ileal segment, which results in compensatory loss of K^+ and HCO_3^-.

Continued

INTERVENTIONS	RATIONALES
Monitor results of serum electrolyte and acid-base studies.	K^+ <3.5 mEq/L signals hypokalemia, and HCO_3^- <24 mEq/L and pH <7.40 signal metabolic acidosis.
If patient is confused or exhibits signs of motor dysfunction, keep bed in lowest position and raise side rails. If convulsions appear imminent, pad side rails. Notify health care provider of significant findings.	Standard safety precautions for patient who has confusion or motor dysfunction.
Encourage oral intake as directed and assess for need for IV management.	To maintain fluid balance, which will help ameliorate acid-base and electrolyte imbalances.
Administer IV fluids with K^+ supplements as prescribed.	To prevent or treat hypokalemia.
If patient is hypokalemic and allowed to eat, encourage foods high in K^+.	Foods high in potassium, such as apricots, avocados, bananas, cantaloupes, mushrooms, oranges, potatoes, prune juice, pumpkin, spinach, sweet potatoes, Swiss chard, tomatoes, and watermelon, will help reverse hypokalemia.
Encourage patient to ambulate by second or third day after surgery.	Mobility will help prevent urinary stasis, which increases risk of electrolyte problems.

●●● **Related NIC and NOC labels:** *NIC:* Seizure Precautions; Vital Signs Monitoring; Neurologic Monitoring *NOC:* Neurologic Status: Consciousness

Nursing Diagnosis:

Risk for Impaired Skin Integrity

related to presence of urine or sensitivity to the appliance material

Desired Outcome: Patient's peristomal skin remains nonerythematous and intact.

INTERVENTIONS	RATIONALES
For patient with significant allergy history, patch-test the skin for a 24-hr period, at least 24 hr before ostomy surgery. If erythema, swelling, bleb formation, itching, weeping, or other indicators of tape allergy occur, document type of tape that caused the reaction and note on the cover of the chart "Allergic to ___ tape."	To assess for and document allergies to different tapes that might be used on the postoperative appliance.
Inspect integrity of peristomal skin with each pouch change and question patient about presence of itching or burning. Change pouch routinely (per agency or surgeon preference) or immediately if leakage is suspected.	Itching or burning can signal leakage of pouch contents on the skin.
Assess for inflamed hair follicles (folliculitis) or a reaction to the tape.	May necessitate a change in the tape used.
Report presence of a rash to health care provider.	A rash can occur with a yeast infection and will require topical medication.
When changing pouch, measure stoma with a measuring guide and ensure that skin barrier opening is cut to the exact size of the stoma.	To protect peristomal area from maceration caused by pooling of urine on the skin.

Continued

INTERVENTIONS	RATIONALES
- For a patient using a two-piece system or pouch with a barrier: Size the barrier to fit snugly around the stoma. If using a barrier and attaching an adhesive pouch, size barrier to fit snugly around stoma and size pouch to clear stoma by at least $1/8$ inch.	
- For a patient using a one-piece "adhesive-only" pouch: If pouch has an antireflux valve, size the pouch to clear stoma and any peristomal creases so that pouch adheres to a flat, dry surface. An antireflux valve prevents pooling of urine on the skin.	
If the pouch does not have an antireflux valve, size the pouch so that it clears the stoma by $1/8$ inch.	Prevents stomal trauma while minimizing amount of exposed skin.
Use a copolymer/nonalcohol film sealant wipe on peristomal skin before applying adhesive-only pouch.	This will provide a moisture barrier and reduce epidermal trauma when the pouch is removed.
Wash peristomal skin with water or a special cleansing solution marketed by ostomy supply companies. Dry the skin thoroughly before applying skin barrier and pouch.	Other products can dry out the skin, which would increase risk of irritation and infection.
When changing pouch, instruct patient to hold a gauze pad on (but not in) stoma.	To absorb urine and keep the skin dry.
After applying pouch, connect it to bedside drainage system if patient is on bedrest.	To facilitate drainage of urine.
When patient is no longer on bedrest, empty pouch when it is one-third to one-half full by opening spigot at the bottom of the pouch and draining urine into patient's measuring container. Instruct patient accordingly.	If the pouch were to become too full, it could break the seal of the appliance with patient's skin.
Change incisional dressing as often as it becomes wet, using sterile technique.	To reduce possibility of infection. Skin that is not intact increases risk of ingress of microorganisms.
Teach patient to treat peristomal skin irritation in the following ways after hospital discharge:	
- Dry skin with a hair dryer on a cool setting.	Eliminates necessity of wiping skin, which would increase the irritation.
- Dust peristomal skin with karaya or Stomahesive powders.	These powders absorb moisture.
- If desired, swab peristomal skin with a protective wipe.	To provide a moisture barrier.
- Use a porous tape.	To prevent moisture trapping.
- Notify health care provider or ET nurse of any severe or nonresponsive skin problems.	To enable skilled intervention.

●●● **Related NIC and NOC labels:** *NIC:* Skin Surveillance; Incision Site Care; Ostomy Care; Skin Care: Topical Treatments *NOC:* Tissue Integrity: Skin and Mucous Membranes

Nursing Diagnosis:

Ineffective Tissue Perfusion: Peripheral (Stomal)

(or risk for same) *related to* altered circulation

Desired Outcomes: Patient's stoma remains pink or bright red and shiny. The stoma of a cutaneous urostomy is raised, moist, and red.

INTERVENTIONS	RATIONALES
Inspect stoma at least q8h and as indicated.	The stoma of an ileal conduit will be edematous and should be pink or red with a shiny appearance. The stoma formed by a cutaneous ureterostomy is usually raised during the first few weeks after surgery, red, and moist. A stoma that is dusky or cyanotic is indicative of insufficient blood supply and impending necrosis and must be reported to health care provider for immediate intervention.
Assess degree of swelling.	The stoma should shrink considerably over the first 6-8 wk and less significantly over the next year.

●●● **Related NIC and NOC labels:** *NIC:* Pressure Management; Skin Surveillance *NOC:* Tissue Integrity: Skin and Mucous Membranes

Nursing Diagnosis:

Impaired Urinary Elimination

related to urinary diversion surgery

Desired Outcome: Patient's urinary output is ≥30 ml/hr.

INTERVENTIONS	RATIONALES
Monitor I&O and record total amount of urine output from the urinary diversion for the first 24 hr postoperatively. Differentiate and record separately amounts from all drains, stents, and catheters. Notify health care provider of an output <60 ml during a 2-hr period.	To assess for discrepancies between intake and output. In the presence of adequate intake a decreased output can signal a ureteral obstruction, a leak in one of the anastomotic sites, or impending renal failure.
Assess for flank pain, costovertebral angle (CVA) tenderness, nausea, vomiting, and anuria.	Other indicators of ureteral obstruction.
Monitor functioning of ureteral stents.	Ureteral stents, which exit from the stoma into the pouch, maintain ureteral patency and assist in healing of the anastomosis. Stents may become blocked with mucus. As long as urine is draining adequately around the stent and the volume of output is adequate, this is not a problem.
Monitor functioning of stoma catheters.	Expect output from stoma catheter to include pink or light red urine with mucus and small red clots for the first 24 hr. Urine should become amber colored with occasional clots within 3 postoperative days. Mucus production will continue but should decrease in volume.
Monitor for decreasing urinary output from stoma or stents, flank or abdominal pain, increasing abdominal distention, and increasing drainage from wound drains. Notify health care provider of significant findings.	These are indicators of anastomotic breakdown/intraabdominal urine leakage that may occur in individuals with intestinal conduit or continent diversion and necessitate prompt notification of health care provider for timely intervention.
Monitor functioning of the drains.	Any urinary diversion may have Penrose drains or closed drainage systems in place to facilitate healing of the ureterointestinal anastomosis. Drainage from drainage systems may be light red to pink for the first 24 hr and then lighten to amber and decrease in amount. Excessive lymph fluid and urine can be removed via these drains to reduce pressure on anastomotic suture lines.

Continued

INTERVENTIONS	RATIONALES
Notify health care provider if signs of an anastomotic leak occur.	In a continent urinary diversion, an increase in drainage after amounts have been low might signal an anastomotic leak.
Monitor drainage from indwelling catheter or urethral drain (if present). Note color, consistency, and volume of drainage, which may be red to pink with mucus.	Patients who have had a cystectomy may have a urethral drain, whereas those with a partial cystectomy will have an indwelling catheter in place.
Report sudden increase or decrease in drainage. Report significant findings to health care provider.	A sudden increase would occur with hemorrhage; a sudden decrease can signal blockage that can lead to infection or, with partial cystectomy, hydronephrosis.
Encourage intake of at least 2-3 L/day in the nonrestricted patient.	To keep the urinary tract well irrigated and help prevent infection that could be caused by urinary stasis.

●●● **Related NIC and NOC labels:** *NIC:* Tube Care: Urinary; Urinary Catheterization *NOC:* Urinary Elimination

Nursing Diagnosis:

Risk for Infection

related to an invasive surgical procedure and risk of ascending bacteriuria with urinary diversion

Desired Outcome: Patient is free of infection as evidenced by normothermia, white blood cell (WBC) count ≤11,000/mm³, and absence of purulent or excessive drainage, erythema, edema, warmth, and tenderness along the incision.

INTERVENTIONS	RATIONALES
Monitor patient's temperature q4h during first 24-48 hr after surgery. Notify health care provider of fever (>101° F).	Elevated temperature is a sign that the body is mounting a defense against infection.
Inspect dressing frequently after surgery. Change dressing when it becomes wet, using sterile technique. Use extra care to prevent disruption of the drains.	Infection is most likely to become evident after the first 72 hr. The presence of purulent or excessive drainage on the dressing signals infection and the need to notify health care provider promptly for timely intervention.
Note condition of the incision. Be alert to erythema, tenderness, local warmth, edema, and purulent or excessive drainage.	Indicators of infection at the incision line.
Monitor and record character of urine at least q8h.	Urine should be yellow or pink tinged during the first 24-48 hr after surgery.
	Mucus particles are normal in urine of patients with ileal conduits and continent urinary diversions because of the nature of the bowel segment used. Cloudy urine, however, is abnormal and can signal infection.
Assess for flank or CVA pain, malodorous urine, chills, and fever.	Other indicators of UTI.
Note position of the stoma relative to the incision. If they are close together, apply pouch first to avoid overlap of the pouch with the suture line.	Overlapping pouch with the suture line can increase risk of infection.
If necessary, cut pouch down on one side or place it at an angle.	To avoid contact with drainage, which may loosen adhesive.
Wash your hands before and after caring for patient.	To help prevent contamination and cross-contamination.

Continued

INTERVENTIONS | RATIONALES

INTERVENTIONS	RATIONALES
Patients with cystectomies without anastomosis to the urethra may have an indwelling urethral catheter to drain serosanguineous fluid from the peritoneal cavity. Do *not* irrigate this catheter.	Irrigation can result in peritonitis.
Encourage a fluid intake of at least 2-3 L/day.	This helps flush urine through the urinary tract, removing mucous shreds and preventing stasis that could result in infection.

●●● **Related NIC and NOC labels:** *NIC:* Infection Control: Intraoperative; Incision Site Care; Skin Surveillance; Wound Care: Closed Drainage; Tube Care: Urinary *NOC:* Infection Status; Wound Healing: Primary Intention

Nursing Diagnosis:

Deficient Knowledge:

Self-care regarding urinary diversion

Desired Outcome: Patient or significant other demonstrates proper care of stoma and urinary diversion within the 24-hr period before hospital discharge.

INTERVENTIONS | RATIONALES

INTERVENTIONS	RATIONALES
Involve ET or wound, ostomy, continence (WOC) nurse in patient teaching if available.	An ET nurse or WOC nurse is specially trained and skilled in teaching urinary diversion care.
Assist patient with organizing equipment and materials needed to accomplish home care.	Usually patient is discharged with disposable pouching systems. Most of these patients continue using disposable systems for the long term. Those who will use reusable systems usually are not fitted for 6-8 wk after surgery.
Teach how to remove and reapply pouch, how to empty it, and how to use gravity drainage system at night, including procedures for rinsing and cleansing drainage system.	These are the basic skills the patient will need to accomplish self-care after hospital discharge.
Teach signs and symptoms of UTI, peristomal skin breakdown, and appropriate therapeutic responses, including maintenance of an acidic urine (if not contraindicated), importance of adequate fluid intake, and techniques for checking urine pH, which should be assessed weekly.	Persons with urinary diversion have a higher incidence of UTI than the general public, so it is important to keep their urinary pH acidic.
Explain that urine pH should remain ≤6.0.	If it is >6.0, patient needs to increase fluid intake and, with health care provider approval, to increase vitamin C intake to 500-1000 mg/day, which will increase urine acidity.
Teach patient with continent diversion the technique for reservoir catheter irrigation.	In continent urinary diversions, a catheter is placed in the reservoir to prevent distention and promote healing of suture lines. This new reservoir (i.e., resected intestine) exudes large amounts of mucus, necessitating catheter irrigation with 30-50 ml of normal saline, which is instilled gently and allowed to empty via gravity.
Teach patient with continent urinary diversion with urethral anastomosis signals of the urge to void.	Feelings of vague abdominal discomfort and abdominal pressure or cramping are sensations of the need to void.

Continued

INTERVENTIONS	RATIONALES
Instruct patient with continent urinary diversion with urethral anastomosis about the procedure to void.	Relaxing the perineal muscles and employing Valsalva's maneuver helps empty the diversion.
Emphasize importance of follow-up visits.	Follow-up visits, particularly for patients with continent urinary diversions who will be taught how to catheterize the reservoir and use a small dressing over the stoma rather than an appliance, helps to ensure that patient can manipulate pouch and facilitates follow-up for questions.
Provide a list of ostomy support groups and ET nurses in the area.	For referral and assistance.
Provide patient with enough equipment and materials for the first week after hospital discharge.	The first postoperative visit is usually 1 wk after hospital discharge.
Remind patient of the importance of proper cleansing of ostomy appliances.	To reduce risk of bacterial growth and UTI.

●●● **Related NIC and NOC labels:** *NIC:* Teaching: Individual; Teaching: Procedure *NOC:* Knowledge: Illness Care

ADDITIONAL NURSING DIAGNOSES/ PROBLEMS:

PATIENT-FAMILY TEACHING AND DISCHARGE PLANNING

When providing patient-family teaching, focus on sensory information, avoid giving excessive information, and initiate a visiting nurse referral for necessary follow-up teaching. Include verbal and written information about the following:

✓ Medications, including drug name, dosage, schedule, drug/drug and food/drug interactions, precautions, and potential side effects.

✓ Indicators that necessitate medical intervention: fever or chills; nausea or vomiting; abdominal pain, cramping or distention; cloudy or malodorous urine; incisional drainage, edema, local warmth, pain or redness; peristomal skin irritation; or abnormal changes in stoma shape or color from the normal bright and shiny red.

✓ Maintenance of fluid intake at least 2-3 L/day to maintain adequate kidney function.

✓ Monitoring of urine pH, which should be checked weekly. Urine pH should remain at ≤6.0. Individuals with urinary diversions have a higher incidence of UTI than the general public, so it is important to keep their urinary pH acidic. If it is >6.0, advise patient to increase fluid intake and, with health care provider approval, to increase vitamin C intake to 500-1000 mg/day, which will increase urine acidity.

✓ Care of stoma and application of urostomy appliances; referrals to local suppliers. The patient should be proficient in application technique before hospital discharge.

✓ Care of urostomy appliances. Remind patient that proper cleansing will reduce risk of bacterial growth, which would contaminate urine and increase risk of UTI.

✓ Importance of follow-up care with health care provider and ET nurse. Confirm date and time of next appointment.

✓ Phone numbers to call should questions or concerns arise about therapy after discharge. In addition, many cities have local support groups. Information for these patients can be obtained by contacting:

United Ostomy Association
19722 MacArthur Blvd., Suite 200
Irvine, CA 92612-2405
(800) 826-0826
www.uoa.org

The American Cancer Society
1599 Clifton Road NE
Atlanta, GA 30329
(800) ACS-2345
www.cancer.org

National Cancer Institute Information Service (CIS)
Bldg. 31, Room 10A16
9000 Rockville Pike
Bethesda, MD 20892
(800) 422-6237
www.nci.nih.gov/cancer_information/

Urinary Tract Obstruction

Urinary tract obstruction usually is the result of blockage from pelvic tumors, calculi, and urethral strictures. Additional causes include neoplasms, benign prostatic hypertrophy, ureteral or urethral trauma, inflammation of the urinary tract, pregnancy, and pelvic or colonic surgery in which ureteral damage has occurred. Obstructions can occur suddenly or slowly, over weeks to months. They can occur anywhere along the urinary tract, but the most common sites are the ureteropelvic and ureterovesical junctions, bladder neck, and urethral meatus. The obstruction acts like a dam, blocking the passage of urine. Muscles in the area contract to push urine around the obstruction, and the structures behind the obstruction begin to dilate. The smaller the site of obstruction, the greater the damage. Obstructions in the lower urinary structures, such as the bladder neck or urethra, can lead to urinary retention and urinary tract infection (UTI). Obstructions in the upper urinary tract can lead to bilateral involvement of the ureters and kidneys, leading to hydronephrosis, renal insufficiency, and kidney destruction. Hydrostatic pressure increases, and filtration and concentration processes in the tubules and glomerulus are compromised.

HEALTH CARE SETTING
Primary care and acute care

ASSESSMENT
Physical assessment: Bladder distention and kettle drum sound over bladder with percussion (absent if obstruction is above the bladder); mass in flank area, abdomen, pelvis, or rectum.

History of: Recent fever (possibly caused by the obstruction); hypertensive episodes (caused by increased renin production from the body's attempt to increase renal blood flow).

Signs and symptoms: Anuria, nausea, vomiting, local abdominal tenderness, hesitancy, straining to start a stream, dribbling, decreased caliber and force of urinary stream, hematuria, oliguria, and uremia. Pain may be sharp and intense or dull and aching; localized or referred (e.g., flank, low back, buttock, scrotal, labial pain).

DIAGNOSTIC TESTS
Serum K^+ and Na^+ levels: To evaluate renal function. Normal range for K^+ is 3.5-5 mEq/L; normal range for Na^+ is 137-147 mEq/L.

Blood urea nitrogen (BUN) and creatinine: To evaluate renal-urinary status. Normally, their values will be elevated with decreased renal-urinary function. **Note:** These values must be considered based on the patient's age and hydration status. For the older adult, serum creatinine level may not be a reliable indicator because of decreased muscle mass and a decreased glomerular filtration rate. Hydration status can affect BUN: fluid volume excess can result in reduced values, whereas volume deficit can cause higher values.

Urinalysis: To provide baseline data on the functioning of the urinary system, detect metabolic disease, and assess for the presence of UTI. A cloudy, hazy appearance; foul odor; pH >8.0; and presence of red blood cells (RBCs), leukocyte esterase, white blood cells (WBCs), and WBC casts are signals of a UTI.

Urine culture: To determine type of bacteria present in the genitourinary tract. To minimize contamination, a sample should be obtained from a midstream collection.

Hgb and Hct: To assess for anemia, which may be related to decreased renal secretion or erythropoietin.

Kidney, ureter, bladder (KUB) radiography: To identify size, shape, and position of the kidneys, ureters, and bladder and abnormalities such as tumors, calculi, or malformations.

Imaging studies: A variety of imaging studies may be used to identify the area and cause of obstructions.

Excretory urography/intravenous pyelogram: To evaluate the cause of urinary dysfunction by visualizing the kidneys, renal pelvis, ureters, and bladder.

Antegrade urography: Involves placement of a percutaneous needle or nephrostomy tube through which radiopaque contrast is injected. Antegrade urography is indicated when the kidney does not concentrate or excrete intravenous dye.

Retrograde urography: Radiopaque dye is injected through ureteral catheters placed during cystoscopy.

Cystogram: Radiopaque dye is instilled via cystoscope or catheter. This allows visualization of the bladder and evaluation of the vesicoureteral reflex.

Computed tomography (CT) scans: To identify the degree and location of obstruction, as well as the cause in many situations.

Maximal urinary flow rate (MUFR): A rate of <15 ml/sec indicates significant obstruction to flow.

Postvoid residual (PVR) volume: Normal is <12 ml. Higher volume signals obstructive process.

Cystoscopy: To determine degree of bladder outlet obstruction and facilitate visualization of any tumors or masses.

Ultrasonography: To reveal areas of ureteral dilation or distention from retained urine.

Nursing Diagnosis:

Risk for Deficient Fluid Volume

related to postobstructive diuresis

Desired Outcomes: Patient is normovolemic as evidenced by HR ≤100 bpm (or within patient's normal range), BP ≥90/60 mm Hg (or within patient's normal range), RR ≤20 breaths/min; no significant changes in mental status; and orientation to person, place, and time (within patient's normal range). Within 2 days after bladder decompression, output approximates input, patient's urinary output is normal for patient (or ≥30-60 ml/hr), and weight becomes stable.

INTERVENTIONS	RATIONALES
Following catheterization for urinary obstruction, monitor I&O hourly for 4 hr and then q2h for 4 hr after bladder decompression.	To monitor for postobstructive diuresis.
Notify health care provider if output exceeds 200 ml/hr or 2 L over an 8-hr period.	This can signal postobstructive diuresis, which can lead to major electrolyte imbalance. If it occurs, anticipate initiation of IV infusion.
Monitor VS for decreasing BP, changes in level of consciousness (LOC), tachycardia, tachypnea, thready pulse.	Signs of shock.
Anticipate need for urine specimens for analysis of electrolytes and osmolality and blood specimens for analysis of electrolytes.	Postobstructive diuresis can lead to major electrolyte imbalance.
Observe for and report the following:	
- Abdominal cramps, lethargy, dysrhythmias.	These are signs of hypokalemia.
- Diarrhea, colic, irritability, nausea, muscle cramps, weakness, irregular apical or radial pulses.	These are signs of hyperkalemia.
- Muscle weakness and cramps, complaints of tingling in fingers, positive Trousseau's and Chvostek's signs.	These are signs of hypocalcemia.
- Excessive itching.	This is a sign of hyperphosphatemia.
Monitor mentation status.	Disorientation can occur with electrolyte disturbance.
Weigh patient daily using the same scale and at the same time of day (e.g., before breakfast).	Weight fluctuations of 2-4 lb (0.9-1.8 kg) normally occur in a patient who is undergoing diuresis. Losses greater than this can result in dehydration and electrolyte imbalances.

●●● **Related NIC and NOC labels:** *NIC:* Electrolyte Management; Electrolyte Monitoring; Laboratory Data Interpretation; Vital Signs Monitoring; Shock Prevention; Intravenous (IV) Insertion *NOC:* Electrolyte and Acid/Base Balance; Fluid Balance; Hydration

Nursing Diagnosis:

Acute Pain

related to bladder spasms

Desired Outcomes: Within 1 hr of intervention, patient's subjective perception of discomfort decreases, as documented by a pain scale. Objective indicators, such as grimacing, are absent or diminished.

INTERVENTIONS	RATIONALES
Assess for and document complaints of pain in suprapubic or urethral area. Devise a pain scale with patient, rating pain from 0 (no pain) to 10 (worst pain).	To establish a baseline for subsequent assessment and determine degree of pain relief obtained. Spasms occur frequently with obstruction.
Medicate with antispasmodics or analgesics as prescribed. Document pain relief obtained, using the pain scale.	To relieve spasms and reduce pain. Belladonna and opium (B&O) suppositories may be specifically prescribed for bladder spasms.
If patient is losing urine around the catheter and has a distended bladder (with or without bladder spasms), check catheter and drainage tubing for evidence of obstruction. Inspect for kinks and obstructions in drainage tubing, compress and roll catheter gently between fingers to assess for gritty matter within catheter, milk drainage tubing to release obstructions, or instruct patient to turn from side to side. Obtain prescription for catheter irrigation if these measures fail to relieve the obstruction.	To detect and manage obstructions in the catheter and tubing.
In nonrestricted patients, encourage intake of fluids of at least 2-3 L/day.	To reduce frequency of spasms
Teach nonpharmacologic methods of pain relief, such as guided imagery, relaxation techniques, and distraction. See relaxation technique described in "Coronary Heart Disease," **Health-Seeking Behaviors, p. 183**	These pain relief techniques augment pharmacologic interventions.

●●● **Related NIC and NOC labels:** *NIC:* Medication Management; Pain Management; Distraction; Progressive Relaxation Therapy, Simple Guided Imagery *NOC:* Comfort Level, Pain Control; Pain Level

Nursing Diagnosis:

Risk for Injury

related to nephrostomy tube complications secondary to its insertion/presence

Desired Outcome: Patient remains free of signs of nephrostomy tube complications as evidenced by urine that is clear and of normal color after the first 24 to 48 hr, a urine output of at least 30 to 60 ml/hr, and absence of discomfort/pain.

INTERVENTIONS	RATIONALES
Report gross hematuria (urine that is bright red, possibly with clots).	Transient hematuria can be expected for 24-48 hr after tube insertion. Gross hematuria, however, can signal that a blood vessel was nicked during tube insertion.
Notify health care provider of leakage around catheter, as well as a sudden decrease in urine output.	Leakage around the catheter can occur with blockage. Decreased urine output can signal a dislodged or blocked catheter.

Continued

INTERVENTIONS	RATIONALES
Report a sudden onset of or increase in pain.	Pain can signal perforation of a body organ by the catheter.
Keep tube securely taped to patient's flank with elastic tape.	To stabilize tube and keep it from becoming dislodged.
If tube accidentally becomes dislodged, cover insertion site with a sterile dressing; notify health care provider immediately.	Protects insertion site from infection until prompt medical intervention can be made.
Before removing nephrostomy tube, the health care provider may request that it be clamped for several hours at a time.	To evaluate if patient's ureteral obstruction has been resolved.
While the tube is clamped, monitor patient for the following: flank pain, diminished urinary output, and fever. Notify health care provider of significant findings.	Indications that ureteral obstruction has not been resolved and that patient will require continued medical intervention.

●●● **Related NIC and NOC labels:** *NIC:* Bleeding Precautions *NOC:* Risk Control

ADDITIONAL NURSING DIAGNOSES/ PROBLEMS:

"Perioperative Care"   p. 47

"Ureteral Calculi" for **Risk for Impaired**   p. 276
    Skin Integrity related to wound drainage

PATIENT-FAMILY TEACHING AND DISCHARGE PLANNING

When providing patient-family teaching, focus on sensory information, avoid giving excessive information, and initiate a visiting nurse referral for necessary follow-up teaching. Include verbal and written information about the following:

✓ Medications, including drug name, dosage, purpose, schedule, drug/drug and food/drug interactions, precautions, and potential side effects.

✓ Indicators that signal recurrent obstruction and require prompt medical attention: pain, fever, and decreased urinary output.

✓ Activity restrictions as directed for patient who has had surgery: avoid lifting heavy objects (>10 lb) for first 6 wk, be alert to fatigue, get maximum rest, and increase activities gradually to tolerance.

✓ Care of drains or catheters if patient is discharged with them; care of surgical incision if present.

✓ Indicators of *wound infection:* persistent redness, local warmth, tenderness, drainage, swelling, and fever.

✓ Indicators of UTI that necessitate medical attention: chills; fever; hematuria; flank, costovertebral angle (CVA), suprapubic, low back, buttock, scrotal, or labial pain; cloudy and foul-smelling urine; frequency; urgency; dysuria; and increasing or recurring incontinence.

General Care of Patients with Neurologic Disorders

Nursing Diagnoses:

Risk for Falls/Risk for Injury

related to weakness, difficulties with balance, or unsteady gait secondary to sensorimotor deficit

Desired Outcomes: Patient does not fall and is free of injury caused by gait unsteadiness. Before discharge from care facility, patient demonstrates proficiency with assistive devices if appropriate.

INTERVENTIONS	RATIONALES
Evaluate gait and assess for weakness, difficulty with balance, tremors, spasticity, or paralysis.	These are indicators of motor deficits.
Document baseline assessments.	This enables changes in status to be detected more readily.
Assist patient as needed when unsteady gait, weakness, or paralysis is noted. Instruct patient to ask or call for assistance with ambulation. Check frequently on patients who may forget to call for assistance. Lock bed or wheelchair.	To minimize risk of falls.
Stand on patient's weak/affected side.	To assist with balance and support.
Use transfer belt when guarding patient. Instruct patient to use stronger side for gripping railing when stair climbing or using a cane.	To promote safety.
Keep necessary items (including water, snacks, phone, call light) within easy reach.	To minimize need to walk to get to these items.
Assess patient's ability to use call light.	Patients who are very weak or partially paralyzed may require a tap bell or specially adapted call light.

Continued

INTERVENTIONS	RATIONALES
Maintain an uncluttered environment with unobstructed walkways. Ensure adequate lighting at night (e.g., a night light). In addition, keep side rails up and bed in its lowest position with bed brakes on.	To minimize risk of tripping, falls in the dark, or injury from falling out of bed.
Encourage patient to use any needed hearing aids and corrective lenses when ambulating.	Promotes safety by ensuring better sensory and visual acuity.
For unsteady, weak, or partially paralyzed patient, encourage use of low-heel, nonskid, supportive shoes for walking.	To promote safety and prevent falls during ambulation.
Teach use of a wide-based gait.	To provide a broader base of support, which will decrease risk of falls.
Instruct patient to note foot placement when ambulating or transferring.	To ensure foot is flat and in a position of support.
Teach, reinforce, and encourage use of assistive device, such as a cane, walker, or crutches.	To provide added stability.
Teach exercises that strengthen arm and shoulder muscles for using walkers and crutches. Teach safe use of transfer or sliding boards. Teach patients in wheelchairs how and when to lock and unlock wheels.	To promote safety.
Demonstrate how to secure and support weak or paralyzed arms.	To prevent subluxation and injury from falling into wheelchair spokes or wheels.
Suggest seat or chest belt, H-straps for leg positioning, and a wheelchair with an antitip device.	These devices likely will help patients with poor sitting balance from falling over or tipping the wheelchair.
Keep wheelchair close to bed.	For easier access, which will promote safety.
Teach patients to maintain sitting position for a few minutes before assuming standing position for ambulating.	To ensure balance and minimize any dizziness that may occur because of rapid position changes. This procedure also gives patients time to get their feet flat and under them.
Monitor spasticity, antispasmodic medications, and their effect on physical function.	Uncontrolled or severe spasms may cause falls, whereas mild to moderate spasms can be useful in activities of daily living (ADL) and transfers if patient learns to control and trigger them.
Review with patient and significant other potential safety needs at home.	Safety measures include adding wall, bath, and toilet hand rails; elevated toilet seat; and nonslip surface in bathtub or shower. Other safety measures include the following: - Removing loose rugs to prevent slipping and falling. - Turning down temperatures on hot water heaters to prevent scalding in event of a fall in the shower or tub. - Moving furniture in the home and strategically placing additional lighting to provide clear, safe pathways that avoid sharp corners on furniture, glass cabinets, or large windows patient might fall against. - Taping edges of steps in the home with bright color strips to provide sufficient contrast so that edges can be recognized and more safely negotiated. - Balancing rest with activity because fatigue tends to increase unsteadiness and potential for falls.
Seek referral for physical therapist (PT) as appropriate.	Patient may have special needs that cannot be met by nursing staff.

●●● **Related NIC and NOC labels:** *NIC:* Fall Prevention; Surveillance: Safety; Environmental Management: Safety; Home Maintenance Assistance; Area Restriction; Risk Identification *NOC:* Safety Status: Falls Occurrence; Safety Status: Physical Injury

Nursing Diagnosis:

Disturbed Sensory Perception: Tactile

related to impaired pain, touch, and temperature sensations secondary to sensory deficit or decreased
level of consciousness (LOC)

Desired Outcomes: Patient is free of symptoms of injury caused by impaired pain, touch, and
temperature sensations. Patient and significant other identify factors that increase potential for
injury.

INTERVENTIONS	RATIONALES
Assess for impaired temperature and pain sensation.	Indicators of sensory deficits.
Document baseline neurologic and physical assessments.	This will enable rapid detection of changes in status, as well as enable development of a care plan specific to patient's needs.
Do not serve scalding hot beverages or foods. Avoid use of hot equipment. Encourage use of sunscreen when outside.	Protects patient from exposure to sun and hot food or equipment that can burn the skin.
Always check temperature of heating devices and bath water before patient is exposed to them. Teach patient and significant other about these precautions.	Patient's tactile senses are altered and would not recognize if water or device is too hot.
Inspect skin twice daily for evidence of irritation. Teach coherent patient to perform self-inspection and provide mirror for inspecting posterior aspects of the body.	Patient would not be able to feel skin irritation.
Use emollient lotion liberally on patient's skin.	Keeps skin soft and pliable and less likely to break down.
Teach patient to inspect placement of limbs that have altered sensation.	To ensure that they are in a safe and supported position and to avoid placing ankles directly on top of each other, which could affect circulation and irritate the skin.
Pad wheelchair seat, preferably with a gel pad.	To evenly distribute patient's weight and decrease pressure areas that could result in skin breakdown.
Teach patient to change position q15-30min by lifting self and shifting position side to side and forward to backward. Encourage frequent turning while in bed and, if tolerated and not contraindicated, periodic movement into prone position.	To promote circulation and prevent pressure ulcers. Patient likely will not feel the need to do this and therefore should do it on a scheduled basis. Spending time in the prone position with hips extended helps prevent hip flexion contractures.
Have patient lift, not drag, self during transfers.	To prevent shearing damage to skin.

●●● **Related NIC and NOC labels:** *NIC:* Peripheral Sensation Management; Skin Surveillance;
Cutaneous Stimulation; Positioning; Pressure Management *NOC:* Sensory Function: Cutaneous

Nursing Diagnosis:

Impaired Corneal Tissue Integrity

(or risk for same) *related to* irritation secondary to diminished blink reflex or inability to close the
eyes

Desired Outcome: Patient's corneas remain clear and intact.

INTERVENTIONS	RATIONALES
If patient has a diminished blink reflex or is stuporous or comatose, assess eyes for irritation or presence of foreign objects.	Normally, blinking occurs every 5-6 sec. Indicators of corneal irritation include red, itchy, scratchy, or painful eye; sensation of foreign object in eye; scleral edema; blurred vision; or mucous discharge.
Instill prescribed eye drops or ointment.	To prevent corneal irritation.
Instruct coherent patients to make a conscious effort to blink eyes several times each minute.	
Apply eye patches or warm, sterile compresses over closed eyes for relief.	
If the eyes cannot be completely closed, use caution in applying eye shield or taping eyes shut. Consider use of moisture chambers (plastic eye bubbles), protective glasses, soft contacts, or humidifiers.	Semiconscious patients may open eyes underneath shield or tape and injure their corneas. Eye bubbles provide moisture to prevent corneal irritation.
	For chronic eye closure problems, special springs or weights on upper lids may be used. Surgical closure (tarsorrhaphy) may be necessary to ensure that eyelids stay closed, which will help maintain intact corneas.
Teach patient to avoid exposing eyes to talc or baby powder, wind, cold air, smoke, dust, sand, or bright sunlight. Instruct patient not to rub eyes.	These are irritants that could harm patient's corneas.
Advise patient to wear glasses when outdoors and tight-fitting goggles when swimming.	To protect against corneal damage caused by wind, dust, and water.

●●● **Related NIC and NOC labels:** *NIC:* Eye Care; Medication Administration: Eye *NOC:* Tissue Integrity: Skin and Mucous Membranes

Nursing Diagnosis:

Imbalanced Nutrition: Less than body requirements

related to inability to ingest food secondary to chewing and swallowing deficits, fatigue, weakness, paresis, paralysis, visual neglect, or decreased LOC

Desired Outcome: Patient has adequate nutrition as evidenced by maintenance of or return to baseline body weight.

INTERVENTIONS	RATIONALES
Assess alertness, ability to cough, and swallow and gag reflexes before all meals. Keep suction equipment at bedside if indicated.	Deficits found during this assessment signal that patient is at risk for aspiration. Aspiration precautions could lead to imbalanced nutrition.
Assess for type of diet that can be eaten safely. Request soft, semisolid, or chopped foods as indicated.	Although a pureed diet may be needed eventually, pureed food can be unappealing and may have a negative impact on self-concept.
Reduce other stimuli in the room (e.g., turn off TV or radio). Minimize conversation and other disruptions such as phone calls. If patient wears glasses, put them on patient; ensure adequate lighting. As needed, redirect patient's attention to eating.	These measures help patient focus on eating.

Continued

INTERVENTIONS	RATIONALES
Provide analgesics, if appropriate, before meals.	Ensures patient is comfortable and can concentrate on eating.
Evaluate food preferences and offer small, frequent servings of nutritious food. Encourage significant other to bring in patient's favorite foods if not contraindicated. Plan meals for times when patient is rested; use a warming tray or microwave oven to keep food warm and appetizing until patient is able to eat. Serve cold foods while they are cold.	Optimally these measures will promote eating.
Provide oral care before feeding. Clean and insert dentures before each meal.	For comfort and to enhance patient's ability to taste and chew.
Cut up foods, unwrap silverware, and otherwise prepare food tray.	This enables patient with a weak or paralyzed arm to manage the tray one-handed.
For patient with visual neglect, place food within unaffected visual field. Return during meal to make sure patient has eaten from both sides of the plate. Turn plate around so that any remaining food is in patient's visual field	To ensure that patient eats most or all of the food on the plate.
Feed or assist very weak or paralyzed patients. If not contraindicated, position patient in a chair or elevate head of bed (HOB) as high as possible.	Raising HOB helps prevent aspiration by promoting gravity drainage into the stomach and through the pylorus. Assisting patient also helps conserve his or her energy and provides social interaction, which may promote eating.
Ensure that patient's head is flexed slightly forward.	To close the airway and prevent aspiration.
Begin with small amounts of food. Encourage chewing food on unaffected side. Do not hurry patient. Be sure that each bite is completely swallowed before giving another. Encourage patient with hemiplegia to consciously sweep paralyzed side of mouth with the tongue to clear it.	These measures help prevent aspiration.
If appropriate, provide assistive devices, such as built-up utensil handles, broad-handled spoons, spill-proof cups, rocker knife for cutting, wrist or hand splints with clamps to hold utensils, stabilized plates, sectioned plates, and other devices.	To promote self-feeding and independence.
Encourage eating of finger foods.	To promote independence and oral intake.
Provide materials for oral hygiene after meals.	To minimize risk of aspiration of food particles. Good oral hygiene will also help maintain integrity of mucous membranes for subsequent oral intake.
Provide oral care for patients unable to do so for themselves.	To minimize risk of stomatitis, which may prevent adequate oral intake.
Document your assessment of patient's appetite. Weigh patient regularly (at least weekly) to assess for loss or gain. If indicated, notify health care provider of potential need for high-protein or high-calorie supplements. Obtain dietitian consultation. For additional information, see "Providing Nutritional Support," p. 589.	Trend of the patient's weight is a good indicator of nutritional status. Calculation of weight enables determination of percentage below ideal weight for patient's height and frame. Patient may need enteral or parenteral nutrition.
For weak, debilitated, or partially paralyzed patient, assess support systems, such as family or friends, who can assist patient with meals. Consider referral to an organization that will deliver a daily meal to patient's home.	To promote patient's optimum nutritional status.
If appropriate for patient's diagnosis (e.g., multiple sclerosis [MS]) consider referral to a speech pathologist.	For exercises that enhance ability to swallow.

Continued

INTERVENTIONS	RATIONALES
For patients with visual problems, assess their ability to see food. Identify utensils and foods and describe their location. Arrange foods in an established pattern.	To promote independence with eating. Poor vision has been associated with lower caloric intake.
For patient with binocular diplopia, consider patching one eye.	Patching one eye may enable better vision.
For patients with chewing or swallowing difficulties, see interventions in **Impaired Swallowing,** p. 308.	

●●● **Related NIC and NOC labels:** *NIC:* Nutrition Management; Weight Gain Assistance; Self-Care Assistance: Feeding; Sustenance Support; Nutrition Therapy; Swallowing Therapy *NOC:* Nutritional Status: Food and Fluid Intake

Nursing Diagnosis:

Risk for Deficient Fluid Volume

related to facial and throat muscle weakness, depressed gag or cough reflex, impaired swallowing, or decreased LOC affecting access to and intake of fluids

Desired Outcome: Patient is normovolemic as evidenced by balanced I&O, stable weight, good skin turgor, moist mucous membranes, BP within patient's normal range, HR ≤100 bpm, normothermia, and urinary output ≥30 ml/hr with a specific gravity ≤1.030.

INTERVENTIONS	RATIONALES
Assess gag reflex, alertness, and ability to cough and swallow before offering fluids.	To determine if patient has intact swallowing and gag reflexes, can cough, and is alert and therefore can safely ingest fluids.
Keep suction equipment at bedside if indicated.	To intervene in the event of aspiration.
Monitor I&O to assess for fluid volume imbalance. Involve patient or significant other with keeping fluid intake records.	Patients with neurologic deficits may have difficulty attaining adequate fluid intake. Involving patient and significant other in record keeping optimally will keep them aware of the need for increased oral intake and influence their participation in fluid intake accordingly.
Perform daily weight assessments if patient is at risk for sudden fluid shifts or imbalances.	Weight is a useful measurement of hydration status, especially in patients with renal or cardiac disease.
Alert health care provider to a significant I&O imbalance.	A deficiency in intake may signal need for enteral or IV therapy to prevent dehydration.
Assess for and teach patient and significant other indicators of dehydration, including thirst, poor skin turgor, decreased BP, increased pulse rate, dry skin and mucous membranes, increased body temperature, concentrated urine (specific gravity >1.030), and decreased urinary output. Advise that conditions such as fever or diarrhea increase fluid loss and increase risk of dehydration.	A knowledgeable person likely will report these indicators promptly for timely intervention and will understand need to increase fluid intake during conditions that promote dehydration.
Evaluate fluid preferences (type and temperature). Offer fluids q1-2h. For nonrestricted patients, encourage a fluid intake of at least 2-3 L/day.	Patients, especially if fatigued, will be more likely to consume preferred fluids in small volumes at frequent intervals. A fluid intake of 2-3 L/day will keep patient well hydrated. Renal and cardiac patients may have fluid restrictions.
Feed or assist very weak or paralyzed patients.	To facilitate oral fluid intake.

Continued

INTERVENTIONS	RATIONALES
Instruct patient to flex head slightly forward. If not contraindicated, assist patient into a high Fowler's position.	Closes the airway and helps prevent aspiration.
	A high Fowler's position facilitates gravity flow into the stomach and through the pylorus.
Begin with small amounts of liquid. Instruct patient to sip rather than gulp fluids. Do not hurry patient.	Sipping small amounts tests and promotes patient's ability to swallow the fluid without choking.
In patients at risk for aspiration, use thickened fluids and maintain appropriate upright position while patient is eating and for at least $\frac{1}{2}$ hr after the meal.	Thickened liquids form a cohesive bolus that can be swallowed more readily. Gravity aids swallowing, and staying upright decreases risk of aspiration.
Provide periods of rest.	To prevent fatigue, which can contribute to decreased oral intake.
Provide oral care as needed.	To enhance taste perception and prevent stomatitis, which could decrease subsequent oral intake.
If appropriate, provide assistive devices (e.g., plastic, unbreakable, special-handled, spill-proof cups or straws).	To promote independence with oral intake, which is likely to increase consumption of fluids.
Teach patient with hemiparalysis or paresis to tilt head toward unaffected side.	Fluids will drain by gravity to the side of the face and throat over which patient has control.
Also see American Dietetic Association's website: www.eatright. org. For patients with chewing or swallowing difficulties, see interventions under **Impaired Swallowing**, p. 308.	

●●● **Related NIC and NOC labels:** *NIC:* Fluid Management; Fluid Monitoring; Vital Signs Monitoring; Bedside Laboratory Testing; Enteral Tube Feeding; Total Parenteral Nutrition Administration; Intravenous Therapy; Oral Health Restoration; Swallowing Therapy; Self-Care Assistance: Feeding *NOC:* Fluid Balance; Nutritional Status: Food and Fluid Intake

Nursing Diagnosis:

Risk for Aspiration

related to facial and throat muscle weakness, depressed gag or cough reflex, impaired swallowing, or decreased LOC

Desired Outcomes: Patient is free of the signs of aspiration as evidenced by RR 12-20 breaths/min with normal depth and pattern (eupnea), O_2 saturation >92%, normal color, normal breath sounds, normothermia, and absence of adventitious breath sounds. Following instruction and on an ongoing basis, patient or significant other relates measures that prevent aspiration.

INTERVENTIONS	RATIONALES
Assess lung sounds before and after patient eats and effectiveness of patient's cough.	New onset of crackles or wheezing can signal aspiration. Patients with a weak cough reflex are at risk for aspiration.
If it is not contraindicated, maintain patient in a right side-lying position with HOB elevated, especially after meals, or upright if possible for at least $\frac{1}{2}$ hr after eating.	To minimize potential for regurgitation and aspiration. This position facilitates flow of ingested food and fluids by gravity from the greater stomach curve to the pylorus.
Provide small, frequent meals. Feed slowly and allow time for chewing/swallowing.	To reduce potential for regurgitation.

Continued

INTERVENTIONS	RATIONALES
Consult health care provider for an upper gastrointestinal (GI) stimulant (e.g., metoclopramide).	Metoclopramide stimulates upper GI tract motility and gastric emptying, which also decreases potential for regurgitation.
Provide oral hygiene after meals.	To prevent aspiration of residual food particles.
Assess frequently for presence of obstructive material or secretions in throat or mouth and suction as needed.	To prevent aspiration of these materials.
If patient has nausea or vomiting, turn on one side.	To facilitate secretion drainage and prevent aspiration.
Anticipate need for artificial airway if secretions cannot be cleared. Teach significant other the Heimlich maneuver.	To facilitate a patent airway.
For other interventions, see this nursing diagnosis in "Older Adult Care," p. 101.	

●●● **Related NIC and NOC labels:** *NIC:* Aspiration Precautions; Vomiting Management; Airway Suctioning; Artificial Airway Management; Positioning; Respiratory Monitoring *NOC:* Aspiration Control

Nursing Diagnosis:

Bathing/Hygiene, Dressing/Grooming, Feeding, Toileting Self-Care Deficit

related to spasticity, tremors, weakness, paresis, paralysis, or decreasing LOC secondary to sensorimotor deficits

Desired Outcome: Within 24 hr of this diagnosis, patient performs care activities independently and demonstrates ability to use adaptive devices for successful completion of ADL. (Totally dependent patients express satisfaction with activities that are completed for them.)

INTERVENTIONS	RATIONALES
Assess patient's ability to perform ADL.	To determine performance barriers and degree to which patient needs assistance with completing ADL. This data will enable development of an individualized care plan.
As appropriate, demonstrate use of adaptive devices. Have patient return the demonstration.	To assist patient in maintaining independent care. Demonstration by nurse and return demonstration by patient are effective tools for learning. Examples of adaptive devices include long- or broad-handled combs; long-handled pickup sticks, brushes, and eating utensils; dressing sticks; stocking helpers; Velcro fasteners; elastic waist bands; nonspill cups; and stabilized plates. A flexor-hinge splint or universal cuff may aid in brushing teeth and combing hair. Electric toothbrush and electric razor also may promote self-care.
Set short-range, realistic goals with patient.	To decrease frustration and improve learning.
Acknowledge progress. Encourage continued effort and involvement (e.g., in selection of meals, clothing).	
Provide care to totally dependent patient; ask for patient's input in planning schedules. Assist those who are not totally dependent according to degree of disability. Encourage patient to perform self-care to the maximum ability as defined by patient. Allow sufficient time for task perform-	Promoting autonomy and positive self-image helps prevent learned helplessness.

Preserving energy by providing sufficient time for the task increases activity to tolerance. |

INTERVENTIONS	RATIONALES
ance; do not hurry patient. Involve significant other with care activities if he or she is comfortable doing so. Supervise activity until patient can safely perform task without help.	
Encourage use of electronically controlled wheelchair and other technical advances (e.g., environmental control system).	To improve mobility and enable independent operation of electronic devices such as lights, radio, door openers, and window shade openers.
Provide privacy and a nondistracting environment. Place patient's belongings within reach. Set out items needed to complete self-care tasks in the order they are to be used. Apply any needed adaptive devices such as hand splints.	Conveys respect, simplifies the task, and increases patient's motivation.
Encourage patient to wear any prescribed corrective eye lenses or hearing aids.	Enhanced vision and hearing may increase participation in self-care.
Provide analgesics.	To relieve pain, which can hinder self-care activity.
Provide a rest period before self-care activity or plan activity for a time when patient is rested.	Fatigue reduces self-care ability.
Encourage patient or significant other to buy shoes without laces; long-handled shoe horns; wide-legged pants; and clothing that is loose fitting with enlarged arm holes, front fasteners, zipper pulls, or Velcro closures. Avoid items with small buttons or tight buttonholes. Lay out clothing in the order it will be put on. Advise patient to sit while dressing.	To facilitate dressing and undressing.
Place stool in shower.	For patients for whom sitting down will promote self-care with bathing.
Make sure bathrooms have nonslip mats and grab bars.	To ensure safety by preventing falls.
Suggest hand-held shower spray, long-handled bath sponge, or a washer mitt with a pocket that holds soap.	To promote autonomy with bathing.
Provide commode chair or elevated toilet seat or male or female urinal.	To facilitate self-care with elimination.
As indicated, teach self-transfer techniques.	These techniques will enable patient to get to commode or toilet independently.
Keep call light within patient's reach. Instruct patient to call as early as possible.	Provides staff time to respond, and patient will not have to rush because of urgency.
Offer toileting reminders q2h, after meals, and before bedtime.	Toileting schedules convey the message that continence is valued, optimally reducing episodes of incontinence.
Suggest use of a long-handled grasper that can hold tissues or washcloth.	May help patient maintain independence with perineal care.
For patient with hemiparesis or hemiparalysis, teach use of stronger or unaffected hand and arm for dressing, eating, bathing, and grooming. Have patient dress weaker side first.	Simplifies the task and conserves energy.
For patients with visual field deficit, avoid placing items on their blind side. Encourage patient to scan environment for needed items by turning head.	To enable vision of the task at hand.
Suggest use of splints, weighted utensils, or wrist weights for patients with tremors.	Adaptive devices increase speed and safety of self-care and decrease exertion. In addition, resting head against a high-backed chair may reduce head tremors.
Obtain referral for occupational therapist (OT) if indicated.	To determine best method for performing activity.
For patients with cognitive defects, use gestures, demonstrations, reminders of next step, and gentle repetition.	Cueing promotes relearning and successful completion of tasks.

Continued

INTERVENTIONS	RATIONALES
Provide consistent caregiver and ADL routine.	To promote familiarity and decrease frustration.
If indicated, teach patient self-catheterization or teach technique to caregiver.	At-home intermittent catheterization usually is done with clean, not sterile, technique and equipment. The catheter is washed after use in warm, soapy water, rinsed, and placed in a clean plastic sack. Catheter insertion guides are available commercially for females with limited upper arm mobility. Crusted catheters are soaked in a solution of half distilled vinegar and half water.
Teach patient to monitor for and notify health professional of cloudy, foul-smelling, or bloody urine; urine with sediment; chills or fever; pain in lower back or abdomen; or a red or swollen urethral meatus.	Indicators of urinary tract infection (UTI), which necessitates timely intervention.
Discuss, as appropriate, changing home environment.	Changing home environment (e.g., with extended sinks, lower closet hooks, wheelchair-accessible shower, modified phones, lowered mirrors, and lever door handles that operate with reduced hand pressure) promotes independence and performance of ADL at home.
Listen and provide opportunities for patient to express self and communicate that it is normal to have negative feelings about changes in autonomy. Discuss with health care team ways to provide consistent and positive encouragement and strategies that increase independence progressively.	Frustration can be decreased and coping skills increased when an individual expresses feelings in a supportive environment.

●●● **Related NIC and NOC labels:** *NIC:* Self-Care Assistance: Bathing/Hygiene, Dressing/Grooming, Feeding, Toileting; Energy Management; Self-Responsibility Enhancement *NOC:* Self-Care: Activities of Daily Living

Nursing Diagnosis:

Oral Hygiene Self-Care Deficit

related to sensorimotor deficit or decreased LOC

Desired Outcome: Following intervention, patient or significant other demonstrates ability to perform patient's oral care.

INTERVENTIONS	RATIONALES
Assess patient's ability to perform mouth care.	To identify performance barriers (e.g., sensorimotor or cognitive deficits) and facilitate development of an individualized care plan.
If patient has decreased LOC or is at risk for aspiration, remove dentures and store them in a water-filled denture cup.	Protects and prevents loss of dentures.
If patient cannot perform mouth care, assist by cleaning teeth, tongue, and mouth at least twice daily with a soft-bristled toothbrush and nonabrasive toothpaste.	Promotes oral hygiene and prevents accumulation of bacteria that can cause oral inflammation.
If patient is unconscious or at risk for aspiration, turn to a side-lying position.	To prevent aspiration of oral solutions.

Continued

INTERVENTIONS	RATIONALES
Swab mouth and teeth with sponge-tipped applicator (Too-thette) moistened with diluted (half-strength) mouthwash solution and irrigate mouth with a large syringe. If patient cannot self-manage secretions, use only a small amount of liquid for irrigation each time and, using a suction catheter or Yankauer tonsil suction tip, remove secretions.	
Perform this oral hygiene regimen as frequently as possible. As appropriate, teach procedure to significant other.	Good oral hygiene helps prevent stomatitis and tooth decay and reduces risk of infections caused by oral mucous membrane that is not intact.
Make toothbrush adaptations for patients with physical disabilities.	For patients with limited hand mobility, enlarging the toothbrush handle by covering it with a sponge hair roller or aluminum foil, attaching with an elastic band, or by attaching a bicycle handle grip with plaster of Paris increases hand mobility.
	For patients with limited arm mobility, extending toothbrush handle by overlapping another handle or rod over it and taping them together increases arm mobility.

●●● **Related NIC and NOC labels:** *NIC:* Self-Care Assistance: Bathing/Hygiene; Oral Health Maintenance; Teaching: Individual; Oral Health Promotion; Oral Health Restoration *NOC:* Self-Care Hygiene

Nursing Diagnosis:

Impaired Verbal Communication

related to facial/throat muscle weakness, intubation, or tracheostomy

Desired Outcome: Following intervention and on an ongoing basis, patient communicates effectively, either verbally or nonverbally, and relates decreasing frustration with communication.

INTERVENTIONS	RATIONALES
Assess patient's ability to speak, read, write, and comprehend.	To help determine patient's communication abilities and interventions that would promote them.
Encourage patient to perform exercises that increase ability to control facial muscles and tongue. If appropriate, obtain referral to a speech therapist or pathologist.	These exercises assist patient in strengthening muscles used in speech and may include holding a sound for 5 sec, singing the scale, reading aloud, and extending tongue and trying to touch chin, nose, or cheek.
Provide a supportive and relaxed environment for those patients who are unable to form words or sentences or who are unable to speak clearly or appropriately. Explain that patience is needed for both patient and caregiver.	Patient likely will be frustrated over inability to communicate. Maintaining a calm, positive, reassuring attitude and continuing to speak to patient using normal volume (unless patient's hearing is impaired) will help ease frustrations.
Maintain eye contact.	To promote focus.
Provide enough time for patient to articulate words. Ask patient to repeat unclear words. Observe for nonverbal cues; watch patient's lips closely. Do not interrupt or finish sentences. Anticipate needs and phrase questions to allow simple answers, such as "yes" or "no."	To decrease patient's frustration.
As indicated, provide a language board, alphabet cards, picture or letter-number board, flash cards, or pad and pencil.	These are alternative methods of communication for patients unable to speak.

Continued

INTERVENTIONS	RATIONALES
	Other systems use eye blinks, tongue clicks, or hand squeezes; bell signal taps; or gestures, such as hand signals, head nods, pantomime, or pointing.
Document method of communication used.	Helps ensure that other health care team members use the same method.
If patient's voice is weak and difficult to hear, reduce environmental noise.	To enhance listener's ability to hear patient's words.
Suggest that patient take a deep breath before speaking; provide a voice amplifier if appropriate.	To project voice.
Remind patients to speak slowly, exaggerate pronunciation, and use facial expressions.	Patient may have flat affect in both pronunciation and facial expression. Exaggerating both may make patient's conversation more engaging.
If patient has swallowing difficulties that result in accumulation of saliva, suction mouth.	To promote clearer speech.
If indicated, massage facial and neck muscles before patient attempts to communicate.	To promote clearer speech in patients with muscle rigidity or spasm.
If patient has a tracheostomy and is therefore unable to speak, ensure that a tap bell is within reach.	Tap bell sounds give patient the means to communicate and increase a sense of self-control and safety.
Explain to patient with a temporary tracheostomy that ability to speak will return.	Provides reassurance about future ability to communicate.
For patient with permanent tracheostomy, discuss learning alternate communication systems.	Alternate communication systems include sign language or esophageal speech, in which a fenestrated tube or covering tracheostomy tube opening with a finger will enable speech.
Establish a method of calling for assistance and ensure that patient knows how to use it. Keep calling device where patient can activate it (e.g., place call bell on nonparalyzed side). Depending on deficit, use a tap bell for weak patients, a pillow pad call light (triggered by arm or head movement), or a sip and puff device (triggered by mouth).	Ensures that patients of varying abilities will be able to call for assistance.
Provide a means of communication for patient regardless of his or her ability.	This will ensure that patient has a means of ventilating feelings and expressing concerns. Patients with ability to write can keep a diary or write letters. If patient has a weak writing arm, a splint may enable holding a pen or pencil. Felt-tip markers also are useful because they require minimal pressure for writing. Large-barrel pens may be easier for grasping and writing, or patient may be able to type. For patient able to speak, a computer voice recognition program may facilitate written and e-mail communication.

●●● **Related NIC and NOC labels:** *NIC:* Active Listening; Communication Enhancement: Speech Deficit; Anxiety Reduction *NOC:* Communication Ability; Communication: Expressive Ability

Nursing Diagnosis:

Constipation

related to inability to chew and swallow a high-roughage diet, side effects of medications, immobility, and spinal cord involvement

Desired Outcome: Within 2-3 days of intervention, patient passes soft, formed stools and regains and maintains his or her normal bowel pattern.

INTERVENTIONS	RATIONALES
Teach patients with chewing and swallowing difficulties that consuming 1 or 2 servings of applesauce with added bran, prune juice, or cooked bran cereal each day may be effective in reversing constipation. Otherwise encourage use of natural fiber laxatives such as psyllium (e.g., Metamucil).	Although a high-roughage diet is ideal for promoting peristalsis in a patient who is immobilized or on prolonged bedrest, individuals with chewing and swallowing difficulties may be unable to consume such a diet.
Encourage/promote the following: setting a regular time of day for attempting a bowel movement, preferably 30 min after eating a meal or drinking a hot beverage; using a commode instead of a bedpan for more natural positioning during elimination; using a medicated suppository 15-30 min before a scheduled attempt; bearing down by contracting abdominal muscles or applying manual pressure to abdomen; and drinking 4 oz of prune juice nightly. Abdominal and pelvic exercise also may be included in patient's morning and evening routine. Keep a call bell within patient's reach.	Elements that may be included in a successful bowel elimination program. For more detail, see **Constipation,** p. 75, in "Prolonged Bedrest."
Assess patient's sitting balance and intervene accordingly.	To ensure safety while on commode.
Caution: Spinal cord injury (SCI) patients with involvement at T8 and above should use extreme caution if using an enema or suppository. If use is unavoidable, liberal application of anesthetic jelly into the rectum should precede their use.	Either measure can precipitate life-threatening autonomic dysreflexia (AD). Large amounts of anesthetic jelly reduce that risk.
In addition, instruct patient at risk of IICP not to bear down with bowel movements.	This action can cause increased intraabdominal pressure, which in turn increases ICP.
Unless contraindicated, encourage fluid intake to >2500 ml/day, including liberal amounts of fresh fruit juices.	Adequate fluid intake helps prevent hard, dry stools that are difficult to evacuate.
If indicated by patient's diagnosis (e.g., MS), provide instructions for anal digital stimulation.	To promote reflex bowel evacuation.
Caution: This intervention is contraindicated for SCI patients with involvement at T8 or above.	It can precipitate life-threatening AD.
For other interventions, see **Constipation,** p. 75, in "Prolonged Bedrest."	

●●● **Related NIC and NOC labels:** *NIC:* Bowel Management; Constipation/Impaction Management; Fluid Management; Medication Management; Self-Care Assistance: Toileting; Nutrition Management *NOC:* Bowel Elimination; Hydration; Symptom Control

Nursing Diagnosis:

Decreased Intracranial Adaptive Capacity

related to altered blood flow with risk of IICP and herniation secondary to positional factors, increased intrathoracic or intraabdominal pressure, fluid volume excess, hyperthermia, or discomfort secondary to brain injury

Desired Outcomes: Patient is free of symptoms of IICP and herniation as evidenced by stable or improving Glasgow Coma Scale score; stable or improving sensorimotor functioning; BP within patient's normal range; HR 60-100 bpm; pulse pressure 30-40 mm Hg (the difference between systolic and diastolic BPs); orientation to person, place, and time; normal vision; bilaterally equal and normoreactive pupils; RR 12-20 breaths/min with normal depth and pattern (eupnea); normal gag, corneal, and swallowing reflexes; and absence of headache, nausea, nuchal rigidity, posturing, and seizure activity.

INTERVENTIONS	**RATIONALES**
Monitor for and report any of the following:	ICP is the pressure exerted by brain tissue, cerebrospinal fluid (CSF), and cerebral blood volume within the rigid, unyielding skull. An increase in any one of these components without a corresponding decrease in another will increase ICP. Normal ICP is 0-10 mm Hg; IICP is >15 mm Hg. Cerebral perfusion pressure (CPP) is the difference between systemic arterial pressure and ICP. As ICP rises, CPP may decrease. Normal CPP is 70-100 mm Hg. If CPP falls below 40-60 mm Hg, ischemia occurs. When CPP falls to 0, cerebral blood flow ceases. Cerebral edema and IICP usually peak 2-3 days after an injury and then decrease over 1-2 wk.
- Early indicators of IICP: declining Glasgow Coma Scale score, alterations in LOC ranging from irritability, restlessness, and confusion to lethargy; possible onset of or worsening of headache; beginning pupillary dysfunction, such as sluggishness; visual disturbances, such as diplopia or blurred vision; onset of or increase in sensorimotor changes or deficits, such as weakness; onset of or worsening of nausea.	
- Late indicators of IICP: continuing decline in Glasgow Coma Scale score; continued deterioration in LOC leading to stupor and coma; projectile vomiting; hemiplegia; posturing; widening pulse pressure, decreased HR, and increased systolic BP; Cheyne-Stokes breathing or other respiratory irregularity; pupillary changes, such as oval shaped, inequality, dilation, and nonreactivity to light; papilledema; and impaired brain stem reflexes (corneal, gag, swallowing).	The single most important indicator of early IICP is a change in LOC. Late indicators of IICP are generally related to brain stem compression and disruption of cranial nerves and vital centers. Brain herniation occurs when IICP causes displacement of brain tissue from one cranial compartment to another. Late indicators of IICP signal impending or actual herniation.
- Brain herniation: deep coma, fixed and dilated pupils (first unilateral and then bilateral), posturing progressing to bilateral flaccidity, lost brain stem reflexes, and continuing deterioration in VS and respirations.	
If the above changes occur, prepare for possible transfer of patient to intensive care unit (ICU).	Insertion of ICP sensors for continuous ICP monitoring, continuous bedside cerebral blood flow (CBF) monitoring, CSF ventricular drainage, vasopressor usage (e.g., dopamine, nitroprusside), intubation, mechanical ventilation, propofol sedation, neuromuscular blocking, or barbiturate coma therapy may be necessary. Continuous cardiac monitoring for dysrhythmias will also be done.
For patients at risk for IICP, ensure a patent airway, deliver O_2 as prescribed, and limit suctioning to 10-15 sec. Monitor arterial blood gas (ABG) or pulse oximetry values.	For patients at risk for IICP, prevention of hypoxia and CO_2 retention is essential for preventing vasodilation of cerebral arteries.
If mechanical hyperventilation is used, monitor CBF and jugular venous oxygen saturation measurements at frequent intervals.	Mechanical hyperventilation via reduced $Paco_2$ levels and cerebral vasoconstriction may be used in cases of acute deterioration to reduce ICP. Ideally, CBF measurements and continuous jugular venous oxygen saturation should be considered if hyperventilation is used as a treatment because hyperventilation produces varied blood flow responses and may cause cerebral ischemia.
Keep HOB elevated at 15-30 degrees (unless otherwise directed); maintain head and neck alignment to avoid hyperextension, flexion, or rotation; ensure that tracheostomy, endotracheal tube ties, or O_2 tubing does not compress the jugular vein; and avoid Trendelenburg position for any reason.	To promote venous blood return to the heart to reduce cerebral congestion.
Ensure that pillows under patient's head are flat.	To maintain head in a neutral rather than flexed position, which prevents backup of jugular venous outflow.
Take precautions against increased intraabdominal and intrathoracic pressure in the following ways:	
- Teach patient to exhale when turning.	Reduces intrathoracic pressure.
- Provide passive range-of-motion (ROM) exercises rather than allow active or assistive exercises.	
- Administer prescribed stool softeners or laxatives; avoid enemas and suppositories.	To prevent straining at stool, which would increase intraabdominal and intracranial pressures.

Continued

INTERVENTIONS	RATIONALES
- Instruct patient not to move self in bed; allow only passive turning; use a pull sheet. Instruct patient to avoid pushing against foot of bed or pulling against side rails. Avoid footboards; use high-top tennis shoes with toes removed to level of the metatarsal heads instead.	These movements involve pushing, which would increase intraabdominal and intrathoracic pressures.
- Assist patient with sitting up and turning.	
- Instruct patient to avoid coughing and sneezing or, if unavoidable, to do so with an open mouth; provide antitussive for cough as prescribed and antiemetic for vomiting.	To avoid increase in intraabdominal and intrathoracic pressures.
- Instruct patient to avoid hip flexion. Do not place patient in a prone position.	Increases intraabdominal pressure.
- Avoid using restraints.	Straining against restraints increases ICP.
- Rather than have patient perform Valsalva's maneuver, to prevent an air embolism during insertion of a central venous catheter, health care provider should use a syringe to aspirate air from the catheter lumen.	Valsalva's maneuver increases intraabdominal and intrathoracic pressures.
Administer IV fluids as prescribed.	To maintain normovolemia and balanced electrolyte status.
Avoid fluid restrictions.	The resulting increased blood viscosity and decreased volume may lead to hypotension, which would decrease CPP.
Administer IV fluids only with an infusion control device. Keep accurate I&O records.	To prevent fluid overload and thus cerebral edema.
When administering additional IV fluids (e.g., IV drugs) avoid using D_5W.	The hypotonicity of D_5W can increase cerebral edema and hyperglycemia, which have been associated with inferior neurologic outcomes.
Help maintain patient's body temperature within normal limits.	Fever increases metabolic requirements (10% for each 1° C) and aggravates hypoxia. Maintaining temperature at normal limits may be achieved by giving prescribed antipyretics, regulating temperature of the environment, limiting/promoting use of blankets, keeping patient's trunk warm to prevent shivering, and administering tepid sponge baths or using hypothermia blanket or convection cooling units to reduce fever.
When using a hypothermia blanket, wrap patient's extremities in blankets or towels.	To prevent shivering, which would increase ICP.
Administer prescribed osmotic and loop diuretics.	To reduce cerebral edema and blood volume, thereby lowering ICP.
Administer BP medications as prescribed.	To keep BP within the prescribed limits that will promote optimal CBF without increasing cerebral edema.
Administer prescribed analgesics promptly and as necessary.	Pain can increase BP and consequently increase ICP.
Recognize that barbiturates and narcotics are usually contraindicated.	These drugs have the potential for masking signs of IICP and causing respiratory depression. However, intubated, restless patients are usually sedated. A continuous propofol or midazolam drip has been demonstrated to decrease IICP.
If indicated/prescribed, administer lidocaine before suctioning an endotracheal tube.	To prevent coughing, which would increase pressures.
Administer antiepilepsy drugs as prescribed.	To prevent or control seizures, which would increase cerebral metabolism, hypoxia, and CO_2 retention, thereby increasing cerebral edema and ICP.
Monitor bladder drainage tubes for obstruction or kinks.	A distended bladder can increase ICP.

Continued

INTERVENTIONS	RATIONALES
Control noise and other environmental stimuli. Use a gentle touch and avoid jarring the bed. Try to limit painful procedures, avoid tension on tubes (e.g., urinary catheter), and consider limiting pain-stimulation testing. Avoid unnecessary touch (e.g., leave BP cuff in place for frequent VS; use automatic recycling blood pressure monitoring devices); and speak softly, explaining procedures before touching to avoid startling patient. Try to avoid situations in which patient may become emotionally upset. Do not say anything in the presence of the patient that you would not say if he or she were awake. Family discussions should take place outside the room. Limit visitors as necessary.	To provide a quiet and soothing environment, which optimally will help keep pressures within therapeutic limits.
Encourage significant other to speak quietly to patient.	Hearing a familiar, soft voice may promote relaxation and decrease ICP.
If possible, arrange for patient to listen to soft favorite music with earphones.	May help decrease ICP.
Individualize care to ensure rest periods and optimal spacing of activities; avoid turning, suctioning, and taking VS all at one time. Plan activities and treatments accordingly so that patient can sleep undisturbed as often as possible.	Multiple procedures and nursing care activities can increase ICP. Rousing patients from sleep also has been shown to increase ICP.

●●● **Related NIC and NOC labels:** *NIC:* Cerebral Edema Management; Cerebral Perfusion Promotion; Intracranial Pressure (ICP) Monitoring; Neurologic Monitoring; Fluid Management; Fluid Monitoring; Medication Administration; Positioning: Neurologic; Vital Signs Monitoring; Seizure Precautions; Anxiety Reduction *NOC:* Neurological Status; Neurological Status: Consciousness

Nursing Diagnosis:

Disturbed Sensory Perception: Visual

related to diplopia secondary to neurologic deficit

Desired Outcome: Immediately following intervention, patient verbalizes that ability to see has improved.

INTERVENTIONS	RATIONALES
Assess for diplopia.	Diplopia may occur in neurologic patients resulting from dysfunction of cranial nerves III, IV, and VI.
If patient has diplopia, provide an eye patch or eyeglasses with a frosted lens.	A temporary means of eliminating this condition.
Teach patient that depth perception will be altered and to use visual cues and scanning.	For safety and to prevent falls.
Advise patient of availability of "talking books" (tapes) and large-type reading materials.	It would be difficult for patient with diplopia to read books with smaller print.
Place a sign over patient's bed that indicates patient's visual impairment.	Communicates to health care staff and visitors that patient may require visual assistance.

●●● **Related NIC and NOC labels:** *NIC:* Environmental Management; Surveillance: Safety; Communication Enhancement: Visual Deficit; Fall Prevention *NOC:* Sensory Function: Vision; Vision Compensation: Behavior

Nursing Diagnosis:

Acute Pain

related to spasms, headache, and photophobia secondary to neurologic dysfunction

Desired Outcomes: Within 1 hr of intervention, patient's subjective perception of discomfort decreases, as documented by a pain scale. Objective indicators, such as grimacing, are absent or diminished.

INTERVENTIONS	RATIONALES
Assess characteristics (e.g., quality, severity, location, onset, duration, precipitating factors) of patient's pain or spasms. Devise a pain scale with patient and document discomfort on a scale of 0 (no pain) to 10 (worst pain).	To determine degree and type of discomfort, trend of the discomfort, and relief obtained following interventions.
Respond immediately to patient's complaints of pain. Administer analgesics and antispasmodics as prescribed. Consider scheduling doses of analgesia. Document effectiveness of the medication, using pain scale. Monitor for untoward effects.	To reduce pain before it becomes less manageable and promote pain relief before painful procedures and moves. Prolonged stimulation of pain receptors results in increased sensitivity to painful stimuli and will increase the amount of drug required to relieve pain.
Teach patient and significant other about importance of timing the pain medication so that it is taken before pain becomes too severe and before major moves.	
Teach patient about relationship between anxiety and pain, as well as other factors that promote pain and spasms (e.g., staying in one position for too long, fatigue, chilling).	Gives patient control over some causes of pain.
Instruct patient and significant other in use of techniques such as repositioning; ROM; supporting painful extremity or part; back rubs, acupressure, massage, warm baths, and other tactile distraction; auditory distraction such as listening to soothing music; visual distraction such as television; heat applications such as warm blankets or moist compresses; cold applications such as ice massage; guided imagery; breathing exercises; relaxation tapes and techniques; biofeedback; and a transcutaneous electrical nerve stimulation (TENS) device, as appropriate. See **Health-Seeking Behaviors:** Relaxation technique effective for stress reduction, p. 183.	These are nonpharmacologic methods of pain management that can be effective when used to supplement pharmacologic treatment. These methods also promote a sense of focus and self-control.
Encourage rest periods. Try to provide uninterrupted sleep time at night.	To facilitate sleep and relaxation. Fatigue tends to exacerbate the pain experience. Pain may result in fatigue, which in turn may cause exaggerated pain and further exhaustion.
If patient has photophobia, provide a quiet and dark environment. Close door and curtains, provide sunglasses, and avoid artificial lights whenever possible.	To eliminate light sources for patients with photophobia.
Recognize that pain in the SCI patient often is poorly localized and may be referred; monitor for it accordingly.	In the SCI patient, intrascapular pain may arise from the stomach, duodenum, or gallbladder. Umbilical pain may stem from the appendix, and testicular or inner thigh pain may originate from the kidneys (e.g., with pyelonephritis).
Evaluate SCI patient for tachycardia, restlessness, urinary incontinence when it was previously controlled, and fever. Report significant findings to health care provider.	These are indicators of infection or inflammatory processes that may result in pain and discomfort and should be reported promptly for timely intervention.

Continued

INTERVENTIONS	RATIONALES
If patient's present complaint of pain varies significantly from previous pain or if interventions are ineffective, notify health care provider.	May signal a new or acute problem and should be reported promptly for timely intervention.

●●● **Related NIC and NOC labels:** *NIC:* Medication Management; Documentation; Pain Management; Environmental Management: Comfort; Simple Relaxation Therapy; Sleep Enhancement; Biofeedback; Cutaneous Stimulation; Distraction; Heat/Cold Application; Simple Guided Imagery; Transcutaneous Electrical Nerve Stimulation *NOC:* Pain Control; Pain: Disruptive Effects

Nursing Diagnosis:

Impaired Swallowing

related to neuromuscular impairment (e.g., decreased or absent gag reflex, decreased strength or excursion of muscles involved in mastication, perceptual impairment, facial paralysis)

Desired Outcome: Before oral foods and fluids are reintroduced, patient exhibits ability to swallow safely without aspirating.

INTERVENTIONS	RATIONALES
Assess for factors that affect ability to swallow safely, including LOC, gag and cough reflexes, and strength and symmetry of tongue, lip, and facial muscles.	Deficits reflect need for aspiration precautions.
Monitor for coughing, regurgitation of food and fluid through the nares, drooling, food oozing from the lips, and food trapped in buccal spaces.	These are signs of impaired swallowing. Development of a weak, "wet," or hoarse voice during or after eating may signal potential for impaired swallowing.
Check swallow reflex by first asking patient to swallow own saliva. Place a finger gently on top of larynx, and if the larynx elevates, this is a sign that the swallow reflex is intact. Next ask patient to swallow 3-5 ml of plain water. Document findings.	Inability to swallow own saliva or small amount of water and presence of a stationary larynx during attempt to swallow signal loss of the swallowing reflex.

The act of swallowing is complex, and interventions vary according to the phase of swallowing that is dysfunctional. Video fluoroscopy may be used to evaluate swallowing, and some patients with swallowing dysfunction are referred to speech therapists for evaluation. |
Recognize that the presence of the cough reflex is essential for the patient to relearn swallowing safely.	The cough reflex protects against aspiration and if delayed may signal silent aspiration.
Encourage patient to practice prescribed exercises.	Exercises such as tongue and jaw ROM, sound phonation such as "gah-gah-gah" to promote elevation of the soft palate, puckering lips, and sticking tongue out to touch nose, chin, and cheeks are prescribed to facilitate swallowing.
Recognize that a nasogastric (NG) tube may hinder patient's ability to relearn to swallow.	NG tubes may desensitize and impair reflexive response to bolus stimulus.
Keep suction equipment and a manual resuscitation bag with face mask at patient's bedside. Suction secretions in patient's mouth as necessary.	To intervene in the event that aspiration occurs.
Ensure that patient is alert and responsive to verbal stimuli before he or she attempts to swallow.	Patients who are drowsy, inattentive, or fatigued have difficulty cooperating and are at risk of aspiration.

Continued

INTERVENTIONS	RATIONALES
Provide a rest period before meals or swallowing attempts.	To help minimize fatigue.
Initiate swallowing attempts with plain water (see earlier). Progressively add easy-to-swallow food and liquids as patient's ability to swallow improves. Add gravy or sauce to dry foods to facilitate swallowing. Determine which foods and liquids are easiest for patient to swallow.	Generally, semisolid foods of medium consistency, such as puddings, hot cereals, and casseroles, tend to be easiest to swallow. Thicker liquids, such as nectars, tend to be better tolerated than thin liquids.
If indicated/prescribed, add commercially available powders (e.g., Thicket) to liquids.	To increase viscosity of liquids and make them easier to swallow.
Avoid or limit foods such as peanut butter, chocolate, or milk.	These foods may stick in the throat or produce mucus.
Avoid nuts, hard candies, or popcorn.	These foods may be aspirated.
Reduce stimuli in the room (e.g., turn off television, lower radio volume, minimize conversation, and limit disruptions from phone calls). Advise patient not to talk while eating.	To help patient focus on swallowing.
If patient must remain in bed, use high Fowler's position if possible. Support shoulders and neck with pillows.	Most patients swallow best when in an upright position. Sitting in a straight-back chair with feet on the floor is ideal.
Ensure that head is erect and flexed forward slightly, with chin at the midline and pointing toward chest (i.e., the "chin tuck").	This head position minimizes risk that food will go into the airway by forcing the trachea to close and the esophagus to open. In addition, stroking anterior neck lightly may help some patients to swallow.
Maintain patient in an upright position for at least 30-60 min after eating.	To prevent regurgitation and aspiration by facilitating flow of foods and fluids by gravity from the stomach to the pylorus.
Break down the act of chewing and swallowing into steps.	Talking patient through the following steps promotes concentration and focus: - Take small bites or sips (approximately 5 ml each). - Place food on tongue. - Use tongue to transfer food so that it is directly under teeth on unaffected side of the mouth. Chew food thoroughly. - Move food to middle of tongue and hold it there. - Flex neck, and tuck chin against the chest. - Hold the breath and think about swallowing. - Without breathing, raise tongue to roof of the mouth and swallow. - Swallow several times if necessary. - When mouth is empty, raise chin and clear the throat or cough purposefully once or twice.
Ensure that each previous bite has been swallowed before patient takes the next bite. Check mouth for pockets of food. After every few bites of solid food, provide a liquid to help clear the mouth.	Food may become pocketed in the affected side.
Avoid using a syringe to clear patient's mouth.	The force of the fluid in the syringe, if sprayed in patient's mouth, may cause aspiration.
Tear a piece out of a Styrofoam cut to make a space for the nose so that patient can drink with neck flexed.	This head position minimizes risk that food will go into the airway by forcing the trachea to close and the esophagus to open.
Teach patient who has food pockets in the buccal spaces to periodically sweep mouth with the tongue or finger or to clean these areas with a napkin.	To prevent later aspiration of food particles, stomatitis, and tooth decay.

Continued

INTERVENTIONS	RATIONALES
Teach patients who have a weak or paralyzed side to place food on side of the face they can control and tilt head to side that promotes optimal swallowing.	Tilting head toward stronger side will allow gravity to help keep food or liquid on side of the mouth they can manipulate. However, some patients may find that rotating head to weak side will close damaged side of the pharynx and facilitate more effective swallowing.
Serve only warm or cool foods to patients with loss of oral sensation.	Patients with loss of oral sensation may be unable to identify foods or fluids of tepid temperature by their tongue or oral mucosa, potentially resulting in oral tissue injury caused by food retention. Verbal cues and use of a mirror may help ensure that these patients keep their mouths clear after swallowing.
For patients with tongue rigidity, encourage repeated swallowing attempts.	Patients with a rigid tongue (e.g., with parkinsonism) have difficulty getting the tongue to move the bolus of food into the pharynx for swallowing.
Evaluate patient's swallowing ability at different times of the day.	This may enable rescheduling mealtimes to times of the day when patient has improved swallowing, or, as appropriate, discussing with health care provider the possibility of changing dose schedule of patient's anti-Parkinson medication.
If decreased salivation is contributing to patient's swallowing difficulties, perform one of the following before feeding: swab patient's mouth with a lemon-glycerin sponge; have patient suck on a tart-flavored hard candy, dill pickle, or lemon slice; teach patient to move tongue in a circular motion against inside of cheek; or use artificial saliva.	To stimulate salivation, which may promote effective swallowing.
Moisten food with melted butter, broth or other soup, or gravy. Dip dry foods such as toast into coffee or other liquid.	To soften the food when salivation is decreased.
Rinse patient's mouth as needed.	To remove particles and lubricate mouth.
Investigate medications that patient is taking for potential side effect of decreased salivation (e.g., anti-Parkinson medications or those with extrapyramidal side effects).	To determine if medication may be contributing to decreased salivation.
Recognize that crushed tablets or opened capsules mix easily into certain soft foods.	Tablets or capsules may be swallowed more easily when added to foods such as puddings or ice cream.
Check with pharmacist before altering a medication.	To ensure that crushing a tablet or opening a capsule does not adversely affect its absorption or duration (i.e., slow-release medications should not be crushed). Liquid forms of medications also may be available through the pharmacy.
Teach significant other the Heimlich or abdominal thrust maneuver.	So he or she can intervene in the event of choking.

●●● **Related NIC and NOC labels:** *NIC:* Aspiration Precautions; Airway Management; Airway Suctioning; Positioning; Risk Identification; Swallowing Therapy; Cough Enhancement; Referral *NOC:* Aspiration Control; Swallowing Status

Nursing Diagnosis:

Risk for Imbalanced Body Temperature

related to illness or trauma affecting temperature regulation and inability or decreased ability to perspire, shiver, or vasoconstrict

Desired Outcome: Following the intervention, patient is normothermic with core temperatures between 36.5° and 37.7° C (97.8° and 100° F).

INTERVENTIONS	**RATIONALES**
Monitor rectal, tympanic, or bladder core temperature q4h or, if patient is in spinal shock, q2h.	Infection and hypothalamic dysfunction as a result of cerebral insult (trauma, edema) are two common causes of hyperthermia. The rapid development of spinal lesions (e.g., in SCI) breaks the connection between the hypothalamus and the sympathetic nervous system (SNS), causing an inability to adapt to environmental temperature. In spinal cord shock, temperatures tend to lower toward the ambient temperature. Inability to vasoconstrict and shiver makes heat conservation difficult; the inability to perspire prevents normal cooling.
Monitor for impaired ability to think, disorientation, confusion, drowsiness, apathy, and reduced HR and RR. Monitor for complaints of being too cold, goose bumps (piloerection), and cool skin (in SCI patients, above level of injury).	Signs of hypothermia.
Monitor for flushed face, malaise, rash, respiratory distress, tachycardia, weakness, headache, and irritability. Monitor for complaints of being too warm, sweating, or hot and dry skin (in SCI patients, above level of injury).	Signs of hyperthermia.
Monitor for parched mouth, furrowed tongue, dry lips, poor skin turgor, decreased urine output, increased concentration of urine (specific gravity >1.030), and weak, fast pulse.	Signs of dehydration that can result from hyperthermia.
For hyperthermia: maintain a cool room temperature (20° C [68° F]). Provide a fan or air conditioning. Remove excess bedding and cover patient with a thin sheet. Give tepid sponge baths. Place cool, wet cloths at patient's head, neck, axilla, and groin. Administer antipyretic agent as prescribed. Use a padded hypothermia blanket (wrap hands and feet in towels or blankets to prevent shivering) or convection cooling device if prescribed. Provide cool drinks. Evaluate for potential infectious cause.	To prevent overheating.
For hypothermia: increase environmental temperature. Protect patient from drafts. Provide warm drinks. Provide extra blankets. Provide warming (hyperthermia) blanket or convection warming device.	To increase body temperature.
Keep feverish patient dry. Change bed linens after diaphoresis. Provide careful skin care when patient is on a hypothermia or hyperthermia blanket.	To prevent skin irritation and potential loss of skin integrity that could result from hyperthermia.
Monitor I&O and maintain adequate hydration accordingly.	Consider insensible water loss from fever, which may affect total hydration, when measuring I&O and promoting hydration. Unless contraindicated, encourage increased fluid intake in febrile patients (e.g., 3000 ml/day).
Increase caloric intake.	Patient will have increased metabolic needs with a fever.

●●● **Related NIC and NOC labels:** *NIC:* Temperature Regulation; Environmental Management; Fever Treatment; Fluid Management; Bathing; Environmental Management: Comfort Heat/Cold Application; Vital Signs Monitoring *NOC:* Thermoregulation

36

Bacterial Meningitis

Bacterial meningitis is an infection that results in inflammation of the meningeal membranes covering the brain and spinal cord. Bacteria in the subarachnoid space multiply and cause an inflammatory reaction of the pia and arachnoid meninges. Purulent exudate is produced, and the inflammation and infection spread quickly through the cerebrospinal fluid (CSF) that circulates around the brain and spinal cord. Bacteria and exudate can create vascular congestion, plugging the arachnoid villi. This obstruction of CSF flow and decreased reabsorption of CSF can lead to hydrocephalus, increased intracranial pressure (IICP), brain herniation, and death.

Meningitis generally is transmitted in one of four ways: (1) via airborne droplets or contact with oral secretions from infected individuals; (2) from direct contamination (e.g., from a penetrating skull wound; a skull fracture, often basilar, causing a tear in the dura; lumbar puncture [LP]; ventricular shunt; or surgical procedure); (3) via the bloodstream (e.g., pneumonia, endocarditis); or (4) from direct contact with an infectious process that invades the meningeal membranes, as can occur with osteomyelitis, sinusitis, otitis media, mastoiditis, or brain abscess. In adults, pneumococcal meningitis, caused by *Streptococcus pneumoniae,* is the most common bacterial meningitis. Any bacteria can cause a meningitis, and some, such as that caused by *Staphylococcus aureus,* can be difficult to treat because of their resistance to antibiotic therapy. The prognosis, however, is good, and complete neurologic recovery is possible if the disorder is recognized early and antibiotic treatment is initiated promptly. Left untreated, the mortality rate is 70%-100%.

HEALTH CARE SETTING

Acute care setting

ASSESSMENT

Cardinal signs: Headache, fever, stiff neck.
Infection: Fever, chills, malaise.
IICP and herniation: Decreased level of consciousness (LOC; irritability, drowsiness, stupor, coma), nausea and vomiting, a decreasing Glasgow Coma Scale score, VS changes (increased BP, decreased HR, widening pulse pressure), changes in respiratory pattern, decreased pupillary reaction to light, pupillary dilation or inequality, severe headache.

Meningeal irritation: Back stiffness and pain, headache, nuchal rigidity.

Other: Generalized seizures and photophobia. In the presence of *Haemophilus influenzae,* deafness or joint pain may occur.

Physical assessment: A positive Brudzinski's sign may be elicited because of meningeal irritation: when the neck is passively flexed forward, both legs flex involuntarily at the hip and knee.

A positive Kernig's sign also may be found: when the thigh is flexed 90 degrees at the hip, the individual cannot extend the leg completely without pain.

In the presence of meningococcal meningitis, a pink, macular rash; petechiae; ecchymoses; purpura; and increased deep tendon reflexes (DTRs) may occur. The rash signals septicemia and is associated with a 40% mortality rate, even with appropriate antibiotics.

DIAGNOSTIC TESTS

LP, CSF analysis, and Gram stain and culture: To identify causative organism. Glucose is generally decreased, and protein is usually increased. Typically, the CSF will be cloudy or milky because of increased white blood cells (WBCs), and CSF pressure will be increased because of the inflammation and exudate, causing an obstruction in outflow of CSF from the arachnoid villi. This test, in the presence of IICP, can cause brain herniation. If CSF pressure is elevated, check neurologic status and VS at frequent intervals for signs of brain herniation (decreased LOC; pupillary changes such as dilation, inequality, or decreased reaction; irregular respirations; hemiparesis).

Culture and sensitivity testing of blood, sputum, urine, and other body secretions: To identify infective organism and/or its source and determine appropriate antibiotic.

Coagglutination tests: To detect microbial antigens in CSF and enable identification of the causative organism. Coagglutination tests have generally replaced counterimmunoelectrophoresis (CIE) because results are obtainable much more rapidly.

Sinus, skull, and chest x-ray examinations: Taken after treatment is started to rule out sinusitis, pneumonia, and cranial osteomyelitis.

Enzyme-linked immunosorbent assay (ELISA): To detect microbial antigens in the CSF and thereby identify the causative organism.

Computed tomography (CT) scan with contrast: To rule out hydrocephalus or mass lesions such as brain abscess and detect exudate in the CSF spaces.

Nursing Diagnosis:

Deficient Knowledge:

Side effects and precautions for the prescribed antibiotics

Desired Outcome: Before beginning the medication regimen, patient and contacts verbalize accurate knowledge about purpose, potential side effects, and precautions for prescribed antibiotics.

INTERVENTIONS	RATIONALES
Explain to patient that he or she likely will receive high doses of parenteral antibiotics immediately.	Meningitis has a high mortality rate when it is left untreated, and therefore treatment cannot be delayed until the results of the culture are known. The antibiotic must penetrate the blood-brain barrier into the CSF. Adjustments in therapy can be made after coagglutination test, CIE, and culture and sensitivity test results are available.
	Antibiotics may include the following (usually in combination): cefotaxime, ceftriaxone, penicillin G, ampicillin, chloramphenicol, gentamicin, or vancomycin.
As appropriate, teach patient that sometimes intrathecal (i.e., in the subarachnoid space) antibiotics are used.	Intrathecal antibiotics may be given if it is believed that systemic antibiotics alone will not be curative in the presence of particular bacteria (e.g., *Pseudomonas, Enterobacter, Staphylococcus*).
For patient's contacts taking prophylactic rifampin explain prescribed dose and schedule. Emphasize importance of taking this drug as a preventative measure against meningitis and describe potential side effects.	Rifampin should be taken 1 hr before or 2 hr after meals for maximum absorption. Side effects include nausea, vomiting, diarrhea, orange urine, headache, and dizziness. If gastrointestinal (GI) symptoms are a problem, rifampin can be taken with food, although doing so will postpone absorption. Other antibiotics that may be used in lieu of rifampin include sulfadiazine or minocycline.
Caution against wearing contact lenses. In addition, caution patients who are pregnant that this drug is contraindicated. Explain precautions to patients taking oral contraceptives.	This drug will permanently color the lenses orange. Rifampin crosses the placenta of pregnant women and also reduces effectiveness of oral contraceptives.
Instruct contacts who are taking rifampin to report onset of jaundice (yellow skin or sclera), allergic reactions, and persistence of GI side effects.	Side effects that should be reported for timely intervention.

●●● **Related NIC and NOC labels:** *NIC:* Teaching: Prescribed Medication *NOC:* Knowledge: Medication

Nursing Diagnosis:

Deficient Knowledge:

Rationale and procedure for Standard and Expanded Precautions

Desired Outcome: Before visitation, patient and significant other verbalize accurate knowledge about the rationale for Standard and Expanded Precautions and comply with the prescribed restrictions and precautionary measures.

INTERVENTIONS	RATIONALES
For patients with meningitis caused by *H. influenzae* or *Neisseria meningitidis,* explain method of disease transmission and rationale for private room and special precautions.	Patients with *N. meningitidis,* with *H. influenzae,* or in whom the causative organism is in doubt require observation with Expanded Precautions: Droplet, for 24 hr after initiation of appropriate antibiotic therapy, and patient should be placed in a private room. Infection may be spread by contact with airborne droplets or oral secretions. Masks should be worn and other Standard Precaution procedures observed.
Provide instructions for covering mouth before coughing or sneezing and properly disposing of tissue.	Infection control/precaution measures to prevent contact of others with airborne droplets.
Instruct patients with Expanded Precautions: Droplet, to stay in their rooms. If they must leave the room for a procedure or test, explain that a mask must be worn.	To protect others from contact with airborne droplets.
For individuals in contact with patient, explain importance of wearing a surgical mask, using good handwashing technique, and wearing gloves when handling patient's body fluid, especially oral secretions.	To reduce risk of infection from airborne droplets and oral secretions.
Reassure patient that special Expanded Precautions: Droplet, are temporary.	They will be discontinued once patient has been taking appropriate antibiotic for 24-48 hr, the amount of time necessary to ensure the antibiotic has penetrated the blood-brain barrier into the CSF.
Instruct individuals in contact with patient that if the symptoms of meningitis develop (e.g., headache, fever, neck stiffness, photophobia), they should be reported rapidly to their health care provider.	To ensure prompt treatment. Mortality is high (70%-100%) in persons in whom meningitis is left untreated. However, in individuals in whom diagnosis and antibiotic treatment are established early, prognosis is good, and complete neurologic recovery is possible.

●●● **Related NIC and NOC labels:** *NIC:* Teaching: Procedure/Treatment; Teaching: Disease Process; Infection Protection; Infection Control *NOC:* Knowledge: Illness Care; Knowledge: Infection Control

Nursing Diagnosis:

Acute Pain

related to headache, photophobia, and neck stiffness secondary to meningitis

Desired Outcomes: Within 1 hr of intervention, patient's subjective perception of discomfort decreases, as documented by a pain scale. Objective indicators, such as grimacing, are absent or diminished.

INTERVENTIONS	RATIONALES
Provide a quiet and dark environment. Restrict visitors and provide sunglasses as indicated.	To provide comfort for patients with headache and photophobia.
Promote bedrest and assist with activities of daily living (ADL) as needed.	To decrease movement that may cause pain.
Apply ice bag to head or cool cloth to eyes.	To help diminish headache by vasoconstricting the blood vessels.
Support patient in a position of comfort.	Many persons with meningitis are comforted in a position with head in extension and body slightly curled. Elevating head of bed (HOB) to 30 degrees may decrease cerebral congestion and edema by promoting venous drainage. Keeping neck in alignment during position changes will help prevent added discomfort for patients with neck stiffness.
Provide gentle passive range of motion (ROM) and massage to neck and shoulder joints and muscles.	To help relieve stiffness.
If patient is afebrile, apply moist heat to neck and back.	To promote muscle relaxation and decrease pain. Using moist heat in a febrile patient would add to patient's hyperthermia.
Implement measures to reduce body temperature for patients with hyperthermia.	Patient may be comforted by tepid bath, cooling blanket, or convection blanket. These are measures that help reduce hyperthermia. Administering acetaminophen as prescribed will reduce cerebral metabolism and help control fever.
Keep communication simple and direct, using a soft, calm tone of voice. Avoid needless stimulation. Consolidate activities. Loosen constricting bed clothing. Avoid restraining patient. Reduce stimulation to the minimal amount needed to accomplish required activity.	Patients tend to be hyperirritable with hyperalgesia. Sounds are loud. Even gentle touching may startle patient.
Administer analgesics, such as acetaminophen or codeine, as prescribed.	To relieve headache, myalgia, and other pain.
Along with antibiotic therapy, administer glucocorticoids if they have been prescribed.	Glucocorticoids (e.g., dexamethasone) may be given to reduce the inflammation and discomfort caused by the toxic by-products released by the bacterial cells as they are killed by the antibiotics.
For other interventions, see **Acute Pain** in "General Care of Patients with Neurologic Disorders," p. 307.	

●●● **Related NIC and NOC labels:** *NIC:* Medication Administration; Environmental Management: Comfort; Pain Management; Positioning; Heat/Cold Application; Simple Massage *NOC:* Comfort Level; Pain Control Pain: Disruptive Effects

ADDITIONAL NURSING DIAGNOSES/ PROBLEMS:

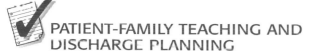

PATIENT-FAMILY TEACHING AND DISCHARGE PLANNING

The extent of teaching and discharge planning will depend on whether the patient has any residual damage. When providing patient-family teaching, focus on sensory information, avoid giving excessive information, and initiate a visiting nurse referral for necessary follow-up teaching. Include verbal and written information about the following:

✓ Referrals to community resources, such as public health nurse, visiting nurses association, community support groups, social workers, psychologic therapy, vocational rehabilitation agency, home health agencies, and extended and skilled care facilities.

✓ Medications, including drug name, purpose, dosage, schedule, precautions, drug/drug and food/drug interactions, and potential side effects for patient's medications, as well as those for the prophylactic antibiotics taken by family and significant other.

✓ For patients with residual neurologic deficits, teach the following as appropriate: exercises that promote muscle strength and mobility; measures for preventing contractures and skin breakdown; transfer techniques and proper body mechanics; safety measures if patient has decreased pain and sensation or visual disturbances; use of assistive devices; indications of constipation, urinary retention, or urinary tract infection (UTI); bowel and bladder training programs; self-catheterization technique or care of indwelling catheters; and seizure precautions if indicated.

✓ Additional information can be obtained by contacting the following organization:

Meningitis Foundation of America
7155 Shadeland Station, Suite 190
Indianapolis, IN 46256
(800) 668-1129
www.musa.org

Cerebrovascular Accident

Acerebrovascular accident (CVA) or stroke is the sudden disruption of O_2 supply to the nerve cells, generally caused by obstruction or rupture in one or more of the blood vessels that supply the brain. *Ischemic CVA* has three main mechanisms: thrombosis, embolism, and systemic hypoperfusion. Thrombosis or embolism results in a blockage of blood supply to the brain tissue. The resulting ischemia, if prolonged, causes brain tissue necrosis (infarction), cerebral edema, and increased intracranial pressure (IICP). Most thrombotic strokes are caused by blockage of large vessels as a result of atherosclerosis. Most embolic strokes are cardiogenic and the result of emboli produced from valve disease or during atrial fibrillation of the heart. Ischemic stroke caused by systemic hypoperfusion usually is the result of decreased cerebral blood flow owing to circulatory failure. Circulatory failure results from too little blood, too low BP, or failure of the heart to pump blood adequately. Hypoxia from any cause also can produce this syndrome.

Hemorrhagic CVA causes neural tissue destruction because of the infiltration and accumulation of blood. Ischemia and infarction may occur distal to the hemorrhage because of interrupted blood supply. Although a cerebral hemorrhage usually results from hypertension or an aneurysm, trauma also can cause hemorrhagic CVA. Bleeding may spread into the brain tissue itself, causing an intracerebral hemorrhage, or into the subarachnoid space. Usually there is a large rise in ICP with a hemorrhagic stroke because of cerebral edema and the mass effect of blood.

A *transient ischemic attack* (TIA), which is a temporary (<24 hr) neurologic deficit that resolves completely without permanent damage, occurs when the artery cannot deliver enough blood to meet the brain's O_2 requirement. TIAs are a warning sign, and treatment may prevent a stroke. Most TIAs last an average of 5-10 min. A reversible ischemic neurologic deficit (RIND) lasts longer than 24 hr but otherwise is similar to a TIA.

A CVA may be classified as a *progressive stroke in evolution*, in which deficits continue to worsen over time, or as a *completed stroke*, in which maximum deficit has been acquired and has persisted for longer than 24 hr. Progressive strokes usually are the result of a thrombus formation and often take 1-3 days to become "completed." CVA is the third most common cause of death and the most common cause of neurologic disability. Half the survivors are left permanently disabled or experience another CVA. Improvement may continue for 1-2 yr, but deficits at 6 mo usually are considered permanent.

HEALTH CARE SETTING

Critical care unit, step-down unit, acute rehabilitation unit, outpatient rehabilitation program

ASSESSMENT

Note: Because of the narrow 3-hr window that may reverse permanent neurologic damage, it is critical to teach patients not to ignore symptoms, which include sudden weakness, numbness (especially on one side of the body), vision loss or dimming, trouble talking or understanding speech, unexplained dizziness, unsteadiness, or severe headache.

General findings: Classically, symptoms appear on the side of the body opposite the damaged site. For example, a CVA in the left hemisphere of the brain will produce symptoms in the right arm and leg. However, when the CVA affects the cranial nerves, the symptoms of cranial nerve deficit will appear on the same side as the site of injury. Similarly, an obstruction of an anterior cerebral artery can produce bilateral symptoms, as will severe bleeding or multiple emboli. Hemiplegia is fairly common. Initially, the patient usually has flaccid paralysis. As spinal cord depression resolves, more normal tone is seen, and hyperactive reflexes occur.

Signs and symptoms: Vary with the size and site of injury and may improve in 2-3 days as the cerebral edema decreases. Changes in mentation, including apathy, irritability, disorientation, memory loss, withdrawal, drowsiness, stupor, or coma; bowel and bladder incontinence; numbness or loss of sensation; weakness or paralysis on part or one side of the body; aphasia; headache; neck stiffness and rigidity; vomiting; seizures; dizziness or syncope; and fever may occur. A brain stem infarct leaving the patient completely paralyzed with intact cortical function is called *locked-in syndrome*.

With *cranial nerve involvement*, visual disturbances may include diplopia, blindness, and hemianopia; inequality or fixation of the pupils, nystagmus, tinnitus, and difficulty chewing and swallowing also occur.

Physical assessment: Papilledema, arteriosclerotic retinal changes, or hemorrhagic retinal areas on ophthalmic examination. Hyperactive deep tendon reflexes (DTRs), decreased superficial reflexes, and positive Babinski's sign also may be present. To check for Babinski's response, stroke the lateral aspect of the sole of the foot (from the heel to the ball of the foot) with a hard object. Dorsiflexion of the great toe with fanning of the other toes is a positive sign. Positive Kernig's or Brudzinski's sign (see "Bacterial Meningitis," p. 313) indicates meningeal irritation.

TIAs: Typical symptoms include temporal episodes of slurred speech, weakness, numbness or tingling, blindness in one eye, blurred or double vision, dizziness or ataxia, and confusion.

History of: TIAs; hypertension; atherosclerosis; high serum cholesterol or triglycerides; diabetes mellitus; gout; smoking; cardiac valve diseases, such as those that may result from rheumatic fever, valve prosthesis, and atrial fibrillation; cardiac surgery; blood dyscrasias; anticoagulant therapy; neck vessel trauma; oral contraceptive use; cocaine or methamphetamine use; family predisposition for arteriovenous malformation (AVM); aneurysm; or previous CVA.

DIAGNOSTIC TESTS

The computed tomography (CT) scan or magnetic resonance imaging (MRI) is the test most likely to be obtained for every patient with a suspected stroke. However, technologic advances have provided numerous diagnostic tests for CVA. The selection, sequence, and urgency of these tests will be determined by the patient's history and symptoms. For example, the patient who has a TIA will have a different set or sequence of tests than the patient who is in a coma.

CT scan: To reveal site of infarction, hematoma, and shift of brain structures. CT scan is of particular value in identifying blood released early during hemorrhagic strokes. CT scan is the test of choice for unstable patients. Generally, identifying ischemic areas is difficult until they start to necrose at around 48-72 hr. Xenon-enhanced CT may be done to study cerebral blood flow; CT angiography may be performed to evaluate blood vessels.

MRI: To reveal site of infarction, hematoma, shift of brain structure, and cerebral edema. MRI diffusion and perfusion weighted studies are of particular value in identifying ischemic strokes early. Other magnetic resonance (MR) techniques include MR angiography to evaluate vessels and MR spectrography.

Phonoangiography/Doppler ultrasonography: To identify presence of bruits if the carotid blood vessels are partially occluded. B-mode imaging and duplex scanning also may be done to evaluate the carotids.

Transcranial Doppler (TCD) ultrasound: To provide information (noninvasively) about pressure and flow in the intracranial arteries; it can be performed at the bedside or in a diagnostic laboratory.

Positron emission tomography (PET): To provide information on cerebral metabolism and blood flow characteristics. This test is useful in identifying ischemic stroke by showing areas of reduced glucose metabolism.

Single photon emission computed tomography (SPECT): To identify cerebral blood flow.

Electroencephalogram (EEG): To show abnormal nerve impulse transmission and indicate the amount of brain wave activity present.

Lumbar puncture (LP) and cerebrospinal fluid (CSF) analysis: Not done routinely, especially in the presence of IICP, but may reveal increase in CSF pressure; clear to bloody CSF, depending on the type of stroke; and presence of infection or other nonvascular cause for bleeding. CSF glutamic oxaloacetic transaminase (GOT) will be increased for 10 days after injury. Blood in the CSF signals that a subarachnoid hemorrhage has occurred.

Cerebral angiography: If surgery is contemplated, this procedure is done to pinpoint site of rupture or occlusion and identify collateral blood circulation, aneurysms, or AVM.

Digital subtraction angiography (DSA): To visualize cerebral blood flow and detect vascular abnormalities, such as stenosis, aneurysm, and hematomas.

Echocardiography (e.g., transthoracic and transesophageal): To evaluate valvular heart structures for thrombus and myocardial walls for mural thrombi that may provide a source of emboli.

Laboratory Tests: To detect and monitor for clotting abnormalities as a source of hemorrhagic stroke and monitor serum or capillary glucose for presence of hyperglycemia, which has been associated with poor outcomes.

Nursing Diagnosis:

Unilateral Neglect

related to disturbed perceptual ability secondary to neurologic insult

Desired Outcome: Following intervention and on an ongoing basis, patient scans the environment and responds to stimuli on affected side.

INTERVENTIONS	RATIONALES
Assess patient's ability to recognize objects to right or left of his or her visual midline; perceive body parts as his or her own; perceive pain, touch, and temperature sensations; judge distances; orient self to changes in the environment; differentiate left from right; maintain posture sense; and identify objects by sight, hearing, or touch. Document specific deficits.	This assessment for disturbed perceptual ability, including unilateral neglect, enables nurse to develop a plan of care individualized for the patient.
Assess for neglect of affected side.	Neglect of and inattention to stimuli on affected side occur more often with right hemisphere injury. Neglect cannot be totally explained on the basis of loss of physical senses (e.g., both ears are used in hearing, but with auditory neglect, patient may ignore conversation or noises that occur on affected side). Types of neglect include the following: *Visual neglect:* Patient does not turn head to see all parts of an object (e.g., may read only half of a page or eat from only one side of plate). When patient exhibits signs of visual neglect, continue to place objects necessary for activities of daily living (ADL) and call bells on unaffected side and approach patient from that side. *Self-neglect:* Patient does not perceive arm or leg as being a part of the body. For example, when combing or brushing hair, patient attends to only one (unaffected) side of the head. Inadequate self-care and injury may occur. *Auditory neglect:* Patient ignores individuals who approach and speak from affected side but communicates with those who approach or speak from unaffected side.
Intervene in the following ways for patients with *visual neglect:*	To shift patient's attention to the neglected side.
- Gradually increase stimuli on affected side (e.g., while communicating with patient, physically move across her or his visual boundary and stand on that side; encourage patient to turn head past the midline and scan entire environment; place patient's food on neglected side and encourage patient to look to neglected side and name the food before eating; place a bright red tape or ribbon on affected side and encourage patient to scan and find it). Continuously clue patient to the environment. Initially place patient's unaffected side toward most active part of room, but as compensation occurs, reverse this. As patient begins to compensate, place additional items out of his or her visual field.	
Intervene in the following ways for patients with *self-neglect:*	
- Encourage patient to touch or massage and look at neglected side and make a conscious effort to care for neglected body parts; also, check for proper position.	To enhance patient's self-recognition of neglected side.
- When patient is in bed or up in a chair, provide safety measures, such as side rails and restraints.	To prevent patient from attempting to get up, which can occur because of unawareness of neglected side.
- Teach patient to use unaffected arm to perform range-of-motion (ROM) exercises on affected side. Position arm on bedside table or wheelchair lap board with hand or arm past the midline, where patient can see it. Teach patient to attend to affected side first when performing ADL, consciously look for affected side, monitor its position, and check for exposure to sharp objects and irritants.	To integrate patient's neglected arm into activities, as well as prevent contractures, skin breakdown, and trauma on that side.

Continued

INTERVENTIONS	RATIONALES
- Provide a mirror.	This will enable patient to watch and attend to both sides when shaving or brushing teeth and hair.
- Instruct patient to take precautions with hot or cold items or when around moving machinery. Stand on patient's affected side when ambulating with patient	Safety measures for patients unaware of affected side.
- Teach use of arm sling.	To support affected arm when patient is out of bed and when in bed to elevate and protect affected arm.
Intervene in the following ways for patients with *auditory neglect:*	
- Move across auditory boundary while speaking, and continue speaking from patient's neglected side to bring patient's attention to that area.	To stimulate patient's attention to affected side.
- Arrange environment by keeping necessary objects, such as call light, on patient's unaffected side.	To maximize performance of ADL.
- If possible, move bed.	To enable patient's unaffected side to face room's largest section.
- Approach and speak to patient from unaffected side. If you must approach affected side, announce yourself.	To avoid startling patient.
- Perform activities on patient's unaffected side.	Unless you are specifically attempting to stimulate patient's neglected side, communicating and performing activities on patient's unaffected side will engage and be less confusing for patient.

●●● **Related NIC and NOC labels:** *NIC:* Unilateral Neglect Management: Body Image Enhancement; Positioning; Self-Care Assistance; Touch; Exercise Promotion; Fall Prevention; Environmental Management: Safety *NOC:* Body Image; Body Positioning: Self-Initiated; Self-Care: Activities of Daily Living

Nursing Diagnosis:

Impaired Physical Mobility

related to neuromuscular impairment with limited use of the upper and/or lower limbs secondary to CVA

Desired Outcome: By at least 24 hr before hospital discharge (or within 24 hr after instruction if patient is not hospitalized), patient and significant other demonstrate techniques that promote safe ambulating and transferring.

INTERVENTIONS	RATIONALES
Teach patient to use stronger extremity to move weaker extremity.	These are safe and effective methods for turning and moving. For example, to move affected leg in bed or when changing from a lying to a sitting position, patient should slide unaffected foot under affected ankle to lift, support, and bring affected leg along in the desired movement.
Encourage patient to make a conscious attempt to look at extremities and check position before moving. Remind patient to make a conscious effort to lift and then extend foot when ambulating.	Safety measures to prevent falling.

Continued

INTERVENTIONS	RATIONALES
Instruct patient with impaired sense of balance to compensate by leaning toward stronger side. As necessary, remind patient to keep body weight forward over feet when standing.	The tendency is to lean toward weaker or paralyzed side.
Recommend wearing well-fitting shoes.	Slippers, for example, tend to slide and can result in falls.
Protect impaired arm with a sling to support arm and shoulder when patient is up. Position patient in correct alignment and provide a pillow or lap board for support.	To help maintain anatomic position.
Encourage active/passive ROM.	To improve muscle tone.
Avoid pulling on patient's shoulders or arms; use a lift sheet to reposition in bed.	To prevent subluxation.
Monitor for subluxation of the shoulder.	Shoulder subluxation manifests as shoulder pain and tenderness, swelling, decreased ROM, and altered appearance of bony prominences.
Follow these general principles when transferring patient:	All are safety measures to compensate for patient's affected side.
- Encourage weight bearing on patient's stronger side.	
- Use a transfer belt during transfers.	Provides support without placing excessive stress on patient's upper extremities.
- Ensure that a helper stands and walks on patient's affected side.	
- Instruct patient to pivot on stronger side and use stronger arm for support.	
- Teach patient to transfer toward unaffected side.	
- Instruct patient to place unaffected side closest to bed or chair to which he or she wishes to transfer.	
- Explain that when transferring, affected leg should be under patient with foot flat on the ground.	
Position a braced chair or locked wheelchair close to patient's stronger side.	
- If patient requires assistance from staff member, teach patient not to support self by pulling on or placing hands around assistant's neck. Staff members should use their own knees and feet to brace feet and knees of patients who are very weak.	
Obtain physical therapy (PT) and occupational therapy (OT) referrals as appropriate. Reinforce special mobilization techniques (e.g., Bobath, constraint-induced movement therapy, proprioceptive neuromuscular facilitation [PNF]) per patient's individualized rehabilitation program.	To help patient maintain mobility and independence with ADL.
Recognize that these techniques may vary from the above general principles.	For example, Bobath focuses on use of affected side in mobility training, so patient would try to bear weight on affected side and move toward affected side to relearn normal movement patterns and position.

●●● **Related NIC and NOC labels:** *NIC:* Exercise Therapy: Ambulation; Body Mechanics Promotion; Fall Prevention; Exercise Promotion *NOC:* Ambulation: Walking; Ambulation: Wheelchair; Joint Movement: Active; Mobility Level; Transfer Performance

Nursing Diagnosis:

Disturbed Sensory Perception

related to altered sensory reception, transmission, and/or integration secondary to neurologic damage

Desired Outcome: Following intervention and on an ongoing basis, patient interacts appropriately with his or her environment and does not exhibit evidence of injury caused by sensory/perceptual deficit.

INTERVENTIONS	RATIONALES
Remind patients who have a dominant (left) hemisphere injury to scan their environment.	These patients usually lack or have decreased pain sensation and position sense and usually have visual field deficit on right side of body, although most have normal awareness of their body and spatial orientation. These patients usually do not exhibit unilateral neglect.
Provide frequent, accurate, and immediate feedback on their performance.	These patients tend to be slow, cautious, and disorganized when approaching an unfamiliar problem. They may respond well to nonverbal encouragement, such as a pat on the back.
Keep conversation on a concrete level (e.g., say "water," not "fluid"; "leg," not "limb"). Give short, simple messages or questions and step-by-step directions.	Because of short attention span and impaired logical reasoning, patient is easily distracted and may have poor abstract thinking.
Enable patient to touch items such as washcloth and comb and have caretaker name these items.	Patient may have difficulty recognizing items by touch alone.
Encourage patients with nondominant (right) hemisphere injury to slow down and check each step or task as it is completed.	Patients with nondominant (right) hemisphere injury may have decreased pain sensation and position sense and visual field deficit, but typically they are unconcerned or unaware of or deny deficits or lost abilities. These patients tend to be impulsive and too quick with movements. Typically, they have impaired judgment about what they can or cannot do and often overestimate their abilities. They also are at risk for burns, bruises, cuts, and falls; may need to be restrained from attempting unsafe activities; and are more likely to have unilateral neglect (see **Unilateral Neglect,** p. 320) than individuals with dominant (left) hemisphere injury.
Be careful what you say because it may be taken literally (e.g., if you say "ate the lion's share," patient may think someone literally ate the lion's portion of the meal).	The patient generally retains ability to think logically but sees specifics rather than the global picture (i.e., can see trees but not the forest). This patient also may have impaired ability to recognize subtle distinctions (e.g., the difference between a fork and spoon may become too subtle to detect).
Have patients with apraxia return your demonstration of the task.	These patients have an inability to carry out previously learned motor tasks, although they may be able to describe them in detail. They may be able to be talked through a task or may be able to talk themselves through a task step-by-step.
Encourage making a conscious effort to scan the rest of the environment by turning head from side to side.	Patients may have visual field deficits in which they can physically see only a portion of the normal visual field.
Patients with nondominant (right) hemisphere injury also may require the following:	
- Direct patient's attention to a particular sound (e.g., if a cat meows on the television, state that it is the sound a cat makes and point to the cat on the screen).	Patient may have impaired ability to recognize, associate, or interpret sounds (e.g., voice quality, animal noises, musical pieces, types of instruments).

Continued

INTERVENTIONS

RATIONALES

INTERVENTIONS	RATIONALES
- Keep a structured, consistent environment. Mark outer aspects of patient's shoes or tag inside sleeve of a sweater or pair of pants with "L" and "R," which may help self-dressing efforts.	Patient may have visual-spatial misconception. For example, patient may underestimate distances and bump into doors or confuse inside and outside of an object, such as an article of clothing. These patients may lose their place when reading or adding up numbers and therefore never complete the task.
- Assist with eating. Monitor environment for safety hazards and remove unsafe objects, such as scissors, from the bedside.	Patient may have difficulty recognizing and associating familiar objects, such as silverware, and may not recognize dangerous or hazardous objects because he or she does not know the object's purpose.
- Provide a restraint or wheelchair belt for support and safety.	Patient may have inability to orient self in space and not recognize if he or she is standing, sitting, or leaning.
- Teach patient to concentrate on body parts (e.g., by watching feet carefully while walking). Provide a mirror to help him or her adjust.	Misconception of body and body parts is common.
- Keep environment simple. Remove distracting stimuli.	Patient has impaired ability to recognize objects by means of senses of hearing, vibration, or touch. These patients rely more on visual cues and could be distracted easily because of sensory overload.

●●● **Related NIC and NOC labels:** *NIC:* Body Image Enhancement; Self-Awareness Enhancement; Self-Care Assistance; Cognitive Stimulation; Environmental Management; Positioning; Surveillance: Safety *NOC:* Body Image; Cognitive Orientation

Nursing Diagnosis:

Impaired Verbal Communication

related to aphasia secondary to cerebrovascular insult

Desired Outcome: At least 24 hr before hospital discharge (or within 24 hr following interventions if patient is not hospitalized), patient demonstrates improved self-expression and relates decreased frustration with communication.

INTERVENTIONS

RATIONALES

INTERVENTIONS	RATIONALES
Evaluate nature and severity of patient's aphasia. When doing so, avoid giving nonverbal cues. Assess patient's ability to point or look toward a specific object, follow simple directions, understand yes/no questions, understand complex questions, repeat both simple and complex words, repeat sentences, name objects that are shown, demonstrate or relate purpose or action of the object, fulfill written requests, write requests, and read. When evaluating for aphasia, recognize that patient may be responding to nonverbal cues and may understand less than you think. Document this assessment with simple descriptions and specific examples of aphasia symptoms. Use it as the basis for a communication plan.	Aphasia is the partial or complete inability to use or comprehend language and symbols and may occur with dominant (left) hemisphere damage and is not the result of impaired hearing or intelligence. There are many different types of aphasia. Generally the patient has a combination of types, which vary in severity. *Fluent aphasia* (e.g., Wernicke's, sensory, or receptive aphasia) is characterized by inability to recognize or comprehend spoken words. It is as if a foreign language were being spoken or patient has word deafness. The patient often is good at responding to nonverbal cues. In *nonfluent aphasia* (e.g., Broca's, motor, or expressive aphasia), the ability to understand and comprehend language is retained, but the patient has difficulty expressing words or naming objects. Gestures, groans, swearing, or nonsense words may be used.

Continued

INTERVENTIONS	RATIONALES
Obtain referral to a speech therapist or pathologist as needed. Provide therapist with a list of words that would enhance patient's independence and/or care. In addition, ask for tips that will help improve communication with patient.	Patient may require expertise of a specialist to facilitate ability to communicate.
When communicating with patient, try to reduce distractions in the environment, such as television or others' conversations.	To focus patient's attention on communication.
Try to ensure that patient is well rested.	Fatigue adversely affects ability to communicate.
Communicate with patient as much as possible. If patient does not understand after repetition, try different words. Use gestures, facial expressions, and pantomime. Give short, simple directions and repeat as needed. Use concrete terms (e.g., "water" instead of "fluid," "leg" instead of "limb").	These are general principles for communicating with patients who may not recognize or comprehend the spoken word. Other suggestions include facing patient and establishing eye contact, speaking slowly and clearly, giving patient time to process your communication and answer, keeping messages short and simple, staying with one clearly defined subject, avoiding questions with multiple choices but rather phrasing questions so that they can be answered "yes" or "no," and using the same words each time you repeat a statement or question (e.g., "pill" vs. "medication," "bathroom" vs. "toilet").
When helping patients regain use of symbolic language, start with nouns first and progress to more complex statements as indicated, using verbs, pronouns, and adjectives. For continuity, keep a record at the bedside of words to be used (e.g., "pill" rather than "medication").	Progression from the simple to the complex helps facilitate comprehension.
Treat patient as an adult. Be respectful.	It is not necessary to raise the volume of your voice unless patient is hard of hearing.
When patients have difficulty expressing words or naming objects, encourage them to repeat words after you. Begin with simple words such as "yes" or "no" and progress to others, such as "cup." Progress to more complex statements as indicated.	For practice in verbal expression.
Listen and respond to patient's communication efforts. Praise accomplishments.	Otherwise, patient may give up.
Be prepared for labile emotions.	These patients become frustrated and emotional when faced with their impaired speech.
When improvement is noted, let patient complete your sentence (e.g., "This is a __"). Keep a list of words that the patient can say and add to list as appropriate. Avoid finishing patient's sentences.	This list can be used when forming questions that the patient can answer.
Avoid labeling patient as belligerent or confused when the problem is aphasia and frustration. Listen for errors in conversation and provide feedback.	Patients who have lost ability to monitor their verbal output may not produce sensible language, but they may think they are making sense and not understand why others do not comprehend or respond appropriately to them.
Avoid instructing patient to "wait 5 minutes."	Patients who have lost ability to recognize number symbols or relationships will have difficulty understanding time concepts or telling time.
Point to an object and clearly state its name. Watch signals the patient gives you.	This facilitates practice in receiving word images.
Bring patients back to the subject by saying, "Let's go back to what we were talking about."	Patients with nondominant (right) hemisphere damage often have no difficulty speaking; however, they may use excessive detail, give irrelevant information, and go off on a tangent. These patients tend to respond better to verbal, rather than nonverbal, encouragement.

Continued

INTERVENTIONS	RATIONALES
If patient makes an error, do not criticize the effort but rather compliment it by saying, "That was a good try." Do not react negatively to emotional displays. Address and acknowledge patient's frustration over the inability to communicate. Maintain a calm and positive attitude. If you do not understand patient, say so. Ask patient to repeat unclear words, ask for more clues, ask patient to use another word, or have patient point to the object.	To provide a supportive and relaxed environment for patients who are unable to form words or sentences or speak clearly or appropriately.
Observe for nonverbal cues and anticipate patient's needs. Allow time to listen if patient speaks slowly and repeat or rephrase it aloud.	To validate patient's message.
Dysarthria can complicate aphasia. For additional interventions for patients with dysarthria, see **Impaired Verbal Communication** in "General Care of Patients with Neurologic Disorders," p. 301.	

●●● **Related NIC and NOC labels:** *NIC:* Communication Enhancement: Speech Deficit; Active Listening; Anxiety Reduction *NOC:* Communication Ability; Communication: Expressive Ability

Nursing Diagnosis:

Deficient Knowledge:

Carotid endarterectomy or carotid angioplasty/stent procedure

Desired Outcome: Before surgery, patient verbalizes accurate understanding of the carotid endarterectomy procedure, including purpose, risks, expected benefits or outcome, and postsurgical care

INTERVENTIONS	RATIONALES
After health care provider has explained procedure to patient, determine patient's level of understanding and reinforce or clarify information as needed	Enables development of an individualized teaching plan and ensures that patient understands procedure in the preoperative stage.
For Patient Undergoing Carotid Endarterectomy:	
As indicated, explain the carotid endarterectomy procedure.	This procedure increases blood supply to the brain by removing plaque in the obstructed artery.
Describe the following postsurgical assessments:	
- Monitoring of VS and neurologic status at least hourly.	Pupils will be checked with a light, and hands and legs will be tested for strength and bilateral equality.
- Explain that patient may be asked to swallow, move the tongue, chew, smile, speak, and shrug shoulders to determine facial drooping, tongue weakness, hoarseness, dysphagia, shoulder weakness, or loss of facial sensation.	Deficits in these abilities are signs of cranial nerve impairment. Stretching of the cranial nerves during surgery can occur, causing edema, and may leave a temporary deficit.
- Patient should report any numbness, tingling, or weakness.	May indicate carotid occlusion.
- In addition, explain that superficial temporal and facial pulses will be palpated for strength, quality, and symmetry.	To evaluate patency of external carotid artery.

Continued

INTERVENTIONS	RATIONALES
- Advise that the neck will be assessed periodically for edema, hematoma, bleeding, or tracheal deviation. Explain that patient should report immediately any respiratory distress, difficulty managing secretions, or sensation of neck tightness.	Any bleeding or excess edema at surgical site can cause neck edema, which can deviate the trachea and compromise the airway. This can result in an emergent situation that necessitates airway management and surgical evacuation of the hematoma.
- Additional O_2 likely will be supplied, even without respiratory distress or airway compromise.	Manipulation of the carotid sinus may cause temporary loss of normal physiologic response to hypoxia.
- Pulse oximetry may be continuously monitored. Readings <92% will be reported to health care providers.	This may signal need for supplemental oxygen.
- Frequent BP checks may be performed.	Temporary carotid sinus dysfunction may cause BP problems (usually hypertension).
- Patient may need vasoactive medications.	To keep systolic BP within a specified range (usually 100-150 mm Hg) to maintain cerebral perfusion while preventing disruption of graft or sutures.
- Explain that head of bed (HOB) must be maintained in prescribed position (flat or elevated). Patient generally is positioned off the operative side.	HOB may be elevated to promote wound drainage, particularly if a closed suction drain is left in place. Positioning also enables visibility of wound site.
- Advise patient that a closed drainage system with suction may be left in the neck for a day. Ice packs may be prescribed for the incision.	To reduce edema formation and pain.
- Teach patient that anticoagulant/antiplatelet therapy (e.g., aspirin, warfarin) may be instituted for 3-6 mo after the procedure.	To help prevent further thromboses.
- Include home instructions on the following: incision care (washing gently with soap and water), signs of infection (incision red or painful, drainage, fever >100.5° F), activity restrictions (no heavy lifting, no driving while neck turning is uncomfortable), changes in neurologic status.	To decrease risk of infection and ensure patient's physiologic safety.
For Patients Undergoing Carotid Angioplasty and Stenting:	
As indicated, teach patient about angioplasty and stenting.	This procedure involves opening of a stenosed artery by passing a slender catheter through the narrow spot and inflating the balloon. A stent may be positioned to hold the newly unblocked vessel open.
Explain that frequent checks of VS and neurologic status (as described earlier) will be performed.	Cranial nerve problems are less frequent with this procedure because nerves have not been stretched, but they still will be included in the neurologic examination.
Advise patient that BP medications will be given.	To keep BP within specified parameters.
Advise patient that groin and distal pulses will be monitored.	The femoral artery is the usual vessel accessed, and it will be monitored for bleeding and patency.
Explain that patients are usually discharged the next day and go home with anticoagulants such as aspirin or ticlopidine.	To prevent platelet aggregation that may lead to thrombus formation in patients who have had ischemic strokes from thrombosis.

●●● **Related NIC and NOC labels:** *NIC:* Preparatory Sensory Information; Teaching: Procedure/Treatment
NOC: Knowledge: Treatment Procedures

ADDITIONAL NURSING DIAGNOSES/ PROBLEMS:

PATIENT-FAMILY TEACHING AND DISCHARGE PLANNING

When providing patient-family teaching, focus on sensory information, avoid giving excessive information, and initiate a visiting nurse referral for necessary follow-up teaching. Include verbal and written information about the following:

✓ Symptoms that necessitate prompt attention: sudden weakness, numbness (especially on one side of the body), vision loss or dimming, trouble talking or understanding speech, unexplained dizziness, unsteadiness, or severe headache.

✓ Interventions for safe swallowing and aspiration prevention.

✓ Importance of minimizing or treating the following risk factors: diabetes mellitus, hypertension, high cholesterol, high Na^+ intake, obesity, inactivity, smoking, prolonged bedrest, and stressful lifestyle.

✓ Interventions that increase effective communication in the presence of aphasia or dysarthria. Additional patient information can be obtained by contacting the following organization:

National Aphasia Association
156 Fifth Ave., Suite 707
New York, NY 10010
(800) 922-4622
www.aphasia.org

✓ Referrals to the following as appropriate: public health nurse, visiting nurses association, psychologic therapy, vocational rehabilitation agency, home health agencies, and extended and skilled care facilities. Also provide the following addresses:

National Stroke Association
9707 E. Easter Lane
Englewood, CO 80112
(303) 649-9229 or (800) 787-6537
www.stroke.org

American Stroke Association
A division of the American Heart Association
7272 Greenville Avenue
Dallas, TX 75231
www.strokeassociation.org

✓ For patient information pamphlets, contact the following organization:

National Institute of Neurological Disorders and Stroke
   (NINDS)
Box 5801 Bethesda, MD 20892
(800) 352-9424
www.ninds.nih.gov

✓ Additional general information can be obtained by contacting the following organizations:

National Center for Cardiac Information
8180 Greensboro Drive #1070
McLean, VA 22102
(703) 356-6568

Stroke Connection/American Heart Association
7272 Greenville Avenue
Dallas, TX 75231
(800) 553-6321
www.amhrt.org/

See also: Teaching and discharge planning (third through tenth entries only) under "Multiple Sclerosis."

Guillain-Barré Syndrome

Guillain-Barré syndrome (GBS) is a rapidly progressing polyneuritis of unknown cause. An inflammatory process causes lymphocytes to enter the perivascular spaces and destroy the myelin sheath covering the peripheral or cranial nerves. Posterior (sensory) and anterior (motor) nerve roots can be affected because of this segmental demyelinization, and the individual may experience both sensory and motor losses. Respiratory insufficiency may occur in as many as half of the individuals affected. Life-threatening respiratory muscle weakness can develop as rapidly as 24-72 hr after onset of initial symptoms. In about 25% of cases, motor weakness progresses to total paralysis. Peak severity of symptoms usually occurs within 1-3 wk after onset of symptoms. A plateau stage follows that usually lasts 1-2 wk. It may take months to years for a full recovery. Full neurologic recovery occurs in about 50% of patients. Five percent of patients may have permanent severe disability. GBS may follow a recent viral illness, such as upper respiratory infection or gastroenteritis, a rabies or influenza vaccination, lupus erythematosus, or Hodgkin's disease or other malignant process. Although the exact cause of GBS is unknown, it is believed to be an autoimmune response to a viral infection.

HEALTH CARE SETTING

The patient is likely to be in acute care (intensive care unit [ICU]) when the neurologic deficit is progressing and in an acute rehabilitation setting during the recovery phase.

ASSESSMENT

Weakness is the most common indicator. Typically, numbness and weakness begin in the legs and ascend symmetrically upward, progressing to the arms and facial nerves. Ascending GBS is more common, but descending GBS, in which cranial nerves are affected first and weakness progresses downward

with rapid respiratory involvement, also can occur. Peak severity usually occurs within 10-14 days of onset. GBS does not affect level of consciousness (LOC), cognitive function, or pupillary function.

Anterior (motor) nerve root involvement: Weakness or flaccid paralysis. Respiratory muscle involvement can be life threatening. There is a loss of reflexes, muscle tension, and tone, but muscle atrophy usually does not occur.

Autonomic nervous system (ANS) involvement: Sinus tachycardia, bradycardia, hypertension, hypotension, cardiac dysrhythmias, facial flushing, diaphoresis, inability to perspire, loss of sphincter control, urinary retention, adynamic ileus, and increased pulmonary secretions may occur. ANS involvement may occur unexpectedly and can be life threatening, but it usually does not persist for longer than 2 wk.

Cranial nerve involvement: Inability to chew, swallow, speak, or close the eyes.

Posterior (sensory) nerve root involvement: Paresthesias, such as numbness and tingling, which usually are minor compared with the degree of motor loss. Ascending sensory loss often precedes motor loss. Muscle cramping, tenderness, or pain may occur.

Physical assessment: Symmetric motor weakness, impaired position and vibration sense, hypoactive or absent deep tendon reflexes, hypotonia in affected muscles, and decreased ventilatory capacity.

DIAGNOSTIC TESTS

Diagnostic tests are performed to rule out other diseases, such as acute poliomyelitis. The diagnosis of GBS is based on clinical presentation, history of recent viral illness, and cerebrospinal fluid (CSF) findings.

Lumbar puncture (LP) and CSF analysis: Usually show an elevated protein (especially immunoglobulin G [IgG]) without an increase in cell count. Although CSF pressure usually is normal, in severe disease it may be elevated.

Electromyography (EMG): Reveals slowed nerve conduction velocities soon after paralysis appears because of demyelinization. Denervation potentials appear later.

Serum complete blood count (CBC): Will show presence of leukocytosis early in illness, possibly as a result of the inflammatory process associated with demyelinization.

Evoked potentials (auditory, visual, brain stem): May be used to distinguish GBS from other neuropathologic conditions.

Nursing Diagnosis:

Ineffective Breathing Pattern

related to neuromuscular weakness or paralysis of the facial, throat, and respiratory muscles (severity of symptoms peaks around wk 1-3)

Desired Outcome: Deterioration in patient's breathing pattern (e.g., PaO_2 <80 mm Hg, vital capacity <800 ml [or <10-12 ml/kg], tidal volume <75% of predicted value, or O_2 saturation ≤92% via oximetry) is detected and reported promptly, resulting in immediate medical treatment.

INTERVENTIONS	RATIONALES
Test for ascending loss of sensation by touching patient lightly with a pin or fingers at frequent intervals (hourly or more frequently initially). Assess from the level of the iliac crest upward toward the shoulders. Measure the highest level at which decreased sensation occurs.	Decreased sensation frequently precedes motor weakness. If it ascends to the T8 dermatome level, anticipate that intercostal muscles (used with respirations) soon will be impaired.
Check patient for presence of arm drift and inability to shrug shoulders. Alert health care provider to significant findings.	Shoulder weakness is present if patient cannot shrug shoulders. Arm drift is detected in the following way: patient holds both arms out in front of the body, level with the shoulders and with palms up; patient closes eyes while holding this position. Arm drift is present when one arm pronates or drifts down or out from its original position. These findings need to be reported promptly for timely intervention because upper arm and shoulder weakness precedes respiratory dysfunction.
Monitor patient's ability to take fluids orally. Assess patient q8h and before oral intake for cough reflexes, gag reflexes, and difficulty swallowing.	To detect changes or difficulties that may indicate ascending paralysis. Impaired swallowing and cough and gag reflexes likely will necessitate parenteral feedings to prevent aspiration until reflexes return to normal.
Monitor patient's respiratory rate, rhythm, and depth. Auscultate breath sounds.	Accessory muscle use, nasal flaring, dyspnea, shallow respirations, diminished breath sounds, and apnea are signs of respiratory deterioration that necessitate prompt notification of health care provider.
Be alert to changes in mental status, LOC, and orientation.	May signal reduced oxygenation to the brain as a result of ineffective breathing pattern.
Monitor patient for breathlessness while speaking. To detect breathlessness, ask patient to take a deep breath and slowly count as high as possible.	Inability to count to a higher number before breathlessness occurs may signal grossly reduced ventilatory function.
Monitor arterial blood gas (ABG) levels and pulse oximetry.	To detect hypoxia or hypercarbia ($PaCO_2$ >45 mm Hg), a signal of hypoventilation. PaO_2 <80 mm Hg or O_2 saturation ≤92% usually signals need for supplemental oxygen.
Raise head of bed (HOB).	To promote optimal chest excursion by taking pressure of abdominal organs off the lungs, which may increase oxygenation.

Continued

INTERVENTIONS	RATIONALES
Alert health care provider to significant findings.	Patient may require tracheostomy, endotracheal intubation, or mechanical ventilation, depending on findings. If patient's respiratory status deteriorates, he or she likely will be transferred to ICU or transition care unit for closer monitoring.
For other interventions, see **Risk for Aspiration** in "Older Adult Care," p. 101.	

●●● **Related NIC and NOC labels:** *NIC:* Respiratory Monitoring; Ventilation Assistance; Aspiration Precautions; Mechanical Ventilation; Oxygen Therapy; Positioning; Acid-Base Monitoring *NOC:* Respiratory Status: Ventilation

Nursing Diagnosis:

Acute Pain

related to muscle tenderness; hypersensitivity to touch; or discomfort in shoulders, thighs, and back

Desired Outcomes: Within 1-2 hr of intervention, patient's subjective perception of discomfort decreases, as documented by a pain scale. Objective indicators, such as grimacing, are absent or diminished.

INTERVENTIONS	RATIONALES
For patients with hypersensitivity, assess amount of touch that can be tolerated and incorporate this information into patient's plan of care.	Facilitates development of an individualized plan of care and helps ensure that patient is not touched more than necessary by all staff members.
For patients with muscle tenderness, consider use of massage, moist heat packs, cold application, or warm baths.	To soothe tender muscles.
Reposition patient at frequent intervals.	To determine optimal positions that decrease muscle tension and fatigue. Some individuals find that a supine "frog-leg" position is particularly comfortable.
Provide passive range of motion (ROM).	To reduce joint stiffness.
Administer analgesics, such as acetaminophen, codeine, or morphine, as prescribed.	To help manage muscle pain.
As prescribed, administer anticonvulsants, such as gabapentin and carbamazepine, and tricyclics, such as amitriptyline.	To relieve uncomfortable paresthesias.
For other interventions, see **Acute Pain,** p. 307, in "General Care of Patients with Neurologic Disorders."	

●●● **Related NIC and NOC labels:** *NIC:* Pain Management; Heat/Cold Applications; Medication Administration; Positioning; Simple Massage *NOC:* Pain Level

Nursing Diagnosis:

Ineffective Cardiopulmonary and Cerebral Tissue Perfusion

(or risk for same) related to interrupted sympathetic outflow with concomitant BP fluctuations secondary to autonomic dysfunction

Desired Outcomes: Patient has optimal cardiopulmonary and cerebral tissue perfusion as evidenced by systolic BP ≥90 mm Hg and ≤160 mm Hg, no significant mental status changes, and orientation to person, place, and time. BP fluctuations, if they occur, are detected and reported promptly.

INTERVENTIONS	RATIONALES
Monitor BP, noting wide fluctuations; report significant findings to health care provider.	Changes in BP that result in severe hypotension or hypertension may occur because of unopposed sympathetic outflow or loss of outflow to the peripheral nervous system, causing changes in vascular tone. These BP findings necessitate prompt reporting to enable timely intervention. Short-acting antihypertensive agents may be required for persistent hypertension.
Monitor carefully for BP changes during activities such as coughing, suctioning, position changes, or straining at stool.	These are events that can trigger BP changes.
For patients with hypotension or postural hypotension, see **Ineffective Cardiopulmonary and Cerebral Tissue Perfusion,** p. 395, in "Spinal Cord Injury."	

●●● **Related NIC and NOC labels:** *NIC:* Medication Administration; Dysrhythmia Management; Emergency Care; Fluid Management; Intravenous Therapy; Vital Signs Monitoring; Neurologic Monitoring; Hypovolemia Management *NOC:* Tissue Perfusion: Cardiac; Tissue Perfusion: Pulmonary; Tissue Perfusion: Cerebral

Nursing Diagnosis:

Imbalanced Nutrition: Less than body requirements

related to adynamic ileus

Desired Outcome: Patient has adequate nutrition as evidenced by maintenance of baseline body weight.

INTERVENTIONS	RATIONALES
Auscultate abdominal sounds, noting presence, absence, or changes from baseline. Notify health care provider of significant findings.	Abdominal distention or tenderness, nausea and vomiting, and absence of stool output are signals of the onset of ileus. Also, GBS has been associated with *Campylobacter jejuni,* an infection that manifests as gastroenteritis. These findings should be reported promptly for timely intervention.
Provide a high-fiber diet if one has been prescribed.	To promote bulk in the stools and help prevent constipation.
Initiate gastric, gastrostomy, or parenteral feedings as prescribed. See "Providing Nutritional Support," p. 589, for more details.	For patients who cannot chew or swallow effectively because of cranial nerve involvement. Patients with adynamic ileus generally require gastric decompression with a nasogastric tube and cannot take foods orally.
Also see **Imbalanced Nutrition,** p. 294, in "General Care of Patients with Neurologic Disorders."	

●●● **Related NIC and NOC labels:** *NIC:* Nutrition Management; Nutrition Monitoring; Enteral Tube Feeding; Total Parenteral Nutrition Administration; Weight Gain Assistance *NOC:* Nutritional Status: Nutrient Intake; Nutritional Status: Food and Fluid Intake

Nursing Diagnosis:

Anxiety

related to threat to biologic integrity and loss of control

Desired Outcome: Within 24 hr of this diagnosis, patient expresses concerns regarding changes in life events, states anxiety is less or under control, and exhibits fewer symptoms of increased anxiety (e.g., heart and respiratory rates return to patient's normal range).

INTERVENTIONS	RATIONALES
For patients in whom neurologic deficit is still progressing, arrange for a transfer to a room close to the nurses' station.	To help alleviate the anxiety of being suddenly incapacitated and helpless.
Be sure call light is within easy reach. Frequently assess patient's ability to use it.	For patient's safety and to allay anxiety.
Provide continuity of patient care through assignment of staff and use of care plan.	Familiarity may help reduce anxiety.
Perform assessments at frequent intervals, letting patient know you are there. Provide care in a calm and reassuring manner.	Calm begets calm. Frequent assessments also reassure patient that he or she is being watched out for.
Allow time for patient to vent concerns; provide realistic feedback regarding what patient may experience. Determine past effective coping behaviors.	Unexpressed concerns can contribute to frustration and stress. Information helps reduce anxiety caused by lack of knowledge. Knowing past effective coping behaviors facilitates problem solving for ways in which these methods and others may prove useful in the current situation.
For other interventions, see **Anxiety**, p. 82, and **Fear**, p. 86, in "Psychosocial Support."	

●●● **Related NIC and NOC labels:** *NIC:* Anxiety Reduction; Active Listening; Calming Technique; Coping Enhancement; Presence; Environmental Management *NOC:* Anxiety Control

Nursing Diagnosis:

Deficient Knowledge:

Therapeutic plasma exchange procedure

Desired Outcome: Before scheduled date of each procedure, patient verbalizes accurate information about the plasma exchange procedure.

INTERVENTIONS	RATIONALES
Before plasma exchange procedure, patient's health care provider explains the reason for the procedure, its risks, and anticipated benefits or outcome. Determine patient's level of understanding of this explanation.	Provides an opportunity to clarify or reinforce information accordingly.
Determine patient's experience with plasmapheresis, positive or negative effects, and nature of any fears or concerns. Document and communicate this information to other caregivers.	To clarify or reinforce patient's knowledge about this procedure, which optimally will decrease fears and concerns.

Continued

INTERVENTIONS	**RATIONALES**
Explain in words patient can understand that the goal of plasma exchange is to remove autoimmune factors from the blood to decrease patient's symptoms.	The procedure is similar to hemodialysis. Blood is removed from patient and separated into its components. Patient's plasma is discarded; other blood components (e.g., red blood cells [RBCs], white blood cells [WBCs], platelets) are saved and returned to patient with donor plasma or replacement fluid. Multiple exchanges over a period of weeks can be expected.
Explain that if started within 1-2 wk of GBS symptoms, the exchange process seems to decrease duration and severity of the disease.	Antibodies to patient's peripheral and cranial nerve tissue are reduced by removal of the blood's plasma portion, which contains the circulating antibodies.
Answer any questions regarding complications.	Although rare, patient is at risk for the following complications during this procedure: deficient fluid volume, hypotension, hypokalemia, hypocalcemia, cardiac dysrhythmias, clotting disorders, anemia, phlebitis, infection, hypothermia, and air embolism. Fears and concerns must be addressed throughout all phases of this illness, particularly because these treatments can occur over several weeks.
Explain that although the antecubital vein may be accessed, the health care provider may need to insert a central IV line or a femoral catheter.	This procedure requires good blood flow.
If the antecubital site is used, place a sign alerting others to avoid using this site for routine laboratory sticks.	Patient's access site must be preserved for plasma exchange procedure.
Explain that patient can expect the procedure to take 2-4 hr, although it may take considerably longer.	Length of time will depend on condition of patient's veins, blood flow, and Hct level.
Explain that patient can expect preprocedure and postprocedure blood work.	To assess clotting factors and electrolyte levels, particularly of potassium and calcium, which can be reduced during this exchange procedure.
Advise patient that VS and weight measurements will be taken before and after the procedure, with frequent VS checks during the procedure.	To assess for hypotension and shift in fluid volume.
Explain that patient may be placed on cardiac monitoring.	To assess for dysrhythmias caused by electrolyte imbalance, particularly hypokalemia or hypocalcemia.
Advise that calcium gluconate or potassium chloride (KCl) may be administered.	To correct electrolyte imbalances.
Explain that patient's temperature will be checked during the procedure and warm blankets will be provided if needed.	To prevent or manage chills and hypothermia, which can occur during this procedure for two reasons: (1) the anticoagulant citrate dextrose binds to serum ionized calcium, causing a transient hypocalcemia that increases muscle tension and can cause chills; and (2) the plasma is delivered closer to room temperature than body temperature, and this lowers patient's core temperature.
Encourage patient to report any unusual feelings or symptoms during plasma exchange.	Unusual feelings or symptoms that can occur during plasma exchange include chills, fever, hives, and sweating or light-headedness, thirst, faintness, or dizziness. These symptoms can occur in the presence of hypotension, hypocalcemia, or hypovolemia. To help prevent these problems, patient should take oral fluids during the procedure if possible.
	In addition, patient may experience numbness or tingling around lips or in the hands, arms, and legs; muscle twitching; cramping; or tetany. These symptoms can occur with hypocalcemia.
	Patient also may experience, fatigue, nausea, weakness, or cramping, which signal hypokalemia.

Continued

INTERVENTIONS	RATIONALES
Inform patient that medications may be held until after the procedure.	Medications otherwise would be removed from the blood during the plasma exchange.
If patient does not have a urinary catheter, remind him or her to void before and during the procedure, if necessary.	To avoid any mild hypotension caused by a full bladder.
Explain that patient probably will feel fatigued 1-2 days after the procedure. Encourage extra rest and a high-protein diet during this time.	Fatigue is a result of decreased plasma protein levels that occur during the exchange.
Teach patient to monitor IV access site for warmth, redness, swelling, or drainage and to report significant findings.	Signs of infection.
Teach patient to monitor for signs of bruising or bleeding.	The anticoagulant citrate dextrose is used in the extracorporeal machine circuitry to prevent clotting. This may cause excessive bleeding at the access site.
Advise patient that a pressure dressing may be kept in place over the access site for 2-4 hr after the procedure. Caution patient to avoid cutting self or bumping into objects and to sustain pressure over cuts.	To prevent clotting and bruising.
Inform patient that black, tarry stools may occur and should be reported.	Black, tarry stools signal that bleeding is occurring internally, and this necessitates prompt medical attention.

●●● **Related NIC and NOC labels:** *NIC:* Preparatory Sensory Information; Teaching: Procedure/Treatment; Learning Readiness Enhancement *NOC:* Knowledge: Treatment Procedure

ADDITIONAL NURSING DIAGNOSES/ PROBLEMS:

PATIENT-FAMILY TEACHING AND DISCHARGE PLANNING

Most patients with GBS eventually recover fully, but because the recovery period can be prolonged, the patient often goes home with some degree of neurologic deficit. Discharge planning and teaching will vary according to the degree of disability. When providing patient-family teaching, focus on sensory information, avoid giving excessive information, and initiate a visiting nurse referral for necessary follow-up teaching. Include verbal and written information about the following:

✓ Disease process, expected improvement, and importance of continuing in rehabilitation or physical therapy (PT) program to promote as full a recovery as possible.

✓ Safety measures relative to decreased sensorimotor deficit.

✓ Exercises that promote muscle strength and mobility, measures for preventing contractures and skin breakdown, transfer techniques and proper body mechanics, and use of assistive devices.

✓ Indications of constipation, urinary retention, or urinary tract infection (UTI); implementation of bowel and bladder training programs; and, if appropriate, care of indwelling catheters or self-catheterization technique.

✓Indications of upper respiratory infection (URI); measures for preventing regurgitation, aspiration, and respiratory infection.

✓Medications, including drug name, purpose, dosage, schedule, precautions, drug/drug and food/drug interactions, and potential side effects.

✓Importance of follow-up care, including visits to health care provider, physical therapist, and occupational therapist.

✓Referrals to community resources, such as public health nurse, visiting nurse association, community support groups, social workers, psychologic therapy, home health agencies, and extended and skilled care facilities. Additional general information can be obtained by contacting the following organization:

Guillain-Barré Syndrome Foundation International
Box 262
Wynnewood, PA 19096
(610) 667-0131

Head Injury

Head injuries (HIs) can cause varying degrees of damage to the skull and brain tissue. Primary injuries occur at the time of impact and include skull fracture, concussion, contusion, scalp laceration, brain tissue laceration, and tear or rupture of cerebral vessels. Secondary problems that arise soon after the primary injury and are the result of that injury include hemorrhage and hematoma formation from the tear or rupture of vessels, ischemia from interrupted blood flow, cerebral swelling and edema, infection, and increased intracranial pressure (IICP) or herniation, any of which can interrupt neuronal function. These secondary injuries or events increase the extent of initial injury and result in poorer recovery and higher risk of death. Cervical neck injuries are commonly associated with HIs. Because of the potential for spinal cord injury (SCI), all HI patients should be assumed to have cervical neck injury until it is conclusively ruled out by cervical spine x-ray.

HEALTH CARE SETTING

Acute care (trauma center, intensive care); rehabilitation unit

ASSESSMENT

The Glasgow Coma Scale standardizes observations for objective assessment of a patient's level of consciousness (LOC). This or some other objective scale should be used to prevent confusion with terminology and to detect changes or trends quickly in the patient's LOC. LOC is the most sensitive indicator of overall brain function.

Concussion: Mild diffuse HI in which there is temporary, reversible neurologic impairment typically involving loss of consciousness and possible amnesia of the event. No damage to brain structure is visible on computed tomography (CT) or magnetic resonance imaging (MRI) examination. After the concussion, the patient may have headache, dizziness, nausea, lethargy, and irritability. Although full recovery usually occurs in a few days, a postconcussion syndrome with headaches, dizziness, irritability, emotional lability, lethargy, and decreased judgment, concentration, and memory abilities may continue for several weeks or months.

Diffuse axonal injury (DAI): A diffuse brain injury caused by stretching and tearing of the neuronal projections because of a rotational, shearing type of injury. Diffuse microscopic damage occurs. No distinct focal lesion, such as infarction, ischemia, contusion, or intracerebral bleeding, is noted, but the patient has an immediate and prolonged unconsciousness of at least 6-hr duration. CT scan may show small hemorrhagic areas in the corpus callosum, cerebral edema, and small midline ventricles. Brain stem injury may be associated with DAI, resulting in autonomic dysfunction. The injury may be quite mild with full recovery, or in severe cases the individual may be comatose for months, die, or be left in a vegetative state.

Contusion: Bruising of the brain tissue, which produces a longer-lasting neurologic deficit than concussion. The size and severity of bruising vary widely, and the bruise or small, diffuse venous hemorrhage usually is visible on CT scan. Traumatic amnesia often occurs, causing loss of memory not only of the trauma but also of events occurring before the incident. Loss of consciousness is common, and it is generally more prolonged than that with concussion. Changes in behavior, such as agitation or confusion, can last for several hours to days. Headache, nausea, lethargy, motor paralysis, paresis, and possibly seizures can occur as well. Depending on the extent of damage, there is potential for either full recovery or permanent neurologic deficit, such as seizures, paralysis, paresis, or even coma and death.

Brain laceration: Actual tearing of the cortical surface of the brain, resulting in direct mechanical disruption of neural function, causing focal deficits. Blood vessel tearing causes hemorrhage, resulting in contusion, edema, or hematoma formation. Seizures often occur as well. Brain lacerations usually result from depressed skull fractures, penetrating injuries, missile or impalement injuries, or rotational shearing injury within the skull. A knife or other impalement object should be supported and left in the wound to control bleeding until it can be removed during surgery. Contusions and lacerations often are found together.

Skull fracture: Can be *closed* (simple, with the skin intact) or *open* (compound), depending on whether the scalp is torn, thereby exposing the skull to the outside environment. Skull fractures are further classified as *linear* (hairline), *comminuted* (fragmented, splintered), or *depressed* (pushed inward toward the brain tissue). A blow forceful enough to break the skull is capable of causing significant brain tissue damage, and therefore close observation is essential. With a penetrating wound or basilar fracture (see below), there is potential for cerebrospinal fluid (CSF) leakage, meningitis, encephalitis, brain abscess, cellulitis, or osteomyelitis.

- **Basilar fractures:** Fractures of the base of the skull do not show up easily on skull/cervical x-rays. Indicators include blood from the nose, throat, ears; serous or serosanguineous drainage from the nose (rhinorrhea), throat, ears (otorrhea), eyes; Battle's sign (bruising noted behind the ear); "raccoon's eyes" (bruising around the eyes in the absence of eye injury); and bleeding behind the tympanum (eardrum) noted on otoscopic examination. Basilar fractures may damage the internal carotid artery and the cranial nerves. Hearing loss also may occur.
- **Temporal fractures:** May result in deafness or facial paralysis.
- **Occipital fractures:** May cause visual field and gait disturbances.
- **Sphenoidal fractures:** May disrupt the optic nerve, possibly causing blindness.

Rupture of cerebral blood vessels:

- **Epidural (extradural) hematoma or hemorrhage:** Usually, bleeding between the dura mater (outer meninges) and skull causes hematoma formation. This creates pressure on the underlying brain and produces a local mass effect, causing IICP and shifting of tissue, which leads to brain stem compression and herniation. Indicators are primarily those of IICP: altered LOC, headache, vomiting, unilateral pupil dilation (on same side as the lesion), and possibly hemiparesis. A unilateral dilated fixed pupil is a sign of impending herniation and is a neurosurgical emergency. The patient should not be left alone because respiratory arrest may occur at any time.
- **Subdural hematoma or hemorrhage:** Accumulation of venous blood between the dura mater (outer meninges) and arachnoid membrane (middle meninges) that is not reabsorbed. Hematoma formation creates pressure on the underlying brain and produces a local mass effect, causing IICP and shifting of tissue, leading to brain stem compression and herniation. This type of hematoma is classified as acute, subacute, or chronic depending on how quickly indicators arise. Early indicators can include headache, progressive personality changes, decreased intellectual functioning, slowness, confusion, and drowsiness. Later indicators may include unilateral weakness or paralysis, loss of consciousness, and occasionally seizures. Patients with cerebral atrophy (e.g., older persons, long-term alcohol users) are more prone to subdural hematoma formation.
- **Intracerebral hemorrhage:** Arterial or venous bleeding into the white matter of the brain. Signs of IICP may develop early if the bleeding causes a rapidly expanding space-occupying lesion. If the bleeding is slower, signs of IICP can take 36-72 hr to develop. Indicators depend on location of the hematoma and can include altered LOC, headache, aphasia, hemiparesis, hemiplegia, hemisensory deficits, pupillary changes, and loss of consciousness.
- **Subarachnoid hemorrhage:** Bleeding into the subarachnoid space below the arachnoid membrane (middle meninges) and above the pia mater (inner meninges next to brain). The patient often has a severe headache. Other general indicators include vomiting, restlessness, seizures, and loss of consciousness. Signs of meningeal irritation include nuchal rigidity and positive Kernig's and Brudzinski's signs. This patient may be a candidate for a shunt because of hemorrhagic interference with CSF circulation and reabsorption. The patient is at particular risk of cerebral vasospasm.

Indicators of IICP:

- **Early indicators:** Alteration in LOC ranging from irritability, restlessness, and confusion to lethargy; possible onset or worsening of headache; beginning pupillary dysfunction, such as sluggishness; visual disturbances, such as diplopia or blurred vision; onset of or increase in sensorimotor changes or deficits, such as weakness; onset or worsening of nausea.
- **Late indicators:** Continued deterioration of LOC leading to stupor and coma; projectile vomiting; hemiplegia; posturing; alterations in VS (typically increased systolic BP, widening pulse pressure, decreased pulse rate); respiratory irregularities, such as Cheyne-Stokes breathing; pupillary changes, such as inequality, dilation, and nonreactivity to light; papilledema; and impaired brain stem reflexes (corneal, gag, swallowing). **Note:** The single most important early indicator of IICP is a change in LOC. Late indicators of IICP usually signal impending or occurring brain stem herniation.

Brain herniation: Brain herniation occurs when IICP causes displacement of brain tissue from one cranial compartment to another. See late indicators of IICP, earlier, for signs of impending or initial herniation. In the presence of actual brain herniation, the patient is in a deep coma, pupils become fixed and dilated bilaterally, posturing may progress to bilateral flaccidity, brain stem reflexes generally are lost, and respirations and VS deteriorate and may cease.

Brain death: Criteria for determining brain death are not universally agreed on. Check state and institutional guidelines. General criteria include absent brain stem reflexes (e.g., apnea, pupils nonreactive to light, no corneal reflex, no oculovestibular reflex to ice water calorics), absent cortical activity (e.g., several flat electroencephalogram [EEG] tracings spaced over time), and coma irreversibility continued over a prescribed period (e.g., 24 hr). Brain stem auditory evoked responses and cerebral blood flow studies also may be used to help establish brain death.

DIAGNOSTIC TESTS

Cervical spine and skull x-rays: To locate neck and skull fractures. Because of the close association between HIs and spinal or vertebral injuries, cervical immobilization is essential until cervical x-rays rule out fracture and potential SCI.

CT scan: Used with acute injury to identify type, location, and extent of injury, such as accumulation of blood or a shift of midline structure caused by IICP.

MRI: To identify the type, location, and extent of injury. Although not usually performed in acute, unstable patients, this test is the study of choice for subacute or chronic HI. It is superior to CT scan for detecting isodense chronic subdural hematomas or evaluating contusions and shearing injuries, especially in the brain stem area.

EEG: To reveal abnormal electrical activity indicating neuronal damage caused by ischemia or hemorrhage. EEG may be used to establish brain death in conjunction with other tests and may be done serially to assess development of pathologic waves.

Cerebral blood flow studies (transcranial Doppler [TCD], xenon inhalation with or without CT): To determine focal areas of low blood flow or spasm, possibly indicating ischemic areas, by noninvasively measuring cerebral blood flow velocities.

Positron emission tomography (PET): To evaluate tissue metabolism of glucose and oxygen.

Single photon emission computed tomography (SPECT): To determine low cerebral blood flow and areas at risk for ischemic tissue perfusion.

Evoked response potentials: To evaluate the integrity of the brain's anatomic pathways and connections. Stimulation of a sense organ, such as an ear, triggers a discrete electrical response (i.e., evoked potential) along a neurologic pathway to the brain. Measurement of the brain's response to auditory, visual, and/or somatosensory stimulation also aids in predicting neurologic outcome.

Cerebral angiography: To reveal presence of a hematoma and status of blood vessels secondary to rupture or compression. Angiography usually is performed only if CT scan or MRI is unavailable or to evaluate possible carotid or vertebral artery dissection.

Infrared spectroscopy: To continuously and noninvasively assess cerebral O_2 saturation.

Nursing Diagnosis:

Deficient Knowledge:

Caretaker's responsibilities for observing patient who is sent home with a concussion

Desired Outcomes: Immediately following instruction, caretaker verbalizes accurate knowledge about the observation regimen. Caretaker returns patient to the hospital if neurologic deficits are noted.

INTERVENTIONS	RATIONALES
If patient goes home for observation, provide caretaker with the following verbal and written instructions:	
Do not give patient anything stronger than acetaminophen to relieve headache.	A possible exception is codeine for pain control. Narcotics and other medications that alter mentation are avoided because they can mask neurologic indicators of IICP and cause respiratory depression.
Avoid giving patient aspirin.	Aspirin can prolong bleeding if it occurs.
Check patient at least q1-2h for first 24 hr as follows: awaken patient; ask name, location, and caretaker's name. Be alert for twitching or seizure activity, nausea/vomiting, visual disturbances, drainage from nose or ear, weakness, or neck stiffness.	This assessment gives caretaker the necessary information for returning patient to the hospital immediately, that is, if patient becomes increasingly difficult to awaken; cannot answer questions appropriately; cannot answer at all; becomes confused, restless, or agitated; develops slurred speech; develops twitching or seizures; develops or reports worsening headache or nausea/vomiting; has visual disturbances (e.g., blurred or double vision); develops weakness, numbness, or clumsiness or has difficulty walking; has clear or bloody drainage from nose or ear; or develops a stiff neck.
Ensure that patient rests and eats lightly for first day or so after concussion or until he or she feels well.	Nausea and vomiting can occur with increased ICP.
Over next 2-3 days, ensure that patient avoids alcohol, driving, contact sports, swimming, using power tools, and taking medication for headache or nausea without calling health care provider.	To ensure safety. There is potential for neurologic deterioration at this time. For this reason, patient should return to a full schedule slowly.

Continued

INTERVENTIONS	RATIONALES
Inform patient and significant other about postconcussion syndrome. Explain importance of reporting signs and symptoms of this syndrome to health care provider, especially if they worsen.	Some individuals may continue to have headaches, dizziness, or lethargy for several weeks or months after a concussion. Patient also may experience sleep disturbance, difficulty concentrating, poor memory, irritability, emotional lability, and difficulty with judgment or abstract thinking and be very distractible. These problems should be reported promptly for timely intervention.

●●● **Related NIC and NOC labels:** *NIC:* Teaching: Procedure/Treatment; Teaching: Prescribed Medication; Teaching: Prescribed Diet; Teaching: Disease Process *NOC:* Knowledge: Treatment Regimen

Nursing Diagnosis:

Risk for Infection

related to inadequate primary defenses secondary to basilar skull fractures, penetrating or open head injuries, or surgical wounds

Desired Outcomes: Patient is free of symptoms of infection as evidenced by normothermia, stable or improving LOC, and absence of headache, photophobia, or neck stiffness. Patient verbalizes knowledge about signs and symptoms of infection and importance of reporting them promptly.

INTERVENTIONS	RATIONALES
Monitor injury site or surgical wounds for indicators of infection. Notify health care provider of significant findings.	Erythema, local warmth, pain, hardness, and purulent drainage are indicators of infection, which can occur because of loss of skin integrity.
Be alert to indicators of meningitis or encephalitis.	Indicators of meningitis or encephalitis (fever, chills, malaise, back stiffness and pain, nuchal rigidity, photophobia, seizures, ataxia, sensorimotor deficits) can occur after a penetrating, open HI or cerebral surgical wound.
When examining scalp lacerations and assessing for foreign bodies or palpable fractures, wear sterile gloves and follow sterile technique. Cleanse area gently and cover scalp wounds with sterile dressings.	To reduce possibility of infection, which can become serious if the HI has created a breach directly into the nervous system.
Document drainage and its amount, color, and odor.	If patient has clear or bloody drainage from the nose, throat, or ears, it should be assumed patient has a dural tear with CSF leakage until proven otherwise and health care provider should be notified of findings for prompt intervention. Complaints of a salty taste or frequent swallowing may signal CSF dripping down back of the throat. Bending forward may produce nasal drainage that can be tested for CSF.
Inspect dressing and pillowcases for a halo ring (blood encircling a yellowish stain).	May indicate CSF drainage.
Test clear drainage with a glucose reagent strip. Drainage may be sent to laboratory to test for Cl⁻.	The presence of glucose and Cl^- (CSF Cl^- is > serum Cl^-) in nonsanguineous drainage indicates that the drainage is CSF rather than mucus or saliva.
If CSF leakage occurs, do not clean ears or nose unless prescribed by health care provider. Place a sterile pad over affected ear or under nose to catch drainage but do not pack them. Position patient so that fluids can drain. Change dressings when they become damp, using sterile technique.	To avoid introducing bacteria into the nervous system from the breach created by the HI.

Continued

INTERVENTIONS	RATIONALES
Caution patient to avoid excessive movement. If not contraindicated, place patient on bedrest with head of bed (HOB) in semi-Fowler's position.	To help reduce cerebral congestion and edema and promote venous drainage.
With CSF leakage or possible basilar fracture, avoid nasal suction.	To prevent introduction of bacteria into the nervous system.
Instruct patient to avoid Valsalva's maneuver, straining with bowel movement, and vigorous coughing. Caution patient not to blow nose, sneeze, or sniff in nasal drainage.	May tear the dura and increase CSF flow.
If patient has a nasogastric (NG) tube, visually check back of patient's throat for presence of the tube.	NG tubes have been known to enter the fracture site and curl up into patient's cranial vault during insertion attempts. **Note:** The tube for gastric decompression may be inserted through the mouth. This is often used for patients with basilar skull fractures to avoid passing the tube via the nose through the fracture area and into the brain. If NG tube is placed nasally, the health care provider usually performs the intubation.
Check tube placement, preferably by x-ray, before applying suction.	To help confirm its proper placement and avoid causing harm to patient.
Recognize that individuals with basilar skull fractures generally are placed flat in bed on complete bedrest.	This position helps decrease pressure and amount of CSF draining from a dural tear.
Administer antibiotics as prescribed.	Patients are given antibiotics to prevent or treat infection and observed for healing and sealing of the dural tear, which usually occurs within 7-10 days.
Teach patient to report any indicators of infection promptly.	To monitor for and prevent infections, especially meningeal infection caused by CSF contamination
For more information, see Appendix for "Infection Prevention and Control," p. 831.	

●●● Related NIC and NOC labels: *NIC:* Infection Prevention; Wound Care; Tube Care; Gastrointestinal; Tube Care: Lumbar Drain *NOC:* Infection Status; Wound Care: Primary Intention

Nursing Diagnosis:

Acute Pain

related to headaches secondary to head injury

Desired Outcome: Within 1 hr of intervention, patient's subjective perception of pain decreases, as documented by a pain scale.

INTERVENTIONS	RATIONALES
Monitor and document duration and character of patient's pain, rating it on a scale of 0 (no pain) to 10 (worst pain).	This enables baseline for subsequent comparison and quantifies degree of pain and pain relief obtained.
Administer analgesics as prescribed.	Patients with HIs generally do not have much pain, and it is usually relieved by analgesics, such as acetaminophen. Sometimes codeine is prescribed, but as a rule, other narcotics are contraindicated because they can mask neurologic indicators of IICP and cause respiratory depression.
For additional interventions, see **Acute Pain,** p. 307, in "General Care of Patients with Neurologic Disorders."	

●●● Related NIC and NOC labels: *NIC:* Pain Management; Analgesic Administration *NOC:* Comfort Level

Nursing Diagnosis:

Excess Fluid Volume

related to compromised regulatory mechanisms with increased antidiuretic hormone (ADH) and increased renal resorption secondary to syndrome of inappropriate antidiuretic hormone (SIADH)

Desired Outcome: By hospital discharge (or within 3 days of injury), patient is normovolemic as evidenced by stable weight, balanced I&O, urinary output ≥30 ml/hr, urine specific gravity 1.010–1.030, BP within patient's baseline limits, absence of fingerprint edema over the sternum, and orientation to person, place, and time.

INTERVENTIONS	RATIONALES
Monitor serum Na⁺ levels. Notify health care provider of significant findings.	In the presence of SIADH, a potential secondary complication of HI, the patient will have excessive water retention and hyponatremia. Expect seizure activity when serum Na⁺ level drops below 118 mEq/L. Serum Na⁺ level <115 mEq/L may result in loss of reflexes, coma, and death.
Assess for fingerprint edema over sternum.	Reflects cellular edema. Because fluid is not retained in the interstitium with SIADH, peripheral edema will not necessarily occur.
Depending on serum Na⁺ value, restrict fluids as prescribed to an amount as low as 500-1000 ml/24 hr.	Fluid overload can increase ICP.
Recognize that free use of salt or salty foods may be prescribed for patient's diet.	To help normalize patient's Na⁺ level.
For other interventions, see this nursing diagnosis in "Syndrome of Inappropriate Antidiuretic Hormone," p. 433.	

●●● **Related NIC and NOC labels:** *NIC:* Fluid/Electrolyte Management; Electrolyte Monitoring; Laboratory Data Interpretation; Electrolyte Management: Hyponatremia *NOC:* Electrolyte & Acid/Base Balance

Nursing Diagnosis:

Deficient Knowledge:

Ventricular shunt procedure

Desired Outcome: Within the 24-hr period following teaching (or before procedure), patient verbalizes accurate information about ventricular shunt procedure, including presurgical and postsurgical care.

INTERVENTIONS	RATIONALES
Determine patient's understanding of the procedure after health care provider's explanation, including purpose, risks, and anticipated benefits or outcome. Intervene accordingly.	Enables clarification and reinforcement of previous teaching.
As indicated, explain why the procedure is performed.	The procedure is performed to enable drainage of CSF when flow is obstructed (e.g., because of presence of a tumor or blood).
Explain that patient may have a cranial dressing, as well as a dressing on the neck, chest, or abdomen.	Shunt types vary but can extend from lateral ventricle of the brain to one of the following: subarachnoid space of the spinal canal, right atrium of the heart, a large vein, or the peritoneal cavity.

Continued

INTERVENTIONS	RATIONALES
Explain that it is important to avoid lying on insertion site after the procedure.	To avoid pressure on shunt mechanism, which would decrease CSF drainage.
Advise that the head and neck are kept in alignment.	To prevent kinking and compression of shunt catheter.
Explain that the shunt site will be monitored for redness, tenderness, bulging, or fluid collection, and swelling will be assessed along the shunt's course.	To assess for infection and determine if shunt is functioning properly.
If the shunt has a valve for controlling CSF drainage or reflux, explain that the valve will be pumped or compressed a certain number of times (e.g., 10 × q6h) at prescribed intervals.	To flush system of exudate and prevent plugging.
Explain that the valve, which is usually located behind or above the ear and is the approximate diameter of a pencil, can be felt to empty and then refill.	Malfunction may be noted by failure of the reservoir to refill when pumped or by deterioration in neurologic status.
Reassure patient and significant other that before hospital discharge, specific instructions will be given about shunt care, recognition of shunt site infection and malfunction, and steps to take should they occur. Teach signs and symptoms of IICP (i.e., headache, change in LOC such as drowsiness, lethargy, irritability, nausea, personality changes) that should be reported to health care provider.	Patient teaching and discharge planning considerations that will enable self-care and assessment while at home and the knowledge of signs and symptoms of complications that necessitate prompt medical intervention. Other complications that may occur include movement of the cannula (resulting in inadequate drainage of ventricles) or subdural hematoma formation. For ventriculoatrial shunts, emboli or endocarditis may occur. For ventriculoperitoneal shunts, ascites or ruptured viscus may occur.
For additional interventions, see **Risk for Infection,** earlier, and **Deficient Knowledge:** Surgical procedure, p. 47, in "Perioperative Care."	

●●● **Related NIC and NOC labels:** *NIC:* Preparatory Sensory Information; Teaching: Procedure/Treatment; Teaching: Psychomotor Skill; Learning Facilitation *NOC:* Knowledge: Treatment Procedures

Nursing Diagnosis:

Deficient Knowledge:

Craniotomy procedure

Desired Outcome: Within the 24-hr period following teaching (or before procedure), patient verbalizes accurate understanding of the craniotomy procedure, including presurgical and postsurgical care.

INTERVENTIONS	RATIONALES
After health care provider's explanation of the procedure, determine patient's level of understanding of purpose, risks, and anticipated benefits or outcome. Intervene accordingly.	Enables clarification and reinforcement of previous teaching.
As indicated, explain purpose of patient's craniotomy.	A craniotomy is a surgical opening into the skull to remove a hematoma or tumor, repair a ruptured aneurysm, or apply arterial clips or wrap the involved vessel to prevent future rupture.

Continued

INTERVENTIONS	RATIONALES
As appropriate, explain that the bone flap may be left open postoperatively.	To accommodate cerebral edema and prevent compression. When the bone is removed, the procedure is called a craniectomy.
Explain that before surgery, antiseptic shampoos may be given and patient may be started on corticosteroids, such as dexamethasone, and antiepilepsy drugs.	Hair can be a major source of microorganisms. Dexamethasone may be given for cerebral edema; antiepilepsy drugs may be given prophylactically.
Explain that a baseline neurologic assessment will be performed.	To provide a basis for comparison with postoperative neurologic checks.
During the immediate postoperative period, patient is in intensive care unit (ICU). Explain the considerations and interventions that are likely to occur.	- At least hourly, patient will be asked to perform a variety of assessment measures, including squeezing tester's hand, moving extremities, extending tongue, and answering questions. - Changes in body image can occur. These result from loss of hair, presence of a large head dressing, and potential for and expected duration of facial edema. - There may be need for respiratory and airway support, including O_2, intubation, or ventilation. Typically patients are on a cardiac monitor for 24-48 hr because dysrhythmias are not unusual after posterior fossa surgery or when blood is in CSF. - Patient will be NPO for first 24-48 hr because of risk of vomiting and aspiration and may experience a dry throat at this time. - Periorbital swelling usually occurs within 24-48 hr of supratentorial surgery because of localized edema caused by head positioning during surgery. Relief is obtained with applications of cold or warm compresses around the eyes. Having HOB up with patient lying on nonoperative side also may help reduce edema. - Indwelling urinary catheter will be inserted to enable accurate measurement of I&O and monitor for problems such as diabetes insipidus. - Core temperature (e.g., rectal, tympanic, bladder) will be measured at frequent intervals. A rectal probe or bladder catheter temperature probe may be used for continuous monitoring. Oral temperatures are avoided during the period that cognitive function is decreased.
Teach patient about postsurgical positions as indicated.	Postsurgical positioning is a key factor in patient's recovery. - *Supratentorial craniotomy:* HOB is elevated to 30 degrees or as prescribed. The patient will be assisted with turning and usually will be kept off operative site, especially if the lesion was large. Head and neck will be kept in good alignment. - *Infratentorial craniotomy* (for cerebellar or brain stem surgery): HOB is kept flat or as prescribed. Sitting may increase risk of venous air embolus with posterior fossa surgery. Pressure usually is kept off operative site, especially with a craniectomy, so these patients are kept off their backs for 48 hr. In posterior fossa surgery, the supporting neck muscles are altered. Patient is log-rolled to alternate sides, keeping head in good alignment. A soft cervical collar may be used to prevent anterior or lateral angulation of the neck. A small pillow may be used for comfort.

Continued

INTERVENTIONS	RATIONALES
Teach patients undergoing infratentorial surgery that they are likely to experience the following:	
- A longer period of bedrest.	These patients may experience an extended period of dizziness and hypotension.
- Nausea, which should be reported promptly.	So that antiemetics (e.g., metoclopramide, trimethobenzamide) can be given in a timely manner.
- Possible swallowing difficulties, extraocular movements, or nystagmus, any of which should be reported promptly.	These problems can occur as a result of cranial nerve edema.
Teach patient about precautions that must be taken to prevent increased intraabdominal and intrathoracic pressure.	Increased intraabdominal and intrathoracic pressure can cause increased ICP. These precautions include:
	- Exhaling when being turned.
	- Not straining at stool.
	- Not moving self in bed, but rather letting staff members do all moving.
	- Importance of deep breathing and avoiding coughing and sneezing. If coughing and sneezing are unavoidable, they must be done with an opened mouth.
	- Avoiding hip flexion and lying prone.
For additional precautions against IICP, see **Decreased Intracranial Adaptive Capacity**, p. 303.	
Teach patient that precautions are taken for seizures.	See **Risk for Trauma** related to oral, musculoskeletal, and airway vulnerability secondary to seizure activity, p. 376.
Teach patient wound care and indicators of infection. For more information, see **Risk for Infection,** earlier.	To prevent wound infection at surgical site and promote healing. Generally, a surgical cap is worn after removal of head dressing. Patient must avoid scratching wound, staples, or sutures and must keep the incision dry. When sutures or staples are removed, hair can be shampooed, being careful not to scrub around incision line. Hair dryers are avoided until hair is regrown.
Explain that patients undergoing acoustic neuroma excision may have nausea, hearing loss, facial weakness or paralysis, diminished or absent blinking, eye dryness, tinnitus, vertigo, headache, and occasionally swallowing, throat, taste, or voice problems.	Acoustic neuromas can wrap around cranial nerve VII, and surgery may damage this cranial nerve and cause localized edema. Other cranial nerves whose nuclei are in the brain stem also may be affected.
	Nausea and dizziness may be profound problems after surgery. Patient will be given antiemetics and should be turned and moved slowly. Patient should be spoken to on unaffected side for best hearing, and phone and call light should be placed on that side of bed. Contralateral routing of signal hearing aids may improve hearing by directing sound from deaf ear to hearing ear via a tiny microphone and transmitter. Background music or other white noise may mask tinnitus. Awareness of tinnitus eventually should lessen. Balance exercises and walking with assistance will start compensation process by the functioning vestibular system.
	Watching television or reading may be difficult because of vertigo; books on tape, listening to the radio, or music may be good alternatives.

Continued

INTERVENTIONS	RATIONALES
	Because of impaired eyelid function, eye dryness may require use of eye drops or ointment. An eye bubble, which contains moisture, may be used if patient is unable to blink or close the eye.
For additional interventions, see **Deficient Knowledge: Surgical procedure, p. 47, in "Perioperative Care."**	

●●● **Related NIC and NOC labels:** *NIC:* Preparatory Sensory Information; Teaching: Procedure/ Treatment; Teaching: Psychomotor Skill; Learning Facilitation *NOC:* Knowledge: Treatment Procedures

ADDITIONAL NURSING DIAGNOSES/ PROBLEMS:

PATIENT-FAMILY TEACHING AND DISCHARGE PLANNING

The head-injured patient can have varying degrees of neurologic deficit, ranging from mild to severe. When providing patient-family teaching, focus on sensory information, avoid giving excessive information, and initiate a visiting nurse referral for necessary follow-up teaching. Include verbal and written information about the following:

✓ Safety measures related to decreased sensation, visual disturbances, motor deficits, and seizure activity.

✓ Measures that promote communication in the presence of aphasia.

✓ Wound care and indicators of infection.

✓ Measures that deal with cognitive or behavioral problems. As appropriate, include home evaluation for safety. Caution significant other that personality can change drastically after HI. The patient may demonstrate inappropriate social behavior, inappropriate affect, hallucination, delusion, and altered sleep pattern.

✓ If patient had a concussion, a description of problems that may occur at home and necessitate prompt medical attention (see **Deficient Knowledge,** p. 341).

✓ Referrals to community resources, such as cognitive retraining specialist, head injury rehabilitation centers, visiting nurses association, community support groups, social workers, psychologic therapy, vocational rehabilitation agency, home health agencies, and extended and skilled care facilities. Additional general information can be obtained by contacting the following organization:

Brain Injury Association, Inc.
105 North Alfred Street
Alexandria, VA 22314
(800) 444-6443
www.biausa.org

✓ For other information, see teaching and discharge planning interventions (fourth through tenth entries only) in "Multiple Sclerosis," p. 359, as appropriate.

Intervertebral Disk Disease

The intervertebral disk is a semifluid filled fibrous capsule that facilitates movement of the spine and acts as a shock absorber. The ability of the disk to withstand stressors is not unlimited and diminishes with aging. Pressure on the disk eventually may force elastic material from the center of the disk, called the nucleus pulposus, to break, or herniate, through the fibrous rim of the disk. Herniation usually occurs posteriorly because the posterior longitudinal ligament is inherently weaker than the anterior longitudinal ligament. The rupture or bulging of an intervertebral disk causes its typical symptoms by pressing on and irritating the spinal nerve roots or spinal cord itself. Herniated nucleus pulposus usually is the result of injury or a series of insults to the vertebral column from lifting or twisting. When the disk ruptures without a known discrete injury, it is believed to be caused by degenerative changes. Deterioration can occur suddenly, or it may happen gradually, with symptoms appearing months or years after the initial injury.

HEALTH CARE SETTING

Primary care or acute care

ASSESSMENT

General indicators: Onset can be sudden, with intense unilateral pain or with pain that is dull, diffuse, deep, and aching. Symptoms vary according to the level of injury and nerves involved. Usually, pain is increased with movement or activities that increase intraabdominal or intrathoracic pressure, such as sneezing, coughing, and straining. Often pain is improved by lying down.

Note: Immediate medical attention is essential if there is any paralysis, extreme sensory loss, or altered bowel or bladder function.

Lumbar disk disease: Pain in the lumbosacral area with possible radiculopathy (sciatica) to the buttock, down the posterior surface of the thigh and calf, and to the lateral border of the foot. Frequently, mobility is altered, as evidenced by decreased ability to stand upright, listing to one side, asymmetric gait, limited ability to flex forward, and restricted side movement caused by pain and muscle spasms. The individual walks cautiously, bearing little weight on the affected side, and often finds sitting or climbing stairs particularly painful. Reflex muscle spasms can cause bulging of the back with concomitant flattening of the lumbar curve and possible scoliosis at the level of the affected disk.

Physical assessment: Possible findings include depressed reflexes, muscle atrophy, paresthesias (described as "pins and needles"), or anesthesia (numbness) in the dermatome of the involved nerves. The following tests are two of several that are performed to confirm the presence of lumbar disk disease.

- **Straight leg raise test:** Examiner extends and raises patient's leg. The test is positive if patient has pain on the posterior aspect of the leg. People without injury usually can have a leg raised to 90 degrees without significant discomfort.
- **Sciatic nerve test:** Examiner extends and raises patient's leg until pain is elicited and then lowers the leg to a comfortable level. The examiner then dorsiflexes the foot to stretch the sciatic nerve. If this causes pain, the test is positive for sciatic nerve involvement.

Risk factors: Repetitive bending or lifting involving a twisting motion, continuous vibration, smoking, poor physical condition, obesity, above-average height, osteoporosis, prolonged sitting, depression, severe scoliosis, spondylolisthesis, or genetic predisposition.

DIAGNOSTIC TESTS

In the absence of serious symptoms, diagnostic testing may not be done until a month has passed and symptoms persist (90% of back pain resolves in <1 mo).

Magnetic resonance imaging (MRI): May reveal that the disk is impinging on the spinal cord or nerve root or may reveal a related pathologic condition, such as a tumor or spondylosis. MRI has replaced computed tomography (CT) scan and myelogram as the test of choice in diagnosing herniated nucleus pulposus.

CT scan of the spine: May reveal disk protrusion/prolapse or a related pathologic condition, such as a tumor, spondylosis, or spinal stenosis.

Myelogram: May show characteristic deformity and filling defect or a related pathologic condition; usually done in conjunction with a CT scan.

X-ray examination of the spine: May show narrowing of the vertebral interspaces in affected areas, loss of curvature of the spine, and spondylosis.

Diskography: Identifies degenerated or extruded disks by means of contrast medium injected into the disk space, using fluoroscopy.

Electromyography (EMG): May show denervation patterns of specific nerve roots to indicate the level and site of injury.

Laboratory tests (serum alkaline and acid phosphatase, glucose, calcium, erythrocyte sedimentation rate [ESR], white blood cells [WBCs]): May rule out metabolic bone disease, metastatic tumors, diabetic mononeuritis, and disk space infection.

Nursing Diagnosis:

Health-Seeking Behaviors:

Proper body mechanics and other measures that prevent back injury

Desired Outcome: Within the treatment session (outpatient) or within the 24-hr period before hospital discharge, patient verbalizes accurate knowledge of measures that prevent back injury and demonstrates proper body mechanics accordingly.

INTERVENTIONS	RATIONALES
Teach proper body mechanics: stand and sit straight with chin and head up and pelvis and back straight; bend at knees and hips rather than at the waist (squat), keeping back straight (not stooping forward); when carrying objects, hold them close to the body, avoiding twisting when lifting or reaching. Spread feet for a wider base of support. Lift with legs, not the back. Turn using entire body. Do not strain to reach things. If an object is overhead, raise yourself to its level, or move things out of the way if they are obstructing the object. Avoid lifting anything heavier than 10-20 lb. Encourage use of long-handled pickup sticks to pick up small objects.	Using proper body mechanics avoids movements such as twisting, lifting with the back, and straining to reach that can cause recurrence of back injury.
Teach about the following measures for keeping body in alignment: sit close to pedals when driving a car and use a seat belt and firm back rest to support the back; support feet on a footstool when sitting so that knees are elevated to hip level or higher; obtain a firm mattress or bedboard; use a flat pillow when sleeping to avoid strain on neck, arms, and shoulders; sleep in a side-lying position with knees bent or in a supine position with knees and legs supported on pillows; avoid sleeping in a prone position; avoid reaching or stretching to pick up objects. Avoid sitting on furniture that does not support back.	Keeping the body in proper alignment avoids strain on the back, thereby helping to prevent recurring back injury.

Continued

INTERVENTIONS	RATIONALES
Encourage patient to achieve and/or maintain proper weight for age, height, and gender and continue exercise program prescribed by health care provider.	Being overweight or obese can cause back strain and alteration in center of balance, which can result in back pain and pressure. Exercise strengthens abdominal, thoracic, and back muscles. Using thoracic and abdominal muscles when lifting keeps a significant portion of weight off vertebral disks.
Teach rationale and procedure for Williams' back exercises.	Williams' back exercises are performed to strengthen abdominal muscles, stretch hip muscles, and make a stiff back limber. They are performed while lying on the floor with knees flexed.
	Pelvic tilt (to strengthen abdominal muscles): Stomach and buttock muscles are tightened, and pelvis is tilted with lower spine kept flat against the floor; that is, hips and buttocks are kept on the floor.
	Knee-to-chest raises (to help make a stiff back limber): Starting with a pelvic tilt, each knee is individually raised to chest and returned to starting position. Both knees are then raised to chest and held there (both on chest together).
	Nose-to-knee touch (to stretch hip muscles and strengthen abdominal muscles): Knee is raised to the chest, and then knee is pulled to chest with hands. The patient raises head and tries to touch nose to knee, keeping lower back flat on floor.
	Half sit-ups (to strengthen abdomen and back): Head and neck are slowly raised to top of chest. Both hands reach forward to the knees and hold for a count of 5. This is repeated, keeping lower back flat on floor.
Instruct patient to wear supportive shoes with a moderate heel height for walking.	To maintain proper alignment of back and hips.
Teach the following technique for sitting up at the bedside from a supine position: log-roll to side and then raise to sitting position by pushing against mattress with hands while swinging legs over side of bed. Instruct patient to maintain alignment of the back during procedure.	Prevents strain on back and promotes good body alignment.
Caution patient that pain is the signal to stop or change an activity or position.	Prevents additional back injury.
Encourage patient to continue with a regular exercise and stretching program.	Strengthens abdominal, thoracic, and back muscles to help prevent subsequent back injury. Walking and exercising in water can be included in the exercise program.
Encourage patient to continue physical therapy and graded exercise program.	Strengthens legs, back, and abdominal muscles and teaches correct body mechanics. It is initiated once acute symptoms subside. Physical therapy has become the mainstay of therapy for chronic low back pain.
Teach patient that the following indicators necessitate medical attention: increased sensory loss, increased motor loss/weakness, and loss of bowel and bladder function.	May signal disk herniation, which necessitates timely intervention.
Ask patient to demonstrate proper body mechanics.	To ensure that patient understands principles of proper body mechanics.

●●● **Related NIC and NOC labels:** *NIC:* Health Education; Exercise Promotion; Weight Management
NOC: Health Promoting Behavior

Nursing Diagnosis:

Deficient Knowledge:

Pain control measures

Desired Outcome: Following instruction within outpatient treatment session or within the 24-hr period before hospital discharge, patient verbalizes accurate knowledge about pain control measures and demonstrates ability to initiate these measures when appropriate.

INTERVENTIONS	RATIONALES
Teach methods of controlling pain and their individual applications.	To reduce pain using nonpharmacologic measures, which can be used solely or to augment drug therapy. Methods include distraction, use of counterirritants, massage, hydrotherapy, dorsal column stimulation, use of transcutaneous electrical nerve stimulation (TENS), percutaneous electrical nerve stimulation (PENS), behavior modification, relaxation techniques, hypnosis, music therapy, imagery, biofeedback, and diathermy. In addition, application of local heat (e.g., warm/hot showers or heating pads) or cold massage to painful areas are other methods to attain pain relief. The latter can be achieved by freezing water in a paper cup, tearing off top of cup to expose the ice, and massaging in a circular motion, using remaining portion of cup as a handle. A bag of frozen peas or corn may be used to apply continuous cold to lower back. A layer of cloth should be used so that ice does not touch the skin. A 20-min application 4-6 times/day is recommended.
Suggest that patient use a stool to rest affected leg when standing.	To relieve sciatica.
Advise patient to sit in a straight-back chair that is high enough to get out of easily.	To facilitate ease of movement in and out of chairs and to provide comfort. Raised toilet seats also may be useful. Straddling a straight-back chair and resting arms on the chair back are comfortable for many individuals.
Encourage use of a firm mattress and extra pillows as needed for positioning.	To support normal spinal curvature and to limit spinal flexion.
Instruct patient on bedrest to roll rather than lift off bedpan.	To avoid straining the back. The patient may find a fracture bedpan more comfortable than a regular bedpan.
Caution patient to avoid sudden twisting or turning movements. Explain importance of log-rolling when moving from side to side.	To prevent movement that could induce a back injury.
Advise patient to avoid staying in one position too long, fatigue, chilling, and anxiety.	Factors that promote spasms.
Suggest lying on side with knees bent or lying supine with knees supported on pillows. Advise use of a small pillow supporting nape of the neck for patients with cervical pain. Teach patient to avoid prolonged periods of sitting, which stress the back.	To promote positions of comfort.
Instruct patient to apply a heating pad to the back for 15-30 min before getting out of bed in the morning.	To allay stiffness and discomfort. Heating pads should be used only for short intervals and only if patient's temperature sensations are intact.
Remind patient to place a towel or cloth between heating pad and skin.	To prevent burns.

●●● **Related NIC and NOC labels:** *NIC:* Teaching: Procedure/Treatment; Teaching: Psychomotor Skill; Health Education; Behavior Modification *NOC:* Knowledge: Treatment Procedures; Knowledge: Health Behaviors

Nursing Diagnosis:

Deficient Knowledge:

Diskectomy with laminectomy or fusion procedure

Desired Outcomes: Before surgery, patient verbalizes knowledge about the surgical procedure, preoperative routine, and postoperative regimen. Patient demonstrates activities and exercises correctly.

INTERVENTIONS	RATIONALES
Assess patient's knowledge about the surgical procedure, preoperative routine, postoperative regimen, and potential complications. Provide ample time for instruction and clarification.	To ensure that patient is as informed as possible before the surgical procedure.
	Diskectomy with laminectomy: An incision is made, allowing removal of part of the vertebra (laminectomy) so that the herniated portion of the disk can be removed (diskectomy). If multiple intervertebral disk spaces are explored, a wound drain may be present after surgery. Complications include paralytic ileus, urinary retention, cerebrospinal fluid (CSF) leakage, meningitis, hematoma at the operative site, nerve root injury causing wristdrop or footdrop, arachnoiditis, and postural deformity. Candidates include individuals with motor or sphincter weakness who have not responded to conservative treatment.
	Spinal fusion: Bone chips are harvested from the iliac crest or tibia and placed between the vertebrae in the prepared area of the unstable spine to fuse and stabilize the area. Internal fixation (e.g., rods, wiring, pedicle screws, fusion cages) may be necessary to provide added stability until the fusion has healed fully. Intervertebral body fusion using a threaded titanium cage also relieves nerve root compression and stabilizes the spine. If the patient's own bone quality or quantity is inadequate, allograft bone may be considered. Fusion may be indicated for patients with recurrent low back pain, spondylolisthesis, or subluxation of the vertebrae. Some health care providers promote primary use of fusion for patients who have not responded to conservative therapy.
Teach technique for deep breathing. Also teach patient use of incentive spirometry.	Will be performed immediately after surgery to help expand the alveoli and aid in mobilizing lung secretions. Coughing, if it is allowed, will clear the lungs of the secretions.
Advise that coughing may be contraindicated in immediate postoperative period.	To prevent disruption of fusion or surgical repair.
Explain that baseline VS and neurovascular checks, including color, capillary refill, pulse, warmth, muscle strength, movement, and sensation, will be documented before surgery and continued after surgery. Reassure patient that this is normal and does not indicate that anything is wrong.	VS and neurologic status will be evaluated at frequent intervals after surgery and compared with baseline to monitor trend.
Teach the following signs and symptoms and importance of reporting them promptly: paresthesias, weakness, paralysis, radiculopathy, and changes in bowel or bladder function.	These indicators of impairment necessitate immediate attention by health care staff because they signal presence of autonomic stimulation.
Teach the following signs and symptoms and importance of reporting them promptly: increased HR, thirst, faintness, or dizziness.	These are signs, along with decreased BP, of hypovolemia and may occur because of blood loss. Patients undergoing fusion lose more blood during surgery than those undergoing laminectomy.

Continued

INTERVENTIONS	RATIONALES
Explain that the surgical dressing will be inspected for excess drainage or oozing at frequent intervals and that a closed wound drainage device may be present for 1-3 days postoperatively.	Bleeding with a laminectomy usually is minimal. Patients with fusion may have slight bloody oozing postoperatively. Bulging in the area of the wound may also signal CSF leakage or hematoma formation and should be reported promptly for timely intervention.
	Serous drainage usually is checked with a glucose reagent strip. Presence of glucose is a signal of CSF leakage. The dressing is monitored for increased drainage after patient is up.
Advise that lumbar dressings will be checked after each bedpan use. Inform patients undergoing fusions that they will have a second dressing at the donor site.	Wet or contaminated dressings require prompt changing to prevent infection.
Instruct patient to report any nausea or vomiting.	So that antiemetics can be given promptly.
Explain that patient will be monitored for bowel and bladder dysfunction after the procedure.	Stimulation of the sympathetic nervous system during surgery can contribute to paralytic ileus. The abdomen will be checked for bowel sounds and distention.
	Patient may be asked to void within 8 hr of the procedure to check for urinary retention.
Provide or advise patient to use stool softeners to prevent straining at stool.	Prevents constipation and pain from straining caused by increased intraspinal pressure.
Explain that fever may occur during first few days postoperatively but that this does not necessarily signal an infection.	Early fever may be caused by drainage and contamination of CSF. Patient will be assessed for other indicators of infection, such as heat, erythema, irritation, swelling, or drainage at wound site.
Instruct patient to report headache, neck stiffness, or photophobia.	Possible signs of meningeal irritation.
Inform patient that postoperative pain or tingling (paresthesia) often is caused by nerve root irritation and edema. Spasms are common on the third or fourth postoperative day.	Provides reassurance and allays anxiety when patient knows what to expect. Pain may take days or weeks to resolve and does not indicate that surgery was unsuccessful.
Teach patient to request medication for pain as needed and not let pain get out of control.	Pain is easier to manage before it becomes severe. Prolonged stimulation of pain receptors results in increased sensitivity to painful stimuli and will increase the amount of analgesic required to relieve pain. Patients who have had a fusion may expect significant pain from bone graft donor site (commonly the iliac crest). The donor site may have extra padding. Muscle relaxants may be prescribed to supplement pain control. Patient-controlled analgesia (PCA) and non-steroidal antiinflammatory drugs (NSAIDs) also may be used for postoperative pain control.
Explain that in the immediate postoperative period the patient probably will be required to lie supine for several hours.	To minimize possibility of wound hematoma formation.
	After this period, head of bed (HOB) of laminectomy patient usually can be raised to 20 degrees to facilitate eating and bedpan use.
	The patient undergoing spinal fusion usually is kept flat and on bedrest considerably longer than a patient with laminectomy because spinal fusion is used to stabilize the spine. This necessitates slower activity and promotes better alignment and healing.
Teach patient the following log-rolling technique: position a pillow between legs, cross arms across chest while turning, and contract long back muscles to maintain shoulders and	Log-rolling is the only method used for turning. This method stabilizes the spine and maintains alignment to enable healing and prevent dislodgement of the bone graft if fusion is done.

Continued

INTERVENTIONS	RATIONALES
pelvis in straight alignment. Explain that initially patient will be assisted in this procedure. Use a turning sheet and sufficient help when log-rolling patient.	
Teach the following technique for getting out of bed: log-roll to side, splint back, and rise to a sitting position by pushing against mattress while swinging legs over side of bed.	To facilitate ease of getting out of bed and prevent disruption of the bone graft for fusion patients.
Explain that initially patient will be helped to a sitting position and should not push against mattress. Patients with cervical laminectomy should not pull themselves up with their arms or pull on side rails. When assisting patients with cervical laminectomy to a sitting position, caution them not to put their arms on nurse's shoulders.	While in hospital with an electric bed, the HOB may be raised to facilitate a sitting position. These restrictions prevent neck flexion, extension, and hyperextension and strain on the operative site and incision.
Explain that antiembolism hose and possibly sequential compression sleeves will be applied after surgery.	To promote venous return and prevent thrombus formation.
Teach techniques for ankle circling and calf pumping. Teach patient to report calf pain, tenderness, or warmth.	To promote circulation in legs. Possible signs of deep vein thrombosis.
Advise patient that health care provider will prescribe certain postoperative activity restrictions.	Sitting is commonly restricted or allowed for only limited, prescribed periods in a straight-back chair.
Teach patient not to sit for long periods on edge of mattress.	A mattress does not provide enough support.
Explain that weakness, dizziness, and lightheadedness may occur on a first walk.	These problems may occur secondary to orthostatic hypotension. For management, see discussion in **Ineffective Cerebral Tissue Perfusion,** p. 73, in "Prolonged Bedrest."
Explain that patient will be encouraged to walk progressively longer distances.	To promote endurance
Instruct patient to avoid stretching, twisting, flexing, or jarring spine. Explain that the spine should be kept aligned and in a neutral position.	To prevent vertebral collapse, shifting of bone graft, or a bleeding episode.
If patient is scheduled for cervical laminectomy, explain that a cervical collar will be worn postoperatively.	Aids in immobilizing the cervical spine.
Teach use of braces or corsets if prescribed.	The person undergoing a fusion procedure often wears a supportive brace or corset for ≤3 mo to keep operative site immobile so that the graft will heal and not dislodge. Braces should be applied while in bed.
Explain importance of wearing cotton underwear under brace, powdering skin lightly with cornstarch, or providing additional padding.	These measures will help protect skin under the brace from irritation that could affect its integrity.
Explain that driving or riding in car, sexual activity, lifting and carrying objects, tub bathing (generally, soaking incision is avoided until about 1 wk after sutures are out), going up and down stairs, amount of time to spend in and out of bed, back exercises, and expected time away from work will be discussed by health care provider before patient is discharged.	These guidelines and activity restrictions promote patient safety and an uneventful recovery once he or she is at home.
Teach the following symptoms that require medical attention: swelling, discharge, persistent redness, local warmth, fever, and pain. The incision should be kept dry and open to the air.	These symptoms signal postoperative wound infection and require timely intervention.
For additional interventions, see **Deficient Knowledge:** Surgical procedure, preoperative routine, and postoperative care in "Perioperative Care," p. 47.	

●●● **Related NIC and NOC labels:** *NIC:* Preparatory Sensory Information; Teaching: Procedure/Treatment; Teaching: Psychomotor Skill; Anxiety Reduction; Teaching: Preoperative; Teaching: Prescribed Activity/ Exercise *NOC:* Knowledge: Treatment Regimen; Knowledge: Treatment Procedures

Nursing Diagnosis:

Impaired Swallowing

(or risk for same) *related to* postoperative edema, hematoma formation, or bleeding secondary to anterior cervical fusion

Desired Outcome: Patient regains uncompromised swallowing ability (usually by the third postoperative day) as evidenced by normal breath sounds and absence of food in the oral cavity or choking/coughing.

INTERVENTIONS	RATIONALES
As part of preoperative teaching, caution patient about potential for difficulty with swallowing after anterior cervical fusion. Explain need to report promptly any significant postoperative difficulty with swallowing.	An informed patient likely will report postoperative difficulties with swallowing promptly for timely intervention.
Explain that a soft diet and throat lozenges may be prescribed for 2-3 days postoperatively.	For patient's comfort in swallowing. A sore throat can be expected after this surgery.
Monitor for edema of face or neck and tracheal compression or deviation that could compromise respiratory function. Monitor and rapidly report stridor or respiratory distress.	These may be signs of hematoma or bleeding at the operative site that could cause airway compromise and therefore necessitate immediate intervention.
Listen for hoarseness. Encourage voice rest and facilitate alternative communication (e.g., story boards, pen and pencil, flash cards).	Hoarseness can indicate laryngeal nerve irritation and signal ineffective cough or swallowing difficulty, which would necessitate precautions against choking and aspiration. For patients with hoarseness, the voice will usually return to normal as inflammation around laryngeal nerve subsides.
Report immediately any respiratory distress, inability to speak, worsening hoarseness, or voice change.	These may be signs of aspiration, laryngeal nerve involvement/irritation, or increased edema or hematoma formation affecting the laryngeal nerve and vocal cords, any of which can be life threatening and necessitate prompt intervention.
Monitor for and report diminished breath sounds compared with patient's normal or preoperative status.	This could signal that aspiration has occurred and may result in pneumonia.
As indicated, monitor oximetry as a quantitative measure of systemic oxygenation.	Values ≤92% may signal need for supplemental oxygenation.
Monitor for complaints of excessive pressure in neck or severe, uncontrolled incisional pain.	Can signal excessive bleeding and potential airway compromise.
Monitor closed suction devices and recharge suction device/chamber as indicated.	To facilitate wound drainage.
Check for gag and swallowing reflexes before starting patient on oral intake.	Absence of gag and swallowing reflexes indicates that patient cannot begin oral intake. Begin postoperative diet with clear fluids and progress to more solid foods only after patient demonstrates ability to ingest fluids safely.
Position patient in Fowler's position, or semi-Fowler's position at minimum, when initiating fluid intake.	To minimize risk of aspiration by promoting movement of fluids by gravity to the stomach and into the pylorus.
If not prohibited by surgery, encourage use of chin tuck.	A chin tuck forces the trachea to close and the esophagus to open, which decreases risk of aspiration.
Also see **Risk for Aspiration,** p. 101, in "Older Adult Care."	

●●● **Related NIC and NOC labels:** *NIC:* Aspiration Precautions; Positioning; Risk Identification; Feeding *NOC:* Aspiration Control; Swallowing Status: Oral Phase

Additional Nursing Diagnoses/ Problems:

PATIENT-FAMILY TEACHING AND DISCHARGE PLANNING

When providing patient-family teaching, focus on sensory information, avoid giving excessive information, and initiate a visiting nurse referral for necessary follow-up teaching. Include verbal and written information about the following:

✓ Prescribed exercise regimen, including rationale for each exercise, technique for performing the exercise, number of repetitions of each, and frequency of exercise periods. If possible, ensure that patient demonstrates understanding of exercise regimen and proper body mechanics before hospital discharge.

✓ Wound incision care. Indicators of postoperative wound infection that necessitate medical attention include swelling, discharge, persistent redness, local warmth, fever, and pain.

✓ Review of use and application of cervical collar for patients who have had a cervical fusion. The cervical collar is worn at all times. Patient should be instructed to cleanse neck 1-2 times/day, cleaning incision with mild soap. To accomplish this, patient should request help from a significant other. Patient should lie flat, open front portion of collar, keeping head and neck still and straight while collar is open. The incision should be cleansed and dried and collar replaced and fastened. Then patient should turn on one side with a thin pillow under the head. The posterior portion of the collar is opened, back of the neck is washed and dried, and posterior portion of the collar is replaced and fastened. Men should shave chin and neck beneath collar while lying flat. Whenever collar is released and opened, head and neck should be kept straight and not moved. A silk scarf worn beneath collar may decrease discomfort. A small cervical pillow may be used. Patients should avoid watching wall-mounted television units because of risk of extension, rotation, and flexion of the neck.

✓ Use and care of a brace or immobilizer if appropriate.

✓ Medications, including drug name, rationale, dosage, schedule, precautions, drug/drug and food/drug interactions, and potential side effects.

✓ Anticonstipation routine, which should be initiated during hospitalization.

✓ Pain control measures.

✓ Phone number of a resource person, should questions arise after hospital discharge.

✓ Postsurgical activity restrictions as directed by health care provider. These may affect the following: driving and riding in a car, returning to work, sexual activity, lifting and carrying, tub bathing, going up and down steps, and amount of time spent in or out of bed.

✓ Signs and symptoms of worsening neurologic function and the importance of notifying health care provider immediately if they develop. These include numbness, weakness, paralysis, or bowel and bladder dysfunction.

Multiple Sclerosis

Multiple sclerosis (MS) is an inflammatory disorder causing scattered and sporadic demyelinization of the central nervous system (CNS). This demyelinization interrupts electrical nerve transmission and causes the wide variety of symptoms associated with MS. The course of MS is highly variable, and although the cause of MS is unknown, it is generally believed to result from an environmental insult to the body, such as an earlier viral infection that triggers an autoimmune response in a predisposed individual. MS is more common among people living in cool, temperate climates. Heat and fever tend to aggravate symptoms.

- **Benign:** Attacks are few and mild. Complete or nearly complete clearing of symptoms occurs with little or no disability.
- **Relapsing-remitting:** Characterized by episodes of neurologic impairment followed by complete recovery and stability (remission).
- **Secondary progressive:** Neurologic impairment progresses continuously with or without superimposed relapses.
- **Primary progressive:** Gradual ongoing accumulation of symptoms and deficits with the absence of clear-cut relapses and remissions.

HEALTH CARE SETTING

Primary care or long-term care, with possible hospitalization resulting from complications

ASSESSMENT

Onset of MS can be extremely rapid, or it can be insidious with exacerbations and remissions. Signs and symptoms vary widely, depending on the site and extent of demyelinization, and they can change from day to day. Usually early symptoms are mild, including fatigue, weakness, heaviness, clumsiness, numbness, and tingling. Optic neuritis is sometimes the first symptom.

Damage to motor nerve tracts: Weakness, paralysis, and spasticity. Fatigue is common. Diplopia may occur secondary to ocular muscle involvement.

Damage to cerebellar or brain stem regions: Intention tremor, nystagmus, or other tremors; incoordination, ataxia; weakness of facial and throat muscles resulting in difficulty chewing, dysphagia, and dysarthria. Slurred speech often occurs early, whereas scanning speech (slow speech with pauses between syllables) is usually seen in later stages.

Damage to sensory nerve tracts: Decreased perception of pain, touch, and temperature; paresthesias, such as numbness and tingling; decrease or loss of proprioception; and decrease or loss of vibratory sense. Optic neuritis is an early common symptom, potentially causing partial or total loss of vision, visual clouding or shimmering, and pain with eye movement.

Damage to cerebral cortex (especially frontal lobes): Mood swings, inappropriate affect, euphoria, apathy, irritability, depression, hyperexcitability, poor memory, and poor abstract reasoning.

Damage to motor and sensory control centers: Urinary frequency, urgency, or retention; urinary and fecal incontinence; constipation.

Sacral cord lesions: Impotence; diminished sensations that result in inhibited sexual response.

Physical assessment: Lhermitte's sign may be present in which an electrical sensation runs down the back and legs during neck flexion. Ophthalmoscopic inspection may reveal temporal pallor of optic disks. Reflex assessment may show increased deep tendon reflexes (DTRs) and diminished abdominal skin and cremasteric reflexes.

DIAGNOSTIC TESTS

Note: MS is sometimes called the "great masquerader." Diagnosis of MS usually is made after other neurologic disorders with similar symptoms have been ruled out, when the patient has experienced two or more exacerbations of neurologic symptoms, and when the patient has two or more areas of demyelinization or plaque formation throughout the CNS, as demonstrated by diagnostic tests, such as magnetic resonance imaging (MRI) and evoked potential studies, or by the patient's clinical symptoms.

MRI: Reveals presence of plaques and demyelinization in the CNS. This is the test of choice when MS is suspected. Expanding MRI technology is becoming ever more sensitive in identifying current sites of inflammation and demyelinization, as well as showing changes associated with disease progression.

Evoked potential studies: Responses may be slow or absent because of interference of nerve transmission from demyelinization or plaque formation.

Lumbar puncture (LP) and cerebrospinal fluid (CSF) analysis: Evaluates CSF levels of oligoclonal bands of immunoglobulin G (IgG), protein, γ-globulin, myelin basic protein, and lymphocytes, any of which may be elevated in the presence of MS. Oligoclonal bands of IgG are seen in 85%-95% of patients with MS and help confirm diagnosis. During acute MS attacks, destruction of the myelin sheath will release myelin basic protein into the CSF.

Computed tomography (CT) scan: Demonstrates presence of plaques and rules out mass lesions. This scan is less effective than MRI in detecting areas of plaque and demyelinization.

Electroencephalogram (EEG): Shows abnormal slowing in one third of patients with MS because of altered nerve conduction.

Positron emission tomography (PET): May show altered locations and patterns of cerebral glucose metabolism. This test usually is available only at research centers.

Nursing Diagnosis:

Deficient Knowledge:

Factors that aggravate and exacerbate MS symptoms

Desired Outcome: By day 3 of diagnosis (or before hospital discharge), patient and significant other verbalize accurate knowledge of factors that exacerbate, prevent, or ameliorate symptoms of MS.

INTERVENTIONS	RATIONALES
Teach patient and significant other to avoid heat, both external (hot weather, bath, shower) and internal (fever). Advise use of fans or air conditioning and acetaminophen or aspirin to reduce fever, if present.	Heat tends to aggravate weakness, pain, and other symptoms of MS. Coolants and antipyretics aid in reducing body temperature.
Caution patient to avoid exposure to persons known to have infections of any kind.	Infection often precedes exacerbations.
Teach indicators of common infections (see "Care of the Renal Transplant Recipient," p. 261) and importance of seeking prompt medical treatment should they occur.	An informed patient is likely to seek treatment in a timely manner.
Instruct patients to check body temperature periodically for fever and indications that a urinary tract infection (UTI) has reached the kidneys (e.g., costovertebral angle tenderness, chills, flank pain).	Because of the disease process, the patient may not feel any pain with urination.
Encourage patient to get sufficient rest, stop activity short of fatigue, and schedule activity and rest periods. See "Coronary Heart Disease" for **Health-Seeking Behaviors:** Relaxation technique effective for stress reduction, p. 183.	Avoiding stress and fatigue may prevent exacerbations. Examples of how to do this include sitting while getting dressed, sliding heavy objects along work surfaces rather than lifting, using a wheeled cart to transport items, and having work surfaces at the proper height. In addition, patient could ask health care provider for prescription for medication (e.g., amantadine, pemoline, fluoxetine, modafinil) that combats fatigue.
Provide information about birth control measures to female patients who desire counseling.	There may be an increase in exacerbations postpartum.
Encourage continued activity and normal lifestyle even when limitations are necessary.	Most persons with MS do not become severely disabled.

●●● **Related NIC and NOC labels:** *NIC:* Teaching: Disease Process; Learning Facilitation; Teaching: Prescribed Activity/Exercise; Infection Control; Energy Management *NOC:* Knowledge: Disease Process; Knowledge: Illness Care; Knowledge: Infection Control; Knowledge: Prescribed Activity

Nursing Diagnosis:

Chronic Pain

(and spasms) *related to* motor and sensory nerve tract damage

Desired Outcomes: Within 1-2 hr of intervention, patient's subjective evaluation of pain and spasms improves, as documented by a pain scale. Objective indicators, such as grimacing, are absent or reduced.

INTERVENTIONS	RATIONALES
Provide passive, assisted, or active range of motion (ROM) q2h and periodic stretching exercises. Teach these exercises to patient and significant other and encourage their performance several times daily. Administer antispasmodics as prescribed.	Reduces muscle tightness and spasms.
Suggest sleeping in a prone position.	May decrease flexor spasm of the hips and knees.
For other interventions, see "General Care of Patients with Neurologic Disorders," **Acute Pain,** p. 307.	

●●● **Related NIC and NOC labels:** *NIC:* Pain Management; Exercise Promotion; Stretching; Exercise Promotion: Joint Mobility *NOC:* Pain Control

Nursing Diagnosis:

Deficient Knowledge:

Purpose, precautions, and potential side effects of prescribed medications

Desired Outcome: Immediately following instruction (or before hospital discharge), patient verbalizes accurate information about the prescribed medication.

INTERVENTIONS	RATIONALES
Injectable glatiramer acetate (Copaxone), previously called copolymer I	May be prescribed to reduce frequency of relapses in relapsing-remitting MS. It is a synthetic copy of myelin basic protein and is believed to act as a "decoy" to spare the patient's myelin from immune system attack.
Teach patient to monitor for and report self-limiting reaction of chest tightness, palpitations, flushing, or anxiousness that may last 30 sec–30 min after injection. Injection site reaction (redness, swelling, pain) is also common. Notify health care provider of injection site redness, ongoing chest pain, shortness of breath, or dizziness.	Common side effects.
Explain importance of refrigerating medication.	Ensures its potency.
Caution patient that it is administered by SC route only.	Muscle stiffness may occur via IM route.
Teach patient to rotate injection site daily.	Pain at injection site is common.
Prednisone	May be prescribed during an exacerbation in an attempt to reduce symptoms by decreasing inflammation and associated edema of the myelin, thereby hastening onset of remission.

Continued

INTERVENTIONS	RATIONALES
Advise patient to take antacids, histamine H_2-receptor blockers, potassium (K^+) supplements, diuretics, blood pressure medications, and psychotropic agents as prescribed.	May combat side effects of steroids.
Teach patient to monitor for and report signs of sodium (Na^+) and fluid retention (increased weight and BP), gastric ulcers, stomach upset, weakness, hypokalemia, mood changes, impaired wound healing, and masking of infections.	These are common side effects of steroids.
Advise taking the medication with food, milk, or buffering agents and avoiding aspirin, indomethacin, caffeine, or other gastrointestinal (GI) irritants.	To help prevent gastric irritation.
Caution patient to taper rather than abruptly stop the drug when it is discontinued.	Helps maintain the body's own cortisone sources. Abrupt discontinuation may result in adrenal crisis.
Teach patient to be alert to and report symptoms of K^+ deficiency (anorexia, nausea, and muscle weakness) and to eat foods high in K^+.	Hypokalemia is a common side effect of steroid use.
Suggest patient eat foods low in Na^+ content.	Reduces potential for fluid retention.
Teach patient to monitor for and report black, tarry stools.	May signal occult blood, which can occur because of gastric ulcers.
Baclofen or dantrolene	May be given to decrease spasticity.
Teach patient to monitor for and report drowsiness, dizziness, fatigue, and nausea. In addition, dantrolene can cause diarrhea, muscle weakness, hepatitis, and photosensitivity.	Common side effects.
Advise patient to take the medication with food, milk, or a buffering agent.	Reduces gastric upset or nausea.
Caution patient to avoid alcohol consumption.	Alcohol has additive CNS depression effects.
Teach patient to monitor for and report severe diarrhea if taking dantrolene; avoid exposure to the sun and use sunscreens if exposure is unavoidable.	The drug may cause diarrhea and photosensitivity.
Caution patient to avoid activities that require alertness until the drug's effect on the CNS is known.	Can cause transient drowsiness.
Advise patients susceptible to seizures to use baclofen cautiously.	Baclofen can lower the seizure threshold.
Caution patients with diabetes mellitus who are taking baclofen that they may need an insulin dose adjustment.	Baclofen may raise blood glucose levels.
Advise caution during initial transfers/ambulation.	Some weak patients cannot tolerate the loss in the spasticity that may be permitting them to bear weight.
Teach patients taking dantrolene to monitor for and report fever, jaundice, dark urine, clay-colored stools, and itching.	These symptoms signal hepatitis, a potential side effect of this drug.
Bethanechol chloride	Smooth muscle stimulant that helps prevent urinary retention.
Teach patient to monitor for and report hypotension, diarrhea, abdominal cramps, urinary urgency, and bronchoconstriction.	Common side effects.
Advise that patient take the drug on an empty stomach.	Helps avoid nausea and vomiting.
Teach patient to notify health care provider if lightheadedness occurs.	Can signal hypotension, a potential side effect of this drug.
Caution patient to seek medical attention if an asthmatic attack occurs.	Avoids potentially life-threatening situation that can occur as a result of taking this drug.
Advise patient to make position changes slowly and in stages.	Prevents fainting caused by orthostatic hypotension, a potential side effect.

Continued

INTERVENTIONS	**RATIONALES**
Propantheline bromide, tolterodine, or oxybutynin	Smooth muscle relaxant that decreases urinary frequency and urgency.
Teach patient to monitor for and report dryness of the mouth, blurred vision, constipation, palpitations, increased heart rate, decreased sweating, and urinary retention or overflow incontinence.	Common side effects.
Teach measures that relieve constipation.	Constipation is a side effect.
Teach measures for remaining cool in hot or humid weather.	Heat stroke is more likely to develop while taking this medication.
Advise patient to notify health care provider immediately if urinary retention or overflow incontinence occurs.	Potential side effects that necessitate treatment.
Suggest that patient use sugarless gum, hard candy, or artificial saliva products if patient can chew and swallow effectively.	May reduce mouth dryness.
Encourage slow position changes and monitoring for dizziness.	Postural hypotension may occur when the drug is first started.
Mitoxantrone	Has received Food and Drug Administration (FDA) approval for secondary-progressive or worsening MS. This drug, in addition to being an immunosuppressive, also may cause heart and liver toxicity. Patient will be evaluated for normal cardiac function before starting the drug and will need periodic cardiac monitoring to ensure that there are no toxic cardiac effects. Medication has a lifetime cumulative dose restriction to limit toxicities.
Teach patient to be alert to and report swelling of feet and lower legs and shortness of breath.	Possible side effects.
Explain that risk of infection is increased and that it is important to avoid contact with people with infections, as well as live virus vaccinations. Teach patient to report signs of infection to health care provider (e.g., fever, chills, cough, hoarseness, lower back or side pain, and painful or difficult urination).	This drug decreases white blood cells, which help defend patient against infection.
Teach patient to be alert to and report mouth or lip sores, black tarry stools, and stomach pains.	Possible untoward effects of this drug.
Caution patient to report any jaundice.	This drug may affect liver function.
Teach patient that the following may occur: nausea, temporary hair loss, and menstrual changes. After taking medication, urine may be blue-green in color for about 24 hr.	Common side effects that generally do not require medical attention.
Caution patient that diarrhea should be reported if it continues.	Diarrhea is likely to occur, but if it is prolonged, it can result in dehydration.

●●● **Related NIC and NOC labels:** *NIC:* Teaching: Prescribed Medication *NOC:* Knowledge: Medication

Additional Nursing Diagnoses/Problems:

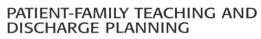

PATIENT-FAMILY TEACHING AND DISCHARGE PLANNING

The patient with MS may have a wide variety of symptoms that cause disability, ranging from mild to severe. When pro-viding patient-family teaching, focus on sensory information, avoid giving excessive information, and initiate a visiting nurse referral for necessary follow-up teaching. Include verbal and written information about the following:

✓ Remission/exacerbation aspects of the disease process.

✓ Safety measures relative to decreased sensation, visual disturbances, and motor deficits.

✓ Medications, including drug name, purpose, dosage, frequency, precautions, drug/drug and food/drug interactions, and potential side effects.

✓ Exercises that promote muscle strength and mobility, measures for preventing contractures and skin breakdown, transfer techniques and proper body mechanics, use of assistive devices and other measures to minimize neurologic deficits.

✓ Measures for relieving pain, muscle spasms, or other discomfort.

✓ Indications of constipation, urinary retention, or UTI; implementation of bowel and bladder training programs; self-catheterization technique or care of indwelling urinary catheters.

✓ Indications of upper respiratory infection; implementation of measures that help prevent regurgitation, aspiration, and respiratory infection.

✓ Dietary adjustments that may be appropriate for neurologic deficit (e.g., soft, semisolid foods for patients with chewing difficulties or a high-fiber diet for patients experiencing constipation).

✓ Importance of follow-up care, including visits to health care provider, physical therapist, and occupational therapist, as well as speech, sexual, or psychologic counseling.

✓ Referrals to community resources, such as local and national Multiple Sclerosis Society chapters, public health nurse, visiting nurse association, community support groups, social workers, psychologists, vocational rehabilitation agencies, home health agencies, extended and skilled care facilities, and financial counseling. Additional general information can be obtained by contacting the following organizations:

National Multiple Sclerosis Society
733 Third Avenue
New York, NY 10017
(800) 344-4867
www.nmss.org

Multiple Sclerosis Foundation
6350 North Andrews Avenue
Fort Lauderdale, FL 33309
(800) 441-7055
www.msfact.org

42

Parkinsonism

arkinson's disease (PD) is a slowly progressive degenerative disorder of the central nervous system (CNS) affecting the brain centers that regulate movement and balance. For unknown reasons, cell death occurs in the substantia nigra of the midbrain. When healthy, the substantia nigra projects dopaminergic neurons into the corpus striatum and releases the neurotransmitter dopamine in that area. Degeneration of these neurons leads to an abnormally low concentration of dopamine in the basal ganglia. The basal ganglia control muscle tone and voluntary motor movement via a balance between two main neurotransmitters, dopamine and acetylcholine. The deficit of dopamine, which has an inhibitory effect, allows the relative excess of acetylcholine. The excitatory effect of acetylcholine causes overactivity of the basal ganglia, which interferes with normal muscle tone and the control of smooth, purposeful movement, causing the characteristic symptoms of PD: muscle rigidity, tremors, and slowness of movement.

Parkinsonism has many possible causes. The majority of PD occurs without an apparent or known cause. Genetic susceptibility is believed to play a role. Parkinsonism is usually progressive, and death can result from aspiration pneumonia or choking. *Parkinsonian crisis,* a medical emergency, is usually precipitated by emotional trauma or failure to take the prescribed medications.

HEALTH CARE SETTING

Primary care with possible acute care hospitalization resulting from complications as the disease progresses

ASSESSMENT

Initially, symptoms are mild and include stiffness or slight hand tremors. They gradually increase and can become disabling. Cardinal features are tremors, rigidity, and bradykinesia. Assessment findings vary in degree and are highly individualized. PD is sometimes categorized as either tremor, predominant type, or postural instability and gait disturbance (PIGD).

Tremors: Increase when the limb is at rest and stop with voluntary movement and during sleep (nonintentional tremor).

"Pill-rolling" tremor of the hands and "to-and-fro" tremor of the head are typical.

Bradykinesia: Slowness, stiffness, and difficulty initiating movement. The patient may have a masklike, blank facial expression; "unblinking" stare; difficulty chewing and swallowing; drooling caused by decreased frequency of swallowing; and a high-pitched, monotonal, weak voice. Speech may be slow and slurred. The patient also has loss of automatic associated movements, such as the ability to swing the arms when walking and episodes of "freezing."

Increased muscle rigidity: Limb muscles become rigid on passive motion. Typically, this rigidity results in jerky ("cogwheel") motions or steady resistance to all movement ("lead-pipe" rigidity).

Loss of postural reflexes: Causes the typical stooped, forward leaning, shuffling, propulsive gait with short, rapidly accelerating steps; stumbling; and difficulty maintaining or regaining balance, which makes the individual prone to stumbling and falling. Abnormal gait in which the body is bent backward (retropulsion) also may be present.

Autonomic Symptoms: Excessive diaphoresis, seborrhea, postural hypotension, decreased libido, hypomotility of the gastrointestinal (GI) tract (causing constipation), and urinary hesitancy. Vision may blur as a result of lost accommodation.

Other: Dementia (e.g., forgetfulness, irritability, paranoia, hallucinations) commonly is associated with PD, particularly if Lewy bodies are present. However, not all patients develop impaired intellectual and mental functioning. Mental status testing may be complicated by the patient's movement disorder. Some patients may experience akathisia, a condition of motor restlessness in which the individual has a compelling need to walk about constantly. Handwriting becomes progressively smaller, cramped, and tremulous. Depression is common.

Physical assessment: Usually a positive blink reflex is elicited by tapping a finger between the patient's eyebrows. Blinking may occur 5-10 times/min instead of the normal 20 times/min. A positive palmomental (palm-chin) reflex can be elicited (muscles of the chin and corner of mouth contract when the patient's palm is stroked). Diminished postural reflexes are present on neurologic examination; however, there is risk of injury with this test because the patient may quickly lose balance and fall.

Parkinsonian crisis: This sudden and severe increase in bradykinesia, muscle rigidity, and tremors can lead to tachycardia, hyperpnea, hyperpyrexia, and muscle paralysis, causing an inability to swallow or maintain a patent airway.

Oculogyric crisis: Fixation of the eyes in one position, generally upward, sometimes for several hours. This is relatively rare.

Unified Parkinson's Disease Rating Scale (UPDRS) or Postural-Locomotor-Manual (PLM) test: May be used as a standardized assessment tool.

Core Assessment Program for Surgical Interventional Therapies in Parkinson's Disease (CAPSIT-PD): May be used for clinical assessment in clinical trials involving transplantation, as well as in therapeutic interventions such as pallidotomy and deep brain stimulation.

DIAGNOSTIC TESTS

Diagnosis usually is made on the basis of physical assessment and characteristic symptoms and after other neurologic problems have been ruled out.

Urinalysis: May reveal decreased dopamine level, which supports the diagnosis.

Medication withdrawal: Long-term therapy with large doses of medications, such as haloperidol or phenothiazines, can produce extrapyramidal side effects known as pseudoparkinsonism. If caused by these medications, symptoms will disappear when the drug is discontinued.

Electroencephalogram (EEG): Often shows abnormalities, such as diffuse, nonspecific slowing of Θ-waves.

Lumbar puncture (LP) with cerebrospinal fluid (CSF) analysis: May show decreased levels of dopamine or its metabolite in the CSF.

Positron emission tomography (PET; e.g., F-Dopa-PET): May reveal areas of decreased dopamine metabolism; usually available only in research settings.

Single photon emission computed tomography (SPECT): Reveals how a radioisotope-tagged drug accumulates in the brain. It may be useful in detecting PD and gauging disease progress.

Tremor studies: Serial measurements of functional activity will show decreased performance.

Cineradiographic study of swallowing: May show abnormal pattern and delayed relaxation of cricopharyngeal muscles.

Nursing Diagnosis:

Risk for Falls

related to unsteady gait secondary to bradykinesia, tremors, and rigidity

Desired Outcome: Within 1 hr following instruction, patient demonstrates safe and effective ambulatory techniques and preventive measures for falls.

INTERVENTIONS	RATIONALES
During ambulation, encourage patient to deliberately swing arms and raise feet.	To assist gait and help prevent falls.
Advise patient to step over imaginary object or line, practice taking long steps, and avoid shuffling.	Helps patient raise feet higher and increase stride.
Have patient practice movements that are especially difficult (e.g., turning). Teach patient to walk in a wide arc ("U-turn") rather than pivot when turning.	To avoid crossing one leg over the other.
Teach head and neck exercises.	To promote good posture.
Remind patient repeatedly to maintain upright posture and look up, not down, especially when walking.	To avoid dizziness and keep the focus on area ahead.
Advise patient to stop occasionally to slow walking speed. Teach patients to count cadence and concentrate on listening to feet as they touch the floor.	To prevent too fast a gait that could result in falls.
Encourage patient to lift toes, walk with heels touching floor first, and maintain a wide-based gait.	To keep soles of feet flat on the floor and avoid tripping.

Continued

INTERVENTIONS	RATIONALES
Provide a clear pathway while patient is walking. Teach patient to avoid crowds, scatter rugs, uneven surfaces, fast turns, narrow doorways, and obstructions. Advise patient to wear shoes with nonskid soles.	To minimize risk of falling.
Encourage patient to perform range-of-motion (ROM) and stretching exercises daily and to exercise for flexibility, strength, gait, and balance.	Routine exercises, along with prescribed medications, may prevent or delay disability. Exercises may be prescribed by a physical therapist.
Advise patient to wear leather-sole or smooth-sole shoes but to test shoes to ensure that they are not too slippery.	Rubber-sole or crepe-sole shoes tend to catch on floors, especially carpeted floors, and may cause falls.
Encourage males to keep a urinal at bedside. A commode at bedside may be helpful for females.	Slowness of gait and inability to get to the bathroom fast enough may cause incontinence. Keeping this equipment at the bedside helps eliminate need to rush to the bathroom, which could result in a fall.
For other interventions, see **Risk for Falls/Risk for Injury,** p. 293, in "General Care of Patients with Neurologic Disorders."	

●●● **Related NIC and NOC labels:** *NIC:* Fall Prevention; Surveillance: Safety; Environmental Management: Safety; Home Maintenance Assistance; Risk Identification; Teaching: Prescribed Activity/Exercise *NOC:* Safety Status: Falls Occurrence

Nursing Diagnosis:

Impaired Physical Mobility

related to difficulty initiating movement

Desired Outcome: Within 1 hr following instruction, patient demonstrates measures that enhance the ability to initiate desired movement.

INTERVENTIONS	RATIONALES
Teach patient measures that may help initiate movement.	Patients with PD often have difficulty initiating movement because their disease affects the brain centers that regulate movement and balance. Rocking from side to side may help initiate leg movement. Marching in place a few steps before resuming forward motion also may be helpful. Other measures that may help are relaxing back on heels and raising toes; tapping hip of the leg to be moved; bending at knees and straightening up; raising arms in a sudden, short motion; or humming a marching tune. If feet remain "glued" to the floor despite these measures, suggest that patient think of something else for a few moments and then try again. It might work to try changing directions (e.g., move sideways if going forward is impossible).
Teach patient measures that will help him or her to get out of a chair.	The deficit of dopamine, which has an inhibitory effect, allows the relative excess of acetylcholine. The excitatory effect of acetylcholine causes overactivity of the basal ganglia, which interferes with normal muscle tone and the control of smooth, purposeful movement, causing the characteristic symptoms of PD: muscle rigidity, tremors, and slowness of movement. These combined problems make it difficult to get out of a chair.

Continued

INTERVENTIONS	RATIONALES
	The following measure is helpful: get to edge of seat, place hands on arm supports, bend forward slightly, move feet back, and then rhythmically rock in the chair a few times before trying to get up.
Advise patient to sit in chairs with backs and arms and to purchase elevated toilet seats or sidebars in the bathroom.	To assist with rising from a sitting position and help prevent falls.
Teach patient measures that may help him or her to get out of bed.	The following measures may help with getting out of bed when at home: place blocks under legs of head of bed (HOB) to elevate it, rock to a sitting position, and tie a rope or sheet to foot of bed to help pull to a sitting position.
Teach patients and significant others to recognize situations that can cause freezing episodes.	"Freezing" is variable and can fluctuate with stress or emotional state. Patient and significant others can anticipate and plan to avoid these situations. For example, attempting two movements simultaneously, such as trying to change direction quickly while walking, can cause freezing. Distracting environmental, visual, or auditory stimuli also can precipitate a freezing episode. Doorways; narrow passages; or a change in floor color, texture, or slope can pose problems for many patients.
Provide a referral to Canine Partners as indicated.	Specially trained dogs (e.g., Canine Partners) can help patients walk or get back up if a fall occurs and are trained to help break a "freeze" by tapping on patient's foot.

●●● **Related NIC and NOC labels:** *NIC:* Positioning; Teaching: Psychomotor Skill; Self-Care Assistance; Teaching: Prescribed Activity/Exercise; Body Mechanics Promotion; Fall Prevention *NOC:* Transfer Performance; Mobility Level

Nursing Diagnosis:

Deficient Knowledge:

Side effects of and precautionary measures for taking anti-Parkinson medications

Desired Outcome: Immediately following instruction or within the 24-hr period before hospital discharge, patient and significant other verbalize accurate knowledge about the side effects of and necessary precautionary measures for taking anti-Parkinson medications.

INTERVENTIONS	RATIONALES
Side Effects Common to Most Anti-Parkinson Medications:	
Stress importance of taking medication on schedule and not forgetting a dose.	Missing a dose may adversely affect mobility. Patient and health care provider can adjust dose schedule so that medication peaks at mealtime or times when patient needs mobility most. Patients having difficulty with self-medicating should have premeasured doses in segmented or separate containers labeled with date/time of dose.
Teach patient to take non–levodopa-containing medications with meals.	To decrease potential for nausea.

Continued

INTERVENTIONS	RATIONALES
Encourage patient with anorexia to eat frequent, small nutritious snacks and meals.	Eating smaller meals rather than 3 larger meals is usually better tolerated in the patient who is anorexic.
Teach patient ways in which to counteract orthostatic hypotension and to report dizziness to health care provider.	Orthostatic hypotension is a potential side effect of these drugs. Patient should make position changes slowly and in stages and dangle legs a few minutes before standing. Antiembolism hose may help by promoting venous return. Males should urinate from a sitting rather than standing position if possible.
Teach ways to ease dry mouth and maintain integrity of oral mucous membrane.	Dry mouth is a common side effect of these drugs. Patient may try sugarless chewing gum or hard candy, frequent mouth rinses with water, or artificial saliva products to counteract this effect.
Advise patient to report any urinary hesitancy or incontinence.	May signal urinary retention. Individuals taking anticholinergics may find that voiding before taking medication relieves this problem.
Teach patient how to counteract constipation. For interventions, see **Constipation,** p. 75, in "Prolonged Bedrest."	Constipation is a common problem with these medications.
Teach patient to report mental status changes to health care provider promptly.	Many of these drugs can cause or aggravate mental status changes, such as confusion, mental slowness or dullness, and even agitation, paranoia, and hallucinations. Many side effects are dose related and can be controlled by an adjustment in the dosage.
Teach safety measures for patient with blurred vision.	Blurred vision is a side effect of many anti Parkinson drugs. Implementing safety measures such as keeping walkways unobstructed and asking for assistance when ambulating may help prevent falls.
Side Effects Specific to Levodopa:	
Teach patient that levodopa should be taken with a full glass of water on an empty stomach.	To facilitate absorption.
Suggest that patient eat 10-15 min after taking medication.	To minimize nausea or GI upset. If patient continues to experience GI upset or nausea, the medication may be taken with food.
Teach patient to avoid vitamin preparations or fortified cereals that contain pyridoxine (vitamin B$_6$) and if prescribed to limit intake of foods high in pyridoxine, such as wheat germ, whole grain cereals, legumes, and liver.	Pyridoxine reduces effectiveness of levodopa.
Teach patient to avoid excessive amounts of meat, eggs, dairy products, and legumes.	Although diet should meet recommended daily allowance of protein (i.e., 0.8 g/kg body weight), a dietary intake high in protein may interfere with effectiveness of levodopa. If dietary supplementation with L-tryptophan has been prescribed, it needs to be calculated into total protein allotment.
Advise patient that if possible, virtually all protein should be eaten at evening meal.	To minimize interaction with levodopa.
Instruct patient to report muscle twitching or spasmodic winking.	Early signs of overdose.
Teach patient to be alert to sudden and severe increase in bradykinesia (slowness of movement and speech), muscle rigidity, and tremors.	These are signs of parkinsonian crisis, which may occur if patient does not take this drug as scheduled or stops taking the drug abruptly.

Continued

INTERVENTIONS	RATIONALES
Emphasize need for immediate medical intervention with this crisis.	Respiratory and cardiac support may be necessary via IM or IV sodium phenobarbital or sodium amobarbital.
Stress importance of taking levodopa as scheduled and not to stop this medication abruptly.	These measures are necessary to avoid parkinsonian crisis.
Teach significant other to place patient in a quiet, calm environment with subdued lighting until medical help arrives if parkinsonian crisis occurs.	These measures are known to help ameliorate the crisis until medical interventions can be taken.
Explain signs of on-off response, wearing-off, other complications of therapy, and interventions and importance of reporting these problems to health care provider.	An informed patient will be more likely to report problems to health care provider, thereby facilitating fine-tuning of the medication regimen.
	On-off response: A rapid fluctuation or change in patient's condition. The individual is "on" one moment, in a state of relative mobility, and "off" the next, in a state of complete or nearly complete immobility. Although the cause is uncertain, it is believed to be related to fluctuating drug levels in the brain.
	"End of dose" wearing-off phenomenon: This is the return of signs and symptoms before next dose is given.
	Other complications of dopamine therapy: Choreiform or involuntary movements (e.g., facial grimacing, tongue protrusion, restlessness) and vivid dreaming
Teach patient and significant other to be alert to and report behavioral changes.	Severe depression with suicidal overtones can be caused by this drug and should be reported immediately. The health care provider may prescribe a dose reduction.
Explain that patient's medication may cause dark-colored urine and sweat.	Knowing what to expect may eliminate anxiety if these problems occur.
Caution patient to avoid alcohol.	Alcohol impairs levodopa's effectiveness.
Explain importance of medical follow-up while taking this drug.	To monitor for and manage such problems as increased intraocular pressure and changes in glucose control.
Side Effects Specific to Amantadine (Symmetrel):	
Teach patient to take this drug earlier in the day.	May help prevent insomnia, which is one of its side effects.
Teach patient and significant other to monitor for and report any shortness of breath, peripheral edema, significant weight gain, problems with urination, or change in mental status.	These are potential side effects.
Instruct patient not to stop taking this medication abruptly.	Doing so may precipitate parkinsonian crisis.
Teach patient to report changes in skin coloration and explain that it is not serious.	A diffuse, rose-colored mottling of the skin, usually confined to lower extremities, may develop. Exposure to cold or standing may make the color more prominent. The condition may subside with continued therapy and will disappear in a few weeks to months after the drug is discontinued. It may be reassuring to know that this condition is more cosmetic than serious.
Instruct patient to be alert for and promptly report to health care provider a loss of seizure control.	Patients with history of seizures may have an increase in the number of seizures.
Caution patient to avoid alcohol and CNS depressants.	These agents potentiate effects of amantadine.
Explain that most side effects of amantadine are dose related.	Many side effects can be controlled by an adjustment in the dosage.

Continued

INTERVENTIONS	RATIONALES
Side Effects Specific to Dopamine Agonists *(pramipexole, ropinirole, bromocriptine, pergolide, andropinirole, cabergoline)*:	
Caution patient to avoid alcohol when taking this medication.	Patient will experience less tolerance to alcohol.
Teach patient to avoid exposure to cold and to report onset of finger or toe pallor.	Bromocriptine can cause digital vasospasm.
Side Effects Specific to Anticholinergic Medications *(e.g., trihexyphenidyl, benztropine mesylate)*:	
Explain that patient should avoid strenuous exercise and keep cool during summer.	To avoid heat stroke. This medication may decrease perspiration.
Teach patient not to stop taking this medication abruptly.	Doing so can result in parkinsonian crisis.
Teach patient to monitor for increased heart rate or palpitations and to report either condition.	Many side effects such as this can be controlled by an adjustment in the dosage.
Side Effects Specific to Selegiline and Lazabemide:	
Stress importance of taking this medication only in prescribed dose and following dietary modifications to reduce intake of tyramine-containing foods.	Selegiline and lazabemide are selective monoamine oxidase (MAO) type B inhibitors and in the recommended dose of ≤10 mg/day do not cause the hypertensive crisis that can occur when tyramine-containing foods (e.g., cheese, red wine, beer, yogurt) are eaten. Dosages >10 mg/day may result in hypertension when tyramine-containing foods are eaten.
Advise patient to avoid meperidine and other opioids if possible.	Fatal drug interactions have occurred with patients taking other nonselective MAO inhibitors and could conceivably occur if higher-than-recommended doses were taken. At recommended doses, however, no drug interactions have been noted.
Teach patient to take the drug earlier in the day.	May prevent insomnia, a side effect of this drug.
Side Effects Specific to Entacapone:	
Teach patient that this medication might cause urine discoloration (brownish orange) but it is not clinically important.	An informed patient is not likely to become anxious if discoloration occurs.
Teach patient that hallucinations, increased dyskinesia, or persistent nausea or diarrhea should be reported promptly.	Many side effects are dose related and can be controlled by adjustment in dosage.

●●● **Related NIC and NOC labels:** *NIC:* Teaching: Prescribed Medication *NOC:* Knowledge: Medication

Nursing Diagnosis:

Health-Seeking Behaviors:

Facial and tongue exercises that enhance verbal communication and help prevent choking

Desired Outcome: Within 1 hr following the demonstration or within the 24-hr period before hospital discharge, patient demonstrates facial and tongue exercises and states the rationale for their use.

INTERVENTIONS	RATIONALES
Explain that special exercises can help strengthen and control facial and tongue muscles.	Routine exercises of facial and tongue muscles, along with prescribed medications, may prevent or delay disability. A speech therapist may need to be consulted to help with verbal communication.
Teach exercises that will improve verbal communication and help prevent choking and have patient return the demonstration.	Teaching, followed by return demonstration, is an effect way of helping patient understand and retain knowledge. Teaching patient how to hold a sound for 5 sec, sing the scale, recite alphabet and days of the week, practice vowel breaths (ah, oh, oo) and nonsense syllables (ma, me, mi, pull, pill, pie), read aloud, and extend tongue and try to touch chin, nose, and cheek will help improve verbal communication skills and help prevent choking.
Encourage patient to practice increasing voice volume.	This exercise will help combat monotone speech while promoting speech quality and understandability. This may be accomplished by having patient take a deep breath before speaking, open mouth to let sound come out more, use shorter sentences, exaggerate sound of every syllable, speak louder than others may think necessary, and use a tape recorder for feedback.
Provide a written handout that lists and describes the preceding exercises.	To reinforce patient's knowledge.
Encourage patient to perform them hourly while awake.	Frequency of performance will enhance patient's verbal communication skills.
Teach importance of stating feelings verbally. Encourage use of a mirror to practice expressing emotions such as happiness and displeasure.	Monotone speech and lack of facial expression impede nonverbal communication.

●●● **Related NIC and NOC labels:** *NIC:* Health Education; Self-Modification Assistance; Exercise Promotion *NOC:* Health Promoting Behavior

ADDITIONAL NURSING DIAGNOSES/ PROBLEMS:

PATIENT-FAMILY TEACHING AND DISCHARGE PLANNING

When providing patient-family teaching, focus on sensory information, avoid giving excessive information, and initiate a visiting nurse referral for necessary follow-up teaching. Include verbal and written information about the following:

✓ Related safety measures for patients with bradykinesia, muscle rigidity, and tremors.

✓ Emphasis that disability may be prevented or delayed through exercises and medications.

✓ Evaluation of home environment and tips for home accident prevention.

✓ Measures to prevent or lessen postural hypotension.

✓ Signs and symptoms of parkinsonian crisis (see p. 366) and the need for immediate medical attention.

✓ Referrals to community resources, such as local and national Parkinson's Society chapters, public health nurse, visiting nurses association, community support groups, social workers, psychologic therapy, vocational rehabilitation agency, home health agencies, and extended and skilled care facilities. Additional general information can be obtained by contacting the following organizations:

American Parkinson Disease Association
1250 Hylan Blvd., Suite 4B
Staten Island, NY 10305
(800) 223-APDA
www.apdaparkinson.com

Parkinson's Disease Foundation, Inc.
Executive Director

William Black Medical Research Building
Columbia Presbyterian Medical Center
710 West 168th Street
New York, NY 10032
(212) 923-4700 or (800) 457-6676
www.pdf.org

National Parkinson Foundation, Inc.
1501 NW 9th Avenue
Miami, FL 33136
(800) 327-4545
www.parkinson.org

✓ For other interventions, see "Patient-Family Teaching and Discharge Planning" (third through tenth entries only), in "Multiple Sclerosis," p. 359.

Seizure Disorders

Seizures result from an abnormal, uncontrolled, electrical discharge from the neurons of the cerebral cortex in response to a stimulus. If the activity is localized in one portion of the brain, the individual will have a partial seizure, but when it is widespread and diffuse, a generalized seizure occurs. Symptoms vary widely, depending on the involved area of the cerebral cortex. Seizures are generally manifested as an alteration in sensation, behavior, movement, perception, or consciousness lasting from seconds to several minutes. *Epilepsy* is a term used for recurrent seizures.

Seizure threshold refers to the amount of stimulation needed to cause the neural activity. The seizure threshold is lowered in some individuals, and this may result in spontaneous seizures. Potential causes for lowered seizure threshold include congenital defects, head injury, subarachnoid hemorrhage, intracranial tumors, infections, exposure to toxins, hypoxia, drug withdrawal, and metabolic and endocrine disorders. Phenothiazine, tricyclic antidepressants, and alcohol usage increase the risk of seizure by lowering the seizure threshold. If a trigger stimulus is identified, the individual has what is termed *reflex epilepsy*.

HEALTH CARE SETTING

Primary care with possible hospitalization for complications of therapy, continuous diagnostic video electroencephalogram (EEG) monitoring during pharmacologic or surgical interventions, or intensive care unit for status epilepticus.

ASSESSMENT

There are many clinical types of seizures, but the following are the most serious or common.

Generalized tonic-clonic (grand mal): Possible prodromal phase of increased irritability, tension, mood changes, or headache preceding the seizure by hours or days. Patient may experience an aura (a sensory warning, such as a sound, odor, or flash of light) immediately preceding the seizure by seconds or minutes. The seizure usually does not last more than 2-6 min and includes the following phases.

- *Tonic (rigid/contracted):* Often lasts only 15 sec, usually subsiding in less than 1 min. Symptoms include loss of consciousness, clenched jaws (potential for tongue to be bitten), apnea (may hear a cry as air is forced out of the lungs), and cyanosis. The patient may be incontinent, and the pupils may dilate and become nonreactive to light.
- *Clonic (rhythmic contraction and relaxation of the extremities and muscles):* May subside in 30 sec but can last 2-5 min. The eyes roll upward, and excessive salivation results in foaming at the mouth. During this phase, the potential is greatest for biting the tongue.
- *Stupor:* May last 5 min. The individual is limp and unresponsive. The pupils begin to react to light and return to their normal size.
- *Postictal:* In the period immediately after the seizure, the patient may be sleepy, semiconscious, confused, unable to speak clearly, and uncoordinated; have a headache; complain of muscle aches; and have no recollection of the seizure event. Temporary weakness, dysphasia, or hemianopia lasting up to 24 hr after the seizure may be experienced.

Generalized absence (petit mal): Patient has momentary loss of awareness with an abrupt cessation of voluntary muscle activity. The patient may appear to be daydreaming, with a vacant stare. Patient may experience facial, eyelid, or hand twitching. The patient usually does not lose general body muscle tone and so does not fall. The individual resumes previous activity when the seizure ends. There is usually no memory of the seizure, and the patient may have difficulty reorienting after the seizure event. This type of seizure can last 1-10 sec and may occur up to 100 times/day. This type of seizure usually resolves by puberty.

Generalized myoclonic: Sudden, very brief contraction or jerking of muscles or muscle groups. The individual may have a very brief, momentary loss of consciousness with some postictal confusion.

Partial simple motor (focal motor seizures): An irritative focus located in the motor cortex of the frontal lobe causes clonic movement in a particular part of the body, such as the hands or face. If the seizure activity spreads or marches in an orderly fashion to an adjacent area (e.g., the hands to the arms to the shoulders), the seizure is termed a *focal motor seizure with jacksonian march*. The seizure usually lasts several seconds to minutes. There is no loss of consciousness. Other simple, partial seizures with somatosensory symptoms (e.g., smells, sounds), autonomic symptoms (e.g., tachycardia, tachypnea, diaphoresis, goose bumps [piloerection], pallor, flushing), or psychic symptoms (e.g., fear, déjà vu) may be experienced.

Partial complex seizure (psychomotor, "temporal lobe"): Generally lasts 1-4 min. Usually there is loss of consciousness and a postictal state of confusion lasting several minutes. However, the individual does not fall to the ground. The patient is able to interact with the environment, exhibits purposeful but inappropriate movements or behavior, and has no memory of the event. The individual will perform such automatisms as lip smacking, chewing, facial grimacing, picking, or swallowing movements. These patients may experience and remember various sensory or emotional hallucinations or sensations that occur immediately before the seizure, such as smells, ringing or hissing sounds, or feelings of déjà vu, fear, or pleasure.

Status epilepticus: State of continuous or rapidly recurring seizures in which the individual does not completely recover baseline neurologic functioning between seizures. Individuals who suddenly stop taking their antiepilepsy medication are likely to develop this condition. This is a medical emergency, especially with tonic-clonic seizures, resulting in such potential complications as cerebral anoxia and edema, aspiration, hyperthermia, and exhaustion. Irreversible damage may occur in 60 min. Death may result.

Other classifications: Seizures also can be classified according to epileptic syndrome, for example, generalized epilepsies, idiopathic with age-related onset. Establishing the correct diagnosis of seizure type and, when possible, epilepsy syndrome will help tailor effective antiepilepsy drugs and treatment.

DIAGNOSTIC TESTS

Because a variety of problems can precipitate seizures, testing may be extensive. Common tests include the following:

Serum glucose and electrolytes: To rule out metabolic causes, such as hypoglycemia, hyponatremia, or hypocalcemia.

EEG—both sleeping and awake: To reveal abnormal patterns of electrical activity, particularly with such stimuli as flashing lights or hyperventilation. Telemetry EEGs may also be performed. Generalized tonic-clonic seizures show up as high, fast-voltage spikes in all leads.

Magnetic resonance imaging (MRI): To show structural lesions causing partial seizures; also may reveal a space-occupying lesion, such as a tumor or hematoma.

Positron emission tomography (PET): To check for areas of cerebral glucose hypometabolism that correlate with the irritative seizure-causing focus. This test is useful in partial seizures but is available only in a few centers.

Computed tomography (CT) scan: To check for presence of a space-occupying lesion, such as a tumor or hematoma.

Skull x-ray examination: To reveal fractures, tumors, calcifications, or congenital anomalies (pineal shift, ventricular deformity).

Lumbar puncture (LP) and cerebrospinal fluid (CSF) analysis: To rule out increased intracranial pressure (IICP) or infection, such as meningitis, as the source of the seizures; also can check brain levels of gamma aminobutyric acid (GABA).

Single photon emission computed tomography (SPECT): To measure cerebral blood flow; may be used to evaluate patients for surgery (e.g., ictal-SPECT).

Nursing Diagnosis:

Risk for Trauma

related to oral, musculoskeletal, and airway vulnerability secondary to seizure activity

Desired Outcomes: Patient exhibits no signs of oral or musculoskeletal tissue injury or airway compromise after the seizure. Patient's significant other verbalizes knowledge of actions necessary during seizure activity.

INTERVENTIONS	RATIONALES
Seizure precautions: Pad side rails with blankets or pillows. Keep side rails up and bed in its lowest position when patient is in bed. Keep bed, wheelchair, or stretcher brakes locked.	To promote safety and protect patient from trauma should a seizure occur.
Tape a soft rubber oral airway to the bedside. Remove wooden tongue depressors (if used, they may splinter). Keep suction and oxygen equipment readily available.	To maintain a patent airway, prevent hypoxia, and protect patient from trauma should a seizure occur.
Consider a heparin lock for IV access for high-risk patient.	Some antiepilepsy drugs must be administered IV, especially as loading doses or in the event of sustained seizure activity.

Continued

INTERVENTIONS	**RATIONALES**
Use electronic tympanic thermometers for patients at high risk for seizure.	Glass or other breakable oral thermometers should be avoided when taking patient's temperature because of the harm they could cause patient should they break.
Caution patient to lie down and push call button if experiencing prodromal or aural warning. Keep call light within reach.	Prodromal or aural warnings precede seizures in many patients.
Encourage patient to empty mouth of dentures or foreign objects when experiencing prodromal or aural warning.	To prevent choking.
Do not allow unsupervised smoking.	To prevent fire damage to patient and surroundings should a seizure occur.
Evaluate need for and provide protective headgear as indicated.	To protect patient's head should a seizure occur.
During the seizure: Remain with patient. Observe for, record, and report type, duration, and characteristics of seizure activity and any postseizure response.	Seizure activity should be documented in detail to aid in management and differentiation of seizure type and identification of triggering factors. Characteristics of seizure and postseizure response should include, as appropriate, precipitating event, aura, initial location and progression, automatisms, type and duration of movement, changes in level of consciousness (LOC), eye movement (e.g., deviation, nystagmus), pupil size and reaction, bowel and bladder incontinence, head deviation, tongue deviation, or teeth clenching.
Prevent or break the fall and ease patient to floor if seizure occurs while patient is out of bed. Keep patient in bed if seizure occurs while there and lower head of bed (HOB) to a flat position.	To promote patient's physical safety.
If patient's jaws are clenched, do not force an object between the teeth. If able to do so safely and without damage to oral tissue, insert an airway.	Forcing objects into patient's mouth could break teeth or lacerate oral mucous membranes.
Avoid use of tongue depressors. A rolled washcloth may be used as an alternative.	Tongue depressors may splinter; a rolled washcloth may be used to prevent lip and tongue biting.
Never put your fingers in patient's mouth.	Patient may bite your fingers.
Protect patient's head from striking the ground. Remove from environment objects (e.g., chairs) patient may strike. Pad floors to protect patient's arms and legs. Remove patient's glasses.	To protect patient's head and extremities from injury during seizure activity. A towel folded flat or hands may be used to cushion patient's head from striking the ground.
Do not restrain patient but rather guide patient's movements gently.	To prevent injury caused by flailing.
Roll patient into a side-lying position. Use head-tilt/chin-lift maneuver. Provide O₂ and suction as needed.	To promote drainage of secretions, maintain a patent airway, and prevent hypoxia.
Loosen tight clothing, collar, or belt.	To prevent injury/hypoxia caused by constrictive clothing.
Maintain patient's privacy. Clear nonessential people from the room.	Seizures likely are embarrassing for the patient.
After the seizure: Reassure and gently reorient patient. Check neurologic status and VS.	During the postictal period that follows the seizure, patient will need to be reoriented and reassured because some memory lapse will have occurred during the event.
Ask patient if an aura preceded the seizure activity. Record this information and postictal characteristics.	An aura is a sensory warning such as a sound, odor, or flash of light. It can be used to warn patient of an impending seizure.

Continued

INTERVENTIONS	RATIONALES
Provide a quiet, calm environment. Keep talk simple and to a minimum. Speak slowly and with pauses between sentences.	Sounds and stimuli can be confusing to the awakening patient. Repetition may be necessary.
Use room light that is behind, not above, patient.	To prevent additional seizures triggered by the light and for patient comfort.
Do not offer food or drink until patient is fully awake.	To prevent vomiting/aspiration.
Check patient's tongue for lacerations and body for injuries. Monitor for weakness or paralysis, dysphasia, or visual disturbances. Document accordingly.	Potential occurrences during a seizure.
Monitor urine for red or cola color.	May signal rhabdomyolysis or myoglobinuria from muscle damage.
If patient vomited during the seizure, notify health care provider.	This is a sign that aspiration can occur with subsequent seizures.
As indicated, check fingerstick blood glucose.	To detect hypoglycemia, a potential metabolic cause of the seizure.
Obtain serum laboratory tests as prescribed.	Electrolyte disorders such as hyponatremia and hypocalcemia can trigger a seizure.
Monitor for status epilepticus (i.e., state of continuous or rapidly recurring seizures in which the individual does not completely recover baseline neurologic functioning). Notify health care provider immediately.	This condition is life threatening and can cause cerebral anoxia and edema, aspiration, hyperthermia, and exhaustion.
Provide significant other with verbal and written information for the preceding interventions.	Significant other is likely to be in patient's presence during subsequent seizures. If well informed, he or she will be able to protect patient from trauma and life-threatening complications.

●●● **Related NIC and NOC labels:** *NIC:* Environmental Management: Safety; Fall Prevention; Home Maintenance Assistance; Vital Signs Monitoring; Seizure Precautions *NOC:* Safety Status: Physical Injury

Nursing Diagnosis:

Deficient Knowledge:

Life-threatening environmental factors and preventive measures for seizures

Desired Outcomes: Before hospital discharge or within 1 hr following teaching, patient verbalizes accurate information about measures that may prevent seizures and environmental factors that can be life threatening in the presence of seizures. Patient exhibits health care measures that reflect this knowledge.

INTERVENTIONS	RATIONALES
Assess patient's knowledge of measures that can prevent seizures and environmental hazards that can be life threatening in the presence of seizure activity.	This assessment enables nurse to provide or clarify information as indicated and facilitates development of an individualized teaching plan.
Advise patient to check into state regulations about automobile operation.	Most states require 1-3 seizure-free years before an individual can obtain a driver's license.

Continued

INTERVENTIONS	**RATIONALES**
Caution patient to refrain from operating heavy or dangerous equipment, swimming, climbing to excessive heights, and possibly even tub bathing until he or she is seizure free for amount of time specified by health care provider. Teach patient never to swim alone, regardless of amount of time he or she has been seizure free.	To prevent injury that could result while performing these activities should a seizure occur.
Caution patient to swim only in shallow water and in the company of a strong swimmer.	To make rescue easier if a seizure occurs.
Advise patient to turn temperature of hot water heaters down.	To prevent scalding if a seizure occurs in the shower or bath.
Encourage stress management, progressive relaxation techniques, biofeedback, and diaphragmatic respiratory training.	To control emotional stress and hyperventilation, which can trigger seizures.
Caution patient who rides a bike, for example, to wear a helmet and avoid heavy traffic.	Some activities, such as climbing or bicycle riding, require careful risk/benefit evaluation.
Encourage vocational assessment and counseling.	The patient's epilepsy may place others at risk in some occupations, such as bus driver or airline pilot.
Advise female patients that seizure activity may change (increase or decrease) during menses or pregnancy. Provide birth control information if requested.	Tonic-clonic seizures have caused fetal death. Antiepilepsy drugs are associated with birth defects; however, 90% of women have normal pregnancies and healthy children. When seizures in women worsen with hormonal changes, suppressing ovulation with medication may be recommended.
Teach that use of stimulants (e.g., caffeine) and depressants (e.g., alcohol) should be avoided.	Withdrawal from stimulants and depressants can increase likelihood of seizures.
Teach patient to get adequate amounts of rest, avoid physical and emotional stress, and maintain a nutritious diet.	Measures that may help prevent seizures.
Recommend a balanced diet spaced evenly throughout the day. A ketogenic diet (high in fats, low in carbohydrates) appears to reduce seizures in children.	To prevent hypoglycemia, which may trigger seizures.
If stimuli such as flashing lights, video or computer games, or loud music appear to trigger seizures, advise patient to avoid environments that are likely to have these stimuli. Explain that poorly adjusted TVs should be fixed, and patient should monitor for and treat fever early during an illness and avoid overhydration.	These are examples of seizure triggers and measures that can prevent them.
Encourage individuals who have seizures that occur without warning to avoid chewing gum or sucking on lozenges.	May be aspirated during a seizure.
Encourage patient to wear a Medic-Alert bracelet or similar identification or to carry a medical information card.	To provide information to health care professionals if patient is unable to.

●●● **Related NIC and NOC labels:** *NIC:* Teaching: Disease Process; Learning Readiness Enhancement; Teaching: Individual; Risk Identification; Health Education; Behavior Modification *NOC:* Knowledge: Disease Process; Knowledge: Health Behaviors; Knowledge: Personal Safety

Nursing Diagnosis:

Deficient Knowledge:

Purpose, precautions, and side effects of antiepilepsy medications

Desired Outcome: Before hospital discharge or following teaching, patient verbalizes accurate knowledge about the prescribed antiepilepsy medication.

INTERVENTIONS	RATIONALES
Stress importance of taking prescribed medication regularly and on schedule and not discontinuing medication without health care provider guidance.	Missing a scheduled dose can precipitate a seizure several days later. Lack of seizures does not mean the drug is unnecessary. Abrupt withdrawal of any antiepilepsy medication can precipitate seizures. Discontinuing these medications is the most common cause of status epilepticus.
Assist patients in finding methods that will help them remember to take the medication and monitor their drug supply to avoid running out.	Drugs may be necessary for duration of patient's life, and a fool-proof method of remembering to take them and keeping them well stocked should be initiated early on.
Explain concept of drug half-lives and steady blood levels.	It is important to maintain a therapeutic blood level of the drug to manage seizures. Drugs differ in amount of time they remain in the body and reach peak activity.
Caution patient to consult health care provider before changing from a trade name to a generic medication.	There are possible differences in bioavailability.
Encourage patient to keep a drug and seizure chart "diary."	To help detect trend of seizures, which will enable health care provider to determine if current treatment is at a therapeutic level.
Stress importance of keeping appointments for periodic laboratory work and informing health care provider about side effects (e.g., bruising, bleeding, jaundice).	To determine whether blood levels are therapeutic and manage side effects. For example, many antiepilepsy medications can cause blood dyscrasias or liver damage.
Explain that vitamin D, vitamin K, and folic acid supplements may be prescribed.	To help counteract bruising, bleeding, or jaundice.
Advise patient to avoid activities that require alertness until central nervous system (CNS) response to the medication has been determined.	Antiepilepsy medications may make people drowsy.
Teach patient to take the drug with food or large amounts of liquid.	To minimize gastric upset. Nausea and vomiting are common side effects of most antiepilepsy medications.
Advise patients taking valproic acid, topiramate, and zonisamide not to chew the medication.	These drugs may irritate the oral mucous membrane.
Also advise patients taking valproic acid that this drug may produce a false-positive test for urine ketones; any vision change should be reported immediately.	A vision change may signal ocular toxicity, which necessities timely intervention.
Instruct patient to notify health care provider if a significant weight gain or weight loss occurs.	May necessitate a change in dose or scheduling.
Teach patient to avoid alcoholic beverages and over-the-counter (OTC) medications containing alcohol.	Long-term alcohol use stimulates the body to metabolize phenytoin (Dilantin) more quickly, thus lowering the seizure threshold because of decreased plasma phenytoin levels.
Caution patients taking phenobarbital (Luminal) or primidone (Mysoline) to avoid alcohol.	Potentiates CNS depressant effects.
Caution patient to avoid OTC medications.	Anticonvulsant agents are potentiated or inhibited by many drugs, including aspirin and antihistamines, and may affect potency of other medications as well.
Instruct patient to report uncoordinated movement (ataxia), double vision (diplopia), involuntary/rhythmic eye movement (nystagmus), and dizziness.	Other side effects common to antiepilepsy medications.
Teach patients who take carbamazepine (Tegretol), ethosuximide (Zarontin), or zonisamide to report immediately fever, mouth ulcers, sore throat, peripheral edema, dark urine, bruising, or bleeding.	Side effects of these drugs.

Continued

INTERVENTIONS	RATIONALES
Advise patients taking phenytoin to perform frequent oral hygiene with gum massage and gentle flossing and brush teeth 3-4 times/day with a soft toothbrush. Teach patient to report immediately any measlelike rash.	This drug can cause gingival hypertrophy and rash.
Caution patients taking phenytoin that there are two types of this drug: Dilantin Kapseal is absorbed more slowly and is longer acting.	It is important not to confuse this extended-release phenytoin with prompt-release phenytoin. Doing so may cause dangerous underdose or overdose.
Caution patient that generic phenytoin should not be substituted for Dilantin Kapseal.	Dilantin Kapseal is the slow-release type and should be maintained to ensure therapeutic form.

●●● **Related NIC and NOC labels:** *NIC:* Teaching: Prescribed Medication; Medication Management
NOC: Knowledge: Medication

Nursing Diagnosis:

Noncompliance: Therapy

related to denial of the illness or perceived negative consequences of the treatment regimen secondary to social stigma, negative side effects of antiepilepsy medications, or difficulty with making necessary lifestyle changes

Desired Outcome: Before hospital discharge or immediately following interventions, patient verbalizes accurate knowledge about the disease process and treatment plan, acknowledges consequences of continued noncompliant behavior, explains the experience that caused patient to alter the prescribed behavior, describes the appropriate treatment of side effects or the appropriate alternatives, and exhibits health care measures that reflect this knowledge, following an agreed-on plan of care.

INTERVENTIONS	RATIONALES
Assess patient's understanding of the disease process, medical management, and treatment plan.	This assessment enables nurse to explain or clarify information as indicated and facilitates development of an individualized care plan.
Assess for causes of noncompliance, such as financial constraints, inconvenience, forgetfulness, medication side effects, or difficulty making significant lifestyle changes or following medication schedule.	Once causes are identified the nurse can then focus the care plan accordingly.
Explain drug half-life and concept of a steady blood level. Explain importance of health care provider guidance if medication is stopped for any reason. Instruct and provide written instructions for patient in how to contact health care provider and importance of health care provider and laboratory follow-up. Explain what to do if a dose is missed and how to refill a prescription if medication is lost or depleted.	Intermittent medication use may be informal experimentation or an effort to gain control. Explanations of consequences helps ensure awareness that stopping medications can be life threatening (e.g., cause status epilepticus).
Promote patient's expression of feelings (e.g., dependence, powerlessness, embarrassment, being different). In addition, determine patient's perception of effectiveness or noneffectiveness of treatment.	To evaluate patient's perception of vulnerability to the disease process and ascertain signs of denial of the illness.
Confront myths and stigmas. Provide realistic assessment of risks.	To determine if a value, cultural, or spiritual conflict is causing noncompliance and thereby counter misconceptions.

Continued

INTERVENTIONS	RATIONALES
Discuss methods of dealing with common problems, such as obtaining insurance and counteracting job or workplace discrimination.	Helping to eliminate problems optimally will promote compliance.
Assess patient's support systems.	To determine whether presence of a family disruption pattern (whether or not it is caused by patient's illness) is making compliance difficult and "not worth it."
After the reason for noncompliance is found, intervene accordingly. If it appears that changing medical treatment plan (e.g., scheduling medications) may promote compliance, discuss this possibility with health care provider. Provide patient with information about interventions that can minimize the drug's side effects (e.g., taking drug with food or large amounts of liquid to minimize gastric distress).	To help facilitate compliance.
Encourage involvement with support systems, such as local epilepsy centers and national organizations.	Many people appreciate the support of others with the same condition. Feeling less alone and supported by others may promote compliance.

●●● **Related NIC and NOC labels:** *NIC:* Patient Counseling; Behavior Modification; Learning Facilitation; Support System Enhancement; Teaching: Disease Process; Family Involvement Promotion; Coping Enhancement; Family Support *NOC:* Compliance Behavior; Adherence Behavior

ADDITIONAL NURSING DIAGNOSES/ PROBLEMS:

Ineffective Coping	p. 87
"Psychosocial Support" for **Disturbed Body Image**	p. 92
"Psychosocial Support for the Patient's Family and Significant Others" for **Interrupted Family Processes**	p. 95

PATIENT-FAMILY TEACHING AND DISCHARGE PLANNING

When providing patient-family teaching, focus on sensory information, avoid giving excessive information, and initiate a visiting nurse referral for necessary follow-up teaching. Include verbal and written information about the following:

✓Reinforcement of knowledge of disease process, pathophysiology, symptoms, and precipitating or aggravating factors.

✓Medications, including drug name, purpose, dosage, schedule, precautions, drug/drug and food/drug interactions, and potential side effects. In addition, patient should wear a Medic-Alert bracelet.

✓Importance of follow-up care and keeping medical appointments. Stress that use of antiepilepsy drugs necessitates periodic monitoring of blood levels to ensure therapeutic medication levels and assessment for side effects. Instruct patient to keep emergency contact numbers for health care provider.

✓An uncomplicated convulsive seizure in an individual known to have epilepsy is not necessarily a medical emergency. On average, these people can continue about their business after a rest period. An ambulance should be called or medical attention sought if the seizure happens in water; if there is any question of the seizure being caused by epilepsy; if the individual is injured, pregnant, or diabetic; if the seizure lasts longer than 5 min; if a second seizure starts; or if consciousness does not begin to return.

✓Environmental factors that can be life threatening in the presence of seizures, measures that may help prevent seizures, and safety interventions during seizures. Review state and local laws that apply to individuals with seizure disorders. Sensible safety precautions should be employed at home or in the work environment related to use of shatterproof glass, uncluttered stairs, handrails, helmets when cycling, adequate sleep, and stress avoidance.

✓Employment or vocational counseling as needed. Discuss need to avoid overprotection and maintain, as possible, normal work and recreation.

✓Risks of antiepilepsy drugs during pregnancy. Provide birth control information or genetic counseling referral as requested.

✓Provide the following address as appropriate:

Epilepsy Foundation of America
4351 Garden City Drive, Suite 406
Landover, MD 20785
(301) 459-3700 or (800) 332-1000
www.efa.org

Spinal Cord Injury

The spinal cord injuries (SCIs) discussed in this section are caused by vertebral fractures or dislocations that sever, lacerate, stretch, or compress the spinal cord and interrupt neuronal function and transmission of nerve impulses. Blood supply to the spinal cord also may be interrupted. The spinal cord swells in response to injury, and this, along with hemorrhage, can cause additional compression, ischemia, and compromised function. Neurologic deficits resulting from compression may be reversible if the resulting edema and ischemia do not lead to spinal cord degeneration and necrosis. SCIs are classified in a number of different ways according to type (open, closed), cause (concussion, contusion, laceration, transection), site (level of spinal cord involved), mechanism of injury (compression, hyperflexion, hyperextension, rotational, penetrating), stability, and degree of spinal cord function loss (complete, incomplete). A *spinal cord concussion* is a transient loss of cord function caused by a traumatic event and resulting in immediate flaccid paralysis that resolves completely in a matter of minutes or hours.

Prognosis: Any evidence of voluntary motor function, sensory function, or sacral sensation below the level of injury indicates an incomplete SCI, with the potential for partial or complete recovery. The level of injury is the lowest level in which motor function and sensation remain intact. After an acute injury, the spinal cord usually goes into a condition called *spinal shock,* in which there can be total loss of spinal cord function below the level of injury. During spinal shock there is no reflex activity. If there is no evidence of returning motor function after local reflexes have returned, the spinal cord is considered irreversibly damaged. Generally, SCI does not cause immediate death unless it is at C1 through C3, which results in respiratory muscle paralysis. Individuals who survive these injuries require a ventilator for the rest of their lives.

HEALTH CARE SETTING

Acute care, subacute care, rehabilitation center

ASSESSMENT

Acute indicators: Loss of sensation, weakness, or paralysis below the level of injury; localized pain or tenderness over the site of injury; headache; hypothermia or hyperthermia; and alterations in bowel and bladder function.

Cervical injury: Possible alterations in level of consciousness (LOC), weakness or paralysis in all four extremities (quadriparesis or quadriplegia), paralysis of respiratory muscles or signs of respiratory problems, such as flaring nostrils and use of accessory muscles for respirations. Any cervical injury can result in a low body temperature (to 96° F [35.5° C]), slowed pulse rate (<60 bpm) caused by vagal stimulation of the heart, hypotension (systolic BP <80 mm Hg) caused by vasodilation, and decreased peristalsis.

Thoracic and lumbar injuries: Paraparesis/paraplegia or altered sensation in the legs; hand and arm involvement in upper thoracic injuries.

Acute spinal shock: Can last 2 days to 4-6 mo but usually resolves in 1-6 wk. Spinal shock results from a loss of sympathetic nerve outflow below the level of injury. Indicators depend on the severity of the injury and include total loss of spinal cord function, loss of skin sensation, flaccid paralysis or absence of reflexes below the level of injury, paralytic ileus and constipation secondary to atonic bowel, bladder distention secondary to atonic bladder, bradycardia, low/falling BP secondary to loss of vasomotor tone and decreased venous return, and anhidrosis (absence of sweating and loss of temperature regulation) below the level of injury. Autonomic instability is more dramatic in higher (e.g., cervical) lesions.

Chronic Indicators: As spinal shock resolves, muscle tone, reflexes, and some function may return, depending on severity and level of injury. The return of reflexes usually results in muscle spasticity. Chronic autonomic dysfunction may be manifested as fever; mild hypotension; anhidrosis; and alterations in bowel, bladder, and sexual function. Chronic neural pain may occur after SCI and tends to occur as either diffuse pain below the level of injury or pain adjacent to the level of injury. Injuries at or below L1 may result in permanent flaccid paralysis. Orthostatic hypotension is more typical of lesions above T7.

Upper motor neuron (UMN) involvement: UMNs are nerve cell bodies that originate in high levels of the central nervous system (CNS) and transmit impulses from the brain down the spinal cord. Injury will interrupt this impulse transmission, causing muscle or organ dysfunction below the level of injury. However, because the injury does not interrupt reflex arcs coming from those muscles or organs to the spinal cord, hypertonic reflexes, clonus paralysis, and spastic paralysis are seen. The patient will have a positive Babinski's reflex.

Lower motor neuron (LMN) involvement: LMNs are anterior horn cell bodies that originate in the spinal cord. LMNs transmit nerve impulses to muscles and organs and are involved in reflex arcs that control involuntary responses. Damage to LMNs will abolish voluntary and reflex responses of muscles and organs, resulting in flaccid paralysis, hypotonia, atrophy, and muscle fibrillations and fasciculations. The patient will have an absent Babinski's reflex.

Bowel and bladder dysfunction: Usually conscious sensation of the need to void or defecate is lost. UMN bowel and bladder involvement results in reflex incontinence. Flaccid LMN bladder involvement causes urinary retention with overflow incontinence. Flaccid LMN bowel involvement causes fecal retention/impaction.

Autonomic dysreflexia (AD): An exaggerated and unopposed sympathetic response to noxious stimuli below the SCI lesion can be life threatening as reflex activity returns. AD is seen most commonly in patients with injuries at or above T6, but it has been reported in patients with injuries as low as T8. Signs and symptoms include gross hypertension (up to 240-300/150 mm Hg), pounding headache, blurred vision, bradycardia, nausea, and nasal congestion. Above the level of the injury, flushing and sweating may occur. Below the level of injury, piloerection (goose bumps) and skin pallor, which signal vasoconstriction, often occur. Seizures, subarachnoid hemorrhage, cerebrovascular accident (CVA), or retinal hemorrhage may occur.

Physical assessment:
- **Acute (spinal shock):** Absence of deep tendon reflexes (DTRs) below level of injury; absence of cremasteric reflex (scratching or light stroking of the inner thigh for male patients causes the testicle on that side to elevate) for T12 and L1 injuries; absence of penile or anal sphincter reflex.
- **Chronic:** Generally, increased DTRs occur if the spinal cord lesion is of the UMN type.

DIAGNOSTIC TESTS

X-ray examination of the spine: To delineate fracture, deformity, or displacement of vertebrae, as well as soft tissue masses, such as hematomas.

Computed tomography (CT) scan: To reveal changes in the spinal cord, vertebrae, and soft tissue surrounding the spine.

Myelography: To show blockage or disruption of the spinal canal; used if other diagnostic examinations are inconclusive. Radiopaque dye is injected into the subarachnoid space of the spine, using a lumbar or cervical puncture.

Magnetic resonance imaging (MRI): To reveal changes in the spinal cord and surrounding soft tissue. MRI evaluation is preferred for evaluation of the degree of injury in patients who can tolerate it.

Arterial blood gas (ABG)/pulmonary function tests: To assess effectiveness of respirations and detect the need for O_2 or mechanical ventilation.

Cystometry: To assess capacity and function of the bladder after resolution of spinal shock for the best type of bladder training program.

Pulmonary fluoroscopy: To evaluate the degree of diaphragm movement and effectiveness in individuals with high cervical injuries.

Evoked potential studies (e.g., somatosensory): To help locate the level of spinal cord lesion by evaluating the integrity of the nervous system's anatomic pathways and connections. Stimulation of a peripheral nerve triggers a discrete electrical response along a neurologic pathway to the brain. Response or lack of response to stimulation is measured in this test.

Nursing Diagnosis:

Risk for Autonomic Dysreflexia

related to exaggerated unopposed autonomic response to noxious stimuli below the level of injury for individuals with SCI at or above T6

Desired Outcomes: On an ongoing basis, patient is free of symptoms of AD as evidenced by BP within patient's baseline range, HR 60-100 bpm, and absence of headache and other clinical indicators of AD. Following instruction, patient and significant other verbalize knowledge of factors that cause AD, treatment and prevention, and when immediate emergency treatment is indicated.

INTERVENTIONS	RATIONALES
Monitor for indicators of AD, including hypertension (>20 mm Hg above baseline but may go as high as 240-300/150 mm Hg), pounding headache, bradycardia, blurred vision, nausea, nasal congestion, flushing and sweating above the level of injury, and piloerection (goose bumps) or pallor below level of injury. Remove antiembolism hose to enable assessment of lower extremities.	AD is a medical emergency that can occur after spinal shock resolution for patients with SCIs at or above T6, although cases have been reported in patients with injuries as low as T8.
If AD is suspected, raise head of bed (HOB) immediately to 90 degrees or assist patient into a sitting position. Remove antiembolism hose and binders.	To lower patient's blood pressure and decrease venous return. Seizures, subarachnoid hemorrhage, myocardial infarction (MI), CVA, or retinal hemorrhage can occur if severe hypertensive episode continues.
Call for someone to notify health care provider; stay with patient, and try to find and ameliorate the noxious stimulus. Speed is essential.	The noxious stimulus (e.g., a distended bladder) must be found and alleviated as quickly as possible.
Monitor BP q3-5min during hypertensive episode.	To assess trend of the BP.
Remain calm and supportive of patient and significant other.	They will be very anxious.
Assess the following sites for causes and implement measures for removing the noxious stimulus:	
Bladder: Distention, urinary tract infection (UTI), calculus and other obstructions, bladder spasms, catheterization, or bladder irrigations performed too quickly or with too cold a liquid.	Problems with the bladder are the most likely causes of AD.
Do not use Credé's method for a distended bladder.	May produce stimuli that would trigger AD.
Catheterize patient (ideally using anesthetic jelly) if there is a possibility or question of bladder distention. Consult health care provider *stat*.	Bladder distention is a potential cause of AD and requires immediate intervention. Anesthetic jelly prevents skin stimulation, which could trigger AD.
If a catheter is already in place, check tubing for kinks and lower drainage bag. For catheter obstruction such as sediment, irrigate catheter as indicated, using no more than 30 ml of normal saline. If catheter patency is uncertain, recatheterize patient using anesthetic jelly.	These interventions check for catheter tube patency. An obstruction is a potential cause of AD.
If the bladder is not distended, check for cloudy urine, hematuria, and positive laboratory or x-ray results.	Signs of UTI and/or urinary calculi.
Obtain urine specimen.	For culture and sensitivity studies as indicated. A UTI may be a potential cause of AD.
Bowel: Constipation, impaction, insertion of suppository or enema, or rectal examination.	Problems with the bowel are the second most likely cause of AD.
Do not attempt rectal examination without first anesthetizing the rectal sphincter and anal canal with anesthetic jelly.	Prevents skin stimulation, which could trigger AD.
Use large amounts of anesthetic jelly in anus and rectum before disimpacting bowel.	A bowel impaction is a potential cause of AD.
Wait 5 min before disimpacting.	To ensure anesthetic jelly has been effective, as manifested by a lower BP
Skin: Pressure, infection, injury, heat, pain, or cold.	These are possible causes of AD.
Loosen clothing and remove antiembolism hose, leg bandages, abdominal binder, or constrictive sheets as appropriate.	Pressure on the skin is a potential cause of AD.
For male patients, check for pressure source on penis, scrotum, or testicles and remove pressure if present.	

Continued

INTERVENTIONS	RATIONALES
Check skin surface below level of injury. Monitor for presence of a pressure area or sore, infection, laceration, rash, sunburn, ingrown toenail, or infected area. Or check skin for contact with a hard object. If indicated, apply a topical anesthetic.	Skin infection, pain, and injury are potential causes of AD.
Observe for and remove source of heat or cold (e.g., ice pack, heating pad).	Topical heat and cold are two potential causes of AD.
Additional causes: Surgical manipulation, incisional pain, sexual activity, menstruation, labor, vaginal infection.	
Administer antihypertensive agents, such as SL nifedipine, hydralazine, or diazoxide as prescribed.	To lower blood pressure for patient's safety.
On resolution of the crisis, answer patient's and significant other's questions about AD. Discuss signs and symptoms, treatment, and methods of prevention. Encourage patient to wear a medical-alert type bracelet or tag.	Prevention is the best way to deal with AD. A good bowel regimen and skin integrity program are key factors in preventing the noxious stimuli that constipation or pressure areas may cause.
Loosen clothing, bed sheets, and constricting bands; turn patient off side. Keep the bed free of sharp objects and wrinkles. Adhere to turning schedules. Institute measures to reduce the potential for UTI and urinary calculi and teach the patient self-inspection of skin and urinary catheter and the importance of using anesthetic jelly for catheterization and disimpaction.	To relieve other possible sources of pressure.

●●● **Related NIC and NOC labels:** *NIC:* Dysreflexia Management; Neurologic Monitoring; Vital Signs Monitoring; Anxiety Reduction; Emergency Care; Infection Control; Medication Administration; Positioning; Surveillance: Safety; Temperature Regulation; Urinary Elimination Management; Bowel Management; Heat Exposure Treatment; Infection Protection; Skin Surveillance; Urinary Catheterization *NOC:* Neurological Status: Autonomic; Symptom Severity; Vital Signs Status

Nursing Diagnosis:

Constipation

related to immobility and decreased peristalsis, atonic bowel, and loss of sensation and voluntary sphincter control secondary to sensorimotor deficit

Desired Outcome: Patient has bowel movements that are soft and formed every 1–3 days or within patient's preinjury pattern.

INTERVENTIONS	RATIONALES
During acute phase of spinal shock, assess patient's bowel function. Notify health care provider of significant findings.	To assess for constipation, ileus, and presence of fecal impaction. During acute phase of spinal shock, which usually resolves in 1-6 wk, constipation and paralytic ileus are common.
In the presence of fecal impaction, ensure gentle manual removal or administer small-volume enema.	The atonic intestine distends easily.
Avoid long-term use of enemas.	May disrupt normal flora and affect peristalsis and sphincter tone.
Administer stool softeners (e.g., docusate sodium) if prescribed.	To keep stool soft and prevent fecal impaction while the bowel is atonic.

Continued

INTERVENTIONS	RATIONALES
Manage a flaccid bowel with increased intraabdominal pressure techniques (see below), manual disimpaction, and small-volume enemas.	Lesions below the conus medullaris (T12) may injure S3, S4, and S5 nerve segments, resulting in disruption of the reflex arc and causing an LMN flaccid bowel and loss of anal tone.
For patient with UMN reflex bowel, once bowel activity returns, explain desirability of attempting bowel movement 30 min after a meal or warm drink.	This regimen will enable patient's gastrocolic and duodenocolic peristalsis reflexes to assist with evacuation. Lesions above the conus medullaris (located at the lower two levels of the thoracic region where the cord begins to taper) generally leave S3, S4, and S5 spinal cord nerve segments intact. If the spinal reflex arc is intact, patient will have a UMN bowel and be capable of stimulating (training) reflex evacuation of the bowel.
In addition, teach patient to bear down, bend forward, or apply manual pressure to the abdomen.	To promote bowel movement by increasing intraabdominal pressure. An abdominal belt may be used if patient is unable to strain at stool. Massaging abdomen in a clockwise, circular motion may help as well.
As prescribed, use a medicated suppository if necessary. If allowed, provide a bedside commode. Check patient's ability to maintain balance on a commode.	To promote bowel evacuation.
If patient is bedridden, turn onto side with a pad to catch bowel movement rather than a bedpan.	To prevent skin breakdown in dependent areas that would be in contact with bedpan's hard surface. Patient is at risk because depression of autonomic nervous system below lesion level affects circulation and muscle tone.
For patients with injuries at T8 or above, promote adequate fluid intake (>2500 ml/day) and use of stool softeners and high-fiber diet.	To promote soft, formed stools.
Use suppositories and enemas only when essential and with extreme caution.	They can precipitate AD.
Use anesthetic jelly liberally when performing a rectal examination or inserting a suppository or an enema.	To decrease potential for AD.
For patients with hand mobility (who are not at risk for AD), teach technique for suppository insertion and digital stimulation of the anus.	To promote reflex bowel evacuation. Suppository inserters and rectal stimulation devices are available for patients with limited hand mobility.
For digital stimulation, insert lubricated finger about 1½-2½ inches into rectum and gently rotate in a circular motion, gently stretching sphincter, for about 30 sec (but no longer than a minute at a time) until the internal sphincter relaxes. Restart circular motion if sphincter tightens and remove finger if bowel movement begins. Stop if sphincter spasms are felt or if signs of AD occur. Repeat q5-10min several times until adequate evacuation occurs. If unsuccessful after 20-30 min of stimulation, insert a suppository.	Digital stimulation stretches and relaxes the internal sphincter to facilitate bowel movement.
Teach patient to keep fingernails cut short.	To prevent injury to the rectal mucosa.
For other interventions, see **Constipation** in "General Care of the Neurologic Patient" p. 302.	

●●● **Related NIC and NOC labels:** *NIC:* Bowel Management; Constipation/Impaction Management; Fluid Management; Medication Management; Nutrition Management; Self-Care Assistance: Toileting
NOC: Bowel Elimination

Nursing Diagnosis:

Ineffective Airway Clearance

related to neuromuscular paralysis/weakness or restriction of chest expansion secondary to halo vest obstruction

Desired Outcome: Within 24 hr following interventions, patient has a clear airway as evidenced by RR of 12-20 breaths/min with normal depth and pattern (eupnea) and absence of adventitious breath sounds.

INTERVENTIONS	RATIONALES
Monitor ventilation capability by checking vital capacity, tidal volume, and pulmonary function tests. Monitor serial ABG values and/or pulse oximetry readings.	If vital capacity is <1 L or if patient exhibits signs of hypoxia (PaO_2 <80 mm Hg, O_2 saturation ≤92%, tachycardia, increased restlessness, mental status changes or dullness, cyanosis), these are indicators of respiratory insufficiency and signal need to notify health care provider immediately.
Monitor for increasing difficulty with secretions, coughing, respiratory difficulties, bradycardia, fluctuating BP, and increased motor and sensory losses at a higher level than baseline findings.	These signs may signal ascending cord edema secondary to effects of contusion or bleeding. Patient may require increased respiratory support.
Monitor for loss of previous ability to bend arms at the elbows (C5-C6) or shrug shoulders (C3-C4). If these findings are noted, notify health care provider immediately.	Changes from baseline or previous assessment may signal problems such as contusion, compression, bleeding, or damage to blood supply and necessitate prompt intervention.
Keep patient's head in neutral position and suction as necessary. Be aware that suctioning may cause severe bradycardia in the patient with AD. If indicated, prepare patient for a tracheostomy, endotracheal intubation, and/or mechanical ventilation. If appropriate, arrange for a transfer to intensive care unit (ICU) for continuous monitoring.	To maintain a patent airway and support respiratory function.
If patient is wearing halo vest traction, assess respiratory status at least q4h or more frequently as indicated.	To ensure that vest is not restricting chest expansion.
Teach use of incentive spirometry.	To promote adequate ventilation and assess for quality of patient's inspiratory capability.
Be alert to the following: shortness of breath, hemoptysis, tachycardia, and diminished breath sounds.	Indicators of pulmonary embolus (PE), which is a common complication because of impaired ventilation, altered vascular tone, and decreased mobility. Pain may or may not be present with PE, depending on level of SCI. Sudden shoulder pain may be referred pain from PE.
If patient's cough is ineffective, implement the following technique, known as "assisted coughing": place palm of your hand under patient's diaphragm (below xiphoid process and above navel). As patient exhales forcibly, push up into diaphragm.	To assist in producing a more forceful cough. Assisted coughing may be contraindicated in patients with spinal instability.
Feed patients in Stryker frames, Foster beds, or similar mechanical beds in prone position. Raise stable patients in halo traction to high Fowler's position if it is not contraindicated.	To minimize potential for aspiration.
For additional information, see **Risk for Aspiration,** p. 101, in "Older Adult Care."	

●●● **Related NIC and NOC labels:** *NIC:* Airway Management; Respiratory Monitoring; Vital Signs Monitoring; Ventilation Assistance; Airway Suctioning; Aspiration Precautions; Positioning; Cough Enhancement; Artificial Airway Management; Mechanical Ventilation; Laboratory Data Interpretation *NOC:* Respiratory Status: Ventilation; Respiratory Status: Gas Exchange; Respiratory Status: Airway Patency; Aspiration Control

Nursing Diagnosis:

Risk for Disuse Syndrome

related to paralysis, immobilization, or spasticity secondary to SCI

Desired Outcomes: After stabilization of the injury, patient exhibits complete range of motion (ROM) of all joints. By time of discharge from care facility, patient demonstrates measures that promote mobility, reduce spasms, and prevent complications.

INTERVENTIONS	RATIONALES
Once injury is stabilized, assist patient with position changes on a regular schedule.	To alternate sites of pressure relief and decrease risk for contracture formation. For example, a prone position, if not contraindicated, helps prevent sacral decubiti and hip contractures.
For patients with spasticity, use hand splints or cones, keeping fingers extended.	To assist with maintaining a functional grasp.
If patient has spasticity, fit him or her with splints or high-top tennis shoes that are cut off at the toes so that each shoe ends just proximal to the metatarsal head.	To help prevent foot contractures for patients with spasticity. These shoes help keep feet dorsiflexed but prevent contact of balls of feet with a hard surface, which can cause spasticity.
Avoid footboards for these patients.	The hard surface may trigger spasticity and promote plantar flexion.
Teach patient that some factors that trigger spasms are cold, anxiety, fatigue, emotional distress, infections, bowel or bladder distention, ulcers, pain, tight clothing, and lying too long in one position.	Controlling these factors may reduce number of spasms experienced.
Teach patients with spasticity proper positioning, ROM, and daily sustained stretching exercises.	Steady, continuous, directional stretching several times daily is especially important because it may decrease spasticity for several hours. Cooling and icing techniques, heat, vibration therapy, and transcutaneous electrical nerve stimulation (TENS) of spastic muscles also may be helpful.
Limit touching of patient by caregivers. When touch is necessary, do it in a firm, gentle, steady manner.	Tactile stimulation may trigger spasms.
For additional interventions, see **Risk for Disuse Syndrome,** p. 69, in "Prolonged Bedrest."	

●●● **Related NIC and NOC labels:** *NIC:* Exercise Promotion: Stretching; Positioning; Teaching: Prescribed Activity/Exercise; Pressure Ulcer Prevention *NOC:* Immobility Consequences: Physiological

Nursing Diagnosis:

Risk for Injury

related to incorrect neck position, irritation of cranial nerves, impaired lateral vision secondary to presence of halo vest traction, and lack of access for external cardiac compression

Desired Outcome: At time of discharge from care facility (and ongoing during use of halo traction), patient exhibits no adverse changes in motor, sensory, or cranial nerve function and is free of symptoms of injury caused by impaired vision.

INTERVENTIONS	RATIONALES
Assess position of patient's neck in relation to the body. Alert health care provider to presence of flexion or hyperextension.	To ensure proper alignment, patient's neck should be in a neutral position.
Assess any difficulty with swallowing.	May signal improper position of neck and chin.
Keep a torque screwdriver in a secure place.	To ensure that health care provider can readily adjust tension on bars to return patient's neck position to neutral.
Evaluate degree of sensation and movement of upper extremities and assess cranial nerve function. Notify health care provider of sudden changes in motor, sensory, or cranial nerve function (e.g., weakness, paresthesias, ptosis, difficulty chewing or swallowing).	Changes in cranial nerve function can occur if cranial pins compress or irritate a nerve.
Never use superstructure of halo traction in turning or moving patient.	This could cause misalignment of patient's affected area.
Assess pins, bolts, and vest structure for looseness at least daily. Notify health care provider if pins or vest become loose or dislodged. Stabilize patient's head as necessary.	Clicking sounds may signal a loose pin, and if this occurs, it will be necessary to stabilize patient's head to prevent misalignment.
Instruct patient to avoid pulling clothes over top of halo apparatus but rather step into and pull clothes up over feet and legs. Advise patient to buy strapless bras, tube tops, or clothes that are several sizes larger or to modify neck openings (e.g., with Velcro closures, ties).	To prevent loosening pins.
Avoid loosening a buckle without health care provider's directive.	The device must be worn correctly to maintain alignment, prevent skin breakdown, and prevent nerve injury. Buckle holes should be marked so that they are always cinched correctly to appropriate snugness.
If patient is ambulatory, teach how to survey environment while walking, either by using a mirror, by turning eyes to their extreme lateral positions, or by turning entire body. Suggest use of a cane to help determine height of curbs and detect unseen objects or uneven walking surfaces.	The halo vest impairs lateral vision.
Explain that trunk flexibility is limited and achieving balance can be difficult. Suggest ambulating with a walker initially to help patient learn to adjust. Advise abdominal- and back-strengthening exercises to aid balance and walking. Caution patient that bending over can be hazardous.	The vest's weight is top-heavy.
Advise patient to walk only in low-heel shoes. Caution that extra space allowance may be needed when passing through doorways and to avoid bumping into objects. Advise wearing slip-on shoes and using long-handled assistive devices to reach or pick up objects.	To prevent falls and other injuries caused by wearing the vest.
Suggest use of a shower chair that rolls and usually can fit over a toilet seat, providing an extra 3-6 inches in height.	This is the best method to promote safety and avoid straining to raise and lower body onto toilet seat.
To get out of bed, teach patients to roll onto their side at edge of bed and then drop their legs over side of bed while pushing up their trunk sideways.	To promote alignment and good body mechanics.
Recommend backing into car seat with body bent forward for getting into a car.	Prevents hitting pins and device on car door frame.
Caution patient against driving.	Patient will have limited field of vision when wearing the vest.
Teach patient to use high tables and swivel chairs at home.	A high table will help bring objects into better view, and a swivel chair will permit easier visualization of the entire environment while wearing the vest.

Continued

INTERVENTIONS	RATIONALES
Explain that patient will need assistance of another person to shampoo hair.	Promotes safety and helps prevent falling should water spill on floor.
Advise that shampooing a short haircut is easiest and that hair should be blown dry.	Toweling hair dry may loosen pins.
Teach caregivers and significant other how to release vest in an emergency.	For example, this may be necessary if patient were to require external cardiac compression.

●●● **Related NIC and NOC labels:** *NIC:* Fall Prevention; Surveillance: Safety; Emergency Care; Environmental Management: Safety; *NOC:* Safety Status: Physical Injury

Nursing Diagnosis:

Risk for Impaired Skin Integrity and/or Impaired Tissue Integrity

related to altered circulation and mechanical factors secondary to presence of halo vest traction or tongs

Desired Outcome: At time of discharge and on an ongoing basis, patient's skin is nonerythemic and unbroken; tissue underlying and surrounding the halo vest blanches appropriately.

INTERVENTIONS	RATIONALES
Inspect skin around vest edges for erythema and other signs of irritation. Keep skin dry.	To detect signs of impaired circulation caused by the vest. Skin is kept dry to prevent irritation.
Gently massage nonerythematous areas routinely.	To promote circulation.
Teach patient skin inspection, which may require use of a mirror, flashlight, or another person.	If patient detects breakdown, sensitive spots, odor, dirty vest liner, or loose pins, he or she should notify health care provider for timely intervention.
Investigate complaints of discomfort or uncomfortable fit. Pad vest as needed until it can be properly adjusted or trimmed by health care provider. Protect vest from moisture and soiling.	A finger should be able to fit between vest and patient's skin. Weight loss or gain can affect fit.
Be alert to foul odor from in or around cast openings.	Can signal pressure necrosis beneath vest. Serosanguineous drainage on a pillowcase slipped through the vest from one side to another may indicate an area of skin breakdown.
Instruct/assist patient with changing body position q2h. If patient is in bed, support vest and use log-roll technique with sufficient help.	To promote circulation and prevent skin and tissue breakdown by alternating sites of pressure relief.
Use soft padding.	To prevent pressure on prominent body areas such as forehead or shoulder.
Use a small pillow under patient's head or roll under neck at sleep time.	Promotes comfort and provides support for the neck while preventing misalignment of affected area by flexion.
Wash skin under the vest with soap and warm water.	Usually, releasing one vest belt at a time as patient is lying down is allowed for washing.
Avoid use of lotion and powder.	These products can cake under vest.
Replace soiled linens promptly. Dry perspiration with hair dryer on a cool setting.	Prevents skin irritation and breakdown caused by moisture.

Continued

INTERVENTIONS	RATIONALES
Be alert to presence of a rash.	Patient may be allergic to vest's lining. A synthetic liner, knitted body stockinette, or T-shirt may correct this problem.
In event of skin breakdown, keep skin cleansed, dried, and covered with a transparent dressing.	To protect exposed skin from further breakdown and promote healing.
Notify health care provider and orthotist accordingly	Skin breakdown necessitates a brace adjustment.
Place rubber corks over tips of halo device.	To diminish annoying sound vibrations if the apparatus is bumped and to prevent skin lacerations from sharp edges.

●●● **Related NIC and NOC labels:** *NIC:* Pressure Management; Circulatory Precautions; Positioning; Simple Massage; Traction/Immobilization Care; Skin Surveillance; Skin Care: Topical Treatments; Pressure Ulcer Prevention *NOC:* Immobility Consequences: Physiological; Tissue Integrity: Skin & Mucous Membranes

Nursing Diagnosis:

Urinary Retention or Reflex Urinary Incontinence

related to neurologic impairment (spasticity or flaccidity occurring with SCI)

Desired Outcomes: Patient has urinary output without incontinence. Patient empties bladder with residual volumes of <50 ml by time of discharge. Following instruction, patient demonstrates triggering mechanism and gains some control over voiding.

INTERVENTIONS	RATIONALES
General guidelines for individuals with bladder dysfunction	
If intermittent catheterization is used and episodes of incontinence occur or more than 500 ml of urine is obtained, catheterize patient more often.	Bladder dysfunction is complicated and should be assessed by cystometric testing to determine best type of bladder program. Initially patient will have an indwelling urinary catheter or scheduled intermittent catheterizations.
Teach patient and significant other procedure for intermittent catheterization, care of indwelling catheters, and indicators of UTI (e.g., fever, cloudy and/or foul-smelling urine, malaise, anorexia, restlessness, incontinence).	To ensure readiness for self-care on discharge from care facility.
Teach patient and significant other about a habit/bladder scheduling program.	When the bladder can hold 300-400 ml of urine, measures to stimulate voiding are attempted. This program consists of gradually increasing time between catheterizations or periodically clamping indwelling catheter. The goal is a gradual increase in bladder tone.
Make sure that patient takes fluids at even intervals throughout the day.	Promotes adequate hydration and increased bladder tone.
Restrict fluids before bedtime.	To prevent nighttime incontinence. Alcohol and caffeine-containing foods and beverages (e.g., cola, chocolate, coffee, tea) have a diuretic effect and may cause incontinence. In addition, caffeine-containing products may increase bladder spasms and reflex incontinence.
Instruct patients using bladder-emptying techniques to void at least q3h.	To maintain regular schedule and prevent distention. Wristwatches with timer alarms or an alarm clock can help patient maintain this schedule.

Continued

INTERVENTIONS	RATIONALES
Catheterize patient after an attempt to empty bladder.	To obtain postvoid residual urine. Residual amounts >100 ml usually indicate need for return to scheduled intermittent catheterization program.
Guidelines for patients with UMN-involved spastic reflex bladder Explain to these patients that eventually they may be able to empty bladder automatically and may not require catheterization.	Lesions above conus medullaris (located at lower two levels of the thoracic region where the cord begins to taper) generally leave the S2, S3, and S4 spinal cord nerve segments intact. If this spinal reflex arc is intact, the patient will have UMN-involved bladder, resulting in a spastic bladder. This bladder has tone and occasional bladder contractions and periodically will empty on its own, resulting in reflex incontinence. The UMN-involved bladder is "trainable" with techniques that stimulate reflex voiding.
Implement/teach techniques that stimulate the voiding reflex. Perform selected technique for 2-3 min or until a good urine stream has started. Wait 1 min before trying another stimulation technique.	The following techniques stimulate the voiding reflex and should be taught to patient accordingly. - *Bladder tapping:* Position self in a half-sitting position. Tapping is performed over the suprapubic area, and the patient may shift the site of stimulation within that area to find the most effective site. Tapping is performed rapidly (7-8 times/sec) with one hand for approximately 50 single taps. Continue tapping until a good stream starts. When stream stops, wait about 1 min and repeat tapping until bladder is empty. One or two tapping attempts without response indicate that no more urine will be expelled. - *Anal stretch technique (contraindicated in individuals with lesions at T8 or above because of the potential for AD):* Position self on commode or toilet. Lean forward on thighs and insert 1 or 2 lubricated fingers into anus to anal sphincter. Spread anal sphincter gently by spreading fingers apart or pulling in a posterior direction. Maintain stretching position, take a deep breath, and hold breath while bearing down to void. Relax and repeat until bladder is empty.
Teach patients with abdominal muscle control to bear down using Valsalva's maneuver when attempting to trigger voiding.	Increasing intraabdominal pressure may help promote voiding by overcoming sphincter pressure.
Teach patient that incontinence is a possibility and that incontinence briefs will help manage accidents.	Incontinence can occur as a result of stimulating reflex trigger zones.
Avoid plastic or rubber sheets.	These sheets trap heat and moisture, promoting skin breakdown.
Administer baclofen if prescribed.	Baclofen tends to promote more complete emptying of the bladder by reducing tone of external urinary sphincter.
Guidelines for patients with LMN-involved flaccid bladders	Lesions below the conus medullaris (T12) may injure the S2, S3, and S4 nerve segments, which will disrupt the reflex arc, causing an LMN-involved flaccid bladder. This bladder has no tone and will distend until it overflows, resulting in overflow incontinence.
Explain that occasionally patient may be able to empty bladder manually well enough to avoid catheterization.	Need for catheterization can be determined by checking residual urine volume.
Teach patient bladder-emptying techniques, such as straining or Valsalva's maneuver.	These techniques increase intraabdominal pressure, which may overcome sphincter pressure to enable bladder emptying.

Continued

INTERVENTIONS	RATIONALES
If Credé's method is prescribed, teach the technique to patient.	Credé's method is another technique for increasing intraabdominal pressure. It is performed as follows: place ulnar surface of the hand horizontally along umbilicus; while bearing down with abdominal muscles, press hand downward and toward bladder in a kneading motion until urination is initiated; continue 30 sec or until urination ceases.
For either technique, wait a few minutes and repeat the procedure.	To ensure complete emptying of the bladder.
Recognize, however, that use of Credé's method is controversial.	There is potential for reflux past the vesicoureteral junction, and this reflux would increase risk for ascending UTIs.
Suggest alternative measures if patient's bladder cannot be trained to empty completely.	Intermittent catheterization or external collection devices usually are indicated, and patient may be a candidate for an artificial inflatable sphincter device or urinary diversion.

●●● **Related NIC and NOC labels:** *NIC:* Urinary Elimination Management; Urinary Retention Care; Fluid Management; Self-Care Assistance: Toileting; Urinary Catheterization: Intermittent; Urinary Bladder Training; Urinary Habit Training *NOC:* Urinary Elimination

Nursing Diagnosis:

Ineffective Cardiopulmonary and Cerebral Tissue Perfusion

related to relative hypovolemia secondary to decreased vasomotor tone with SCI

Desired Outcomes: By at least 24 hr before hospital discharge (or as soon as vasomotor tone improves), patient has adequate cardiopulmonary and cerebral tissue perfusion as evidenced by systolic BP >90 mm Hg and orientation to person, place, and time. For a minimum of 48 hr before discharge from care facility, patient is free of dysrhythmias.

INTERVENTIONS	RATIONALES
Monitor for hypotension (drop in systolic BP >20 mm Hg, systolic BP <90 mm Hg), lightheadedness, dizziness, fainting, and confusion.	Low/falling BP can occur secondary to loss of vasomotor tone and decreased venous return.
Monitor heart rate and rhythm. Document dysrhythmias.	Sinus tachycardia/bradycardia may develop because of impaired sympathetic innervation or unopposed vagal stimulation.
Monitor I&O.	Adequate hydration and elimination status are necessary to maintain stable hemodynamics.
Give prescribed IV fluids cautiously.	Impaired vascular tone can make patient sensitive to small increases in circulating volume. Intravascular volume expanders or vasopressors may be required for hypotension.
Implement measures that prevent episodes of decreased cardiac output caused by postural hypotension.	Decreased cardiac output compromises cerebral and peripheral circulation. Postural hypotension is seen frequently in SCI, but it can be prevented and managed. These measures include: - Changing position slowly. - Performing ROM exercises q2h.

Continued

INTERVENTIONS	RATIONALES
	- Preventing patient's legs from crossing, especially when in a dependent position to prevent venous pooling.
	- Patients with SCI at higher levels, especially above T6, may require abdominal binder in addition to antiembolic hose and sequential compression devices or pneumatic foot pumps. These individuals are prone to more severe hypotensive reactions, even with minor changes, such as raising HOB.
	- Working with physical therapist (PT) to implement a gradual sitting program that will help patient progress from a supine to an upright position. This may include a bed that can rotate gradually from a horizontal position to a vertical position or a chair that has multiple positions progressing from flat to sitting. The goal is to increase patient's ability to sit upright while avoiding adverse effects, such as hypertension, dizziness, and fainting.
For additional information, see **Ineffective Cerebral Tissue Perfusion** in "Prolonged Bedrest," p. 73.	

●●● **Related NIC and NOC labels:** *NIC:* Cardiac Care: Acute Dysrhythmia Management; Fluid Management; Vital Signs Monitoring; Hypovolemia Management; Neurologic Monitoring; Cerebral Perfusion Promotion; Positioning *NOC:* Cardiac Pump Effectiveness; Tissue Perfusion: Cardiac; Tissue Perfusion: Pulmonary; Vital Signs Status; Tissue Perfusion: Cerebral

Nursing Diagnosis:

Ineffective Peripheral and Cardiopulmonary Tissue Perfusion

related to interrupted blood flow (venous stasis) with corresponding risk of thrombophlebitis and pulmonary emboli (PE) secondary to immobility and decreased vasomotor tone

Desired Outcome: For at least 24 hr before discharge from care facility and on an ongoing basis, patient has adequate peripheral and cardiopulmonary tissue perfusion as evidenced by absence of heat, erythema, and swelling in calves and thighs; HR ≤100 bpm; RR <20 breaths/min with normal depth and pattern (eupnea); and PaO_2 >80 mm Hg or O_2 saturation >92%.

INTERVENTIONS	RATIONALES
Monitor calves and thighs for erythema, warmth, decreased pulses, and swelling over area of inflammation; venous dilation; and coolness, pallor, and edema.	Indicators of thrombophlebitis.
Measure calves and thighs daily while patient is supine or before activity and monitor for increased circumference.	An increase of >2 cm in 1 day is significant, as well as calf diameter >3 cm larger than opposite calf.
Recognize that low-grade fever may be a more reliable signal of thrombophlebitis than pain. Notify health care provider about significant findings.	Pain or tenderness in the lower extremities may not be felt, depending on the level of SCI.
Protect patient's legs from injury during transfers and turning. Avoid IM injections in the legs.	SCI patients are prone to deep vein thrombosis (DVT), which can occur in the lower extremities because of immobility and changes in vascular tone.

INTERVENTIONS	RATIONALES
Provide ROM to legs qid. If not contraindicated, place patient in Trendelenburg position for 15 min q2h or elevate legs 10-15 degrees.	To promote venous drainage.
Monitor for tachycardia, shortness of breath, hemoptysis, decrease in Pao_2, O_2 saturation ≤92%, and decreased or adventitious breath sounds. Notify health care provider about significant findings.	Indicators of PE, which necessitate immediate intervention. Presence of pain depends on level of injury. Sudden shoulder pain may represent referred pain from PE.
Consult health care provider about use of antiembolism hose, sequential compression devices, pneumatic foot pumps, or prophylactic pharmacotherapy (e.g., ASA, warfarin, low-molecular-weight or low-dose heparin).	These measures help prevent PE.
For other interventions, see **Ineffective Peripheral Tissue Perfusion** in "Prolonged Bedrest," p. 71.	

●●● **Related NIC and NOC labels:** *NIC:* Embolus Precautions; Vital Signs Monitoring; Circulatory Care: Venous Insufficiency; Respiratory Monitoring; Circulatory Care: Arterial Insufficiency; Embolus Care: Pulmonary *NOC:* Tissue Perfusion: Cardiac; Tissue Perfusion: Pulmonary; Tissue Perfusion: Cerebral

Nursing Diagnosis:

Sexual Dysfunction

related to altered body function secondary to SCI

Desired Outcome: Patient discusses concerns about sexuality and verbalizes knowledge of alternative methods of sexual expression.

INTERVENTIONS	RATIONALES
Evaluate your own feelings about sexuality. As necessary, refer patient to someone (e.g., knowledgeable staff member, professional sexual therapy counselor) who can address patient's sexual concerns.	Nurses may not be able to answer all of the patient's questions or may be uncomfortable discussing sexuality issues. The nurse's discomfort would add to patient's discomfort.
Provide a supportive, nonjudgmental environment that gives patient permission to have and express sexual concerns.	Using opportunities as they evolve to elicit patient's knowledge, concerns, and questions may be therapeutic for patient. For example, sexuality can be discussed as it relates to an erection that occurs during a bath or to objective findings noted during physical assessment.
Expect acting-out behavior related to patient's sexuality.	This is a normal response to anxiety about sexual response and prognosis. Such behaviors may include asking questions, sexual jokes or innuendos, self-deprecating remarks, or flirting with staff.
Provide information about normal sexual response and changes caused by SCI.	Sexual functioning may be different but still possible with SCI. The general rule for men is the higher the lesion, the greater the chance of retaining the ability to have an erection but with less chance to ejaculate. Women may have problems with lubrication, and orgasm may be difficult to achieve because of decreased sensation. Women may also have a transient loss of ovulation. Ovulation usually returns, and women can become pregnant and deliver vaginally.

Continued

INTERVENTIONS

RATIONALES

INTERVENTIONS	RATIONALES
Provide information about birth control and oral contraception for women who desire it, as indicated. Oral contraceptives may be contraindicated, however.	Uterine contractions of labor in women with an SCI lesion at T8 or above may cause AD. Oral contraceptives can increase risk of thrombophlebitis.
Suggest some or all of the following techniques: oral-genital sex, digital stimulation, cuddling, mutual masturbation, anal eroticism, and massage. Suggest use of erection assistive techniques and devices (e.g., vacuum suction pump, prostaglandin penile injection, penile prosthesis or implant) that may aid men with SCI to attain erections.	Sexual activity may seem impossible to the SCI patient. These specific suggestions may provide gratification.
Suggest that patient decrease fluid intake 2-3 hr before sexual encounter, empty bladder and bowels (if necessary) before a sexual encounter, (for men) fold back indwelling catheter along the penis and hold it in place with a condom, (for women) tape catheter to the abdomen and leave it in place, take a warm bath before sexual activity to reduce spasticity, plan sexual activity for a time of day in which both partners are rested, experiment with a variety of positions, and apply topical anesthetics to areas that are hypersensitive to touch.	Specific guidelines for managing common problems that can occur during a sexual encounter.
Explain that water-soluble lubricants are useful, if needed, but that petroleum-based lubricants should be avoided.	Petroleum-based lubricants can cause UTI.
Explain that adductor spasms in women may pose a barrier but can be overcome if a rear entry is acceptable. Prolonged foreplay with stroking and light massage may also relax muscles. If AD occurs during sexual activity, suggest that patient consult health care provider about preventive measures (e.g., taking a ganglionic blocking agent before having sexual intercourse or applying topical anesthetic).	Specific guidelines for managing less common problems that can occur during a sexual encounter.
Suggest that patient's partner be included in discussion about sexual concerns.	Explaining the physical condition caused by SCI and preparing the partner for scars, lack of muscle tone, atrophy, and presence of a catheter are important and will provide partner with an opportunity to discuss sexual concerns as well.
For additional interventions, see **Ineffective Sexuality Pattern** in "Prolonged Bedrest," p. 78.	

●●● **Related NIC and NOC labels:** *NIC:* Sexual Counseling; Self-Esteem Enhancement; Teaching: Sexuality; Energy Management *NOC:* Sexual Functioning

ADDITIONAL NURSING DIAGNOSES/ PROBLEMS:

PATIENT-FAMILY TEACHING AND DISCHARGE PLANNING

When providing patient-family teaching, focus on sensory information, avoid giving excessive information, and initiate a visiting nurse referral for necessary follow-up teaching. Include verbal and written information about the following:

✓ Spinal cord functioning and the effects trauma has on how the body works.

✓ Safety measures relative to decreased sensation, motor deficits, and orthostatic hypotension and symptoms, preventive measures, and interventions for AD.

✓ Use and care of a brace or immobilizer as appropriate.

✓ What patient can expect if transferred to rehabilitation center.

✓ Techniques and devices for performing activities of daily living (ADL), including bathing, grooming, turning, feeding, and other self-care activities, to patient's maximum potential. The patient may need a home accessibility evaluation and a driving evaluation and training.

✓ Indicators of urinary calculi and dietary measures to prevent their formation (see p. 273).

✓ Indicators of DVT and measures to prevent it (see p. 000).

✓ For additional information, see teaching and discharge planning interventions (the fourth through tenth entries only) in "Multiple Sclerosis," p. 359, as appropriate.

✓ Referrals to community resources, such as public health nurse, visiting nurses association, community support groups, social workers, psychologic therapy, vocational rehabilitation agency, home health agencies, and extended and skilled care facilities. Additional general information can be obtained by contacting the following organizations:

National Spinal Cord Injury Association
6701 Democracy Road, Suite 300
Bethesda, MD 20817
(800) 962-9629
www.spinalcord.org/

Christopher Reeve Paralysis Foundation
500 Morris Avenue
Springfield, NJ 07081
(800) 225-0292
www.apacure.org/

Paralyzed Veterans of America
801 18th Street NW
Washington, DC 20006
(800) 424-8200
www.pva.org

Diabetes Mellitus

Diabetes mellitus (DM) is a chronic disease affecting about 10% of the total U.S. population with metabolic, vascular, and neurologic disorders resulting from dysfunctional glucose transport into body cells. Individuals with DM have impaired glucose transport because of decreased or absent insulin secretion and/or ineffective insulin action. Carbohydrate, fat, and protein metabolism are abnormal, and patients are unable to store glucose in the liver and muscle as glycogen, store fatty acids and triglycerides in adipose tissue, and transport amino acids into cells normally. DM is classified into the following five types of disorders.

Type 1 (formerly called insulin-dependent diabetes mellitus [IDDM]): Complete lack of effective endogenous insulin, causing hyperglycemia and ketosis. Previously this was termed *juvenile,* or *growth onset,* diabetes because a majority of those affected are <30 yr of age. This type of DM is precipitated by altered immune responses, genetic factors, and environmental stressors. These individuals depend on insulin for survival and prevention of life-threatening diabetic ketoacidosis (DKA).

Type 2 (formerly called non–insulin-dependent diabetes mellitus [NIDDM]): Moderate to severe lack of effective endogenous insulin, causing severe hyperglycemia without ketosis. Previously it was termed *adult,* or *maturity onset,* diabetes, and it is precipitated by obesity and aging. Two subgroups of patients with type 2 DM are distinguished by the presence or absence of obesity.

Other types (formerly termed secondary diabetes):
- *Pancreatic diseases that destroy the beta islet cells* (e.g., pancreatitis, cystic fibrosis, hemochromatosis)
- *Liver disease* (e.g., cirrhosis, hemochromatosis)
- *Muscle disorders* (e.g., myotonic dystrophies)
- *Adipose tissue disorders* (e.g., lipoatrophy, lipodystrophy, truncal obesity)
- *Drug-induced by insulin antagonists* (e.g., phenytoin [Dilantin], steroids [hydrocortisone, dexamethasone], hormones [estrogen])
- *Endocrine dysfunction/hormonal diseases* (e.g., acromegaly, Cushing's syndrome, pheochromocytoma)
- *Insulin resistance:* caused by dysfunctional insulin receptors
- *Genetic syndromes:* those that predispose individuals to DM (e.g., human leukocyte antigen [HLA] genetic system defects)
- *Defective insulin molecule production:* caused by mutation of the insulin gene

Gestational diabetes: Intolerance to glucose, which develops during pregnancy in 2%-3% of pregnant women, resulting in increased perinatal risk to the child and increased risk of the mother developing chronic DM during the next 10-15 yr. See "Diabetes in Pregnancy," p. 715, for more information.

Malnutrition-related diabetes: Type of DM added by the World Health Organization (WHO) for a syndrome with onset in individuals 10-40 yr of age in underdeveloped countries. This type requires insulin for control of blood glucose. Ketosis does not occur. The role of malnutrition as a cause currently is unknown.

HEALTH CARE SETTING

Primary care, with possible hospitalization resulting from complications

ASSESSMENT

Signs and symptoms:

- **Metabolic:** Fatigue, weakness, weight loss, paresthesias, mild dehydration, and symptoms of hyperglycemia (polyuria, polydipsia, polyphagia). These indicators are seen in the early stages of illness.
- **Impending type 1 crisis:** Profound dehydration and hyperglycemia, electrolyte imbalance, metabolic acidosis caused by ketosis, altered mental status, Kussmaul's respirations (paroxysmal dyspnea), acetone breath, possible hypovolemic shock (hypotension, weak and rapid pulse), abdominal pain, and possible strokelike symptoms.
- **Impending type 2 crisis:** Severe dehydration, hypovolemic shock (hypotension, weak and rapid pulse), severe hyperglycemia, shallow respirations, altered mental status, slight lactic acidosis or normal pH, possible strokelike symptoms.

COMPLICATIONS

Potential for acute crisis: *For type 1,* include DKA and hypoglycemia; *for type 2,* include hyperosmolar hyperglycemic nonketotic (HHNK) syndrome and hypoglycemia. These complications should be preventable in individuals diagnosed with DM and are discussed later in this section.

Long-term complications: The most important factor in delaying progression to long-term complications is the stabilization of blood glucose levels to normal range.

- **Macroangiopathy:** Vascular disease affecting the coronary arteries and the larger vessels of the brain and lower extremities. Risk factors are hyperglycemia, hypertension, hypercholesterolemia, smoking, aging, and extended duration of DM. Macroangiopathy may result in myocardial infarction, cerebrovascular accident, and peripheral vascular disease.

- **Microangiopathy:** Thickening of capillary basement membranes resulting in retinopathy and nephropathy. Early symptoms include increased leakage of retinal vessels and microalbuminuria. Late manifestations are blindness and renal failure.

- **Neuropathy:** Affects the peripheral and autonomic nervous systems, resulting in impaired or slowed nerve transmission, for example, numbness or lack of sensation, particularly in the feet (peripheral), and orthostatic hypotension, neurogenic bladder, and impaired gastric emptying (autonomic).

Morning hyperglycemia: Blood glucose elevation found on awakening. Causes include each of the following or a combination of the effects of their interactions:

- **Insufficient insulin:** The most common cause of hyperglycemia before breakfast is probably inadequate levels of circulating insulin. The patient may need a higher dosage, a mixture of insulins, or longer-acting insulin.

- **Dawn phenomenon:** Glucose remains normal until approximately 3 AM, when the effect of nocturnal growth hormone may elevate glucose in type 1 diabetes. It may be corrected by changing the time of the evening dose of intermediate-acting insulin injection to bedtime instead of dinnertime.

- **Somogyi phenomenon:** The patient becomes hypoglycemic during the night. Compensatory mechanisms to raise glucose levels are activated and result in overcompensation. It may be corrected by decreasing the evening dose of intermediate-acting insulin and/or eating a more substantial bedtime snack.

Problems with insulin:

- **Insulin resistance:** A problem experienced by most individuals with DM and other diseases at some point in the illness, when the daily insulin requirement to control hyperglycemia and prevent ketosis exceeds 200 U. Typically, it results from profound or complete insulin deficiency in type 1 DM and obesity in type 2 DM.

- **Local allergic reactions:** Soreness, erythema, or induration at the insulin injection site within 2 hr after injection. Reactions are decreasing in frequency with the evolution of more purified insulins.

- **Systemic allergic reactions:** Rare occurrence that begins with a localized skin reaction, which evolves into generalized urticaria or anaphylaxis. Patients must be desensitized to insulin by progression from minuscule to more normal doses over the course of 1 day, using a series of SC injections.

- **Lipodystrophy:** Local disturbance in fat metabolism resulting in loss of fat (lipoatrophy) or development of abnormal fatty masses at the injection sites (lipohypertrophy). Lipoatrophy rarely has been seen since the development of ^{100}U and human source insulins. Rotation of injection sites helps to prevent lipohypertrophy. Individuals experiencing lipohypertrophy should use alternate injection sites until the condition resolves.

DIAGNOSTIC TESTS

WHO defines the following diagnostic criteria for DM in nonpregnant adults.

Fasting blood sugar: A value >126 mg/dl is indicative of glucose intolerance if found on at least two occasions.

Oral glucose tolerance test: The 2-hr sample during the test is >200 mg/dl on at least two occasions.

Random plasma glucose: Value >200 mg/dl on at least two occasions is diagnostic of DM, as is this value on one occasion in the presence of other signs and symptoms of DM.

Glycosylated hemoglobin (glycohemoglobin or hemoglobin A1C): Normal range is 4%-7%. Individuals with DM will have values >7%. This value is measured to assess control of blood glucose over a preceding 2- to 3-mo period. The larger the percentage of glycosylated Hgb, the poorer the blood glucose control. Kits are now available to monitor this value in the home.

Diagnostic procedures under investigation

Immunoassay for islet cell antibodies: Kits to detect these antibodies are undergoing clinical trials. Islet cell antibodies have been identified in 85% of patients within the first few weeks after DM was diagnosed.

Serum fructosamine: Fructosamine is used to reflect glycemic control over the previous 2 weeks before the testing. Normal value is 1.5-2.4 mmol/L when albumin is 5 g/dl. Because this test is not affected by abnormal hemoglobin or hemolytic conditions, it may be used in place of glycohemoglobin, which is unreliable in these conditions.

Nursing Diagnosis:

Ineffective Tissue Perfusion: Peripheral, Cardiopulmonary, Renal, Cerebral, and GI

(or risk for same) *related to* interrupted blood flow secondary to development and progression of macroangiopathy and microangiopathy

Desired Outcomes: Optimally, patient has adequate tissue perfusion as evidenced by warmth, sensation, brisk capillary refill time (<2 sec), and peripheral pulses >2+ on a 0-4+ scale in the extremities; BP within his or her optimal range; urinary output ≥30 ml/hr; baseline vision; good appetite; and absence of nausea and vomiting. Patient does not exhibit evidence of injury as a result of peripheral and autonomic neuropathies.

INTERVENTIONS	RATIONALES
Check blood glucose before meals and at bedtime.	To monitor effectiveness of blood glucose control when patient's glucose is not increased by food being digested.
Encourage patient to perform regular home blood glucose monitoring.	Compliance with the therapeutic regimen is essential for promoting optimal tissue perfusion. Progression of vascular disease, including blindness and kidney failure, is the root cause of all complications of DM. By keeping serum glucose in a more normal range, the vascular endothelium receives better nourishment within the cells and will be less likely to deteriorate. Urine glucose testing is less reliable and should not be used by patients with reduced renal function.
Check BP q4h. Alert health care provider about values outside patient's normal range. Administer antihypertensive agents as prescribed and document response.	Hypertension is a common complication of diabetes. Careful control of BP is critical in preventing or limiting development of heart disease, retinopathy, or nephropathy.
In addition to sensation, assess capillary refill, temperature, peripheral pulses, and color in the extremities.	To monitor peripheral perfusion.
Protect patients with impaired peripheral perfusion from injury with sharp objects or heat (e.g., avoid use of heating pads).	Patients may experience decreased sensation in extremities because of peripheral neuropathy.
Teach patient to avoid pressure at the back of the knees (e.g., by not crossing legs or "gatching" bed under the knees) and to avoid wearing constricting garments on the extremities and lower body. For additional information, see **Risk for Impaired Skin Integrity**, p. 403.	To prevent venous stasis and any reduction in arterial perfusion in patients with macroangiopathy or impending peripheral vascular disease.
As indicated, orient patient to the location of such items as water, tissues, glasses, and call light.	Provides necessary information and a safe environment for patients with diminished eyesight caused by diabetic retinopathy.
Monitor laboratory values for changes in renal function.	Laboratory values that would signal changes in renal function include increases in blood urea nitrogen (BUN; [>20 mg/dl]) and creatinine (>1.5 mg/dl in men and >1.2 mg/dl in women) along with altered urine output. Approximately half of all persons with type 1 DM develop chronic renal failure (CRF) and end-stage renal disease. Proteinuria (protein >8 mg/dl in a random sample of urine) and microalbuminuria have been recognized as indicators of developing CRF. Current American Diabetes Association (ADA) recommendations indicate that patients should see a nephrologist when creatinine is increased.

Continued

INTERVENTIONS	RATIONALES
Ensure that patients who will receive contrast medium are well hydrated and possibly receive several doses of oral acetyl-cysteine (Mucomyst) to protect the kidneys from contrast-related deterioration. Observe these patients for indicators of acute renal failure (ARF).	Individuals with DM and with reduced renal function are at significant risk for dehydration and development of ARF after exposure to contrast medium. See "Acute Renal Failure," p. 223, and "Chronic Renal Failure," p. 243, for more information.
Monitor for the following:	Individuals with DM may experience multiple problems resulting from autonomic neuropathy.
Orthostatic hypotension:	
- Check BP while patient is lying down, sitting, and then standing. Alert health care provider to significant findings.	BP decreased from patient's normal, along with lightheadedness, dizziness, diaphoresis, pallor, tachycardia, and syncope, are signals of orthostatic hypotension. A drop in systolic BP ≥20 mm Hg signals the need to return patient to a supine position.
- Assist patients when getting up suddenly or after prolonged recumbency.	To prevent falls caused by orthostatic hypotension.
Impaired gastric emptying with nausea, vomiting, and diarrhea:	Nausea, vomiting, and anorexia can signal developing uremia in patients with progressive renal failure.
- Administer metoclopramide before meals if prescribed.	Metoclopramide is an antiemetic that also promotes gastric emptying.
- Keep a record of all stools.	Diarrhea is a potential problem in patients with DM who have autonomic neuropathy.
Neurogenic bladder:	
- Encourage patients to void q3-4h during the day.	If patient has difficulty voiding, intermittent catheterization may be necessary.

●●● **Related NIC and NOC labels:** *NIC:* Circulatory Care: Arterial Insufficiency; Circulatory Care: Venous Insufficiency; Vital Signs Monitoring; Laboratory Data Interpretation; Neurologic Monitoring; Hypovolemia Management; Nausea Management; Foot Care; Pressure Management; Skin Surveillance *NOC:* Tissue Perfusion: Cardiac; Tissue Perfusion: Cerebral; Tissue Perfusion: Abdominal Organs; Tissue Perfusion: Peripheral; Tissue Integrity: Skin and Mucous Membranes

Nursing Diagnosis:

Risk for Infection

related to chronic disease process (e.g., hyperglycemia, neurogenic bladder, poor circulation)

Desired Outcome: Patient is free of signs of infection as evidenced by normothermia, negative cultures, and white blood cell (WBC) count <11,000/mm^3.

INTERVENTIONS	RATIONALES
Monitor temperature q4h. Alert health care provider to elevations.	Infection is the most common cause of DKA. Fever can signal presence of an infection.
Ensure good handwashing and maintain meticulous sterile technique when changing dressings, performing invasive procedures, or manipulating indwelling catheters.	To minimize risk of infection. Nonintact skin and invasive procedures and catheters place patient at risk for ingress of bacteria.
Monitor for fever, chills, cough productive of sputum, crackles, rhonchi, dyspnea, inflamed pharynx, and sore throat.	Indicators of upper respiratory infection.

Continued

INTERVENTIONS	RATIONALES
Monitor for burning or pain with urination, cloudy or malodorous urine, tachycardia, diaphoresis, nausea, vomiting, and abdominal pain.	Indicators of urinary tract infection.
Monitor for hypothermia, flushed skin, and hypotension.	Indicators of systemic sepsis.
Monitor for erythema, swelling, purulent drainage, and warmth at IV sites.	Indicators of localized infection.
Consult health care provider about obtaining culture specimens for blood, sputum, and urine during temperature spikes or for wounds that produce purulent drainage.	Infection can be present in blood (sepsis), urine, sputum (lungs/respiratory tract), or wounds. Specimens reveal these sources. Occult infection also can be present outside these sources.
For more information, see Appendix for "Infection Prevention and Control," p. 831.	

●●● **Related NIC and NOC labels:** *NIC:* Infection Control; Infection Prevention; Specimen Management; Vital Signs Monitoring; Wound Care *NOC:* Infection Status

Nursing Diagnosis:

Risk for Impaired Skin Integrity

related to altered circulation and sensation secondary to peripheral neuropathy and vascular pathology

Desired Outcomes: Patient's skin remains intact. Within 1 hr of instruction, patient verbalizes and demonstrates accurate knowledge of proper foot care.

INTERVENTIONS	RATIONALES
Assess integrity of the skin, particularly of the lower extremities (LE), and evaluate LE reflexes by checking knee and ankle deep tendon reflexes, proprioceptive sensations, two-point discrimination, and vibration sensation (using a tuning fork on the medial malleolus).	To monitor presence/degree of neuropathy and vascular pathology. Although all skin is at risk, especially that on extremities and pressure points, skin on the LE is at highest risk and typically is the first to exhibit problems. If sensations are impaired, anticipate patient's inability to respond appropriately to harmful stimuli.
Monitor peripheral pulses, comparing the quality bilaterally.	Peripheral pulses ≤2+ on a 0-4+ scale signal poor circulation that could compromise skin integrity.
Use foot cradle on bed, space boots for ulcerated heels, elbow protectors, and pressure-relief mattress.	To prevent pressure points and promote patient comfort.
Minimize patient activities and incorporate progressive passive and active exercises into daily routine. Discourage extended rest periods in the same position.	To alleviate acute discomfort while preventing hemostasis.
Teach patient the following steps for foot care:	
- Wash feet daily with mild soap and warm water; check water temperature with water thermometer or elbow.	Patients with decreased sensation are at risk for burns if they are unaware that water temperature is too hot. Hot water and strong soaps also can promote dry skin, which can become irritated and break down.
- Inspect feet daily for presence of redness, discoloration, or trauma, using mirrors as necessary for adequate visualization.	These are signs that the skin needs vigilant assessment and preventive care. When the skin is no longer intact, the patient is at risk for infection that eventually can lead to amputation.

Continued

INTERVENTIONS	RATIONALES
- Alternate between at least two pairs of properly fitted shoes.	To avoid potential for pressure points that can occur by wearing one pair only.
- Change socks or stockings daily and wear only cotton or wool blends.	Decreases risk of infection from moisture or dirt in contact with broken skin.
- Use gentle moisturizers.	To soften and lubricate dry skin.
- Visit a podiatrist to get toenails cut. If this is not possible, cut toenails straight across after softening them during bath. File nails with an emery board.	To prevent ingrown toenails, which could lead to infection.
- Do not self-treat corns or calluses; visit podiatrist regularly. Do not go barefoot indoors or outdoors.	To minimize risk for trauma, which can lead to infection and ultimately to amputation.
- Attend to any foot injury immediately and seek medical attention.	To avoid potential complications discussed above.

●●● **Related NIC and NOC labels:** *NIC:* Pressure Management; Skin Surveillance; Bathing; Foot Care; Infection Protection; Positioning; Wound Care; Bed Rest Care *NOC:* Tissue Integrity: Skin and Mucous Membranes

Nursing Diagnosis:

Deficient Knowledge:

Proper insulin administration and dietary precautions for promoting normoglycemia

Desired Outcome: Within 1 hr of instruction, patient verbalizes and demonstrates accurate knowledge of proper insulin administration, hypoglycemia and hyperglycemia, and the prescribed dietary regimen.

INTERVENTIONS	RATIONALES
Teach patient to check expiration date on insulin vial and to avoid using it if outdated.	Insulin may lose potency if the bottle has been open for >30 days.
Also teach proper storage of insulin and importance of avoiding temperature extremes.	Extreme temperatures destroy insulin.
Explain that intermediate- and long-acting insulins require mixing (contraindicated for the intermediate/rapid).	Insulin separates when the bottle sits, and the molecules must be remixed to ensure appropriate concentration throughout the vial.
Demonstrate rolling insulin vial between palms to mix the contents. Caution patient to avoid shaking vial.	Vigorous shaking produces air bubbles that can interfere with accurate dose measurement.
Explain that regular insulin should be injected 30 min before mealtime; newer insulin analogs (e.g., Humalog) need to be injected immediately before eating.	Time of onset/peak of older, regular insulins is slightly delayed compared with the newer insulins.
Explain that either making a change in insulin type or withholding a dose of insulin may be required in some instances.	These instances include the following: when fasting for studies or surgery, when not eating because of nausea/vomiting, or when hypoglycemic. Stress from illness or infection can increase insulin requirements (or necessitate insulin therapy for one who is normally controlled with oral hypoglycemics), and increased exercise will necessitate additional food intake to prevent hypoglycemia when no change is made in insulin dose. Adjustments are always individually based and require clarification with patient's health care provider.

Continued

INTERVENTIONS	RATIONALES
Provide a chart that depicts rotation of the injection sites. Explain that injection sites should be at least 1 inch apart.	Injections in or near the same site each time may result in development of hard lumps or extra fatty deposits. Both of these problems are unsightly and make the insulin action less reliable.
Explain importance of inserting needle perpendicular to the skin rather than at an angle. Very thin persons may need to use a 45-degree angle.	To ensure deep SC administration of insulin.
Ensure that patient understands and demonstrates the technique and timing for home monitoring of blood glucose.	A commercial kit provides ongoing data reflecting degree of control and may identify necessary changes in diet and medication before severe metabolic changes occur. Self-monitoring by patients has proved to be extremely useful in reducing complications, especially in type 1 DM patients who require more stringent control of serum glucose levels. Self-monitoring also enables patient's self-control and psychologic security.
Caution patient about importance of following prescribed diet.	Adequate nutrition and controlled calories are essential to maintaining normoglycemia in persons with DM. A diet low in fat and high in fiber is an effective means of controlling blood fats, especially cholesterol and triglycerides. Diet is the sole method of control for many individuals with type 2 DM.
For patients who experience low blood glucose at night, discuss availability of commercially available long-acting carbohydrate sources.	Long-acting carbohydrate sources may decrease risk of nighttime low blood glucose levels.
Instruct patient to be alert to changes in mentation, apprehension, erratic behavior, trembling, slurred speech, staggering gait, seizure activity.	Indicators of hypoglycemia.
Teach patient to treat hypoglycemia as prescribed. Explain that oral hypoglycemics should be omitted several days before planned surgery.	Hypoglycemia involving oral hypoglycemics can be severe and persistent. Monitoring must be diligent. Any condition, situation, or medication that enhances the hypoglycemic effects of these drugs requires close monitoring of blood glucose when symptoms of hypoglycemia arise. Common factors in the development of hypoglycemia are fasting for diagnostic purposes, skipping meals, unplanned increase in activity, malnourishment related to illness or nausea and vomiting, and other medication therapy (any of which adds to the hypoglycemic action of the oral hypoglycemics).
Teach patient signs and symptoms of hyperglycemia.	Hyperglycemia can occur with increased food intake, too little insulin, decreased exercise, infection or illness, and emotional stress. Signs and symptoms of hyperglycemia (polydipsia, polyuria, polyphagia, fatigue, fruity-smelling breath) can appear within hours or even several days. Hyperglycemia will be detected during routine self-testing of blood glucose.

●●● **Related NIC and NOC labels:** *NIC:* Teaching: Disease Process; Teaching: Prescribed Diet; Teaching: Prescribed Medication; Hyperglycemia Management; Hypoglycemia Management; Medication Administration: Subcutaneous; Teaching: Psychomotor Skill *NOC:* Knowledge: Diabetes Management

ADDITIONAL NURSING DIAGNOSES/ PROBLEMS:

PATIENT-FAMILY TEACHING AND DISCHARGE PLANNING

When providing patient-family teaching, avoid giving excessive information and initiate a visiting nurse referral for necessary follow-up teaching. Part of the initial assessment should include asking about existing knowledge of the disease, ability for self-management, and psychologic acceptance. Include verbal and written information about the following:

✓ Importance of carrying a diabetic identification card and wearing Medic-Alert bracelet or necklace and identification card outlining diagnosis and emergency treatment. Contact the following organization:

Medic Alert
323 Colorado Avenue
Turlock, CA 95382
(209) 668-3333

✓ Recognizing warning signs of both hyperglycemia and hypoglycemia, treatment, and factors that contribute to both conditions. Emphasize importance of disclosing all alternative and complementary health practices being used because some may affect blood glucose or possibly lead to adverse drug reactions. Remind patient that stress from illness or infection can increase insulin requirements (or necessitate insulin therapy for one who is normally controlled with oral hypoglycemics) and that increased exercise will necessitate additional food intake to prevent hypoglycemia when no change is made in insulin dosage under normoglycemic conditions. Blood glucose at a level >250 mg/dl at the beginning of exercise will make the exercise a stressor that elevates the glucose level rather than decreasing it.

✓ Drugs that potentiate **hyperglycemia:** estrogens, corticosteroids, thyroid preparations, diuretics, phenytoin, glucagon, and drugs containing sugar (e.g., cough syrup). Drugs that potentiate **hypoglycemia:** salicylates, sulfonamides, tetracyclines, methyldopa, anabolic steroids, acetaminophen, monoamine oxidase (MAO) inhibitors, ethanol, haloperidol, and marijuana. Propranolol and other β-adrenergic agents may mask the signs of and inhibit recovery from hypoglycemia.

✓ Home monitoring of blood glucose using commercial kits and possibly daily urine testing for ketones, which provide ongoing data reflecting the degree of control and may identify necessary changes in diet and medication before severe metabolic changes occur. These tests also provide a means for patient's self-control and psychologic security. In addition, kits for monitoring glycohemoglobin (HbA1C) are available for home use and may assist patients in determining the overall effectiveness of their diabetes management regimen. New, smaller lancets allow more frequent blood glucose testing by decreasing pain from fingersticks. Stress need for careful control of blood glucose as a means of decreasing risk of or minimizing long-term complications of DM. Encourage patient to rotate fingerstick sites as much as possible to avoid possibility of injuring any one site.

✓ Importance of daily exercise, maintenance of normal body weight, and yearly medical evaluation. Explain that exercise is as important as diet in treating DM. It lowers blood glucose, helps maintain normal cholesterol levels, and increases circulation. These effects increase the body's ability to metabolize glucose and help reduce the therapeutic dose of insulin for most patients. Stress that each exercise program must be individualized (especially for persons with type 1 DM) and implemented consistently. The patient should have a complete physical examination and then be encouraged to incorporate acceptable exercise activities into his or her daily routine.

✓ Diet that is low in fat and high in fiber as an effective means of controlling blood fats, especially cholesterol and triglycerides. Stress that diet is the sole method of control for many individuals with type 2 DM. Adequate nutrition and controlled calories are essential to maintaining normoglycemia in these individuals. Patients who gained weight before developing type 2 DM are sometimes able to normalize their blood glucose by losing weight and regaining ideal body weight. When treatment also includes oral hypoglycemic medications or insulin, increased amounts of carbohydrates are required to offset the hypoglycemic effects of these medications. Individuals with type 1 DM require day-to-day consistency in diet and exercise to prevent hypoglycemia. Typically, three daily meals and an evening snack are prescribed. Some fat and protein should be present in all meals and snacks to slow down the elevation of postprandial blood glucose. Adding 10-15 g of fiber will slow the digestion of monosaccharides and disaccharides. For all types of diabetes, refined and simple sugars should be reduced and complex carbohydrates (breads, cereals, pasta, beans) should be encouraged. Various artificial sweeteners are used in "diet" products. Some contribute calories, which must be accounted for in a calorie-restricted diet. Exchange lists commonly are used for meal planning.

✓ Necessity for individuals with type 1 to use ^{100}U syringes with ^{100}U insulin. Various *types/sources* of insulin (beef, pork, biosynthetic) should not be mixed. When mixing various *acting* insulins, draw up the regular first, followed by the intermediate- or long-acting insulin. Some insulin analogs (e.g., Novolog) are not mixed with other insulin preparations.

✓ Availability of syringe magnifiers that can be used for patients with poor visual acuity. Other products that permit safe and accurate filling of syringes are also available.

✓ Necessity of rotating injection sites and injecting insulin at room temperature. Provide a chart showing possible injection sites and describe the system for rotating the sites. Complications related to insulin injections, including lipodystrophy, insulin resistance, and allergic reactions, should be discussed thoroughly.

✓ Importance of meticulous skin, wound, and foot care.

✓ Importance of annual eye examinations for early detection and treatment of retinopathy.

✓ Importance of regular dental checkups because periodontal disease poses a major problem for individuals with DM. The mouth often is the primary site of origination for low-grade infections.

✓ Importance of inserting the needle perpendicular to the skin rather than at an angle to ensure deep SC administration of insulin. Individuals who are very thin may need to use a 45-degree angle.

✓ Name, purpose, dosage, schedule, precautions, drug/drug and food/drug interactions, and potential side effects for any supplemental medications used.

✓ Identification of available resources for ongoing assistance and information, including nurses, dietitian, patient's health care provider, and other individuals with DM in patient care unit. Other resources include the local chapter of the ADA and the local library for free access to current materials on diabetes. The following is a list of resources available to patients:

> American Diabetes Association
> 1660 Duke Street
> Alexandria, VA 22314
> (800) 232-3472
> www.diabetes.org
>
> Canadian Diabetes Association
> 15 Toronto Street, Suite 1001
> Toronto, Ontario M5C2F3
> (416) 363-3373
> www.diabetes.ca
>
> Juvenile Diabetes Foundation
> 120 Wall Street
> New York, NY 10005
> (800) JDF-CURE
> www.jdfcure.com

> Joslin Diabetes Center
> Director, Joslin Clinic
> 1 Joslin Place
> Boston, MA 02215
> (617) 732-2501
> www.joslin.org
>
> National Diabetes Information Clearinghouse
> One Information Way
> Bethesda, MD 20892-3560
> (800) 860-8747
> (301) 654-3327
> www.niddk.nih.gov/health/diabetes/ndic.htm
>
> American Heart Association
> 7272 Greenville Avenue
> Dallas, TX 75231
> (800) 242-8721
> www.americanheart.org
>
> Can-Am-Care
> (diabetes care store brand availability guide)
> (800) 461-7448

✓ The following is a list of journals available for patients:
- *Diabetes 95,* American Diabetes Association Subscription Department, 1660 Duke Street, Alexandria, VA 22314
- *Diabetes Forecast,* American Diabetes Association Membership Center, Box 2055, Harlan, IA 51593-0238
- *Diabetes in the News,* Ames Center for Diabetes Education, Miles Inc., Box 3105, Elkhart, IN 46515
- *Diabetes Self-Management,* Box 51125, Boulder, CO 80321-1125
- *Health-O-Gram,* SugarFree Center, 13725 Burbank Blvd., Van Nuys, CA 91401
- *Living Well with Diabetes,* Diabetes Center, 13911 Ridgedale Drive, Suite 250, Minnetonka, MN 55343
- *Diabetes Interview,* 3715 Balboa Street, San Francisco, CA 94121

Diabetic Ketoacidosis

Diabetic ketoacidosis (DKA) is a life-threatening condition caused by severe lack of effective insulin, resulting in abnormal carbohydrate, fat, and protein metabolism. The intracellular environment is unable to receive necessary glucose for oxidation and energy production without insulin to facilitate transport of glucose from the bloodstream across the cell membrane. The impairment of glucose uptake results in hyperglycemia, while the intracellular environment continues to lack necessary nutrients. Hyperglycemia acts as an osmotic diuretic, causing severe fluid and electrolyte losses that can lead to hypovolemic shock if untreated.

HEALTH CARE SETTING

Acute care (intensive care unit)

ASSESSMENT

Neurologic: Altered level of consciousness (LOC; confusion, lethargy, irritability, coma); strokelike symptoms (unilateral/bilateral weakness, paralysis, numbness, paresthesia); fatigue.

Respiratory: Deep, rapid Kussmaul's respirations.

Cardiovascular: Tachycardia, hypotension, electrocardiogram (ECG) changes.

Metabolic/gastrointestinal (GI)/endocrine: Polyuria, polyphagia, polydipsia, fruity "acetone" breath, abdominal pain, weight loss, fatigue, generalized weakness, nausea, vomiting.

Integumentary: Dry, flushed skin; poor turgor; dry mucous membranes.

VS monitoring:

BP: low (>20% below normal)

HR: >100 bpm

CVP: <2 mm Hg (<5 H_2O)

Temperature: normal

History/risk factors for development of crisis: Undiagnosed diabetes mellitus (DM), infections, acute pancreatitis, uremia, insulin resistance.

DIAGNOSTIC TESTS

Values reflect dehydration/metabolic acidosis (ketosis) secondary to hyperglycemia, abnormal lipolysis, and osmotic diuresis; fluid loss ≥6.5 L.

Hgb/Hct: Elevated.

Serum blood urea nitrogen (BUN)/creatinine: Elevated.

Serum electrolytes: Initially elevated, then decreased.

Serum glucose: 250-800 mg/dl (+ ketones).

Arterial blood gases (ABGs): pH 6.8-7.3; HCO_3^- 12-20 mEq/L; CO_2 15-25 mEq/L.

Serum osmolality: 300-350 mOsm/L.

Urine glucose/acetone: Positive/positive.

Nursing Diagnosis:

Deficient Fluid Volume

related to failure of regulatory mechanisms or decreased circulating volume secondary to hyperglycemia with osmotic diuresis

Desired Outcome: Patient becomes normovolemic within 10 hr of treatment/interventions, as evidenced by BP ≥90/60 mm Hg (or within patient's normal range), HR 60-100 bpm, central venous pressure (CVP) 2-6 mm Hg (5-12 cm H_2O), good skin turgor, moist and pink mucous membranes, specific gravity <1.020, balanced I&O, and urinary output ≥30 ml/hr.

INTERVENTIONS	RATIONALES
Monitor VS q15min until stable for 1 hr. Notify health care provider of significant findings.	Hyperglycemia acts as an osmotic diuretic, causing severe fluid and electrolyte losses that can lead to hypovolemic shock if untreated. HR >120 bpm, BP <90/60 or decreased ≥20 mm Hg from baseline, and CVP <2 mm Hg (or <5 cm H_2O) are signs of hypovolemia and necessitate notifying health care provider for timely intervention.
Monitor patient for poor skin turgor, dry mucous membranes, sunken and soft eyeballs, tachycardia, and orthostatic hypotension.	Physical indicators of hypovolemia.
Weigh patient daily and measure I&O accurately. Monitor urinary specific gravity and report findings >1.020 in the presence of other indicators of dehydration. Report to health care provider urine output <30 ml/hr for 2 consecutive hr.	Decreasing urinary output may signal diminishing intravascular fluid volume or impending renal failure. Loss of weight and output that exceeds intake may signal dehydration.
Administer IV fluids as prescribed. Be alert to indicators of fluid overload.	To ensure adequate rehydration. Usually normal saline or 0.45% saline is administered until plasma glucose falls to 200-300 mg/dl. Initially, IV fluids are administered rapidly to enable rapid rehydration that will correct hypovolemia (i.e., 2000 ml infused during the first 2 hr of treatment and 200-300 ml/hr thereafter). After administration of saline fluids, dextrose-containing solutions usually are given to prevent rebound hypoglycemia. Indicators of fluid overload (jugular vein distention, dyspnea, crackles, CVP >6 mm Hg [>12 cm H_2O]) can occur with rapid infusion of fluids.
Administer insulin as prescribed. As directed, maintain patient on 5-10 U/hr, or 0.1 U/kg/hr as a continuous infusion. Administer insulin through a separate IV tubing using an infusion control device. When initiating insulin administration, flush 50 ml of the IV insulin solution through the tubing.	Insulin is given to correct or stabilize the existing hyperglycemia and is usually given IV. The initial dose may vary from 10-25 U, or about 0.3 U/kg. IV route provides rapid action, and, in addition, poor tissue perfusion caused by dehydration makes SC route less effective. Dosage is adjusted based on serial glucose levels and resolution of ketosis. To facilitate maximal accuracy in dosing and avoid inadvertent dosage alteration, it is best to use a separate IV system for insulin infusion. To saturate adsorption sites in the walls of the plastic tubing, where the initial insulin molecules may adhere rather than be delivered to the patient. **Note:** Insulin analogs (i.e., Humalog) may be used in place of regular insulin to lower blood glucose levels. Newer insulin analogs are equally as effective as regular insulin. They are made via recombinant DNA technology rather than from an animal source.
Monitor laboratory results for trend. Report abnormalities.	Serum K^+ should decline until it reaches normal levels. Health care provider should be alerted to serum K^+ levels <3.5 mEq/L. Serum Na^+ levels will increase gradually with appropriate IV saline replacement.
Observe for clinical manifestations of electrolyte, glucose, and acid-base imbalances.	The following imbalances are associated with DKA: - *Hyperkalemia:* lethargy, nausea, hyperactive bowel sounds with diarrhea, numbness or tingling in extremities, muscle weakness. - *Hypokalemia:* muscle weakness, hypotension, anorexia, drowsiness, hypoactive bowel sounds.

Continued

INTERVENTIONS	RATIONALES
	- *Hyponatremia:* headache, malaise, muscle weakness, abdominal cramps, nausea, seizures, coma.
	- *Hypophosphatemia:* muscle weakness, progressive encephalopathy possibly leading to coma.
	- *Hypomagnesemia:* anorexia, nausea, vomiting, lethargy, weakness, personality changes, tetany, tremor or muscle fasciculations, seizures, confusion progressing to coma.
	- *Hypochloremia:* hypertonicity of muscles, tetany, depressed respirations.
	- *Hypoglycemia:* headache, impaired mentation, agitation, dizziness, nausea, pallor, tremors, tachycardia, diaphoresis.
	- *Metabolic acidosis:* lassitude, nausea, vomiting, Kussmaul's respirations, lethargy progressing to coma.
As prescribed, replace K^+ and phosphorus.	Use of phosphorus replacement is controversial, but if phosphorus levels remain low, potassium phosphate solutions can be used to assist with K^+ and phosphate replacement. Studies suggest there is no difference in the outcome of patients who receive phosphorus replacement and those who do not.
	K^+ must be monitored and corrected carefully. Before treatment there is a risk of hyperkalemia from excess transport of intracellular K^+ to extracellular spaces. After initiation of treatment, K^+ returns to the intracellular compartment through accelerated transport into cells via insulin and following correction of acidosis, and therefore patient is at risk for becoming hypokalemic.
Administer IV bicarbonate as prescribed.	For pH <7.10. Its use is limited because acidosis will be corrected by insulin therapy. Excessive use of sodium bicarbonate can produce alkalosis, hyperosmolality, and respiratory depression.

●●● **Related NIC and NOC labels:** *NIC:* Fluid/Electrolyte Management; Acid/Base Management; Intravenous Therapy; Laboratory Data Interpretation; Neurologic Monitoring; Vital Signs Monitoring
NOC: Electrolyte and Acid/Base Balance; Fluid Balance

Nursing Diagnosis:

Risk for Infection

related to inadequate secondary defenses (suppressed inflammatory response) secondary to protein depletion

Desired Outcome: Patient is free of infection as evidenced by normothermia, HR ≤100 bpm, BP within patient's normal range, white blood cell (WBC) count ≤11,000/mm^3, and negative culture results.

INTERVENTIONS	RATIONALES
Monitor patient for indicators of infection. Monitor laboratory results and culture purulent drainage as prescribed.	Infection is the most common cause of DKA. Indicators of infection include fever, chills, pain with urination, vomiting, erythema and swelling around IV sites, and increased WBC count.
Ensure good handwashing technique when caring for patient. Limit use of invasive lines. Rotate peripheral IV sites q48-72h, depending on agency policy. Central lines should be discontinued as soon as feasible and when in place should be handled carefully. Schedule dressing changes according to agency policy and inspect site(s) for erythema, swelling, or purulent drainage. Document presence of any of these indicators and notify health care provider.	Patient is at increased risk for bacterial infection because of suppressed inflammatory response. Signs of local infection that should be reported for timely intervention.
Provide good skin care.	To maintain skin integrity, which is a first line of defense against infection.
Use pressure-relief mattress on the bed.	To help prevent skin breakdown that could lead to infection. Air circulation beds are recommended for severe skin breakdown.
Use meticulous sterile technique when caring for or inserting indwelling catheters.	To minimize risk of bacterial entry via these sites.
Limit use of indwelling urethral catheters to patients who are unable to void in a bedpan or when continuous assessment of urine output is essential.	There is increased risk of infection with indwelling catheters.
Provide incentive spirometry and encourage its use, along with deep-breathing and coughing exercises, hourly while patient is awake.	Deep inhalations with incentive spirometry along with deep-breathing exercises expand alveoli and aid in mobilizing secretions to the airways. Coughing further mobilizes and clears the secretions. These exercises help prevent pulmonary infection.
For more information, see Appendix for "Infection Prevention and Control," p. 831.	

●●● **Related NIC and NOC labels:** *NIC:* Infection Protection; Incision Site Care; Urinary Catheterization; Cough Enhancement; Tube Care: Urinary *NOC:* Infection Status

Nursing Diagnosis:

Ineffective Protection

related to altered cerebral function secondary to dehydration or cerebral edema associated with DKA

Desired Outcomes: Patient verbalizes orientation to person, place, and time and does not demonstrate significant change in mental status; normal breath sounds are auscultated over the patient's airway; and patient's oral cavity and musculoskeletal system remain intact and free of injury.

INTERVENTIONS	RATIONALES
Monitor patient's mental status, orientation, LOC, and respiratory status, especially airway patency, at frequent intervals. Keep an appropriate-size oral airway, manual resuscitator and mask, and supplemental oxygen at the bedside.	With DKA, patient's cerebral function may be altered because of dehydration or cerebral edema.

Continued

INTERVENTIONS	RATIONALES
Maintain bed in lowest position, keep side rails up at all times, and use soft restraints as necessary.	To reduce likelihood of injury from falls resulting from patient's altered cerebral function.
Insert gastric tube in comatose patients as prescribed. Attach gastric tube to low, intermittent suction and assess patency q4h.	To decrease likelihood of aspiration.
Elevate head of bed (HOB) to 45 degrees.	To minimize risk of aspiration.
Initiate seizure precautions. For details, see "Seizure Disorders," p. 375.	

●●● **Related NIC and NOC labels:** *NIC:* Environmental Management: Safety; Aspiration Precautions; Seizure Precautions; Positioning *NOC:* Neurological Status: Consciousness

Nursing Diagnosis:

Ineffective Tissue Perfusion: Peripheral

(or risk for same) *related to* interrupted venous or arterial flow secondary to increased blood viscosity, increased platelet aggregation and adhesiveness, and patient immobility

Desired Outcomes: Optimally, patient has adequate peripheral perfusion as evidenced by peripheral pulses ≥2+ on a 0-4+ scale; warm skin; brisk capillary refill (<2 sec); and absence of swelling, bluish discoloration, erythema, and discomfort in the calves and thighs. Alternatively, if signs of altered peripheral tissue perfusion occur, they are detected and reported promptly.

INTERVENTIONS	RATIONALES
Monitor Hct results.	Normal values are 40%-54% (male) or 37%-47% (female). With proper fluid replacement, results should return to normal within 24-48 hr.
Assess BUN value.	Normal value is 6-20 mg/dl. A falling BUN value is an indicator of improved tissue perfusion and renal function.
Assess peripheral pulses q2-4h.	Any decrease in amplitude or absence of pulse(s) should be reported to health care provider promptly as it would signal deep vein thrombosis (DVT) or other cause of perfusion deficit (e.g., hypovolemia, advancing peripheral vascular disease).
Be alert to erythema, pain, tenderness, warmth, and swelling over the area of thrombus and bluish discoloration, paleness, coolness, and dilation of superficial veins in the distal extremities, especially the lower extremities.	Indicators of DVT. For more information, see "Venous Thrombosis/Thrombophlebitis," p. 217.
Also be alert to pain, paresthesia (especially loss of sensation of light touch and two-point discrimination), cyanosis with delayed capillary refill, mottling, and coolness of the extremity.	These are indicators of arterial thrombosis, which can lead to profound limb ischemia and tissue hypoxia and eventually to tissue anoxia and death. When untreated, limb ischemia may result in loss of limbs and and/or digits.
Report significant findings to health care provider immediately.	To avoid loss of limb and/or digits (fingers/toes).
Encourage active exercises to all extremities q2h. Encourage calf pumping and ankle circles qh in patients susceptible to DVT.	To increase blood flow to the tissues, which decreases likelihood of DVT.

Continued

INTERVENTIONS	RATIONALES
Unless contraindicated, encourage fluid intake to >2500 ml/day.	To decrease potential for hemoconcentration, which could lead to DVT.
Apply antiembolic hose, Ace wraps, pneumatic alternating pressure stockings, or pneumatic foot pumps as prescribed.	To promote venous return and aid in prevention of thrombosis.

●●● **Related NIC and NOC labels:** *NIC:* Circulatory Care: Arterial Insufficiency; Circulatory Care: Venous Insufficiency; Circulatory Precautions; Fluid Management; Embolus Care: Peripheral; Pneumatic Tourniquet Precautions; Laboratory Data Interpretation *NOC:* Tissue Integrity: Skin and Mucous Membranes; Tissue Perfusion: Peripheral

Nursing Diagnosis:
Deficient Knowledge:

Cause, prevention, and treatment of DKA

Desired Outcome: Immediately following instruction, patient verbalizes accurate understanding of the cause, prevention, and treatment of DKA.

INTERVENTIONS	RATIONALES
Determine patient's knowledge about DKA and its treatment.	This will enable, as needed, further explanation of disease process of DM and DKA and common early symptoms of worsening hyperglycemia, including polyuria, polydipsia, polyphagia, dry and flushed skin, and increased irritability.
Assess patient's ability to engage in self-management of blood glucose monitoring and control. Explore whether patient psychologically accepts the disease as a significant health challenge.	This information will enable individualized teaching that will facilitate compliance with the prescribed management regimen designed to maintain normoglycemia.
Stress importance of maintaining a regular diet, exercise, and insulin regimen.	To ensure optimal control of serum glucose levels and prevention of adverse physical effects of DM, such as peripheral neuropathies and increased atherosclerosis.
Explain importance of testing urine ketone and blood glucose levels consistently and increasing the frequency of assessment during episodes of illness, injury, and stress. As indicated, review testing procedure. Caution that DKA necessitates professional medical management and cannot be self-treated.	Blood glucose >200 mg/dl and appearance of large amounts of urine ketones should be reported to health care provider so that insulin dose can be increased.
Teach patient that insulin or insulin analog must be taken every day and that lifetime insulin therapy is necessary. Explain that insulin is administered 1-4 times/day as prescribed.	To achieve control of blood glucose.
Explain that insulin may require adjustment during periods of illness or stress.	Increased stress impacts metabolism of carbohydrates, fats, and proteins, causing increased blood glucose.
Remind patient of importance of maintaining adequate oral fluid intake during illness.	Anorexia or nausea may limit food intake, but patient should make every effort to continue fluid intake to avoid dehydration, hypovolemia, and possible hypotension.
Teach patient necessity of reporting to health care provider such indicators as dizziness, impaired mentation, irritability, pallor, and tremors.	These are signs of insulin or insulin analog excess (hypoglycemia).

Continued

INTERVENTIONS	**RATIONALES**
Teach patient necessity of reporting to health care provider such indicators as increased polyuria and polydipsia and dry and flushed skin.	These are signs of insulin deficiency (hyperglycemia).
Teach importance of receiving prompt treatment if any of these indicators occurs.	If untreated, these conditions may lead to coma and death.
Explain importance of dietary changes as prescribed by health care provider.	Typically, patient is put on a fixed-calorie American Diabetes Association (ADA) diet composed of 60% carbohydrates, 20%-30% fats, and 12%-20% proteins.
Explain that fats should be polyunsaturated and proteins chosen from low-fat sources.	Reduction in saturated fat intake reduces risk of development of coronary artery and peripheral vascular disease.
Teach importance of eating three meals per day at regularly scheduled times and a bedtime snack.	To afford the best opportunity for maintaining a physiologically normal blood glucose level rather than "roller coaster" values of alternating hyperglycemia and hypoglycemia. Meals and insulin administration must be linked together, especially when insulin analogs such as Humalog or Novalog are given before meals and in conjunction with snacks. Analogs are quicker acting than regular insulins.
Explain causes for adjustments in insulin dose.	Causes for adjustments in insulin dose include increased or decreased food intake and any physical (e.g., exercise) or emotional stress. Exercise and emotional stress increase release of glucose from the liver, which may increase insulin demand.
Instruct patient to monitor blood glucose and urine ketone levels closely during periods of increased emotional stress and periods of increased or decreased exercise.	These assessments give patient data that will determine need for insulin dose adjustment.
Remind patient that alternative and complementary health strategies may alter blood glucose levels and prompt a need for adjustment of medications.	For example, certain herbal preparations can alter metabolism and may increase or decrease blood glucose. All methods used should be reported to health care provider.
Explain that measures that prevent infection, such as good hygiene and meticulous daily foot care, are necessary.	Persons with diabetes are susceptible to infection because of decreased inflammatory response.
Stress importance of avoiding exposure to communicable diseases.	
Describe indicators of infection that necessitate prompt medical treatment.	Indicators of infection include fever, chills, increased HR, diaphoresis, nausea, and vomiting. In addition, patient and significant other should be alert to wounds or cuts that do not heal, burning or pain with urination, and a productive cough.
Instruct patient to implement the following therapy when ill for any reason:	
- Do not alter insulin, insulin analog (Humalog), biguanide, sulfonylurea, or other antihyperglycemic medication dosage unless health care provider has prescribed a supplemental regimen to be implemented by individuals with type 1 DM for hyperglycemia secondary to illness.	Patient may not effectively alter insulin regimen and may put self at risk for hypoglycemia if medication dosage is increased.
- Perform blood glucose monitoring q3h and promptly report glucose >300 mg/dl to health care provider.	The stress associated with illness alters metabolism and glucose uptake. Hyperglycemia can ensue quickly when patient becomes ill.
- Eat small, frequent meals of soft, easily digestible, nourishing foods if regular meals are not tolerated.	If carbohydrate intake falls significantly, insulin dosage may need alteration to avoid hypoglycemia. Smaller meals may help maintain more normal intake.

Continued

INTERVENTIONS	RATIONALES
- Maintain adequate hydration, particularly if diarrhea, vomiting, or fever is persistent.	Dehydration can lead to hypovolemia, which in turn can lead to shock if left untreated.
- Balance intake of regular sodas or juices with water.	Intake of carbohydrates must be maintained unless insulin dose is altered to avoid hypoglycemia. Water must be drunk to maintain intravascular volume. There may be too much carbohydrate in juice or soda to use either as a primary source of volume.
- Report any of the above conditions to the health care provider.	If carbohydrate intake is not appropriately balanced with water intake, glucose will fluctuate and patient may be at risk for hypovolemia, which can lead to shock.
Provide the following address of the ADA: American Diabetes Association, Inc. 1660 Duke Street Alexandria, VA 22314 (800) 232-3472	For acquisition of pamphlets and magazines related to the disease, its complications, and appropriate treatment.

●●● **Related NIC and NOC labels:** *NIC:* Teaching: Disease Process; Learning Facilitation; Learning Readiness Enhancement; Teaching: Prescribed Diet; Teaching: Prescribed Medication; Hyperglycemia Management; Hypoglycemia Management; Teaching: Prescribed Activity/Exercise; Referral; Medication Management *NOC:* Knowledge: Diabetes Management

ADDITIONAL NURSING DIAGNOSES/ PROBLEMS:

"Psychosocial Support"   p. 81

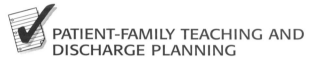

PATIENT-FAMILY TEACHING AND DISCHARGE PLANNING

See **Deficient Knowledge:** Cause, prevention, and treatment of DKA, p. 414.

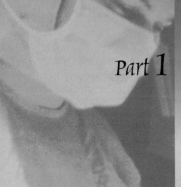

47

Hyperthyroidism

Hyperthyroidism is a clinical syndrome caused by excessive circulating thyroid hormone. Because thyroid activity affects all body systems, excessive thyroid hormone exaggerates normal body functions and produces a hypermetabolic state. Family history of hyperthyroidism is a significant factor for development of this disorder. Hyperthyroidism also can be caused by nodular toxic goiters in which one or more thyroid adenomas hyperfunction autonomously.

Graves' disease (diffuse toxic goiter) accounts for approximately 85% of reported cases of hyperthyroidism. It is characterized by spontaneous exacerbations and remissions that appear to be unaffected by therapy. The cause of Graves' disease is unknown, but recent advances in diagnostic techniques have isolated an immunoglobulin known as long-acting thyroid stimulator in a majority of patients with this disorder, suggesting that Graves' disease is an autoimmune response.

The most severe form of hyperthyroidism is thyrotoxic crisis, or thyroid storm, which results from a sudden surge of large amounts of thyroid hormones into the bloodstream, causing an even greater increase in body metabolism. This is a medical emergency.

HEALTH CARE SETTING

Primary care with possible hospitalization resulting from complications

ASSESSMENT

Signs and symptoms: Rapid pulse (usually noted by patient), menstrual irregularities, weight loss, fatigue, heat intolerance, increased perspiration, frequent defecation, anxiety, restlessness, tremor, and insomnia.

Physical assessment: Tachycardia, palpitations, widened pulse pressure, hyperpyrexia, enlargement of the thyroid gland, muscle weakness, hyperreflexia, fine tremor, fine hair, thin skin, hypercholesterolemia, impaired glucose tolerance, and stare and/or lid lag. Occasionally, males may present with gynecomastia.

Thyrotoxic crisis (thyroid storm): Acute exacerbation of some or all the above signs, marked tachycardia, hyperpyrexia, central nervous system (CNS) irritability, and sometimes coma or heart failure.

DIAGNOSTIC TESTS

Serum thyroid-stimulating hormone (TSH; thyrotropin): Decreased in the presence of disease.

Serum free thyroxine triiodothyronine (free T_3): Elevated in the presence of disease.

Radioiodine (^{131}I) uptake and thyroid scan: Clarifies size of gland and detects presence of hot or cold nodules.

^{131}I scintiscan: Defines functional characteristics of the gland.

Nursing Diagnosis:

Imbalanced Nutrition: Less than body requirements

related to hypermetabolic state and/or inadequate nutrient absorption

Desired Outcomes: By a minimum of 24 hr before hospital discharge (or within a week after intervention/treatment if patient is not hospitalized), patient has adequate nutrition as evidenced by stable weight and a positive nitrogen balance. Within 24 hr of instruction, patient lists types of foods that are necessary to restore a normal nutritional state.

INTERVENTIONS	RATIONALES
Teach patient about and provide foods high in calories, protein, carbohydrates, and vitamins.	These are foods that will help restore a normal nutritional state for patients with hyperthyroidism.
Provide between-meal snacks.	To maximize patient's consumption.
Administer vitamin supplements as prescribed and explain their importance to patient.	Vitamins provide essential nutrients to facilitate appropriate digestion/absorption of foods that contribute to energy production.
Administer prescribed antidiarrheal medications.	These medications increase absorption of nutrients from the gastrointestinal (GI) tract.
Weigh patient daily and report significant losses to health care provider.	Weight assessment is a useful indicator of nutritional status.

●●● **Related NIC and NOC labels:** *NIC:* Nutrition Management; Weight Gain Assistance; Teaching: Prescribed Diet; Medication Management *NOC:* Nutritional Status: Nutrient Intake

Nursing Diagnosis:
Disturbed Sleep Pattern

related to accelerated metabolism

Desired Outcome: Within 48 hr of interventions/treatment, patient relates the attainment of sufficient rest and sleep.

INTERVENTIONS	RATIONALES
Adjust care activities to patient's tolerance.	It may be necessary to alter care regimen to comply with patient's rest/sleep disturbance.
Provide frequent rest periods of at least 90-min duration.	Patients will have difficulty relaxing. Therefore all efforts must be made to provide a calm, quiet environment to promote rest/sleep. If possible, patient should have bedrest in a quiet, cool room with nonexertional activities, such as reading, watching television, working crossword puzzles, or listening to soothing music.
As necessary, assist with walking up stairs or other exertional activities.	If patient is tired, more assistance is needed until rest/sleep pattern normalizes.
Administer short-acting sedatives (e.g., lorazepam [Ativan]) as prescribed.	To promote rest.
After administering these agents, raise side rails and caution patient not to smoke in bed.	To protect patient, who will be drowsy after taking these sedatives.

●●● **Related NIC and NOC labels:** *NIC:* Energy Management; Sleep Enhancement; Self-Care Assistance; Environmental Management; Medication Management *NOC:* Rest; Sleep

Nursing Diagnosis:
Risk for Injury

related to potential for thyrotoxic crisis (thyroid storm) secondary to emotional stress, trauma, infection, or surgical manipulation of the gland

Desired Outcomes: Patient is free of symptoms of thyroid storm as evidenced by normothermia; BP ≥90/60 mm Hg (or within patient's baseline range); HR ≥100 bpm; and orientation to person, place, and time. If thyroid storm occurs, it is detected promptly and reported immediately.

INTERVENTIONS	RATIONALES
Measure and report rectal or core temperature >38.3° C (101° F).	An increased temperature often is the first sign of impending thyroid storm.
In patients in whom thyroid storm is suspected, monitor VS hourly.	To be alert for evidence of hypotension and increasing tachycardia and fever, which occur with thyroid storm.
Monitor patient for signs of heart failure. Immediately report any significant findings to health care provider and prepare to transfer patient to intensive care unit (ICU) if they are noted.	Signs of heart failure (jugular vein distention, crackles, decreased amplitude of peripheral pulses, peripheral edema, and hypotension) can occur as an effect of thyroid storm. If not aggressively monitored and managed, thyroid storm can lead to lethal cardiac and hemodynamic compromise.
Provide a cool, calm, protected environment. Reassure patient and explain all procedures before performing them. Limit the number of visitors.	To minimize emotional and physical stress, including fevers, which can precipitate thyroid storm.
Ensure good handwashing and meticulous aseptic technique for dressing changes and invasive procedures. Advise visitors who have contracted or been exposed to a communicable disease either not to enter patient's room or to wear a surgical mask, if appropriate.	To reduce risk of infection, which is a precipitating factor in development of thyroid storm.
In the Presence of Thyroid Storm:	
As prescribed, administer acetaminophen.	To decrease temperature secondary to the fever associated with thyroid storm.
Caution: Avoid giving aspirin.	Aspirin is contraindicated because it releases thyroxine from protein-binding sites and increases free thyroxine levels, which would exacerbate symptoms of thyroid storm.
Provide cool sponge baths or apply ice packs to patient's axilla and groin areas. If high temperature continues, obtain a prescription for a hypothermia blanket.	To decrease fever caused by thyroid storm.
Administer propylthiouracil (PTU) as prescribed.	To prevent further synthesis and release of thyroid hormones. The most severe side effect of this drug is leukopenia. Leukopenia increases the possibility that patient may acquire an infection. Patients should discontinue the drug at the first sign of infection and obtain a complete blood count (CBC). If the blood count is normal, medication is promptly resumed. Rash, another side effect, can be treated easily with antihistamines.
Administer propranolol as prescribed.	To block sympathetic nervous system (SNS) effects. Propranolol reduces HR and BP, which are elevated as a result of hyperthyroidism.
Administer IV fluids as prescribed.	To provide adequate hydration and prevent vascular collapse.
Carefully monitor I&O hourly.	To prevent fluid overload or inadequate fluid replacement. Fluid volume deficit may occur because of increased fluid excretion by the kidneys or excessive diaphoresis. Decreasing output with normal specific gravity may indicate decreased cardiac output, whereas decreasing output with increased specific gravity can signal dehydration.

Continued

INTERVENTIONS	RATIONALES
Administer sodium iodide as prescribed, 1 hr after administering PTU.	To attempt to provide iodine necessary for subsequent production of thyroid hormones following resolution of the crisis.
	Caution: If given before PTU, sodium iodide can exacerbate symptoms in susceptible persons.
Administer small doses of insulin as prescribed.	To control hyperglycemia. Hyperglycemia can occur as an effect of thyroid storm because of the release of stress hormones as part of the body's response to the hypermetabolic state.
Administer prescribed supplemental O₂ as necessary.	O₂ demands are increased as metabolism increases.

●●● **Related NIC and NOC labels:** *NIC:* Emergency Care; Environmental Management; Risk Identification *NOC:* Safety Status: Physical Injury

Nursing Diagnosis:

Anxiety

related to excessive amounts of thyroid hormones stimulating the SNS

Desired Outcomes: Within 24 hr of interventions/treatment, patient is free of harmful anxiety as evidenced by HR ≤100 bpm, RR 12-20 breaths/min with normal depth and pattern (eupnea), and absence of or decrease in irritability and restlessness. Immediately following teaching, patient and significant others verbalize knowledge about the causes of patient's behavior.

INTERVENTIONS	RATIONALES
In the presence of signs of anxiety administer short-acting sedatives as prescribed.	Short-acting sedatives (e.g., alprazolam [Xanax] or lorazepam [Ativan]) reduce anxiety.
Provide a quiet, stress-free environment away from loud noises or excessive activity.	To reduce stress and anxiety.
Limit number of visitors and the amount of time they spend with patient. Advise significant others to avoid discussing stressful topics and refrain from arguing with the patient.	To reduce stress and anxiety.
Administer propranolol as prescribed.	To reduce symptoms of anxiety, tachycardia, and heat intolerance.
Administer mild tranquilizers as prescribed.	To minimize anxiety and promote rest.
Reassure patient that anxiety symptoms are related to the disease process and that treatment decreases their severity.	Reassurance helps patient regain emotional control/reduce emotional stress through better understanding of the cause and treatment.
Inform significant others that patient's behavior is physiologic and should not be taken personally.	Reassuring family members helps them regain emotional control/reduce their stress regarding patient's unusual behaviors.

●●● **Related NIC and NOC labels:** *NIC:* Anxiety Reduction; Counseling; Medication Administration; Environmental Management *NOC:* Anxiety Control

Nursing Diagnosis:

Impaired Tissue Integrity (Corneal)

related to dryness that can occur with exophthalmos in persons with Graves' disease

Desired Outcome: Within 24 hr of interventions/treatment, patient's corneas are moist and intact.

INTERVENTIONS	RATIONALES
As appropriate, apply eye shields or tape the eyes shut at bedtime.	Hyperthyroidism can result in severe exophthalmos that prevents eyelids from closing fully, making the corneas vulnerable to injury.
Teach patient to wear dark glasses.	To protect the corneas. Dark glasses also protect those individuals who are photosensitive.
Administer lubricating eyedrops as prescribed.	To supplement lubrication and decrease SNS stimulation, which can cause lid retraction.
Administer thioamides as prescribed.	To maintain normal metabolic state and halt progression of exophthalmos.

●●● **Related NIC and NOC labels:** *NIC:* Eye Care; Medication Administration: Eye *NOC:* Tissue Integrity: Skin and Mucous Membranes

Nursing Diagnosis:

Disturbed Body Image

related to exophthalmos or surgical scar

Desired Outcome: Following teaching, patient verbalizes measures for disguising exophthalmos or surgical scar and exhibits self-acceptance.

INTERVENTIONS	RATIONALES
Encourage patient to communicate feelings of frustration.	To help patients relieve stress that can further stimulate the hypophyseal/thyroid/adrenal axis.
Advise patient to wear dark glasses.	To disguise exophthalmos while also protecting corneas from photosensitivity.
Suggest measures that can disguise the scar.	Customized jewelry, high-necked clothing such as turtlenecks, or loose-fitting scarves are examples of measures that will help disguise the scar.
Suggest that after incision has healed, patient can use makeup colored in his or her skin tone.	To decrease visibility of the scar.
Caution patient that creams are contraindicated until the incision has healed completely, and even then they may not minimize scarring.	Standard postoperative teaching for most surgical procedures.
Suggest that patient increase vitamin C intake.	Patients are advised by some physicians to increase vitamin C intake up to 1 g/day to promote healing.

Continued

INTERVENTIONS	RATIONALES
As directed by physician, advise against direct sunlight to the operative site.	Some surgeons advise against direct sunlight to the operative site for 6-12 mo to avoid hyperpigmentation of the incision.
For additional information, see this nursing diagnosis in "Psychosocial Support," p. 81.	

●●● **Related NIC and NOC labels:** *NIC:* Body Image Enhancement; Active Listening; Coping Enhancement; Counseling; Emotional Support *NOC:* Body Image

Nursing Diagnosis:

Deficient Knowledge:

Potential for side effects from iodides and thioamides or stopping thioamides abruptly

Desired Outcome: Immediately following teaching, patient verbalizes knowledge about potential side effects of prescribed medications, signs and symptoms of hypothyroidism and hyperthyroidism, and importance of following the prescribed medical regimen.

INTERVENTIONS	RATIONALES
Explain importance of taking antithyroid medications daily, in divided doses, and at regular intervals as prescribed.	A knowledgeable patient is more likely to comply with the treatment regimen.
Teach indicators of hypothyroidism and the signs and symptoms that necessitate medical attention.	Indicators of hypothyroidism (e.g., early fatigue, weight gain, anorexia, constipation, menstrual irregularities, muscle cramps, lethargy, inability to concentrate, hair loss, cold intolerance, and hoarseness) may occur from excessive medication. Signs and symptoms that necessitate medical attention because the medications that cause them may require dose adjustment include cold intolerance, fatigue, lethargy, and peripheral or periorbital edema.
Teach side effects of thioamides that necessitate medical attention.	Appearance of a rash, fever, or pharyngitis can occur in the presence of agranulocytosis, a recognized side effect of thioamides. This necessitates medical attention to adjust the dose or change the medication.
Alert patients taking iodides to signs of worsening hyperthyroidism. Stress importance of reporting these signs promptly to health care provider.	Signs of worsening hyperthyroidism (high body temperature, palpitations, rapid HR, irritability, anxiety, and feelings of restlessness or panic) may signal need for medication dosage adjustment to manage worsening hyperthyroidism and should be reported promptly for timely intervention.

●●● **Related NIC and NOC labels:** *NIC:* Teaching: Prescribed Medication *NOC:* Knowledge: Medication; Knowledge: Treatment Regimen

Nursing Diagnosis:

Acute Pain

related to surgical procedure

Desired Outcomes: Within 2 hr following surgery, patient's subjective perception of pain decreases, as documented by a pain scale. Objective indicators, such as hesitation before turning or moving the head, are absent or diminished.

INTERVENTIONS	RATIONALES
Devise a pain scale with patient, rating pain on a scale of 0 (no pain) to 10 (worst pain). Document degree and character of patient's pain, including precipitating events.	This will enable nurse to determine trend of the pain and degree of pain relief obtained.
Inform patient to clasp hands behind neck when moving.	To minimize stress on the incision.
After health care provider has removed surgical clips and drain, teach patient to perform gentle range-of-motion (ROM) exercises for the neck.	While the surgical clips and drain are in place, mobility of the neck is limited, leading to tight neck muscles. Following removal of these devices, gentle ROM is done to help relax the neck muscles and decrease pain.
For other interventions, see "Pain," p. 41, and "Perioperative Care," p. 47.	

●●● **Related NIC and NOC labels:** *NIC:* Pain Management; Positioning *NOC:* Comfort Level; Pain Control

Nursing Diagnosis:

Impaired Swallowing

(or risk for same) *related to* edema or laryngeal nerve damage resulting from thyroidectomy

Desired Outcomes: Patient reports ability to swallow with minimal difficulty, has minimal or absent hoarseness, and is free of symptoms of respiratory dysfunction as evidenced by RR 12-20 breaths/min with normal depth and pattern (eupnea) and absence of inspiratory stridor. Laryngeal nerve damage, if it occurs, is detected promptly and reported immediately.

INTERVENTIONS	RATIONALES
Monitor respiratory status for dyspnea, choking, inspiratory stridor, and inability to swallow.	These are signs of postsurgical edema. Edema in the neck may impinge on the pharynx or esophagus, making swallowing more difficult.
Also assess patient's voice.	Although slight hoarseness is normal after surgery, hoarseness that persists should be reported to health care provider promptly. Persistent hoarseness is indicative of laryngeal nerve damage. If bilateral nerve damage is present, upper airway obstruction and dysphagia can occur.
Elevate head of bed (HOB) 30-45 degrees.	Elevating HOB enables gravity to facilitate swallowing and promotes edema reduction.
Support patient's head with flat or cervical pillows so that it is in a neutral position with the neck (does not flex or hyperextend).	To minimize incisional stress and reduce chance of choking and dysphagia.
Keep tracheostomy set and O_2 equipment at the bedside at all times.	For emergency treatment in the event upper airway obstruction occurs.
Suction upper airway as needed, using gentle suction.	Patients can aspirate retained secretions if edema and/or laryngeal nerve problems are present. Using gentle, rather than aggressive, suctioning avoids stimulating laryngospasm.
Administer analgesics promptly and as prescribed.	To minimize pain and anxiety and enhance patient's ability to swallow.
See this nursing diagnosis in "Perioperative Care," p. 47.	

●●● **Related NIC and NOC labels:** *NIC:* Airway Suctioning; Positioning; Surveillance *NOC:* Aspiration Control; Swallowing Status; Swallowing Status: Esophageal Phase; Swallowing Status: Pharyngeal

PATIENT-FAMILY TEACHING AND DISCHARGE PLANNING

When providing patient-family teaching, focus on sensory information, avoid giving excessive information, and initiate a visiting nurse referral for necessary follow-up teaching. Part of the initial assessment should include asking about existing knowledge of the disease, ability for self-management, and psychologic acceptance. Include verbal and written information about the following:

✓ Diet high in calories, protein, carbohydrates, and vitamins. Inform patient that as a normal metabolic state is attained, the diet may change.

✓ Medications, including drug name, purpose, dosage, schedule, precautions, drug/drug and food/drug interactions, and potential side effects.

✓ Changes that can occur as a result of therapy, including weight gain, normalized bowel function, increased strength of skeletal muscles, and a return to normal activity levels.

✓ Importance of continued and frequent medical follow-up; confirm date and time of next appointment.

✓ Indicators that necessitate medical attention, including fever, rash, or sore throat (side effects of thioamides), and symptoms of hypothyroidism (see p. 425) or worsening hyperthyroidism.

✓ For patients receiving radioactive iodine, the importance of not holding children to the chest for 72 hr following therapy, because they are more susceptible to the effects of radiation. Explain that there is negligible risk for adults.

✓ Importance of avoiding physical and emotional stress early in the recuperative stage and maximizing coping mechanisms for dealing with stress. See **Health-Seeking Behaviors:** Relaxation technique effective for stress reduction, p. 183.

48

Hypothyroidism

Hypothyroidism is a condition in which there is an inadequate amount of circulating thyroid hormone, causing a decrease in metabolic rate that affects all body systems.

- *Primary hypothyroidism* accounts for ≥90% of cases of hypothyroidism and is caused by pathologic changes in the thyroid itself. There are several possible causes, including dietary iodine deficiency, thyroiditis, thyroid atrophy or fibrosis of unknown cause, radiation therapy to the neck (e.g., with treatment for hyperthyroidism), surgical removal of all or part of the gland, drugs that suppress thyroid activity including propylthiouracil (PTU) and iodides, or a genetic dysfunction resulting in the inability to produce and secrete thyroid hormone.
- *Secondary hypothyroidism* is caused by dysfunction of the anterior pituitary gland, which results in decreased release of thyroid-stimulating hormone (TSH). It can be caused by pituitary tumors, postpartum necrosis of the pituitary gland, or hypophysectomy.
- *Tertiary hypothyroidism* is caused by a hypothalamic deficiency in the release of thyrotropin-releasing hormone (TRH).

When hypothyroidism is untreated, or when a stressor such as infection affects an individual with hypothyroidism, a life-threatening condition known as *myxedema coma* can occur. The clinical picture of myxedema coma is that of exaggerated hypothyroidism, with dangerous hypoventilation, hypothermia, hypotension, and shock.

HEALTH CARE SETTING

Primary care with possible hospitalization resulting from complications

ASSESSMENT

Signs and symptoms can progress from mild early in onset to life threatening. They may include early fatigue, weight gain, anorexia, lethargy, cold intolerance, menstrual irregularities, depression, and muscle cramps.

Physical assessment: Possible presence of goiter, bradycardia, hypothermia, deepened voice or hoarseness, hypercholesterolemia, and obesity. The skin may be dry, cool, and coarse, and the hair may be thin, coarse, and brittle. The tongue may be enlarged (macroglossia), and the reflexes may be slowed.

Myxedema coma: Hypoventilation, hypoglycemia, hypothermia, hypotension, bradycardia, and shock.

DIAGNOSTIC TESTS

TSH: Elevated unless the disease is long standing or severe.

Free thyroxine Index (FTI) and thyroxine (T_4) levels: Decreased.

^{131}I scan and uptake: Will be <10% in a 24-hr period. In secondary hypothyroidism, uptake increases with administration of exogenous TSH.

Thyroperoxidase antibodies: Positive test signals chronic autoimmune thyroiditis.

Nursing Diagnosis:

Ineffective Breathing Pattern

(or risk for same) *related to* upper airway obstruction occurring with enlarged thyroid gland and/or decreased ventilatory drive caused by greatly decreased metabolism

Desired Outcomes: Patient has an effective breathing pattern as evidenced by RR 12-20 breaths/min with normal depth and pattern (eupnea), normal skin color, normal O_2 saturation (≥95%), and absence of adventitious breath sounds. Alternatively, if an ineffective breathing pattern occurs, it is detected, reported, and treated promptly.

INTERVENTIONS	RATIONALES
Assess quality of breath sounds.	This enables nurse to be alert to presence of adventitious sounds (e.g., from developing pleural effusion) or decreasing or crowing sounds (e.g., from swollen tongue or glottis).
Be alert to and immediately report signs of ventilatory insufficiency.	Decreased respiratory rate, shallow breathing, and circumoral or peripheral cyanosis are signs of inadequate ventilation. Ventilatory insufficiency in a patient with hypothyroid condition can indicate onset of heart failure secondary to impending myxedema coma/hypothyroid crisis.
Measure O_2 saturation intermittently or continuously in patients with decreased ventilatory drive.	Decreasing O_2 saturation may signal need for oxygen supplementation in symptomatic patients.
Teach patient coughing, deep breathing, and use of incentive spirometer. Suction upper airway prn.	To help clear secretions that may increase with hypoventilation.
For a patient experiencing respiratory distress, be prepared to assist health care provider with intubation or tracheostomy and maintenance of mechanical ventilatory assistance or transfer patient to intensive care unit (ICU).	Patient likely will need emergency treatment and intensive care.

●●● **Related NIC and NOC labels:** *NIC:* Airway Management; Airway Insertion and Stabilization; Cough Enhancement; Respiratory Monitoring; Emergency Care; Mechanical Ventilation; Oxygen Therapy; Ventilation Assistance *NOC:* Respiratory Status: Airway Patency; Respiratory Status: Ventilation

Nursing Diagnosis:

Excess Fluid Volume

related to compromised regulatory mechanisms occurring with hypothyroid crisis that can lead to adrenal insufficiency

Desired Outcome: Within 24 hr after interventions/treatment, patient is normovolemic as evidenced by urinary output ≥30 ml/hr, stable weight, nondistended jugular veins, presence of eupnea, and peripheral pulse amplitude ≥2+ on a 0-4+ scale.

INTERVENTIONS	RATIONALES
Monitor I&O hourly for evidence of decreasing output.	Decreasing output signals fluid retention leading to hypervolemia.
Weigh patient at the same time every day, with the same clothing and using the same scale. Report increasing weight gain to health care provider.	Increasing weight gain signals fluid retention leading to hypervolemia/volume overload.
Monitor for indicators of heart failure. Report significant findings to health care provider.	Indicators of heart failure include jugular vein distention, crackles, shortness of breath, dependent edema of extremities, and decreased amplitude of peripheral pulses. Lack of thyroid hormones can decrease the heart rate and force of contractions, leading to heart failure. Associated fluid retention worsens the problem.
Restrict fluid and Na^+ intake as prescribed.	To prevent fluid retention leading to volume overload.
Administer IV fluids using a rate control device.	To prevent accidental fluid overload.

●●● **Related NIC and NOC labels:** *NIC:* Fluid Monitoring; Fluid/Electrolyte Management; Hypervolemia Management; Vital Signs Monitoring; Cardiac Care: Acute *NOC:* Fluid Balance

Nursing Diagnosis:

Activity Intolerance

related to weakness and fatigue secondary to slowed metabolism and decreased cardiac output caused by pericardial effusions, atherosclerosis, and decreased adrenergic stimulation

Desired Outcome: During activity patient rates perceived exertion at ≤3 on a 0-10 scale and exhibits cardiac tolerance to activity as evidenced by HR ≤20 bpm over resting HR, systolic BP ≤20 mm Hg over or under resting systolic BP, warm and dry skin, and absence of crackles (rales), murmurs, chest pain, and new dysrhythmias.

INTERVENTIONS	RATIONALES
Monitor VS and apical pulse, urine output, and mentation status at frequent intervals.	This enables nurse to be alert to hypotension, slow pulse, dysrhythmias, decreasing urine output, and changes in mentation, which along with complaints of chest pain or discomfort may signal heart failure/impending pulmonary edema.
Ask patient to rate perceived exertion (RPE). See this diagnosis in "Prolonged Bedrest," p. 67, for details.	RPE >3 on a 0-10 scale is a signal of cardiac intolerance during exertion and also a sign that patient should stop or modify the activity causing the exertion.
Promptly report significant changes to health care provider.	To avoid progression of heart failure to cardiac arrest.
Balance activity with adequate rest.	To decrease workload of the heart.
As prescribed, administer IV isotonic solutions such as normal saline.	To help prevent hypotension. Hypotension ensues as a result of reduced sympathetic nervous system (SNS) stimulation, which causes decreased cardiac output and hypotension.
Assist patient with range-of-motion (ROM) and other in-bed exercises and consult with physician about implementation of exercises that require greater cardiac tolerance. For details, see **Risk for Activity Intolerance,** p. 67, and **Risk for Disuse Syndrome,** p. 69.	To prevent problems of immobility.

●●● **Related NIC and NOC labels:** *NIC:* Energy Management; Exercise Promotion *NOC:* Energy Conservation

Nursing Diagnosis:

Risk for Infection

related to compromised immunologic status secondary to alterations in adrenal function

Desired Outcome: Patient is free of infection as evidenced by normothermia, absence of adventitious breath sounds, normal urinary pattern and characteristics, and well-healing wounds.

INTERVENTIONS	RATIONALES
Be alert to early indicators of infection. Notify health care provider of significant findings.	Fever; erythema, swelling, or discharge from wounds or IV sites; urinary frequency, urgency, or dysuria; cloudy or malodorous urine; presence of adventitious sounds on auscultation of lung fields; and changes in color, consistency, and amount of sputum are early indicators of infection.

Continued

INTERVENTIONS	RATIONALES
	Prompt assessment and treatment can halt their progression to prevent complications such as myxedema coma, a life-threatening condition.
Provide meticulous care of indwelling catheters.	To minimize risk of urinary tract infection.
Ensure good handwashing and use sterile technique when performing dressing changes and invasive procedures.	To minimize risk of wound and other infections. Nonintact skin and invasive procedures can lead to bacterial ingress.
Provide good skin care.	To maintain skin integrity and prevent pressure ulcers. Open sores are sites of ingress for bacteria.
Advise visitors who have contracted or been exposed to a communicable disease not to enter patient's room or to wear a surgical mask, if appropriate.	To minimize risk of infection.
For more information, see Appendix for "Infection Prevention and Control," p. 831.	

●●● **Related NIC and NOC labels:** *NIC:* Infection Protection; Risk Identification; Surveillance; Infection Control; Environmental Management; Incision Site Care; Wound Care *NOC:* Immune Status; Infection Status

Nursing Diagnosis:

Risk for Imbalanced Nutrition: More than body requirements of calories

related to slowed metabolism

Desired Outcomes: Optimally, patient does not experience weight gain. Immediately following teaching, patient verbalizes accurate understanding of the rationale and measures for the dietary regimen.

INTERVENTIONS	RATIONALES
Provide a diet that is high in protein and low in calories.	To promote weight loss.
As prescribed, restrict or limit Na^+ and foods high in Na^+ content.	To decrease edema caused by fluid retention.
Teach patient about foods to augment and limit or avoid.	Foods high in protein and low in calories/Na^+ will help with weight control while patient is in a hypometabolic/fluid-retaining state.
Provide small, frequent meals of appropriate foods that the patient particularly enjoys.	To promote weight control and decrease chance of patient overeating if allowed to get too hungry.
Encourage foods that are high in fiber content (e.g., fruits with skins, vegetables, whole grain breads and cereals, nuts).	To improve gastric motility, which will help elimination that may be decreased as a result of slowed metabolism.
Administer vitamins as prescribed.	For patients whose diets require supplementation because of inability to consume appropriate recommended daily allowance (RDA) minimum requirements on their restricted diet.

●●● **Related NIC and NOC labels:** *NIC:* Nutrition Management; Teaching: Prescribed Diet; Weight Management *NOC:* Nutritional Status: Food and Fluid Intake; Weight Control

Nursing Diagnosis:

Constipation

related to inadequate dietary intake of roughage and fluids, prolonged bedrest, and/or decreased peristalsis secondary to slowed metabolism

Desired Outcome: Within 48-72 hr of interventions/treatment, patient relates the attainment of his or her normal pattern of bowel elimination.

INTERVENTIONS	RATIONALES
Ask patient about current bowel function; document changes.	To be alert to or help prevent constipation.
Monitor for decreasing bowel sounds and the presence of distention and increases in abdominal girth.	Can occur with ileus or fecal impaction leading to an obstructive process, which is fairly common in hypothyroidism, especially in older adults.
Encourage patient to maintain a diet with adequate roughage, fluids, and protein.	To help prevent constipation by increasing bulk in and softening stools. Protein is digested more slowly and provides an energy source that lasts longer than energy from carbohydrates and fats.
Provide examples of foods high in bulk. Ensure that fluid intake in persons without underlying cardiac or renal disease is at least 2-3 L/day.	Such foods as fruits with skins, fruit juices, cooked fruits, vegetables, whole grain breads and cereals, and nuts provide bulk, which will promote bowel elimination by increasing peristalsis and, coupled with increased fluid intake, add moisture to keep stool moving through the intestines/colon.
Administer stool softeners and laxatives as prescribed.	To minimize constipation by moistening stool and increasing peristalsis.
Caution: Avoid use of suppositories.	When administering them, there is risk of stimulating the vagus nerve, which would further decrease HR and BP.
Advise patient to increase amount of exercise.	To promote regularity by increasing peristalsis. Exercise also tones gastrointestinal (GI) muscles to hold intestines/colon in place, which seems to facilitate bowel elimination.

●●● **Related NIC and NOC labels:** *NIC:* Bowel Management; Exercise Promotion; Fluid Management; Nutrition Management; Medication Administration *NOC:* Bowel Elimination; Hydration

Nursing Diagnosis:

Disturbed Sensory Perception

related to altered sensory reception, transmission, or integration secondary to cerebral retention of water

Desired Outcomes: Optimally, patient verbalizes orientation to person, place, and time. Alternately, if signs of myxedema coma appear, they are detected, reported, and treated promptly.

INTERVENTIONS	RATIONALES
Monitor patient's mental status at frequent intervals by assessing orientation to person, place, and time. Report significant findings to health care provider.	Increasing lethargy or confusion can signal onset of myxedema coma, which necessitates immediate medical attention.

Continued

INTERVENTIONS	RATIONALES
Reorient patient frequently. Have a clock and calendar visible and use radio or television for orientation.	To ensure that patient has information necessary to answer neurologic assessment questions appropriately.
Clearly explain all procedures to patient before performing them. Provide adequate time for patient to ask questions.	To promote better understanding of procedures to a patient who may have memory impairment.
If necessary, remind patient to complete activities of daily living (ADL) such as bathing and brushing hair.	Same as above.
Encourage visitors to discuss topics of special interest to patient.	To enhance patient's alertness.
Administer thyroid replacement hormones, such as oral thyroid hormone (i.e., levothyroxine), as prescribed.	To increase metabolic rate, which in turn will promote cerebral blood flow. Patients are started on low doses that are increased gradually, based on serial laboratory tests (TSH and T_4), and adjusted until the TSH is in a normal range. This dose titration prevents hyperthyroidism caused by too much exogenous hormone. Therapy is continued for the patient's lifetime.

Note: For patients with secondary hypothyroidism, thyroid supplements can promote acute symptoms and therefore are contraindicated. |

●●● **Related NIC and NOC labels:** *NIC:* Cognitive Stimulation; Reality Orientation; Medication Management *NOC:* Cognitive Orientation

Nursing Diagnosis:

Risk for Injury (myxedema coma)

related to inadequate response to treatment of hypothyroidism or stressors such as infection

Desired Outcomes: Patient is free of symptoms of myxedema coma as evidenced by HR ≥60 bpm, BP ≥90/60 mm Hg (or within patient's normal range), RR ≥12 breaths/min with normal depth and pattern (eupnea), and orientation to person, place, and time. Alternately, if myxedema coma occurs, it is detected, reported, and treated promptly.

INTERVENTIONS	RATIONALES
Monitor for signs of heart failure.	Jugular vein distention, crackles, shortness of breath, peripheral edema, and weakening peripheral pulses are signs of heart failure that can occur secondary to hypothyroidism and lead to myxedema coma.
Monitor VS at frequent intervals. Report systolic BP <90 mm Hg, HR <60 bpm, or RR <12 breaths/min.	Bradycardia, hypotension, and decrease in RR are signals of impending cardiac arrest.
Monitor patient for circumoral or peripheral cyanosis and decrease in level of consciousness (LOC).	Signs of hypoxia, which is a signal that patient may be about to experience cardiac arrest.
Immediately report significant findings to health care provider.	Patient may experience cardiac arrest. At minimum, patient likely will need an increased dosage of the medication.
Monitor serum electrolytes and glucose levels.	In myxedema coma, patient may have decreasing Na^+ (<137 mEq/L) and glucose (<80 mg/dl) levels.

Continued

INTERVENTIONS	RATIONALES
In the presence of myxedema coma, implement the following:	
- Restrict fluids or administer hypertonic saline as prescribed.	To correct hyponatremia.
- Use an infusion control device.	To maintain accurate infusion rate of IV fluids.
- As prescribed, administer IV thyroid replacement hormones with IV hydrocortisone and IV glucose.	To treat hypoglycemia. Rapid IV administration of thyroid hormone can precipitate hyperadrenalism. This can be avoided by concomitant administration of IV hydrocortisone.
Prepare to transfer patient to ICU. Keep an oral airway and manual resuscitator at the bedside in the event of seizure, coma, or the need for ventilatory assistance.	Emergency treatment for decreased ventilatory drive.

●●● **Related NIC and NOC labels:** *NIC:* Risk Identification; Emergency Care *NOC:* Safety Status: Physical Injury

PATIENT-FAMILY TEACHING AND DISCHARGE PLANNING

When providing patient-family teaching, focus on sensory information, avoid giving excessive information, and initiate a visiting nurse referral for necessary follow-up teaching. Part of the initial assessment should include asking about existing knowledge of the disease, ability for self-management, and psychologic acceptance. Include verbal and written information about the following:

✓ Medications, including drug name, purpose, dosage, schedule, precautions, drug/drug and food/drug interactions, and potential side effects. Remind patient that thioamides, iodides, and lithium are contraindicated because they decrease thyroid activity. Be sure patient is aware that thyroid replacement medications are to be taken for life.

✓ Dietary requirements and restrictions, which may change as hormone replacement therapy takes effect.

✓ Expected changes that can occur with hormone replacement therapy: increased energy level, weight loss, and decreased peripheral edema. Neuromuscular problems should improve as well.

✓ Importance of continued, frequent medical follow-up; confirm date and time of next medical appointment

✓ Importance of avoiding physical and emotional stress and ways for patient to maximize coping mechanisms for dealing with stress. See **Health-Seeking Behaviors:** Relaxation technique effective for stress reduction, p. 183.

✓ Signs and symptoms that necessitate medical attention, including fever or other symptoms of upper respiratory, urinary, or oral infections and signs and symptoms of hyperthyroidism, which may result from excessive hormone replacement.

Syndrome of Inappropriate Antidiuretic Hormone

Syndrome of inappropriate antidiuretic hormone (SIADH) is caused by release of antidiuretic hormone (ADH) from the pituitary gland without regard to serum osmolality, plasma volume, or blood pressure, resulting in excessive water retention and hyponatremia. The action of ADH increases reabsorption of water in the last segment of the distal tubules and collecting ducts of the kidney. ADH secretion usually is stimulated by one of three mechanisms: (1) increased serum osmolality, (2) decreased plasma volume, or (3) decreased BP. SIADH requires differential diagnosis from other problems that prompt elevation of vasopressin and resultant hyponatremia because of an appropriate response to hypovolemic or hypotensive stimuli. SIADH is seen in postoperative, multiorgan dysfunction syndrome, and oncology patients. Sometimes it is present but not diagnosed because of mild or transient symptoms. Water intoxication, cerebral edema, and severe hyponatremia cause altered neurologic/mental status, which if untreated may lead to death.

HEALTH CARE SETTING

Acute care

ASSESSMENT

Signs and symptoms: Decreased urine output with concentrated urine. Signs of water intoxication may appear, including altered level of consciousness (LOC), fatigue, headache, diarrhea, anorexia, nausea, vomiting, and seizures. **Note:** Because of the loss of Na^+, edema will not accompany the fluid volume excess.

Physical assessment: Weight gain without edema, elevated BP, altered mental status.

History of: Cancers of the lung, pancreas, duodenum, and prostate, which can secrete a biologically active form of ADH. Other common causes include pulmonary disease (e.g., tuberculosis, pneumonia, chronic obstructive pulmonary disease), acquired immunodeficiency syndrome (AIDS), head trauma, brain tumor, intracerebral hemorrhage, meningitis, and encephalitis. Positive-pressure ventilation, physiologic stress, chronic metabolic illness, and a wide variety of medications (chlorpropamide, acetaminophen, oxytocin, narcotics, general anesthetic, carbamazepine, thiazide diuretics, tricyclic antidepressants, neuroleptics, angiotensin-converting enzyme [ACE] inhibitors, cancer chemotherapy agents) all have been linked to SIADH.

DIAGNOSTIC TESTS

Serum Na^+ level: Decreased to <137 mEq/L.

Plasma osmolality: Decreased to <275 mOsm/kg.

Urine osmolality: Elevated disproportionately relative to plasma osmolality.

Urine Na+ level: Increased to >200 mEq/L. Urine Na+ level (e.g., increased) is best evaluated in comparison with serum Na+ level (e.g., decreased).

Urine specific gravity: >1.030.
Plasma ADH level: Elevated.

Nursing Diagnosis:

Excess Fluid Volume

related to compromised regulatory mechanisms resulting in increased serum ADH level, renal water reabsorption, and renal Na+ excretion

Desired Outcome: Patient becomes normovolemic (and normonatremic) within 7 days of onset of symptoms, as evidenced by orientation to person, place, and time; intake that approximates output plus insensible losses; stable weight; central venous pressure (CVP) 2-6 mm Hg; BP 90-140/60-85 mm Hg or within patient's normal range; and HR 60-100 bpm.

INTERVENTIONS	RATIONALES
Assess LOC, VS, and I&O at least q4h; measure weight daily. Promptly report significant findings or changes to health care provider.	Decreasing LOC, elevated BP and CVP, urine output <30 ml/hr, and weight gain are signs of excess fluid volume that occur with SIADH.
Monitor laboratory results, including those for serum Na+, urine and serum osmolality, and urine specific gravity. Report significant findings to health care provider.	Normal values are as follows: urine specific gravity, 1.010-1.020; serum Na+, 137-147 mEq/L; urine osmolality, 300-1090 mOsm/kg; and serum osmolality, 280-300 mOsm/kg. Decreased serum Na+ and plasma osmolality, urine osmolality elevated disproportionately in relation to plasma osmolality, and increased urine Na+ are values that are seen with SIADH. Water retention secondary to increased ADH secretion dilutes blood and results in reduced amounts of more concentrated urine.
Maintain fluid restriction as prescribed. Explain necessity of this treatment to patient and significant other. Do not keep water or ice chips at the bedside. Ensure precise delivery of fluid administered IV by using a monitoring device.	Restricting fluids to the amount manageable by the kidneys will allow restoration of normal serum Na+ levels and osmolality without complications from drug therapy.
Elevate head of bed (HOB) 10-20 degrees.	To promote venous return and thus reduce ADH release. Excess fluid volume can sometimes result in cerebral edema that may add to problems with neural regulation of ADH secretion.
Administer demeclocycline, lithium, furosemide, or bumetanide as prescribed; carefully observe and document patient's response.	These drugs promote water excretion.
Administer hypertonic (3%) NaCl or isotonic (0.9%) solution as prescribed.	May be given if the patient has severe hyponatremia. Rate of administration usually is based on serial serum Na+ levels.
	Supplemental Na+ solutions may be administered with IV furosemide (Lasix) or bumetanide (Bumex) or osmotic diuretics, such as mannitol, to promote water excretion.
Ensure that specimens for laboratory tests are drawn on time and results are reported to health care provider promptly.	To assess serum blood levels of sodium to ensure that patient does not have hypernatremia as a result of aggressive treatment.

Continued

INTERVENTIONS	RATIONALES
Institute seizure precautions as indicated.	Padded side rails, supplemental oxygen, and oral airway at the bedside, as well as side rails up at all times when staff member is not present, prevent patient injury in the event of seizure. Seizures can occur in the presence of hyponatremia, which results from the excess fluid volume present in SIADH.

●●● **Related NIC and NOC labels:** *NIC:* Fluid/Electrolyte Management; Electrolyte Management: Hyponatremia; Fluid Monitoring; Laboratory Data Interpretation; Neurologic Monitoring; Vital Signs Monitoring; Cerebral Edema Management; Medication Administration *NOC:* Electrolyte and Acid/Base Balance; Fluid Balance

Nursing Diagnosis:

Ineffective Protection

related to potential for increased intracranial pressure (IICP), diabetes insipidus (DI), cerebrospinal fluid (CSF) leak, hemorrhage, and infection secondary to transsphenoidal hypophysectomy

Desired Outcomes: Optimally, patient demonstrates normal level of mental acuity; verbalizes orientation to person, place, and time; and is free of indicators of injury caused by complications of transsphenoidal hypophysectomy. Immediately after instruction, patient and significant other verbalize accurate understanding of the importance of avoiding Valsalva type of maneuvers; describe the signs and symptoms of IICP, DI, and infection; and verbalize the importance of notifying staff of postnasal drip or excessive swallowing.

Note: Transsphenoidal hypophysectomy is performed if medical management cannot correct the SIADH or if patient has a pituitary tumor.

INTERVENTIONS	RATIONALES
Be alert to indicators of IICP.	Indicators of IICP include change in mental status or LOC, sluggish or unequal pupils, and changes in respiratory rate or pattern and can occur as a complication of transsphenoidal hypophysectomy.
Monitor patient for decreased vision, eye muscle weakness, abnormal extraocular eye movement, double vision, and airway obstruction. Report significant findings to health care provider.	The surgery may interfere with cranial nerves governing eye movements and visual acuity—II, III, IV, VI.
Measure I&O hourly for 24 hr and monitor urine specific gravity q1-2h. Monitor weight daily for evidence of loss.	Output >200 ml/hr for 2 consecutive hr or a total of 500 ml/hr and specific gravity <1.007 are found with DI. Weight loss can occur with excessive urinary output.
Explain signs of DI to the patient, including polydipsia, polyuria, and decreased urine specific gravity.	DI often occurs as a result of the edema caused by manipulating the pituitary stalk and usually is transitory.
Notify health care provider of significant findings.	The presence of DI necessitates fluid replacement to correct for excessive fluid loss.
Inspect nasal packing at frequent intervals. Note the number of times the mustache dressing is changed.	To determine presence of frank bleeding or CSF leakage. Expect nasal packing removal in about 3-4 days.

Continued

INTERVENTIONS	RATIONALES
Test serous/*non*sanguineous drainage for the presence of CSF using a glucose reagent strip.	CSF contains glucose. However, because blood also contains glucose, testing should be done only on drainage that appears to be clear.
Monitor for complaints of postnasal drip or excessive swallowing and explain relevance to patient.	May signal CSF drainage down the back of patient's throat.
Elevate HOB and immediately report any suspicious drainage.	To minimize potential for bacteria entering the brain. Presence of CSF represents a serious breach in cranial integrity.
Elevate HOB 30 degrees.	To decrease ICP and swelling.
Administer dexamethasone if it is prescribed.	To reduce cerebral swelling.
Explain that coughing, sneezing, and other Valsalva type of maneuvers must be avoided.	These actions can stress the operative site and increase ICP, causing CSF leakage.
Teach patient to cough or sneeze with an open mouth if either is unavoidable. Remind patient that nose blowing should be avoided until the nasal mucosa is healed (about 1 mo).	Pressure is high in the nasopharynx and sinuses if the mouth is closed when the patient coughs or sneezes. Opening the mouth will reduce this pressure and hence stress on incisional area.
Advise patient about importance of mouth breathing and possibility of having a soft nasal airway.	Nasal passages may not be patent. Patient likely would be more comfortable breathing through the mouth.
Obtain prescription for a mild cathartic or stool softener if indicated.	To prevent straining with bowel movements, which would increase ICP.
Do not allow patient to brush teeth. Provide mouthwash (e.g., hydrogen peroxide diluted with water to half strength) and sponge-tipped applicator for oral hygiene. Remind patient that front teeth should not be brushed until incision has healed (about 10 days). Advise patient that diet will be liquid initially but quickly will progress to soft.	To prevent disturbance in integrity of the operative site.
Monitor for extreme erythema or swelling at the suture line. Be alert to and teach patient the importance of monitoring for the following: fever, nuchal rigidity, headache, and photophobia.	Signs of infection, which can lead to meningitis and must be reported promptly.
Teach patient that he or she may have periorbital edema, headache, and tenderness over the sinuses for 2-3 days, which may be helped with cold compresses to the eyes. Also explain that the transsphenoidal donor site for fat or muscle packing usually is the thigh or abdomen, and the patient should expect a small dressing there. Advise patient that sense of smell usually returns in about 2-3 wk.	Postoperative teaching.

●●● **Related NIC and NOC labels:** *NIC:* Cerebral Perfusion Promotion; Neurologic Monitoring; Postanesthesia Care; Respiratory Monitoring; Airway Management; Surveillance; Vital Signs Monitoring; Positioning *NOC:* Neurological Status: Consciousness

ADDITIONAL NURSING DIAGNOSES/ PROBLEMS:

"Diabetic Ketoacidosis" for **Ineffective**   p. 412
Protection related to altered cerebral
function

PATIENT-FAMILY TEACHING AND DISCHARGE PLANNING

When providing patient-family teaching, focus on sensory information, avoid giving excessive information, and initiate a visiting nurse referral for necessary follow-up teaching. Include verbal and written information about the following:

✓ Importance of fluid restriction for the prescribed period. Assist patient with planning permitted fluid intake (e.g., by saving liquids for social and recreational situations as indicated).

✓ How to safely enrich the diet with Na^+ and K^+ salts, particularly if ongoing diuretic use is prescribed.

✓ Obtaining daily weight measurements as an indicator of hydration status.

✓ Indicators of water intoxication and hyponatremia, including altered LOC, fatigue, headache, nausea, vomiting, and anorexia, any of which should be reported promptly to health care provider.

✓ Medications, including drug name, dosage, route, purpose, precautions, drug/drug and food/drug interactions, and potential side effects. Encourage patient to report to health care provider all alternative and complementary health strategies being used.

✓ Importance of continued medical follow-up; confirm date and time of next medical appointment.

✓ Importance of obtaining a Medic-Alert bracelet and identification card outlining diagnosis and emergency treatment. Contact the following organization:

Medic Alert
2323 Colorado Avenue
Turlock, CA 95382
(209) 668-3333

Abdominal Trauma

Abdominal trauma may cause serious injury to major organs. It is essential to understand the nature of the injury (blunt or penetrating) and abdominal organs affected to avoid complications in the recovery period. Astute assessment skills in the posttraumatic period may prevent serious consequences and avoid life-threatening situations. Common injuries to abdominal organs may be predicted with knowledge of the nature and location of the injury. Gradual or sudden changes in vital signs may be the heralding signs of hemorrhage following trauma, with tachycardia and hypotension key indicators of bleeding or shock.

Blunt trauma most commonly affects the spleen, especially in the presence of left lower rib fractures. Rupture may be delayed for several days, again reinforcing the need for astute assessment. Other organs that may be affected by blunt trauma include the liver and kidneys and, infrequently, the pancreas and small and large intestines. Bleeding is the most common complication, resulting in increased morbidity and mortality.

Penetrating trauma most commonly affects the liver, with control of bleeding and bile drainage from liver lacerations being the major concern. If the lower esophagus and stomach are injured by penetration, complications from the release of irritating gastric fluids into the peritoneum and free air below the diaphragm may present. Penetrating injuries also may occur to the small intestine and mesentery. Decreased intestinal perfusion may result in infarction, with serious consequences.

HEALTH CARE SETTING

Emergency care, trauma center, acute care surgical unit, rehabilitation center

ASSESSMENT

Pain: Mild tenderness to severe abdominal pain may be present, with the pain either localized to the site of injury or diffuse. Blood or fluid collection within the peritoneum causes irritation, resulting in involuntary guarding, distention, rigidity, and rebound tenderness. Fluid or air under the diaphragm may cause referred shoulder pain. Kehr's sign (left shoulder pain caused by splenic bleeding) also may be noted.

Gastrointestinal (GI) symptoms: Nausea and vomiting may be present following blunt or penetrating trauma secondary to bleeding or obstruction. The absence of signs and symptoms, especially in the patient who has sustained head or spinal cord injury, does not exclude the presence of major abdominal injury.

Inspection: Abrasions and ecchymoses are suggestive of underlying injury (e.g., ecchymosis over left upper quadrant [LUQ] suggests splenic rupture; ecchymotic areas on the flank are suggestive of retroperitoneal bleeding; erythema and ecchymosis across the lower abdomen suggest intestinal injury caused by lap belts). Ecchymoses may take hours to days to develop, depending on the rate of blood loss. Abdominal distention may signal bleeding, free air, or inflammation.

Auscultation: Auscultate before palpation and percussion to avoid stimulating the bowel and confounding assessment findings. Bowel sounds may be decreased or absent with abdominal organ injury, intraperitoneal bleeding, or recent surgery. However, the presence of bowel sounds does not exclude significant abdominal injury. Bowel sounds should be auscultated frequently, especially in the first 24-48 hr after injury. Absence of bowel sounds is suggestive of ileus or other complications, such as bleeding, peritonitis, or bowel infarction.

Palpation: Tenderness or pain to palpation suggests abdominal injury. Blood or fluid in the abdomen can result in signs and symptoms of peritoneal irritation, such as generalized abdominal pain or tenderness, guarding of abdomen, abdominal wall rigidity, rebound tenderness, abdominal pain with movement or coughing, abdominal distention, and decreased or absent bowel sounds.

Percussion: Tympany suggests the presence of gas. Percussion may reveal unusually large areas of dullness over ruptured blood-filled organs (e.g., a fixed area of dullness in the LUQ suggests a ruptured spleen).

Vital signs and hemodynamic measurements: Ventilatory excursion may be diminished because of pain, thoracic injury, or limited diaphragmatic movement caused by abdominal distention. Tachycardia and hypotension suggest fluid deficit or bleeding. Vital signs should be assessed frequently to detect changes early.

DIAGNOSTIC TESTS

White blood cell (WBC) count: Leukocytosis is expected immediately after injury. Splenic injuries, in particular, result in rapid development of a moderate to high WBC count. A later increase in WBCs or a shift to the left reflects an increase in the number of neutrophils, which signals an inflammatory response and possible intraabdominal infection. In the patient with abdominal trauma, ruptured abdominal viscera must be considered as a potential source of infection.

Platelet count: Mild thrombocytosis is seen immediately after traumatic injury. After massive hemorrhage, thrombocytopenia may be noted. Platelet transfusion usually is not required unless spontaneous bleeding is present.

Glucose: Glucose is initially elevated because of catecholamine release and insulin resistance associated with major trauma. Glucose metabolism is abnormal after major hepatic resection, and patients should be monitored to prevent hypoglycemic episodes.

Amylase: Elevated serum levels are associated with pancreatic or upper small bowel injury, but values may be normal even with severe injury to these organs.

Aspartate aminotransferase (AST), alanine aminotransferase (ALT): Elevations of these enzymes reflect hepatic injury.

X-ray examinations: Initially, flat and upright chest x-rays exclude chest injuries (frequently associated with abdominal trauma) and establish a baseline. Subsequent chest x-rays aid in detecting complications, such as atelectasis and pneumonia. In addition, chest, abdominal, and pelvic x-rays may reveal fractures, missiles, foreign bodies, free intraperitoneal air, hematoma, or hemorrhage.

Occult blood: Gastric contents, urine, and stool should be tested for blood because bleeding can occur as a result of both direct injury and later complications.

Diagnostic peritoneal lavage (DPL): DPL involves insertion of a peritoneal dialysis catheter into the peritoneum to check for intraabdominal bleeding. It is indicated for confirmed or suspected blunt abdominal trauma for the following patients: (1) those in whom signs and symptoms of abdominal injury are obscured by intoxication, head or spinal cord trauma, opioids, or unconsciousness; (2) those about to undergo general anesthesia for repair of other injuries (e.g., orthopedic, facial); and (3) any patient with equivocal assessment findings. DPL is unnecessary for patients who have obvious intraabdominal bleeding or other indications for immediate laparotomy.

Ultrasound: Ultrasound is a rapid, noninvasive assessment tool for detecting intraabdominal hemorrhage. The Focused Assessment Sonogram for Trauma (FAST) has a sensitivity, specificity, and accuracy rate of >93% in the detection of intraabdominal blood. Although it is not organ specific, it has found popularity as an inexpensive assessment tool.

Computed tomography (CT) scan: CT can detect intraperitoneal and retroperitoneal bleeding and free air (associated with rupture of hollow viscera). It is most useful in assessing injury to solid abdominal organs. **Caution:** A patient in unstable condition should be accompanied by a nurse during the CT scan.

Angiography: Angiography is performed selectively with blunt trauma to evaluate injury to the spleen, liver, pancreas, duodenum, and retroperitoneal vessels when other diagnostic findings are equivocal. **Caution:** Because of the large amount of contrast material used during this procedure, ensure adequate hydration and monitor urine output closely for 24-48 hr, especially in older patients or patients with preexisting cardiovascular or renal disease. Decreased urinary output and increased blood urea nitrogen (BUN) and creatinine may indicate contrast-associated acute tubular necrosis.

Abdominal injuries often are associated with multisystem trauma. See also diagnostic test discussions under "Spinal Cord Injury," p. 383, and "Head Injury," p. 339.

Nursing Diagnosis:

Deficient Fluid Volume

related to active loss secondary to bleeding/hemorrhage

Desired Outcomes: Within 4 hr of admission or following definitive repair (e.g., surgery), patient is normovolemic as evidenced by systolic BP ≥90 mm Hg (or within patient's baseline range), HR 60-100 bpm, central venous pressure (CVP) 2-6 mm Hg (5-12 cm H_2O), urinary output ≥30 ml/hr, warm extremities, brisk capillary refill (<2 sec), distal pulses >2+ on a 0-4+ scale, and absence of orthostasis.

INTERVENTIONS	**RATIONALES**
In *recently injured patients,* monitor BP hourly or more frequently in the presence of obvious bleeding or unstable VS. Be alert to increasing diastolic BP and decreasing systolic BP. In the *stable* postoperative patient, perform routine VS assessment.	Even a small but sudden decrease in systolic BP signals need to notify health care provider, especially with a trauma patient in whom extent of injury is unknown. Most trauma patients are young, and excellent neurovascular compensation results in a near normal BP until there is large intravascular volume depletion.
Be alert to clinical indicators of fluid volume deficit. Report them accordingly.	Clinical indicators of fluid volume deficit, including decreasing BP; tachycardia (>100 bpm); tachypnea (>20 breaths/min); anxiety (early); and confusion, lethargy, and coma (later) should be reported promptly for timely intervention.
Monitor HR and cardiovascular status hourly until patient's condition is stable. Note and report sudden increases or decreases in HR, especially if associated with indicators of fluid volume deficit, as noted above.	Tachycardia and hypotension occur with fluid volume deficit or bleeding. VS should be assessed frequently to detect changes early.
Monitor for diaphoresis, cool and pale extremities, delayed capillary refill ≥2 sec, and absent or decreased strength of distal pulses.	Physical indicators of fluid volume deficit.
Measure CVP q1-4h if indicated.	Low or decreasing values are likely. Sudden decreases in CVP, especially if associated with other indicators of fluid volume deficit, as just noted, are signs of significant volume depletion.
Measure urinary output q4h (or when patient voids). Be alert to decreasing urinary output and/or infrequent voidings.	Low urine output usually reflects inadequate intravascular volume in the patient with abdominal trauma.
Measure all bloody drainage from drainage tubes or catheters, noting drainage color (e.g., coffee ground, burgundy, bright red). Monitor for, and measure when possible, bloody stools.	Provides estimate for ongoing blood loss.
Note frequency of dressing changes because of saturation with blood. Note and report significant increases in amount of drainage, especially if it is bloody.	To estimate amount of blood lost via wound site.
In patient with evidence of volume depletion or active blood loss, administer prescribed fluids rapidly through one or more large-caliber (16-gauge or larger) IV catheters. **Caution:** Evaluate patency of IV catheters frequently during rapid volume resuscitation.	Massive blood loss is frequently associated with abdominal injuries. Restoration and maintenance of adequate volume are essential. Initially, Ringer's lactate or similar balanced salt solution is given. Packed red blood cells (RBCs) are given to replace blood loss, especially with Hgb <9.0.
Monitor patient closely.	To avoid fluid volume overload and complications such as heart failure (see p. 196).

●●● **Related NIC and NOC labels:** *NIC:* Fluid Management; Fluid Monitoring; Hypovolemia Management; Fluid Resuscitation; Intravenous Insertion; Intravenous Therapy; Vital Signs Management; Blood Products Administration; Invasive Hemodynamic Monitoring; Shock Prevention *NOC:* Fluid Balance

Nursing Diagnosis:

Acute Pain

related to irritation caused by intraperitoneal blood or secretions, actual trauma or surgical incision, and manipulation of organs during surgery

Desired Outcomes: Patient's subjective perception of pain decreases, as documented by a pain scale. Nonverbal indicators, such as grimacing, are absent or diminished.

INTERVENTIONS	**RATIONALES**
Evaluate for presence, character, and location of preoperative and postoperative pain. Devise a pain scale with patient, rating discomfort from 0 (no pain) to 10 (worst pain).	Preoperative pain is anticipated and is a vital diagnostic aid. Location and character of postoperative pain also can be important. For example, incisional and some visceral pain can be anticipated, but intense or prolonged pain, especially when accompanied by other peritoneal signs, can signal bleeding, bowel infarction, infection, or other complications. Recognize that autonomic nervous system (ANS) response to pain can complicate assessment of abdominal injury and hypovolemia. A pain scale helps quantify pain and determine subsequent relief obtained.
Administer analgesics as prescribed. Avoid administering analgesics preoperatively until patient has been evaluated thoroughly by a trauma surgeon. Administer postoperatively prescribed analgesics on a continual or regular schedule promptly with additional analgesia as needed, or provide patient-controlled analgesia (PCA).	Analgesics are helpful in relieving pain, as well as aiding the recovery process by promoting greater ventilatory excursion. IV analgesics are recommended for management of pain, usually via patient-controlled pumps. As the severity of pain lessens, alternate analgesics such as nonsteroidal antiinflammatory drugs (NSAIDs; e.g., ketorolac, ibuprofen) may be prescribed if not contraindicated by patient history or gastric bleeding.
Encourage patient to request analgesic before pain becomes severe.	To promote better pain control. Prolonged stimulation of pain receptors results in increased sensitivity to painful stimuli and will increase amount of drug required to relieve pain.
Recognize that drug and alcohol use may precipitate traumatic events. In addition, narcotic analgesics can decrease GI motility and may delay return to normal bowel function. Document degree of relief obtained, using pain scale.	Patients may be drug or alcohol users, with a higher-than-average tolerance for opioids, requiring adjusted dosage for adequate pain relief. Symptoms of alcohol withdrawal (tremors, weakness, tachycardia, elevated BP, delusions, agitation, hallucinations) or narcotic withdrawal (lacrimation, rhinorrhea, anxiety, tremors, muscle twitching, mydriasis, nausea, abdominal cramps, vomiting) necessitate prompt recognition and treatment.
Supplement analgesics with nonpharmacologic maneuvers (e.g., positioning, back rubs, distraction). Provide these instructions to patient and family members.	Nonpharmacologic maneuvers support analgesia therapy in reducing pain.
For more details, see discussion in "Pain," p. 41.	

●●● **Related NIC and NOC labels:** *NIC:* Pain Management; Medication Management: Patient-Controlled Analgesia (PCA) Assistance; Teaching: Procedure/Treatment; Distraction; Simple Massage; Positioning *NOC:* Comfort Level; Pain Control; Pain: Disruptive Effects; Pain Level

Nursing Diagnosis:

Risk for Infection

related to inadequate primary defenses secondary to disruption of the GI tract (particularly of the terminal ileum and colon) and traumatically inflicted open wound; multiple indwelling catheters and drainage tubes; and compromised immune state caused by blood loss and metabolic response to trauma

Desired Outcome: Patient remains free of infection as evidenced by temperature <37.7° C (100° F); HR ≤100 bpm; no significant changes in mental status; orientation to person, place, and time; and absence of unusual erythema, edema, tenderness, warmth, or drainage at surgical incisions or wound sites.

INTERVENTIONS	RATIONALES
Monitor VS, noting temperature increases and associated increases in heart and respiratory rates. Notify health care provider of sudden temperature elevations.	Indicators of infection.
Evaluate mental status, orientation, and level of consciousness (LOC) q8h.	Mental status changes, confusion, or deterioration from baseline LOC can signal infection.
Ensure patency of all surgically placed tubes or drains. Irrigate or attach to low-pressure suction as prescribed. Maintain continuity of closed drainage systems; use sterile technique when emptying drainage and recharging suction containers. Promptly report loss of tube patency.	Blocked drainage systems may promote infection and abscess formation. Maintaining a closed drainage system and using sterile technique decrease risk of infection.
Evaluate incisions and wound sites for unusual erythema, warmth, tenderness, edema, delayed healing, and purulent or unusual drainage.	Evidence of infection.
Note amount, color, character, and odor of all drainage.	Presence of foul-smelling or abnormal drainage can occur with infection.
Administer antibiotics in a timely fashion. Reschedule parenteral antibiotics if a dose is delayed >1 hr.	Failure to administer antibiotics on schedule may result in inadequate blood levels and treatment failure.
As prescribed, administer pneumococcal vaccine to patients with total splenectomy.	To minimize risk of postsplenectomy sepsis.
Administer tetanus immune globulin and tetanus toxoid as prescribed.	Risk for tetanus following trauma increases if patient has not been immunized within the past 10 years.
Change dressings as prescribed, using sterile technique. Change one dressing at a time.	To prevent cross-contamination from various wounds.
Use drains, closed drainage systems, or drainage bags to remove and collect GI secretions.	To avoid contamination of surgical incision site.
If patient has or develops evisceration, do not reinsert tissue or organs. Place a sterile, saline-soaked gauze over evisceration and cover with a sterile towel until the evisceration can be evaluated by the surgeon. Keep patient on bedrest with bed in semi-Fowler's position with knees bent. Maintain NPO status for patient and anticipate need for emergency surgery.	This is an emergent, life-threatening situation. Maintaining homeostasis is essential until surgical intervention can be made.
For more information, see Appendix for "Infection Prevention and Control," p. 831.	

●●● **Related NIC and NOC labels:** *NIC:* Environmental Management; Incision Site Care; Infection Control: Intraoperative; Vital Signs Monitoring; Wound Care; Tube Care: Gastrointestinal; Immunization/Vaccination Management; Infection Protection; Laboratory Data Interpretation; Medication Administration *NOC:* Infection Status; Immune Status

Nursing Diagnosis:

Ineffective Breathing Pattern

related to pain from injury or surgical incision; chemical irritation of blood or bile on pleural tissue; and diaphragmatic elevation caused by abdominal distention

Desired Outcome: Within 24 hr of admission or surgery, patient is eupneic with RR 12-20 breaths/min and clear breath sounds.

INTERVENTIONS	RATIONALES
Note quality of breath sounds, RR, presence/absence of cough, and sputum characteristics.	Individuals sustaining abdominal trauma are likely to be tachypneic, with the potential for poor ventilatory effort. If not reversed, this could result in atelectasis and pneumonia.
Monitor oximetry readings q2-4h and report O_2 saturation ≤92%.	O_2 saturation ≤92% usually signals need for supplemental oxygen.
Administer supplemental oxygen as prescribed. Monitor and document effectiveness.	Supplemental O_2 is delivered until patient's arterial blood gas (ABG) or oximetry values while breathing room air are acceptable.
Encourage and assist patient with coughing, deep breathing, incentive spirometry, and turning q2-4h.	To prevent atelectasis.
Administer analgesics at dose and frequency that relieves pain and associated impaired chest excursion.	To reduce pain and enable full chest excursion for better oxygenation.
Instruct patient in methods to splint abdomen.	To reduce pain on movement, coughing, and deep breathing.
For additional interventions, see **Impaired Gas Exchange**, p. 54, "Perioperative Care."	

●●● **Related NIC and NOC labels:** *NIC:* Respiratory Monitoring; Oxygen Therapy; Cough Enhancement; Pain Management; Teaching: Procedure/Treatment *NOC:* Respiratory Status: Ventilation; Vital Signs Status

Nursing Diagnosis:

Ineffective Tissue Perfusion: Gastrointestinal

(or risk for same) *related to* interrupted blood flow to abdominal viscera secondary to vascular disruption or occlusion or related to moderate to severe hypovolemia caused by hemorrhage

Desired Outcomes: Optimally within 72 hr of surgery or admission, patient has adequate GI tissue perfusion as evidenced by normoactive bowel sounds; soft, nondistended abdomen; and return of bowel elimination. Gastric secretions, drainage, and excretions are negative for occult blood.

INTERVENTIONS	RATIONALES
Auscultate for bowel sounds hourly in recently injured patients and q8h during recovery phase.	Absent or diminished bowel sounds may be anticipated for up to 72 hr after trauma or surgery.
Report prolonged or sudden absence of bowel sounds.	May signal bowel ischemia or infarction.
Evaluate patient for signs of peritoneal irritation.	Signs of peritoneal irritation (generalized abdominal pain or tenderness, guarding of abdomen, abdominal wall rigidity, rebound tenderness, abdominal pain with movement or coughing, abdominal distention, and decreased or absent bowel sounds) may occur acutely secondary to injury or may not develop until days or weeks later if complications caused by slow bleeding or other mechanisms occur.
Ensure adequate intravascular volume (see discussion in **Deficient Fluid Volume,** earlier).	Adequate intravascular volume optimizes organ perfusion.

Continued

INTERVENTIONS	RATIONALES
Evaluate laboratory data for evidence of bleeding (e.g., serial Hct) or organ ischemia (e.g., AST, ALT).	Optimal values are Hct >30%; AST 5-40 IU/L; ALT 5-35 IU/L. Decreases in Hct occur with bleeding. Increases in AST or ALT are especially reflective of hepatic injury.
Document amount and character of GI secretions, drainage, and excretions. Report significant findings.	A sudden change in character or amount of drainage may signal presence of a complication that necessitates timely intervention.

●●● **Related NIC and NOC labels:** *NIC:* Hypovolemia Management; Intravenous Therapy; Laboratory Data Interpretation; Vital Signs Monitoring; Bleeding Reduction: Gastrointestinal; Bowel Management *NOC:* Tissue Perfusion: Abdominal Organs

Nursing Diagnoses:

Risk for Impaired Skin Integrity

related to risk of exposure to irritating GI drainage; *and*

Impaired Tissue Integrity

(or risk for same) *related to* direct trauma and surgery, catabolic posttraumatic state, and altered circulation

Desired Outcome: Patient exhibits wound healing, and skin remains nonerythemic and intact.

INTERVENTIONS	RATIONALES
Promptly change all dressings that become soiled with drainage or blood.	Gastric and intestinal secretions and drainage are irritating and can lead to skin excoriation.
Protect skin surrounding tubes, drains, or fistulas, keeping the areas clean and free from drainage. If necessary, apply ointments, skin barriers, or drainage bags to protect surrounding skin.	
Apply reusable dressing supports such as Montgomery straps or Surginet gauze. Consult enterostomal therapy (ET) nurse for complex or involved cases.	To prevent excessive injury to surrounding skin.
Identify infected and devitalized tissue. Aid in their removal by irrigation, wound packing, or preparing patient for surgical debridement.	Removal of devitalized tissue is essential for wound healing to progress.
Ensure adequate protein and calorie intake (see **Imbalanced Nutrition,** next).	To ensure optimal tissue healing.
For more information, see "Managing Wound Care," p. 583.	

●●● **Related NIC and NOC labels:** *NIC:* Skin Surveillance; Infection Protection; Skin Care: Topical Treatments; Wound Care; Nutrition Management; Incision Site Care; Wound Irrigation *NOC:* Tissue Integrity: Skin and Mucous Membranes

Nursing Diagnosis:

Imbalanced Nutrition: Less than body requirements

related to decreased intake secondary to disruption of GI tract integrity (traumatic or surgical) and increased need secondary to hypermetabolic posttrauma state

Desired Outcome: By at least 24 hr before hospital discharge, patient has adequate nutrition as evidenced by maintenance of baseline body weight and positive or balanced nitrogen (N) state.

INTERVENTIONS	RATIONALES
Collaborate with health care provider, dietitian, and pharmacist to estimate patient's metabolic needs, based on type of injury, activity level, and nutritional status before injury.	For example, patients with hepatic or pancreatic injury may have difficulty with blood sugar regulation; patients with trauma to upper GI tract may be fed enterally, but feeding tube must be placed distal to the injury; patients with disruption of GI tract may require feeding gastrostomy or jejunostomy tube; patients with major hepatic trauma may have difficulty with protein tolerance.
Ensure patency of gastric or intestinal tubes. Use caution and consult surgeon before irrigating nasogastric (NG) or other tubes that have been placed in or near recently sutured organs.	To maintain decompression and encourage healing and return of bowel function.
Confirm placement of feeding tube before each tube feeding. After initial insertion, check x-ray for position of feeding tube. Mark to determine tube migration, secure tubing in place, and reassess q4h and before each feeding.	Insufflation with air and aspiration of stomach contents do not always confirm placement of small-bore feeding tubes.
Assess aspirate for pH.	A pH <5 signals gastric placement.
Proceed slowly with enteral feedings initially to ensure absorption.	Peristalsis is often decreased following trauma/surgery.
Consider administration of prescribed nonnarcotic analgesics (e.g., ketorolac).	Opioid analgesics decrease GI motility and may contribute to nausea, vomiting, abdominal distention, and ileus.
For more information, see "Providing Nutritional Support," p. 589.	

●●● **Related NIC and NOC labels:** *NIC:* Enteral Tube Feeding; Gastrointestinal Intubation
NOC: Nutritional Status

Nursing Diagnosis:

Post-Trauma Syndrome

related to life-threatening accident or event resulting in trauma

Desired Outcomes: By at least 24 hr before hospital discharge, patient no longer exhibits signs of severe stress reaction, such as display of inconsistent affect, suicidal or homicidal behavior, or extreme agitation or depression. Patient cooperates with treatment plan.

INTERVENTIONS	RATIONALES
Evaluate mental status at regular intervals. Be alert to display of affect inconsistent with statements or behavior, suicidal or homicidal statements or actions, extreme agitation or depression, and failure to cooperate with instructions related to care, which are indicators of severe stress reaction.	Many victims of major abdominal trauma sustain life-threatening injury. The patient is often aware of the situation and fears death. Even after the physical condition stabilizes, the patient may have a prolonged or severe reaction triggered by recollection of the trauma.
Consult specialists such as psychiatrist, psychologist, psychiatric nurse practitioner, or pastoral counselor if patient displays signs of severe stress reaction described previously.	The patient likely needs specialized intervention.
Consider organic causes that may contribute to posttraumatic response. Report significant findings to health care provider.	Severe pain, alcohol intoxication or withdrawal, electrolyte imbalance, metabolic encephalopathy, and impaired cerebral perfusion are potential contributors to the posttraumatic response and should be treated accordingly.

●●● **Related NIC and NOC labels:** *NIC:* Coping Enhancement; Spiritual Support; Counseling
NOC: Coping

ADDITIONAL NURSING DIAGNOSES/ PROBLEMS:

PATIENT-FAMILY TEACHING AND DISCHARGE PLANNING

Anticipate extended physical and emotional rehabilitation for the patient and significant other. When providing patient-family teaching, focus on sensory information, avoid giving excessive information, and initiate a visiting nurse referral for necessary follow-up teaching. Include verbal and written information about the following:

✓ Self-management: assessment of patient's ability to manage own care should be completed before hospital discharge. Identification of support persons to assist with care should be initiated early.

✓ Probable need for emotional care, even for patients who have not required extensive physical rehabilitation. Provide referrals to support groups for trauma patients and family members.

✓ Availability of rehabilitation programs, extended care facilities, and home health agencies for patients unable to accomplish self-care on hospital discharge.

✓ Availability of rehabilitation programs for substance abuse, as indicated. Immediately after the traumatic event, patient and family members are very impressionable, making this period an ideal time for the substance abuser to begin to resolve the problem.

✓ Medications, including drug name, purpose, dosage, schedule, precautions, drug/drug and food/drug interactions, and potential side effects. Encourage patients taking antibiotics to take medications for prescribed length of time, even though they may be asymptomatic. If patient received tetanus immunization, ensure that he or she receives a wallet-size card documenting the immunization.

✓ Wound and catheter care. Have patient or caregiver describe and demonstrate proper technique before hospital discharge.

✓ Activity: Restrictions and recommendations should be reviewed thoroughly with patient and caregivers. An at-home assessment may be necessary if activity is severely limited or adaptations are necessary. Consider referral to occupational therapist (OT) or physical therapist (PT).

✓ Diet/nutrition: Review diet recommendations with patient/family. If enteral or parenteral feeding is necessary, have patient or caregiver describe and demonstrate correct technique before hospital discharge. Home health care services may be warranted for support and evaluation.

✓ Importance of seeking medical attention if indicators of infection or bowel obstruction occur (e.g., fever, severe or unusual abdominal pain, nausea and vomiting, unusual drainage from wounds or incisions, a change in bowel habits).

✓ Injury prevention. Following traumatic injury, patient and family members are especially likely to respond to injury prevention education. Provide instructions on proper seat-belt applications (across pelvic girdle rather than across soft tissue of lower abdomen), safety for infants and children, and other factors suitable for individuals involved.

Appendicitis

Appendicitis is the most frequently occurring inflammatory lesion of the bowel and one of the most common reasons for abdominal surgery. Appendicitis occurs most often in adolescents and young adults, especially males. The appendix is a blind, narrow tube that extends from the inferior portion of the cecum and does not serve any known useful function. Appendicitis is usually caused by obstruction of the appendiceal lumen by a fecalith (hardened bit of fecal material), inflammation, a foreign body, or a neoplasm. Obstruction prevents drainage of secretions that are produced by epithelial cells in the lumen, thereby increasing intraluminal pressure and compressing mucosal blood vessels. This tension eventually impairs local blood flow, which can lead to necrosis and perforation. Inflammation and infection result from normal bacteria invading the devitalized wall. Mild cases of appendicitis can heal spontaneously, but severe inflammation can lead to a ruptured appendix, which can cause local or generalized peritonitis.

HEALTH CARE SETTING

Acute care surgical unit

ASSESSMENT

Signs and symptoms vary because of differences in anatomy, size, and age.

Signs and symptoms:

- **Early stage:** The onset of abdominal pain usually occurs in either the epigastric or umbilical area and may be vague and diffuse or associated with mild cramping. Abdominal discomfort is accompanied by fever, nausea, and vomiting.
- **Intermediate (acute) stage:** Over a period of a few hours, pain shifts from the midabdomen or epigastrium to the right lower quadrant (RLQ) at McBurney's point (approximately 2 inches from the anterior superior iliac spine on a line drawn from the umbilicus) and is aggravated by walking, coughing, and movement. The pain may be accompanied by a sensation of constipation (gas-stoppage sensation). Anorexia, malaise, occasional diarrhea, and diminished peristalsis also can occur.

On physical assessment the patient experiences pain in the RLQ elicited by *light* palpation of the abdomen; presence of rebound tenderness; RLQ guarding, rigidity, and muscle spasms; tachycardia; low-grade fever; absent or diminished bowel sounds; and pain elicited with rectal examination. A palpable, tender mass may be felt in the peritoneal pouch if the appendix lies within the pelvis.

Note: Physical assessment is done in four steps: inspection, auscultation, percussion, and palpation, in that order, to avoid stimulating the abdomen by palpation and percussion, which can affect bowel sounds.

Acute appendicitis with perforation: Increasing, generalized pain; recurrence of vomiting.

On *physical assessment* the patient usually exhibits temperature increases >38.5° C (101.4° F) and generalized abdominal rigidity. Typically, the patient remains rigid with flexed knees. Presence of abscess can result in a tender, palpable mass. The abdomen may be distended.

DIAGNOSTIC TESTS

White blood cell (WBC) count with differential: Reveals presence of leukocytosis and an increase in neutrophils. A shift to the left with more than 75% neutrophils is found in ≥90% of cases.

Urinalysis: To rule out genitourinary conditions mimicking appendicitis; may reveal microscopic hematuria and pyuria.

Abdominal x-ray: May reveal presence of a fecalith. About half of these patients may have x-ray findings of localized air-fluid levels, increased soft tissue density in the RLQ, and indications of localized ileus. If perforation has occurred, the presence of free air is noted. Barium enemas do not aid in diagnosis.

Intravenous pyelogram: May be performed to rule out ureteral stone or pyelitis.

Abdominal ultrasound: May be done to rule out appendicitis or conditions that mimic it, such as Crohn's disease, diverticulitis, or gastroenteritis.

Abdominal computed tomography (CT) scan: May reveal an appendiceal abscess or acute appendicitis.

Nursing Diagnosis:

Risk for Infection

related to inadequate primary defenses (danger of rupture, peritonitis, abscess formation) secondary to inflammatory process

Desired Outcomes: Patient is free of infection as evidenced by normothermia, HR <100 bpm, BP >90/60 mm Hg, RR 12-20 breaths/min with normal depth and pattern (eupnea), absence of chills, soft and nondistended abdomen, and bowel sounds 5-34/min in each abdominal quadrant. Immediately following teaching, patient verbalizes rationale for not administering enemas or laxatives preoperatively and enemas postoperatively and demonstrates compliance with the therapeutic regimen.

INTERVENTIONS	RATIONALES
Assess and document quality, location, and duration of pain. Be alert to pain that becomes accentuated and generalized or to presence of recurrent vomiting and note whether patient assumes side-lying or supine position with flexed knees.	Any of these signs can signal worsening appendicitis, which can lead to rupture and peritonitis.
Be alert to pain that worsens and then disappears.	A signal that rupture may have occurred.
Monitor for ambulation with a limp or pain with hip extension.	Retrocecal abscess may irritate the psoas muscle as it traverses the area of posterior RLQ of the abdomen and result in pain with hip extension.
Monitor VS for elevated temperature, increased pulse rate, hypotension, and shallow/rapid respirations and assess abdomen for presence of rigidity, distention, and decreased or absent bowel sounds. Report significant findings to health care provider.	Any of these indicators can occur with rupture.
Caution patient about the danger of preoperative self-treatment with enemas and laxatives.	Enemas and laxatives increase peristalsis, which increases risk of perforation and hence peritonitis and sepsis. Enemas should be avoided until approved by health care provider (usually several weeks after surgery). If constipation occurs postoperatively, health care provider may prescribe laxatives/stool softeners at bedtime after the third day.
Teach postoperative incisional care, as well as care of drains if patient is to be discharged with them.	Maintaining a clean incision and avoiding contamination of drains help prevent infection in areas in which the skin is broken.
Provide instructions about prescribed antibiotics if patient is to be discharged with them. See "Peritonitis" for more information (p. 501).	To prevent systemic infection.
For more information, see Appendix for "Infection Prevention and Control," p. 831.	

●●● **Related NIC and NOC labels:** *NIC:* Infection Protection; Incision Site Care; Vital Signs Monitoring; Health Education; Teaching: Procedure/Treatment *NOC:* Infection Status; Wound Healing: Primary Intention

Nursing Diagnoses:

Acute Pain/Nausea

related to the inflammatory process

Desired Outcomes: Within 1-2 hr of pain/nausea-relieving interventions, patient's subjective perception of pain/nausea decreases, as documented by a pain scale. Objective indicators, such as grimacing, are absent or diminished.

INTERVENTIONS	RATIONALES
Assess and document quality, location, and duration of pain. Devise a pain scale with patient, rating discomfort from 0 (no pain) to 10 (worst pain).	These characteristics of discomfort may be seen during the following stages of appendicitis: *Early stage:* abdominal pain (either epigastric or umbilical) that may be vague and diffuse; nausea and vomiting; fever; and sensitivity over appendix area. *Intermediate (acute) stage:* pain that shifts from epigastrium to RLQ at McBurney's point (approximately 2 inches from anterior superior iliac spine on a line drawn from umbilicus) and is aggravated by walking or coughing. The pain may be accompanied by a sensation of constipation (gas-stoppage sensation). Anorexia, malaise, occasional diarrhea, and diminished peristalsis also can occur. *Acute appendicitis with perforation:* increasing, *generalized* pain; recurrence of vomiting; increasing abdominal rigidity.
Medicate with antiemetics, sedatives, and analgesics as prescribed; evaluate and document patient's response, using the pain scale.	To reduce nausea and pain. Opioids are avoided until diagnosis is certain because they mask clinical signs and symptoms.
Encourage patient to request medication *before* symptoms become severe.	Prolonged stimulation of pain receptors results in increased sensitivity to painful stimuli and will increase the amount of drug required to relieve pain.
Keep patient NPO before surgery.	After surgery, nausea and vomiting usually disappear.
If prescribed, insert gastric tube.	For decompression in preoperative patients with severe nausea and vomiting.
Teach technique for slow, diaphragmatic breathing.	To reduce stress and promote comfort by relaxing tense muscles.
Help position patient for optimal comfort.	Many patients find comfort from a side-lying position with knees bent, whereas others find relief when supine with pillows under knees (avoiding pressure on popliteal area).

●●● **Related NIC and NOC labels:** *NIC:* Medication Management; Pain Management; Positioning; Progressive Muscle Relaxation *NOC:* Comfort Level; Pain Control; Pain Level

ADDITIONAL NURSING DIAGNOSES/ PROBLEMS:

"Perioperative Care" for other nursing   p. 47
diagnoses and interventions

PATIENT-FAMILY TEACHING AND DISCHARGE PLANNING

When providing patient-family teaching, focus on sensory information, avoid giving excessive information, and initiate a visiting nurse referral for necessary follow-up teaching. Include verbal and written information about the following:

✓ Medications, including drug name, dosage, purpose, schedule, precautions, drug/drug and food/drug interactions, and potential side effects.

✓ Care of incision, including dressing changes and bathing restrictions if appropriate.

✓ Indicators of infection: fever, chills, incisional pain, redness, swelling, and purulent drainage.

✓ Postsurgical activity precautions: avoid lifting heavy objects (>10 lb) for the first 6 wk or as directed, be alert to and rest after symptoms of fatigue, get maximum rest, and gradually increase activities to tolerance.

✓ Importance of avoiding enemas for the first few postoperative weeks. Caution patient about need to check with health care provider before having an enema.

Cholelithiasis, Cholecystitis, and Cholangitis

Cholelithiasis is characterized by the presence of stones in the gallbladder. Gallstones may cause pain or other symptoms or remain asymptomatic for years. *Choledocholithiasis* is the term used to describe gallstones in the common bile duct. Gallstones are classified as cholesterol or pigment stones. Precipitating factors for stone formation include disturbances in metabolism, biliary stasis, obstruction, hypertriglyceridemia, and infection. Gallstones are especially prevalent in women who are multiparous, are taking estrogen therapy, or use oral contraceptives. Other risk factors include obesity, dietary intake of fats, sedentary lifestyle, and familial tendencies. Cholelithiasis is frequently seen in disease states such as diabetes mellitus, regional enteritis, and certain blood dyscrasias. Usually cholelithiasis is asymptomatic until a stone becomes lodged in the cystic tract. If the obstruction is unrelieved, biliary colic (intermittent painful episodes) and cholecystitis can ensue.

Cholecystitis is most commonly associated with cystic duct obstructions caused by impacted gallstones; however, it may result also from stasis, bacterial infection, or ischemia of the gallbladder. Cholecystitis involves acute inflammation of the gallbladder and is associated with pain, tenderness, and fever. With obstruction, structural changes can occur, such as swelling and thickening of the gallbladder walls.

Cholangitis is the most serious complication of gallstones and more difficult to diagnose. It is caused by an impacted stone in the common bowel duct, resulting in bile stasis, bacteremia, and septicemia if left untreated. It is more likely to occur when an already infected bile duct becomes obstructed. The mortality rate is high if not recognized and treated early.

HEALTH CARE SETTING

Primary care; acute care

ASSESSMENT

Cholelithiasis: History of intolerance to fats and occasional discomfort after eating. As the stone moves through the duct or becomes lodged, a sudden onset of mild, aching pain occurs in the midepigastrium after eating (especially after a high-fat meal) and increases in intensity during a colic attack, potentially radiating to the right upper quadrant (RUQ) and right subscapular region. Nausea, vomiting, tachycardia, and diaphoresis also can occur. Many individuals with gallstones are entirely asymptomatic.

Cholecystitis: History of intolerance to fats and discomfort after eating, including regurgitation, flatulence, belching, epigastric heaviness, indigestion, heartburn, chronic upper abdominal pain, and nausea. Amber-colored urine, clay-colored stools, pruritus, jaundice, steatorrhea, and bleeding tendencies can be present if there is bile obstruction. Symptoms may be vague. An acute attack may last 7-10 days, but it usually resolves in several hours.

Cholangitis: Fever is present in nearly all patients with bacterial cholangitis. Jaundice, chills, mild and transient pain, mental confusion, and lethargy are part of the presenting symptoms. Leukocytosis and elevated bilirubin are present in 80% of cases.

Physical assessment:

- **Cholelithiasis:** Palpation of RUQ reveals a tender abdomen during colic attack. Otherwise, between attacks, the examination is usually normal.

- **Cholecystitis:** Palpation elicits tenderness localized behind the inferior margin of the liver. With progressive symptoms, a tender, globular mass may be palpated behind the lower border of the liver. Rebound tenderness and guarding may also be present. With the patient taking a deep breath, palpation over the RUQ elicits Murphy's sign (pain and inability to inspire when the examiner's hand comes in contact with the gallbladder).
- **Cholangitis:** RUQ tenderness is present in 90% of cases. Peritoneal signs are not common and only occur in 15% of patients. Hypotension and mental confusion are present in severe cases.

DIAGNOSTIC TEST

Ultrasonography: Preferred test for confirming the presence of gallstones, as well as their number and size. Ultrasonography of the gallbladder and biliary tract may be used to determine the location of gallstones and detect tumors.

Radiologic studies: For example, oral cholangiogram, IV cholangiogram, nuclear scans, and percutaneous transhepatic cholangiogram, may be performed to determine the patency of the biliary or cystic ducts and help rule out other conditions that mimic gallstone disease. Chest, abdominal, upper gastrointestinal (GI), and barium enema x-rays often are used to rule out pulmonary or other GI disorders.

Hepatoiminodiacetic acid (HIDA; lidofenin) scan: Radioisotopic scan that is highly sensitive for diagnosis of acute cholecystitis.

Oral cholecystogram: Measures gallbladder function and demonstrates the number and size of gallstones. This test requires ingestion of iodine-based tablets (i.e., Telepaque) at night, with x-ray films taken the following morning. In 25% of cases, a second dose the next night may be needed for adequate visualization. As an alternative, the patient may be given a double dose of contrast on the initial night. Failure to visualize the gallbladder indicates a nonfunctioning gallbladder, usually because of complete obstruction of the cystic duct or chronic irritation of the gallbladder wall. Diarrhea may be caused by the iodine tablets and sometimes results in nonvisualization of the gallbladder.

Computed tomography (CT) scan: To detect dilated bile ducts and the presence of gallbladder cysts, tumors, abscesses, perforated gallbladder, and other complications of gallbladder disease.

Endoscopic retrograde cholangiopancreatography (ERCP): Visualization and evaluation of the biliary tree or pancreatic duct. This is the gold standard for diagnosing choledocholithiasis.

Electrocardiogram (ECG): To rule out cardiac disease.

Complete blood count (CBC) with differential: To assess for presence of infection or blood loss.

Prothrombin time: To assess for a prolonged clotting time secondary to faulty vitamin K absorption.

Bilirubin tests (serum and urine) and urobilinogen tests (urine and fecal): To differentiate between hemolytic disorders, hepatocellular disease, and obstructive disease. Usually there is an increase of bilirubin in the plasma and urine with biliary disease.

Serum liver enzyme test: Usually normal in cholecystitis but often becomes abnormal in the presence of prolonged cholecystitis or common duct stones.

Nursing Diagnosis:

Acute Pain

related to spasms, nausea, and itching secondary to obstructive or inflammatory process

Desired Outcomes: Patient's subjective perception of discomfort decreases within 1 hr of intervention, as documented by a pain scale. Nonverbal indicators, such as grimacing, are absent or diminished.

INTERVENTIONS	RATIONALES
Monitor patient for pain or other discomfort. Devise a pain scale with patient, rating discomfort on a scale of 0 (no pain) to 10 (worst pain).	Enables more precise measurement of discomfort and relief obtained.
Explain that a bent-knee position will minimize pressure in the RUQ.	This position decreases tension on abdominal contents to promote comfort.
Teach patient to avoid fatty and rough or fibrous foods.	To prevent nausea and spasms. Diet varies according to the patient's condition. During an acute attack, NPO status with IV fluids may be instituted. With severe nausea and vomiting, a gastric tube is inserted and attached to low, intermittent suction. Diet advances to patient's tolerance, and small, frequent feedings of a low-fat diet are recommended for both the acute and chronic conditions.

Continued

INTERVENTIONS	RATIONALES
Administer antiemetics (e.g., hydroxyzine, ondansetron, prochlorperazine, promethazine) as prescribed.	To prevent or treat nausea and vomiting.
Administer bile salt binding agent (e.g., cholestyramine) as prescribed.	To provide relief from pruritus caused by prolonged obstructive jaundice. Cholestyramine (Questran) and colestipol (Colestid) bind with bile salts in the intestine to facilitate their excretion.
Administer analgesics as prescribed.	Nonsteroidal antiinflammatory drugs (NSAIDs) or opioid analgesics may be indicated, depending on severity of the pain. For the postoperative patient, epidural, continuous IV, and patient-controlled infusions of opioid analgesics are used with increasing frequency and superior efficacy. Recently, IV ketorolac (Toradol) q6h for 4-8 doses has shown benefit in controlling postoperative pain with these patients, reducing need for opioid analgesics. It should not be used for >3-5 days because of its toxic effects.
Administer acid suppression therapy if prescribed.	To neutralize gastric hyperacidity and reduce associated pain.
Provide cool Alpha Kori baths and cold water or ice for topical application and use soft linens on the bed.	To help control itching.
For additional interventions, see "Pain," p. 41.	

●●● **Related NIC and NOC labels:** *NIC:* Pain Management; Analgesic Administration; Positioning; Cold Application; Environmental Management: Comfort *NOC:* Comfort Level; Pain Control; Pain Level

Nursing Diagnosis:

Risk for Injury

related to potential for postsurgical perforation or recurrence of biliary obstruction

Desired Outcomes: Patient is free of symptoms of postsurgical perforation as evidenced by diminishing dark brown drainage of <1000 ml/day and presence of a soft and nondistended abdomen. Patient is free of symptoms of recurring biliary obstruction as evidenced by normal skin color, brown-colored stools, and straw-colored urine.

INTERVENTIONS	RATIONALES
Note and record color, amount, odor, and consistency of drainage from T-tube or wound drain q2h on day of surgery and at least every shift thereafter.	Initially drainage will be dark brown with small amounts of blood and can amount to 500-1000 ml/day. Greater amounts of blood or drainage should be reported to health care provider inasmuch as it could signal a perforation. The amount should subside gradually as swelling diminishes in common duct and drainage into duodenum normalizes.
Monitor color of the skin, sclera, urine, and stool.	Brown color should return to stools once bile begins to drain normally into the duodenum. If obstruction recurs and bile is forced back into the bloodstream, jaundice will be present, urine will be amber, and stools will be clay colored (clay color is normal if bile is drained via a T-tube).
Ensure that drainage collection devices are positioned lower than the level of the common bile duct.	To prevent reflux of drainage when patient is ambulating.

Continued

INTERVENTIONS	RATIONALES
Be alert to abdominal distention, rigidity, and complaints of diaphragmatic irritation along with cessation or significant decrease in amount of drainage. If these signs occur, notify health care provider immediately and anticipate tube replacement with a 14 Fr catheter.	These are indicators of a dislodged or clogged drainage tube causing bile leakage into the abdomen or backup of bile and necessitating timely intervention.
See also "Perioperative Care," p. 47, for perioperative care plans and "Hepatitis" for **Risk for Impaired Skin Integrity** related to pruritus, p. 485.	

●●● **Related NIC and NOC labels:** *NIC:* Surveillance: Safety; Risk Identification *NOC:* Safety Status: Physical Injury

PATIENT-FAMILY TEACHING AND DISCHARGE PLANNING

When providing patient-family teaching, focus on sensory information, avoid giving excessive information, and initiate a visiting nurse referral for necessary follow-up teaching. Include verbal and written information about the following:

✓ Notifying health care provider if the following indicators of recurrent biliary obstruction occur: dark urine, pruritus, jaundice, and clay-colored stools. Inform patient that loose stools may occur for several months as the body adjusts to the continuous flow of bile.

✓ Medications, including drug name, dosage, schedule, purpose, precautions, drug/drug and food/drug interactions, and potential side effects.

✓ Care of dressings and tubes if patient is discharged with them and monitoring of incision and drain sites for signs of infection (e.g., fever, persistent redness, pain, purulent discharge, swelling, increased local warmth).

✓ Importance of maintaining a diet low in fat and eating frequent, small meals for medically managed patients.

✓ Importance of follow-up appointments with health care provider; reconfirm time and date of next appointment.

✓ Avoiding alcoholic beverages during first 2 postoperative mo to minimize risk of pancreatic involvement.

✓ Necessity of postsurgical activity precautions: avoid lifting heavy objects (>10 lb) for first 4-6 wk or as directed, rest after periods of fatigue, get maximum amounts of rest, and gradually increase activities to tolerance.

✓ Postsurgical patients may experience fatty food intolerance (e.g., flatulence, cramps, diarrhea) for several months postoperatively until the body acclimates to loss of the gallbladder.

✓ For more information, contact the following organization:

National Digestive Diseases Information Clearinghouse, National Institute of Diabetes and Digestive and
Kidney Diseases
Project Officer
2 Information Way
Bethesda, MD 20892
(302) 468-6344
www.aerie.com/nihdb/ddbase.htm

53

Cirrhosis

Cirrhosis is a chronic, serious disease in which normal configuration of the liver is changed, resulting in cell death. When new cells are formed, the resulting scarring causes disruption of blood and lymph flow. Although pathologic changes do not occur for many years, structural changes gradually lead to total liver dysfunction. Manifestations of cirrhosis are related to hepatocellular necrosis and portal hypertension. Complications caused by cellular failure are similar to those of acute hepatitis and include inability to metabolize bilirubin and resultant jaundice; difficulty producing serum proteins, including albumin and certain clotting factors; hyperdynamic circulation and decreased vasomotor tone; pulmonary changes (ventilation-perfusion mismatch) and sometimes cyanosis; changes in nitrogen (N) metabolism (e.g., inability to convert ammonia to urea); and difficulty metabolizing some hormones (especially the sex hormones). Complications related to portal hypertension include development of ascites, bleeding esophageal and gastric varices, portal-systemic collaterals, encephalopathy, and splenomegaly.

Alcoholic (Laënnec's) cirrhosis: Associated with long-term alcohol abuse; accounts for 50% of all cases. Changes in liver structure caused by cirrhosis are irreversible, but compensation of liver function can be achieved if the liver is protected from further damage by alcohol cessation and proper nutrition. The histologic definition of this form of cirrhosis is micronodular cirrhosis.

Postnecrotic cirrhosis: Associated with history of viral hepatitis or hepatic damage from drugs or toxins; accounts for 20% of all cases. This type appears to predispose the patient to the development of a hepatoma. The histologic definition of this form of cirrhosis is macronodular cirrhosis.

Biliary cirrhosis: Associated with chronic retention of bile and inflammation of bile ducts; accounts for 15% of all cases. The histologic definition of this form of cirrhosis is mixed nodular cirrhosis; it may be further classified as follows:

- **Primary biliary cirrhosis (PBC; nonsuppurative destructive cholangitis):** Results from cholestasis from an unknown cause. This progressive disease has other findings, including steatorrhea, xanthomatous (yellow tumors) neuropathy, osteoporosis, and portal hypertension. Hypercholesterolemia, hyperlipidemia, and hepatomegaly are found in about 85% of patients with PBC.
- **Secondary biliary cirrhosis:** Results from chronic obstruction to bile flow, usually from an obstruction outside the liver, such as calculi, neoplasms, or biliary atresia.

HEALTH CARE SETTING

Primary care with possible hospitalization for complications

ASSESSMENT

Signs and symptoms: Weakness, fatigability, weight loss, pruritus, fever, anorexia, nausea, occasional vomiting, abdominal pain, diarrhea, menstrual abnormalities, sterility, impotence, loss of libido, and hematemesis. Urine may be dark (brownish) because of the presence of urobilinogen, and stools may be pale and clay colored because of the absence of bilirubin.

Physical assessment: Jaundice, hepatomegaly, ascites, peripheral edema, pleural effusion, and fetor hepaticus (a musty, sweetish odor on the breath). There may be slight changes in personality and behavior, which can progress to coma (a result of hepatic encephalopathy); spider angiomas, testicular atrophy, gynecomastia, pectoral and axillary alopecia (a result of hormonal changes); splenomegaly; hemorrhoids (a result of portal hypertension complications); spider nevi; purpuric lesions; and palmar erythema. Asterixis may be present in advanced cirrhosis, that is, jerking movements of the hands and wrists when the wrists are dorsiflexed with the fingers extended.

History of: Excessive alcohol ingestion; hepatitis B, C, or D infection; exposure to hepatotoxic drugs, such as 5-aminosalicylic acid derivatives and corticosteroids or chemicals; biliary or metabolic disease; poor nutrition.

DIAGNOSTIC TESTS

Hematologic: Red blood cells (RBCs) are decreased in hypersplenism and decreased with hemorrhage. White blood cells (WBCs) are decreased with hypersplenism and increased with infection. Platelet counts are less than normal.

Serum biochemical tests:

- **Bilirubin levels:** Elevated because of failure in hepatocyte metabolism and obstruction in some instances. Very high or persistently elevated levels are considered a poor prognostic sign.
- **Alkaline phosphatase levels:** Normal to mildly elevated in most cases; in PBC it is elevated 2-3 × normal.
- **Aspartate aminotransferase (AST) and alanine aminotransferase (ALT) levels:** Usually elevated >300 U with acute failure and normal or mildly elevated with chronic failure. ALT is more specific for hepatocellular damage.
- **Albumin levels:** Reduced, especially with ascites. Persistently low levels suggest a poor prognosis.
- **Na$^+$ levels:** Normal to low. Na$^+$ is retained but is associated with water retention, which results in normal serum Na$^+$ levels or even a dilutional hyponatremia. Often severe hyponatremia is present in the terminal stage and is associated with tense ascites and hepatorenal syndrome.
- **K$^+$ levels:** Slightly reduced unless patient has renal insufficiency, which would result in hyperkalemia. Chronic hypokalemic acidosis is common in patients with chronic alcoholic liver disease.
- **Glucose levels:** Hypoglycemia possible because of impaired gluconeogenesis and glycogen depletion in patients with severe or terminal liver disease.
- **Blood urea nitrogen (BUN) levels:** May be slightly decreased because of failure of Krebs cycle enzymes in the liver or elevated because of bleeding or renal insufficiency.
- **Ammonia levels:** Elevation expected because of inability of the failing liver to convert ammonia to urea and shunting of intestinal blood via collateral vessels. Gastrointestinal (GI) hemorrhage or an increase in intestinal protein from dietary intake increases ammonia levels. **Note:** Keep patient NPO except for water for 8 hr before drawing the ammonia level. Notify laboratory of all antibiotics taken by patient because they may lower the ammonia level.

Coagulation: Prothrombin time (PT) is prolonged and, in severe liver disease, unresponsive to vitamin K therapy. Coagulation abnormalities usually include factor V, but also factors II, VII, IX, and X.

Urine tests: Urine bilirubin is increased; urobilinogen is normal or increased. There may be proteinuria.

Liver biopsy: Obtains a specimen of liver for microscopic analysis and diagnosis of cirrhosis, hepatitis, or other liver disease. Percutaneous liver biopsy is contraindicated in patients with markedly prolonged PT or very low platelet counts because of the risk of hemorrhage. In these patients a transvenous biopsy via the jugular and hepatic vein may be attempted instead. Open liver biopsy, or minilaparotomy, may also be done for liver biopsy.

Barium swallow: Used in nonemergency situations (i.e., for patients without active bleeding) to verify the presence of gastroesophageal varices. **Note:** The patient should be NPO from midnight until completion of the test. Because of the constipating effects of barium, enemas should be given on the patient's return from the procedure.

Radiologic studies: Ultrasound differentiates hemolytic and hepatocellular jaundice from obstructive jaundice and shows hepatomegaly and intrahepatic tumors. Computed tomography (CT) scan of the liver/spleen is done to evaluate size and location of tumors and to rule out gallbladder disease. Percutaneous transhepatic cholangiography reveals the extent of obstruction via contrast dye. Endoscopic retrograde cholangiopancreatography (ERCP) is a fiberoptic technique used to show obstructions of the common bile and pancreatic ducts as potential causes of jaundice. Liver scans enable visualization of the spleen and liver via injection of radioisotopes.

Angiographic studies: Establish patency of the portal vein and visualize the portosystemic collateral vessels to determine cause and effective treatment for variceal bleeding. Portal venous anatomy must be established before such operations as portal systemic shunt or hepatic transplantation. In patients with previously constructed surgical shunts, loss of patency may be confirmed as a factor leading to the present bleeding episode.

- The most common procedure is portal venography by indirect angiography. The femoral artery is catheterized, and contrast material is injected into the splenic artery. Contrast material flows through the spleen into the splenic and portal veins.
- Hepatic vein wedge pressure is measured by introducing a balloon catheter into the femoral vein and threading it into a hepatic vein branch.
- Direct access to the portal vein may be achieved through transhepatic portography. During this procedure, varices may be obliterated by injection of thrombin or gel foam into veins that supply the varices. **Note:** Transhepatic portography involves a direct puncture through the liver and has many of the same risks as liver biopsy. Patients returning from this procedure should be positioned on their right side and monitored closely.

Esophagoscopy: Visualizes the esophagus and stomach directly via a fiberoptic esophagoscope. Varices in the esophagus and upper portion of the stomach are identified, and attempts are made to identify the exact source of bleeding. Variceal bleeding may be treated by sclerotherapy, electrocautery, laser, vasoconstrictive agents, or other methods during the endoscopic procedure.

Peritoneoscopy or laparoscopy: Visualizes the liver (to identify characteristic "hobnailed" appearance in cirrhosis) and allows for biopsy.

Electroencephalogram (EEG): Traces the electrical impulses of the brain to detect or confirm encephalopathy. EEG changes occur very early, usually before behavioral or biochemical alterations.

Psychometric testing: Evaluates for hepatic encephalopathy. A common test is the Reitan number connection (trailmaking) test. The patient's speed and accuracy at connecting a series of numbered circles are evaluated at intervals. A daily handwriting test is an easy check of intellectual deterioration or improvement.

Nursing Diagnosis:

Imbalanced Nutrition: Less than body requirements

related to anorexia, nausea, or malabsorption

Desired Outcome: By at least 24 hr before hospital discharge (or within 1-2 wk if not hospitalized), patient demonstrates stable weight and adequate progression toward balanced or positive nitrogen state, scrum protein 6-8 g/dl, and serum albumin 3.5-5.5 g/dl.

INTERVENTIONS	RATIONALES
Explain dietary restrictions. Encourage patient to eat foods that are permitted within dietary restrictions.	With fluid retention and ascites, Na^+ and fluids are restricted. Usually half the calories are supplied as carbohydrates to provide adequate energy when liver damage may prevent efficient liver metabolism and storage of carbohydrates.
Restrict protein as prescribed.	The action of intestinal bacteria on protein increases blood ammonia levels, which causes or worsens the coma state. Protein is restricted in hepatic coma or precoma. If the ammonia level rises (normal levels are whole blood 70-200 µg/dl and plasma 56-150 µg/dl), protein and foods high in ammonia also will be restricted.
Administer parenteral or enteral nutrition as prescribed	Parenteral nutrition is administered in the presence of GI dysfunction. Enteral nutrition may be used in patients with intact guts who are not eating adequately or at all. Either route is used to maintain adequate nutrient intake in patients who cannot or will not eat by mouth.
Monitor I&O; weigh patient daily.	To assess adequacy of diet/nutritional intake.
Encourage small, frequent meals.	To ensure adequate nutrition without causing bloating from large meals.
Encourage significant other to bring desirable foods as permitted.	Patients are more likely to consume foods they like.
Administer vitamin and mineral supplements as prescribed.	For example, folic acid may be given for macrocytic anemia and vitamin K for a prolonged PT.
Administer suppression agents, antiemetics, and cathartics as prescribed.	To decrease gastric distress, which may facilitate intake.
Implement prescribed measures such as diuretics, colloid replacement, paracentesis.	To relieve/mobilize ascites and decrease pressure on intraabdominal structures, which may facilitate intake
Promote bedrest.	To reduce metabolic demands on the liver.
Provide soft diet if patient has esophageal varices that are not bleeding.	To minimize risk of bleeding/hemorrhage. Patients with bleeding esophageal varices are NPO.
Encourage abstinence of alcohol in patients with alcoholic cirrhosis.	This remains the primary intervention in patients with alcohol-induced cirrhosis. Abstinence can result in healing of reversible factors of alcoholic liver disease over a period of months. Continued use of alcohol will further damage the liver to the point of irreversibility.

●●● **Related NIC and NOC labels:** *NIC:* Nutrition Management; Nutrition Therapy; Teaching: Prescribed Diet; Enteral Tube Feeding; Gastrointestinal Intubation; Sustenance Support; Total Parenteral (TPN) Administration *NOC:* Nutritional Status; Nutritional Status: Nutrient Intake; Nutritional Status: Food & Fluid Intake

Nursing Diagnosis:

Impaired Gas Exchange

related to alveolar hypoventilation secondary to shallow breathing occurring with ascites or pleural effusion; altered oxygen-carrying capacity of the blood secondary to erythrocytopenia; and possible ventilation–perfusion mismatching

Desired Outcome: Within 24 hr of intervention/treatment, patient has adequate gas exchange as evidenced by $PaCO_2$ ≤45 mm Hg, PaO_2 <80 mm Hg, O_2 saturation ≥92%, and RR 12-20 breaths/min with normal depth and pattern (eupnea).

INTERVENTIONS	RATIONALES
During complaints of dyspnea or orthopnea, assist patient into semi-Fowler's or high Fowler's position.	To promote gas exchange, which is likely to be altered by pressure of ascitic fluid on the diaphragm that restricts respirations.
Monitor arterial blood gas (ABG) values and pulse oximetry; notify health care provider of PaO_2 <80 mm Hg or O_2 saturation ≤92%. Administer oxygen as prescribed.	These values usually signal need for supplemental oxygen.
Obtain baseline abdominal girth measurement and measure girth either daily or every shift. Measure around same circumferential area each time; mark site with indelible ink. Report significant findings to health care provider.	An increase in abdominal girth indicates increased ascitic fluid accumulation, which can cause pressure on the diaphragm with subsequent dyspnea.
Encourage patient to change positions and deep-breathe at frequent intervals. If secretions are present, ensure that patient coughs frequently.	Deep breathing expands the alveoli and aids in mobilizing secretions to the airway. Coughing further promotes secretion mobilization and clears them.
Notify health care provider of spiking temperatures, chills, diaphoresis, and adventitious breath sounds.	These are indicators of respiratory infection and can lead to complications such as pneumonia and respiratory distress. Patients with severe cirrhosis are weak and with poor maintenance of secretions can become more susceptible to infections.
Position patient in a side-lying position during episodes of vomiting.	To prevent aspiration, which could result in respiratory complications such as pneumonia.

●●● **Related NIC and NOC labels:** *NIC:* Oxygen Therapy; Airway Management; Chest Physiotherapy; Positioning; Respiratory Monitoring; Aspiration Precautions; Cough Enhancement; Laboratory Data Interpretation *NOC:* Respiratory Status: Gas Exchange

Nursing Diagnosis:

Ineffective Protection

related to increased risk of esophageal bleeding secondary to portal hypertension and altered clotting factors

Desired Outcome: Patient is free of esophageal bleeding as evidenced by BP >90/60 mm Hg; HR ≤100 bpm; warm extremities; distal pulses >2+ on a 0-4+ scale; brisk capillary refill (<2 sec); and orientation to person, place, and time.

INTERVENTIONS	RATIONALES
Monitor VS q4h (or more frequently if VS are outside of patient's baseline values).	Upper GI hemorrhage is common in patients with chronic liver disease and can result from esophageal varices, portal hypertensive gastropathy, duodenal or gastric ulcers, or Mallory-Weiss tear (mucosal laceration at the juncture of the distal esophagus and proximal stomach). Early diagnosis is essential to enable appropriate intervention. Hypotension and increased HR, as well as cool extremities, delayed capillary refill, decreased amplitude of distal pulses, mental status changes, and decreasing level of consciousness (LOC), are physical indicators of hypovolemia and hemorrhage.
Teach patient to avoid swallowing foods that are chemically or mechanically irritating.	Rough or spicy foods, hot foods, hot liquids, and alcohol may be injurious to the esophagus and result in bleeding.
Teach patient to avoid, if possible, coughing, sneezing, lifting, and vomiting.	These actions increase intraabdominothoracic pressure, which can result in bleeding.
Administer stool softeners as prescribed.	To help prevent straining with defecation, which puts patient at risk for bleeding.
Inspect stools for presence of blood; perform stool occult blood test as indicated.	To monitor for bleeding within the GI tract.
Monitor PT.	Normal range is 10.5-13.5 sec; a PT that is prolonged signals that patient is at risk for bleeding.
Assess patient for altered VS, irritability, air hunger, pallor, weakness, melena, and hematemesis	Signs of bleeding.
As appropriate, encourage intake of foods rich in vitamin K (e.g., spinach, cabbage, cauliflower, liver).	To help decrease PT.
As often as possible, avoid invasive procedures such as giving injections and taking rectal temperatures.	If patient's clotting is altered, invasive procedures could result in prolonged bleeding.
Monitor patient undergoing sclerotherapy for increased HR, decreased BP, pallor, weakness, and air hunger.	Signs of esophageal perforation caused by sclerotherapy, whether by injection, cautery, or the scope itself.
If signs of perforation occur, notify health care provider immediately, keep patient NPO, and prepare for gastric suction.	NPO status and gastric suction prevent leakage of fluid, secretions, or food through the perforation into the mediastinum. This emergency situation necessities immediate intervention.

●●● **Related NIC and NOC labels:** *NIC:* Bleeding Precautions; Emergency Care; Hemorrhage Control
NOC: Coagulation Status

Nursing Diagnosis:

Disturbed Sensory Perception: Kinesthetic

related to increased risk of neurosensory changes secondary to hepatic coma occurring with cerebral accumulation of ammonia or GI bleeding

Desired Outcome: Patient verbalizes orientation to person, place, and time; exhibits intact signature; and is free of symptoms of injury caused by neurosensory changes.

INTERVENTIONS	RATIONALES
Perform a baseline assessment of patient's personality characteristics, LOC, and orientation. Enlist aid of significant other.	Having a baseline assessment will help determine changes in patient's personality or behavior, which could progress to hepatic coma if left unchecked.
Reorient at frequent intervals.	Because of patient's encephalopathy and resulting neurosensory changes, reminders and reorientation are necessary to help ensure patient's safety.
Have patient demonstrate signature daily.	If writing deteriorates, ammonia levels may be increasing. The diseased liver cannot convert ammonia to urea, and buildup of ammonia adds to progression of hepatic encephalopathy.
Be alert to generalized muscle twitching and asterixis (flapping tremor induced by dorsiflexion of wrist and extension of fingers). Report significant findings to health care provider.	Asterixis may be present in advanced cirrhosis.
Remind patient to avoid protein and foods high in ammonia, such as gelatin, onions, and strong cheeses.	Buildup of ammonia adds to progression of hepatic encephalopathy.
Monitor for indicators of GI bleeding, including melena or hematemesis (for details, see **Ineffective Protection,** earlier). Report bleeding promptly to health care provider and obtain prescription for cleansing enemas if indicated.	GI bleeding can precipitate hepatic coma.
Keep side rails up and bed in its lowest position and assist patient with ambulation when need is determined.	Protects patient against injury that could be precipitated by confused state.
Use caution when administering sedatives, antihistamines, and other agents affecting central nervous system. Avoid opiate analgesics and phenothiazines.	Opioids and sedatives are metabolized by the liver and therefore are contraindicated. Small doses of benzodiazepines with a short half-life, such as oxazepam (Serax), may be administered if absolutely necessary.

●●● **Related NIC and NOC labels:** *NIC:* Reality Orientation; Environmental Management; Neurologic Monitoring: Surveillance: Safety; Nutrition Management *NOC:* Cognitive Orientation; Muscle Function

Nursing Diagnosis:

Excess Fluid Volume

related to compromised regulatory mechanism with sequestration of fluids secondary to portal hypertension and hepatocellular failure

Desired Outcome: By at least 24 hr before discharge from care facility, patient becomes normovolemic as evidenced by stable or decreasing abdominal girth, RR 12-20 breaths/min with normal depth and pattern (eupnea), HR ≤100 bpm, edema ≤1+ on a 0-4+ scale, and absence of crackles (rales).

INTERVENTIONS	RATIONALES
Obtain baseline abdominal girth measurement. Measure girth daily or every shift as appropriate.	Enables comparison for subsequent assessment. Girth measurements indicate amount of ascitic fluid in the abdomen and provide information regarding effectiveness of medical treatment.
Place patient in supine position and mark abdomen with indelible ink.	To ensure accurate serial measurements from same circumferential site.

Continued

INTERVENTIONS	RATIONALES
Monitor weight and I&O.	Output should be equal to or exceed intake. Weight loss should not exceed 0.23-0.5 kg/day ($\frac{1}{2}$-1 lb), except in the presence of massive edema, which would permit a greater loss. Rapid diuresis from diuretics can lead to loss or shifts in electrolytes, particularly sodium, leading to encephalopathy and elevated creatinine.
Assess degree of edema, from 1+ (barely detectable) to 4+ (deep, persistent pitting) and document accordingly.	The presence of edema signals excess sodium intake or low serum albumin. Severe hyponatremia is often present in the terminal stage and is associated with tense ascites and hepatorenal syndrome. Low albumin levels are associated with ascites; persistently low levels suggest a poor prognosis.
Be alert to dyspnea, basilar crackles that do not clear with coughing, orthopnea, and tachypnea.	These are clinical indicators of pulmonary edema, which occurs from excess fluid volume in the circulatory system. Symptoms also may be present with pleural effusion caused by a small defect in the right hemidiaphragm, which develops with acute, rapid shortness of breath as the abdomen decompresses.
Give frequent mouth care and provide ice chips.	To help minimize thirst while not compounding problems with fluid volume excess.
Monitor serum Na^+ and K^+ values and report abnormalities to health care provider.	Optimal values are serum Na^+ 137-147 mEq/L and serum K^+ 3.5-5 mEq/L. Na^+ is retained but is associated with water retention, which results in normal serum Na^+ levels or even a dilutional hyponatremia. Severe hyponatremia is present in the terminal stage and is associated with tense ascites and hepatorenal syndrome. K^+ may be slightly reduced unless patient has renal insufficiency, which would result in hyperkalemia. Chronic hypokalemic acidosis is common in patients with chronic alcoholic liver disease.
Restrict Na^+ and replace K^+ as prescribed.	Sodium may be restricted because of retention by the kidneys; potassium may be replaced because of loss with diuretic use.
Remind patient to avoid food and nonfood items that contain Na^+, such as antacids, baking soda, and some mouthwashes.	To help keep Na^+ levels as low as possible.
Elevate extremities.	To decrease peripheral edema.
Apply antiembolism hose (AEH), support stockings, sequential compression devices, or pneumatic foot compression devices as prescribed.	Decreases peripheral edema by external compression of the extremities.
Monitor for variceal hemorrhage (see **Ineffective Protection,** p. 460).	Rapid increases in intravascular volume can precipitate variceal hemorrhage in susceptible patients.
Teach patient to inhale against resistance, using a blow bottle (if a LeVeen peritoneovenous or Denver shunt is in place). In addition, provide instructions about the following: importance of lifestyle changes such as low-Na^+ diet, abstinence from alcohol, practicing breathing exercises, obtaining daily weight and abdominal girth measurements, and monitoring I&O and edema.	Inhaling against resistance raises intraperitoneal pressure sufficiently to enable ascitic fluid to flow through the shunt.

●●● **Related NIC and NOC labels:** *NIC:* Fluid/Electrolyte Management; Laboratory Data Interpretation; Nutrition Management; Respiratory Monitoring *NOC:* Fluid Balance

ADDITIONAL NURSING DIAGNOSES/ PROBLEMS:

"Hepatitis" for **Deficient Knowledge:** Causes p. 485 of hepatitis and modes of transmission

PATIENT-FAMILY TEACHING AND DISCHARGE PLANNING

When providing patient-family teaching, focus on sensory information, avoid giving excessive information, and initiate a visiting nurse referral for necessary follow-up teaching. Include verbal and written information about the following:

✓ Medications, including drug name, purpose, dosage, schedule, precautions, drug/drug and food/drug interactions, and potential side effects.

✓ Dietary restrictions, in particular that of Na^+, protein, and ammonia.

✓ Potential need for lifestyle changes, including avoiding alcoholic beverages. Stress that alcohol cessation is a major factor in survival of this disease. Include appropriate referrals (e.g., to Alcoholics Anonymous, Al-Anon, and Al-Ateen). As appropriate, provide referrals to community nursing support agencies.

✓ Awareness of hepatotoxic agents, especially over-the-counter (OTC) drugs, including acetaminophen and aspirin.

✓ Importance of breathing exercises (see p. 460) when ascites is present.

✓ Indicators of variceal bleeding/hemorrhage (i.e., vomiting blood, change in LOC) and need to inform health care provider should they occur.

✓ Phone numbers to call should questions or concerns arise about therapy or disease after discharge. Additional general information can be obtained by contacting the following organization:

National Digestive Diseases Information
   Clearinghouse, National Institute of Diabetes
   and Digestive and Kidney Diseases
Project Officer
2 Information Way
Bethesda, MD 220892-3570
(301) 654-3810
www.niddk.nih.gov

✓ For patients awaiting transplantation, provide the following information as appropriate:

United Network for Organ Sharing
UNOS Communication Department
P.O. Box 13770
Richmond, VA 23225
(804) 330-8561 or (800) 243-6667 (voice mail) =
www.unos.org

✓ As an additional information source, refer patients to the following organization:

American Liver Foundation
1425 Pompton Ave.
Cedar Grove, NJ 07009
(800) 223-0179
www.liverfoundation.org

Crohn's Disease

Crohn's disease, also known as *regional enteritis, granulomatous colitis,* or *transmural colitis,* is a chronic inflammatory disease that can involve any part of the gastrointestinal (GI) tract from the mouth to the anus. Usually the disease occurs segmentally, demonstrating discontinuous areas of disease with segments of healthy bowel in between. The terminal ileum is the most frequent site of involvement, followed by the colon. The disease affects all layers of the bowel: the mucosa, submucosa, circular and longitudinal muscles, and serosa. A family history of this disease or ulcerative colitis occurs in 15%-20% of affected patients. The cause is unknown, but theories include infection, immunologic factors, environmental factors, and genetic predisposition.

HEALTH CARE SETTING

Primary care, with possible hospitalization resulting from complications

ASSESSMENT

Signs and symptoms: Clinical presentation varies as a direct reflection of the location of the inflammatory process, its extent, severity, and relationship to contiguous structures. Sometimes the onset is abrupt, and the patient can appear to have appendicitis, ulcerative colitis, intestinal obstruction, or a fever of obscure origin. Acute symptoms include right lower quadrant (RLQ) pain, tenderness, spasm, flatulence, nausea, fever, and diarrhea. A more typical picture is insidious onset with more persistent but less severe symptoms, such as vague abdominal pain, unexplained anemia, and fever. Diarrhea—liquid, soft, or mushy stools—is the most common symptom. The presence of gross blood is rare. Abdominal pain is a frequent symptom, and it may be colicky or crampy, initiated by meals, centered in the lower abdomen, and relieved by defecation because of the chronic partial obstruction of the small intestine, colon, or both. As the disease progresses, anorexia, malnutrition, weight loss, anemia, lassitude, malaise, and fever can occur in addition to fluid, electrolyte, and metabolic disturbances.

Physical assessment: In the early stages the examination is often normal but may demonstrate mild tenderness in the abdomen over the affected bowel. In more advanced disease, a palpable mass may be present, especially in the RLQ with terminal ileum involvement. Persistent rectal fissure, large ulcers, perirectal abscess, or rectal fistula is the first indication of disease in 15%-25% of patients with small bowel involvement and in 50%-75% of patients with colonic involvement. Rectovaginal, abdominal, and enterovesical fistulas also can occur. Extraintestinal manifestations characteristic of ulcerative colitis do occur, but less frequently (10%-20%).

DIAGNOSTIC TESTS

Stool examination: Usually reveals occult blood; frank blood may be noted in stools of patients with colonic involvement or with ulcerations and fistulas of the rectum. A few patients present with bloody diarrhea. Stool cultures and smears rule out bacterial and parasitic disorders. Specimens are also examined for fecal fat.

Sigmoidoscopy: Evaluates possible colonic involvement and obtains rectal biopsy. The finding of granulomas on mucosal biopsy argues strongly for the diagnosis of Crohn's disease. However, because granulomas are more numerous in the submucosa, suction biopsy of the rectum provides deeper, larger, and less traumatized specimens for a better diagnostic yield than mucosal biopsy obtained through an endoscope.

Colonoscopy: May help differentiate Crohn's disease from ulcerative colitis. Characteristic patchy inflammation (skip lesions) rules out ulcerative colitis. However, colonoscopy usually does not add useful diagnostic information in the presence of positive findings from sigmoidoscopy or radiologic examination. When the diagnosis is unclear and there is a question of malignancy, colonoscopy provides the means of directly visualizing mucosal changes and obtaining biopsies, brushings, and washings for cytologic examination. Colonoscopy also may assist in planning for surgery by documenting the extent of colonic disease. **Note:** This procedure may be contraindicated because of the risk of perforation in patients with acute phases of Crohn's colitis or when deep ulcerations or fistulas are known to be present.

Endoscopic ultrasonography: Aids in the diagnosis of perirectal fistula and abscesses and in detecting the transmural depth of inflammation in the bowel or esophagus, using an endoscopically placed ultrasound probe.

Small bowel enteroscopy: Permits visualization of the upper GI tract to identify areas of inflammation and bleeding to the level of the midjejunum.

Barium enema and upper GI series with small bowel follow-through: Contribute to the diagnosis of Crohn's disease. Involvement of only the terminal ileum or segmental involvement of the colon or small intestine almost always indicates Crohn's disease. Thickened bowel wall with stricture (string sign) separated by segments of normal bowel, cobblestone appearance, and presence of fistulas and skip lesions are common findings. A double-contrast barium enema technique may increase sensitivity in detecting early or subtle changes. **Note:** Barium enema may be contraindicated in patients with acute phases of Crohn's colitis because of the risk of perforation. Upper GI barium series is contraindicated in patients in whom intestinal obstruction is suspected.

Computed tomography (CT) scan: Complements information gathered via endoscopy and conventional radiography. In advanced disease, CT scanning clearly delineates extraluminal complications (e.g., abscess, phlegmon, bowel wall thickening, mesenteric inflammation). CT has been used also to percutaneously drain fistulas (colovesicular, enterovesicular, colovaginal, enterocolonic) and to evaluate perirectal disease, enterocutaneous fistula, and sinus tracts.

Radionuclide imaging: Intravenous indium-111- or technetium-99-labeled leukocytes migrate to areas of active inflammation and are then identified by scans done after 4 and 24 hr. This procedure aids in differentiating Crohn's disease from ulcerative colitis and evaluating abscess and fistula formation.

Blood tests: Are nonspecific for the diagnosis of Crohn's disease but help determine whether the inflammatory process is active and evaluate the patient's overall condition. Anemia may be present and may be (1) microcytic because of iron deficiency from chronic blood loss and bone marrow depression secondary to chronic inflammatory process or (2) megaloblastic because of folic acid or vitamin B_{12} deficiency (usually seen only in patients with extensive ileitis causing malabsorption). Increased white blood cell (WBC) count and sedimentation rate reflect disease activity and inflammation. Hypoalbuminemia corresponds with the disease activity and results from decreased protein intake, extensive malabsorption, and significant enteric loss of protein. Hypokalemia is seen in patients with chronic diarrhea; hypophosphatemia and hypocalcemia are seen in patients with significant malabsorption. Liver function studies may be abnormal in the presence of pericholangitis.

Urinalysis and urine culture: May reveal urinary tract infection secondary to enterovesicular fistula.

Tests for malabsorption: Because patients with active, extensive disease (especially when it involves the small intestine) may develop malabsorption and malnutrition, the following tests are clinically significant: D-xylose tolerance test (for upper jejunal involvement); Schilling's test (for ileal involvement); serum albumin, carotene, calcium, and phosphorus levels; and fecal fat (steatorrhea).

Nursing Diagnosis:

Deficient Fluid Volume

related to active loss secondary to diarrhea or presence of GI fistula

Desired Outcomes: Patient becomes normovolemic within 24 hr as evidenced by balanced I&O, urinary output >30 ml/hr, specific gravity 1.010-1.030, BP >90/60 mm Hg (or within patient's normal range), RR 12-20 breaths/min, stable weight, good skin turgor, and moist mucous membranes. Patient states that diarrhea is controlled and reports no signs of electrolyte imbalance.

INTERVENTIONS	RATIONALES
Monitor I&O, weigh patient daily, and monitor laboratory values of electrolytes. Keep a stool count and measure volume of liquid stools.	To monitor for fluid loss and electrolyte imbalance. GI fluid losses (nasogastric [NG] suction, vomiting, diarrhea, fistula) can lead to hyponatremia, hypokalemia, and hypochloremia. Optimal electrolyte values are serum K^+ 3.5-5 mEq/L, serum Na^+ 137-147 mEq/L, and serum Cl^- 95-108 mEq/L.
Monitor frequency, character, and consistency of stools.	To assess and record presence and amount of blood, mucus, fat, and undigested food, which occur secondary to the underlying inflammatory process.

Continued

INTERVENTIONS	**RATIONALES**
Monitor for thirst, poor skin turgor, dryness of mucous membranes, fever, and concentrated (specific gravity >1.030) and decreased urinary output.	Indicators of dehydration.
Maintain patient on parenteral replacement of fluids, electrolytes, blood, and vitamins as prescribed.	To promote anabolism and healing. Parenteral replacement of fluids, electrolytes, and blood products is maintenance therapy for acute exacerbation as indicated by laboratory test results.
When patient is taking food by mouth, provide bland, high-protein, high-calorie, low-fat, low-residue diet, as prescribed. Assess tolerance to diet by determining incidence of cramping, diarrhea, and flatulence.	Bland diets low in residue, roughage, and fat but high in protein, calories, carbohydrates, and vitamins provide good nutrition and reduce excessive stimulation of the bowel. A diet free of milk, milk products, gas-forming foods, alcohol, and iced beverages reduces cramping and diarrhea.
Modify diet plan accordingly.	Elemental diets (e.g., Vivonex, Ensure) that are free of bulk and residue, low in fat, and digested in the upper jejunum provide good nutrition with low fecal volume to enable bowel rest in selected patients. Use of elemental diets is being investigated for effectiveness as primary therapy, as an alternative to steroids and bowel rest, in treating patients with acute Crohn's disease.

●●● **Related NIC and NOC labels:** *NIC:* Fluid Management; Electrolyte Monitoring; Intravenous Therapy; Laboratory Data Interpretation; Diarrhea Management; Blood Products Administration
NOC: Fluid Balance; Bowel Elimination; Electrolyte & Acid/Base Balance

Nursing Diagnoses:

Risk for Infection/Risk for Injury

related to complications caused by intestinal inflammatory disorder

Desired Outcomes: Patient is free from indicators of infection and intraabdominal injury as evidenced by normothermia; HR 60-100 bpm; RR 12-20 breaths/min; normal bowel sounds; absence of abdominal distention, rigidity, or localized pain and tenderness; absence of nausea and vomiting; negative culture results; no significant change in mental status; and orientation to person, place, and time. Patient or significant other verbalizes accurate knowledge of reportable signs and symptoms of infection.

INTERVENTIONS	**RATIONALES**
Monitor for abdominal distention and rigidity and increased episodes of nausea and vomiting.	These are indicators of intestinal obstruction. Contributing factors to development of intestinal obstruction include use of opiates and prolonged use of antidiarrheal medication.
Monitor for fever, increased RR and HR, chills, diaphoresis, and increased abdominal discomfort.	Can occur with intestinal perforation, abscess or fistula formation, or generalized fecal peritonitis and septicemia. **Note:** Systemic therapy with corticosteroids and antibiotics can mask development of preceding complications.
Evaluate mental status, orientation, and level of consciousness (LOC) q4h.	Mental cloudiness, lethargy, and increased restlessness can occur with peritonitis and septicemia.
Obtain cultures of blood, urine, and fistulas as prescribed if patient has a sudden temperature elevation. Monitor culture reports and notify health care provider promptly of any positive results.	Abscesses or fistulas to abdominal wall, bladder, or vagina are common in Crohn's disease and are potential sources of infection, as are abscesses or fistulas to other loops of small bowel and colon.

Continued

INTERVENTIONS	RATIONALES
If draining fistulas or abscesses are present, change dressings and pouching system or irrigate tubes or drains as prescribed. Note color, character, and odor of all drainage.	Presence of foul-smelling or abnormal drainage, which can signal infection, or loss of tube/drain patency should be reported to health care provider promptly.
Administer antibiotics as prescribed and on prescribed schedule.	To control suppurative complications (e.g., bacterial overgrowth) and perianal fistulas in patients with mild-to-moderate colonic or ileocolonic Crohn's disease. In patients who are allergic, intolerant, or unresponsive to sulfasalazine, metronidazole (Flagyl) appears to be effective in colonic disease and in promoting healing of perianal disease. Long-term use of metronidazole is limited because of potential for peripheral neuropathy and other side effects. Patients with bacterial overgrowth in the small intestine may be treated with broad-spectrum antibiotics. Ciprofloxacin (Cipro) may be useful in treating patients who are intolerant or unresponsive to metronidazole therapy.
Ensure good handwashing technique before and after caring for patient and dispose of dressings and drainage using proper infection control techniques.	To prevent transmission of potentially infectious organisms.
For more information, see Appendix for "Infection Prevention and Control," p. 831.	

●●● **Related NIC and NOC labels:** *NIC:* Infection Control; Infection Protection; Medication Administration; Specimen Management; Wound Care *NOC:* Infection Status

Nursing Diagnoses:

Acute Pain/Nausea

related to intestinal inflammatory process

Desired Outcomes: Patient's subjective perception of discomfort decreases within 4 hr of intervention, as documented by a pain scale. Objective indicators, such as grimacing, are absent or diminished.

INTERVENTIONS	RATIONALES
Monitor and document characteristics of discomfort and determine triggering factor. Devise a pain scale with patient, rating discomfort from 0 (no discomfort) to 10 (worst discomfort). Document relief obtained, using pain scale. Eliminate foods that cause cramping and discomfort.	The discomfort of pain, nausea, and abdominal cramping may be associated with certain foods or emotional stress. A pain scale will help determine degree of relief obtained after interventions have been implemented.
As prescribed, keep patient NPO and provide parenteral nutrition.	To allow bowel rest, which will help alleviate discomfort.
Administer antidiarrheal medications and analgesics as prescribed.	These medications are given to reduce abdominal discomfort. Codeine or loperamide often reduces diarrhea with a concomitant decrease in abdominal cramping. Anticholinergics are not recommended because they may mask obstructive symptoms and precipitate toxic megacolon. For these reasons, antidiarrheal medications should be administered with caution.
Instruct patient to request analgesic before pain becomes severe.	Prolonged stimulation of pain receptors results in increased sensitivity to painful stimuli and will increase the amount of drug required to relieve discomfort.

Continued

INTERVENTIONS	RATIONALES
Assess patient's response to these medications. Report significant findings to health care provider.	If a patient does not respond appropriately to standard antidiarrheal medications and mild sedation, the presence of obstruction, bowel perforation, or abscess formation is suspected.
Provide nasal and oral care at frequent intervals.	To lessen discomfort from NPO status and presence of NG tube.
Administer antiemetic medications before meals.	To enhance appetite when nausea is a problem.
Administer sedatives and tranquilizers as prescribed.	To promote rest and reduce anxiety, which may reduce symptoms.
For additional information, see "Pain," p. 41.	

●●● **Related NIC and NOC labels:** *NIC:* Medication Management; Pain Management; Anxiety Reduction, Bowel Management *NOC:* Comfort Level

Nursing Diagnosis:

Diarrhea

related to intestinal inflammatory process

Desired Outcome: Patient reports a reduction in frequency of stools and a return to more normal stool consistency within 3 days of this diagnosis.

INTERVENTIONS	RATIONALES
If patient is experiencing frequent and urgent passage of loose stools, provide covered bedpan or commode or be sure bathroom is easily accessible and ready to use at all times.	Providing easy access to bedpan, commode, or bathroom reduces stress and enables patient to cope with diarrhea more effectively.
Empty bedpan or commode promptly.	To control odor and decrease patient's anxiety and self-consciousness.
Administer antidiarrheal medication as prescribed.	To decrease fluidity and number of stools.
Administer cholestyramine as prescribed.	To control diarrhea if bile salt deficiency (because of ileal disease or resection) is contributing to this problem.

●●● **Related NIC and NOC labels:** *NIC:* Diarrhea Management; Anxiety Reduction; Bowel Management; Medication Administration *NOC:* Symptom Severity

Nursing Diagnosis:

Activity Intolerance

related to generalized weakness secondary to intestinal inflammatory process

Desired Outcome: Patient adheres to prescribed rest regimen and sets appropriate goals for self-care as the condition improves (optimally within 3-7 days of this diagnosis).

INTERVENTIONS	RATIONALES
Keep patient's environment quiet.	To facilitate rest.
Assist patient with activities of daily living (ADL) and plan nursing care to provide maximum rest periods.	Adequate rest is necessary to sustain remission.
Facilitate coordination of health care providers. Allow 90 min for undisturbed rest.	To allow rest periods between care activities.
As prescribed, administer sedatives and tranquilizers.	To promote rest and reduce anxiety.
As patient's physical condition improves, encourage self-care to greatest extent possible and assist patient with setting realistic, attainable goals.	Enables patient to increase endurance incrementally to his or her tolerance and prevents problems associated with prolonged bedrest.
For additional information, see **Risk for Activity Intolerance,** p. 67, in "Prolonged Bedrest."	

●●● **Related NIC and NOC labels:** *NIC:* Energy Management; Self-Care Assistance; Environmental Management; Mutual Goal Setting *NOC:* Energy Conservation; Self-Care: Activities of Daily Living; Endurance

Nursing Diagnosis:

Deficient Knowledge:

Drugs used during exacerbations of Crohn's disease

Desired Outcome: Immediately following teaching, patient verbalizes accurate information about drugs used during exacerbations of Crohn's disease.

INTERVENTIONS	RATIONALES
Teach Patient About the Following Drugs:	
Sulfasalazine	Given to treat acute exacerbations of colonic and ileocolonic disease.
– Sulfasalazine does not prevent recurrence of Crohn's disease.	Although sulfasalazine does not prevent recurrence of Crohn's disease, patients who respond tend to benefit from long-term therapy and relapse when the agent is discontinued.
– It appears to be more effective in patients with mild-to-moderate disease limited to the colon than in those with disease limited to the small bowel.	
– Folic acid supplements are necessary during treatment.	Sulfasalazine impairs folate absorption.
– Have blood count done within first 4 mo of treatment.	WBCs may be lowered with this drug, and anemia can occur (uncommon).
– Have liver enzymes checked within first year of treatment.	Hepatitis, though uncommon, has occurred.
– Males may want to check for infertility by sperm analysis.	Infertility has occurred in some men, though it reverses when patient stops taking the drug.
– Be alert to the following side effects: fever, skin rash, joint pain, nausea, headache, or fatigue when dose exceeds 4 tablets/day.	Most side effects are sulfa related and caused by the sulfa component of the drug.

Continued

INTERVENTIONS	RATIONALES
5-Aminosalicylic acid (5-ASA) preparations	Slow-release mesalamine (Pentasa) and enteric-coated mesalamine (Asacol) have demonstrated effectiveness in maintenance therapy for preventing recurrence of Crohn's disease. These agents are undergoing clinical trials to determine their effectiveness in preventing recurrence in patients after surgical resection.
- Patients on prolonged treatment must have annual kidney profile and urine examination, including blood urea nitrogen (BUN) and creatinine.	There is risk of kidney damage with high doses (above 4000 mg/day).
Corticosteroids	Reduce the active inflammatory response, decrease edema in moderate-to-severe forms, and control exacerbations.
- Check BP during each clinic/office visit.	Hypertension is a side effect.
- Test blood glucose after 1 mo of therapy, then q3mo.	Increased blood glucose level can occur.
- Schedule eye examination q6mo and bone density evaluation every few years for patients taking steroids >12 mo.	There is potential for cataract formation and osteoporosis with long-term treatment.
- Be alert to rounding of face (moon face), acne, increased appetite and weight gain, red marks/blotches on skin, facial hair, severe mood swings, weakness, and leg cramps.	Typical side effects with steroids.
- As active disease subsides, prednisone is tapered.	The goal is eventual elimination of the drug.
- In some cases of chronic disease, continuous corticosteroid therapy may be necessary.	Many patients with Crohn's disease become steroid dependent, meaning they are symptomatic with low-dose therapy (5-15 mg/day) or with total discontinuation of the drug.
- A new steroidal agent, budesonide, is undergoing clinical trials.	It shows promise for providing benefits of traditional therapy without the side effects.
- Topical therapy is an effective route.	Topical therapy with hydrocortisone has controlled inflammation via retention enemas for patients with proctosigmoiditis (involvement to 40 cm); suppositories have been used for patients with Crohn's proctitis.
Immunosuppressive agents	To allow dosage reduction or withdrawal of corticosteroids in steroid-dependent patients, for maintenance therapy with a lower relapse rate, and to aid in healing and reduce drainage of perianal fistulas. Oral immunosuppressive agents include azathioprine and 6-mercaptopurine (6-MP).
- If taking 6-MP, check blood cell counts every other week until dose has been stable for 6 mo. Then monitor every month for 3 mo, then once every 3 mo.	Lowered WBC count can occur, as can anemia (rare).
- Be alert to the following when taking 6-MP: allergic reaction (fever, skin rash, joint aches) and inflammation of the pancreas.	Possible side effects.
- IV cyclosporine has been used to treat refractory Crohn's disease and treatment-resistant fistulas.	Oral cyclosporine has not proved to be effective for maintenance therapy because relapse occurs when dosage is reduced or stopped. Because of the frequency and severity of toxicity and side effects, short-term IV administration is the best method for cyclosporine.
- If taking cyclosporine, check BP at 2-wk intervals.	Elevated BP can occur.
- Monitor kidney function, including BUN and creatinine.	Decreased kidney function can occur.
- Parenteral (IM, SC) methotrexate provides both immunosuppressive and antiinflammatory effects and allows for reduction or cessation of steroid therapy in some patients with chronically active Crohn's disease. However, long-term	

Continued

INTERVENTIONS	RATIONALES
efficacy, incidence of side effects, and toxicity need to be determined.	
- Methotrexate is used with extreme caution in people who consume significant quantities of alcohol. Blood cell counts and liver enzymes are checked monthly for first 3 mo, then at 3-mo intervals.	This drug can affect the liver.
- Methotrexate is contraindicated in pregnancy or in women anticipating pregnancy.	May cause fetal death and congenital abnormalities; can be transferred via breast milk.
Antibodies: infliximab (Remicade)	To block tumor necrosis factor (TNF)-alpha, a protein that escalates inflammation.
- Has shown great promise since being approved for use in Crohn's disease in 1998. Clinical benefits last from a few weeks to many months; repeat infusions may be necessary to control the disease.	Infliximab reduces symptoms in patients with moderately to severely active disease.
- Patient should be alert to sore throat, upper respiratory infection, abscesses, sinusitis, and bronchitis.	Signs of infection. There is risk of altered immune response with this drug.
- There is risk of malignancy.	Lymphoma has occurred in some patients.
- Complications that occur during or shortly after the drug is given include headache, low BP, rash, muscle and joint pain, itching, and shortness of breath.	These complications usually are of short duration and almost always respond to treatment with diphenhydramine and/or acetaminophen.
Ensure that patient verbalizes accurate knowledge about purpose, precautions, and potential side effects of any prescribed drug he or she will be taking.	A knowledgeable individual is more likely to comply with therapy and promptly report untoward side effects to health care provider.

●●● **Related NIC and NOC labels:** *NIC:* Teaching: Prescribed Medication *NOC:* Knowledge: Medication

ADDITIONAL NURSING DIAGNOSES/ PROBLEMS:

PATIENT-FAMILY TEACHING AND DISCHARGE PLANNING

When providing patient-family teaching, focus on sensory information, avoid giving excessive information, and initiate a visiting nurse referral for necessary follow-up teaching. Include verbal and written information about the following:

✓ Medications, including drug name, rationale, dosage, schedule, route of administration, precautions, drug/drug and food/drug interactions, and potential side effects.

✓ Signs and symptoms that necessitate medical attention, including fever, nausea and vomiting, abdominal discomfort, any significant change in appearance and frequency of stools, or passage of stool through the vagina or stool mixed with urine, any of which can signal recurrence or complications of Crohn's disease.

✓ Importance of dietary management to promote nutritional and fluid maintenance and prevent abdominal cramping, discomfort, and diarrhea.

✓ Importance of perineal/perianal skin care after bowel movements.

✓ Importance of balancing activities with rest periods, even during remission, because adequate rest is necessary to sustain remission.

✓ Importance of follow-up medical care, including supportive psychotherapy, because of the chronic and progressive nature of Crohn's disease.

✓ Referral to community resources, including the following organization:

Crohn's and Colitis Foundation of America
386 Park Ave. South, 17th Floor
New York, NY 10016-8804
(800) 932-2423
www.ccfa.org

In addition, if the patient has a fecal diversion:

✓ Care of incision, dressing changes, and bathing.

✓ Care of stoma and peristomal skin, use of ostomy equipment, and method for obtaining supplies.

✓ Gradual resumption of ADL, excluding heavy lifting (>10 lb), pushing, or pulling for 6-8 wk to prevent incisional herniation.

✓ Importance of reporting signs and symptoms that require medical attention, such as change in stoma color from the normal bright and shiny red; lesions of stomal mucosa that may indicate recurrence of disease; peristomal skin irritation; diarrhea or constipation, fever, chills, abdominal pain, distention, nausea, and vomiting; and incisional pain, local increased temperature, drainage, swelling, or redness.

✓ Referral to community resources, including home health care agency; wound, ostomy, continence (WOC)/enterostomal therapy (ET) nurse; and local chapter of the United Ostomy Association.

United Ostomy Association
19722 MacArthur Blvd., Suite 200
Irvine, CA 92612-2405
(800) 826-0826
www.uoa.org

Fecal Diversions

For a discussion of ulcerative colitis, see p. 507, for Crohn's disease, see p. 465.

SURGICAL INTERVENTIONS

It is sometimes necessary to interrupt the continuity of the bowel because of intestinal disease or its complications. A fecal diversion may be necessary to divert stool around a diseased portion or, more commonly, out of the body. A fecal diversion can be located anywhere along the bowel, depending on location of the diseased or injured portion, and it can be permanent or temporary. The most common sites for fecal diversion are the colon and ileum.

Colostomy

Created when the surgeon brings a portion of the colon to the surface of the abdomen. An opening in the exteriorized colon permits elimination of flatus and stool through the stoma. Any part of the colon may be diverted into a colostomy.

Transverse colostomy: Most frequently created stoma to divert feces on a temporary basis. Surgical indications include relief of bowel obstruction before definitive surgery for tumors, inflammation, or diverticulitis and colon perforation secondary to trauma. Stool can be liquid to pastelike or soft and unformed, and bowel elimination is unpredictable. A temporary colostomy may be double barreled, with a proximal stoma through which stool is eliminated and a distal stoma adjacent to the proximal stoma called a *mucous fistula*. More commonly, a loop colostomy is created with a supporting rod placed beneath it until the exteriorized loop of colon heals to the skin.

Descending or sigmoid colostomy: Usually a permanent fecal diversion. Cancer of the rectum is the most common cause for surgical intervention. Stool is usually formed, and some individuals may have stool elimination at predictable times. In a permanent colostomy, the surgeon brings the severed end of the colon to the abdominal skin surface. The diseased or injured portion of the colon and/or rectum is resected and removed. To create the stoma, the colon above the skin surface is rolled back on itself to expose the mucosal surface of the intestine.

The end of the cuff is sutured to the skin with absorbable sutures to hold it in place as it heals.

Temporary colostomy: Typically created when there is significant inflammation in the diseased portion of the bowel (e.g., perforated diverticulum or ulcerative colitis). When a temporary colostomy is created, the severed end of the colon is brought through the abdominal wall as for a permanent colostomy. The diseased or injured portion of the colon is resected and removed. The remaining rectum or rectosigmoid is oversewn, left in the peritoneal cavity, and is referred to as Hartmann's pouch. After the inflammatory process has resolved (e.g., 3-6 mo), the colostomy is taken down and reattached to the Hartmann's pouch, thus reconstructing continuity of the bowel and normal bowel elimination.

Cecostomy or ascending colostomy: Not a commonly seen procedure. A temporary diverting colostomy is most commonly used to bypass an unresectable tumor. The stool from an ascending colostomy is soft, unformed, pastelike, semiliquid, or liquid, and bowel elimination is unpredictable. Surgical procedure is similar to that with transverse colostomies.

Ileostomy

Conventional (Brooke) ileostomy: Created by bringing a distal portion of the resected ileum through the abdominal wall. A permanent ileostomy is created by the same procedure discussed with a permanent colostomy. Surgical indications include ulcerative colitis, Crohn's disease, and familial adenomatous polyposis (FAP) requiring excision of the entire colon and rectum. For any ileostomy, the output is usually liquid (or more rarely, pastelike) and is eliminated continually. The more proximal the ileostomy, the more active are digestive enzymes within the effluent (stool) and the greater their potential for irritation to exposed skin around the stoma. A collection pouch is worn over the stoma on the abdomen to collect gas and fecal discharge.

Temporary ileostomy: Usually a loop stoma with or without a supporting rod in place beneath the loop of the ileum until the exteriorized loop of ileum heals to the skin. The purpose is to divert the fecal stream away from a more distal anastomotic site or fistula repair until healing has occurred.

Continent (Kock pouch) ileostomy: An intraabdominal pouch constructed from approximately 30 cm of distal ileum. Intussusception of a 10-cm portion of ileum is done to form an outlet nipple valve from the pouch to the skin of the abdomen, where a stoma is constructed flush with the skin. The intraabdominal pouch is continent for gas and fecal discharge and is emptied approximately qid by inserting a catheter through the stoma. No external pouch is needed, and a Band-Aid or small dressing is worn over the stoma to collect mucus. Surgical indications include ulcerative colitis and FAP requiring removal of the colon and rectum. Crohn's disease is a contraindication for this procedure because the disease can recur in the pouch, necessitating its removal.

Ileoanal reservoir (or restorative proctocolectomy)

A two-stage surgical procedure developed to preserve fecal continence and prevent the need for a permanent ileostomy.

During the first stage after total colectomy and removal of the rectal mucosa, an ileal reservoir is constructed and lowered into position in the pelvis just above the rectal cuff. Then the ileal outlet from the reservoir is brought down through the cuff of the rectal muscle and anastomosed to the anal canal. The anal sphincter is preserved, and the resulting ileal reservoir provides a storage place for feces. A temporary diverting ileostomy is required for 2-3 mo to allow healing of the anastomosis. The second stage occurs when the diverting ileostomy is taken down and fecal continuity is restored. Initially, the patient experiences fecal incontinence and 10 or more bowel movements per day. After 3-6 mo, the patient experiences a decrease in urgency and frequency with 4-8 bowel movements per day. This procedure is an option for patients requiring colectomy for ulcerative colitis or FAP. It is contraindicated in patients with Crohn's disease and incontinence problems.

Nursing Diagnoses:

Risk for Impaired Peristomal Skin Integrity

related to exposure to effluent or sensitivity to appliance material; *and*

Impaired Stomal Tissue Integrity

(or risk for same) *related to* improperly fitted appliance resulting in impaired circulation

Desired Outcomes: Patient's stomal and peristomal skin and tissue remain nonerythemic and intact. Before hospital discharge (or immediately following teaching if patient is not hospitalized), patient or significant other demonstrates appropriate peristomal/perianal/perineal skin care for prevention and/or management of breakdown. Patient or significant other identifies and reports signs and symptoms of impaired skin and/or tissue integrity.

INTERVENTIONS	RATIONALES
After Colostomy or Conventional Ileostomy (Permanent or Temporary):	
Apply a pectin, gelatin, methylcellulose-based, or synthetic, solid-form skin barrier around stoma.	To protect peristomal skin from irritation caused by contact with stool.
Cut an opening in skin barrier the exact circumference of stoma or as recommended by manufacturer. Remove release paper, and apply sticky surface directly to peristomal skin. As indicated, use pectin-based paste to "caulk" around the barrier and compensate for irregular surfaces on peristomal skin.	For some pouching systems, the skin barrier may be a separate barrier to be used with an adhesive-backed pouch, part of a two-piece system, or an integral part of a one-piece pouch system. A pectin-based paste may prevent undermining of barrier with effluent and protect skin immediately adjacent to stoma.
Remove skin barrier and inspect skin q3-4 days. Monitor peristomal skin for changes (e.g., erythema, erosion, serous drainage, bleeding, induration). Carefully document	These indicators may signal presence of infection, irritation, or sensitivity to materials placed on skin.

Continued

INTERVENTIONS	**RATIONALES**
abnormal findings and report them to health care provider. Patch-test patient's abdominal skin. Discontinue use of irritating materials and substitute other materials.	To determine sensitivity to materials used and eliminate those materials accordingly.
Recalibrate skin barrier opening to size of stoma with each change.	Stomas become less edematous over a period of weeks after surgery, necessitating changes in size of skin barrier opening.
Ensure skin barrier opening is the exact circumference of the stoma.	To prevent contact of stool with skin. Burning, itching, and odor are signs that effluent has had contact with the skin.
Use a commercial template if one is available.	To aid in estimating size of the opening needed for the skin barrier.
Apply a two-piece pouch system or a pouch with access cap.	Enables inspection of stoma for viability q12-24h in the immediate postoperative period.
Assess color and character of the stoma.	A mature stoma will be red in color with overlying mucus. A nonmature stoma will be red and moist where the mucous membrane is exposed but can be a darker, mottled, grayish red with a transparent or translucent film of serosa elsewhere.
Cleanse skin with warm water when removing skin barrier and pouch for routine care. Dry peristomal skin completely.	This ensures skin will retain its normal integrity and that skin barrier and pouch materials adhere well.
Empty pouch when it is one-third to one-half full of stool or gas.	To maintain a secure pouch seal. A pouch with a larger amount of stool could break the seal.

After Continent Ileostomy (Kock Pouch):

Avoid stress on ileostomy catheter and its securing suture.	To prevent tissue destruction and catheter dislodgement.
As prescribed, maintain catheter on low, continuous suction or gravity drainage.	The catheter was inserted through the stoma into the continent ileostomy pouch during surgery to prevent stress on nipple valve and maintain pouch decompression so that suture lines are allowed to heal without stress or tension.
Monitor site for erythema, induration, drainage, or erosion around the stoma. Report significant findings to health care provider.	These are signs of infection, irritation, or sensitivity to materials placed on skin.
Check catheter q2h for patency and irrigate with sterile saline (30 ml). Notify health care provider if solution cannot be instilled, if there are no returns from catheter, or if leakage of irrigating solution or pouch contents appears around catheter.	To check for and help prevent catheter obstruction. Instilling 30 ml of saline will clear the catheter and liquefy the secretions/effluent without adding unnecessary pressure on the pouch walls and areas of anastomosis.
Change 4 × 4 dressing around stoma q2h or as often as it becomes wet. Report presence of frank bleeding to health care provider.	To prevent peristomal skin irritation. Normally drainage will be serosanguineous at first and mixed with mucus.
Assess stoma for viability with each dressing change.	The stoma should be red in color and moist and shiny with mucus. A stoma that is pale or dark purple to black or dull in appearance may indicate circulatory impairment and should be reported to health care provider immediately and documented.

After Ileoanal Reservoir:

Perform routine care for diverting ileostomy (see earlier discussion).	
If indicated, irrigate mucus out of reservoir daily with 60 ml of water or gently cleanse the area with water and cotton balls or soft tissues.	To maintain perineal/peristomal skin integrity. After the first stage of the operation, patient may have incontinence of mucus. **Note:** Pouch irrigation to remove mucus rarely is indicated now because of new reservoir configurations that allow spontaneous emptying of reservoir.

Continued

INTERVENTIONS	RATIONALES
Avoid soap.	Can cause itching or irritation.
Use absorbent pad at night.	To absorb oozing mucus.
After second stage of the operation (when ileostomy is taken down), monitor patient's defecation pattern.	Expect patient to experience frequency and urgency of defecation during this stage.
Wash perineal/perianal area with warm water or commercial perianal/perineal cleansing solution, using squeeze bottle, cotton balls, or soft tissues.	To promote comfort and cleanse the perineal/perianal area.
Do not use toilet paper.	Toilet paper can cause irritation.
If desired, dry the area with hair dryer on a cool setting.	To prevent skin irritation that would be caused by materials used for drying.
Provide sitz baths.	To promote comfort and help clean perineal/perianal area.
Apply protective skin sealants or ointments. Avoid use of skin sealants on irritated or eroded skin.	Skin sealants have a high alcohol content, which would cause a painful burning sensation.

●●● **Related NIC and NOC labels:** *NIC:* Skin Surveillance; Circulatory Precautions; Incision Site Care; Ostomy Care; Skin Care: Topical Treatments; Self-Care Assistance: Bathing/Hygiene *NOC:* Tissue Integrity: Skin and Mucous Membranes

Nursing Diagnosis:

Bowel Incontinence

related to disruption of normal function with fecal diversion

Desired Outcomes: Within 2-4 days after surgery, patient has bowel sounds and eliminates gas and stool via the fecal diversion. Within 3 days after teaching has been initiated, patient verbalizes accurate understanding of measures that will maintain normal elimination pattern and demonstrates care techniques specific to the fecal diversion.

INTERVENTIONS	RATIONALES
After Colostomy and Conventional Ileostomy (Permanent and Temporary):	
Empty stool from pouch's bottom opening and assess quality and quantity of stool. Record volume of liquid stool and its color and consistency.	To document return of normal bowel function and its quality and quantity.
If colostomy is not eliminating stool after 3-4 days and bowel sounds have returned, gently insert a gloved, lubricated finger into the stoma.	To determine presence of stricture at skin or fascial levels and note presence of any stool within reach of examining finger.
If health care provider prescribes colostomy irrigation, see **Deficient Knowledge:** Colostomy irrigation procedure, p. 480.	
After Continent Ileostomy (Kock Pouch):	
Monitor I&O and record amount, color, and consistency of output.	Expect bright red blood or serosanguineous liquid drainage from Kock pouch during early postoperative period.
As gastrointestinal (GI) function returns after 3-4 days, monitor and document color and character of output.	Expect drainage to change from blood-tinged to greenish brown liquid. When ileal output appears, suction (if used) is discontinued and pouch catheter is connected to or maintained on gravity drainage.

INTERVENTIONS	RATIONALES
Check and irrigate catheter q2h and as needed.	To maintain catheter patency. As patient's diet progresses from clear liquids to solid food, ileal output thickens. If patient reports abdominal fullness in area of pouch along with decreased fecal output, catheter placement and patency should be assessed.
When patient is alert and taking food by mouth, teach catheter irrigation procedure, which should be performed q2h; demonstrate how to empty pouch contents through the catheter into the toilet.	Irrigation liquefies effluent for easier flow through the catheter. Frequent irrigations prevent overdistention of the pouch.
Before hospital discharge, teach patient how to remove and reinsert catheter. Have patient return the demonstration.	Teaching, followed by return demonstration, helps ensure that learning has occurred and facilitates retention of that information.
After Ileoanal Reservoir:	
Monitor I&O.	To assess quantity, quality, and consistency of output from diverting ileostomy and reservoir.
Monitor patient for temperature elevation accompanied by perianal pain and discharge of purulent, bloody mucus from drains and anal orifice. Report significant findings to health care provider.	These are signs of infection or anastomotic leak.
If drains are present, irrigate them as prescribed.	To maintain patency, decrease stress on suture lines, and decrease incidence of infection.
Advise patient to wear a small pad in undergarment.	To avoid soiling outer garments. After first stage of the operation, patient may experience oozing of mucus.
After second stage of the operation (when ileostomy is taken down), monitor patient's output.	Expect incontinence and 15-20 bowel movements per day with urgency when patient is on a clear-liquid diet.
Assist with perianal care and apply protective skin care products.	To maintain perineal/perianal skin integrity. If nocturnal incontinence is especially troublesome, the catheter can be placed in the reservoir and connected to gravity drainage bag overnight.
Monitor output after patient starts eating solid foods.	Expect number of bowel movements to decrease to 6-12/day and consistency to thicken when patient is eating solid foods.
Administer hydrophilic colloids and antidiarrheal medications as prescribed.	To decrease frequency and fluidity of stools.
Provide diet consultation if indicated.	Patient can learn about foods that cause liquid stools (spinach, raw fruits, highly seasoned foods, green beans, broccoli, prune and grape juices, alcohol) and increase intake of foods that cause thick stools (cheese, ripe bananas, applesauce, creamy peanut butter, gelatin, pasta).
Reassure patient that frequency and urgency are temporary and that as the reservoir expands and absorbs fluid, bowel movements should become thicker and less frequent.	This may decrease anxiety about the disruption of usual bowel pattern.

●●● **Related NIC and NOC labels:** *NIC:* Bowel Management; Ostomy Care; Nutrition Management
NOC: Bowel Elimination; Tissue Integrity: Skin and Mucous Membranes

Nursing Diagnosis:

Disturbed Body Image

related to presence of fecal diversion

Desired Outcomes: Within 5-7 days after surgery, patient demonstrates actions that reflect beginning acceptance of the fecal diversion and incorporates changes into self-concept as evidenced by acknowledging body changes, viewing the stoma, and participating in the care of the fecal diversion. Patient resumes activities of daily living (ADL), social activities, and role-related responsibilities.

INTERVENTIONS	RATIONALES
Monitor patient for expressed fears about the fecal diversion.	Many fears may be expressed by patients experiencing a fecal diversion. Some patients view incontinence as a return to infancy. The following fears may be expected: physical, social, and work activities will be curtailed significantly; rejection, isolation, and feelings of uncleanliness will occur; everyone will know about the altered pattern of fecal elimination; and loss of voluntary control may occur.
Encourage patient to discuss feelings and fears. Involve family members in discussions because they too may have anxieties and misconceptions.	Fears and anxieties about body image may be reduced by talking about them. Such discussions also enable clarification about misconceptions.
Provide a calm and quiet environment for patient and significant other to discuss the surgery. Initiate an open, honest discussion.	An open discussion enables understanding of patient's perspective of the impact the diversion will have and assists in development of an individualized plan of care that will help patient.
Monitor carefully for and listen closely to expressed or nonverbalized needs.	Each patient will react differently to the surgical procedure.
Have patient participate in care. Assure patient that education offers a means of control.	To encourage patient's acceptance of the fecal diversion and rebuild a sense of independence and self-esteem.
Assure patient that physical, social, and work activities will not be affected by presence of a fecal diversion.	Assisting patient with resuming previous lifestyle with minimal disruption is an essential component of the patient's rehabilitation.
Expect patient to have fears about sexual acceptance. If you are uncomfortable talking about sexuality with patients, be aware of these potential concerns and arrange for a consultation with someone who can speak openly and honestly about these problems.	Although these fears usually are not expressed overtly, concerns center on change in body image; fears about odor and the ostomy appliance interfering with intercourse; conception, pregnancy, and discomfort from perianal wound and scar in women; and impotence and failure to ejaculate in men, especially after more radical dissection of the pelvis in patients with cancer.
Consult patient's health care provider about a visit by another person with an ostomy.	Patients gain reassurance and build positive attitudes and body image by seeing a healthy, active person who has undergone the same type of surgery, and it expands patient's support system as well.

●●● **Related NIC and NOC labels:** *NIC:* Active Listening; Anxiety Reduction; Coping Enhancement; Emotional Support; Ostomy Care; Support Group; Body Image Enhancement *NOC:* Body Image

Nursing Diagnosis:

Deficient Knowledge:

Colostomy irrigation procedure

Desired Outcome: Within 3 days after initiation of teaching, patient demonstrates proficiency with the procedure for colostomy irrigation.

INTERVENTIONS	**RATIONALES**
Instruct patient about the following steps.	The prescribed colostomy irrigation is taught to patient with permanent descending or sigmoid colostomy. Colostomy irrigation is performed daily or every other day so that wearing a pouch becomes unnecessary. An appropriate candidate is a patient who has one or two formed stools each day at predictable times (same as normal stool elimination pattern before illness). In addition, the patient must be able to manipulate the equipment, remember the technique, and be willing to spend approximately 1 hr/day performing the procedure. It may take 4-6 wk for the patient to have stool elimination regulated with irrigation.
Position irrigating sleeve over colostomy, centering stoma in opening. Secure sleeve in place with adhesive disk on the sleeve or with a sleeve belt.	The irrigation sleeve provides controlled diversion of stool and irrigation solution into the toilet.
Fill enema/irrigation container with 500-1000 ml (1-2 pints) warm water. With patient in a sitting position on toilet or on a chair facing toilet, position sleeve so that it empties into toilet. Hang enema/irrigation container so that bottom surface is at patient's shoulder level.	Volume of water must be titrated for each patient to affect colon distention without causing cramping or excessive stretching of colon wall.
Open slide or roller clamp and flush tubing with the water; reclamp tubing.	To remove air from tubing.
Gently dilate stoma with a gloved finger lubricated with water-soluble lubricant.	This enables patient to identify direction of intestinal lumen and presence or absence of obstructing stool or stomal stenosis.
Lubricate cone or catheter with shield and slowly insert into stoma. If using catheter with shield, insert catheter no more than 3 inches.	To prevent bowel perforation. **Note:** Use of cone tip rather than catheter and shield is recommended because of the potential of bowel perforation with the catheter.
Hold cone or shield on catheter gently, but firmly, in place against stoma.	To prevent backflow of irrigant.
Allow water to slowly enter stoma from the container through the tubing; allow 15 min for fluid to enter the colon.	To prevent cramping. **Note:** If cramping occurs while water is flowing, stop the flow and leave cone in place until cramping passes; then flow of water may be resumed. If cramping does not resolve, the colon is probably ready to evacuate and should be allowed to do so.
After water has entered colon, advise patient to hold cone in place for a few seconds and then gently remove it.	To ensure complete infusion of water.
Leave sleeve in place for 30-40 min.	To enable water and stool to be eliminated.
When elimination is complete, remove irrigation sleeve and cleanse and dry peristomal area.	Cleaning and drying the skin help prevent skin irritation.
Apply a small dressing or security pouch over colostomy between irrigations.	To collect mucus drainage from stoma. **Note:** During initial adaptation period, a drainable pouch is worn between irrigations to collect expected spillage of stool.
For the next irrigation, have patient demonstrate and explain each step.	A return demonstration with explanation for each step will enable nurse to determine patient's knowledge level and facilitate learning retention for the patient.

●●● **Related NIC and NOC labels:** *NIC:* Teaching: Procedure *NOC:* Knowledge: Treatment Regimen

ADDITIONAL NURSING DIAGNOSES/ PROBLEMS:

PATIENT-FAMILY TEACHING AND DISCHARGE PLANNING

When providing patient-family teaching, focus on sensory information, avoid giving excessive information, and initiate a visiting nurse referral for necessary follow-up teaching. Include verbal and written information about the following:

✓ Medications, including drug name, rationale, dosage, schedule, route of administration, precautions, drug/drug and food/drug interactions, and potential side effects.

✓ Importance of dietary management to promote nutritional and fluid maintenance.

✓ Care of incision, dressing changes, and permission to take baths or showers once sutures and drains are removed.

✓ Care of stoma and peristomal/perianal skin; use of ostomy equipment; and method for obtaining supplies.

✓ Gradual resumption of ADL, excluding heavy lifting (>10 lb), pushing, or pulling for 6-8 wk to prevent development of incisional herniation.

✓ Importance of follow-up care with health care provider and wound, ostomy, continence (WOC)/enterostomal therapy (ET) nurse; confirm date and time of next appointment.

✓ Importance of reporting signs and symptoms that require medical attention, such as change in stoma color from normal bright and shiny red; peristomal or perianal skin irritation; any significant changes in appearance, frequency, and consistency of stools; fever, chills, abdominal pain, or distention; and incisional pain, increased local warmth, drainage, swelling, or redness.

✓ Referral to community resources, including home health care agency, WOC/ET nurse, and local chapter of the United Ostomy Association.

United Ostomy Association
19722 MacArthur Blvd., Suite 200
Irvine, CA 92612-2405
(800) 826-0826
www.uoa.org

Hepatitis

Viral hepatitis may be caused by one of five viruses that are capable of infecting the liver: hepatitis A (HAV), B (HBV), C (HCV), D (HDV), or E (HEV). A sixth virus, hepatitis G (HGV), has been isolated in a few cases of hepatitis caused by other viruses of the five common strains. It is not known what the role of HGV is in liver disease, nor are clinical manifestations, natural history, or pathogenesis known. However, it has been found in a significant proportion of blood donors, sometimes along with other hepatotropic viruses and sometimes alone.

Chronic hepatitis is inflammation of the liver for more than 6 mo. The term is used to describe a spectrum of inflammatory liver diseases ranging from mild chronic persistent hepatitis to severe chronic active hepatitis. Forms of chronic hepatitis are associated with infection from HBV, HCV, or HDV; viral infections such as cytomegalovirus (CMV); excessive alcohol consumption; inflammatory bowel disease; and autoimmunity (chronic active lupoid hepatitis).

Alcoholic hepatitis occurs as a result of tissue necrosis caused by alcohol abuse; it is nonviral and noninfectious. Generally it is a precursor to cirrhosis (see p. 457), but it may occur simultaneously with cirrhosis.

Jaundice is discoloration of body tissues from increased serum levels of bilirubin (total serum bilirubin >2.5 mg/dl). Jaundice may be seen in any patient with impaired hepatic function and occurs as the bilirubin begins to be excreted through the skin. There is also an increased excretion of urobilinogen and bilirubin by the kidneys, resulting in darker, almost brownish, urine. Jaundice is classified as follows:

- **Prehepatic (hemolytic):** Caused by increased production of bilirubin following erythrocyte destruction. Prehepatic jaundice is implicated when the indirect (unconjugated) serum bilirubin is >0.8 mg/dl.
- **Hepatic (hepatocellular):** Caused by the dysfunction of the liver cells (hepatocytes), which reduces their ability to remove bilirubin from the blood and form it into bile. Hepatic jaundice is also implicated with indirect serum bilirubin and is associated with hepatitis.
- **Posthepatic (obstructive):** Caused by an obstruction of the flow of bile out of the liver and resulting in backed-up bile through the hepatocytes to the blood. Posthepatic jaundice is implicated when the direct serum bilirubin is >0.3 mg/dl.

HEALTH CARE SETTING

Primary care, with possible brief hospitalization resulting from complications

ASSESSMENT

Signs and symptoms: Nausea, vomiting, malaise, anorexia, muscle or joint aches, fatigue, irritability, slight to moderate temperature increases, epigastric discomfort, dark urine, clay-colored stools, pruritus, aversion to smoking

Acute hepatic failure: Nausea, vomiting, and abdominal pain tend to be more severe. Jaundice is likely to appear earlier and deepen more rapidly. Mental status changes (possibly progressing to encephalopathy), coma, seizures, ascites, sharp rise in temperature, significant leukocytosis, coffee-ground emesis, gastrointestinal (GI) hemorrhage, purpura, shock, oliguria, and azotemia all may be present.

Physical assessment: Presence of jaundice; palpation of lymph nodes and abdomen may reveal lymphadenopathy, hepatomegaly, and splenomegaly. Liver size usually is small with acute hepatic failure.

History of: Clotting disorders, multiple blood transfusions, excessive alcohol ingestion, parenteral drug use, exposure to hepatotoxic chemicals or medications, travel to developing countries.

DIAGNOSTIC TESTS

Hematologic tests: Anti-HAV immunoglobulin M (IgM) is present with HAV, as is hepatitis B surface antigen (HBsAg) with HAV. Anti-HCV is present approximately 15 wk after infection with HCV. Aspartate aminotransferase (AST) and alanine aminotransferase (ALT) are elevated initially and then drop. Total bilirubin is elevated, and prothrombin time (PT) is prolonged. Differential white blood cell (WBC) count reveals leukocytosis, monocytosis, and atypical lymphocytes; λ-globulin levels are increased.

Urine tests: Reveal elevation of urobilinogen, mild proteinuria, and mild bilirubinuria.

Liver biopsy: Performed percutaneously or via laparoscopy to collect a specimen for histologic examination to confirm differential diagnosis.

Nursing Diagnosis:

Fatigue

related to decreased metabolic energy production secondary to liver dysfunction, which causes faulty absorption, metabolism, and storage of nutrients

Desired Outcome: By at least 24 hr before hospital discharge (or within 3 days of intervention/treatment), patient relates decreasing fatigue and increasing energy.

INTERVENTIONS	RATIONALES
Provide or restrict protein as prescribed.	Protein is moderately restricted, or eliminated, depending on degree of mental status changes (i.e., with encephalopathy). If no mental status changes are noted, normal amounts of high-biologic-value protein are indicated to provide energy and facilitate tissue healing.
Encourage small, frequent feedings and provide emotional support during meals.	Smaller and more frequent meals are usually better tolerated in patients who are fatigued, nauseated, and anorexic.
Consult dietitian regarding increased intake of carbohydrates or other high-energy food sources within prescribed dietary limitations.	High-energy foods may help eliminate fatigue.
Maintain bedrest and provide rest periods of at least 90 min before and after activities and treatments.	Bedrest and rest periods allow recovery after the body has experienced stress and may be indicated when symptoms are severe, with a gradual return to normal activity as symptoms subside.
Avoid activity immediately after meals.	Exercise after meals increases potential for nausea and vomiting, which could cause loss of nutrients and exacerbate fatigue.
Keep frequently used objects within easy reach.	To conserve energy.
Decrease environmental stimuli, provide back massage and relaxation tapes, and speak with patient in short, simple terms.	To promote rest and sleep.
Administer acid suppression therapy, antidiarrheal medications, and cathartics as prescribed.	To minimize gastric distress and promote absorption of nutrients, which will help provide energy and reverse feelings of fatigue.
Administer antiemetics such as hydroxyzine and ondansetron as prescribed.	These antiemetics are good for nausea, but phenothiazines, such as prochlorperazine (Compazine), are avoided because they cause excessive sedation and would exacerbate fatigue.

●●● **Related NIC and NOC labels:** *NIC:* Energy Management; Nutrition Management; Sleep Enhancement; Simple Relaxation Therapy; Nutrition Therapy: Environmental Management *NOC:* Energy Conservation; Nutritional Status: Energy

Nursing Diagnosis:

Deficient Knowledge:

Causes of hepatitis and modes of transmission

Desired Outcome: Immediately following teaching, patient verbalizes accurate knowledge about
the causes of hepatitis and measures that help prevent transmission.

INTERVENTIONS	RATIONALES
Assess patient's knowledge about disease process and educate as necessary.	Determining patient's level of knowledge will facilitate development of an individualized teaching plan.
Avoid making moral judgments about alcohol/drug use or sexual behavior.	This will promote patient's confidence in you.
Teach patient and significant other importance of wearing gloves and good handwashing if contact with body fluids such as urine, blood, wound exudate, and feces is possible.	To prevent spread of infection.
If appropriate, advise patients with HAV to avoid crowded living conditions with poor sanitation.	To prevent recurrence.
Remind patients with HBV and HCV that they should modify sexual behavior as directed by health care provider. Explain that blood donation is no longer possible.	For patients with HBV and HCV, contact with blood is a likely mode of transmission, and blood contact can occur with some types of sexual activity. For patients with HBV, sexual contact is a likely mode.
Advise patients with HBV that their sexual partners should receive HBV vaccine.	For patients with HBV, sexual contact is a likely mode of transmission.

●●● **Related NIC and NOC labels:** *NIC:* Teaching: Disease Process; Risk Identification; Health Education;
Teaching: Safe Sex; Behavior Modification; Infection Protection; Substance Use Prevention; Infection Control;
Immunization/Vaccination Management *NOC:* Knowledge: Disease Process; Knowledge: Health Behaviors;
Knowledge: Infection Control

Nursing Diagnosis:

Risk for Impaired Skin Integrity

related to pruritus secondary to hepatic dysfunction

Desired Outcome: Patient's skin remains intact.

INTERVENTIONS	RATIONALES
Use tepid water, avoid alkaline soap, and apply emollient lotions at frequent intervals.	Hot water and alkaline soaps can dry the skin and may cause irritation in patients with sensitive skin. Emollients and lipid creams (i.e., Eucerin) are used to keep patient's skin moist and supple.
Encourage patient not to scratch skin and to keep nails short and smooth. Suggest use of knuckles if patient must scratch. Wrap or place gloves on patient's hands (especially comatose patients).	To prevent skin breakdown and infection. Knuckles are less traumatic to the skin and tissue than fingernails.
Treat any skin lesion promptly.	To prevent infection. Pathogens can enter the body through nonintact skin.

Continued

INTERVENTIONS	RATIONALES
Administer antihistamines (diphenhydramine) as prescribed; observe closely for excessive sedation.	For symptomatic relief of pruritus. Antihistamines and tranquilizers, if used, are administered with caution and in low doses because they are metabolized by the liver.
Encourage patient to wear loose, soft clothing; provide soft linens (cotton is best).	To avoid abrasions caused by tight clothing or rough material on skin that is already compromised.
Keep environment cool.	To avoid further skin irritation by perspiration.
Change soiled linen as soon as possible.	To avoid further irritation by waste products or fluids having constant skin contact.

●●● **Related NIC and NOC labels:** *NIC:* Skin Surveillance; Bathing; Skin Care: Topical Treatments; Nail Care *NOC:* Tissue Integrity: Skin & Mucous Membranes

Nursing Diagnosis:

Ineffective Protection

related to increased risk of bleeding secondary to decreased vitamin K absorption or thrombocytopenia

Desired Outcome: Patient is free of bleeding as evidenced by negative tests for occult blood in the feces and urine, absence of ecchymotic areas, and absence of bleeding at the gums and injection sites.

INTERVENTIONS	RATIONALES
Monitor PT daily.	To be alert for prolonged PT; optimal range for PT is 10.5-13.5 sec. In hepatitis, PT is prolonged because of inability of the liver to produce coagulation factors.
Monitor platelet count daily.	For evidence of thrombocytopenia. Optimal range is 150,000-400,000/mm^3. In hepatitis, platelet count is decreased because of decrease in production of thrombopoietin or platelet pooling caused by splenomegaly and portal hypertension.
Monitor Hct and Hgb daily.	To detect decreases that may indicate occult bleeding; optimal ranges are Hct 40%-54% (male) and 37%-47% (female) and Hgb 14-18 g/dl (male) and 12-16 g/dl (female).
Handle patient gently (e.g., when turning or transferring).	To minimize risk of bleeding within the tissues.
Rotate sites and use small-gauge needles.	To minimize bleeding caused by large-bore needles. Rotating sites prevents tissue damage caused by frequent injections in same tissue.
Apply moderate pressure after an injection but do not massage site.	To minimize bleeding at injection site while preventing excessive pressure on tissue.
Administer medications orally or intravenously when possible.	To minimize IM injections with subsequent risk for bleeding caused by tissue trauma.
Observe for ecchymotic areas. Inspect gums and test urine and feces for bleeding. Report significant findings to health care provider.	To detect early signs of bleeding potential and abnormal coagulation factors.

Continued

INTERVENTIONS	RATIONALES
Teach patient to use electric razor and soft-bristle toothbrush.	To minimize risk of bleeding from cuts or abrasions caused by razor or hard bristles.
Administer vitamin K as prescribed.	For patients with prolonged PT, vitamin K is a cofactor that modifies clotting factors to provide a site for calcium binding—an essential part of the clotting function. Patients with severe hepatic failure may not respond to vitamin K and may require transfusions of fresh frozen plasma.

●●● **Related NIC and NOC labels:** *NIC:* Bleeding Precautions; Bleeding Reduction; Blood Products Administration *NOC:* Coagulation Status

ADDITIONAL NURSING DIAGNOSES/ PROBLEMS:

"Cirrhosis" **for Ineffective Protection**   p. 460

PATIENT-FAMILY TEACHING AND DISCHARGE PLANNING

When providing patient-family teaching, focus on sensory information, avoid giving excessive information, and initiate a visiting nurse referral for necessary follow-up teaching. Include verbal and written information about the following:

✓ Importance of rest and getting adequate nutrition. When appropriate, provide a list of high-biologic-value protein food sources or protein foods to avoid and sample menus to demonstrate how these foods may be incorporated into or excluded from the diet. Instruct patient to eat frequent, small meals; to eat slowly; and to chew all food thoroughly. Teach patient to rest for 30-60 min after meals.

✓ Importance of avoiding hepatotoxic agents, including over-the-counter (OTC) drugs.

✓ Prescribed medications (e.g., multivitamins), including drug name, purpose, dosage, schedule, drug/drug and food/drug interactions, potential side effects, and precautions.

✓ Importance of informing health care providers, dentists, and other health care workers of hepatitis diagnosis.

✓ Potential complications, including delayed healing, skin injury, and bleeding tendencies.

✓ Importance of avoiding alcohol during recovery.

✓ Referral to alcohol/drug treatment programs as appropriate.

Pancreatitis

The pancreas serves both endocrine (hormonal) and exocrine (nonhormonal) functions. The exocrine portion comprises 98% of the tissue mass of the pancreas. Its function is the secretion of potent enzymes that act to reduce proteins, fats, and carbohydrates into simpler chemical substances.

Acute pancreatitis occurs when pancreatic ductal flow becomes obstructed and digestive enzymes escape from the pancreatic duct into surrounding tissue. Self-destruction of the pancreas produces edema, hemorrhage, and necrosis of pancreatic and surrounding tissue. Complications of acute pancreatitis include pancreatic abscess, hemorrhage, pancreatic pseudocyst, fistula formation, and transient hypoglycemia. Acute, life-threatening complications include renal failure, hemorrhagic pancreatitis, septicemia, acute respiratory distress syndrome (ARDS), shock, and disseminated intravascular coagulation (DIC).

Chronic pancreatitis is characterized by varying degrees of pancreatic insufficiency, which results in decreased production of enzymes and bicarbonate and malabsorption of fats and proteins. The digestion of fat is affected most severely. As a result, a high fat content in the bowel stimulates water and electrolyte secretion, which produces diarrhea. The action of bacteria on fecal fat produces flatus, fatty stools (steatorrhea), and abdominal cramps. Often diabetes mellitus occurs as a result of chronic pancreatitis because of damage to the insulin-producing beta cells and resultant deficient insulin production. Chronic pancreatitis is associated with complications of diabetes mellitus, chronic pain, maldigestion, pseudocysts, and bleeding.

HEALTH CARE SETTING

Primary care with hospitalization for acute pancreatitis and complications of chronic pancreatitis

ASSESSMENT

Acute pancreatitis: Sudden onset of constant, severe epigastric pain, often after a large meal or alcohol intake. The pain frequently radiates to the back or left shoulder and is somewhat relieved by a sitting position. Nausea and vomiting, sometimes with persistent retching, usually occur. Jaundice suggests biliary tree obstruction. Extreme malaise, restlessness, respiratory distress, and diminished urinary output may be present. Hypovolemic shock may be present with hemorrhagic events, or distributive shock may occur secondary to systemic inflammatory response syndrome.

Physical assessment: Diminished or absent bowel sounds, suggesting presence of ileus; mild to moderate ascites; generalized abdominal tenderness, tachypnea, crackles (rales) at the lung bases related to atelectasis, and interstitial fluid accumulation; diminished ventilatory excursion related to splinting and guarding with pain; low-grade fever (37.7°-38.8° C [100°-102° F]) or pronounced fever with abscess or sepsis; and agitation, confusion, and altered mental status may occur because of electrolyte/metabolic abnormalities or acute alcohol withdrawal. Gray-blue discoloration of the flank (Grey Turner's sign) or around the umbilicus (Cullen's sign) sometimes is present with pancreatic hemorrhage.

Chronic pancreatitis: Constant, dull epigastric pain; steatorrhea resulting from malabsorption of fats and protein; severe weight loss; and onset of symptoms of diabetes mellitus: polydipsia, polyuria, and polyphagia. In addition, chemical addiction is often seen because of the chronic pain.

History of: Biliary tract disease, chronic excessive alcohol consumption, physical trauma to the abdomen (especially in young people), peptic ulcer disease, viral infection, endoscopic retrograde cholangiopancreatography (ERCP), cystic fibrosis, neoplasms, shock, and use of certain medications, such as estrogen-containing oral contraceptives, glucocorticoids, sulfonamides, chlorothiazides, and azathioprine.

DIAGNOSTIC TESTS

Serum amylase: When significantly elevated (>500 U/dl), rules out acute abdomen conditions, such as cholecystitis, appendicitis, bowel infarction/obstruction, and perforated peptic ulcer, and confirms presence of pancreatitis. These levels return to normal 48-72 hr after the onset of acute symptoms, even though clinical indicators may continue.

Serum lipase: Rises more slowly than serum amylase and persists longer. Both lipase and amylase levels reflect the degree of necrotic pancreatic tissue.

Hyperglycemia: Occurs because of interference with beta cell function. It is transient with acute pancreatitis but common with chronic pancreatitis, during which diabetes mellitus is likely to develop.

Serum calcium and magnesium: May be lower than normal. On electrocardiogram (ECG), hypocalcemia is evidenced by prolonged QT segment with a normal T wave.

Complete blood count (CBC): Elevated white blood cells (WBCs) caused by inflammatory process. Polymorphonuclear bodies may increase if bacterial peritonitis is present secondary to duodenal rupture.

Blood urea nitrogen (BUN) and serum creatinine: To evaluate renal function

Urinalysis: May show presence of glycosuria, which can signal the onset of diabetes mellitus. Elevated urine amylase levels are useful diagnostically when serum levels have dropped off. An elevated specific gravity reflects the presence of dehydration.

Abdominal x-ray examination: May show dilation of the small or large bowel and presence of pancreatic calcification in chronic pancreatitis.

Ultrasound, magnetic resonance imaging (MRI), or computed tomography (CT) scan: May reveal an enlarged and edematous pancreatic head or abscess, pseudocyst, or calcification.

Magnetic resonance cholangiopancreatography (MRCP): Used to visualize pancreatic and common bile ducts and may be used if an ERCP is not feasible.

ERCP: A combined endoscopic-radiographic tool that is used to study the degree of pancreatic disease via assessment of biliary-pancreatic ductal systems. It allows direct visualization of the ampulla of Vater, diagnoses biliary stones and duct stenosis, and distinguishes cancer of the pancreas from pancreatic calculi. ERCP is not performed until the acute episode has subsided.

Secretin stimulation test: To diagnose chronic pancreatitis.

Nursing Diagnosis:

Deficient Fluid Volume

related to active loss secondary to nasogastric (NG) suctioning, vomiting, diaphoresis, or pooling of fluids in the abdomen and retroperitoneum

Desired Outcome: Patient is normovolemic within 8 hr of intervention/treatment as evidenced by HR 60-100 bpm, central venous pressure (CVP) 2-6 mm Hg (5-12 cm H_2O), brisk capillary refill (<2 sec), peripheral pulse amplitude >2+ on a 0-4+ scale, urinary output ≥30 ml/hr, and stable weight and abdominal girth measurements.

INTERVENTIONS	RATIONALES
Monitor VS q2-4h.	To be alert to falling BP and increasing HR, which can occur with moderate to severe fluid loss.
Measure I&O and CVP, if available, q2-4h. Be alert to and report I&O imbalances. Weigh daily and note trends. Correlate weights with I&O ratios. Report significant findings.	CVP <2 mm Hg can occur with volume-related hypotension, and output > intake signals fluid loss. Weight decreases when fluid is lost or intake is insufficient. Fluid loss requires immediate replacement to prevent shock and acute renal failure. Approximately 1 kg weight = 1 L fluid.
Measure orthostatic VS initially and q8h. Report significant findings.	To be alert to decreasing BP and increasing HR on standing, which suggests need for crystalloid and/or colloid volume expansion.
Administer plasma volume expanders as prescribed.	To maintain adequate circulating blood volume.
Monitor closely for adventitious breath sounds, increased weight, and drop in Hct without concomitant blood loss.	These are signs of fluid overload and potentially of pulmonary edema as a result of overly aggressive fluid resuscitation. In cases of severe, acute pancreatitis, patients develop a profound loss of circulating blood volume and need adequate fluid resuscitation quickly, sometimes as much as 5-6 L/day. This increases risk for fluid overload, especially if patient has been hypotensive and the kidneys are not functioning well enough to handle the large amounts of

Continued

INTERVENTIONS

RATIONALES

INTERVENTIONS	RATIONALES
	fluid. The fluid overload can lead to pulmonary edema and respiratory failure. In fact, respiratory dysfunction is the most frequent complication of severe, acute pancreatitis and one of the main causes of early death.
Be alert to positive Chvostek's sign (facial muscle spasm) and Trousseau's sign (carpopedal spasm), muscle twitching, tetany, or irritability.	Indicators of hypocalcemia, which can occur with electrolyte loss.
Monitor values of the following for irregularities: Hct, Hgb, Ca^{++}, glucose, BUN, creatinine, K$^+$, and WBCs. Report significant findings.	Irregularities can occur in patients with infection, inflammatory response, and bleeding caused by necrotic pancreas and would be outside the following normal values: Hct 40%-54% (male) and 37%-47% (female); Hgb 14-18 g/dl (male) and 12-16 g/dl (female); Ca^{++} 8.5-10.5 mg/dl (4.3-5.3 mEq/L); glucose <145 mg/dl (2-hr postprandial) and 65-110 mg/dl (fasting); BUN 6-20 mg/dl; K$^+$ 3.5-5 mEq/L; and WBCs 4500-11,000 mm^3.
Replace electrolytes (i.e., K$^+$, Ca^{++}) as prescribed.	To prevent cardiac dysrhythmias, tetany, and other problems caused by decrements of specific electrolytes.

●●● **Related NIC and NOC labels:** *NIC:* Fluid/Electrolyte Management; Electrolyte Monitoring; Laboratory Data Interpretation; Vital Signs Monitoring; Blood Products Administration *NOC:* Electrolyte and Acid/Base Balance; Fluid Balance

Nursing Diagnosis:

Acute Pain

related to inflammatory process of the pancreas

Desired Outcomes: Within 6 hr of intervention, patient's subjective perception of discomfort decreases, and it is controlled within 24 hr, as documented by a pain scale. Nonverbal indicators, such as splinting of abdominal muscles, are absent or diminished.

INTERVENTIONS

RATIONALES

INTERVENTIONS	RATIONALES
Assess for and document degree and character of patient's discomfort. Devise a pain scale with patient, rating discomfort on a scale of 0 (no pain) to 10 (worst pain).	Pain characteristics may signal different problems (see Assessment section). Baseline and subsequent use of pain scale helps determine effectiveness of pain relief.
Assess patient's previous responses to pain and previously effective pain relief measures. Consider possible cultural and spiritual influences.	Patient's previous history of pain and how well it was managed influence perceptions and trust in present pain relief measures. Some cultures allow less outward show of pain, whereas others do not prohibit expressions of pain.
Ensure that patient maintains limited activity or bedrest.	To minimize pancreatic secretions and pain and to maximize needed rest.
Maintain NPO status. Monitor NG tube function and maintain patency.	To minimize stimulation of pancreatic secretions.
Administer analgesics, histamine H$_2$-receptor blockers (such as cimetidine, ranitidine, famotidine, and nizatidine), antiemetics, and other medications as prescribed; be alert to patient's response to medications, using pain scale. Instruct patient to request analgesic before pain becomes severe.	To reduce discomfort associated with pancreatitis. Pain is more easily managed when it is treated before it becomes severe. Prolonged stimulation of pain receptors results in increased sensitivity to painful stimuli and will increase the amount of drug required to relieve pain.

Continued

INTERVENTIONS	RATIONALES
If analgesic is ineffective, notify health care provider. Optimally, analgesics are administered via patient-controlled pumps. Avoid IM injections in individuals with clotting or bleeding complications.	Patient may require another intervention. Transdermal analgesic or small, frequent doses of IV opiates usually are more effective than IM injections, which also increase the risk of bleeding in individuals with bleeding/clotting complications.
Assist patient in attaining a position of comfort.	To promote comfort by relaxing abdominal muscles. A sitting or supine position with knees flexed often helps.
Emphasize nonpharmacologic pain interventions (e.g., relaxation techniques, distraction, guided imagery, massage). See **Health-Seeking Behaviors:** Relaxation technique effective for stress reduction, p. 183.	These interventions are especially important for patients who develop chronic pancreatitis and are prone to chemical dependence.
Prepare significant other for personality changes and behavioral alterations associated with extreme pain and opioid analgesia. Reassure them that these are normal responses.	Pancreatitis can be very painful. Family members sometimes misinterpret patient's lethargic or unpleasant disposition and may even blame themselves.
Monitor patient's respiratory pattern and level of consciousness (LOC) closely.	Both may be depressed by the large amount of opioids usually required to control pain.
Monitor oxygen saturation and report values ≤92%.	Continuous pulse oximetry identifies decreasing oxygen saturation associated with hypoventilation. Values ≤92% often signal need for supplemental oxygen.
Consider referral to a pain management team.	To manage conventional pain control measures during acute pain situations in patients with chronic or frequent bouts of pancreatitis or with low pain tolerance. Less conventional measures such as nerve blocks that interfere with transmission of pain sensations along visceral nerve fibers are effective in the relief of pancreatic pain. Bilateral splanchnic nerve or left celiac ganglion blocks may be performed as well.
For additional pain interventions, see "Pain," p. 41.	

●●● **Related NIC and NOC labels:** *NIC:* Pain Management; Medication Management; Analgesic Administration; Positioning; Patient-Controlled Analgesia Assistance; Simple Massage; Simple Relaxation Therapy; Distraction; Family Support *NOC:* Comfort Level; Pain Control; Pain: Disruptive Effects

Nursing Diagnosis:

Impaired Gas Exchange

(or risk for same) *related to* ventilation–perfusion mismatching secondary to atelectasis or accumulating pulmonary fluid

Desired Outcome: Patient has adequate gas exchange as evidenced by RR 12-20 breaths/min with normal depth and pattern (eupnea); oxygen saturation >92%; no significant changes in mental status; orientation to person, place, and time; and breath sounds that are clear and audible throughout the lung fields.

INTERVENTIONS	RATIONALES
Monitor and document RR q2-4h as indicated by patient's condition. Report significant deviations from baseline to health care provider.	Irregular pattern, decreased chest excursion, and use of accessory muscles of respiration occur with impending respiratory compromise (can occur with ARDS and respiratory failure) and may be a sign of inadequate pain control or worsening pancreatitis.

Continued

INTERVENTIONS	RATIONALES
Auscultate both lung fields q4-8h.	Presence of abnormal (crackles, rhonchi, wheezes) or diminished breath sounds can occur with fluid overload (see discussion in **Deficient Fluid Volume,** earlier) or atelectasis.
Monitor sputum production and promptly report to health care provider an increase in respiratory secretions.	Indicates respiratory tract infection or pulmonary edema.
Be alert to changes in mental status, restlessness, agitation, and alterations in mentation.	Early signs of hypoxia.
Monitor pulse oximetry q8h or as indicated (report oxygen saturation ≤92%). Monitor arterial blood gas (ABG) results as available (report Pao_2 <80 mm Hg).	These decreased values usually signal need for supplementary oxygen.
In the presence of hypoxemia, administer oxygen as prescribed. Monitor oxygen delivery system at regular intervals.	Hypoxemia is an early sign of impending respiratory failure and necessitates oxygen delivery.
Elevate head of bed (HOB) 30 degrees or higher, depending on patient comfort.	To maintain body position that optimizes ventilation and oxygenation.
If pleural effusion or other defect is present on one side, position patient with unaffected lung dependent.	To maximize ventilation-perfusion relationship, which optimizes oxygenation.
Avoid overaggressive fluid resuscitation.	Can lead to hypoxemia, heart failure, pleural effusions, and respiratory failure. See discussion with **Deficient Fluid Volume,** earlier.
Explain to patient and significant other that patient is at risk for hypostatic pneumonia.	Pancreatitis results in decreased production of surfactant, and pain limits adequate respiratory excursion, increasing potential for hypostatic pneumonia.
Teach use of hyperinflation device (e.g., incentive spirometer) followed by coughing exercise. Explain that emphasis of this therapy is on inhalation to expand the lungs maximally. Ensure that patient inhales slowly and deeply 2× normal tidal volume and holds the breath at least 5 sec at end of inspiration. Monitor patient's progress and document in nurses' notes.	Deep breathing expands alveoli and aids in mobilizing secretions to the airways; coughing further mobilizes and clears secretions. Ten breaths/hr is recommended to maintain adequate alveolar inflation.
When appropriate, teach methods of splinting wounds or upper abdomen.	To reduce pain and enable effective cough.
Instruct patients who cannot cough effectively in cascade cough, that is, a succession of shorter and more forceful exhalations.	Helps keep lung expanded when abdominal pain would not otherwise enable deep cough.
Encourage activity as prescribed.	To help mobilize secretions and promote effective airway clearance.

●●● **Related NIC and NOC labels:** *NIC:* Oxygen Therapy; Chest Physiotherapy; Positioning; Respiratory Monitoring; Cough Enhancement; Pain Management *NOC:* Respiratory Status: Gas Exchange; Tissue Perfusion: Pulmonary

Nursing Diagnosis:

Risk for Infection

related to risk of tissue destruction with resulting necrosis secondary to release of pancreatic enzymes

Desired Outcome: Patient remains free of infection as evidenced by body temperature <37.7° C (<100° F); negative culture results; HR 60-100 bpm; RR 12-20 breaths/min; BP within patient's normal range; and orientation to person, place, and time.

INTERVENTIONS	RATIONALES
Check patient's temperature q4h.	To assess for increase that may signal infection. **Note:** Hypothermia may precede hyperthermia in some individuals, particularly older adults.
Monitor VS along with temperature.	To detect increases in HR and RR associated with temperature elevations.
If there is a sudden elevation in temperature, obtain specimens for culture of blood, sputum, urine, wound, drains, and other sites as indicated. Monitor culture reports and report findings promptly to health care provider.	Cultures enable detection of developing necrotic pancreas or presence of abscess.
Evaluate patient's mental status, orientation, and LOC q4-8h. Document and report significant deviations from baseline.	Impairments may occur with alcohol withdrawal, hypotension, electrolyte imbalance, and hypoxemia.
Administer parenteral antibiotics in a timely fashion. Reschedule antibiotics if a dose is delayed for >1 hr.	To maintain bacteriocidal serum levels. Failure to administer antibiotics on schedule can result in inadequate blood levels and treatment failure.
Observe all secretions and drainage for changes in appearance or odor.	May signal infection. Sputum, for example, can become more copious and change in color from clear to white to yellow to green.
Use good handwashing technique before and after caring for patient and dispose of dressings and drainage carefully.	To prevent transmission of potentially infectious agents.
For more information, see Appendix for "Infection Prevention and Control," p. 831.	

●●● **Related NIC and NOC labels:** *NIC:* Infection Control; Infection Protection; Laboratory Data Interpretation; Medication Administration; Respiratory Monitoring; Vital Signs Monitoring *NOC:* Infection Status

Nursing Diagnosis:

Imbalanced Nutrition: Less than body requirements

related to anorexia, dietary restrictions, and digestive dysfunction

Desired Outcome: Patient maintains baseline body weight and exhibits a positive or balanced nitrogen (N) state on N studies by 24 hr before hospital discharge or within 3 days of this diagnosis if patient is not hospitalized.

INTERVENTIONS	RATIONALES
Monitor capillary blood sugar levels for presence of hyperglycemia and be alert to dysphagia, polydipsia, and polyuria.	These indicators of a hyperglycemic state reflect need for health care provider evaluation and intervention to ensure proper metabolism of carbohydrates if endocrine function is impaired.
Initiate parenteral nutrition and adjust insulin amounts according to capillary blood glucose levels, as prescribed.	Laboratory values of fasting blood sugar and bedside monitoring of blood glucose will reveal abnormalities in blood glucose levels and direct the appropriate insulin therapy (see "Diabetes Mellitus," p. 399, for more information).
Provide oral hygiene at frequent intervals.	To enhance appetite and minimize nausea.

Continued

INTERVENTIONS	RATIONALES
When the gastric tube is removed, provide diet as prescribed.	Small, high-carbohydrate, low-fat meals at frequent intervals (six per day) with protein added according to patient's tolerance is the usual diet for patients with pancreatitis.
Instruct patient to avoid coffee, tea, alcohol, and nicotine.	These are stimulants that increase pancreatic enzyme secretion.
Weigh patient daily to assess gain or loss.	Progressive weight loss may signal need to change diet or provide enzyme replacement therapy.
Note and document amount and degree of steatorrhea (foamy, foul-smelling stools high in fat content).	This is an indicator of fat intolerance, which is common with chronic pancreatitis.
As prescribed, administer pancreatic enzyme supplements before introducing fat into the diet.	To enable digestion of fats.
If prescribed, administer other dietary supplements that support nutrition and caloric intake.	These supplements, which may include products that consist of medium chain triglycerides (MCTs) such as MCT oil, do not require pancreatic enzymes for absorption.
Avoid administering pancreatin with hot foods or drinks.	Heat deactivates enzyme activity.
Provide meals in small feedings throughout the day.	Smaller, more frequent meals may help alleviate bloating, nausea, and cramps experienced by some patients.

●●● **Related NIC and NOC labels:** *NIC:* Nutrition Management; Nutrition Therapy; Teaching: Prescribed Diet; Sustenance Support *NOC:* Nutritional Status; Nutritional Status: Food & Fluid Intake

ADDITIONAL NURSING DIAGNOSES/ PROBLEMS:

"Perioperative Care"	p. 17
"Pain"	p. 41

PATIENT-FAMILY TEACHING AND DISCHARGE PLANNING

When providing patient-family teaching, focus on sensory information, avoid giving excessive information, and initiate a visiting nurse referral for necessary follow-up teaching. Include verbal and written information about the following:

✓ Cause for current episode of pancreatitis, if known, so that recurrence may be avoided.

✓ Alcohol consumption, which can cause or exacerbate chronic pancreatitis.

✓ Diet: frequent, small meals that are high in carbohydrates and protein. Food should be bland until gradual return to normal diet is prescribed. Remind patient to avoid enzyme stimulants, such as coffee, tea, nicotine, and alcohol.

✓ Medications, including drug name, purpose, dosage, schedule, precautions, drug/drug and food/drug interactions, and potential side effects.

✓ Signs and symptoms of diabetes mellitus, including fatigue, weight loss, polydipsia, polyuria, and polyphagia.

✓ Necessity of medical follow-up; confirm time and date of next medical appointment.

✓ Potential for recurrence of steatorrhea as evidenced by foamy, foul-smelling stools that are high in fat content. Steatorrhea can indicate recurrence of disease process or ineffectiveness of drug therapy and should be reported to health care provider.

✓ Weighing daily at home; importance of reporting weight loss to health care provider.

✓ If surgery was performed, the indicators of wound infection: redness, swelling, discharge, fever, pain, or increased local warmth.

✓ Availability of chemical dependency programs to prevent/ treat drug dependence, which is a common occurrence with chronic pancreatitis, or to treat alcoholism. Availability of community support groups, such as the following:

Alcoholics Anonymous
www.alcoholics-anonymous.org/

Narcotics Anonymous
www.na.org

✓ For more information contact the following organization:

National Digestive Diseases Information Clearinghouse, National Institute of Diabetes and Digestive and Kidney Diseases Project Officer
2 Information Way
Bethesda, MD 20892
(302) 468-6344
www.niddk.nih.gov

58

Peptic Ulcers

Peptic ulcers are erosions of the upper gastrointestinal (GI) tract mucosa. They may occur anywhere the mucosa is exposed to the erosive action of gastric acid and pepsin. Commonly, ulcers are gastric or duodenal, but the esophagus, surgically created stomas, and other areas of the upper GI tract may be affected. Autodigestion of mucosal tissue and ulceration are associated with an increase in acidity of the stomach juices or an increased sensitivity of the mucosal surfaces to erosion. Erosions can penetrate deeply into the mucosal layers and become a chronic problem, or they can be more superficial and manifest as an acute problem resulting from severe physiologic or psychologic trauma, infection, or shock (stress ulceration of the stomach or duodenum). Both duodenal and gastric ulcers can occur in association with high-stress lifestyle, smoking, use of irritating drugs, and presence of *Helicobacter pylori,* as well as secondary to other diseases. Ulceration may occur as a part of Zollinger-Ellison syndrome, in which gastrinomas (gastrin-secreting tumors) of the pancreas or other organs develop. Gastric acid hypersecretion and ulceration subsequently occur.

Serious and disabling complications, such as hemorrhage, GI obstruction, perforation, peritonitis, or intractable ulcer pain, are common. With treatment, ulcer healing usually occurs within 4-6 wk (gastric ulcers can take as long as 12-16 wk to heal), but there is potential for recurrence in the same or another site.

HEALTH CARE SETTING

Primary care; acute care for complications

ASSESSMENT

Signs and symptoms: Burning, gnawing, dull pain typically 1-3 hr after eating. Discomfort occurs more frequently between meals and at night. With duodenal ulcer, eating usually alleviates discomfort; with gastric ulcer, pain often worsens after meals. Hematemesis, melena, dizziness, and syncope are associated with an actively bleeding ulcer. Sudden, severe epigastric pain, often radiating to the right shoulder, suggests perforation of an ulcer. Pain described as piercing through to the back suggests penetration of the ulcer into adjacent posterior structures in the abdomen.

Physical assessment: Tenderness over the involved area of the abdomen. With perforation, there will be severe pain (see "Peritonitis" for more information) and rebound tenderness. With penetration the pain is usually altered by changes in back position (extension or flexion).

History of: Nonsteroidal antiinflammatory drug (NSAID) use; chronic or acute stress; smoking; use of irritating agents such as caffeine, alcohol, corticosteroids, salicylates, reserpine, indomethacin, or phenylbutazone; disorders of the endocrine glands, pancreas, or liver; and hypersecretory conditions, such as Zollinger-Ellison syndrome.

DIAGNOSTIC TESTS

Barium swallow: Uses contrast agent (e.g., barium) to detect abnormalities. Patient should maintain NPO status and not smoke for at least 8 hr before the test. Postprocedure care involves administration of prescribed laxatives and enemas to facilitate passage of the barium and prevent constipation and fecal impaction.

Endoscopy: Allows visualization of the stomach (gastroscopy), duodenum (duodenoscopy), both stomach and duodenum (gastroduodenoscopy), or the esophagus, stomach, and duodenum (esophagogastroduodenoscopy) via passage of a lighted, flexible tube. A biopsy may be performed as part of the endoscopy procedure. Biopsied tissue may be sent for histologic examination and for culture and sensitivity to identify *Helicobacter pylori* infection.

Gastric secretion analysis: Is helpful in differentiating gastric ulcer from gastric cancer. A nasogastric (NG) tube is passed, and the stomach contents are aspirated and analyzed for the presence of blood and free hydrochloric acid. Achlorhydria (absence of free hydrochloric acid) suggests gastric cancer, whereas mildly elevated levels suggest gastric ulcer. Excessive elevation of free hydrochloric acid occurs with Zollinger-Ellison syndrome. A tubeless gastric analysis involves administration of a gastric stimulant followed by a resin dye. A urine specimen is obtained 2 hr later and analyzed for the presence of dye. Absence of dye indicates achlorhydria.

Complete blood count (CBC): Reveals a decrease in Hgb, Hct, and red blood cells (RBCs) when acute or chronic blood loss accompanies ulceration.

Helicobacter pylori ***testing:*** Serum antigen testing identifies exposure to *H. pylori* bacteria; this is the least expensive means of identifying *H. pylori* infection. A breath test is available to identify *H. pylori* infection by detecting carbon dioxide and ammonia as by-products of the action of the bacterium's urease in the patient's expired air.

Stool for occult blood: Is positive if bleeding is present.

Nursing Diagnosis:

Ineffective Protection

related to potential for bleeding, obstruction, and perforation secondary to ulcerative process

Desired Outcome: Patient is free of signs and symptoms of bleeding, obstruction, perforation, and peritonitis as evidenced by negative results for occult blood testing, passage of stool and flatus, soft and nondistended abdomen, good appetite, and normothermia.

INTERVENTIONS	RATIONALES
Assess for hematemesis and melena. Check all NG aspirate, emesis, and stools for occult blood. Report positive findings.	Indicators of bleeding that can occur with an ulcerative process.
Monitor results of CBC studies. Report significant findings.	Hct <40% (male) or <37% (female) and Hgb <14 g/dl (male) or <12 g/dl (female) are indicators of bleeding and should be reported promptly.
Also check coagulation study results if indicated.	The incidence of peptic ulcers is increased in cirrhosis patients, in whom clotting factors are altered. Be alert to partial thromboplastin time (PTT) >70 sec or prothrombin time (PT) >12.5 sec, which are longer than normal clotting times.
If indicated, insert gastric tube.	To evacuate blood from stomach, monitor for bleeding, and perform gastric lavage as prescribed.
Do not use gastric tubes in patients who have or are suspected of having esophageal varices.	Trauma from tube insertion could result in hemorrhage.
Monitor O$_2$ saturation via oximetry.	To evaluate systemic oxygenation status. Usually patients with O$_2$ saturation ≤92% require oxygen supplementation.
If patient is actively bleeding or if Hct or Hgb is low, administer O$_2$.	A low Hct or Hgb indicates an anemic state, which means there is less available Hgb for oxygen transport.
Monitor and note abdominal pain, abnormal (increased peristalsis, "rushes," or "tinkles") or absent bowel sounds, distention, anorexia, nausea, vomiting, and inability to pass stool or flatus.	Indicators of obstruction, a serious complication of peptic ulcers.
Be alert to sudden or severe abdominal pain, distention and abdominal rigidity, fever, nausea, and vomiting. Notify health care provider immediately of significant findings. For more information, see "Peritonitis," p. 501.	Indicators of perforation and peritonitis, serious complications of peptic ulcers.
Teach the previously mentioned signs and symptoms of GI complications and importance of reporting them promptly to staff or health care provider if they occur.	A knowledgeable patient likely will report these signs promptly, which will enable rapid treatment.

●●● **Related NIC and NOC labels:** *NIC:* Bleeding Precautions *NOC:* Coagulation Status

Nursing Diagnosis:

Impaired Tissue Integrity

related to exposure to chemical irritants (gastric acid, pepsin)

Desired Outcomes: Immediately following teaching, patient verbalizes knowledge of necessary
lifestyle alterations and demonstrates compliance with medical recommendations for peptic ulcer.
Gastric and duodenal mucosal tissues heal and remain intact as evidenced by reduced or absent
pain and absence of bleeding.

INTERVENTIONS	RATIONALES
Encourage patient to avoid foods that seem to cause pain or increase acid secretion.	Although this response is highly individualized, foods that cause pain or increase acid secretion worsen mucosal erosion.
Advise patient to avoid the following foods and drugs: coffee, caffeine, alcohol, aspirin, and ibuprofen and other NSAIDs.	These are associated with increased acidity and GI erosions.
If applicable, recommend strategies for smoking cessation.	Smoking impairs ulcer healing and has been associated with a higher incidence of complications and the need for surgical repair of the ulcer.
Administer *H. pylori* eradication therapy (e.g., amoxicillin, tetracycline, metronidazole, bismuth subsalicylate) as prescribed.	Indicated for patients in whom *H. pylori* is cultured. Highest eradication rates are obtained with one of the following regimens: (1) proton pump inhibitor (PPI), clarithromycin 500 mg bid, and either amoxicillin or metronidazole for 2 wk; (2) ranitidine bismuth citrate, clarithromycin 500 mg bid, and amoxicillin, metronidazole, or tetracycline for 2 wk; or (3) PPI, bismuth, metronidazole, and tetracycline for 1-2 wk.
Administer acid suppression therapies as prescribed:	For acute episodes of ulceration.
Histamine H_2-receptor blockers (e.g., cimetidine [Tagamet], ranitidine [Zantac], nizatidine [Axid], famotidine [Pepcid])	Administered PO or IV to suppress secretion of gastric acid and facilitate ulcer healing. They also can be used prophylactically for limited periods of time, especially in patients susceptible to stress ulceration. They are administered with meals at least 1 hr apart from antacids because antacids can reduce their absorption.
Sucralfate (Carafate)	An antiulcer agent that coats the ulcer with a protective barrier so that healing can occur. This drug must be taken before meals and at bedtime. It should not be taken within 30 min of antacids because acid facilitates adherence of sucralfate to the ulcer.
Antacids	Administered orally or through an NG tube to provide symptomatic relief, facilitate ulcer healing, and prevent further ulceration; can be administered prophylactically in patients who are especially susceptible to ulceration. They are administered after meals and at bedtime or give periodically via NG tube for patients who are intubated.
Omeprazole (Prilosec)	Deactivates the enzyme system that pumps hydrogen ions (H^+) from the parietal cells, thus inhibiting gastric acid secretion; used for short-term treatment of active duodenal and gastric ulcers and for long-term treatment of hypersecretory conditions.
Misoprostol (Cytotec)	Synthetic prostaglandin E_1 analog that enhances the body's normal mucosal protective mechanisms and decreases acid secretion. The drug is used in the healing and prevention of NSAID-induced ulcers.

Continued

INTERVENTIONS	RATIONALES
	This drug is used with caution in women of childbearing years who could be pregnant because it can cause abortion.
Stress importance of taking medications at prescribed intervals, not just for symptomatic relief of pain.	Initial pain relief does not mean the ulcer is completed healed.

●●● **Related NIC and NOC labels:** *NIC:* Bleeding Reduction: Gastrointestinal; Nutrition Management; Medication Management *NOC:* Tissue Integrity: Skin and Mucous Membranes

ADDITIONAL NURSING DIAGNOSES/ PROBLEMS:

PATIENT-FAMILY TEACHING AND DISCHARGE PLANNING

When providing patient-family teaching, focus on sensory information, avoid giving excessive information, and initiate a visiting nurse referral for necessary follow-up teaching of skilled needs. Include verbal and written information about the following:

✓ Importance of following prescribed diet to facilitate ulcer healing, prevent exacerbation or recurrence, or control postsurgical dumping syndrome. If appropriate, arrange consultation with dietitian.

✓ Medications, including drug name, rationale, dosage, schedule, precautions, drug/drug and food/drug interactions, and potential side effects.

✓ Signs and symptoms of exacerbation and recurrence, as well as potential complications.

✓ Care of incision line and dressing change technique, as necessary.

✓ Signs of wound infection, including persistent redness, swelling, purulent drainage, local warmth, fever, and foul odor.

✓ Role of lifestyle alterations in preventing exacerbation or recurrence of ulcer, including smoking cessation, stress reduction (see **Health-Seeking Behaviors:** Relaxation technique effective for stress reduction, p. 183), decreasing or eliminating consumption of alcohol, and avoidance of irritating foods and drugs. In addition, histamine H_2-receptor blockers are more effective in individuals who are nonsmokers.

✓ Referral to health care specialist for assistance with stress reduction as necessary.

✓ Referrals to community support groups, such as Alcoholics Anonymous.

Peritonitis

Peritonitis is the inflammatory response of the peritoneum to offending chemical and bacterial agents invading the peritoneal cavity. The inflammatory process can be local or generalized and acute or chronic, depending on the pathogenesis of the inflammation. Common causes include abdominal trauma; postoperative leakage of gastrointestinal (GI) content or blood into the peritoneal cavity; intestinal ischemia; ruptured or inflamed abdominal organs; poor sterile techniques (e.g., with peritoneal dialysis); and direct contamination of the bloodstream. As the disease progresses, paralytic ileus occurs, and intestinal fluid, which then cannot be reabsorbed, leaks into the peritoneal cavity. As a result of the fluid shift, cardiac output and tissue perfusion are reduced, leading to impaired cardiac and renal function. If infection or inflammation continues, respiratory failure and shock can ensue. Peritonitis frequently is progressive and can be fatal. It is the most common cause of death following abdominal surgery.

HEALTH CARE SETTING

Acute care surgical unit, critical care unit

ASSESSMENT

Signs and symptoms:
- **Early findings:** acute abdominal pain with movement, anorexia, nausea, vomiting, chills, fever, rigor, malaise, weakness, hiccoughs, diaphoresis, and abdominal distention and rigidity (often described as *boardlike*).
- **Later findings** may include those of dehydration (e.g., thirst, dry mucous membranes, oliguria, concentrated urine, poor skin turgor).

Physical assessment: Presence of tachycardia, hypotension, and shallow and rapid respirations caused by abdominal distention and discomfort. Often the patient assumes a supine position with the knees flexed or side-lying with the knees drawn up toward the chest. Palpation usually reveals peritoneal irritation as shown by distention, abdominal rigidity with general or localized tenderness, guarding, and rebound or cough tenderness. However, as many as one fourth of these patients will have minimal or no indications of peritoneal irritation. Auscultation findings include hyperactive bowel sounds during the gradual development of peritonitis and an absence of bowel sounds or infrequent high-pitched sounds ("tinkling" or "squeaky") during later stages if paralytic ileus occurs. Mild ascites may be present as demonstrated by shifting areas of dullness on percussion.

History of: Abdominal surgery, peptic ulcer disease, cholecystitis, acute necrotizing pancreatitis, GI disorders, acute salpingitis, ruptured appendix or diverticulum, trauma, peritoneal dialysis.

DIAGNOSTIC TESTS

Serum tests: May reveal the presence of leukocytosis (usually with a shift to the left), hemoconcentration, elevated blood urea nitrogen (BUN), and electrolyte imbalance, particularly hypokalemia. Hypoalbuminemia and prolonged prothrombin time, in combination with leukocytosis, are especially characteristic.

Arterial blood gas (ABG) values: May reveal hypoxemia (PaO_2 <80 mm Hg) or acidosis (pH <7.40).

Urinalysis: Often performed to rule out genitourinary involvement (e.g., pyelonephritis).

Paracentesis for peritoneal aspiration with culture and sensitivity: May be performed to determine the presence of blood, bacteria, bile, pus, and amylase content and identify the causative organism. Gram stain of ascitic fluid is positive in only about 25% of these patients.

Abdominal x-ray examination: May be performed to determine the presence of distended loops of bowel and abnormal levels of fluid and gas, which usually collect in the large and small bowel in the presence of a perforation or obstruction. "Free air" under the diaphragm also may be visualized, which indicates a perforated viscus.

Chest x-ray examination: Abdominal distention may elevate the diaphragm. Pain from peritonitis may limit respiratory excursion and lead to associated infiltrates in the lower lobes. In later stages, changes in serum osmolality allow for pleural effusions to occur.

Contrast x-ray examination: May be used to identify specific intestinal pathologic conditions. Water-soluble contrast (e.g., meglumine diatrizoate [Gastrografin]) may be used to evaluate suspected upper GI perforation.

Computed tomography (CT) scan and ultrasound: May be used to evaluate abdominal pain and more clearly delineate nondistinct areas found by plain abdominal x-rays. Magnetic resonance imaging (MRI) has not been an effective adjunct in abdominal surveys because of motion artifacts.

Radionuclide scans: Such as gallium, hepatoiminodiacetic acid (HIDA; lidofenin), and liver-spleen scans, may be used to identify intraabdominal abscess.

Nursing Diagnoses:

Acute Pain/Nausea

related to inflammatory process, fever, and tissue damage

Desired Outcomes: Patient's subjective perception of discomfort decreases within 1 hr of intervention, as documented by a pain scale. Nonverbal indicators, such as grimacing and abdominal guarding, are absent or diminished.

INTERVENTIONS	RATIONALES
Assess and document character and severity of discomfort q1-2h. Devise a pain scale with patient, rating discomfort on a scale of 0 (no pain) to 10 (worst pain).	This assessment will not only define the type of discomfort, but it will monitor relief of discomfort obtained to determine effectiveness of the treatment.
After diagnosis has been made, administer opioids, other analgesics, and sedatives as prescribed. Encourage patient to request analgesic *before* pain becomes severe. Document relief obtained, using the pain scale.	To relieve severe pain and discomfort once the diagnosis has been confirmed. Because potent analgesics can mask diagnostic symptoms, opioids should not be administered until surgical evaluation has been completed. Pain management is more effective when analgesia is given before pain becomes too severe. Prolonged stimulation of pain receptors results in increased sensitivity to painful stimuli and will increase the amount of drug required to relieve pain.
Keep patient on bedrest. Provide a restful and quiet environment.	To minimize pain, which can be aggravated by activity and stress.
Instruct patient in methods to splint abdomen.	To reduce pain on movement, coughing, and deep breathing.
Keep patient in a position of comfort, usually semi-Fowler's or high Fowler's position with knees bent.	To promote fluid shift to the lower abdomen, which will reduce pressure on the diaphragm and enable deeper and easier respirations. Raising the knees will lower stress on the abdominal wall.
Explain all procedures.	To help minimize anxiety, which can exacerbate discomfort.
Offer mouth care and lip moisturizers at frequent intervals.	To help relieve discomfort from continuous or intermittent suction, dehydration, and NPO status.
Administer antiemetics (e.g., hydroxyzine, ondansetron, prochlorperazine, promethazine) as prescribed; instruct patient to request medication *before* nausea becomes severe.	To combat nausea and vomiting in a timely fashion before they become more difficult to control.

●●● **Related NIC and NOC labels:** *NIC:* Medication Management; Anxiety Reduction; Environmental Management: Comfort; Medication Administration; Positioning; Splinting; Nausea Management
NOC: Comfort Level

Nursing Diagnosis:

Impaired Gas Exchange

related to alveolar hypoventilation and decreased depth of respirations secondary to guarding with abdominal pain or distention

Desired Outcomes: Patient has an effective breathing pattern as evidenced by PaO_2 ≥80 mm Hg, oxygen saturation >92%, BP ≥90/60 mm Hg (or within patient's baseline range), HR ≤100 bpm, and orientation to person, place, and time. Eupnea occurs within 1 hr after pain-relieving intervention.

INTERVENTIONS	RATIONALES
Monitor VS, mental status, and ABG and oximetry results.	The following are indicators of hypoxemia and usually signal the need for supplemental oxygen: PaO_2 <80 mm Hg, low oxygen saturation (≤92%), hypotension, tachycardia, tachypnea, restlessness, confusion or altered mental status, central nervous system (CNS) depression, and possibly cyanosis.
Auscultate lung fields. Note and document presence of decreased or adventitious breath sounds.	To assess ventilation and detect pulmonary complications, such as pleural effusion. Pleural effusion, an accumulation of fluid in the pleural space, can develop in later stages of peritonitis because of changes in serum osmolality. Decreased breath sounds and pleural friction rub are diagnostic of pleural effusion.
Keep patient in semi-Fowler's or high Fowler's position. Instruct patient in splinting abdomen to facilitate respiratory hygiene.	To aid respiratory effort and promote deep breathing to enhance oxygenation and coughing to clear pulmonary secretions.
Administer oxygen as prescribed.	To support increased metabolic needs and treat hypoxia.

●●● **Related NIC and NOC labels:** *NIC:* Laboratory Data Interpretation; Oxygen Therapy; Chest Physiotherapy; Positioning; Respiratory Monitoring; Cough Enhancement *NOC:* Respiratory Status: Gas Exchange

Nursing Diagnoses:

Risk for Injury/Risk for Infection

related to potential for worsening/recurring peritonitis or development of septic shock secondary to inflammatory process

Desired Outcome: Patient is free of symptoms of worsening/recurring peritonitis or septic shock as evidenced by normothermia, BP ≥90/60 mm Hg (or within patient's normal range), HR ≤100 bpm, absence of chills, presence of eupnea, urinary output ≥30 ml/hr, central venous pressure (CVP) 2-6 mm Hg (5-12 cm H_2O), decreasing abdominal girth measurements, and minimal tenderness to palpation.

INTERVENTIONS	RATIONALES
Assess abdomen q1-2h during acute phase and q4h once patient is stabilized. Measure abdominal girth.	To monitor for increasing distention, which would signal development of ascites.
Use a permanent marker to identify placement of tape measure.	To ensure consistent measurement area by caregivers.

Continued

INTERVENTIONS	RATIONALES
Auscultate bowel sounds.	To assess motility. Bowel sounds often are frequent during the beginning phase of peritonitis but are absent in the presence of paralytic ileus.
Lightly palpate abdomen for evidence of increasing rigidity or tenderness. Notify health care provider of significant findings.	Increasing rigidity or tenderness indicates disease progression. If patient experiences increased pain on removal of your hand, rebound tenderness is present.
Administer antibiotics as prescribed; ensure close adherence to schedules.	Combination broad-spectrum antibiotic therapy is rapidly begun to ensure treatment of gram-negative bacilli and anaerobic bacteria. Common agents include cephalosporins (cefotaxime, cefepime), aminoglycosides (gentamicin), ampicillin, floxacin (Floxin), and metronidazole. Antibiotics are commonly administered IV and may also be directly instilled into the peritoneal cavity via surgically placed catheters.
Draw peak and trough antibiotic serum levels as prescribed.	Peak and trough levels are drawn at specific times around the antibiotic dose. Peak levels indicate if there is enough drug in the bloodstream and the dose is high enough. The trough level indicates if the kidneys/liver are clearing the drug adequately.
Monitor complete blood count (CBC) for presence of leukocytosis (increased white blood cells [WBCs]) and hemoconcentration (increased Hct and Hgb). Notify health care provider of significant findings.	Normal values are as follows: WBC count 4500-11,000/mm^3; Hgb 14-18 g/dl (male) or 12-16 g/dl (female); and Hct 40%-54% (male) or 37%-47% (female). Leukocytosis signals infection. With peritonitis, WBC count usually is >20,000/mm^3. Hemoconcentration occurs with a decrease in plasma volume, which may be present as a result of fluid shift into the peritoneum.
Maintain sterile technique with dressing changes and all invasive procedures.	To reduce spread of infection.
Teach signs and symptoms of recurring peritonitis and importance of reporting them promptly if they occur: fever, chills, abdominal pain, vomiting, and abdominal distention.	An informed individual likely will report these signs promptly for rapid treatment.

●●● **Related NIC and NOC labels:** *NIC:* Risk Identification; Infection Control; Infection Protection; Vital Signs Monitoring; Medication Administration; Tube Care: Gastrointestinal *NOC:* Infection Status

Nursing Diagnosis:

Imbalanced Nutrition: Less than body requirements

related to vomiting and intestinal suctioning

Desired Outcome: By at least 24 hr before hospital discharge, patient demonstrates optimal progress toward adequate nutritional status as evidenced by stable weight, balanced or positive nitrogen (N) state, serum protein 6-8 g/dl, and serum albumin 3.5-5.5 g/dl.

INTERVENTIONS	RATIONALES
Keep patient NPO as prescribed during acute phase of the disorder.	Oral fluids are not resumed until patient has passed flatus and the gastric/intestinal tube has been removed.
Reintroduce oral fluids gradually once motility has returned, as evidenced by presence of bowel sounds, decreased distention, and passage of flatus.	To ensure that patient will tolerate fluids through the intestines, which may have become irritated from the inflammatory process.

Continued

INTERVENTIONS	RATIONALES
Maintain gastric/intestinal tube as prescribed; closely monitor amount and consistency of drainage.	An increased volume of output would signal presence of an ileus and continued need for the tube.
Support patient with peripheral parenteral nutrition (PPN) or total parenteral nutrition (TPN), as prescribed, depending on duration of the acute phase of peritonitis.	If the GI tract is nonfunctioning, TPN usually is initiated in the early stages to promote nutrition and protein replacement.
Administer replacement fluids, electrolytes, and vitamins as prescribed.	To maintain hydration and restore electrolytes and nutrients lost in gastric/intestinal tube output and fluid shifts.
Instruct patient in rationale for tube placement and NPO status, underlying pathologic condition (as appropriate), need for close monitoring of fluid intake and output, and, eventually, diet advancement.	A knowledgeable patient likely will adhere to the treatment regimen and report symptoms that would necessitate timely intervention.

●●● **Related NIC and NOC labels:** *NIC:* Nutrition Therapy; Nutritional Monitoring; Teaching: Prescribed Diet; Enteral Tube Feeding; Fluid/Electrolyte Management; Gastrointestinal Intubation; Total Parenteral Nutrition Administration; Intravenous Therapy; Laboratory Data Interpretation *NOC:* Nutritional Status; Nutritional Status: Food and Fluid Intake; Nutritional Status: Nutrient Intake

ADDITIONAL NURSING DIAGNOSES/ PROBLEMS:

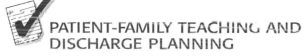

PATIENT-FAMILY TEACHING AND DISCHARGE PLANNING

When providing patient-family teaching, focus on sensory information, avoid giving excessive information, and initiate a visiting nurse referral for necessary monitoring of wound care and follow-up teaching. Include verbal and written information about the following:

✓ Medications, including drug name, dosage, schedule, purpose, precautions, drug/drug and food/drug interactions, and potential side effects.

✓ Activity alterations as prescribed by health care provider, such as avoiding heavy lifting (>10 lb), resting after periods of fatigue, getting maximum amounts of rest, and gradually increasing activities to tolerance.

✓ Notifying health care provider of the following indicators of recurrence: fever, chills, abdominal pain, vomiting, and abdominal distention.

✓ If patient has undergone surgery, indicators of wound infection: fever, pain, chills, incisional swelling, persistent erythema, and purulent drainage.

✓ Importance of follow-up medical care; confirm date and time of next medical appointment.

Ulcerative Colitis

Ulcerative colitis is a nonspecific, chronic inflammatory disease of the mucosa and submucosa of the colon. Generally the disease begins in the rectum and sigmoid colon, but it can extend proximally and uninterrupted as far as the cecum. In some instances, a few centimeters of distal ileum are affected. This is sometimes referred to as *backwash ileitis,* and it occurs in only about 10% of patients with ulcerative colitis involving the entire colon.

The cause of ulcerative colitis is unknown, but theories posit an interaction of external agents, host responses, and genetic immunologic factors creating the pathogenic responses. Factors that have been associated with ulcerative colitis include infection, allergy, immunologic abnormalities, psychosomatic factors, and heredity. The most firmly established risk factor for developing inflammatory bowel disease is a positive family history.

HEALTH CARE SETTING

Primary care; acute care for complications

ASSESSMENT

Signs and symptoms: Bloody diarrhea (the cardinal symptom). The clinical picture can vary from acute episodes with frequent discharge of watery stools mixed with blood, pus, and mucus, accompanied by fever, abdominal pain, rectal urgency, and tenesmus, to loose or frequent stools, to formed stools coated with a little blood. However, nearly two thirds of patients have cramping abdominal pain and varying degrees of fever, vomiting, anorexia, weight loss, and dehydration. Remissions and exacerbations are common. Extracolonic manifestations also can occur, including polyarthritis, skin lesions (erythema nodosum, pyoderma gangrenosum), liver impairment, and ophthalmic complications (iritis, uveitis). Extracolonic manifestations may precede overt bowel disease, and their clinical activity may be related or unrelated to the clinical activity of the bowel disease.

Physical assessment: With severe disease, the abdomen will be tender, especially in the left lower quadrant (LLQ); distention and a tender, spastic anus also may be present. With rectal examination, the mucosa may feel gritty, and the examining gloved finger may be covered with blood, mucus, or pus.

Risk factors: Duration of active disease >10 yr, pancolitis, and family history of colonic cancer.

DIAGNOSTIC TESTS

Stool examination: Reveals the presence of frank or occult blood. Stool cultures and smears rule out bacterial and parasitic disorders. **Note:** Collect specimens *before* barium enema is performed.

Sigmoidoscopy: Reveals red, granular, hyperemic, and extremely friable mucosa; strips of inflamed mucosa undermined by surrounding ulcerations, which form pseudopolyps; and thick exudate composed of blood, pus, and mucus. **Note:** Enemas should not be given before the examination because they can produce hyperemia and edema and may cause exacerbation of the disease.

Colonoscopy: Will help determine extent of the disease and differentiate ulcerative colitis from Crohn's disease through both endoscopic appearance and histologic examination of biopsy tissues. Serial colonoscopy is also done to monitor patients with chronic ulcerative colitis at risk for colon carcinoma. **Note:** This test may be contraindicated in patients with acute disease because of the risk of perforation or hemorrhage.

Rectal biopsy: Aids in differentiating ulcerative colitis from carcinoma and other inflammatory processes.

Barium enema: Reveals mucosal irregularity from fine serrations to ragged ulcerations, narrowing and shortening of the colon, presence of pseudopolyps, loss of haustral markings, and the presence of spasms and irritability. Double-contrast technique may facilitate detection of superficial mucosal lesions. With a double-contrast technique, barium is instilled into the colon as with a conventional barium enema, but most of the barium is then withdrawn and the colon is inflated with air, which causes a thin coating of barium to line the intestinal wall. The double-contrast technique has become the "gold standard" for evaluating patients for colitis. **Note:** Irritant cathartics and enemas should not be given before the examination because they produce hyperemia and edema and may cause exacerbation of the disease.

Abdominal plain films (flat plate): An important tool for screening severely ill patients when colonoscopy and barium enema are contraindicated. An abdominal flat plate may reveal fecal residue, the appearance of mucosal margins, widening or thickening of visible haustra, and the diameter of the colonic wall. In patients with suspected ileus, obstruction, or perforation, the flat plate film reveals abnormal gas and fluid levels or the presence of free air in the peritoneal cavity.

Computed tomography (CT): Used to identify suspected complications of ulcerative colitis (i.e., toxic megacolon, pneumatosis coli).

Serum antibody testing: Several serum antibodies are being evaluated for aiding in the development of noninvasive diagnostic techniques for ulcerative colitis.

Radionuclide imaging: To identify the extent of disease activity, especially when colonoscopy and barium enema are contraindicated. Injections of indium-111–labeled autologous leukocytes are used to identify areas of active inflammation.

Blood tests: Anemia, with hypochromic microcytic red blood indices in severe disease, usually is present because of blood loss, iron deficiency, and bone marrow depression. White blood cell (WBC) count may be normal to markedly elevated in severe disease. Sedimentation rate is usually increased according to the severity of illness. Hypoalbuminemia and negative nitrogen (N) state occur in moderately severe to severe disease and result from decreased protein intake, decreased albumin synthesis in the debilitated condition, and increased metabolic needs. Electrolyte imbalance is common; hypokalemia is often present because of colonic losses (diarrhea) and renal losses in patients taking high doses of corticosteroids. Bicarbonate may be decreased because of colonic losses and may signal metabolic acidosis.

Nursing Diagnosis:

Deficient Fluid Volume

related to active loss secondary to diarrhea and gastrointestinal bleeding/hemorrhage

Desired Outcome: Patient is normovolemic within 24 hr of intervention/treatment as evidenced by balanced I&O, urine output ≥30 ml/hr, urine specific gravity <1.030, good skin turgor, moist mucous membranes, stable weight, BP ≥90/60 mm Hg (or within patient's normal range), and RR 12-20 breaths/min.

INTERVENTIONS	RATIONALES
Monitor I&O and urine specific gravity, weigh patient daily, and monitor laboratory values.	To evaluate fluid, electrolyte, and hematologic status. Optimal values are serum K^+ ≥3.5 mEq/L; Hct 40%-54% (male) and 37%-47% (female); Hgb 14-18 g/dl (male) and 12-16 g/dl (female); and red blood cells (RBCs) 4.5-6 million/mm^3 (male) and 4-5.5 million/mm^3 (female). Hypokalemia is common because of the prolonged diarrhea. Prolonged anemia may result in decreased Hct, Hgb, and RBCs.
Monitor frequency and consistency of stool. For frequent bowel movements, keep a stool count; measure liquid stools. Assess and record presence of blood, mucus, fat, and undigested food.	Although bloody diarrhea is most commonly seen, the patient may experience acute episodes with frequent discharge of watery stools mixed with blood, pus, and mucus, accompanied by fever, abdominal pain, rectal urgency, and tenesmus; loose or frequent stools; or formed stools coated with a little blood.
Monitor for thirst, poor skin turgor (may not be a reliable indicator of hydration in the older adult), dryness of mucous membranes, fever, and concentrated (specific gravity >1.030) and decreased urinary output.	Indicators of dehydration.
Monitor for decreased BP, increased HR and RR, pallor, diaphoresis, and restlessness. Assess stool for quality (e.g., Is it grossly bloody and liquid?) and quantity (e.g., Is it mostly blood or mostly stool?). Report significant findings to health care provider.	Signs of hemorrhage.

Continued

INTERVENTIONS	RATIONALES
Administer parenteral fluids, electrolytes, and vitamins as prescribed.	To maintain acutely ill patient, as indicated by laboratory test results.
Administer blood products and iron as prescribed.	To correct existing anemia and losses caused by hemorrhage.
Provide bland, high-protein, high-calorie, low-residue diet, as prescribed when patient is taking food by mouth. Assess tolerance to diet by determining incidence of cramping, diarrhea, and flatulence.	In severely ill patients, total parenteral nutrition (TPN) along with NPO status is prescribed to replace nutritional deficits while allowing complete bowel rest and improving patient's nutritional status before surgery. For less severely ill patients, a low-residue elemental diet provides good nutrition with low fecal volume to allow bowel rest. A bland, high-protein, high-calorie, low-residue diet with vitamin and mineral supplements and excluding raw fruits and vegetables provides good nutrition and decreases diarrhea. Milk and wheat products are restricted to reduce cramping and diarrhea in patients with lactose and gluten intolerance.

●●● **Related NIC and NOC labels:** *NIC:* Fluid Management; Electrolyte Monitoring; Fluid Management; Laboratory Data Interpretation; Vital Signs Monitoring; Diarrhea Management; Blood Products Administration; Total Parenteral Nutrition; Hemorrhage Control *NOC:* Fluid Balance

Nursing Diagnoses:

Risk for Injury/Risk for Infection

related to potential for perforation secondary to deeply inflamed colonic mucosa

Desired Outcome: Patient is free of signs of perforation as evidenced by normothermia; HR 60–100 bpm; RR 12–20 breaths/min with normal depth and pattern (eupnea); normal bowel sounds; absence of abdominal distention, tympany, or rebound tenderness; negative culture results; no mental status changes; and orientation to person, place, and time. **Note:** Patients with severe ulcerative colitis can have markedly elevated WBC counts: >20,000/mm^3 and occasionally as high as 50,000/mm^3.

INTERVENTIONS	RATIONALES
Monitor for fever, chills, increased respiratory and heart rates, diaphoresis, and increased abdominal discomfort.	Can occur with perforation of the colon and potentially result in localized abscess or generalized fecal peritonitis and septicemia. **Note:** Systemic therapy with corticosteroids and antibiotics can mask the development of this complication.
Evaluate mental status, orientation, and level of consciousness (LOC) q2-4h.	Mental cloudiness, lethargy, and increased restlessness can signal impending or actual septic shock.
Report any evidence of sudden abdominal distention associated with preceding symptoms.	These symptoms can signal toxic megacolon. Factors contributing to development of this complication include hypokalemia, barium enema examinations, and use of opiates and anticholinergics.
If patient has a sudden temperature elevation, culture blood and other sites as prescribed. Monitor culture reports, notifying health care provider promptly of any positive cultures.	A temperature spike can signal septicemia; a culture will identify causative organism if present.
Administer antibiotics as prescribed and in a timely fashion.	To ensure optimal blood levels of effective therapeutic dose in order to kill the bacteria and control the infection.

●●● **Related NIC and NOC labels:** *NIC:* Infection Protection; Laboratory Data Interpretation; Medication Administration; Specimen Management; Vital Signs Monitoring *NOC:* Infection Status; Safety Status: Physical Injury

Nursing Diagnoses:

Acute Pain/Nausea

related to intestinal inflammatory process

Desired Outcomes: Within 4 hr of intervention, patient's subjective perception of discomfort decreases as documented by a pain scale. Objective indicators, such as grimacing, are absent or diminished.

INTERVENTIONS	RATIONALES
Monitor and document characteristics of discomfort and assess whether it is associated with ingestion of certain foods or medications or with emotional stress. Devise a pain scale with patient, rating discomfort from 0 (no pain) to 10 (worst pain). Eliminate foods that cause cramping and discomfort. Document degree of relief obtained, rating it according to the pain scale.	To determine discomfort trigger and degree to which discomfort is alleviated following intervention.
As prescribed, maintain patient on NPO or TPN.	To provide bowel rest, which should help alleviate symptoms.
Provide nasal and oral care at frequent intervals.	To lessen discomfort from NPO status, nausea, or presence of nasogastric (NG) tube.
Keep patient's environment quiet. Facilitate coordination of health care providers to provide rest periods between care activities. Allow 90 min for undisturbed rest.	To promote rest and healing.
Administer sedatives and tranquilizers as prescribed.	To promote rest and reduce anxiety, which optimally will lessen symptoms.
Administer hydrophilic colloids, anticholinergics, and antidiarrheal medications as prescribed.	To relieve cramping and diarrhea.
Instruct patient to request medication before discomfort becomes severe.	Cramping and diarrhea are more easily controlled if they are treated before they become severe.
Note: Administer opiates and anticholinergics with extreme caution.	These drugs contribute to the development of toxic megacolon.
Observe for intensification of symptoms. Notify health care provider of significant findings.	Can indicate presence of complications that should be treated promptly.

●●● **Related NIC and NOC labels:** *NIC:* Medication Management; Bowel Management; Sleep Enhancement; Nausea Management *NOC:* Comfort Level

Nursing Diagnosis:

Diarrhea

related to inflammatory process of the intestines

Desired Outcome: Patient's stools become normal in consistency, and frequency is lessened within 3 days of intervention/treatment.

INTERVENTIONS	RATIONALES
Monitor and record amount, frequency, and character of stools. When possible, measure liquid stools.	Although bloody diarrhea is the cardinal symptom, the clinical picture can vary from acute episodes with frequent discharge of watery stools mixed with blood, pus, and mucus, accompanied by fever, abdominal pain, rectal urgency, and tenesmus, to loose or frequent stools, to formed stools coated with a little blood.
Provide covered bedpan, commode, or bathroom that is easily accessible and ready to use at all times.	To decrease patient's anxiety about incontinence.
Empty bedpan and commode.	To control odor and decrease patient's anxiety and self-consciousness.
Administer hydrophilic colloids, anticholinergics, and antidiarrheal medications as prescribed.	To decrease fluidity and number of stools.
Administer topical corticosteroid preparations and antibiotics via retention enema, as prescribed.	To relieve mucosal inflammation.
If patient has difficulty retaining the enema for the prescribed amount of time, consult health care provider about use of corticosteroid foam.	Corticosteroid foam is easier to retain and administer.
Monitor serum electrolytes, particularly K⁺, for abnormalities. Alert health care provider to K⁺ <3.5 mEq/L.	Hypokalemia is often present because of colonic losses (diarrhea) and renal losses in patients taking high doses of corticosteroids.

●●● **Related NIC and NOC labels:** *NIC:* Fluid/Electrolyte Management; Diarrhea Management; Electrolyte Management: Hypokalemia; Laboratory Data Interpretation; Anxiety Reduction; Medication Administration *NOC:* Electrolyte and Acid/Base Balance; Symptom Severity

Nursing Diagnosis:

Risk for Impaired Perineal/Perianal Skin Integrity

related to presence of persistent diarrhea

Desired Outcome: Patient's perineal/perianal skin remains intact with no erythema.

INTERVENTIONS	RATIONALES
Provide materials or assist patient with cleansing and drying perineal area after each bowel movement. Use a nonirritating cleansing agent.	To help keep skin clean and intact.
Apply protective skin care products (skin preparations, gels, or barrier films).	To prevent irritation caused by frequent liquid stools.
Administer hydrophilic colloids, anticholinergics, and antidiarrheal medications as prescribed.	To decrease fluidity and number of stools.

●●● **Related NIC and NOC labels:** *NIC:* Bathing; Bowel Incontinence Care; Skin Care: Topical Treatments; Diarrhea Management; Perineal Care; Self-Care Assistance: Bathing/Hygiene *NOC:* Tissue Integrity: Skin & Mucous Membranes

Nursing Diagnosis:

Deficient Knowledge:

Purpose and precautions for medications used with ulcerative colitis

Desired Outcome: Immediately following teaching (if patient is not hospitalized) or within the 24-hr period before hospital discharge, patient verbalizes accurate information about the drugs used with ulcerative colitis, including their purpose and necessary precautions.

INTERVENTIONS	RATIONALES
Teach Patient the Following:	
Antiinflammatory agents	Corticosteroids reduce mucosal inflammation.
Dosage and routes of administration vary with the severity and extent of the disease.	In patients with mild disease limited to the rectum and sigmoid colon, rectal instillation of steroids (enema or suppository) may induce or maintain remission. In patients with more extensive (pancolonic) or more active disease, oral corticosteroid therapy with prednisone or prednisolone usually is initiated. In severely ill patients, IV corticosteroids are given. Budesonide, a new steroidal agent, shows promise for providing the benefits of traditional therapy without the side effects.
Once clinical remission is achieved, IV and oral corticosteroids are tapered until discontinuation.	These medications have not been shown to prolong remission or prevent future exacerbations.
Sulfasalazine	To help maintain remissions. This drug generally is effective in the treatment of mild to moderate attacks of ulcerative colitis and appears to decrease frequency of subsequent relapse. Sulfasalazine is considered inferior to corticosteroids in the treatment of severe attacks of disease; once remission has been attained by use of corticosteroid therapy, sulfasalazine appears to be superior to systemic corticosteroids in the maintenance of remission.
To avoid side effects of sulfapyridine, several agents have been developed using a variety of delivery mechanisms that allow release of the active agent in the colon or ileum. These agents include the 5-aminosalicylic acid (5-ASA) derivatives: mesalamine (in enteric-coated and time-release forms), olsalazine, and balsalazide. These three agents are useful alternatives to patients unable to tolerate sulfapyridine; however, these agents have their own side effects.	When administered orally, sulfasalazine is broken down by colonic bacteria into its two constituents: 5-ASA, which is considered the active therapeutic component, and sulfapyridine, which is the carrier and responsible for the side effects experienced by more than one third of the individuals treated with this therapy.
Immunosuppressive therapy	To reduce inflammation in patients not responding to steroids and sulfasalazine; in patients unwilling or unable to undergo colectomy; or as an alternative to steroid dependency. Azathioprine and 6-mercaptopurine (6-MP) have been used alone and in combination with steroids.
Immunosuppressive therapy has been used to maintain remission in patients with frequent relapses.	These agents may have steroid-sparing and steroid-enhancing effects and are used with the goal of gradually withdrawing, or substantially reducing, the dosage of corticosteroids.
Patients need to be closely monitored for hematologic toxicity.	Therapy may be necessary for 3-6 mo to achieve therapeutic response, and this amount of time can result in hematologic toxicity.
IV cyclosporine has been used cautiously in severe, intractable ulcerative colitis. If there is no response within 4-7 days, cyclosporine is unlikely to be effective.	Cyclosporine is toxic and associated with many side effects and thus is used with caution.

●●● **Related NIC and NOC labels:** *NIC:* Teaching: Prescribed Medication *NOC:* Knowledge: Medication

ADDITIONAL NURSING DIAGNOSES/ PROBLEMS:

PATIENT-FAMILY TEACHING AND DISCHARGE PLANNING

When providing patient-family teaching, focus on sensory information, avoid giving excessive information, and initiate a visiting nurse referral for necessary follow-up teaching. Include verbal and written information about the following:

✓ Medications, including drug name, rationale, dosage, schedule, route of administration, precautions, drug/drug and food/drug interactions, and potential side effects. **Note:** Caution patients receiving high-dose steroid therapy about abrupt discontinuation of steroids to prevent precipitation of adrenal crisis. Withdrawal symptoms include weakness, lethargy, restlessness, anorexia, nausea, and muscle tenderness. Instruct patient to notify health care provider if these symptoms occur.

✓ Signs and symptoms that necessitate medical attention, including fever, nausea and vomiting, diarrhea or constipation, and any significant change in appearance and frequency of stools—any of which can signal exacerbation of the disease.

✓ Dietary management to promote nutritional and fluid maintenance and prevent abdominal cramping, discomfort, and diarrhea.

✓ Importance of perineal care after bowel movements.

✓ Enteral or parenteral feeding instructions if patient is to supplement diet or is NPO.

✓ Importance of follow-up medical care, particularly for patients with long-standing disease because so many of them develop colonic adenocarcinoma.

✓ Referral to a mental health specialist if recommended by the health care provider.

✓ Referral to community resources, including the following organization:

Crohn's and Colitis Foundation of America
386 Park Ave. South, 17th Floor
New York, NY 10016-8804
(800) 932-2423
www.ccfa.org

In addition, if patient has a fecal diversion:

✓ Care of incision, dressing changes, and permission to take baths or showers once sutures and drains are removed.

✓ Care of stoma, peristomal/perianal skin, or perineal wound; use of ostomy equipment; and method for obtaining supplies. Sitz baths may be indicated for perineal wound.

✓ Medications that are contraindicated (e.g., laxatives) or that may not be well tolerated or absorbed (e.g., antibiotics, enteric-coated tablets, long-acting tablets).

✓ Gradual resumption of activities of daily living (ADL), excluding heavy lifting (>10 lb), pushing, or pulling for 6-8 wk to prevent incisional herniation.

✓ Importance of reporting signs and symptoms that require medical attention, such as change in stoma color from the normal bright and shiny red; peristomal or perianal skin irritation; diarrhea; incisional pain, local increased temperature, drainage, swelling, or redness; signs and symptoms of fluid and electrolyte imbalance; and signs and symptoms of mechanical or functional obstruction.

✓ Referral to community resources, including home health care agency; wound, ostomy, continence (WOC)/enterostomal therapy (ET) nurse; and the local chapter of the United Ostomy Association.

United Ostomy Association
19722 MacArthur Blvd., Suite 200
Irvine, CA 92612-2405
(800) 826-0826
www.uoa.org

61

Disseminated Intravascular Coagulation

Disseminated intravascular coagulation (DIC) is an acute coagulation disorder characterized by paradoxic clotting and hemorrhage. The sequence usually progresses from massive clot formation, depletion of the clotting factors, and activation of diffuse fibrinolysis to hemorrhage. DIC occurs secondary to widespread coagulation factors in the bloodstream caused by extensive surgery, burns, shock, neoplastic diseases, or abruptio placentae; extensive destruction of blood vessel walls caused by eclampsia, anoxia, or heat stroke; or damage to blood cells caused by hemolysis, sickle cell disease, or transfusion reactions. DIC is also associated with sepsis. Prompt assessment of the disorder can result in a good prognosis. Usually, affected patients are transferred to the intensive care unit (ICU) for careful monitoring and aggressive therapy. DIC may be classified as low grade (compensated or chronic) or fulminant (acute).

HEALTH CARE SETTING
Acute care/critical care unit

ASSESSMENT
Signs and symptoms: Bleeding of abrupt onset; oozing from venipuncture sites or mucosal surfaces; bleeding from surgical sites; the presence of hematuria, blood in the stool (melena or hematochezia), spontaneous ecchymosis (bruising), petechiae, purpura fulminans, pallor, or mottled skin. The patient also may bleed from the vagina (menometrorrhagia), nose (epistaxis), and mucous membranes. Joint pain and swelling may signal bleeding into the joints. Complaint of headache or mental status changes may indicate intracranial hemorrhage. Symptoms of hypoperfusion can occur, including decreased urine output and abnormal behavior.

Physical assessment: Abdominal assessment may reveal signs of gastrointestinal (GI) bleeding, such as guarding; distention (increasing abdominal girth measurements); hyperactive, hypoactive, or absent bowel sounds; and a rigid, boardlike abdomen. With significant hemorrhage, patients may exhibit the following: systolic BP <90 mm Hg and diastolic BP <60 mm Hg; HR >100 bpm; peripheral pulse amplitude <2+ on a 0-4+ scale; RR >22 breaths/min; shortness of breath; urinary output <30 ml/hr; secretions and excretions positive for blood; cool, pale, clammy skin; lack of orientation to person, place, and time; or changes in mental status.

Risk factors: Infection, burns, trauma, hepatic disease, hypovolemic shock, severe hemolytic reaction, obstetric complications, and hypoxia.

DIAGNOSTIC TESTS
Serum fibrinogen: Low because of abnormal consumption of clotting factors in the formation of fibrin clots.

Platelet count: Significantly reduced (usually <120,000/mm^3) because of platelets' role in clot formation.

Fibrin split products (FSPs), also known as fibrin degradation products (FDPs): Increased, indicating widespread dissolution of clots. Fibrinolysis produces FSPs as an end product.

Prothrombin time (PT): Increased because of depletion of clotting factors.

Partial thromboplastin time (PTT): High because of depletion of clotting factors.

Peripheral blood smear: Will show fragmented red blood cells (RBCs).

Bleeding time: Prolonged because of decreased platelets.

Nursing Diagnosis:

Ineffective Cardiopulmonary, Peripheral, Renal, and Cerebral Tissue Perfusion

related to interrupted blood flow secondary to coagulation/fibrinolysis processes

Desired Outcome: Within the 24-hr period following interventions/treatment, patient has adequate cardiopulmonary, peripheral, renal, and cerebral perfusion as evidenced by BP ≥90/60 mm Hg and HR ≤100 bpm (or within patient's baseline range); peripheral pulse amplitude >2+ on a 0-4+ scale; urinary output ≥30 ml/hr; equal and normoreactive pupils; normal/baseline motor function; orientation to person, place, and time; and no mental status changes.

INTERVENTIONS	RATIONALES
Monitor VS and assess peripheral pulses.	To evaluate peripheral perfusion. Decreased BP, increased HR, or decreased amplitude of peripheral pulses may signal that coagulation and thrombus formation are occurring.
Monitor I&O.	To evaluate renal perfusion. Urinary output <30 ml/hr in the presence of adequate intake may signal renal vessel thrombosis.
Perform neurologic checks, including orientation, mental status assessments, pupillary reaction to light, and motor response and assess mental status and level of consciousness (LOC).	To evaluate cerebral perfusion. Deficits may signal that cerebral perfusion is ineffective and should be reported promptly.
If signs of impaired cerebral perfusion occur, institute measures such as keeping bed in lowest position and side rails up.	To protect patient from injury caused by cerebral impairment.
Monitor for hemorrhage from surgical wounds, GI and genitourinary (GU) tracts, and mucous membranes.	Can occur after fibrinolysis.
Monitor laboratory test results.	Low serum fibrinogen (<200 mg/dl), low platelet count (<250,000/mm^3), increased FSPs (>8 μm/ml), increased PT (>11-15 sec), and increased PTT (>40-100 sec) are common with DIC.
Monitor O$_2$ saturation via pulse oximetry q4h or as indicated.	Oxygen saturation ≤92% suggests need for supplemental oxygen.
Report significant findings to patient's health care provider; prepare for transfer to ICU if condition persists or worsens.	Patient will need careful monitoring and aggressive therapy.

●●● **Related NIC and NOC labels:** *NIC:* Bleeding Precautions; Embolus Precautions; Laboratory Data Interpretation; Oxygen Therapy; Vital Signs Monitoring; Emergency Care; Neurologic Monitoring
NOC: Circulation Status; Tissue Perfusion: Cardiac; Tissue Perfusion: Pulmonary; Vital Signs Status; Tissue Perfusion: Cerebral; Tissue Perfusion: Abdominal Organs; Tissue Perfusion: Peripheral

Nursing Diagnosis:

Ineffective Protection

related to increased risk of bleeding secondary to hemorrhagic component of DIC

Desired Outcome: Patient is free of signs of bleeding as evidenced by systolic BP ≥90 mm Hg; HR ≤100 bpm (or within patient's normal range); RR 12-20 breaths/min with normal depth and pattern (eupnea); urinary output ≥30 ml/hr; secretions and excretions negative for blood; stable abdominal girth measurements; orientation to person, place, and time; and no changes in mental status.

INTERVENTIONS	RATIONALES
Monitor VS and LOC at frequent intervals; report significant changes	Hypotension, tachycardia, dyspnea, disorientation, and changes in mental status can signal hemorrhage.
Be cautious of pressure used with BP cuffs. Rotate arm use.	Frequent BP readings may cause bleeding under the cuff. Rotation reduces repeated tissue trauma.
Monitor coagulation studies.	Increased PT (>11-15 sec) is a sign that clotting factors are depleted and patient is at risk for hemorrhage.
Use a reagent screening agent to check stool, urine, emesis, and nasogastric drainage for blood.	A positive test signals presence of blood in the GI/GU tracts and should be reported to health care provider promptly.
Monitor for internal bleeding.	Abdominal pain, abdominal distention, changes in bowel sounds, and a boardlike abdomen are signs of GI bleeding.
Assess puncture sites regularly for oozing or bleeding. When possible, treat bleeding sites with ice, pressure, rest, and elevation.	To assess for and reduce external bleeding or oozing if it occurs. Some health care providers promote use of thrombin-soaked gauze, such as Gelfoam, or topical thrombin powder.
Be alert to other signs of bleeding.	Visual changes may signal retinal hemorrhage. Joint pain and headache are other signs that bleeding may be occurring.
Avoid giving IM injections or performing venipunctures for blood drawing.	To avoid additional risk of bleeding.
Administer blood products (fresh frozen plasma, packed RBCs, platelets) and IV fluids as prescribed.	To help counteract deficiencies and support blood volume.
Teach patient to use electric shaver and soft-bristle toothbrush.	To reduce the risk of bleeding. Razors and hard bristles could break the skin and mucous membranes, causing bleeding.

●●● **Related NIC and NOC labels:** *NIC:* Bleeding Precautions; Blood Products Administration; Bleeding Reduction *NOC:* Coagulation Status

Nursing Diagnosis:

Risk for Impaired Skin Integrity *or* Impaired Tissue Integrity

related to altered circulation secondary to hemorrhage and thrombosis

Desired Outcome: Patient's skin and tissue remain nonerythemic and intact.

INTERVENTIONS	RATIONALES
Assess patient's skin.	Erythema that does not clear after removal of pressure or changes in color, sensation, and temperature may signal decreased perfusion and can lead to tissue damage.
Ensure that patient turns q2h. Use sheepskin on elbows and heels and enhanced pressure-distribution mattress padding. Do not pull on extremities when turning patient.	To eliminate or minimize pressure points.
Encourage active range of motion (ROM) of all extremities q2h.	To reduce pressure and enhance circulation.
Keep patient's extremities warm.	To prevent tissue hypoxia, which would increase risk of tissue damage/necrosis.
Use alternatives to tape to hold dressings in place, such as gauze wraps or net gauze.	Tape removal could damage fragile skin and tissue.
If patient has areas of breakdown, see "Managing Wound Care," p. 583.	

●●● **Related NIC and NOC labels:** *NIC:* Pressure Management; Skin Surveillance; Circulatory Precautions *NOC:* Tissue Integrity: Skin and Mucous Membranes

ADDITIONAL NURSING DIAGNOSES/ PROBLEMS:

"Pulmonary Embolus" for **Ineffective Protection** related to increased risk of bleeding or hemorrhage secondary to anticoagulant therapy. Although anticoagulant therapy is controversial with DIC, heparin may be administered. Heparin interferes with the coagulation process and activation of the fibrinolytic system in an p. 155 attempt to prevent clot formation within organs. Heparin dose is regulated and determined by the PTT. Warfarin may be used in compensated DIC.

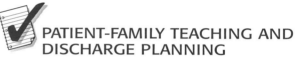

PATIENT-FAMILY TEACHING AND DISCHARGE PLANNING

See patient's primary diagnosis.

Erythropoietin Deficiency Anemia

Erythropoietin (EPO) is a naturally occurring protein hormone produced and released by the kidneys (90%) and liver (10%). EPO stimulates stem cells in the bone marrow to develop and produce RBCs. The kidneys are stimulated to release EPO in response to low blood oxygenation. Patients with decreased renal function (e.g., chronic renal failure) often become anemic because their kidneys cannot produce EPO. Development of recombinant human erythropoietin (epoetin alpha) has provided dramatic benefits for patients with chronic renal failure, patients receiving chemotherapy for cancer, and patients receiving azidothymidine (AZT) for treatment of human immunodeficiency virus (HIV) infection.

HEALTH CARE SETTING

Primary care; acute care for blood transfusion or treatment for sequelae of chronic renal failure

ASSESSMENT

Chronic indicators: The patient may be asymptomatic or have brittle hair and nails. In the presence of severe and chronic disease, dysphagia, stomatitis, and inflammation of the tongue may be present. Patient may have a history of chronic renal disease, dialysis therapy, cancer chemotherapy, or AZT therapy for HIV infection.

Acute indicators: Fatigue, decreased ability to concentrate, cold sensitivity, menstrual irregularities, and loss of libido.

Physical assessment: Tachycardia, palpitations, tachypnea, exertional dyspnea, pale mucous membranes, pale nail beds, vertigo.

DIAGNOSTIC TESTS

Blood count: Usually red blood cells (RBCs) and Hgb are decreased; Hct usually is low because the percentage of RBCs in the total blood volume is decreased.

Peripheral blood smear to examine RBC indices: Morphology may be normal, or there may be microcytosis or hypochromia.

Total iron-binding capacity: Decreased.

Reticulocyte count: Normal to slightly elevated.

Serum iron levels: Decreased.

Nursing Diagnosis:

Activity Intolerance

related to imbalance between oxygen supply and demand secondary to decreased oxygen–carrying capacity of the blood because of anemia

Desired Outcome: Within 24 hr after treatment, patient rates perceived exertion at ≤3 on a 0-10 scale and exhibits tolerance to activity as evidenced by RR 12-20 breaths/min with normal depth and pattern (eupnea), HR ≤100 bpm, and absence of dizziness and headaches.

INTERVENTIONS	RATIONALES
Monitor patient during activities of daily living (ADL). Ask patient to rate perceived exertion (RPE). See "Prolonged Bedrest" for **Risk for Activity Intolerance,** p. 67.	Dyspnea on exertion, dizziness, palpitations, headaches, and verbalization of increased exertion level (RPE >3) are signs of activity intolerance and decreased tissue oxygenation, and patient should stop or modify the activity until signs of increased exertion are no longer present with the activity.
Facilitate coordination of care providers, allowing time for at least 90 min of undisturbed rest.	To provide rest periods as needed between care activities.
As indicated, monitor pulse oximetry.	O$_2$ saturation ≤92% may signal need for supplementary oxygen.
Administer oxygen as prescribed and encourage deep breathing.	To augment oxygen delivery to the tissues.
Administer blood components (usually RBCs) as prescribed.	To increase the number of circulating RBCs, which will increase the oxygen-carrying capacity of the blood.
Double-check type and crossmatching with a colleague and monitor for and report signs of transfusion reaction.	To reduce risk of delivering wrong type of blood to the patient.
Encourage gradually increasing activities to tolerance as patient's condition improves.	To promote endurance and prevent problems caused by prolonged bedrest. Setting mutually agreed on goals with patient (e.g., "Let's plan this morning's activity goals. Do you feel you could walk up and down the hall once, or twice?" [or appropriate amount, depending on patient's tolerance]) is an effective measure.
Reassure patient that symptoms are usually relieved and tolerance for activity increased with therapy such as recombinant EPO (epoetin alfa).	Administering EPO stimulates production of RBCs. With more circulating RBCs, there is increased oxygen-carrying capacity of the blood, which will aid in overcoming activity intolerance.

●●● **Related NIC and NOC labels:** *NIC:* Activity Therapy; Energy Management; Exercise Promotion; Oxygen Therapy; Mutual Goal Setting *NOC:* Endurance; Energy Conservation; Activity Tolerance

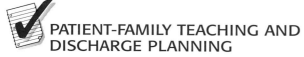

PATIENT-FAMILY TEACHING AND DISCHARGE PLANNING

When providing patient-family teaching, focus on sensory information, avoid giving excessive information, and initiate a visiting nurse referral for necessary follow-up teaching. Include verbal and written information about the following:

✔ Importance of a well-balanced diet, especially iron intake, which is found in foods such as red meat, dark green vegetables, legumes, and certain fruits (apricots, figs, raisins).

✔ Special instructions for taking iron, depending on type prescribed. Therapy may need to be continued for 4-6 mo to adequately replace iron stores.

✔ EPO replacement therapy will need to be continued for life, unless underlying condition (e.g., cancer chemotherapy) is corrected.

✔ When self-administering EPO, patients should understand the need to *avoid* shaking medication vial before administration. Shaking the vial may denature glycoprotein in the solution and render it biologically inactive. Any discolored solution or solution with particulate matter should not be used.

Polycythemia

Polycythemia is a chronic disorder characterized by excessive production of red blood cells (RBCs), platelets, and myelocytes. As these increase, blood volume, blood viscosity, and Hgb concentration increase, causing excessive workload for the heart and congestion of some organ systems (e.g., liver, kidney).

Secondary polycythemia results from an abnormal increase in erythropoietin production (e.g., because of hypoxia that occurs with chronic lung disease or prolonged living in altitudes >10,000 ft) or with renal tumors.

Polycythemia vera is a primary disorder of unknown cause affecting men of Jewish descent, with onset in late midlife. Polycythemia vera results in increased RBC mass, leukocytosis, and slight thrombocytosis. Because of increased viscosity and decreased microcirculation, mortality is high if the condition is left untreated. In addition, there is a potential for this disorder to evolve into other hematopoietic disorders, such as acute leukemia.

HEALTH CARE SETTING

Primary care; acute care for complications

ASSESSMENT

Signs and symptoms: Headache, dizziness, paresthesias, visual disturbances, dyspnea, thrombophlebitis, joint pain, pruritus, night sweats, fatigue, chest pain, and a feeling of "fullness," especially in the head.

Physical assessment: Hypertension, engorgement of retinal blood veins, crackles (rales), weight loss, cyanosis, ruddy complexion (especially palmar aspects of hands and plantar surfaces of feet), and hepatosplenomegaly.

DIAGNOSTIC TESTS

Complete blood count (CBC): Increased RBC mass (8-12 million/mm^3), Hgb (18-25 g/dl), Hct (>54% in men and >49% in women), and leukocytes; overproduction of thrombocytes.

Platelet count: Elevated as a result of increased production.

Bone marrow aspiration: Reveals RBC proliferation.

Uric acid levels: May be increased because of increased nucleoprotein, an end product of RBC breakdown.

Erythropoietin levels: Elevated in secondary polycythemia and decreased in polycythemia vera.

Nursing Diagnosis:

Acute Pain

related to headache, angina, and abdominal and joint discomfort secondary to altered circulation because of hyperviscosity of the blood

Desired Outcomes: Within 1 hr of intervention, patient's subjective perception of discomfort decreases, as documented by a pain scale. Objective indicators, such as grimacing, are absent or diminished. Lifestyle behaviors are not compromised because of discomfort.

INTERVENTIONS	RATIONALES
Assess for presence of headache, angina, abdominal pain, and joint pain. Devise a pain scale with patient, rating discomfort from 0 (no pain) to 10 (worst pain). Document degree of pain relief using pain scale.	Use of a pain intensity scale allows more accurate documentation of discomfort and subsequent relief obtained after analgesia has been administered. The patient provides a personal baseline report, enabling nurse to more effectively monitor subsequent increases and decreases in pain.
In the presence of joint pain, rest joint and elevate extremity. Apply moist heat or ice.	To ease discomfort. Elevation may help increase circulation and prevent pooling of hyperviscous blood in the joint. Moist heat helps to increase circulation and decrease pain. Ice is used (short term) to decrease severe joint pain.
Administer analgesics as prescribed. Avoid analgesics containing aspirin or nonsteroidal antiinflammatory drugs (NSAIDs).	To reduce pain. May exacerbate bleeding associated with thrombocytosis.
Instruct patient to request analgesic before pain becomes too intense.	Pain is easier to control before it becomes severe. Prolonged stimulation of pain receptors results in increased sensitivity to painful stimuli and will increase the amount of drug required to relieve pain.
Encourage use of nonpharmacologic pain control, such as relaxation and distraction.	To incorporate pain measures that potentiate analgesics and do not have side effects.
Be alert to and report calf pain and tenderness.	Indicators of peripheral thrombosis.
Report significant findings to patient's health care provider.	To ensure prompt treatment if indicated.

●●● **Related NIC and NOC labels:** *NIC:* Pain Management; Analgesic Administration; Positioning; Simple Relaxation Therapy; Distraction; Heat/Cold Application *NOC:* Comfort Level

Nursing Diagnosis:

Ineffective Renal, Peripheral, and Cerebral Tissue Perfusion

related to interrupted blood flow secondary to hyperviscosity of the blood

Desired Outcome: Within the 24-hr period following interventions/treatment, patient has adequate renal, peripheral, and cerebral perfusion as evidenced by urinary output ≥30 ml/hr, peripheral pulses >2+ on a scale of 0-4+, distal extremity warmth, adequate (baseline) muscle strength, no mental status changes, and orientation to person, place, and time.

INTERVENTIONS	RATIONALES
Monitor I&O.	To assess renal perfusion. Urine output <30 ml/hr in the presence of adequate intake can signal renal congestion and decreased perfusion.
If fluid intake is inadequate and in the absence of signs of cardiac and renal failure, encourage fluid intake.	Inadequate hydration can increase blood viscosity and contribute adversely to polycythemia.
Monitor peripheral perfusion by palpating peripheral pulses.	Amplitude ≤2+ on a scale of 0-4+ and coolness in distal extremities signal disruption of peripheral tissue perfusion secondary to hyperviscosity of the blood.
Encourage patient to change position qh when in bed or to exercise and ambulate to tolerance.	To promote circulation.

Continued

INTERVENTIONS	RATIONALES
Instruct patient to avoid tight or restrictive clothing.	Could impede blood flow/circulation.
Monitor for muscle weakness and decreases in sensation and level of consciousness (LOC).	Indicators of impending neurologic damage.
If these indicators are present, protect patient by assisting with ambulation or raising side rails on bed, depending on degree of deficit.	To protect patient from injury caused by declining neurologic status.
Administer myelosuppressive agents, as prescribed.	To inhibit proliferation of RBCs. Alkylating and nonalkylating agents, for example, hydroxyurea (preferred), busulfan, chlorambucil, and/or radioactive phosphorus (especially for older persons and those refractive to other agents) inhibit bone marrow function.
If patient smokes, encourage enrollment in a smoking cessation program.	Smoking significantly increases potential of a thromboembolic event.
Report significant findings to patient's health care provider.	To ensure prompt treatment.

●●● **Related NIC and NOC labels:** *NIC:* Embolus Precautions; Circulatory Precautions; Hypovolemia Management; Neurologic Monitoring; Medication Administration *NOC:* Circulation Status; Neurological Status; Tissue Perfusion: Cerebral; Tissue Perfusion: Abdominal Organs; Tissue Perfusion: Peripheral; Tissue Perfusion: Renal

Nursing Diagnosis:

Imbalanced Nutrition: Less than body requirements

related to anorexia secondary to feelings of fullness occurring with organ system congestion

Desired Outcome: By at least 24 hr before hospital discharge (or during weekly follow-up if patient is not hospitalized), patient exhibits adequate nutrition as evidenced by maintenance of or return to baseline body weight or a 1- to 2-lb weight gain.

INTERVENTIONS	RATIONALES
Weigh patient daily.	To identify trend.
Encourage patient to eat small, frequent meals. Document intake.	Smaller, more frequent meals usually are better tolerated than larger, less frequent meals.
Request that significant other bring in patient's favorite foods if they are unavailable in the hospital.	Promotes likelihood that patient will eat.
Advise patient to avoid spicy foods and to eat mild foods.	Mild foods are better tolerated.
Teach patient to avoid intake of iron.	To help minimize abnormal RBC proliferation.
As indicated, obtain a dietary consultation.	For more detailed instruction/discussion about foods to eat and those to avoid.
Teach patient or significant other how to record and maintain a fluid and food intake diary.	To follow trends in food intake and ensure monitoring of hydration status.

●●● **Related NIC and NOC labels:** *NIC:* Nutritional Monitoring; Fluid Monitoring; Weight Gain Assistance; Teaching: Prescribed Diet; *NOC:* Nutritional Status; Nutritional Status: Food & Fluid Intake

Nursing Diagnosis:

Ineffective Cerebral and Cardiopulmonary Tissue Perfusion

(or risk for same) *related to* hypovolemia secondary to phlebotomy

Desired Outcome: Patient has adequate cerebral and cardiopulmonary perfusion as evidenced by no
mental status changes; orientation to person, place, and time; HR ≤100 bpm; BP ≥90/60 mm Hg
(or within patient's baseline range); absence of chest pain; and RR ≤20 breaths/min. **Note:** If a
phlebotomy has been prescribed, 500 ml (250–300 ml in older adults) of blood will be withdrawn every 2-3 days to decrease blood volume and decrease Hct to 40%–45%.

INTERVENTIONS	RATIONALES
During procedure, keep patient recumbent.	To prevent dizziness or hypotension as a result of phlebotomy.
Assess for tachycardia, hypotension, chest pain, or dizziness during procedure; notify patient's health care provider of significant findings.	Signs of deficient fluid volume.
After the procedure, assist patient with sitting position for 5-10 min before ambulation.	To prevent orthostatic hypotension. For more information about orthostatic hypotension, see "Prolonged Bedrest" for **Ineffective Cerebral Tissue Perfusion,** p. 73.
Teach patients, especially those who are older and chronically ill, about potential for orthostatic hypotension and need for caution when standing for at least 2-3 days after phlebotomy.	To help protect against injury caused by falling as a result of orthostatic hypotension.

●●● **Related NIC and NOC labels:** *NIC:* Fluid Monitoring; Hypovolemia Management; Vital Signs
Monitoring; Positioning *NOC:* Circulation Status; Vital Signs Status; Tissue Perfusion: Cerebral

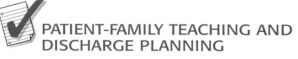

PATIENT-FAMILY TEACHING AND DISCHARGE PLANNING

When providing patient-family teaching, focus on sensory
information, avoid giving excessive information, and initiate a
visiting nurse referral for necessary follow-up teaching. Include
verbal and written information about the following:

✓ Need for continued medical follow-up, including
potential for phlebotomy every 1-3 mo.

✓ Medications, including drug name, purpose, dosage,
schedule, precautions, drug/drug and food/drug interactions,
and potential side effects.

✓ Importance of augmenting fluid intake (e.g., >2.5 L/day)
to decrease blood viscosity.

✓ Signs and symptoms that necessitate medical attention:
angina, muscle weakness, numbness and tingling of extremities,
decreased tolerance to activity, mental status changes, and joint
pain.

✓ Nutrition: importance of maintaining balanced diet to
increase resistance to infection and limiting dietary or
supplemental intake of iron to help minimize abnormal RBC
proliferation.

Thrombocytopenia

Thrombocytopenia is a common coagulation disorder that results from a decreased number of platelets. It can be congenital or acquired, and it is classified according to cause. Common causes include deficient formation of thrombocytes, as occurs with bone marrow disease or destruction; accelerated platelet destruction, loss, or increased use, as in hemolytic anemia, diffuse intravascular coagulation, or damage by prosthetic heart valves; and abnormal platelet distribution, as in hypersplenism and hypothermia. Potential triggers include autoimmune disorder, severe vascular injury, and spleen malfunction. In addition, thrombocytopenia can occur as a side effect of certain drugs. Regardless of the cause or trigger, the disorder affects coagulation and hemostasis. With chemical-induced thrombocytopenia, prognosis is good after withdrawal of the offending drug. Prognosis for other types depends on the form of thrombocytopenia and the individual's baseline health status and response to treatment. **Note:** Thrombocytopenia may be the first sign of systemic lupus erythematosus (SLE) or human immunodeficiency virus (HIV) infection.

Thrombotic thrombocytopenic purpura (TTP) is an acute, often fatal disorder. The cause is presumed to be the absence of a factor in the plasma or the presence of a platelet-stimulating factor. Platelets become sensitized and clump in blood vessels, occluding them.

Idiopathic thrombocytopenic purpura (ITP) is believed to be an immune disorder specifically involving antiplatelet immunoglobulin G (IgG), which destroys platelets. The acute form is most often seen in children (2-6 yr of age) and may be related to a previous viral infection. The chronic form is seen more often in adults (18-50 yr of age) and is of unknown origin. This type also may be referred to as immune thrombocytopenic purpura when it is related to the process of autoreactive antibodies binding to platelets and shortening their lifespan. There are four main causes: drug-induced, viral/infection-induced, pregnancy-induced, and hypersplenism with chronic liver dysfunction (blood pools in the splenic sinuses). Drugs associated with this type include quinidine, quinine, rifampin, amphotericin, methyldopa, vancomycin, acetaminophen, digoxin, amiodarone, cimetidine, chlorothiazide, tamoxifen, amrinone, lithium, diazepam, haloperidol, and minoxidil.

HEALTH CARE SETTING

Primary care; hospitalization for complications

ASSESSMENT

Chronic indicators: Long history of mild bleeding or hemorrhagic episodes from the mouth, nose, gastrointestinal (GI) tract, or genitourinary (GU) tract. Increased bruising (ecchymosis) and petechiae also have been noted.

Acute indicators: Fever, splenomegaly, acute and severe bleeding episodes, weakness, lethargy, malaise, hemorrhage into mucous membranes, gum bleeding, and GU or GI bleeding. Prolonged bleeding can lead to a shock state with tachycardia, shortness of breath, and decreased level of consciousness (LOC). Optic fundal hemorrhage decreases vision and may precede potentially fatal intracranial hemorrhage. **Note:** With TTP, the individual may exhibit signs associated with platelet thrombus formation and ischemic organs, such as decreased renal function or neurologic changes.

History of: Recent infection; recent vaccination; binge alcohol consumption; positive family history of thrombocytopenia; or use of chlorothiazide, digitalis, quinidine, rifampin, sulfisoxazole, chloramphenicol, phenytoin, or heparin.

DIAGNOSTIC TESTS

Platelet count: Can vary from only slightly decreased to nearly absent. Less than $100,000/mm^3$ is significantly decreased; $<20,000/mm^3$ results in a serious risk of hemorrhage.

Peripheral blood smear: Reveals megathrombocytes (large platelets), which are present during premature destruction of platelets.

Complete blood count (CBC): Low Hgb and Hct levels because of blood loss; white blood cell (WBC) count usually is within normal range.

Coagulation studies:
- **Bleeding time:** Increased because of decreased platelets
- **Partial thromboplastin time (PTT):** Increased
- **Prothrombin time (PT):** Increased
- **International Normalized Ratio (INR):** Increased
- **International Sensitivity Index (ISI):** Increased

Bone marrow aspiration: Reveals increased number of megakaryocytes (platelet precursors) in the presence of ITP but may be decreased with certain causes of thrombocytopenia.

Platelet antibody screen: May be positive because of the presence of IgG antibodies.

Nursing Diagnosis:

Ineffective Protection

related to increased risk of bleeding secondary to decreased platelet count

Desired Outcome: Patient is free of the signs of bleeding as evidenced by secretions and excretions negative for blood, BP ≥90/60 mm Hg or within patient's baseline range, HR ≤100 bpm, RR 12-20 breaths/min with normal depth and pattern (eupnea), and absence of bruising or active bleeding.

INTERVENTIONS	RATIONALES
Monitor for hematuria, melena, epistaxis, hematemesis, hemoptysis, menometrorrhagia, bleeding gums, or severe ecchymosis. Teach patient to be alert to and report these indicators promptly.	Signs of bleeding that could occur as a result of thrombocytopenia. These signs should be reported promptly for timely intervention.
When appropriate, pad and keep up side rails.	To protect patient from injury that could result in bleeding.
When possible, avoid venipuncture. If performed, apply pressure on site for 5-10 min or until bleeding stops.	Patient is at risk for prolonged bleeding because of the decreased platelet count.
Avoid IM injections. If injections are necessary, preferably use SC route and small-gauge needle when possible.	Same as above.
Monitor platelet count daily.	Optimal range is 150,000-400,000/mm³. Less than 100,000/mm³ is significantly decreased; <20,000/mm³ results in a serious risk of hemorrhage.
Advise patient to avoid straining at stool and coughing.	Straining increases intracranial pressure and can result in intracranial hemorrhage.
Obtain prescription for stool softeners, if indicated. Teach patient anticonstipation routine as described in "Prolonged Bedrest" for **Constipation,** p. 75.	To prevent constipation, which will minimize need to strain at stool.
Administer corticosteroids as prescribed.	To help minimize platelet destruction.
Teach patient to use electric razor and soft-bristle toothbrush.	Minimizes risk of injury and hence bleeding.
Caution patient to avoid alcohol consumption, smoking, and use of aspirin and nonsteroidal antiinflammatory drugs (NSAIDs).	All increase risk of bleeding.
Administer platelets as prescribed.	Platelet administration provides only temporary relief because the half-life of platelets is only 3-4 days; it may be even shorter with ITP (i.e., minutes to hours).
Double-check type and crossmatching with a colleague.	To ensure that patient receives correct blood product and type, which otherwise could result in transfusion reaction.
Monitor for and report chills, back pain, dyspnea, hives, and wheezing.	Signs of transfusion reaction.
Administer intravenous immunoglobulin (IVIg) as prescribed.	IVIg induces rapid increase in platelet count that lasts for 3-4 wk.

Continued

INTERVENTIONS	RATIONALES
Keep epinephrine nearby.	In the event of anaphylactic reaction. IVIg is contraindicated in patients known to have sensitivity to immune globulins.
Check blood urea nitrogen (BUN)/creatinine before infusing.	These values may increase up to 2 days after infusion of IVIg.
Monitor BP q30min-1h during initial infusion.	Patient may become hypotensive (or develop headache and nausea) during initial infusion, which may necessitate slowing rate of infusion or stopping it until BP returns to baseline or normal.
Do not give IVIg within 3 mo of administration of live viruses (measles, mumps, rubella). Instruct patient not to take these vaccines within 3 mo of having taken IVIg infusion.	Increased toxicity to IVIg is noted with administration of live viruses.
Be alert to and teach patient the following symptoms: flushing of face, tachycardia, hypotension, chest tightness, angioedema, chills, dizziness, fever, headache, lethargy, aseptic migraine syndrome, urticaria, nausea, vomiting, myalgia, nephritic syndrome, renal failure, dyspnea, diaphoresis, hypersensitivity reactions, and anaphylaxis.	Potential adverse reactions to IVIg.
Alert patient's health care provider to significant findings.	To ensure prompt treatment.

●●● **Related NIC and NOC labels:** *NIC:* Bleeding Precautions; Blood Products Administration
NOC: Coagulation Status

Nursing Diagnosis:

Ineffective Cerebral, Peripheral, and Renal Tissue Perfusion

(or risk for same) *related to* interrupted blood flow secondary to presence of thrombotic component, which results in sensitization and clumping of platelets in the blood vessels

Desired Outcome: Patient's cerebral, peripheral, and renal perfusion are adequate as evidenced by no mental status changes; orientation to person, place, and time; normoreactive pupillary responses; absence of headaches, dizziness, and visual disturbances; peripheral pulses >2+ on a 0-4+ scale; and urine output ≥30 ml/hr.

INTERVENTIONS	RATIONALES
Assess for changes in mental status, LOC, and pupillary response.	These changes are indicators of ineffective cerebral tissue perfusion.
Monitor for headaches, dizziness, or visual disturbances.	Same as above.
Palpate peripheral pulses on all extremities. Compare distal extremities for color, warmth, and character of pulses.	Pulse amplitude ≤2+ on a 0-4+ scale is a signal of ineffective peripheral tissue perfusion (thrombosis), as are differences in color, warmth, and pulse character when comparing one extremity to the other.
Assess urine output.	Adequate renal perfusion is reflected by urine output ≥30 ml/hr for 2 consecutive hr.
Monitor I&O. Ensure that patient is well hydrated (2-3 L/day).	To increase perfusion to the small vessels.

●●● **Related NIC and NOC labels:** *NIC:* Neurologic Monitoring; Embolus Care: Peripheral; Fluid Management
NOC: Tissue Perfusion: Cerebral; Tissue Perfusion: Peripheral; Tissue Perfusion: Abdominal Organs

Nursing Diagnosis:

Acute Pain

related to joint discomfort secondary to hemorrhagic episodes or blood extravasation into the tissues

Desired Outcomes: Within 1 hr of intervention, patient's subjective perception of discomfort decreases, as documented by a pain scale. Objective indicators, such as grimacing, are absent or diminished.

INTERVENTIONS	RATIONALES
Monitor patient for presence of joint pain and concomitant problems, including malaise and fatigue. Devise a pain scale with patient, rating discomfort on a scale of 0 (no pain) to 10 (worst pain).	To determine degree and type of discomfort. The pain scale also will help assess degree of relief obtained after treatment/intervention.
Maintain a calm, restful environment.	To promote rest, which will help decrease discomfort and fatigue.
Facilitate coordination of care providers, allowing time for periods of undisturbed rest.	To provide rest periods as needed between care activities.
Elevate legs. Support legs with pillows.	To minimize joint discomfort in lower extremities.
Avoid "gatching" bed at the knee.	To prevent occlusion of popliteal vessels.
Choose chairs with, or provide, padding on seats.	To prevent occlusion of popliteal vessels.
Use a bed cradle; ensure that patient wears socks for warmth.	To decrease pressure on tissues of lower extremities. Decreased circulation results in extremity coolness.
Administer analgesics as prescribed. Document relief obtained, using the pain scale.	To reduce pain.
Caution: Avoid aspirin and other NSAIDs.	These drugs inhibit platelet aggregation, which increases risk of bleeding.
Instruct patient to request analgesic before pain becomes severe.	Pain is more readily controlled when it is treated before it gets severe. Prolonged stimulation of pain receptors results in increased sensitivity to painful stimuli and will increase the amount of drug required to relieve pain.

●●● **Related NIC and NOC labels:** *NIC:* Management; Analgesic Administration; Environmental Management: Comfort; Positioning *NOC:* Comfort Level; Pain Control; Pain: Disruptive Effects; Pain Level

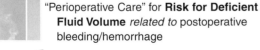

ADDITIONAL NURSING DIAGNOSES/ PROBLEMS:

"Perioperative Care" for **Risk for Deficient**   p. 56
  Fluid Volume *related to* postoperative
  bleeding/hemorrhage

PATIENT-FAMILY TEACHING AND DISCHARGE PLANNING

When providing patient-family teaching, focus on sensory information, avoid giving excessive information, and initiate a visiting nurse referral for necessary follow-up teaching. Include verbal and written information about the following:

✓ Importance of preventing trauma, which can cause bleeding.

✓ Seeking medical attention for *any* signs of infection, especially in patients who are taking steroids or have undergone splenectomy. Steroids suppress the immune response, leaving the patient susceptible to infection, and the spleen is a vital organ in fighting infection. Review signs and symptoms of common infections, such as upper respiratory, urinary tract, and wound infections. Signs and symptoms of common infections are described in "Care of the Renal Transplant Recipient," **Risk for Infection,** p. 268. Also teach patient to assess for signs of bleeding, including hematuria, melena, hematemesis, hemoptysis, menometrorrhagia, oozing from mucous membranes, and petechiae.

✓ Importance of regular medical follow-up for platelet counts.

✓ If patient is discharged taking corticosteroids: side effects of steroids, including weight gain, headache, capillary fragility, hypertension, moon facies, thinning of arms and legs, mood changes, acne, buffalo hump, edema formation, risk of GI hemorrhage, delayed wound healing, and increased appetite. Review need to take medication with food, to immediately take missed doses, and not to precipitously discontinue medication.

✓ Other medications, including drug name, dosage, purpose, schedule, precautions, drug/drug and food/drug interactions, and potential side effects.

✓ Importance of obtaining a Medic-Alert bracelet and identification card outlining diagnosis and emergency treatment. Contact the following organization:

Medic Alert
2323 Colorado Avenue
Turlock, CA 95382
(209) 668-3333
www.medicalert.org

Amputation

Amputation, the removal of part or all of a limb through bone, is now less frequently performed as an orthopaedic surgical intervention than it was before advances in antibiotic therapy, treatment for musculoskeletal neoplasms, and microsurgery/limb salvage techniques. Lower extremity amputation may still be the treatment of choice for complications of diabetes mellitus (DM), such as peripheral vascular disease, and for osteomyelitis or severe trauma. On rare occasions, amputation may be necessary because of congenital limb deficiencies in infants and children.

HEALTH CARE SETTING

Critical care unit, acute care surgical unit, orthopaedic rehabilitation unit

ASSESSMENT

Chronic disease: The patient with advanced peripheral vascular disease often complains of pain and may have gangrene, a chronic venous stasis ulcer, or an infected wound that fails to heal. The affected limb is often a dark red color (rubor) when it is dependent; atrophy of skin and subcutaneous tissue may be apparent.

Trauma: A mangled extremity is common with high-energy injuries. The patient may have multiple injuries, and surgical priority must be given to those injuries that may be life threatening. Trauma may result in a complete amputation, a near or partial amputation, or a segmental amputation of an extremity.

DIAGNOSTIC TESTS

Doppler ultrasound: The most commonly used diagnostic method to document lack of perfusion.

Transcutaneous O_2 pressure: Measured after oxygen sensors are applied to the skin. By determining oxygen tension (desired value is 30-50 mm Hg), the surgeon can map out areas of lesser perfusion in the affected extremity. This test offers the most accurate assessment of blood supply and the best prediction of residual limb healing potential.

Plethysmography: Enables evaluation of arterial flow through performance of segmental systolic blood pressure measurements.

Angiography: Confirms circulatory impairment to determine the appropriate level for amputation. This invasive study involves radiographic imaging after injection of a radiopaque substance into a blood vessel. It is most useful if the patient is a candidate for angioplasty or arterial reconstruction.

Xenon-133: A radioactive isotope injected intradermally at the midpoint of the intended incision for amputation. Skin clearance of this agent reflects skin blood flow as a measure of the appropriate level of amputation.

Fluorescein fluorometry: Determines nutritive blood flow to an affected area through monitoring by a fiberoptic fluorometer after systemic injection with fluorescein (fluorescent) dye.

Nursing Diagnosis:

Risk for Disuse Syndrome

related to severe pain and immobility secondary to amputation

Desired Outcomes: Within 24 hr of instruction, patient verbalizes accurate understanding of the prescribed exercise regimen and performs exercises independently. Patient is free of symptoms of contracture as evidenced by complete range of motion (ROM) of joints and maintenance of muscle mass.

INTERVENTIONS	RATIONALES
Manage patient's pain.	To encourage optimal movement. Early movement and ambulation help in the prevention of flexion contractures. An early return to activity also prevents loss of muscle strength and increases local circulation to improve wound healing.
If prescribed, elevate affected extremity for first 24 hr postoperatively.	During the first 24 hr after surgery, elevation decreases swelling. Elevation is discontinued after this period to prevent hip flexion contracture.
Caution: Do *not* elevate a residual limb with deficient vascular supply.	Elevating a limb with deficient vascular supply would compromise circulation even further.
Assist in performance of ROM exercises.	To promote mobility of proximal joints.
On the second postoperative day, ensure that patient keeps residual limb flat when at rest. Assist patient with lying prone for 1 hr qid and teach patient to perform prescribed exercises.	These are strategies for preventing contracture formation and increasing strength of muscle extensors. Prescribed exercises may include the following: - Above-knee amputation (AKA): Patient attempts to straighten hip from a flexed position against resistance or perform gluteal setting exercises. - Below-knee amputation (BKA): Patient attempts to straighten knee against resistance or perform quadriceps exercises. Patient also should perform exercises for AKA.

●●● **Related NIC and NOC labels:** *NIC:* Exercise Therapy: Joint Mobility; Exercise Therapy: Muscle Control; Positioning; Pain Management; Teaching: Prescribed Activity/Exercise *NOC:* Immobility Consequences: Physiological; Mobility Level

Nursing Diagnosis:

Deficient Knowledge:

Care of the residual limb and prosthesis; signs and symptoms of skin irritation or pressure necrosis

Desired Outcomes: Within 24 hr of hospital discharge, patient verbalizes accurate knowledge about care of the residual limb and prosthesis and independently returns demonstration of wrapping the residual limb. Patient verbalizes knowledge about indicators of pressure necrosis and irritation from the shrinkage device or prosthesis.

INTERVENTIONS	RATIONALES
Explain to patient the importance of elevating the residual limb as prescribed for the first 24 hr after surgery.	To reduce edema.
Explain that after the first 24 hr, the lower residual limb should be kept flat when patient is at rest in bed.	To reduce risk of flexion contracture.
Teach application of a shrinkage device such as an elastic wrap or sock.	A shrinkage device molds the residual limb in patients for whom prosthesis fitting is prescribed. Application of elastic wrap is begun with a recurrent turn over distal end of residual limb; then diagonal circumferential turns are made, overlapping to two-thirds the width of the wrap.

Continued

INTERVENTIONS	RATIONALES
Caution patient to wrap the shrinkage device snugly but not tightly.	If the device were wrapped too tightly, it would impede circulation and healing.
Teach patient that all tissue must be contained by the elastic wrap.	If any tissue is allowed to bulge, proper fitting of prosthesis will be difficult.
Demonstrate use of extra padding with moleskin or lamb's wool.	Extra padding prevents irritation to areas that are susceptible to pressure.
Teach patient to remove the shrinkage device q4h and monitor residual limb for abrasions, blisters, and hair follicle infection.	These are indicators of skin irritations or pressure necrosis caused by shrinkage device or prosthesis.
Explain that if erythema persists, patient should notify health care provider.	Persistent erythema may be an early sign of pressure sore development.
As indicated, instruct patient to leave any open areas on residual limb exposed to air for 1-hr periods qid.	To facilitate healing. While some surgeons request that the wound remain covered, others leave the wound exposed to air after the original dressing has been removed.
Teach a daily routine of skin cleansing with soap and water.	Soap and water have adequate antibacterial effects. Washing also helps toughen skin on the residual limb in preparation for wearing the prosthesis.
Instruct patient to dry residual limb thoroughly before any shrinkage device is applied.	Retained moisture can cause skin maceration, which would contribute to fungal growth.
Explain that the shrinkage device must be changed daily, washed with mild soap and water, and dried thoroughly before reapplication.	Use of a soiled shrinkage device can contribute to wound infection.
Instruct patient to begin to massage residual limb 3 wk postoperatively.	To desensitize the area. Massage will break up adherent scar tissue and prepare skin for stress of prosthesis wear.
Ensure that patient receives complete instructions in care of prosthesis by a certified prosthetist-orthotist or nurse expert.	Patient needs to be encouraged to accept the residual limb and become adept at self-care to be independent as quickly as possible.

●●● **Related NIC and NOC labels:** *NIC:* Teaching: Procedure/Treatment; Teaching: Psychomotor Skill
NOC: Knowledge: Treatment Procedures; Knowledge: Treatment Regimen

Nursing Diagnosis:

Acute Pain or Chronic Pain

related to amputation surgery and postoperative phantom limb sensation

Desired Outcome: Within 24 hr of intervention, patient's subjective perception of pain decreases as documented by a pain intensity rating scale.

INTERVENTIONS	RATIONALES
Ensure adequate pain management before elective surgery.	To decrease likelihood that phantom limb sensation will develop. Patient with unrelieved preoperative pain is more likely to experience phantom limb sensation.
Explain that continued sensations often arise postoperatively from amputated part and may be painful, irritating, or simply disconcerting.	To provide knowledge, which will help patient prepare for the experience of phantom limb sensation.

Continued

INTERVENTIONS	RATIONALES
Assist in use of a pain intensity rating scale to evaluate pain and analgesic relief on a scale of 0 (no pain) to 10 (worst pain imaginable).	Enables more accurate documentation of pain and subsequent relief obtained after analgesia has been administered.
Administer prescribed medications (usually not opioids) and document their effectiveness using pain intensity rating scale.	Although opioids provide effective treatment of incisional pain, they may be ineffective for phantom limb sensation because they do not alter response of afferent nerves to noxious stimuli.
Administer β-blockers such as propranolol as prescribed.	May be used to control a constant dull ache by increasing serotonin levels and thus preventing pain transmission to the brain.
Administer anticonvulsants such as phenytoin and carbamazepine as prescribed.	May be used to treat stabbing pain.
Administer baclofen as prescribed.	May be used to control spasms and cramps in the phantom limb.
Administer tricyclic antidepressants (e.g., amitriptyline, doxepin) as prescribed.	May be used to elevate mood and alleviate insomnia.
Apply Capsaicin cream near the surgical wound if prescribed.	May be used as a topical analgesic.
Teach patient to use counterirritation (e.g., transcutaneous electrical nerve stimulation [TENS]) as indicated.	May provide effective short-term management of phantom limb sensation.
Also consider interventions such as distraction, guided imagery, relaxation, and biofeedback.	Nonpharmacologic methods that augment pharmacologic pain relief.
Instruct patient to begin to massage residual limb 3 wk postoperatively.	To desensitize the area in preparation for prosthesis. Early prosthesis may reduce incidence of phantom limb sensation.
	After surgical wound healing is complete, vigorous stimulation of end of residual limb may be prescribed. This can be accomplished by hitting end of the limb with a rolled towel.
Encourage patient to consider other modalities, including sympathetic blocking agents, acupuncture, ultrasound, and injection with local anesthetics.	To decrease phantom limb sensation.
If indicated, refer patient to a pain clinic.	For a comprehensive program to manage chronic phantom limb sensation.
Explore impact that phantom limb pain can have on patient's ability to function on the job or in interpersonal relationships.	Attempts to cope with chronic pain can deplete patient's resources, leaving little energy for job and relationships.
As indicated, encourage patient to discuss possible surgical interventions (e.g., cordotomy, deep brain stimulation, spinal cord stimulation, sympathectomy) with health care provider.	For patients in whom conservative measures are exhausted and phantom limb sensations continue.

●●● **Related NIC and NOC labels:** *NIC:* Medication Management; Pain Management; Biofeedback; Positioning; Simple Guided Imagery; Simple Massage; Simple Relaxation Therapy; Transcutaneous Electrical Nerve Stimulation; Cutaneous Stimulation; Distraction *NOC:* Comfort Level; Pain Control; Pain: Disruptive Effects; Depression Control

Nursing Diagnoses:

Disturbed Body Image and/or Ineffective Role Performance

related to loss of limb

Desired Outcome: Within 72 hr of surgery, patient begins to show adaptation to loss of limb and demonstrates interest in resuming role–related responsibilities.

INTERVENTIONS	RATIONALES
Perform a psychologic assessment. Support patient in psychosocial recovery following amputation.	Whether the amputation is the result of trauma, chronic illness, or cancer, the patient is likely to experience a period of grieving. Disbelief and anger often mark the initial response. The patient may believe attainment of independence and future goals is impossible. Insomnia and somatic complaints are common. Later, as the patient begins to adjust to the amputation, sadness and tears are often observed.
Gently encourage patient to look at and touch residual limb and verbalize feelings about the amputation. Provide privacy for patient and significant other to express feelings regarding the amputation.	The patient typically will have a stereotyped image of disability and unattractiveness following amputation. Sometimes these emotions are suppressed during rehabilitation and reemerge as time passes. Addressing stereotypical thinking early in recovery and actively involving patient in education will help provide patient with a sense of participation and control. All caregivers must show an accepting attitude and encourage significant other to accept patient's new appearance.
Encourage use of a prosthesis if prescribed immediately after surgery.	To enable patient to be fully ambulatory (and thus "whole").
Introduce patient to others who have successfully adapted to a similar amputation.	This strategy assists patients with adapting to loss of limb while maintaining a sense of what is perceived as the normal self. Teaching aids such as books, pamphlets, audiovisuals, and videotapes can be used to demonstrate how others have adapted to amputation.
Discuss ways that patient may alter task performance to continue to function in vocational and interpersonal roles.	Assistive devices may be needed for continued functioning in current vocational role. If patient's health status precludes continued performance in the current vocational role, referral and counseling for retraining may be needed.
For patient who continues to have difficulty adapting to the amputation, provide a referral to an appropriate resource person such as a psychologist or psychiatric nurse.	Trained professionals can help explore the impact that amputation and phantom limb sensation are having on patient's life and review strategies for adaptation.

●●● **Related NIC and NOC labels:** *NIC:* Body Image Enhancement; Amputation Care; Coping Enhancement; Grief Work Facilitation; Counseling; Support Group; Role Enhancement; Normalization Promotion *NOC:* Body Image; Psychosocial Adjustment: Life Change; Coping; Role Performance

ADDITIONAL NURSING DIAGNOSES/ PROBLEMS:

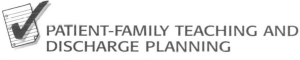

PATIENT-FAMILY TEACHING AND DISCHARGE PLANNING

When providing patient-family teaching, focus on sensory information, avoid giving excessive information, and make appropriate referrals (e.g., visiting or home health nurse, community health resources) for follow-up teaching. Include verbal and written information about the following:

✓ Medications and supplements, including name, dosage, purpose, schedule, precautions, drug/drug and food/drug interactions, and potential side effects.

✓ How and where to purchase necessary supplies and equipment for self-care.

✓ Care of residual limb and prosthesis.

✓ Indicators of wound infection that require medical attention such as swelling, persistent redness, purulent discharge, local warmth, systemic fever, and pain.

✓ Use of a small hand mirror if needed to examine incision and residual limb.

✓Prescribed exercise regimen, including rationale for each exercise, number of repetitions for each, and frequency of exercise periods.

✓Ambulation with assistive devices and prosthesis on level and uneven surfaces and on stairs. Patient should demonstrate independence before hospital discharge. For patient with upper extremity amputation, independence with performance of activities of daily living (ADL) should be demonstrated before discharge.

✓Importance of follow-up care, date of next appointment, and a telephone number to call if questions arise.

✓Referral to visiting/public health or home health nurses as necessary for ongoing care after discharge. Also consider referral to appropriate resource person if patient has continued difficulty with grief or body image disturbance.

✓Referral to community resources, including local amputation support activities.

Amputee Resource Foundation of America
6480 Wayzata Blvd.
Golden Valley, MN 55426
(612) 812-7875
www.amputeeresource.org

Fractures

A fracture is a break in the continuity of a bone. It occurs when stress is placed on the bone that exceeds the bone's biologic loading capacity. Most commonly, the stress is the result of trauma. Pathologic fractures can occur when the bone's decreased loading capacity cannot tolerate even normal stress, as with osteoporosis.

HEALTH CARE SETTING

Emergency care, acute care, primary care

PHYSICAL ASSESSMENT

Physical findings: Include loss of normal bony or limb contours, edema, ecchymosis, limb shortening, decreased range of motion (ROM) of adjacent joints, and false motion (occurs outside a joint). The patient may describe crepitus, but this should not be elicited by the health care provider because of risk of injury to surrounding soft tissues and bone fragments. Complicated or complex fractures can present with signs and symptoms of perforated internal organs, neurovascular dysfunction, joint effusion, or excessive joint laxity. Open fractures involve a break in the skin and will demonstrate a wound in the area of suspected fracture, or bone may be exposed in the wound.

Acute indicators: Fractures may cause insidious and progressive pain. Sudden onset of severe pain usually is associated with trauma or physical stress, such as jogging, strenuous exercise, or a fall. In the event of pathologic fracture, the patient typically describes signs and symptoms associated with the underlying pathologic condition.

Complications: Chronic fracture can result from *delayed union,* which is failure of bone fragments to unite within the normally accepted time frame for that bone's healing. *Nonunion* is demonstrated by nonalignment and lost function secondary to lost bony rigidity. *Pseudoarthrosis* is a state in which the fracture fails to heal and a false joint develops at the fracture site. *Avascular necrosis* occurs when the fracture interrupts the blood supply to a segment of bone, which eventually dies. *Myositis ossificans* involves heterotrophic bone formation (abnormal, out of the normal area) and occurs most commonly in the arms, thighs, and hips. *Complex regional pain syndrome* (formerly known as reflex sympathetic dystrophy) is an incompletely understood process that results in chronic pain out of proportion to the injury, reduced function, joint stiffness, and trophic changes in soft tissue and skin following a traumatic event such as a fracture. Other fracture complications include altered sensation, limb length discrepancies, and chronic lymphatic or venous stasis. **Note:** Any patient with a suspected fracture should be treated as though a fracture is present until it is ruled out. Interventions should include immobilization of the affected area and careful monitoring of neurovascular function distal to the injury. Any restrictions to swelling (e.g., rings, wristwatches, bracelets) should be removed before they can contribute to neurovascular dysfunction.

DIAGNOSTIC TESTS

Most fractures are identified easily with standard anteroposterior (AP) and lateral x-rays. Occasionally, special radiographic views are needed, such as the mortise view with bimalleolar ankle fractures (showing the joint spaces between the fibula, tibia, and talus) or x-rays through the open mouth to identify fractures of the odontoid process. Magnetic resonance imaging (MRI) may be useful in evaluating complicated fractures, but its ability to identify different bone densities is limited. Intraarticular fractures may be diagnosed with arthroscopy. Bone scans, computed tomography (CT) scans, tomograms, stereoscopic films, and arthrograms can also be used.

Nursing Diagnosis:

Dressing/Grooming, Bathing/Hygiene Self-Care Deficit

related to physical limitations secondary to cast, immobilizer, or orthotic devices

Desired Outcome: Within 48 hr of initiation of immobilization, patient demonstrates independence with activities of daily living (ADL).

INTERVENTIONS	RATIONALES
Incorporate a structured exercise regimen that will increase strength and endurance. Direct the regimen toward development of those muscle groups needed for patient's specific activity deficit.	Patients with insufficient strength to manipulate immobilized extremities need planned exercise to assist them in managing self-care while in a cast or immobilizer. Increased strength and endurance contribute to independence in self-care.
Use assistive devices liberally.	Use of appropriate assistive devices maximizes patient's ability to be independent in self-care. These may include a sock donner, long-handled reacher, enlarged handles on eating utensils, and elevated toilet seat.
As appropriate, use adaptive clothing (e.g., garments with Velcro fasteners).	Adaptive clothing accommodates a cast or external fixator and also makes dressing easier.
As indicated, refer patient to occupational therapy.	The occupational therapist is able to evaluate patient's need for dressing/grooming aids. Sock donners, long-handled reachers and brushes, raised toilet seats, and other devices may help minimize stress on joints. Clothing also can be adapted to encourage independence in dressing (e.g., zipper pulls, Velcro closures).
As indicated, refer to care management/social services department of hospital.	Patient may require assistance with funding for purchasing assistive equipment or arranging home help. Care management/social services staff are also aware of community agencies that loan equipment or have other volunteer services.
Ensure that patient receives appropriate treatment as prescribed for pain.	Unrelieved pain can severely limit patient's mobility in a cast or immobilizer, making performance of self-care tasks difficult or impossible.
When needed, teach significant other how to assist patient with self-care activities.	Although independence with self-care is the goal, involvement of the significant other can minimize need for skilled home services. A knowledgeable significant other also can reinforce professional health instructions given to patient.

●●● **Related NIC and NOC labels:** *NIC:* Self-Care Assistance: Bathing/Hygiene; Self-Responsibility Facilitation; Exercise Promotion: Muscle Control; Self-Care Assistance: Dressing/Grooming; Pain Management *NOC:* Self-Care Activities of Daily Living

Nursing Diagnoses:

Risk for Impaired Skin Integrity and/or Impaired Tissue Integrity

related to irritation and pressure secondary to presence of an immobilization device (e.g., cast, splint)

Desired Outcomes: Within 8 hr of immobilization device application, patient verbalizes knowledge about indicators of pressure necrosis. Patient relates the absence of discomfort under immobilization device and exhibits intact skin when the device is removed.

INTERVENTIONS	RATIONALES
When assisting with application of cast or other immobilization device, ensure that adequate padding is put on bony prominences of affected extremity.	Bony prominences are at risk for skin breakdown. Padding decreases pressure over these areas.
While a cast is drying, handle it only with palms of the hands.	Handling a wet cast with fingers can cause indentations that create pressure points on underlying skin. Using palms of the hands ensures a smooth surface as the cast dries and decreases likelihood of underlying pressure points.
Petal edges of plaster casts with tape or moleskin.	Petalling prevents cast crumbs from falling into cast. These crumbs can cause pressure areas or skin irritation/impairment.
Pad surfaces of other immobilization devices.	Padding decreases pressure on skin underneath the devices.
Instruct patient never to insert anything between immobilization device and skin (e.g., coat hanger or stick). In presence of severe itching, advise patient to notify health care provider, who may prescribe a medication to relieve itching.	Use of a coat hanger or stick can cause skin irritation that leads to infection. It also may cause bunching of the cotton material placed between the cast and skin, which would result in pressure points under the cast.
Teach indicators of pressure necrosis under immobilization device such as pain, numbness/tingling, burning sensation, foul odor from opening, or drainage on the device.	An informed individual is more likely to report these findings quickly, which will enable prompt treatment to avoid further impairment.

●●● **Related NIC and NOC labels:** *NIC:* Pressure Management; Skin Surveillance; Circulatory Precautions; Cast Care Management; Traction/Immobilization Care *NOC:* Tissue Integrity: Skin and Mucous Membranes

Nursing Diagnosis:

Deficient Knowledge:

Function of external fixation, performance of pin care, and signs and symptoms of pin site infection

Desired Outcomes: By at least 24 hr before hospital discharge, patient verbalizes accurate knowledge of rationale for the external fixator and indicators of pin site infection. Patient also demonstrates performance of pin care.

INTERVENTIONS	RATIONALES
Teach rationale for use of fixator with type of fracture or injury, emphasizing patient benefits.	A patient who is knowledgeable about essential parts of the device and their purposes is more likely to handle the device judiciously to ensure bone fragment immobilization. External fixation consists of skeletal pins that penetrate the fracture fragments and are attached to universal joints. These joints are in turn attached to rods, which provide stabilization and form a frame around the fractured limb for immobilization.
Instruct patient and significant other in pin care as prescribed by health care provider. If prescribed, teach patient and significant other how to apply antibacterial ointments and small dressings to pin sites.	For external fixator pins, some health care providers require daily cleansing with dilute hydrogen peroxide or other skin preparation solution; iodine-based mixtures may cause corrosion of some fixation devices. Some health care providers request that buildup of crusts from serous drainage be removed when cleansing pin sites, whereas others request that crusts be left intact to minimize risk of infection.

Continued

INTERVENTIONS	RATIONALES
Instruct patient and significant other to avoid using external fixator as a handle or support for moving extremity.	Repeated use of external fixator in this manner may lead to loosening of skeletal pins and loss of bone fragment immobilization.
Teach patient and significant other to support extremity with pillows, two hands, slings, and other devices as necessary.	Adequate support of the extremity prevents stress on skeletal pins. Stress on pins can contribute to loosening and loss of bone fragment immobilization.
Teach patient to monitor pin sites for persistent redness, swelling, drainage, increasing pain, and local warmth. Explain that monitoring should also include systemic indicator of temperature >101° F (38.3° C).	Patient and/or significant other must recognize signs of infection and report them to health care provider for prompt evaluation and treatment.
If an orthotic is used with the external fixator, teach patient and/or significant other its purpose and care.	Orthotics may be added to the external fixator to prevent wristdrop, footdrop, contracture, or other joint dysfunction. Device should be kept clean and dry to decrease risk for infection at pin sites.
Advise patient of need for maintaining adequate immobilization of the fracture and for follow-up care to ensure that device is functioning properly.	Failure to immoblize the fracture adequately may lead to delayed union, malunion, or nonunion. Follow-up assessment of the device will ensure that fracture immobilization is maintained.

●●● **Related NIC and NOC labels:** *NIC:* Teaching: Procedure/Treatment; Teaching: Individual
NOC: Knowledge: Illness Care

Nursing Diagnosis:

Constipation

related to decreased mobility and use of opioid analgesics

Desired Outcomes: Within 8 hr of immobilization device application, patient verbalizes accurate understanding of strategies to maintain normal bowel elimination. Patient maintains bowel elimination in his/her normal pattern.

INTERVENTIONS	RATIONALES
Teach patient about current influences on bowel elimination.	Decreased mobility, use of opioid analgesics, and inconsistent food intake are examples of situations that can adversely influence bowel elimination.
Encourage choice of diet items that will facilitate normal bowel elimination.	Such high-fiber foods as bran, whole grains, nuts, raw and coarse vegetables, and fruits with skins add bulk to stool to promote bowel elimination.
If not contraindicated, encourage patient to drink ample fluids.	Fluid intake helps to promote soft stool.
If patient desires, request prescription for stool softener and/or bulk-forming laxative.	Pharmacologic intervention may be needed to maintain normal bowel elimination.
Encourage mobility to the extent of prescribed activity parameters.	Mobility promotes peristalsis and hence improves bowel elimination. Because of this, the patient should not be left in bed or allowed to use a bedside commode if he or she can tolerate additional mobility.

●●● **Related NIC and NOC labels:** *NIC:* Bowel Management; Exercise Promotion; Fluid Management;
Nutrition Management *NOC:* Bowel Elimination; Hydration

Nursing Diagnosis:

Acute Pain

related to surgical repair and rehabilitation therapy

Desired Outcomes: Within 1–2 hr of intervention, patient's subjective perception of pain decreases as documented by a pain intensity rating scale. Patient demonstrates ability to perform ADL with minimal complaints of discomfort.

INTERVENTIONS	RATIONALES
Assist in use of a pain intensity rating scale to evaluate pain and analgesic relief on a scale of 0 (no pain) to 10 (worst pain imaginable).	Use of a pain intensity scale allows more accurate documentation of pain and subsequent relief obtained after analgesia has been administered. The patient provides a personal baseline report, enabling nurse to more effectively monitor subsequent increases and decreases in pain.
If intraarticular anesthetic or opioid was administered intraoperatively, advise patient that lack of pain in the immediate postoperative period should *not* be mistaken for ability to move the joint excessively.	Patients with minimal postoperative pain may be tempted to become overly active, thereby putting unnecessary stress on the fracture site. Prescribed activity must be carefully followed to avoid additional injury to the affected extremity.
If appropriate, instruct hospitalized surgical patient in use of patient-controlled analgesia (PCA) or epidural analgesia. Verify with another nurse that PCA or epidural pump contains prescribed medication and concentration with prescribed settings for patient dosing, continuous infusion, and/or clinician-activated bolus.	Understanding principles of PCA or epidural analgesia will help patient obtain better pain management. Verification of the pump settings is critical to the safe delivery of the analgesia.
If PCA or epidural analgesia is used, monitor effectiveness of patient's pain management while observing for excessive sedation, respiratory depression, and decreased level of consciousness. Keep appropriate reversal agent readily available.	Excessive sedation may necessitate administration of appropriate reversal agent. Most commonly, naloxone is used for opioid-induced side effects, and ephedrine is given for hypotensive crisis associated with epidural administration of anesthetics such as bupivacaine.
As prescribed, administer nonsteroidal antiinflammatory drugs (NSAIDs) and monitor effectiveness of patient's pain management, as well as adverse effects.	Because of potential for excessive bleeding following NSAID administration, it is important to monitor for hemorrhage at surgical site.
Avoid giving NSAIDs if patient is receiving epidural analgesia.	NSAIDs should not be prescribed during administration of epidural analgesia because of risk of bleeding into the epidural space, which may cause lower extremity impairment through pressure on spinal nerves.
Advise patient to coordinate time of peak effectiveness of analgesics with periods of exercise or ambulation.	Careful timing of analgesics enables patient to achieve optimal pain relief before exercise or ambulation. Participation in the exercise regimen contributes to expediency of patient's recovery.
Teach patient to use nonpharmacologic methods of pain management, including guided imagery, relaxation, massage, distraction, biofeedback, heat or cold therapy, and music therapy.	Nonpharmacologic methods can augment pharmacologic pain management strategies. These methods may be critical for a patient who is resistant to use of analgesics.
Supplement other pain management strategies with traditional nursing interventions such as back rubs and repositioning. Encourage patient to verbalize feelings regarding pain experience and impact of the injury.	Traditional nursing interventions augment the effects of analgesics or nonpharmacologic pain management strategies. In addition, verbalization helps patient examine strategies for coping with pain following injury.

●●● **Related NIC and NOC labels:** *NIC:* Medication Management: Pain Management; Analgesic Administration; Biofeedback; Patient-Controlled Analgesic Assistance; Simple Guided Imagery; Simple Massage; Simple Relaxation Therapy; Distraction; Heat/Cold Application; Music Therapy *NOC:* Comfort Level; Pain Control; Pain Level

Nursing Diagnosis:

Risk for Peripheral Neurovascular Dysfunction

related to interruption of capillary blood flow secondary to increased pressure within the myofascial compartment (compartment syndrome)

Desired Outcomes: Patient has adequate peripheral neurovascular function in the involved extremity as evidenced by normal muscle tone, brisk (<2 sec) capillary refill (or capillary refill consistent with the contralateral extremity), normal tissue pressures (<15 mm Hg), minimal edema or tautness, and absence of paresthesia. Patient verbalizes understanding of the importance of reporting symptoms indicative of impaired neurovascular function.

INTERVENTIONS	RATIONALES
Monitor neurovascular status at regular intervals by checking temperature (circulation), movement, and sensation in affected extremity.	The most reliable physical indicators of compartment syndrome include sensory deficits (loss of two-point discrimination), decreased sensation to light touch or pinprick, and decreased proprioception. Edema is occasionally visible, and muscles are stiff on palpation. Distal to the injury the extremity may be pale and cool. Weakness in affected muscle groups may precede pseudoparalysis, which is caused by patient's avoidance of movements that stress the involved compartment. Pulselessness and true paralysis are late findings.
Apply ice and elevate affected extremity when prescribed.	A fractured limb is elevated to promote venous return. Ice is applied to cause vasoconstriction in the area of injury, which decreases edema and aids in pain management. Because edema can contribute to development of compartment syndrome, these interventions may be critical.
Caution: When acute compartment syndrome is suspected, however, avoid use of ice and elevation.	Ice and elevation may further compromise vascular supply in an extremity that is already experiencing ischemia secondary to developing compartment syndrome.
Teach patient and significant other symptoms of neurovascular compromise that should be immediately reported.	Any changes in temperature, sensation, or ability to move digits of affected extremity are indicators of neurovascular compromise. Awareness of the risk of compartment syndrome will enable patient to respond more quickly to possible symptoms and reduce delay in treatment.
Monitor tissue pressures as prescribed if an intracompartmental pressure device is available. Alert health care provider to pressures >15 mm Hg.	Sustained high pressures may indicate developing compartment syndrome; if pressures exceed systolic BP, perfusion to the extremity is threatened. Continued monitoring of high-risk patients should be done to avoid possible complications (e.g., adolescents or young adults with traumatic injury; confused or developmentally disabled patients who cannot accurately report symptoms).
In response to changes in neurovascular condition, contact health care provider promptly. Adjust constricting device as prescribed (e.g., bivalving cast, loosening elastic wrap around splint) to relieve pressure over affected extremity.	When swelling places patient at risk for acute compartment syndrome, the constricting device (e.g., cast, splint, circumferential dressing) must be loosened down to skin level to prevent further swelling and compromise to the affected extremity.
Wrap a dressing carefully around the split cast.	Dressings maintain adequate immobilization until further interventions can be made.

●●● **Related NIC and NOC labels:** *NIC:* Peripheral Sensation Management; Positioning: Neurologic; Risk Identification; Circulatory Care: Venous Insufficiency; Circulatory Precautions; Pressure Management
NOC: Neurological Status: Spinal Sensory/Motor Function; Tissue Perfusion: Peripheral

Nursing Diagnosis:

Impaired Physical Mobility

related to musculoskeletal pain and use of immobilization devices

Desired Outcomes: By at least 24 hr before hospital discharge, patient maintains appropriate body alignment with external fixation devices in place or demonstrates setup and use of home traction device. Patient verbalizes accurate understanding of use of analgesics and adjunctive methods to decrease pain.

INTERVENTIONS	RATIONALES
Teach patient proper body alignment when applying and using external fixation device, most commonly with joints in neutral position.	Maintenance of neutral position decreases risk of contracture formation, which would affect patient's mobility.
If orthotic devices are used to maintain position, teach exercises and ROM to do when the device is removed.	Prolonged use of the orthotic can cause impaired joint mobility. Exercise at regular intervals will help maintain joint flexibility.
Teach patient and significant other active and/or passive ROM of adjacent joints q8h as appropriate.	ROM exercises help preserve joint mobility and decrease risk of contracture formation.
When appropriate, teach patient and significant other principles of traction and signs and symptoms of complications (e.g., pressure necrosis, impaired neurovascular function).	A knowledgeable patient should be able to identify basic problems associated with the fixator, demonstrate performance of prescribed exercises while in fixator, demonstrate and describe assessment of neurovascular status of the limb, and describe and assess pin sites for signs of infection. Knowledge in these areas will help to ensure optimal healing and prompt treatment in the event of problems.
Instruct patient and significant other in care of an extremity in external fixator.	A knowledgeable patient should be able to identify basic problems associated with the fixator, demonstrate performance of prescribed exercises while in fixator, demonstrate and describe assessment of neurovascular status of the limb, and describe and assess pin sites for signs of infection. Knowledge in these areas will help to ensure optimal healing and prompt treatment in the event of problems.
Instruct patient and significant other in care of casted extremity.	A knowledgeable patient should be able to demonstrate cast care, demonstrate and describe assessment of neurovascular status of the distal extremity, describe assessment of evidence of pressure necrosis beneath cast, demonstrate performance of prescribed exercises, and describe prevention of skin maceration and disuse osteoporosis to ensure optimal healing and prompt treatment in the event of problems.
Instruct patient and significant other in use of analgesics and nonpharmacologic pain management methods.	Effective pain management will increase patient's ability to participate in appropriate exercise and activity.

●●● **Related NIC and NOC labels:** *NIC:* Exercise Therapy: Joint Mobility; Exercise Therapy: Muscle Control; Body Mechanics Promotion; Teaching: Prescribed Activity/Exercise; Pain Management; Positioning; Traction/Immobilization Care; Cast Care: Maintenance; Circulatory Precautions; Neurologic Monitoring; Pressure Management; Skin Surveillance *NOC:* Mobility Level

PATIENT-FAMILY TEACHING AND DISCHARGE PLANNING

When providing patient–family teaching, focus on sensory information, avoid giving excessive information, and make appropriate referrals (e.g., visiting or home health nurse, community health resources) for follow-up teaching. Include verbal and written information about the following:

✓ Medications and supplements, including name, dosage, purpose, schedule, precautions, drug/drug and food/drug interactions, and potential side effects.

✓ Use of nonpharmacologic methods of pain management.

✓ Appropriate use of elevation and thermotherapy.

✓ Importance of performing prescribed exercises.

✓ Rationale for therapy (i.e., casting, external fixation, internal fixation).

✓ Precautions of therapy:

- *Casts:* caring for cast, monitoring neurovascular function of distal extremity and for evidence of pressure necrosis beneath cast, preventing skin maceration, preventing disuse osteoporosis.

- *Internal fixation devices:* caring for wound, noting signs of wound infection and monitoring for delayed infection, following appropriate weight-bearing prescription for lower extremity fracture.

- *External fixator:* demonstrating pin care, monitoring pin sites for signs of infection, knowing when to notify health care provider of problems with fixator, using prescribed orthotics, monitoring neurovascular function of distal extremity.

✓ Use of assistive devices/ambulatory aids. Ensure that patient can perform return demonstration and is independent with devices/aids before hospital discharge.

✓ Materials necessary for wound care at home, with names of agencies that can provide additional supplies.

✓ Importance of follow-up care, date of next appointment, and telephone number to call if questions arise.

✓ For all patients who receive allograft bone for bone graft and who have questions about these grafts, resources for information include the following organizations:

American Red Cross
Tissue Services
(888) 4-TISSUE
Local chapter contact information is available on national website.
www.redcross.org/services/biomed/tissue/

AlloSource
6278 S. Troy Circle
Centennial, CO 80111
(888) 873-8330
www.allosource.org

Osteoarthritis

Osteoarthritis (OA) is the most prevalent articular disease in adults 65 and older. Formerly known as degenerative joint disease (DJD) or degenerative arthritis, OA is now viewed as a process in which all joint structures produce new tissue in response to joint injury or cartilage destruction. It is a chronic, progressive disease characterized by increasing pain, deformity, and loss of function.

OA may be classified as either *idiopathic or secondary*. Previously known as primary OA, idiopathic osteoarthritis occurs in individuals with no history of joint injury or disease or of systemic illness that might contribute to the development of arthritis. Aging is probably one influence on the deterioration of cartilage in arthritic joints, but additional evidence suggests the existence of an autosomal recessive trait for gene defects that causes premature cartilage destruction. In contrast, secondary osteoarthritis has an identifiable cause. Any condition or event that directly damages or overloads articular cartilage or causes joint instability can result in arthritic changes. Secondary OA typically occurs in younger individuals because of congenital processes (e.g., Legg-Calvé-Perthes disease), trauma, repetitive occupational stress, joint hemorrhage, or infection.

HEALTH CARE SETTING

Primary care

ASSESSMENT

Signs and symptoms: Joint pain and stiffness are typically the dominant symptoms and the most common reasons for seeking medical evaluation. However, because the onset of pain is typically insidious, the patient may not be able to recall exactly when it began, often describing an "aching" asymmetric pain that increases with joint use and is relieved by rest, especially in early stages of OA. As the disease progresses, night pain or pain at rest is likely to occur. The patient may also confirm that pain increases with the fall in barometric pressure that precedes inclement weather. Joint stiffness ranges from slowness to pain with initial movement. Early morning stiffness is common but typically lasts <30 min. Stiffness after periods of rest or inactivity *(articular gelling or gel phenomenon)* is also characteristic of OA but resolves within several minutes. The patient may describe a squeaking, creaking, or grating with movement *(crepitus)* caused by loose cartilage particles in the joint capsule.

Physical assessment: Pairs of joints should be compared for symmetry, size, shape, color, appearance, temperature, and pain. Affected joints are likely to be tender to palpation. Reduced range of motion (ROM) is extremely common in osteoarthritic joints and contributes to the patient's overall disability. Limited movement or locking during movement may be accentuated by mild effusion and soft tissue swelling; large effusions are uncommon in OA. Crepitation during passive movement is present in >90% of patients with knee OA and indicates loss of cartilage integrity. Almost 50% of patients with knee OA have a varus deformity resulting from cartilage loss in the medial compartment. Leg length discrepancy may be noted as a result of loss of joint space in advanced hip OA. In addition, muscular atrophy may be seen in advanced disease secondary to joint splinting for pain relief. Deformities may include Heberden's nodes on the distal interphalangeal (DIP) joints and Bouchard's nodes on the proximal interphalangeal (PIP) joints of the hands.

DIAGNOSTIC TESTS

OA almost always can be diagnosed by history and physical examination.

Laboratory tests: To rule out other arthropathic conditions (e.g., rheumatoid arthritis, septic arthritis) and to establish baselines before starting therapy.

- **Complete blood count (CBC):** Suggested for patients who will be taking nonsteroidal antiinflammatory drugs (NSAIDs) for arthritis symptom management, with additional CBCs prescribed periodically to screen for anemia caused by occult gastrointestinal (GI) bleeding.
- **Renal and liver function tests:** For older adults starting aspirin or NSAID therapy, with further testing

done every 6 mo to monitor for occasional side effects such as electrolyte imbalance, hepatitis, or renal insufficiency.

- **Rheumatoid factor (RF) and erythrocyte sedimentation rate (ESR):** Neither excludes a diagnosis of OA in the older patient. About 20% of healthy older adults are in fact RF positive, and ESR tends to rise with age. ESR evaluation is useful to rule out chronic conditions such as polymyalgia rheumatica.

- **Synovial fluid analysis:** Another reliable method for differentiating OA from other arthritic disorders.

X-ray studies: Radiographic findings do not always correlate with severity of the patient's clinical symptoms. With disease progression, x-rays reveal joint space narrowing, osteophytes ("joint mice") at joint margins, subchondral cysts, and an altered shape of bone ends that suggests bone remodeling.

Magnetic resonance imaging (MRI): Much more sensitive than x-rays in marking progression of joint destruction.

Nursing Diagnosis:

Chronic Pain or Acute Pain

related to arthritic joint changes and associated therapy

Desired Outcomes: Within 1-2 hr of intervention, patient's subjective perception of pain decreases as documented by a pain intensity scale. Patient demonstrates ability to perform activities of daily living (ADL) with minimal discomfort.

INTERVENTIONS	RATIONALES
Assist in use of a pain intensity rating scale to evaluate pain and analgesic relief on a scale of 0 (no pain) to 10 (worst pain imaginable).	Use of a pain intensity scale allows more accurate documentation of pain and subsequent relief obtained after analgesia has been administered. The patient provides a personal baseline report, enabling the nurse to more effectively monitor subsequent increases and decreases in pain.
Administer analgesics as prescribed and document their effectiveness using the pain intensity rating scale.	Acetaminophen is recommended by the American College of Rheumatology as the initial treatment for OA pain, with doses up to 1000 mg qid. If acetaminophen proves ineffective, low-dose over-the-counter ibuprofen (up to 400 mg qid) or nonacetylated salicylates are recommended for patients with normal renal function and no prior history of GI problems. Prescriptive NSAID doses are indicated if pain persists or worsens. Traditional NSAIDs such as ibuprofen or naproxen sodium may increase patient's risk of gastric ulceration or renal impairment because of their inhibition of cyclooxygenase-1 (COX-1), which reduces prostaglandin levels in the stomach and kidneys. Because newer NSAIDs (e.g., celecoxib, rofecoxib) have COX-2 selectivity, less GI toxicity is likely. An opioid analgesic can be safely added to acetaminophen or NSAID therapy for up to 2 wk if pain is unremitting.
Apply topical analgesics as prescribed.	Application provides some pain relief for the OA patient. Capsaicin cream in particular has shown to reduce knee pain significantly when used along with regular arthritis medications. Necessity for several applications daily often leads to poor adherence to treatment.
Teach patient about use and purpose of biologic agents.	Glucosamine sulfate and chondroitin sulfate have rapidly gained popularity because of perceived effects on cartilage regeneration. Neither supplement is directly incorporated into the extracellular matrix, so their rapid action suggests an anti-inflammatory effect. The dietary supplement S-adenosylmethionine (SAM-e) is believed to play a role in cell growth and repair and also may provide arthritis pain relief.

Continued

INTERVENTIONS	RATIONALES
Advise patient to coordinate time of peak effectiveness of analgesic or NSAID with periods of exercise or other use of arthritic joints.	Careful timing of analgesics enables patient to achieve optimal pain relief before exercise or ambulation. Participation in the exercise regimen expedites patient's recovery.
Teach patient to use nonpharmacologic methods of pain management, including guided imagery, relaxation, massage, distraction, biofeedback, heat or cold therapy, and music therapy.	Nonpharmacologic methods can augment pharmacologic pain management strategies. These methods may be critical for a patient who is resistent to the use of analgesics. Thermal therapy in particular may lessen pain and stiffness. Ice can be helpful during episodes of acute inflammation, whereas heat therapy may be beneficial for stiffness. Heat therapy is delivered via numerous modalities, including hot packs, ultrasound, whirlpool, paraffin wax, and massage.
Supplement other pain management strategies with traditional nursing Interventions such as back rubs and repositioning. Encourage patient to verbalize feelings regarding pain experience and impact of the chronic disease.	Traditional nursing interventions augment the effects of analgesics or nonpharmacologic pain management strategies. In addition, verbalization helps patient examine strategies for coping with arthritis pain.
Encourage patient to use principles of joint protection, which include a balance of rest and activity.	An affected joint should be rested during periods of acute inflammation and weight bearing restricted to protect the joint and decrease the potential for pain.
Caution patient to avoid joint immobilization for more than a week.	Additional stiffness and discomfort can result from prolonged rest.
Suggest liberal use of assistive devices and modification of occupational and recreational activity.	A variety of devices are available to support small joints during routine occupational and recreational activities. Patients who use appropriate assistive devices are also generally able to continue with routine activities and avoid social isolation.

●●● **Related NIC and NOC labels:** *NIC:* Medication Management; Analgesic Administration; Biofeedback; Emotional Support; Patient-Controlled Analgesia Assistance; Positioning; Simple Guided Imagery; Simple Massage; Distraction; Heat/Cold Application; Music Therapy; Simple Relaxation Therapy; Splinting *NOC:* Comfort Level; Pain Control; Pain: Disruptive Effects

Nursing Diagnosis:

Deficient Knowledge:

Potential interaction between NSAIDs and herbal products

Desired Outcome: Within 1–2 hr of instruction, patient verbalizes accurate understanding of potential interactions between NSAIDs and herbal products that potentiate bleeding.

INTERVENTIONS	RATIONALES
Determine patient's use of NSAIDs and herbal products that potentiate bleeding (e.g., ginkgo, ginger, turmeric, chamomile, kelp, horse chestnut, garlic, dong quai).	Herbal supplements, particularly ginger and turmeric, have been shown to reduce the pain and inflammation of arthritis. However, these herbs can potentiate bleeding, and patient needs to be aware of this potential.
Teach bleeding risk associated with concomitant use of NSAIDs and herbal products.	Bleeding risk may be increased when both NSAIDs and herbal products are used for treatment of arthritis symptoms.
Teach signs of occult bleeding such as black or tarry stools, hematuria, and coughing up or vomiting blood.	A knowledgeable patient is more likely to recognize and report signs of occult bleeding in order to get prompt treatment.

Continued

INTERVENTIONS	RATIONALES
Advise patient to discuss with health care provider use of herbal products while taking NSAIDs for arthritis symptom management.	Health care provider should be aware of any products that increase patient's bleeding risk.

●●● **Related NIC and NOC labels:** *NIC:* Teaching: Prescribed Medication; Health Education; Risk Identification; Medication Management *NOC:* Knowledge: Medication; Knowledge: Personal Safety; Knowledge: Treatment Regimen

Nursing Diagnosis:

Impaired Physical Mobility

related to musculoskeletal impairment and adjustment to new walking gait with an assistive device

Desired Outcomes: Within 1 wk of instruction, patient demonstrates adequate upper body strength for use of an assistive device. Patient demonstrates appropriate use of an assistive device on flat and uneven surfaces.

INTERVENTIONS	RATIONALES
Before beginning gait training, ensure that patient has necessary strength of upper extremities.	Many older adults in particular have impaired upper body strength. Upper extremities must be strong enough to support patient's body weight and allow safe use of prescribed assistive devices such as crutches or walker.
As indicated, teach armchair push-ups.	Armchair push-ups target the triceps muscles, which are critically important for safe ambulation with crutches or walker. The patient should be encouraged to do 10 repetitions several times daily if possible to improve triceps muscle strength.
Be sure that height of the walker, crutches, or cane enables patient to have approximately 15 degrees of elbow flexion when ambulating.	The assistive device must be appropriately sized to the patient to allow safe use.
Ensure that crutch tops rest 1-1½ inches (width of 2 fingers) below axillae.	This position avoids upper extremity paresthesia caused by pressure of crutch tops on the brachial plexus.
Describe and demonstrate use of prescribed assistive device, supervising return demonstration.	Return demonstration and supervised practice ensure that patient will be able to use the device safely on different surfaces and in multiple settings. Ambulation should begin in small increments on a flat surface and progress to all surfaces that the patient is expected to encounter; ensure that patient can safely get in and out of a motor vehicle.

●●● **Related NIC and NOC labels:** *NIC:* Exercise Therapy: Ambulation; Body Mechanics Promotion; Exercise Promotion: Strength Training; Teaching: Prescribed Activity/Exercise *NOC:* Ambulation: Walking; Mobility Level

ADDITIONAL NURSING DIAGNOSES/PROBLEMS:

"Rheumatoid Arthritis" for **Fatigue** related   p. 558
    to state of discomfort, effects of
    prolonged immobility, and psychoemotional
    demands of chronic illness

Dressing/Grooming Self-Care Deficit   p. 559
    related to pain and limitations in joint
    range of motion

✓ PATIENT-FAMILY TEACHING AND DISCHARGE PLANNING

When providing patient-family teaching, focus on sensory information, avoid giving excessive information, and initiate a visiting/home health nurse or community services referral for necessary follow-up teaching whenever possible. Include verbal and written information about the following:

✓ Medications and supplements, including name, dosage, purpose, schedule, precautions, drug/drug and food/drug interactions, and potential side effects.

✓ Importance of laboratory follow-up (e.g., blood or urine testing) for needed monitoring while patient is taking selected medications.

✓ Proper use of heat or cold therapy, as appropriate to joint condition.

✓ Importance of joint protection, with balance of rest and activity.

✓ Use, care, and replacement of orthotics and assistive devices.

✓ Weight reduction, if appropriate.

✓ Importance of follow-up care, date of next appointment, and a telephone number to call if questions arise.

✓ Referral to community resources, including local arthritis support activities:

Arthritis Foundation
1330 West Peachtree Street
Atlanta, GA 30309
(404) 872-7100
www.arthritis.org

✓ Additional information on arthritis may be available through the following:

National Institute of Arthritis and Musculoskeletal and Skin Diseases (NIAMS)
Information Clearinghouse, Information Specialist
1 AMS Circle
Bethesda, MD 20892
(877) 22-NIAMS
www.niams.nih.gov

68

Osteoporosis

Osteoporosis ("porous bone") is the most common metabolic bone disease. It is characterized by reduction in both bone mass and bone strength, while bone size remains constant. These changes make bone more brittle and susceptible to fractures. Osteoporosis, which affects 25-35 million people in the United States, is responsible for up to 1.5 million fractures annually. One in three women and one in six men have the disease. Three types of osteoporosis have been identified: postmenopausal, senile, and secondary.

- **Postmenopausal osteoporosis:** Affects females primarily; clinical symptoms appear 10-15 yr after menopause as a result of lack of estrogen.
- **Senile osteoporosis:** Affects both males and females, more commonly after 70 yr of age; related to poor nutritional status and decreased physical activity.
- **Secondary osteoporosis:** Affects both males and females, results from another disease process (e.g., chronic renal failure/liver disease, diabetes, rheumatoid arthritis), nutritional abnormalities (e.g., malnutrition, hypercalciuria, protein deficiency), medications and therapies (e.g., glucocorticosteroids, anticoagulants, anticonvulsants, cyclosporines, excessive thyroid replacement therapy, radiation therapy), and disuse (e.g., spinal cord injury/loss of biomechanical function, long-term bedrest).

HEALTH CARE SETTING

Primary care; acute care for complications. Individuals with osteoporosis are seen in all health care settings for primary diagnoses other than osteoporosis.

ASSESSMENT

Signs and symptoms: Vertebral compression fractures can develop gradually, resulting in back discomfort and loss of height. Severe chronic flexion of the thoracic spine (kyphosis or "dowager's hump") may inhibit function of multiple organ systems (e.g., gastrointestinal, respiratory). With severe spinal deformities, the patient often describes difficulty in obtaining clothes that fit well.

Risk factors:
- **Unchangeable factors:** Gender, age, family history, body size (small frame, slight build), ethnicity (Caucasian, Asian)
- **Changeable factors:** Hormone levels (surgical or physiologic menopause, hypogonadism), diet (lifelong low-calcium intake, increased protein intake, increased caffeine intake)
- **Lifestyle factors:** Smoking, alcohol use, sedentary activity level
- **Other influences:** Medications, hyperthyroidism, hyperparathyroidism, multiple myeloma, transplantation, chronic diseases

DIAGNOSTIC TESTS

Laboratory tests: Cannot accurately determine bone density but can help in determining cause. For example, urinalysis may reveal elevated calcium in individuals with secondary osteoporosis. Biochemical markers of bone resorption may be useful for both initial assessment and for monitoring treatment effectiveness for confirmed disease.

Standard anteroposterior (AP) and lateral x-ray examinations of the spine: Provide a diagnosis for osteoporotic fractures or kyphosis. They have limited use in diagnosing disease before a fracture, however, because changes are not evident on plain films until at least 30% of bone mineral density has been lost.

Bone mineral density (BMD) tests: Can measure the amount of bone in specific areas of the skeleton to predict risk of fracture. Dual energy x-ray absorptiometry (DEXA) is the most common method for measuring bone density by testing bone mass in the spine, hip, and wrist. Quantitative computed tomography (QCT) measures bone density at sites throughout the body but is most often used in the spine. In the heel, quantitative ultrasound compares favorably with density measurements obtained by DEXA. It is also an easy, low-cost, radiation-free diagnostic aid.

Bone biopsy: Useful in the differential diagnosis of metabolic bone diseases such as osteoporosis and osteomalacia. It can also be useful for diagnosis in individuals with early onset of osteoporosis (age less than 50 yr) or those with severe demineralization.

Nursing Diagnosis:

Health-Seeking Behaviors:

Osteoporosis prevention and treatment and importance of adequate dietary calcium intake/supplementation

Desired Outcome: Within 48 hr of instruction, patient verbalizes knowledge of the disease process, possible treatments, and importance of adequate calcium intake.

INTERVENTIONS	RATIONALES
Ensure that patient understands the silent nature of osteoporosis and realizes that treatment may be less effective if not initiated until symptoms arise.	Because of the insidious onset of osteoporosis, most individuals are not diagnosed until they experience an acute fracture or receive radiographic evidence from x-rays obtained for other conditions (e.g., chest x-ray to confirm pneumonia).
Ensure that instruction on osteoporosis prevention is a routine part of health teaching for children, adolescents, and adults.	Adults need to recognize factors that increase their risk for osteoporosis. Childen and adolescents are still experiencing bone growth, and their bone quality can be improved through awaress of osteoporosis prevention strategies.
Teach patient about appropriate nutrition in relation to calcium intake.	A knowledgeable patient is more likely to comply with prevention and treatment strategies. Appropriate nutrition is the foundation of osteoporosis prevention and treatment, and consistent calcium intake is especially important.
Ensure that health care provider has recommended or approves use of calcium supplements for patient.	Although calcium is important to bone health, excessive calcium intake can lead to nephrolithiasis in susceptible individuals.
Teach patient that calcium supplements come in numerous forms and that calcium carbonate should be purchased.	The most effective form is calcium carbonate (e.g., OsCal), which delivers approximately 40% calcium. Bone meal and dolomite should be avoided because they may contain high amounts of lead or other toxic substances.
Instruct patient to avoid vitamin D supplementation if dietary intake is adequate.	Supplements may be needed by the institutionalized elderly, persons living in high northern or southern latitudes, and people with limited sun exposure. Excessive intake is discouraged because of risk of toxicity. Recommended amounts of vitamin D include 200 IU through age 50 yr, 400 IU for ages 51-70 yr, and 600 IU for those 71 yr or older.
Remind patient of need for sunlight, 15 min/day.	Exposure to sunlight is needed for cutaneous synthesis of vitamin D, but prolonged exposure does not necessarily increase the amount of vitamin D that is synthesized. An average of 15 minutes of exposure to hands, face, arms, and legs typically meets the vitamin D requirement for most people.
Teach patient not to take calcium and iron supplements at the same time.	The two elements bind with each other, and absorption of both will be impaired.
Evaluate patient's medication profile.	Because calcium may reduce absorption of other medications, the nurse should carefully time administration of all medications to ensure maximal absorption.

Continued

INTERVENTIONS	RATIONALES
Teach patient to take calcium 2 hr before or after meals. Calcium is best absorbed at night and should be taken at bedtime.	Foods such as red meats, spinach, colas, bran, or whole grain products may inhibit calcium absorption.
Caution patient to avoid taking more than 500-600 mg of calcium at one time and to spread doses over entire day.	Excessive intake can lead to hypercalcemia, which may cause muscle weakness, constipation, and heart block.
Remind patient to drink a full glass of water with each supplement.	Adequate hydration minimizes risk of developing renal calculi.
Teach patient about importance of weight-bearing exercise and associated precautions.	Weight-bearing exercise contributes to increased bone density and prevents bone loss. Individuals who have established osteoporosis should avoid vigorous unsupervised exercise. In particular, their exercise regimen should avoid spinal flexion through activities such as toe touches and sit-ups. Rotational exercises such as golf and bowling may lead to vertebral injury by creating excessive compressive forces. Walking is generally considered a safe weight-bearing exercise.
If hormone replacement therapy (HRT) has been prescribed, explain its purpose, action, and precautions.	HRT is not routinely recommended for treatment of chronic disease and is prescribed only after risks and benefits have been evaluated for each patient.
	Historically estrogen therapy has been shown to stabilize bone loss if prescribed within 3 yr of the onset of menopause or initiated preventively in women who have experienced surgical menopause. Estrogen improves calcium absorption and increases the number of vitamin D receptor sites on osteoblasts. Because of the increased risk of endometrial hyperplasia with use of unopposed estrogens, the woman with an intact uterus should receive both estrogen and progesterone as hormone replacement. Effects of hormone replacement therapy are experienced only as long as treatment continues. Because a family or personal history of breast cancer may be a contraindication to estrogen therapy, the patient should consider genetic counseling to delineate specific personal risk.
Teach patient about all antiresorptive drugs prescribed for treatment of osteoporosis: indications for use, possible side effects, administration time and method, and need for follow-up laboratory tests.	A knowledgeable patient is likely to comply with the drug therapy and report necessary signs and symptoms to ensure prompt treatment of untoward side effects.
- Anabolic steroids	These medications improve bone density, but masculinizing side effects are usually prohibitive.
- Calcitonin-salmon	Calcitonin exerts a powerful inhibitory effect on osteoclasts to prevent bone resorption. It has also been used prophylactically in patients with low bone mineral density but no other symptoms of osteoporosis. It should be taken in conjunction with a high-calcium diet or with calcium supplementation and adequate amounts of vitamin D.
- Alendronate (Fosamax)	The most effective biphosphonate, it is a nonhormonal oral preparation taken once a day. Its highly selective inhibition of osteoclast activity is greater than that of calcitonin and accomplished without disturbing normal bone formation. Although alendronate is only taken once a day, dosing restrictions may make adherence to the treatment regimen difficult. It must be taken with plain water on first rising, and the patient must refrain from eating or drinking for at least 30 min after taking it and remain in an upright position during this time to avoid regurgitation.

Continued

INTERVENTIONS	RATIONALES
- Raloxifene (Evista)	In the class of medications known as selective estrogen receptor modulators (SERMs), raloxifene has had consistently positive effects on bone mineral density without stimulating the endometrium and contributing to cancer risk. Studies have also documented decreased fracture risk in post-menopausal women, including those with prior osteoporotic fracture. Raloxifene can be given at any time of day without regard to meals. The patient should be taught to avoid prolonged immobility during travel because of the increased risk for venous thromboembolism.

●●● **Related NIC and NOC labels:** *NIC:* Health Education; Risk Identification; Teaching: Individual; Health Screening; Nutrition Management *NOC:* Health Promoting Behavior

Nursing Diagnoses:

Risk for Falls and/or Risk for Injury

related to decreased bone density secondary to osteoporosis

Desired Outcome: Within 24 hr of instruction, patient describes strategies to decrease risk for fall or fracture.

INTERVENTIONS	RATIONALES
Identify personal factors that can contribute to falls via a fall risk assessment tool. Refer to health care provider for additional evaluation of any identified deficits as necessary.	Confusion/dementia, cardiovascular disorders, decreased mobility, generalized weakness, abnormal elimination needs, impaired vision or hearing, and use of medications that affect blood pressure or balance are problems that can result in falls and hence fracture in a patient with decreased bone density.
Instruct patient and family about need to reduce/eliminate environmental hazards that may increase risk for falls in the home.	Patient and family need to assess home for poor lighting, scatter rugs, electrical cords or oxygen tubing that cross floors or halls, and narrow stairs without adequate railing.
Encourage patient to avoid unnecessarily limiting activity because of fear of falling.	Inactivity can place individual at greater risk for fractures by further decreasing bone density and contributing to muscle atrophy.
Instruct patient to avoid lifting objects greater than 5-10 lb. The patient interested in holding a young grandchild should be encouraged to have child crawl, climb, or be placed in adult's lap.	Lifting places patient with osteoporosis at risk for vertebral compression fractures. The patient needs strategies to maintain routine without increasing risk for vertebral injury.
Teach exercise regimen that improves balance.	Aerobic walking and strength training via upper and lower body exercises have been shown to improve standing balance, which will help decrease risk of falls.
Teach patient to take prescribed calcium and vitamin D supplements and antiresorptive medications.	Calcium and vitamin D contribute to bone health and minimize risk of injury should a fall occur. Other prescribed medications such as alendronate or raloxifene must be consistently taken as prescribed for optimal bone health.

●●● **Related NIC and NOC labels:** *NIC:* Environmental Management: Safety; Risk Identification; Fall Prevention: Surveillance: Safety; *NOC:* Safety Behavior: Home Physical Environment; Safety Status: Falls Occurrence

Nursing Diagnosis:

Imbalanced Nutrition: Less than body requirements

for calcium and vitamin D

Desired Outcome: Within 24 hr of instruction, patient demonstrates adequate intake of calcium
and vitamin D and plans a 3-day menu that provides sufficient intake of both.

INTERVENTIONS	RATIONALES
Teach purpose and recommended daily intake for calcium and vitamin D.	Premenopausal women need 1000 mg of calcium daily. After menopause, requirements rise to 1500 mg daily. Adolescents need 1200-1500 mg of calcium daily to maintain bone health. Oral calcium supplements (as calcium carbonate) may help perimenopausal women who have inadequate dietary intake and may compensate for inadequate intestinal absorption of calcium in postmenopausal women. Vitamin D is needed for adequate intestinal absorption and usage of calcium. Dietary sources include dairy products and vitamin-enriched cereals.
Verify patient's ability to select foods high in calcium, including cheese and milk.	If patient is unable to tolerate dairy products, it is important to explore other food choices that can ensure adequate calcium intake (e.g., broccoli, sardines).
Provide sample menus that include adequate daily amounts of calcium and vitamin D. Guide patient in developing a 3-day menu that includes appropriate intake of foods containing calcium and vitamin D.	Sample menus demonstrate easy ways in which adequate calcium and vitamin D can be incorporated into the daily diet.
Teach necessity for appropriate exposure to sunlight.	Even casual sun exposure can prevent vitamin D deficiency. Patient should be outside 15 minutes daily but can achieve this by walking into and out of stores during normal routine.
If patient has limited exposure to sunlight (e.g., resident of a long-term care facility), discuss vitamin D supplementation.	Supplementation will ensure adequate vitamin D intake.

●●● **Related NIC and NOC labels:** *NIC:* Nutritional Counseling; Teaching: Prescribed Diet
NOC: Nutritional Status

ADDITIONAL NURSING DIAGNOSES/ PROBLEMS:

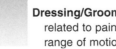

PATIENT-FAMILY TEACHING AND DISCHARGE PLANNING

When providing patient-family teaching, focus on sensory
information, avoid giving excessive information, and make
appropriate referrals (e.g., visiting or home health nurse, community health resources) for follow-up teaching. Include verbal
and written information about the following:

✓ Description of disease process and recommended treatment.

✓ Medications and supplements, including name, dosage,
purpose, schedule, precautions, drug/drug and food/drug interactions, and potential side effects.

✓ Prescribed dietary regimen, including rationale for food choices.

✓ Prescribed exercise regimen, including need to avoid movements that twist or compress the spine (e.g., sit-ups).

✓ Importance of establishing fall prevention measures in the home (e.g., placing handrail in tub or shower, installing night lights, avoiding use of throw rugs). Arrange for home visit from a nurse or physical therapist as necessary.

✓ Importance of reporting to health care provider any indicators of pathologic fracture (i.e., deformity, pain, edema, ecchymosis, limb shortening, false motion, decreased range of motion [ROM], or crepitus). Stress need to promptly report any indicators of vertebral fractures (e.g., paresthesias, weakness, paralysis, or loss of bowel or bladder function) because of risk for possible spinal cord or nerve compression.

✓ Importance of follow-up care, date of next appointment, and telephone number to call if questions arise.

✓ Referral to community resources, including local osteoporosis support activities.

National Osteoporosis Foundation
1232 22nd Street NW
Washington, DC 20037-1292
(202) 223-2226
www.nof.org

National Institute of Arthritis and Musculoskeletal and Skin Diseases (NIAMS)
Information Clearinghouse, Information Specialist
1 AMS Circle
Bethesda, MD 20892
(877) 22-NIAMS
www.niams.nih.gov

Rheumatoid Arthritis

Rheumatoid arthritis (RA) is a chronic systemic disease associated with severe morbidity and functional decline caused by inflammation of connective tissue, primarily in the synovial joints. RA is a direct cause of death more often than has been appreciated; life expectancy is shortened by an average of 7 yr in affected males and 3 yr in females. Women are affected 3 times more often than men. Although no single known cause exists for RA, theory suggests that it occurs in a susceptible host who initially experiences an immune response to an antigen. Because complex genetic factors appear to be involved, the antigen is probably not the same in all patients. No microorganism has been cultured from blood and synovial tissue or fluid with enough reproducibility to determine an infectious etiology for RA.

HEALTH CARE SETTING
Primary care, acute care for complications

ASSESSMENT
Signs and symptoms: The patient often complains of joint pain and swelling, especially in the hands and wrists, accompanied by fatigue, lethargy, and weight loss. Complaints also may include the knee, ankle, and metatarsophalangeal (MTP) joint. Morning stiffness lasting at least 1 hr is typical, but it may in fact last as long as 4 hr. The patient describes increasing difficulty with mobility and performance of activities of daily living (ADL).

Physical assessment: During early disease, examination may reveal spindle-shaped fingers. Swan-neck and boutonniere deformities become apparent because of flexion contractures that occur with disease progression. Ulnar deviation, a "zigzag" deformity of the wrist, is also likely. Affected symmetric (bilateral) joints are typically swollen, red, warm, and tender, with decreased range of motion (ROM). Subcutaneous nodules may be noted over bony prominences, extensor surfaces, or juxtaarticular areas; hoarseness may be evident if nodules have invaded the vocal cords. The patient also may exhibit guarded movement and gait abnormalities because of joint changes.

DIAGNOSTIC TESTS
Diagnosis of RA is based primarily on physical findings and patient history. Radiographic studies are not usually necessary to make a diagnosis. Laboratory results are helpful in confirming diagnosis and monitoring disease progression.

Rheumatoid factor: Positive in approximately 80% of patients. Titers are higher in active disease.

Antinuclear antibodies: Elevated titers are seen in 5%-20% of patients.

Erythrocyte sedimentation rate (ESR), C-reactive protein (CRP): Elevation is a general indicator of active inflammation.

Synovial fluid analysis: Fluid is opaque with cloudy yellow appearance, with elevated white blood cells (WBCs) and polymorphonuclear leukocytes in the presence of RA. Glucose level will be lower than serum glucose.

X-ray studies of affected joints: Radiographs may be inconclusive in early disease but baseline films, especially of the hands, aid in monitoring disease progression. Presence of erosions also helps to determine prognosis. With advanced disease, loss of articular cartilage leads to narrowed joint space. Subluxation and joint malalignment can be identified on x-rays, reflecting changes noted on physical examination. Osteopenia or osteoporosis may be evident in the RA patient who has been treated with corticosteroids.

Bone scan: Detects early synovial changes.

Arthroscopy: Reveals pale, hypertrophic synovium with destruction of cartilage and formation of fibrous scar tissue.

Nursing Diagnosis:

Fatigue

related to state of discomfort, effects of prolonged immobility, and psychoemotional demands of chronic illness

Desired Outcome: Within 24 hr of instruction and interventions, patient verbalizes a reduction in fatigue.

INTERVENTIONS	RATIONALES
Investigate patient's sleep pattern and suggest strategies that facilitate adequate rest (e.g., warm bath at bedtime).	Adequate rest helps patient maintain a more normal routine and decreases risk of disease exacerbation.
Assist patient to evaluate food preparation methods that may contribute to fatigue.	Minimizes impact or facilitates changes in food preparation methods. For example, patient might set table for next day's breakfast before going to bed at night, use convenience foods whenever possible, or prepare food while seated on a stool at the kitchen counter.
Encourage patient to pace activities and allow adequate rest periods during the day.	Balance of rest and activity keeps patient from becoming fatigued. Fatigue contributes to stress and possible disease exacerbations.
Assess patient's stress or psychoemotional distress. Suggest coping strategies or refer patient to an appropriate clinical specialist in psychiatric nursing. Encourage verbalization to family/significant other of stress caused by living with chronic illness.	Stress and psychoemotional distress may increase fatigue and exacerbate disease symptoms. By understanding patient's response to chronic illness, family/significant other are more likely to support efforts to maintain routine activities. If patient is unable to develop and use effective coping strategies independently, referral may be warranted.
Discuss rationale for a stepped approach to exercise. Encourage patient to set realistic exercise goals and share them with associated health care providers.	Endurance and strength should be increased gradually. An aggressive exercise program may cause fatigue and exacerbation of disease symptoms.
Instruct patient in use of assistive devices.	A variety of devices are available to support small joints during routine activities and to assist with ambulation, thus minimizing stress and fatigue. The patient who uses appropriate assistive devices is also generally able to continue with routine activities and avoid social isolation.
Assist patient to evaluate time that fatigue occurs, its relationship to necessary activities, and activities that relieve or aggravate symptoms.	With planning, patient should be able to optimize ability to participate in routine and recreational activities. Patient also can anticipate fatigue-producing activities and plan rest periods accordingly.

●●● **Related NIC and NOC labels:** *NIC:* Activity Therapy; Exercise Promotion; Energy Management; Sleep Enhancement; Coping Enhancement; Mood Management; Pain Management *NOC:* Endurance; Energy Conservation; Psychomotor Energy

Nursing Diagnosis:

Disturbed Body Image

related to development of joint deformities

Desired Outcome: Within 1 month of intervention, patient verbalizes positive adjustment to body image changes.

INTERVENTIONS	RATIONALES
Provide anticipatory counseling about possible joint deformities/body image changes following initial diagnosis, including ways for patient to prepare for reaction of others.	Awareness of the likelihood of deformity will enable patient to develop strategies that make routine encounters and regular activities easier. Patient also can anticipate times when RA deformities may be especially apparent and respond in ways that will minimize potential embarrassment or inconvenience. For example, the nurse may tell the patient, "As the disease progresses, you will notice deformities in your hands that affect your ability to write a check. To make this process easier and to minimize negative reactions of cashiers and other customers, you can write your check before you enter the store and fill in the purchase amount at the cash register."
Routinely assess patient for negative body image.	Manifestations of negative body image may be different in each patient. Examples may include refusal to discuss or participate in care, withdrawal from social contacts, and avoidance of intimate relationships. Early identification of changing body image provides opportunity for overcoming isolating effects of the disease.
Assess patient for negative feelings about body image linked specifically to use of assistive devices/mobility aids. Encourage involvement in a support group.	The nurse can assist in selection of the least obtrusive aids that will help patient maintain a more normal body image. Support group members can be good role models for successfully using assistive devices in public.
Ask patient to complete the Baird Body Image Assessment Tool or other self-assessment survey. Use survey results along with patient statements in planning care.	This tool encourages patient to consider meaning and impact of any physical changes and helps the nurse advise on strategies to cope with those changes.
Demonstrate positive regard for patient and acceptance of any physical changes associated with chronic illness.	The nurse's consistent positive regard will help patient avoid equating self with the disease process. It is critical that the patient recognize the disease as a separate entity rather than the defining element of his/her life.

●●● **Related NIC and NOC labels:** *NIC:* Body Image Enhancement; Active Listening; Coping Enhancement; Counseling; Emotional Support; Anticipatory Guidance; Behavior Modification *NOC:* Body Image; Psychosocial Adjustment: Life Change

Nursing Diagnosis:

Dressing/Grooming Self-Care Deficit

related to pain and limitations in joint range of motion

Desired Outcome: Within 1 wk of instruction, patient exhibits increased independence in dressing/grooming.

INTERVENTIONS	RATIONALES
Determine impact of pain and limitations in joint ROM on independent performance of dressing/grooming activities.	Recognition of extent to which the disease has affected patient's ability to perform dressing/grooming activities independently enables nurse and patient to develop an individualized care/teaching plan for dressing/grooming.

Continued

INTERVENTIONS	RATIONALES
Assess pain and ROM in joints used in dressing/grooming (e.g., small joints in hands; elbows, shoulders, knees).	Independence in dressing/grooming can be quickly lost as small joints become affected by the disease. Strategies for self-care must take into consideration any limitations in the small joints.
Teach patient to coordinate time of peak effectiveness of pre-scribed analgesics and antiinflammatory drugs with periods of joint use for dressing/grooming.	Careful timing of analgesics enables patient to achieve optimal pain relief before initiating dressing/grooming activities that can stress small joints.
Teach patient to perform exercises that increase joint flexibility and decrease pain during joint use for dressing/grooming.	Joint flexibility is critical to patient's ability to perform dressing/grooming acitivities independently. Pain should be minimized to facilitate joint use for dressing/grooming.
Refer patient to occupational therapist as indicated.	The occupational therapist is able to evaluate need for dressing/grooming aids. Sock donners, long-handled reachers and brushes, raised toilet seats, and other devices may help minimize stress on joints. Clothing also can be adapted to encourage independence in dressing (e.g., zipper pulls, Velcro closures).

●●● **Related NIC and NOC labels:** *NIC:* Self-Care Assistance: Dressing/Grooming; Exercise Therapy: Joint Mobility; Pain Management *NOC:* Self-Care: Activities of Daily Living; Self-Care: Dressing; Self-Care: Grooming

Nursing Diagnosis:

Deficient Knowledge:

Drugs used in RA treatment

Desired Outcome: Immediately following teaching, patient verbalizes accurate information about prescribed RA drugs.

INTERVENTIONS	RATIONALES
Teach patient about all drugs prescribed for treatment of arthritis: indications for use, possible side effects, adminis-tration time and method, and need for follow-up laboratory tests.	A knowledgeable patient is likely to comply with the drug therapy and report necessary signs and symptoms to ensure prompt treatment of untoward side effects.
Disease-modifying antirheumatic drugs (DMARDs)	DMARDs have been shown to slow the erosive course of RA and are now considered to be an important first-line therapy in disease treatment. Nonsteroidal antiinflammatory drugs (NSAIDs) are often prescribed along with DMARDs to allow optimal management of pain and swelling until the slower acting disease-modifying agent begins to exert its effect.
	- Methotrexate is most frequently prescribed by rheumatologists in the United States in doses of 7.5-25 mg weekly PO or IM.
	- Gold has been a standard therapy for more than 60 yr (25-50 mg IM every 1-4 wk or 3-6 mg PO daily).
	- Other DMARDs include sulfasalazine (2000-3000 mg daily), hydroxychloroquine (200-400 mg daily), penicillamine (250-1000 mg daily), cyclosporin (1.5-2.5 mg/kg daily), and cyclophosphamide (1-2 mg/kg daily).

Continued

INTERVENTIONS	RATIONALES
	- Leflunomide was approved in this class in 1998 for RA treatment in adults. If a positive response has not occurred within 4-6 wk after initiation of leflunomide therapy, the patient is unlikely to benefit from continued administration of this drug. Leflunomide has been shown to reduce symptoms and slow joint erosions while demonstrating fewer destructive effects on bone marrow than methotrexate.
Teach patient that laboratory monitoring of renal and liver function is necessary with all DMARDs.	Because the potential is great for renal and hepatic toxicity with DMARDs, patient should be instructed to complete all follow-up laboratory tests as prescribed.
Biologic response modifiers (BRMs)	BRMs interfere with cell surface antigens of modulating cytokines to manage RA symptoms in patients with moderate-to-severe disease who have not responded to DMARDs.
Explain that because medications such as etanercept are given by injection, BRMs may not be appropriate for all RA patients.	Self-administration by RA patients may be problematic because of muscle weakness and joint deformity. If patient does not have a family member/significant other who can be taught the injection technique, the nurse may need to request a home health visit or determine patient's ability to return to an outpatient clinic for medication administration.
NSAIDs	A number of over-the-counter (OTC) and prescriptive strength NSAIDs provide largely equal analgesic and antiinflammatory effects in the treatment of RA. They do not affect disease progression and their use in alleviating RA symptoms may in fact delay initiation of DMARD therapy or referral to a rheumatologist.
Teach patient that traditional NSAIDs such as cyclooxygenase-1 (COX-1) inhibitors are linked to increased risk for gastrointestinal (GI) toxicity, and patient should recognize signs and symptoms of internal bleeding or GI ulceration.	The patient must be able to seek prompt medical attention for any suspected bleeding or ulceration.
Advise that approval of COX-2 inhibitors such as celecoxib and rofecoxib offer an alternative to traditional NSAIDs.	Myocardial infarction (MI), transient ischemic attack (TIA), or stroke patients who require antiplatelet therapy can safely use celecoxib because it has no effect on bleeding time or platelet aggregation.
Corticosteroids	Injection of corticosteroids directly into affected joints can temporarily relieve the pain and inflammation of RA exacerbations. Low-dose oral prednisone may be useful in selected patients to minimize disease activity until the prescribed DMARD becomes therapeutic.
Explain that caution is necessary in long-term use of oral corticosteroids.	Corticosteroids have been associated with development of avascular necrosis or osteoporosis and therefore should not be a mainstay of treatment for the patient with RA. Patients who take corticosteroids should receive additional instruction on risks associated with long-term use.
Future drug therapies	Research on underlying causes of inflammation associated with RA may lead to development of new medications or new uses for previously marketed medications. The nurse should listen carefully to patient's stated interest in any other pharmacologic therapies and inform health care provider of patient's willingness to try additional treatments.
	These drugs may include:
	- Calcitonin (down-regulates monocyte function)

Continued

INTERVENTIONS	RATIONALES
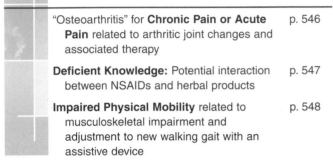	- Rifampin (antitubercular drug acting on ribonucleic acid [RNA] synthesis)
	- Retinoid compounds (multiple effects on biologic systems)
	- Antitumor necrosis factor and monoclonal antibodies (delay abnormal cartilage and bone growth)

ADDITIONAL NURSING DIAGNOSES/ PROBLEMS:

"Osteoarthritis" for **Chronic Pain or Acute Pain** related to arthritic joint changes and associated therapy   p. 546

Deficient Knowledge: Potential interaction between NSAIDs and herbal products   p. 547

Impaired Physical Mobility related to musculoskeletal impairment and adjustment to new walking gait with an assistive device   p. 548

PATIENT-FAMILY TEACHING AND DISCHARGE PLANNING

When providing patient-family teaching, focus on sensory information, avoid giving excessive information, and make appropriate referrals (e.g., visiting or home health nurse, community health resources) for follow-up teaching. Include verbal and written information about the following:

✓ Treatment regimen, including physical therapy and exercises, systemic rest/principles of joint protection, and thermotherapy.

✓ Importance of laboratory follow-up (e.g., blood or urine testing) for needed monitoring while patient is taking selected medications.

✓ Medications and supplements, including name, dosage, schedule, precautions, drug/drug and food/drug interactions, and potential side effects.

✓ Potential complications of disease and therapy, as well as need to recognize and seek medical attention promptly if they occur.

✓ Potential concurrent pathologic conditions, such as pericarditis and ocular lesions, and need to report them promptly to health care provider.

✓ Use, care, and replacement of splints, orthotics, and assistive devices.

✓ Use of adjunctive aids as appropriate, including long-handled reacher, long-handled shoehorn, elastic shoelaces, Velcro fasteners, crutches, walker, and cane.

✓ Referral to visiting/public health or home health nurses as necessary for ongoing care after discharge.

✓ Importance of follow-up care, date of next appointment, and telephone number to call if questions arise.

✓ Referral to community resources, including local arthritis support activities.

Arthritis Foundation
1330 West Peachtree Street
Atlanta, GA 30309
404-872-7100
www.arthritis.org

American Academy of Pediatrics
141 Northwest Point Boulevard
Elk Grove Village, IL 60007-1098
847-434-4000
www.aap.org

National Institute of Arthritis and Musculoskeletal and Skin Diseases (NIAMS)
Information Clearinghouse, Information Specialist
1 AMS Circle
Bethesda, MD 20892
877-22-NIAMS
www.niams.nih.gov

Total Hip Arthroplasty

otal hip arthroplasty (THA) involves surgical resection of the hip joint and its replacement with an endoprosthesis. THA may be necessary for conditions such as osteoarthritis, rheumatoid arthritis, Legg–Calvé–Perthes disease, avascular necrosis (AVN), and benign or malignant bone tumors. Because conservative treatments usually fail to decrease the impact of disease on the patient's functional ability, surgery becomes the next best alternative. Arthroscopy, osteotomy, excision, or arthrodesis (joint fusion) may be considered before the patient and surgeon choose THA.

Early complications of infection, breakage, and loosening now occur less frequently because of improved surgical techniques. Infection risk has been substantially decreased with administration of prophylactic antibiotics. However, potential complications still include dislocation and aseptic loosening of components. The patient is also at risk for deep vein thrombosis (DVT).

HEALTH CARE SETTING

Acute care surgical unit; rehabilitation unit

DIAGNOSTIC TESTS

Various tests are combined with patient history and physical findings to confirm presence of conditions that necessitate THA. X-rays are commonly required, with patient bearing weight for the anteroposterior (AP) view, to enable assessment of bone shape and quality.

Nursing Diagnosis:

Deficient Knowledge:

Appropriate activity precautions to decrease risk for dislocation of the operative hip

Desired Outcome: Within the 24-hr period before surgery, patient verbalizes accurate knowledge about the potential for dislocation of the operative hip and activity precautions that decrease risk for dislocation.

Note: THA is performed most often using a posterolateral approach. However, the anterolateral approach is gaining popularity partly because of its decreased risk for dislocation. The following discussion relates to the posterolateral approach for THA; the anterolateral approach requires different positional restrictions.

INTERVENTIONS	RATIONALES
During preoperative instruction, advise patient of the potential for postoperative dislocation.	A knowledgeable patient is more likely to understand the rationale for and comply with activity and positional restrictions. Risk of dislocation remains high until the periarticular tissues heal around the endoprosthesis (approximately 6 wk). If dislocation occurs once, the potential for recurrence is increased because of stretching of the periarticular tissues. A confirmed dislocation is treated with closed reduction using general anesthesia. Recurrent dislocations may require revision arthroplasty or surgery to tighten periarticular tissues.
Show patient an endoprosthesis and describe how it can be dislocated when positional restrictions are not followed (i.e., flexion of the hip past 90 degrees, internal rotation, or adduction).	Actually seeing how certain positions result in dislocation will help patient understand need for and adhere to positional restrictions.
During preoperative instruction, explain and demonstrate use of ambulatory aids and activities of daily living (ADL) assistive devices that enable independence without violating positional restrictions.	Preoperative introduction to ambulatory aids and ADL assistive devices makes their postoperative use easier because of patient familiarity with devices and techniques for use.
After surgery, reinforce position restrictions and discuss activities that may violate restrictions, including pivoting on the operative leg, sitting on a toilet seat of regular height, bending over to tie shoelaces, or crossing legs.	Following a THA, using the posterolateral approach, the patient may use an abduction wedge to prevent internal rotation and keep the hip in an abducted position. Avoidance of flexion past 90 degrees is required to decrease risk of dislocation.
Also discuss weight bearing as indicated.	For the patient with a cemented prosthesis, the surgeon may prescribe full weight bearing or weight bearing as tolerated. The patient is able to become mobile within 1-2 days because of the immediate fixation of the components. The patient with a noncemented prosthesis will have restricted weight bearing for approximately 6 wk until bony ingrowth into the components has been shown on x-ray.
As indicated, refer patient to occupational or physical therapy. Provide contact information for businesses that sell assistive devices and other necessary equipment. Ensure that patient verbalizes and demonstrates understanding of the positional restrictions based on surgical approach (posterior vs. anterior) and can perform ADL independently using appropriate assistive devices.	Occupational therapy focuses on self-care tasks such as dressing, bathing, and toileting through use of assistive devices that may include a long-handled reacher and sock donner. The patient with posterior precautions will need bathroom equipment such as an elevated toilet seat. Physical therapy generally includes a prescription for muscle-strengthening exercises and gait training with a walker or crutches to maximize patient's mobility. Exercises also target the upper extremities because their weakness can make it difficult for patient to use walker or crutches.
Instruct patient to report pain in hip, buttock, or thigh or prolonged limp.	These symptoms may indicate prosthesis loosening.
See "Perioperative Care," p. 47, for other surgical care plans.	

●●● **Related NIC and NOC labels:** *NIC:* Teaching: Procedure/Treatment; Teaching: Psychomotor Skill; Teaching: Individual; Teaching: Prescribed Activity/Exercise *NOC:* Knowledge: Treatment Regimen

Nursing Diagnosis:

Risk for Peripheral Neurovascular Dysfunction

related to interrupted arterial blood flow secondary to compression from abduction wedge

Desired Outcomes: Patient maintains adequate peripheral neurovascular function distal to operative site as evidenced by warmth, normal color, and ability to dorsiflex the foot and feel sensations with testing of the area enervated by the peroneal nerve. Patient verbalizes accurate knowledge about peripheral neurovascular complications and importance of promptly reporting signs of impairment.

INTERVENTIONS	RATIONALES
Monitor neurovascular condition at regular intervals by checking temperature (circulation), movement, and sensation in affected extremity.	Pressure from the abductor wedge can interrupt arterial blood flow and compress the peroneal nerve. The peroneal nerve runs superficially by the fibular neck; it is assessed by testing sensation in the first web space between the great and second toes and by having patient dorsiflex the foot.
When assessing the peroneal nerve, promptly report loss of sensation or movement to health care provider.	This signals impaired peroneal nerve function. Peroneal nerve damage can lead to severe disability with footdrop and paresthesias.
Ensure that patient is aware of potential for neurovascular impairment and importance of promptly reporting alterations in sensation, strength and movement, temperature, and color of operative extremity.	Patient's awareness of signs of impairment leads to prompt reporting, enabling health care providers to initiate appropriate treatment in a timely way.
Encourage patient to perform prescribed exercises.	Exercises stimulate circulation to distal extremity and decrease risk for neurovascular dysfunction.

●●● **Related NIC and NOC labels:** *NIC:* Peripheral Sensation Management; Surveillance; Traction/Immobilization Care; Exercise Promotion; Circulatory Care: Arterial Insufficiency, Circulatory Precautions; Pressure Management *NOC:* Muscle Function; Tissue Perfusion: Peripheral

Nursing Diagnosis:

Ineffective Tissue Perfusion: Peripheral

(or risk for same) *related to* possible development of deep vein thrombosis

Desired Outcome: Optimally patient demonstrates adequate tissue perfusion in lower extremities as evidenced by maintenance of normal skin temperature and color and absence of calf pain and/or swelling.

INTERVENTIONS	RATIONALES
In the absence of signs of thrombosis (see last intervention in this diagnosis), encourage patient to perform calf-pumping/ankle-circle exercises.	These exercises cause calf muscle contraction. As the contracted muscles tighten on the veins, blood return to the heart is promoted, and risk for thrombus development is decreased.
Encourage patient to perform prescribed exercises and participate fully in physical therapy program.	Early mobilization decreases risk of thrombus formation.
Discuss use of prescribed anticoagulants.	Because of increased risk of DVT with THA, the surgeon typically prescribes anticoagulant therapy.

Continued

INTERVENTIONS	RATIONALES
	Low-molecular-weight heparin is administered by SC injection, or oral warfarin is prescribed. The patient should be knowledgeable about risks associated with anticoagulant use in order to report adverse effects in a timely way. Review **Ineffective Protection** in "Pulmonary Embolus," p. 155.
Encourage patient to wear antiembolic stockings, intermittent pneumatic compression devices, or venous foot pump compression devices whenever in bed or chair.	External modalities such as antiembolism stockings, intermittent pneumatic compression devices, or venous foot pump compression devices may be used. These devices compress the leg muscles and encourage blood return to the heart, decreasing risk for thrombus development.
Assess for and promptly report to health care provider patient's complaints of swelling, warmth, or pain/tenderness along vein tracts in lower extremities. Teach these indicators to patient.	Close monitoring for these signs of thrombosis is imperative to ensure timely treatment. Patient awareness of indicators also contributes to early identification and treatment of potential thrombotic complications.

●●● **Related NIC and NOC labels:** *NIC:* Circulatory Care: Venous Insufficiency; Circulatory Precautions; Skin Surveillance *NOC:* Tissue Perfusion: Peripheral

Nursing Diagnosis:

Acute Pain

related to surgical repair and rehabilitation therapy

Desired Outcomes: Within 1-2 hr of intervention, patient's subjective perception of pain decreases as documented by a pain intensity rating scale. Patient demonstrates ability to perform ADL with minimal complaints of discomfort.

INTERVENTIONS	RATIONALES
Assist in use of a pain intensity rating scale to evaluate pain and analgesic relief on a scale of 0 (no pain) to 10 (worst pain imaginable).	Use of a pain intensity scale allows more accurate documentation of pain and subsequent relief obtained after analgesia has been administered. The patient provides a personal baseline report, enabling nurse to more effectively monitor subsequent increases and decreases in pain.
If intraarticular anesthetic or opioid was administered intraoperatively, advise patient that lack of pain in the immediate postoperative period should *not* be mistaken for ability to move the joint excessively.	Patients with minimal postoperative pain may be tempted to become overly active, thereby putting unnecessary stress on the operative site. Prescribed activity must be carefully followed to avoid additional injury to the affected extremity.
If appropriate, instruct hospitalized surgical patient in use of patient-controlled analgesia (PCA) or epidural analgesia. Verify with another nurse that PCA or epidural pump contains prescribed medication and concentration with prescribed settings for patient dosing, continuous infusion, and/or clinician-activated bolus.	Postoperative protocols often call for use of PCA in an attempt to achieve more consistent pain management for the THA patient. Epidural analgesia has become popular as a pain management strategy, enabling adequate pain relief without some of the side effects of IV medications. Verification of pump settings is critical to the safe delivery of analgesia.
If PCA or epidural analgesia is used, monitor effectiveness of patient's pain management while observing for excessive sedation, respiratory depression, and decreased level of consciousness. Keep appropriate reversal agent readily available.	Excessive sedation may necessitate administration of appropriate reversal agent. Most commonly, naloxone is used for opioid-induced side effects, and ephedrine is given for hypotensive crisis associated with epidural administration of anesthetics such as bupivacaine.

Continued

INTERVENTIONS	RATIONALES
As prescribed, administer nonsteroidal antiinflammatory drugs (NSAIDs) and monitor effectiveness of patient's pain management, as well as adverse effects.	Within 1-2 days after surgery, patient should be taking oral analgesics. Once hemostasis has been achieved, NSAIDs may be prescribed for less severe postoperative pain or for concomitant arthritis pain in other joints.
Closely observe for hemorrhage at surgical site.	There is potential for increased bleeding following NSAID administration.
Avoid giving NSAIDs if patient is receiving epidural analgesia.	NSAIDs should not be prescribed during administration of epidural analgesia because of risk of bleeding into the epidural space, which may cause lower extremity impairment through pressure on spinal nerves.
Advise patient to coordinate time of peak effectiveness of analgesics with periods of exercise or ambulation.	Careful timing of analgesics allows patient to achieve optimal pain relief before exercise or ambulation. Participation in the exercise regimen expedites patient's recovery
Teach patient to use nonpharmacologic methods of pain management, including guided imagery, relaxation, massage, distraction, biofeedback, heat or cold therapy, and music therapy.	Nonpharmacologic methods can augment pharmacologic pain management strategies. These methods may be critical for a patient who is resistant to the use of analgesics.
Supplement other pain management strategies with traditional nursing interventions such as back rubs and repositioning.	Traditional nursing interventions augment effects of analgesics or nonpharmacologic pain management strategies.

●●● **Related NIC and NOC labels:** *NIC:* Medication Management, Biofeedback; Emotional Support; Patient-Controlled Analgesia Assistance; Positioning; Simple Guided Imagery; Simple Massage; Simple Relaxation Therapy; Heat/Cold Application; Music Therapy *NOC:* Comfort Level; Pain Control

Nursing Diagnosis:

Impaired Physical Mobility

related to postoperative musculoskeletal pain and immobilization devices

Desired Outcomes: By at least 24 hr before hospital discharge, patient demonstrates appropriate use of ambulatory aids. Patient verbalizes understanding of use of analgesics and adjunctive methods to decrease pain when performing prescribed exercises or activity.

INTERVENTIONS	RATIONALES
Teach use and care of ambulatory aids such as walker or crutches.	Patient needs to be aware of equipment maintenance and techniques for their safe use to avoid injury.
Teach patient and significant other exercises that improve muscle strength and increase joint flexibility.	Improved muscle strength and joint flexibility contribute to earlier mobilization and safe use of ambulatory aids. Both lower extremity and upper extremity exercises should be included in the prescribed regimen.
Instruct patient and significant other in use of analgesics and nonpharmacologic pain management methods.	Effective pain management will enable patient to become mobile more quickly, decreasing risk of complications associated with impaired physical mobility.

●●● **Related NIC and NOC labels:** *NIC:* Exercise Therapy: Ambulation; Exercise Therapy: Joint Mobility; Exercise Therapy: Muscle Control; Body Mechanics Promotion; Fall Prevention; Pain Management; Teaching: Prescribed Activity/Exercise *NOC:* Mobiity Level; Joint Movement: Active; Ambulation: Walking

PATIENT-FAMILY TEACHING AND DISCHARGE PLANNING

When providing patient-family teaching, focus on sensory information, avoid giving excessive information, and make appropriate referrals (e.g., visiting or home health nurse, community health resources) for follow-up teaching. Include verbal and written information about the following:

✓ Medications and supplements, including name, dosage, purpose, schedule, precautions, drug/drug and food/drug interactions, and potential side effects.

✓ Any precautions related to wound care and signs of infection (i.e., persistent redness or pain, swelling or localized warmth, fever, purulent drainage) or other complications of surgery.

✓ Need to consult health care provider about possible prophylactic antibiotics before any minor surgical procedure (e.g., dental surgery).

✓ Activity and weight-bearing restrictions related to surgical approach and choice of prosthesis.

✓ Use of prescribed immobilization device such as abductor wedge.

✓ Prescribed exercise regimen, including how exercise is performed, number of repetitions, frequency of exercise, and rationale for exercise performance. Ensure that patient independently demonstrates each exercise.

✓ For ADL and ambulation, ensure that patient demonstrates independence in use of ambulatory aids and assistive devices before hospital discharge.

✓ Assessment of neurovascular status at least qid, including need to report symptoms such as numbness and tingling or coolness in extremity to health care provider immediately.

✓ Importance of follow-up care, date of next appointment, and a telephone number to call if questions arise.

Caring for Individuals with Human Immunodeficiency Virus Disease

Acquired immunodeficiency syndrome (AIDS) is a life-threatening illness caused by the human immunodeficiency virus (HIV). AIDS is characterized by the disruption of cell-mediated immunity. This breakdown of the immune system is manifested by opportunistic infections such as *Pneumocystis carinii* pneumonia (PCP) or tumors such as Kaposi's sarcoma (KS).

Confirmed routes of transmission of HIV infection include:

- **Blood:** Exposure by sharing of unsterile needles or other drug paraphernalia, unsterile invasive instruments, occupational exposure to needlesticks or sharps, transfusion with contaminated blood, mucocutaneous exposure to blood or other infected body fluids.
- **Semen:** Exposure during male-to-male or male-to-female sexual activity through the exchange of infected semen. Anal receptive sex is the greatest risk for exposure to the virus.
- **Vaginal fluid:** Exposure during sexual activity; has lower risk of HIV transmission.
- **Breast milk:** From infected woman to infant.
- **Perinatal transmission:** From infected woman to fetus, which can occur during all stages of pregnancy and during labor and delivery.

It is estimated that the average time span between infection with HIV and seroconversion (development of a positive HIV antibody test) is 6-8 wk, although antibody response may be absent for 1 yr or more. Therefore a negative test result does not guarantee the absence of infection. Individuals with a recent history of high-risk behavior and a negative HIV antibody test should be retested at 6-mo intervals for 1 yr and follow guidelines for safer sex practices. Anyone with a positive HIV antibody test must be considered infectious and capable of transmitting the virus.

Epidemiologic focus no longer is on groups but on high-risk behaviors. HIV infection has transcended all racial, social, sexual, and economic barriers, and it is primarily high-risk behaviors that are responsible for its transmission.

To a minimal extent, health care workers who come into contact with infected body fluids of patients also are at some risk. Understanding and practicing stringent infection control is essential for all health care workers. All patients must be considered infectious because the health care worker cannot tell by looking at patients about their HIV status.

AIDS is the advanced phase of HIV infection. It is a chronic viral disease that covers a wide spectrum of illnesses and symptoms for a variable course of time. There is no classic disease progression (e.g., some individuals proceed from an asymptomatic, seropositive state to AIDS, whereas others may experience the symptoms for many years). Therefore HIV disease should be considered a continuum of infection. The stages of illness are described under "Assessment."

Since the introduction of highly active antiretroviral treatment (HAART), there has been a dramatic reduction in HIV-related morbidity and mortality. This treatment includes antiretroviral agents that slow viral replication at different points in the life cycle of HIV within the CD4 cell. Use of combinations of these antiretroviral agents reduces the amount of circulating virus (viral load). This viral load reduction has been shown to enable immune system recovery and slow progression of the disease, resulting in reduction in symptoms and opportunistic diseases and prolonged survival time.

Maintenance of a positive attitude by the patient and caregivers is an essential element in the therapeutic plan, but an honest approach to the realities of any life-threatening illness also must prevail.

HEALTH CARE SETTING

Primary care, hospice, and home care with possible hospitalization resulting from complications or occurrence of opportunistic diseases

ASSESSMENT

HIV risk assessment: Because of continued transmission of HIV infection and incidence of new infections in women, racial and ethnic minorities, and adolescents and the continuing transmission among men who have sex with men, continuous HIV risk assessment and prevention education within all clinical settings are essential. Health care providers have a responsibility to assess each patient's risk for HIV infection. Risk assessment should be sensitive to issues of sexual orientation and practices, as well as cultural values, norms, and traditions. A risk assessment should be used not only to elicit risk behaviors for the purpose of recommending testing but also for development of a "patient-centered" risk reduction plan.

Key components of conducting a sexual history:
- Focus on sexual "behaviors" rather than on categories or labels.
- Avoid making assumptions about individuals.
- Ask about specific sexual behavior rather than asking general questions.
  - For example, "How many sexual partners have you had?" "In the last 5 years?" "In the last month?"
  - "Do you have sex with men, women, or both?"
  - "When is the last time you had sex while under the influence of drugs or alcohol?"
- Ask nonjudgmentally about sexual practices.
  - "What type of sexual intercourse (vaginal, anal, oral) do you have with your partner?"
  - "When you have intercourse, are you the insertive or receptive partner?"

Key components of conducting a drug history:
- Focus on specific drug-using behaviors. Examples of specific questions include:
  - "Do you use alcohol or tobacco?" "If so, how much?"
  - "Have you ever injected any kind of drug?"
  - "What drugs do you ingest?" "What drugs to you inject?"
  - "When did you last inject drugs?" "Share needles?"
  - "Do you clean your works?" "How do you do this?"
- Avoid making assumptions about individuals because drug use occurs in all socioeconomic groups.
- Convey a nonjudgmental attitude.

Four stages of HIV disease (for untreated individuals):
- **Acute or primary infection:** Period of rapid viral replication during which the person may experience flulike symptoms, particularly at the time of seroconversion.
- **Asymptomatic stage:** Immune system continues to mount a massive response to HIV, causing a drop in viral load, but viral replication continues. It may last 10 yr or more and the person may remain free of symptoms or opportunistic infections.
- **Early symptomatic stage:** Rate of viral replication remains relatively constant; however, the immune system's gradual failure results in inability to control the virus, causing increased viral load.
- **Advanced stage, AIDS:** The immune mechanism for virus control fails, resulting in large amounts of circulating virus (viral load) and significant destruction of CD4 cells. Clinical manifestations include wasting and opportunistic diseases such as neoplasms and viral, bacterial, and fungal infections. Dementia also can occur, characterized by cognitive impairment and mood changes.

Physical assessment: The following indicators are seen frequently with HIV infection:
- **General:** Fever, cachexia, weight loss
- **Cutaneous:** Herpes zoster or simplex infection(s), seborrheic or other dermatitis, fungal infections of the skin (moniliasis, candidiasis) or nail beds (onychomycosis), KS lesions, petechiae
- **Head/neck:** "Cotton-wool" spots visualized on funduscopic examination; oral KS; candidiasis (thrush); hairy leukoplakia; aphthous ulcers; enlarged, hard, and occasionally tender lymph nodes
- **Respiratory:** Tachypnea, dyspnea, diminished or adventitious breath sounds (crackles [rales], rhonchi, wheezing)
- **Cardiac:** Tachycardia, friction rub, gallops, murmurs
- **Gastrointestinal (GI):** Enlargement of liver or spleen, diarrhea, constipation, hyperactive bowel sounds, abdominal distention
- **Genital/rectal:** KS lesions, herpes, candidiasis, fistulas
- **Neuromuscular:** Flattened affect, apathy, withdrawal, memory deficits, headache, muscle atrophy, speech deficits, gait disorders, generalized weakness, incontinence, neuropathy

DIAGNOSTIC TESTS

A variety of diagnostic tests are used for specific reasons in the course of HIV disease. Typically the enzyme-linked immunosorbent assay (ELISA) test with a confirmatory Western blot (WB) are used to determine if the individual is HIV infected. Given that it can take up to 6 mo to develop enough antibodies to test positive on these HIV antibody tests, the person may be

HIV infected while testing negatively. This is often referred to as the "window period" for HIV infection. Individuals who test negative on the HIV antibody test should be retested in 6 mo to confirm seronegativity.

ELISA: The initial test for HIV is the ELISA, which tests for presence of HIV antibody. A positive ELISA with a confirmatory WB signals infection with HIV. In an initially reactive ELISA, the test should be repeated on the same specimen. If one or two repeats are reactive, the confirmatory WB is performed.

Western blot: A confirmatory test used to detect immune response to the specific viral proteins of HIV. A reactive WB is defined by a specific pattern of protein bands separated by electrophoresis on a strip of nitrocellulose paper; three of the following bands must be present for reactivity: p24 (see below), gp41, and gp210 or gp160.

p24 Antigen test: Detects HIV p24 antigen in serum, plasma, and cerebrospinal fluid (CSF) of infected individuals. Its advantage is that it detects viral antigen (HIV p24) early in the course of infection before seroconversion.

Immunofluorescence assay: Tests for HIV antibody; has three distinct advantages over the WB test: more sensitive, less expensive, and less technically demanding.

Monitoring tests

With the use of HAART in the clinical management of HIV disease, monitoring tests have become increasingly important and essential in making appropriate clinical treatment decisions.

These clinical decisions are based not only on clinical symptoms but also on the person's CD4 count and viral load. Based on the current Department of Health and Human Service HIV treatment guidelines, asymptomatic persons, depending on these measurements, are appropriate candidates for initiation of HAART.

CD4 count: A measure of the amount of CD4 cells per milliliter in the blood and a marker for the impact of HIV infection on the immune system. With increased viral load there is a reduction in CD4 counts because of destruction of these lymphocytes by HIV.

Viral load testing: Only 3%-4% of the virus is located in the plasma. The remaining 90%+ is located in lymphoid tissues and other blood cells. The viral load test measures the free virus in the plasma but not in these other areas. It is used to determine response of antiretroviral treatment, monitor development of drug resistance, and determine need to change antiretroviral treatment.

Viral resistance testing: A measure that indicates whether the virus is resistant to specific antiretroviral drugs. It is used to determine, before initiating treatment, if the person is already resistant to a specific agent. It is also used to assess treatment failure and assist in determining appropriate changes in the introduction of new or alternative antiretroviral agents. There are two different types of resistance testing: (1) genotypic tests, which look for genetic mutations that have been linked to drug resistance, and (2) phenotypic tests, which assess which drugs can stop HIV growing in a lab setting.

Nursing Diagnosis:

Risk for Infection

related to inadequate secondary defenses of the immune system, malnutrition, or side effects of chemotherapy

Desired Outcome: Patient is free of additional infections as evidenced by negative cultures or biopsies.

INTERVENTIONS	RATIONALES
Assess for persistent fevers, night sweats, fatigue, involuntary weight loss, persistent and dry cough, persistent diarrhea, and headache.	These are indicators of opportunistic infections. Common opportunistic infections and organisms that infect individuals with HIV disease include herpes (1 and 2), cytomegalovirus, varicella, Epstein-Barr virus, and hepatitis. Enterically transmitted hepatitis (A and E) is spread by men having sex with men and using drugs (both injecting and noninjecting). Parenterally transmitted hepatitis (B, C, D, and G) is transmitted through injection drug use. Coinfection with HIV and hepatitis C virus (HCV) is on the rise among injection drug users.
Monitor laboratory data, especially complete blood count (CBC), white blood cell (WBC) count with differential, erythrocyte sedimentation rate (ESR), and cultures. Notify health care provider of significant findings.	Increased/positive values may signal presence/type of infection.

Continued

INTERVENTIONS	RATIONALES
Maintain strict sterile technique for all invasive procedures.	To prevent introduction of new pathogens.
Assist patient in maintaining meticulous body hygiene.	To prevent spread of organisms from body secretions into skin breaks, especially if patient has diarrhea.
Monitor temperature and VS at frequent intervals. Perform a complete physical assessment at least q8h.	To identify changes from baseline assessment that signal fever or sepsis. In addition to increased temperature, other signs include diaphoresis, confusion or mental status changes, decrease in level of consciousness (LOC), increased HR, and decreased BP secondary to the vasodilator effect of the increased body temperature.
Assess for changes in breath sounds.	Diminished or adventitious sounds may indicate opportunistic disease and/or an increasing level of pulmonary infiltrates. PCP is commonly seen in HIV disease when the immune system is extremely compromised (i.e., when there has been a destruction of CD4 cells and rise in viral load). It is most often seen in later stages of HIV disease. Other opportunistic infections that can manifest with pulmonary signs and symptoms include *Mycobacterium tuberculosis* (MTB) and bacterial pneumonia.
Encourage patient to engage in frequent breathing or incentive spirometry exercises.	To promote pulmonary toilet, which will help prevent respiratory infections.
Use caution when performing postural drainage and chest physiotherapy, if prescribed.	Patients may be too ill to tolerate these activities.
Monitor sites of invasive procedures for erythema, swelling, local warmth, tenderness, and purulent exudate.	Signs of local infection.
Enforce good handwashing techniques before contact with patient.	To minimize risk of transmitting infectious organisms from staff and other patients.
Teach patient home care considerations for infection prevention (see "Patient-Family Teaching and Discharge Planning," p. 581).	
For more information, see Appendix for "Infection Prevention and Control," p. 831.	

●●● **Related NIC and NOC labels:** *NIC:* Infection Protection; Laboratory Data Interpretation; Risk Identification; Surveillance; Communicable Disease Management; Environmental Management; Incision Site Care; Vital Signs Monitoring; Bathing; Chest Physiotherapy; Perineal Care *NOC:* Immune Status; Infection Status

Nursing Diagnosis:

Impaired Gas Exchange

related to altered oxygen supply secondary to presence of pulmonary infiltrates, hyperventilation, and sepsis

Desired Outcomes: Optimally within 24 hr after treatment/intervention, patient has adequate gas exchange as evidenced by RR 12-20 breaths/min with normal depth and pattern (eupnea) and absence of adventitious sounds, nasal flaring, and other clinical indicators of respiratory dysfunction. Patient's oximetry reveals O_2 saturation >92% or arterial blood gas (ABG) results as follows: PaO_2 ≥80 mm Hg; $PaCO_2$ 35-45 mm Hg; pH 7.35-7.45.

INTERVENTIONS	RATIONALES
Assess respiratory status q2h during patient's awake period, noting rate, rhythm, depth, and regularity of respirations.	Use of accessory muscles, flaring of nares, presence of adventitious sounds, cough, changes in color or character of sputum, or cyanosis occur with respiratory dysfunction. See discussion in previous nursing diagnosis about adventitious sounds that can occur with opportunistic infections that have pulmonary signs and symptoms.
As indicated, assess O_2 saturation via oximetry.	O_2 saturation ≤92% may signal need for supplementary oxygen and should be reported to health care provider.
Monitor ABG results closely.	Decreased $Paco_2$ (<35 mm Hg) and increased pH (>7.40) can occur with hyperventilation.
As prescribed, initiate or adjust oxygen therapy.	To attain optimal oxygenation, as determined by ABG values.
Deliver humidified oxygen to patient.	To prevent convective losses of moisture and relieve mucous membrane irritation, which can predispose patient to coughing spells.
Instruct patient to report changes in cough, as well as dyspnea that increases with exertion.	May be seen with opportunistic respiratory disease.
Provide chest physiotherapy as prescribed; encourage use of incentive spirometry at frequent intervals.	To maintain adequate tidal volume.
Reposition patient q2h.	To help prevent stasis of lung fluids.
Obtain sputum for culture and sensitivity as indicated.	Changes in color and character of patient's sputum may signal infection; a culture would confirm infection type.
Group nursing activities to provide periods of rest, optimally 90-120 min at a time.	To facilitate uninterrupted rest, which will promote optimum chest excursion.
When administering sulfa for PCP, monitor closely for rash or bone marrow suppression (leukopenia, neutropenia).	Side effects of sulfa.
If administering pentamidine, be alert to side effects such as hypotension or hypoglycemia.	These side effects necessitate frequent BP checks and fingersticks for blood sugar levels.
Administer sedatives and analgesics judiciously.	To help prevent or minimize respiratory depression.
When caring for patients diagnosed as having active tuberculosis, wear respiratory protection consistent with Centers for Disease Control (CDC) and Occupational Safety and Health Administration (OSHA) guidelines. See "Pulmonary Tuberculosis," p. 159, for more information.	To prevent spread of disease.

●●● **Related NIC and NOC labels:** *NIC:* Acid/Base Monitoring; Oxygen Therapy; Chest Physiotherapy; Energy Management; Respiratory Monitoring; Laboratory Data Interpretation; Vital Signs Monitoring; Medication Management *NOC:* Respiratory Status: Gas Exchange; Vital Signs Status; Tissue Perfusion: Pulmonary

Nursing Diagnosis:

Imbalanced Nutrition: Less than body requirements

related to diarrhea and nausea associated with side effects of medications, malabsorption, anorexia, dysphagia, and fatigue

Desired Outcomes: Optimally within 72 hr of this diagnosis, patient exhibits adequate nutrition as evidenced by stable weight, serum albumin 3.5-5.5 g/dl, transferrin 180-260 mg/dl, thyroxine-binding prealbumin 20-30 mg/dl, retinol-binding protein 4-5 mg/dl, and a state of nitrogen (N) balance or a positive N state. Within 24 hr, patient states that nausea and other GI side effects associated with antiretroviral treatment are controlled.

INTERVENTIONS	RATIONALES
Assess nutritional status daily, noting weight, caloric intake, and protein and albumin values.	Progressive weight loss, wasting of muscle tissue, loss of skin tone, and decreases in both total protein and albumin can adversely affect wound healing and impair patient's ability to withstand infection.
Provide small, frequent, high-caloric, high-protein meals, allowing sufficient time for patient to eat. Offer supplements between feedings.	As a rule, these patients are kept in a slightly positive N state (after resolution of the critical phases of this illness) by ensuring daily caloric intake equal to 50 kcal/kg of ideal body weight with an additional 1.5 g of protein per kilogram (e.g., a man weighing 70 kg should receive 3500 kcal plus 105 g of protein per day).
Provide supplemental vitamins and minerals as prescribed.	To replace deficiencies.
Provide oral hygiene before and after meals.	To minimize anorexia and help treat stomatitis, which can occur as a side effect of chemotherapy.
If patient feels isolated socially, encourage significant other to visit at mealtimes and bring patient's favorite high-caloric, high-protein foods from home.	Patient will benefit from socialization at mealtime, which also may promote intake of these high-caloric, high-protein foods.
If patient is nauseated, provide instructions for deep breathing and voluntary swallowing.	To help decrease stimulation of vomiting center.
Administer antiemetics as prescribed. Encourage patients to request medication before discomfort becomes severe.	To help prevent or minimize nausea.
If patient is dysphagic, encourage intake of fluids that are high in calories and protein; provide different flavors and textures for variation.	Fluids may be better tolerated than foods when the patient has dysphagia because they are less irritating; fluids that contain supplemental nutrients will help ensure optimal intake.
As prescribed, deliver isotonic tube feeding for patients unable to eat.	Isotonic fluids will help prevent diarrhea associated with hypertonic or hypotonic fluids.
Check placement of gastric tube before each feeding.	To prevent instillation of fluids into respiratory tract.
Evaluate amount of residual feeding q4h.	To assess degree of feeding that has not been absorbed. Usually feedings are not delivered if residual is >50-100 ml.
Keep head of bed (HOB) elevated 30 degrees while feeding, and position patient in a right side-lying position.	To facilitate gastric emptying and help prevent aspiration.
If indicated, discuss potential need for total parenteral nutrition (TPN) with health care provider.	If patient's caloric intake is insufficient.

●●● **Related NIC and NOC labels:** *NIC:* Nutrition Management; Nutritional Monitoring; Enteral Tube Feeding; Total Parenteral Nutrition Administration; Sustenance Support *NOC:* Nutrition Status; Nutritional Status: Food and Fluid Intake; Nutritional Status: Nutrient Intake

Nursing Diagnosis:

Diarrhea

related to GI infection, chemotherapy, or tube feeding intolerance

Desired Outcome: Within 3 days of this diagnosis, patient has formed stools and a bowel elimination pattern that is normal for him or her.

INTERVENTIONS	RATIONALES
Ensure minimal use of antidiarrheal medications.	Antidiarrheal medications promote intestinal concentration of infectious organisms.
Teach patient to avoid large amounts (>300 mg/day) of caffeine.	Caffeine increases peristalsis and can promote diarrhea.
Maintain accurate I&O records.	To monitor changes in fluid volume status.
Be alert to cool and clammy skin, increased HR (>100 bpm), increased RR (>20 breaths/min), and decreased urinary output (<30 ml/hr).	Signs of hypovolemia that could result from prolonged diarrhea.
Monitor stool cultures.	For evidence of infectious organisms that could be causing the diarrhea.
Monitor for anxiety, confusion, muscle weakness, cramps, dysrhythmias, weak pulse, and decreased BP.	Indicators of electrolyte imbalance that could occur because of fluid loss.
If patient is being given enteral feedings, dilute strength or decrease rate of infusion to prevent "solute drag" (concentrated solutions that pull water into bowel lumen).	Solute drag may be the cause of the diarrhea.
Encourage foods high in potassium (K^+) and sodium (Na^+).	To replace any decrements of these ions.
Protect anorectal area by keeping it cleansed and using compounds such as zinc oxide.	To prevent or retard skin excoriation caused by diarrhea.

●●● **Related NIC and NOC labels:** *NIC:* Diarrhea Management; Medication Management; Electrolyte Management: Hypokalemia; Electrolyte Management: Hyponatremia; Specimen Management; Skin Care: Topical Treatments; Perineal Care *NOC:* Electrolyte and Acid/Base Balance; Bowel Elimination; Symptom Severity

Nursing Diagnosis:

Impaired Tissue Integrity

(or risk for same) *related to* cachexia and malnourishment, diarrhea, side effects of chemotherapy, KS lesions, negative N state, and decreased mobility caused by arthralgia and fatigue

Desired Outcome: Patient's tissue shows signs of healing within 3 days of this diagnosis.

INTERVENTIONS	RATIONALES
Assess and document temperature, moisture, color, vascularity, texture, lesions, and areas of excoriation or poor wound healing. Evaluate KS lesions for location, dissemination, weeping, or significant changes.	A thorough baseline assessment of patient's skin integrity should be performed to which subsequent assessments are compared to determine improving or worsening condition.
Document presence of herpes lesions, especially those that are perirectal.	To enable appropriate systemic treatment and management of pain.
Encourage patient to change position frequently.	To avoid prolonged pressure on dependent body parts, which could cause breakdown in skin that is already at risk.
As indicated, use mattress such as foam, low air loss, alternating air, gel, or water.	These mattresses reduce pressure on body tissues.
Teach patient to use mild, hypoallergenic, nondrying soaps or lanolin-based products for bathing and to rinse thoroughly. When appropriate, use lotions and emollients.	To soften and prevent/relieve itching of dry, flaky skin.
Use soft sheets on the bed, avoiding wrinkles. If patient is incontinent, use some type of rectal device (e.g., fecal incontinence bags, rectal tube).	To protect skin and prevent perirectal excoriation and skin breakdown.

Continued

INTERVENTIONS	RATIONALES
Assist patient toward a positive N state by promoting adequate amounts of protein and carbohydrates (see discussion under **Imbalanced Nutrition,** p. 573).	To promote skin and tissue healing.
Ensure that patient receives minimum daily requirements of vitamins and minerals; supplement them as necessary.	To promote skin and tissue healing.
Encourage range of motion (ROM) and weight-bearing mobility, when possible.	To increase circulation to skin and tissue, which will improve skin/tissue integrity.

●●● **Related NIC and NOC labels:** *NIC:* Wound Care; Nutrition Management; Pressure Management; Bathing; Diarrhea Management; Perineal Care *NOC:* Tissue Integrity: Skin and Mucous Membranes

Nursing Diagnosis:

Acute Pain

related to physical and chemical factors associated with prolonged immobility, side effects of chemotherapy, infections, peripheral neuropathy, and frequent venipunctures

Desired Outcomes: Within 1 hr of intervention, patient's subjective perception of pain decreases, as documented by a pain scale. Nonverbal indicators of discomfort, such as grimacing, are absent or diminished.

INTERVENTIONS	RATIONALES
Assess and record the following: location, onset, duration, and factors that precipitate and alleviate patient's pain. With patient, establish a pain scale, rating pain from 0 (no pain) to 10 (worst pain). Use the scale to evaluate degree of pain and to document degree of relief achieved.	Competent pain management requires frequent and thorough assessment of these factors. Using a pain scale provides an objective measurement that enables assessment of pain management strategies.
Administer analgesic as prescribed. Encourage patient to request medication before the pain becomes severe.	Pain that is allowed to become severe is more difficult to control. Prolonged stimulation of pain receptors results in increased sensitivity to painful stimuli and will increase the amount of drug required to relieve pain.
Provide heat or cold applications to affected areas (e.g., apply heat to painful joints and cold packs to reduce swelling associated with infections or multiple venipunctures).	Heat and cold applications are effective nonpharmacologic measures that reduce pain, as well as augment effects of analgesics.
Encourage patient to engage in diversional activities. Examples include soothing music; quiet conversation; reading; slow, rhythmic breathing.	Diversion is a means of increasing pain tolerance and decreasing its intensity.
Teach techniques such as deep breathing, biofeedback, and relaxation exercises (see **Health-Seeking Behaviors:** Relaxation technique effective for stress reduction, p. 183).	These techniques reduce pain intensity by decreasing skeletal muscle tension.
Discuss with health care provider the desirability of a capped venous catheter for long-term blood withdrawal.	For patients in whom frequent venipunctures cause discomfort.
Administer anticonvulsant agents as prescribed.	For relief of peripheral neuropathy.
Use back rubs and massage.	To promote relaxation and comfort.

●●● **Related NIC and NOC labels:** *NIC:* Pain Management; Medication Management; Biofeedback; Simple Massage; Simple Relaxation Therapy; Distraction; Heat/Cold Application; Music Therapy *NOC:* Comfort Level; Pain Control; Pain: Disruptive Effects

Nursing Diagnosis:

Activity Intolerance

related to generalized weakness secondary to fluid and electrolyte imbalance, arthralgia, myalgia, dyspnea, fever, pain, hypoxia, and effects of chemotherapy

Desired Outcome: Patient rates perceived exertion (RPE) at ≤3 on a 0-10 scale and exhibits tolerance to activity as evidenced by HR ≤20 bpm over resting HR, RR ≤20 breaths/min, and systolic BP ≤20 mm Hg over or under resting systolic BP.

INTERVENTIONS	RATIONALES
Assess HR, RR, and BP before and immediately after activity and ask patient to rate his or her perceived exertion. See "Prolonged Bedrest" for **Activity Intolerance,** p. 67, for details about perceived exertion.	To determine patient's tolerance to activity. If patient's RPE is >3 or he or she exhibits signs of activity intolerance, the activity should be stopped or modified.
Plan adequate (90- to 120-min) rest periods between scheduled activities. Adjust activities as appropriate.	To reduce patient's energy expenditure.
As much as possible, encourage regular periods of exercise.	To help prevent cardiac intolerance to activities, which can occur quickly after periods of prolonged inactivity.
Monitor electrolyte levels.	To determine if muscle weakness is caused by hypokalemia.
Monitor oximetry or ABG values.	Oxygen saturation ≤92% may signal need for supplemental oxygen or an increase in oxygen delivery.
Advise patient to keep anecdotal notes (perhaps in journal format) on exacerbation and remission of signs and symptoms.	A useful tool for self-examination, as well as for reporting to health care provider, who may use this information to alter or modify treatment or develop new strategies.

●●● **Related NIC and NOC labels:** *NIC:* Energy Management; Exercise Promotion; Oxygen Therapy
NOC: Activity Tolerance; Endurance; Energy Conservation

Nursing Diagnoses:

Anxiety and Fear

related to threat of death and social isolation

Desired Outcome: Within 3 hr following intervention, patient expresses feelings and is free of harmful anxiety and fears as evidenced by HR ≤100 bpm, RR ≤20 breaths/min with normal depth and pattern (eupnea), and BP within patient's normal range.

INTERVENTIONS	RATIONALES
Monitor for verbal or nonverbal expressions of anxiety/fear.	Inability to cope, apprehension, guilt for past actions, uncertainty, concerns about rejection and isolation, and suicidal ideation are likely signs of anxiety/fear or depression.
Spend time with patient and encourage expression of feelings and concerns.	Before patients can learn effective coping strategies, they must first clarify their feelings. Verbalizing feelings in a nonthreatening, nonjudgmental environment can help patients deal with unresolved/unrecognized issues that may be contributing to the current stressor.

Continued

INTERVENTIONS	RATIONALES
Support effective coping patterns (e.g., by allowing patient to cry or talk rather than denying his or her legitimate fears and concerns).	To promote healthy behaviors and help build trust.
Provide accurate information about HIV disease, related diagnostic procedures, and emerging treatments.	Some fears and anxieties may be realistic, whereas others may necessitate clarification based on current treatment information.
If patient hyperventilates, teach him or her to mimic your normal respiratory pattern (eupnea).	An effective calming technique.

●●● **Related NIC and NOC labels:** *NIC:* Anxiety Reduction; Active Listening; Calming Technique; Coping Enhancement; Presence *NOC:* Anxiety Control; Coping; Fear Control

Nursing Diagnosis:

Disturbed Body Image

related to biophysical changes secondary to KS lesions, chemotherapy, emaciation, and HAART

Desired Outcome: Within 24 hr of this diagnosis, patient expresses positive feelings about self to family, significant other, and primary nurse.

INTERVENTIONS	RATIONALES
Encourage patient to express feelings, especially the way he or she views or feels about self. Provide patient with positive feedback; help patient focus on facts rather than myths or exaggerations about self.	Provides an environment conducive to free expression and promotes patient's understanding of health status, which may clarify misconceptions that may be contributing to the disturbed body image.
Provide patient with access to clergy, psychiatric nurse, social worker, psychologist, or HIV counselor as appropriate.	Patient may require specialized counseling, especially if he or she is at risk for self-harm.
Encourage patient to join and share feelings with HIV support group.	Many people benefit from support groups and sharing experiences with others who are having similar experiences.
For additional information, see "Psychosocial Support" for **Disturbed Body Image,** p. 92.	

●●● **Related NIC and NOC labels:** *NIC:* Body Image Enhancement; Active Listening; Coping Enhancement; Emotional Support; Counseling; Support Group *NOC:* Body Image; Psychosocial Adjustment: Life Change

Nursing Diagnosis:

Deficient Knowledge:

Disease process, prognosis, lifestyle changes, health maintenance, and treatment plan

Desired Outcome: Within the 24-hr period following instruction/intervention, patient verbalizes accurate information about the disease process, prognosis, behaviors that increase risk of transmitting the virus to others, and treatment plan.

INTERVENTIONS	RATIONALES
Assess knowledge about HIV disease, including pathophysiologic changes that will occur, ways the disease is transmitted, necessary behavioral changes, and side effects of treatment. Provide literature that explores myths and realities of HIV disease process.	This information enables nurse to formulate an individualized teaching plan and correct misinformation and misconceptions as necessary.
Inform patient of private and community agencies that are available to help with tasks such as handling legal affairs, cooking, house cleaning, and nursing care. Provide telephone numbers and addresses for HIV support groups and self-help groups.	Lack of knowledge about these services and groups may add unnecessary stress to patient's illness.
Teach importance of informing sexual partners of HIV condition and modifying high-risk behaviors known to transmit the virus.	To reduce risk of transmitting virus to others.
Involve significant other in the teaching and learning process.	Anxiety often filters information being given. Involving the significant other in the teaching process not only provides information to him or her but enables the significant other to reinforce teaching for the patient as well.
Provide patient and significant other with names and addresses or phone numbers of HIV resources (see "Patient-Family Teaching and Discharge Planning," p. 581).	These resources provide information about current therapies, support services, and funding for medications.

●●● **Related NIC and NOC labels:** *NIC:* Teaching: Disease Process; Behavior Modification, Teaching: Safe Sex; Discharge Planning; Health Care Information Exchange *NOC:* Knowledge: Health Behaviors; Knowledge: Health Resources; Knowledge: Illness Care; Knowledge: Infection Control; Knowledge: Disease Process: Knowledge: Treatment Regimen

Nursing Diagnosis:

Social Isolation

related to altered state of wellness, societal rejection, loss of support system, feelings of guilt and punishment, fatigue, and changed patterns of sexual expression

Desired Outcome: Within 24 hr of this diagnosis, patient begins to communicate and interact with others.

INTERVENTIONS	RATIONALES
Keep patient and significant other well informed about patient's status and treatment plan.	To reduce sense of isolation.
Provide private periods of time for patient to communicate and interact with significant other.	To facilitate communication with significant other.
Encourage significant other to share in care of patient. Encourage physical closeness between patient and significant other. Provide privacy as much as possible.	To increase amount of time for interaction and communication with significant other.
Involve patient in unit or group activities as appropriate.	To reduce sense of isolation and promote socialization.

Continued

INTERVENTIONS	RATIONALES
Explain significance of transmission precautions to patient.	Understanding rationale for these precautions may help patient cope with them better and develop new approaches to life with HIV infection.
Provide link with community support services.	Provides contact with others, psychosocial support, resources, and care.

●●● **Related NIC and NOC labels:** *NIC:* Socialization Enhancement; Support System Enhancement; Active Listening; Presence; Therapy Group; Touch; Visitation Facilitation; Support Group *NOC:* Loneliness; Social Involvement; Social Support

Nursing Diagnosis:

Impaired Environmental Interpretation Syndrome

related to physiologic changes and impaired judgment secondary to infection, space-occupying lesion in the central nervous system (CNS), or HIV dementia

Desired Outcomes: Immediately following intervention, patient verbalizes orientation to person, place, and time. Optimally, within 1 mo patient correctly completes exercises in logical reasoning, memory, perception, concentration, attention, and sequencing of activities.

INTERVENTIONS	RATIONALES
Assess for minor alterations in personality traits that cannot be attributed to other causes, such as stress or medication.	May help rule out medication side effects or opportunistic diseases.
Assess for a slowing of all cognitive functioning, with problems of attention, concentration, memory, perception, logical reasoning, and sequencing of activities.	Signs of dementia.
Encourage patient to report persistent headaches, dizziness, or seizures.	May signal CNS involvement.
Note any cranial nerve involvement that differs from patient's past medical history.	Most commonly the fifth (trigeminal), seventh (facial), and eighth (acoustic) nerves are involved in infectious processes of the CNS.
Assess for signs of mental aberration, blindness, aphasia, hemiparesis, or ataxia.	May signal presence of a demyelinating disease. Blindness, for example, can occur with an opportunistic infection.
Divide activities into small, easily accomplished tasks.	Pacing activities decreases frustration and increases likelihood of completion.
Maintain a stable environment (i.e., do not change location of furniture in room).	Helps patient familiarize self with immediate surroundings.
Write notes as reminders; maintain calendar of appointments. Provide some mechanism (e.g., pill box) to ensure that patient takes medications as prescribed.	Patient will require these reminders to complete tasks, take medications, and make appointments as independently as possible.
Teach importance of reporting changes in neurologic status (e.g., increasing severity of headaches, blurred vision, gait disturbances, or blackouts). Notify health care provider of all significant findings.	Identifies changes that necessitate treatment intervention.

●●● **Related NIC and NOC labels:** *NIC:* Dementia Management; Reality Orientation; Environmental Management; Learning Facilitation; Medication Management *NOC:* Cognitive Orientation; Information Processing; Memory; Safety Behavior: Home Physical Environment

Additional Nursing Diagnoses/ Problems:

PATIENT-FAMILY TEACHING AND DISCHARGE PLANNING

When providing patient-family teaching, focus on sensory information, avoid giving excessive information, and initiate a visiting nurse referral for necessary follow-up teaching. Include verbal and written information about the following:

✓ Importance of avoiding use of recreational drugs, which are believed to potentiate immunosuppressive process, lower resistance to infection, and cause poor judgment that may lead to high-risk behavior.

✓ Significance and importance of refraining from donating blood.

✓ Necessity of modifying high-risk sexual behaviors.

✓ Principles and importance of maintaining a balanced diet; ways to supplement diet with multivitamins and other food sources, such as high-caloric substances (e.g., Isocal, Ensure). Because of increased susceptibility to foodborne opportunistic organisms, fruits and vegetables should be washed thoroughly; meats should be cooked thoroughly at appropriate temperatures; and raw eggs, raw fish (sushi), and unpasteurized milk should be avoided.

✓ Because of decreased resistance to infection, the importance of limiting contact with individuals known to have active infections. In addition, pets may harbor various fungal, protozoal, and bacterial organisms in their excrement. Therefore contact with bird cages, cat litter, and tropical fish tanks should be avoided.

✓ Necessity for meticulous hygiene to prevent spread of any extant or new infectious organisms. To avoid exposure to fungi, damp areas in bathrooms (e.g., shower) should be cleaned with solutions of bleach, refrigerators should be cleaned thoroughly with soap and water, and leftover foodstuffs should be disposed of within 2-3 days.

✓ Techniques for self-assessment of early signs of infection (e.g., erythema, tenderness, local warmth, swelling, purulent exudate) in all cuts, abrasions, lesions, or open wounds.

✓ Care of venous access device, including technique for self-administration of TPN or medications; care of gastric tube and administration of enteral tube feedings if appropriate (see "Providing Nutritional Support," p. 589).

✓ Importance of avoiding fatigue by limiting participation in social activities, getting maximum amounts of rest, and minimizing physical exertion.

✓ Prescribed medications, including drug name, food/drug and drug/drug interactions, dosage, purpose, and potential side effects. Instruct patient and significant other in the necessity of taking antiretroviral medications as prescribed to avoid viral resistance (especially in the case of protease inhibitors).

✓ Importance of maintaining medical follow-up appointments.

✓ Advisability of keeping anecdotal notes (perhaps in journal format) on exacerbation and remission of signs and symptoms.

✓ Importance of reporting changes in neurologic status (e.g., increasing severity of headaches, blurred vision, gait disturbances, blackouts).

✓ Advisability of sharing feelings with significant other or within a support group.

✓ Referral to hospice or agency that provides home help. This should occur before discharge planning begins to ensure continuity of care between hospital and home or hospice.

✓ Patient adherence to treatment education. HIV treatment adherence has become increasingly important to persons with HIV disease and the clinicians providing and monitoring their care. Data from HIV drug clinical trials indicate that adherence to medication regimens is critical to successful treatment. Interruptions in drug treatment can lead to development of viruses resistant to specific antiretroviral drugs, which can result in treatment failure and limit future treatment options. Health care provider and patient partnerships characterized by shared decision making has been identified as a key component in successful HIV treatment.

✓ Strategies for promoting HIV treatment adherence. These must be customized to meet needs of each patient. The approach must be patient-centered and include ongoing education, psychosocial and community support, and resources that involve both patient-directed and provider directed strategies.

✓ Phone numbers to call if questions or concerns arise about hospice after discharge. Information for these patients can be obtained by contacting the following organization:

National Hospice and Palliative Care Organization
1901 North Moore St., Suite 901
Arlington, VA 22209
(703) 243-5900
Fax: (703) 525-5762
www.nhpco.org

✓ In addition, provide the following information regarding HIV resources:

Public Health Service AIDS Hotline
(800) 342-AIDS or (800) 342-2437

National Gay Task Force AIDS Information Hotline
(800) 221-7044

National Sexually Transmitted Diseases Hotline/American Social Health Association
(800) 227-8922

Local chapter of American Red Cross
American Red Cross AIDS Education Office
1730 D Street NW
Washington, DC 20006
(202) 737-8300

CDC National Prevention Information Network
(NPIN)
P.O. Box 6003
Rockville, MD 20849-6003
(800) 243-7012
www.cdcnpin.org

National AIDS Network
729 Eighth Street SE, Suite 300
Washington, DC 20003
(202) 546-2424

Association of Nurses in AIDS Care (ANAC)
11250 Roger Bacon Drive, Suite 8
Reston, VA 20190-5202
(703) 437-4377
www.anacnet.org

National AIDS Education and Training Centers
Health Resources and Services Administration (HRSA)
HIV/AIDS Bureau
5600 Fishers Lane
Parklawn Building, Room 7-99
Rockville, MD 20857
(301) 443-6364

72

Managing Wound Care

A wound is a disruption of tissue integrity caused by trauma, surgery, or an underlying medical disorder. Wound management is directed at preventing infection and deterioration in wound status and promoting healing.

WOUNDS CLOSED BY PRIMARY INTENTION

Clean, surgical, or traumatic wounds whose edges are closed with sutures, clips, tissue glue, or sterile tape strips are referred to as wounds closed by primary intention. Impairment of healing most frequently manifests as dehiscence, evisceration, or infection. Individuals at high risk for disruption of wound healing include those who are obese, diabetic, elderly, malnourished, receiving steroids, or undergoing chemotherapy or radiation therapy.

HEALTH CARE SETTING

Primary care, acute care

ASSESSMENT

Optimal healing: Warm, reddened, indurated, tender incision line immediately after injury. After 1 or 2 days, epithelial cells migrate across the incision line and seal the wound. Over time, a pink scar is visible. After 7-9 days, a healing ridge—a palpable accumulation of scar tissue—forms. In patients who undergo cosmetic surgery, the healing ridge is purposely avoided to minimize scar formation. Healing is complete when structural and functional integrity are reestablished.

Impaired healing: Lack of an adequate inflammatory response manifested by absence of initial redness, warmth, and induration or inflammation that persists or occurs after the fifth postinjury day; continued drainage from the incision line 2 days after injury (when no drain is present); absence of a healing ridge by the ninth day after injury; presence of purulent exudate.

DIAGNOSTIC TESTS

White blood cell (WBC) count with differential: To assess for infection.

Gram stain of drainage: If infection is suspected, to identify the offending organism and aid in the selection of preliminary antibiotics.

Culture and sensitivity of tissue by biopsy or swab: To determine optimal antibiotic. Infection is said to be present when there are $\geq 10^5$ organisms/g of tissue or when fever and drainage are present.

Nursing Diagnosis:

Impaired Tissue Integrity: Wound

related to altered blood flow, metabolic disorders (e.g., diabetes mellitus [DM]), alterations in fluid volume and nutrition, and medical therapy (chemotherapy, radiation therapy, steroid administration)

Desired Outcome: Patient exhibits the following signs of wound healing: well-approximated wound edges; good initial postinjury inflammatory response (erythema, warmth, induration, pain); no inflammatory response past the fifth day after injury; no drainage (without drain present) 48 hr after closure; healing ridge present by postoperative day 7-9.

INTERVENTIONS	RATIONALES
Assess wound for absence of a healing ridge, presence of drainage or purulent exudate, and delayed or prolonged inflammatory response.	Indications of impaired healing.
Monitor VS for elevated temperature and HR. Document findings.	Signs of infection, a manifestation of impaired wound healing.
Follow sterile technique when changing dressings. If a drain is present, keep it sterile, maintain patency (e.g., empty drainage reservoir and recharge suction on closed drainage systems as needed), and handle it gently to prevent it from becoming dislodged. If wound care will be necessary after hospital discharge, teach dressing change procedure to patient and significant other.	Sterile technique eliminates introduction of nosocomial organisms to prevent infection. Most outpatient wound care is done with clean technique. Clean technique is used at home because most people have antibodies to familiar organisms. For immunosuppressed patients, however, sterile technique likely is used at home.
Perform serial monitoring of capillary glucose for persons with DM and administer insulin to keep glucose level ≤150 mg/dl.	To maintain blood glucose within normal range for persons with DM. Hyperglycemia increases risk for infection and impairs blood flow and oxygen release, thereby adversely affecting wound healing.
Explain to patient that deep breathing promotes oxygenation. Encourage deep breathing q2h while awake. Splint incision as needed. If indicated, provide incentive spirometry.	Oxygen enhances wound healing.
Stress importance of position changes and activity as tolerated.	To promote ventilation and circulation and hence oxygenation.
As indicated, monitor pulse oximetry.	Oxygen saturation ≤92% often signals need for supplemental oxygen. After injury, wound Po_2 is low, and administration of O_2 may promote healing.
Monitor BP, HR, and capillary refill time in tissue adjacent to incision.	To determine if blood flow to the area is adequate for healing. BP and HR optimally should be within patient's normal limits; capillary refill should be <2 sec, which signals adequate tissue perfusion to the area.
Assess peripheral pulses, moisture of mucous membranes, skin turgor, volume and specific gravity of urine, and I&O to monitor hydration status.	Hypovolemia adversely affects wound healing.
For nonrestricted patients, ensure a fluid intake of at least 30 ml/kg body weight/day.	To ensure that patient has adequate hydration to assist with healing.
Provide a diet with adequate protein, vitamin C, and calories. If patient complains of feeling full with three meals per day, give more frequent small feedings. Encourage between-meal high-protein supplements (e.g., yogurt, milk shakes).	This diet promotes positive nitrogen balance and nutrients needed for wound healing. Smaller, more frequent meals are often more easily tolerated.
Monitor serum albumin and total lymphocyte counts and report decreases; consult health care provider about high-protein nutrition supplements.	Serum albumin <3.5 g/dl and total lymphocyte count <1800/mm³ can be indications of malnutrition and may necessitate supplemental protein, vitamins, and minerals.

●●● **Related NIC and NOC labels:** *NIC:* Incision Site Care; Wound Care; Fluid Management; Infection Protection *NOC:* Wound Healing: Primary Intention

PATIENT-FAMILY TEACHING AND DISCHARGE PLANNING

When providing patient-family teaching, focus on essential information, avoid giving excessive information, and initiate a home health referral for necessary follow-up care and teaching. Include verbal and written information about the following:

✓Local wound care, including type of equipment necessary, wound care procedure, and therapeutic and negative side effects of topical agents used. Have patient or significant other demonstrate dressing change procedure before hospital discharge.

✓Signs and symptoms of improvement in wound status.

✓Signs and symptoms of deterioration in wound status, including those that necessitate notification of health care provider or clinic.

✓ Diet that promotes wound healing. Discuss importance of adequate protein and calorie intake. See "Providing Nutritional Support," p. 589. Involve dietitian, patient, and significant other as necessary.

✓ Importance of taking multivitamins, antibiotics, and supplements of iron and zinc as prescribed. For all medications to be taken at home, provide the following: drug name, purpose, dosage, schedule, precautions, drug/drug and food/drug interactions, and potential side effects.

✓ Importance of follow-up care with health care provider; confirm time and date of next appointment if known.

✓ If needed, arrange for a visit by a home health nurse before hospital discharge.

SURGICAL OR TRAUMATIC WOUNDS HEALING BY SECONDARY INTENTION

Wounds healing by secondary intention are those with tissue loss or heavy contamination that form granulation tissue, contract, and epithelialize in order to heal. Most often, impairment of healing is caused by contamination and inadequate blood flow, oxygenation, and nutrition. Individuals at risk for impaired healing include those who are obese, diabetic, malnourished, elderly, taking steroids, or undergoing radiation therapy or chemotherapy.

HEALTH CARE SETTING

Acute care, primary care, long-term care, home care

ASSESSMENT

Optimal healing: In the first 3-5 days after surgery, the tissue surrounding the incision is inflamed, indurated, and tender. New granulation tissue is pink and becomes red as its blood supply increases. Wound size decreases as healing progresses.

When a drain is in place, the volume, color, and odor of the drainage should be evaluated. The time frame for healing depends on the size and location of the wound and on the patient's physical and psychologic status. Epithelialization occurs to close the wound. Healing is complete when structure and function have been reestablished.

Impaired healing: Exudate on the floor and walls of the wound signals increased bacterial burden. Occasionally a wound has a tract or sinus that decreases in size gradually as healing occurs.

DIAGNOSTIC TESTS

Complete blood count (CBC) with white blood cell (WBC) differential: Increased WBC count signals infection, whereas a decrease occurs with immunosuppression. Watch the differential for a shift to the left, which indicates infection. Monitor the lymphocyte count and serum albumin: $<1800/mm^3$ and <3.5 g/dl, respectively, may be signs of malnutrition. For optimal healing, the Hct should be $>25\%$.

Gram stain: To determine the characteristics of the offending organism, if present, and aid in selection of the preliminary antibiotic.

Tissue biopsy: To determine presence of infection and the optimal antibiotic, if appropriate.

Nursing Diagnosis:

Impaired Tissue Integrity: Wound

related to presence of contaminants, metabolic disorders (e.g., DM), medical therapy (e.g., chemotherapy, radiation therapy), altered perfusion, or malnutrition

Desired Outcomes: Granulation tissue develops and the wound decreases in size. The wound is free of slough, necrotic tissue, and odor. Patient or significant other successfully demonstrates wound care procedure before hospital discharge, if appropriate.

INTERVENTIONS	RATIONALES
Monitor for the following: decreased inflammatory response in the first 3 days or inflammation that lasts >5 days; granulation tissue that remains pale or excessively dry or moist; presence of odor, exudate, and/or necrotic tissue; and disrupted or slow epithelialization.	Signs of impaired healing.
Cleanse drainage or secretions from skin surrounding wound with a mild disinfectant (e.g., soap and water).	To help prevent contamination.
Cleanse wound with each dressing change using 100-150 ml normal saline or a commercial wound cleanser via a 35-ml syringe and 18-gauge angiocatheter.	To dislodge and remove bacteria and loosen necrotic tissue, foreign bodies, and exudate.

Continued

INTERVENTIONS	RATIONALES
When topical enzymes are prescribed, use them on necrotic tissue only and follow package directions carefully.	To remove necrotic tissue and spare healthy tissue.
Apply hydrophilic agent such as dextranomer (Debrisan) as prescribed.	To remove contaminants and excess exudate.
Remove hydrophilic agents with high-pressure irrigation.	If removed with a 4 × 4 or surgical sponge, the friction would disrupt capillary budding and delay healing.
Apply prescribed dressings, such as moist to moist, transparent, hydrocolloid, hydrogel, alginate, foam, hypertonic, and silver dressings, following meticulous infection control procedures.	Depending on patient's individual need, these dressings keep healthy wound tissue moist. Silver dressings decrease surface bacterial counts.
Insert dressing into all tracts.	To promote gradual closure of those areas.
Ensure good handwashing before and after dressing changes and dispose of contaminated dressings appropriately.	To prevent spread of infection both to patient and others.
When a drain is used, maintain its patency, prevent kinking of the tubing, and secure tubing to prevent the drain from becoming dislodged.	Drains remove excess tissue fluid or purulent drainage.
Use sterile technique when caring for drains.	Drains are inserted directly into tissue.
	Organisms may move into tissue by way of the drain. Sterile technique reduces risk of contamination and ingress of organisms.
With closed drainage systems, empty drainage reservoir and maintain suction as needed.	Suction aids in removal of excess fluid.
Teach patient or significant other prescribed wound care procedure, if indicated.	Wound care may be required after patient is discharged.
See discussion of diet, supplemental oxygen, insulin, hydration, and supplemental vitamins in **Impaired Tissue Integrity**, p. 583, in "Wounds Closed by Primary Intention."	

●●● **Related NIC and NOC labels:** *NIC:* Wound Care; Fluid Management; Infection Control; Infection Protection; Nutrition Management; Wound Care: Closed Drainage; Wound Irrigation *NOC:* Wound Healing: Secondary Intention

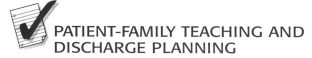

PATIENT-FAMILY TEACHING AND DISCHARGE PLANNING

See teaching and discharge planning interventions in "Wounds Closed by Primary Intention," p. 583.

PRESSURE ULCERS

Pressure ulcers result from a disruption in tissue integrity and are caused by external pressure, friction, and shear.

HEALTH CARE SETTING

Primary care, acute care, long-term care, assisted care, home care

ASSESSMENT

High-risk individuals should be identified with initial assessment, at regularly planned assessments, and when patient's condition changes. When pressure ulcers are present, their severity can be staged on a scale of I to IV as follows:

- **Stage I:** Observable pressure-related alteration of intact skin that appears as persistent redness in lightly pigmented skin, whereas in darker skin tones the ulcer may exhibit persistent red, blue, or purple hues
- **Stage II:** Partial-thickness skin loss that involves epidermis or dermis or both; seen as an abrasion, blister, or shallow crater
- **Stage III:** Full-thickness skin loss that involves subcutaneous tissue but does not extend through the fascia
- **Stage IV:** Full-thickness injury that involves muscle, bone, or supporting structures

See also "Surgical or Traumatic Wounds Healing by Secondary Intention," p. 585, for other assessment data.

DIAGNOSTIC TESTS

See "Diagnostic Tests," p. 585, in "Surgical or Traumatic Wounds Healing by Secondary Intention."

Nursing Diagnoses:

Risk for Impaired Skin Integrity and/or Impaired Tissue Integrity

related to potential for excessive external pressure, friction, and shear, especially in at-risk individuals

Desired Outcomes: Patient's skin and tissue remain intact. Patient or significant other participates in preventive measures and verbalizes accurate understanding of the rationale for these interventions.

INTERVENTIONS	RATIONALES
Identify individuals at risk and systematically assess skin over bony prominences daily; document.	High-risk patients include older persons and those who have decreased mobility, decreased level of consciousness (LOC), impaired sensation, debilitation, incontinence, sepsis/elevated temperature, or malnutrition.
Establish and post a position-changing schedule.	Increases awareness of turning and position-changing schedule for staff and patient/family.
Assist patient with position changes as follows:	There is an inverse relationship between pressure and time in ulcer formation; therefore heavier patients need to change position more frequently.
Turn bed-bound patients q1-2h and have wheelchair-bound patients (who are able) perform push-ups in the chair q15min.	To alternate sites of pressure relief.
Use pillows or foam wedges to pad and position.	To maintain alternative positions and pad bony prominences.
In addition, for patients with history of previous pressure ulcers, provide pressure-relief measures more frequently.	Healed pressure ulcers have a lower pressure tolerance than uninjured skin.
Position patient using the 30-degree rule: head of bed (HOB) <30 degrees; lateral position <30 degrees.	Having HOB <30 degrees minimizes shearing of tissues caused by sliding down in bed. Keeping lateral position <30 degrees prevents high pressures on the trochanter.
For immobile patients, raise heels off the bed surface.	To totally relieve pressure on heels.
Lift rather than drag patient during position changes and transferring.	To minimize friction and shear on tissue during activity.
Use a draw sheet.	To facilitate patient movement.
Do not massage over bony prominences.	This can result in skin/tissue damage.
Cleanse skin at the time of soiling and at routine intervals. Use moisture barriers and disposable briefs as needed.	To minimize skin exposure to moisture and chemical irritants.
Use a mattress such as foam, low air loss, alternating air, gel, or water.	These mattresses reduce pressure on body tissues.
Encourage patient to maintain or increase current level of activity.	To promote blood flow, which helps prevent impaired skin and tissue integrity.

●●● **Related NIC and NOC labels:** *NIC:* Bed Rest Care; Pressure Management; Circulatory Precautions; Positioning; Positioning: Wheelchair; Pressure Ulcer Prevention; Skin Surveillance; Bathing; *NOC:* Immobility Consequences: Physiological; Tissue Integrity: Skin and Mucous Membranes

Nursing Diagnosis:

Impaired Tissue Integrity:

Presence of pressure ulcer, with increased risk for further breakdown *related to* altered circulation and presence of contaminants or irritants (chemical, thermal, or mechanical)

Desired Outcomes: Stages I and II show progressive healing over days to weeks; stages III and IV heal within months. Immediately following intervention and instruction, patient or significant other verbalizes causes and preventive measures for pressure ulcers and successfully participates in the plan of care to promote healing and prevent further breakdown.

INTERVENTIONS	RATIONALES
Evaluate stage of pressure ulcer and wound status (see this nursing diagnosis in "Wounds Healing by Secondary Intention").	To provide data on healing status.
Maintain a moist physiologic environment. Change dressings as needed, using meticulous infection control procedure.	To promote tissue repair and minimize contaminants.
Be sure that patient's skin is kept clean with regular bathing and be especially conscientious about washing urine and feces from the skin. Use soap and thoroughly rinse it from the skin.	Incontinence causes chemical irritation to the skin and reduces tissue tolerance to external pressure.
Apply heel and elbow protection as needed.	To prevent shearing when patient moves.
Avoid use of a heat lamp.	A heat lamp dries tissues and increases tissue metabolic rate, resulting in increased demand for blood flow in an area with impaired perfusion. As a result, ulcer diameter and depth can be increased.
Teach patient and significant other the importance of and measures for preventing excess pressure as a means of preventing pressure ulcers.	Knowledgeable individuals are more likely to comply with prevention measures.
Provide wound care as needed (described under "Surgical or Traumatic Wounds Healing by Secondary Intention," earlier).	

●●● **Related NIC and NOC labels:** *NIC:* Wound Care; Pressure Ulcer Prevention; Infection Protection; Pressure Management; Bathing; Diarrhea Management; Pressure Ulcer Care; Urinary Incontinence Care *NOC:* Tissue Integrity: Skin and Mucous Membranes; Wound Healing: Secondary Intention

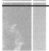

ADDITIONAL NURSING DIAGNOSES/ PROBLEMS:

"Surgical or Traumatic Wounds Healing   p. 585
   by Secondary Intention" for **Impaired Tissue Integrity**

PATIENT-FAMILY TEACHING AND DISCHARGE PLANNING

When providing patient-family teaching, focus on essential information, avoid giving excessive information, and initiate a home health referral for necessary follow-up teaching and care. Consider including verbal and written information about the following:

✓ Location of local medical supply stores that have pressure-reducing mattresses and wound care supplies.

✓ Planning a schedule for changing patient positions.

✓ See also: "Wounds Closed by Primary Intention," p. 584, for other teaching and discharge planning interventions.

Providing Nutritional Support

Hospitalized patients are at high risk for developing protein-energy malnutrition. Studies have shown that 40%-50% of hospitalized surgical patients have insufficient nutrient intake. This situation may be seen in surgical patients who are given IV dextrose/electrolyte solutions alone for extended periods and in patients kept fasting for diagnostic procedures. If this state lasts longer than 5-7 days or if the duration of illness without oral intake is expected to last longer than 10-14 days, nutritional support should be given.

HEALTH CARE SETTING

Acute care

ASSESSMENT

Dietary history: A dietary history is compiled to reveal adequacy of usual and recent food intake. Be alert to excesses or deficiencies of nutrients and any special eating patterns (e.g., various types of vegetarian or prescribed diets), use of fad diets, and excessive supplementation. Note anything that impairs adequate selection, preparation, ingestion, digestion, absorption, and excretion of nutrients. Include the following:

- Three-day review (including a weekend day) of patient's usual dietary intake. Identify any food allergies/intolerances, food aversions, and use of nutritional supplements.
- Recent unplanned weight loss or gain.
- Chewing or swallowing difficulties.
- Nausea, vomiting, or pain with eating.
- Altered pattern of elimination (e.g., constipation, diarrhea).
- Chronic disease affecting use of nutrients (e.g., malabsorption, pancreatitis, diabetes mellitus).
- Surgical resection; disease of the gut or accessory organs of digestion (i.e., pancreas, liver, gallbladder).

- Use of medications (e.g., laxatives, antacids, antibiotics, antineoplastic drugs) or alcohol. Long-term use of drugs that may affect appetite, digestion, or use or excretion of nutrients.

Physical assessment: Most physical findings are not specific to a particular nutritional deficiency. Compare current assessment findings with past assessments, especially related to the following:

- Loss of muscle and adipose tissue
- Work and muscle endurance
- Changes in hair, skin, or neuromuscular function

Anthropometric data

Anthropometric science entails measuring the body or its parts. It is helpful to remember that 1 L of fluid equals approximately 2 lb. To convert pounds and inches to metric measurements, use the following formulas:

Divide pounds *(lb)* by 2.2 to convert to *kilograms (kg)*
Divide inches *(in)* by 39.37 to convert to *meters (m)*

Height: Used to determine ideal weight and body mass index (BMI). If the patient's height is unavailable or impossible to measure, obtain an estimate from family or significant other. When height is unavailable in an adult, arm span or knee height measurement can be obtained using a tape measure. Arm span is measured with arms extended out from the body at a 90-degree angle and the distance from the tip of the longest finger on one hand to the longest finger on the other hand is obtained. With the leg bent at a 90-degree angle, knee height measurement can be obtained by measuring the distance from under the heel of the foot to the anterior surface of the thigh. The knee height measurement is calculated by using the following equations:

Men: Height (cm) = 64.19 − (0.04 × Age [year]) + (2.02 × Knee height [cm])

Women: Height (cm) = 84.88 − (0.24 × Age [year]) + (1.83 × Knee height [cm])

Weight: Used by many to determine nutritional status, but fluctuations may be a result of an amputation, dehydration, diuresis, fluid retention (renal failure, edema, third spacing), fluid resuscitation, wound dressings, or clothing. More reliable information may be obtained by asking the patient to recall usual weight, weight changes (gain and losses), and the time frame in which these occurred. An unintentional loss in weight of >10% over a 6-mo period is considered a significant weight loss and may be associated with severe malnutrition.

Most dietitians use the Hamwi "rule of thumb" calculation to determine ideal body weight:

Men: 106 lb for the first 5 ft and add 6 lb for each inch over 5 ft; *or* 48 kg for the first 1.5 cm and add 2.7 kg for each 2.54 cm over 1.5 cm

Women: 100 lb for the first 5 ft and add 5 lb for each inch over 5 ft; *or* 45 kg for the first 1.5 cm and add 2.3 kg for each 2.54 cm over 1.5 cm

Body mass index: Used to evaluate the weight of adults. One calculation and one set of standards are applicable to both men and women:

$$BMI\ (kg/m^2) = \frac{Weight}{Height\ (m^2)}$$

BMI values of 19-25 are appropriate for ages 19-34, whereas a BMI between 21-27 is appropriate for individuals >35 yr of age. Obesity is defined as BMI >27.5, with severe or morbid obesity >40. A BMI between 16-18.5 is considered mild to moderate malnutrition, whereas a BMI <16 indicates severe malnutrition.

Biochemical data

In an individual who is ill, these biochemical data are more accurate as predictors of outcome or recovery than as indicators of nutritional state.

Protein status: Evaluated via the following tests, with normal values in parentheses: serum albumin (3.5-5 g/dl), transferrin (200-400 mg/dl), thyroxine-binding prealbumin (20-30 mg/dl), and retinol-binding protein (4-5 mg/dl). Normal values may vary somewhat with different laboratory procedures and standards. Albumin and transferrin have relatively long half-lives of 14-20 days and 8-10 days, respectively; whereas thyroxine-binding prealbumin and retinol-binding protein have very short half-lives of 48-72 hr and 12 hr, respectively. If hydration status is normal and anemia is absent, albumin and transferrin levels can be used as baseline indicators of adequacy of protein intake and synthesis. For evidence of response to nutritional therapy, values for the short turnover proteins (although very expensive)—thyroxine-binding prealbumin and retinol-binding protein—are the most useful when the patient has normal renal function.

Iron status: Measurement of red blood cell (RBC) size, that is, mean corpuscular volume (MCV) (normal: 80-95 μm³), aids in determining the type of nutrient anemia. In iron–deficiency

anemia, RBCs are smaller than normal, whereas in folate or vitamin B_{12} deficiencies, RBCs are larger than normal.

Estimating nutritional requirements

The primary goal of nutritional support is to meet the needs for body temperature, metabolic processes, and tissue repair. Having collected all the data, energy needs may be estimated using the following options.

Harris-Benedict equations: To determine basal energy expenditure (BEE). The following equations can be used to calculate BEE:

BEE (male): 66.5 + (13.8 × Weight) + (5 × Height) − (6.8 × Age)
BEE (female): 655.1 + (9.6 × Weight) + (1.9 × Height) − (4.7 × Age)

Weight = weight in kilograms; *Height* = height in centimeters; and *Age* = age in years.

Calorie estimation: To prevent overfeeding, calculation of the total calorie intake can be obtained by the following equations:

Average nourished patient:	25 total calories per kilogram of body weight
Mildly stressed patient:	30 total calories per kilogram of body weight
Severely stressed patient:	35 total calories per kilogram of body weight
Morbid obesity patient:	18 total calories per kilogram of body weight

Distribution of calories: A relatively normal distribution of calories is adequate. Percentages of total calories from carbohydrates, protein, and fat should equal approximately 60%, 15%-20%, and 15%-25%, respectively.

- **Protein requirements:** Usually 0.8-1.5 g/kg/24 hr. (Protein will be restricted if patient has hepatic or renal failure that is not being treated with dialysis.)

  1 g protein = 4 kcal
  1 g nitrogen = 6.25 g protein

- **Carbohydrate (CHO) requirements:** Daily glucose administration of 9-15 g/kg/24 hr is an adequate range. Excess amounts of CHO are not used or tolerated. Overfeeding of CHO may lead to hyperglycemia, ↑ CO_2 production, hypophosphatemia, and fluid overload in short-term use or fatty liver syndrome in long-term use.

  1 g dextrose IV = 3.4 kcal
  1 g CHO in food = 4 kcal

- **Fat requirements:** Fat can be administered in minimal quantities to satisfy needs for essential fatty acids but should not exceed 1 g fat/kg/24 hr because of the potential for suppression of the immune system.

  1 g fat = 9 calories

Special diets for organ-specific pathologic conditions: Commercially available oral supplements and enteral formulas are available for patients with respiratory disease, diabetes, renal failure, hepatic failure, or immune compromise. Well-designed clinical trials may not be available to support the suggested indication.

Vitamin and essential trace mineral requirements: In general, follow the recommended daily allowances (RDAs) to provide minimum quantities of vitamins, minerals, and essential fatty acids. For specific patients, supplement specific vitamins or minerals needed in increased amounts for existing disease states (e.g., burns: zinc, vitamins A and C; chronic alcohol ingestion: thiamine, folate, vitamin B_{12}).

Fluid requirements: Many factors affect fluid balance. Under usual circumstances, an estimate of fluid needs can be made by providing 1 ml of free water for each calorie provided, or 30-50 ml/kg body weight. The daily loss of water includes approximately 1400 ml in urine (60 ml/hr), 350 ml via respiration, 600 ml as evaporation through skin, and about 200 ml in feces. Fluid losses are 100-150 ml/day for each degree of temperature increase above 37° C. If loss by any of these routes is increased, fluid needs increase; if loss by any of these routes is impaired, fluid restriction may be necessary.

NUTRITIONAL SUPPORT MODALITIES

Specialized nutritional support refers to the provision of an artificial formulation of nutrients via the oral, enteral, or parenteral route for the treatment or prevention of malnutrition. Oral supplements are the preferred route because they are less invasive, more natural, and less costly, and enteral nutrition is preferred over parenteral.

Types of feeding tubes

Small-bore nasal tubes: Defined as ≤12 Fr tube; require abdominal x-ray for confirmation of placement. Composition may be polyurethane, silicone, or polyvinyl chloride. Usual length of tube is 36-45 inches, and it may or may not require a stylet for insertion. The physician should determine if the distal tip ends in the stomach or small intestines. Insertion by a nurse is determined by hospital policy. It may also be inserted using fluoroscopy in radiation or endoscopy room. Because of their diameter and composition, these tubes are easily dislocated proximally in the GI tract without any external signs.

Large-bore nasal tubes: Defined as >12 Fr tube; do not require x-ray for confirmation of placement. Composition is either polyurethane or polyvinyl chloride. Usual length of tube is 36 inches. Stylet is not required for insertion. Insertion may be by a nurse. Placement is confirmed by withdrawal of gastric fluid.

Gastrostomy tubes: Exit stomach directly through abdominal wall and usually anchored with either a balloon or disc on the inside of the stomach. Usually ≥12 Fr size. Composition may be polyurethane, silicone, or rubber and may contain multiple ports for insertion of air into the balloon, delivery of medications, and the main lumen. Initially, a physician in radiology, endoscopy, or surgery performs the insertion. When placed by a physician in radiology or endoscopy, the common term used to describe the tube is *percutaneous endoscopic gastrostomy* (PEG). Reinsertion by a nurse is determined by hospital policy.

Gastrostomy button: Placed into a mature gastrostomy stoma. It fits into the stoma tract flush with the outer abdominal wall. The button contains an antireflux valve to prevent leakage, but gastric samples or residuals cannot be obtained via the button.

Jejunostomy tubes: Placed by a physician either surgically or percutaneously (percutaneous endoscopic jejunostomy [PEJ]). Diameter is usually about a 12-18 Fr. Anchoring the tube inside the jejunum presents a problem because a balloon >5 ml might cause bowel obstruction. Confirmation of position requires x-ray with contrast. No residuals should be obtained from this tube. If the tube becomes displaced, the entry site into the jejunum will close down rapidly (approximately 20-30 min). Reinsertion by a nurse is determined by hospital policy, but it is not recommended without special training.

Gastrostomy-jejunostomy tubes: Exit stomach directly through the abdominal wall with a small-bore jejunostomy tube placed through the main lumen of the gastrostomy with the distal tip positioned in the jejunum.

Feeding sites

Stomach: Simulates normal GI functions; may be used for bolus, intermittent, or continuous feedings; indicated for patients who have intact gag or cough reflexes.

Duodenum, jejunum: Must be used only for continuous feedings to prevent dumping syndrome and diarrhea. Small-bore diameter tube is recommended.

TOTAL PARENTERAL NUTRITION

Total parenteral nutrition (TPN) provides some or all nutrients by the intravenous route. TPN is used to provide complete nutrition for patients who cannot receive enteral nutrition or to supplement nutritional needs of patients who are unable to absorb sufficient calories via the GI tract. TPN is more expensive than enteral nutrition and has the potential for developing severe complications more rapidly.

Parenteral solutions

Intravenous solutions are customized combinations of dextrose (CHO), amino acids (protein), intralipids (fat), electrolytes, vitamins, and trace metals.

Carbohydrates (CHO): Dextrose provides the bulk of the calories and energy needs, with concentrations ranging from 5%-70%. The percentage of dextrose selected is based on the available administration site and the volume status of the patient. All solutions that use >12.5% dextrose solution must be administered via a central venous catheter. The average amount of CHO calories delivered is approximately 60% of the total. The more CHO delivered, the greater the potential for complications, which include fatty liver syndrome, increased CO_2 production, and hyperglycemia.

Protein: Synthetic crystalline essential and nonessential amino acid formulations are available in concentrations of 3%-10%. Special amino acid formulations are available that have varied the ratio of essential to nonessential amino acids for specific disorders (e.g., liver disease, renal disease). The amount of protein delivered depends on the patient's renal and hepatic function.

Fat: Intralipid (10%, 20%, or 30%) is an isotonic solution providing essential fatty acids and a source of concentrated calories.

10% Intralipids = 1.1 calories/ml
20% Intralipids = 2 calories/ml
30% Intralipids = 3 calories/ml

When fats are mixed in the same infusion bag with the CHO and amino acids, the solution is referred to as a total nutrient admixture (TNA) or 3:1 solution (all three nutrient components in one bag). The intralipids may be given piggyback into the amino acid/dextrose infusion to infuse over 8-12 hr. The amount of intralipids administered may be reduced or removed for patients who have hypertriglyceridemia (e.g., patients receiving antirejection medication following an organ transplant, patients with coronary heart disease, AIDS patients). Determine if the patient has an egg allergy because the long-chain triglycerides in the lipids may originate from the phospholipids in egg yolks. If a patient develops a rash during the infusion of lipids, consider an allergy immediately. If the ratio of the protein, CHO, and fats in the admixture is not stable, separation of the lipids from the emulsion may occur, which is called "cracking" of the solution. The lipids may float on top of the mixture or appear yellow, much like an egg yolk floating in the solution. In addition, "oiling out" may occur, which looks like an oil slick on top of the solution. Return any solution that appears "different" to the pharmacy and do not use it.

Selection of administration site

Central venous catheter (CVC): Used for all solutions containing >12.5% dextrose or a solution with an osmolality ≥800 mOsm/L. CVC use requires a large, central vein with the distal tip of the catheter in the superior vena cava. The flow of blood through the large vessels rapidly dilutes the hypertonic solutions and decreases the potential for thrombophlebitis.

Peripheral venous catheter: Reserved for individuals with a need for nutritional support for short-term periods, with small nutritional requirements, and for whom CVC access is unavailable. Only a low-osmolality solution (<800 mOsm/L) can be used. To reduce osmolality of the base solution, dilution of the components is usually required. The large volume limits the number of patients in whom this admixture can be administered.

Transitional feeding

A transition is necessary before discontinuing nutritional support. Taper nutritional supplements for patients receiving enteral nutrition as oral intake increases to 60%-70% of estimated needs. Similarly, patients who have received TPN for more than 2-3 wk may have some mucosal atrophy of the bowel and will need a period of adjustment before the bowel can fully resume its usual functions of digestion and absorption. The best diet advancement includes starting with clear liquids and then advancing to a soft diet. Because these individuals have been ill, the lactase in their stomach has decreased, placing them at higher risk for lactose deficiency; therefore they should not receive a full liquid diet because of the increased incidence of bloating, nausea, and diarrhea associated with lactose deficiency.

Nursing Diagnosis:

Imbalanced Nutrition: Less than body requirements

related to inability to ingest, digest, or absorb nutrients

Desired Outcome: Patient has adequate nutrition as evidenced by stabilization of weight at desired level or steady weight gain of 1/2-1 lb/wk, presence of wound granulation (i.e., pinkish white tissue around wound edges; wound edges approximating together), and absence of infection (see **Risk for Infection,** p. 000).

INTERVENTIONS	RATIONALES
For Oral Nutrition:	
Ensure nutritional screening and assessment of patient within 24 hr of admission; document and reassess weekly.	Hospitalized patients are at risk for developing protein-energy malnutrition. Baseline assessment enables comparison with subsequent assessments, which may reveal problems that may require interventions. Because no single sensitive and comprehensive nutritional assessment factor exists, multiple sources of information are used, including any of the following: historical data, nutritional history, anthropometric data, biochemical analysis of blood and urine, and duration of the disease process.

Continued

INTERVENTIONS	RATIONALES
Position patient in high Fowler's position for eating.	Promotes normal position for eating and decreases risk of aspiration.
Assist with preparation of food tray for eating as needed.	To ensure that all packages are opened and patient can access all food.
Involve significant other in meal rituals for companionship.	People who eat alone tend to eat less.
Assess for food allergies/intolerances and avoid these foods.	Individuals with celiac disease, for example, will have severe reactions that may result in malabsorption when exposed to even minute quantities of wheat and other glutens.
Provide small, frequent feedings of diet compatible with disease state and patient's ability to ingest foods.	After an illness, early satiety may be a problem. Small, frequent meals are likely to increase intake.
Respect food aversions, religious guidelines, and food preferences.	Individuals will eat more readily and frequently when consuming preferred foods that are within dietary allowances.
If appropriate, allow family and friends to bring food from home.	Patients may prefer home-cooked meals to those prepared at the hospital.
Provide liquid nutritional supplements as prescribed.	To increase calories consumed and help meet RDAs for vitamins and minerals needed for recovery.
Serve them cold or over ice.	To enhance palatability.
Obtain weight measurement weekly.	Stabilizing weight or weight gain of $\frac{1}{2}$-1 lb/wk is the usual goal if weight gain is desired. This assessment also tracks maintenance of weight.
Provide psychologic support.	Emotional health influences appetite.
For Enteral or Parenteral Nutrition:	
Ensure nutritional screening and assessment within 24 hr of physician directive; document and reassess weekly.	Hospitalized patients are at risk for developing protein-calorie malnutrition. Baseline assessment enables comparison with subsequent assessments, which may reveal problems that may require intervention. Because no single sensitive and comprehensive nutritional assessment factor exists, multiple sources of information are used, including any of the following: historical data, nutritional history, anthropometric data, biochemical analysis of blood and urine, and duration of the disease process.
Administer continuous enteral feedings using a pump at the prescribed rate.	Using a continuous rate provides food at a steady infusion rate, which decreases feelings of fullness and early satiety and avoids peaks in patient's energy needs.
Check infused volume and rate q4h.	To ensure accuracy.
Administer TPN using a volumetric pump at prescribed rate.	Because of potential for complications such as hyperglycemia, a continuous rate for volume is better tolerated by the patient.
Check infused volume and rate q4h.	Checking volume and rate prevents volume overload and other complications that could occur when using the pump.
Monitor laboratory data every day until stable for TPN and enteral feedings, then at least weekly: electrolytes, blood glucose, blood urea nitrogen, creatinine, phosphorus, magnesium, and calcium.	Values outside the normal range may signal intracellular shift, which is associated with refeeding syndrome.
Monitor other laboratory data initially and then at least weekly: liver function tests including albumin, triglycerides (if patient is at risk, i.e., pancreatitis, transplant antirejection medications, AIDS).	These laboratory values provide data about tolerance, clearance, and metabolism by organs and stabilization of the disease process.
Record I&O carefully.	To track fluid balance trends.

Continued

INTERVENTIONS	RATIONALES
Weigh patient initially and daily during an acute illness; then advance to weekly.	Stabilized weight or weight gain of ½-1 lb/wk is the usual goal if weight gain is an intended goal. Weight trend also assesses fluid status and disease process.
Ensure that patient receives prescribed caloric intake.	As a general rule, percentages of total calories from carbohydrates, protein, and fat should equal approximately 60%, 15%-20%, and 15%-25%, respectively. Protein is burned for calories during the recovery phase if enough carbohydrates and fats are not eaten, enabling protein to be used for healing and rebuilding.
Assess for fluid imbalance.	Patient may be especially prone to fluid excess because low protein levels in the blood cause a decrease in oncotic pressure in the vessels, resulting in fluid retention.
	Fluid excess may be manifested by peripheral edema, adventitious breath sounds (especially crackles), and weight gain (1 kg = 1000 ml).

●●● **Related NIC and NOC labels:** *NIC:* Nutrition Management; Weight Gain Assistance; Nutrition Therapy; Nutritional Monitoring; Enteral Tube Feeding; Total Parenteral Nutrition Administration; Intravenous Therapy; Laboratory Data Interpretation *NOC:* Nutritional Status; Nutritional Status: Food and Fluid Intake; Nutritional Status: Nutrient Intake; Weight Control

Nursing Diagnosis:

Risk for Aspiration

related to enteral feeding or delayed gastric emptying

Desired Outcome: Patient is free of aspiration problems as evidenced by auscultation of clear lung sounds, VS within normal limits for the patient, and no signs of respiratory distress.

INTERVENTIONS	RATIONALES
Mark tube to determine length exiting from the body. Check this mark.	The nasogastric (NG) tube can easily slide out of the nose because of nasal discharge, sweat, and loosening of the tape or tube holder.
Secure tubing in place per agency policy; reassess q4h and before each feeding.	To determine tube migration, which if it occurs would necessitate x-ray to confirm placement or tube reinsertion.
Assess respiratory status q4h, including respiratory rate, effort, and adventitious breath sounds.	Patient's lung sounds should be clear, and there should be no signs of respiratory distress before infusing a feeding.
Monitor temperature q4h. Report significant findings.	Temperature outside of parameters as defined by health care provider should be reported. An increased temperature occurs with aspiration pneumonia.
Auscultate bowel sounds q8h. Report significant findings.	High-pitched or absent bowel sounds, abdominal distention, or nausea can occur with ileus, decreased tolerance to the feeding, and small bowel obstruction.
	These problems can lead to vomiting and aspiration and therefore should be reported promptly.

Continued

INTERVENTIONS	RATIONALES
Depending on patient's medical condition, raise head of bed (HOB) ≥30 degrees or place patient in a right side-lying position during and for 1 hr after administration of a bolus or intermittent feeding.	These positions promote gravity flow from the greater stomach curvature through the pylorus into the duodenum and decrease risk for aspiration.
Stop the tube feeding ½-1 hr before chest physical therapy or placing patient supine.	To enable complete emptying of the stomach and decrease potential for aspiration.
Check residuals per agency policy.	The best practice is to hold the feeding if residuals are >200 ml from an NG or orogastric tube or >100 ml from a gastrostomy. High-volume residuals may be a sign of intolerance because of ileus or small bowel obstruction, either of which can lead to vomiting and aspiration.
Recognize that patient should have zero residual or minimal volume from a tube placed into the small intestine.	Unlike the stomach, the small intestine does not function as a reservoir and therefore normally will not hold volume because of forward peristalsis.

●●● **Related NIC and NOC labels:** *NIC:* Aspiration Precautions; Gastrointestinal Intubation; Positioning; Respiratory Monitoring; Enteral Tube Feeding *NOC:* Aspiration Control

Nursing Diagnosis:

Constipation

related to inadequate fluid and fiber in diet

Desired Outcome: Patient states he or she has had a soft bowel movement within 3-4 days of this diagnosis (or within patient's usual pattern).

INTERVENTIONS	RATIONALES
If patient is receiving a formula that contains fiber and is on fluid restriction or receiving large amounts of diuretics, consider changing formula to an isotonic formula without fiber.	Fiber pulls more fluid into the intestines. When a patient is "dry" from medical therapy, there is no extra water to pull, and if no extra water is available, constipation will occur.
If patient is receiving a formula that contains fiber, assess intake of free water.	Optimally water intake should be 1 ml/calorie of intake or 30-50 ml/kg body weight in order to compensate for losses that occur normally via respirations, urination, fever, and so on.
Give free water q4h or as prescribed and after each medication.	To maintain fluid balance and patency of feeding tube, as well as promote soft stools and prevent constipation.
If medically indicated, consider a reduction in the amount of narcotics being administered.	Opioid medications are constipating.
Consider a stool softener, especially if patient regularly uses a laxative at home.	If patient is unable to increase water needs effectively, a stool softener will prevent straining and decrease risk of constipation.

●●● **Related NIC and NOC labels:** *NIC:* Bowel Management; Constipation/Impaction Management; Fluid Management; Medication Management; Nutritional Monitoring; Enteral Tube Feeding *NOC:* Bowel Elimination; Hydration

Nursing Diagnosis:

Impaired Swallowing

related to decreased or absent gag reflex, facial paralysis, mechanical obstruction, fatigue, weight loss, or decreased strength or excursion of muscles involved in mastication

Desired Outcome: Before food or fluids are initiated, patient demonstrates adequate cough and gag reflexes and the ability to ingest foods via the phases of swallowing as instructed.

INTERVENTIONS	RATIONALES
Assess oral motor function within 24 hr of admission or on patient's progression to oral diet.	If patient has adequate oral motor functioning, oral intake can be increased. Otherwise, tube feedings should be considered to prevent aspiration.
Assess cough and gag reflexes before first feeding.	Patients who develop gastric reflux or vomit can aspirate if their cough and gag reflexes are not intact.
Offer semisolid foods and progress to thicker textures as tolerated.	If patient is likely to have difficulty with swallowing, liquids will be the most difficult and most likely to be aspirated.
Coach patient through phases of ingesting food: opening mouth, inserting food, closing lips, chewing, transferring food from side to side in the mouth and then to the back of the oral cavity, elevating tongue to roof of mouth (hard palate), and swallowing between breaths.	With illness, muscles may become weaker, and this may result in bad habits of rushing swallowing and moving food into the trachea rather than into the esophagus, where they are less likely to be aspirated.
If indicated, order extra sauces, gravies, or liquids.	To moisten each bite of food for patients in whom dryness of the oral cavity impairs swallowing ability.
If tolerated, keep patient in high Fowler's position for ½ hr after eating.	To minimize risk of aspiration by promoting gravity flow through the stomach and into the duodenum.
Provide mouth care before and after meals and dietary supplements.	To ensure that all traces of food are removed, preventing subsequent aspiration.
Provide small, frequent meals.	Six smaller feedings per day may increase muscle strength needed for swallowing and be less likely to result in rushing, which could cause aspiration.
Provide foods at temperatures acceptable to patient.	Foods that are too hot or too cold could rush swallowing and lead to aspiration.
If indicated, provide a referral to speech, physical, or occupational therapist.	To assist in retraining or facilitating patient's swallowing.

●●● **Related NIC and NOC labels:** *NIC:* Aspiration Precautions; Positioning; Risk Identification; Swallowing Therapy; Feeding; Referral *NOC:* Aspiration Control; Swallowing Status

Nursing Diagnosis:

Risk for Infection

related to invasive procedures, malnutrition, and suppression of the immune system

Desired Outcome: Patient is free of infection as evidenced by temperature, pulse, and respirations within patient's normal range; and absence of clinical signs of sepsis: erythema, swelling at catheter insertion site, chills, fever, and glucose intolerance.

INTERVENTIONS	RATIONALES
Weekly and prn, monitor white blood cell (WBC) count with differential for values outside the normal range.	A higher value signals infection. Infection requires extra calories.
Monitor bedside glucose for values outside the normal range.	Glucose intolerance is a sign of sepsis. An increase in glucose also promotes bacterial growth and increases risk of infection.
Assess catheter insertion site (if using a transparent dressing) q12h for erythema, swelling, or purulent discharge. If using a gauze dressing, assess site at time of dressing change.	Signs of local infections.
Use meticulous sterile technique when changing central line dressing, containers, or administration lines. Follow agency policy for central line dressing changes.	To reduce possibility of infection.
Restrict use of lumen being used for administration of TPN, if possible. Avoid drawing blood specimens or other fluids, pressure monitoring, or medication administration, if possible.	There is an increased infection rate in catheter lumens used for drawing or administering blood or multiple infusions. Blood adheres to the inside of the lumen; then when TPN is infused with increased carbohydrates, bacteria tends to grow faster.
Change all administration sets as recommended by Centers for Disease Control and Prevention (CDC).	When TPN is being administered, most infections of catheters and blood are related to insertion site or tubing sets.
For more information, see Appendix for "Infection Prevention and Control," p. 831.	

●●● **Related NIC and NOC labels:** *NIC:* Infection Protection; Laboratory Data Interpretation; Risk Identification; Infection Control; Incision Site Care; Nutrition Management; Tube Care: Gastrointestinal; Venous Access Devices Maintenance *NOC:* Immune Status; Infection Status

Nursing Diagnosis:

Risk for Imbalanced Fluid Volume

related to failure of regulatory mechanisms, hyperglycemia, medications, fever, infection, fluid administration, or immobility

Desired Outcome: Patient's hydration status is adequate, as evidenced by baseline VS, serum glucose <200 mg/dl, balanced I&O, weight maintenance or 1-2 lb weight gain per week (if needed), and serum electrolyte and WBC values within normal limits.

INTERVENTIONS	RATIONALES
Assess rate and volume of nutritional support q4h.	To ensure prescribed rate and volume and prevent volume overload or deficiency.
Weigh patient daily initially; then advance to weekly.	Baseline will determine weight goals; subsequent assessments will determine efficacy of those goals.
Monitor I&O q8h or more frequently if medically indicated.	To assess for imbalances and trends toward overhydration or dehydration.
Monitor for signs of circulatory overload during fluid replacement.	Signs of circulatory overload may occur during fluid replacement, including peripheral edema, bounding pulse, jugular distention, and adventitious lung sounds (especially crackles).

Continued

INTERVENTIONS	RATIONALES
	Circulatory overload is more likely to occur in older adults or individuals with heart failure or other chronic medical conditions such as renal insufficiency in which output is decreased, even if fluids are delivered properly.
If medically indicated, provide 1 ml of free water for each calorie of enteral formula provided (or 30-50 ml/kg of body weight).	This is the amount of water needed for normal metabolism and organ functioning per day.
Monitor for hyperglycemia: • In patient who is not diabetic: q6h for 24-48 hr; then discontinue. • In patient who is glucose intolerant: q4h, with sliding scale regular insulin prescribed. • In patient who is diabetic: q4h, with sliding scale regular insulin prescribed; consult with a health care provider who specializes in care of patients with diabetes.	Hyperglycemia may occur because of increased carbohydrate intake or response to the stress of illness or in the presence of type 1 diabetes. Along with hyperglycemia, volume deficits may occur because of osmotic diuresis that accompanies increased glucose.

●●● **Related NIC and NOC labels:** *NIC:* Fluid/Electrolyte Management; Electrolyte Monitoring; Intravenous Therapy; Laboratory Data Interpretation *NOC:* Electrolyte and Acid/-Base Balance; Fluid Balance

Nursing Diagnosis:

Diarrhea

(or risk for same) *related to* medications, dumping syndrome, bacterial contamination, formula intolerance, or side effect of disease

Desired Outcome: Patient has formed stools within 2-3 days of intervention.

INTERVENTIONS	RATIONALES
Determine patient's normal stool pattern.	To establish a baseline and reference point from which current trend can be compared.
Assess abdomen, bowel sounds, and frequency of bowel movements.	Hyperactive bowel sounds may occur with increased stooling, along with signs and symptoms of distention, cramping, and nausea.
Ask patient to define diarrhea.	One loose stool does not mean that patient has diarrhea. Liquid intake normally produces a pasty stool, and patient may misinterpret this as diarrhea.
If indicated, confer with health care provider about stopping prokinetic medication (e.g., Reglan).	These drugs stimulate the bowels.
Suggest a review of medications by pharmacy.	Pharmacists are knowledgeable about drugs that cause diarrhea.
Suggest stopping any stool softeners being administered.	Stool softeners may stimulate the bowels.
Consider giving yogurt or the medication equivalent.	To replace normal flora removed by antibiotics and diarrhea.
Evaluate route of delivery if giving yogurt.	Yogurt will clog a small-bore feeding tube.
Confer with health care provider about administering binding bile salts if diarrhea occurs secondary to uncontrolled diabetes.	Increased bile salts secondary to uncontrolled diabetes is a cause of diarrhea.

INTERVENTIONS	RATIONALES
Contact pharmacy about elixirs being administered. Discuss with health care provider and pharmacist changing form of medication or switching to another medication within the same class.	The majority of elixirs contain sorbitol, which will increase transit time in the intestines and cause diarrhea.
Collect a stool sample for bacterial culture and sensitivity.	Diarrhea may be caused by bacteria.
Do not administer an antidiarrheal medication until stool culture is confirmed as negative.	Giving this medication when stool culture is positive increases risk for toxic megacolon and bowel perforation.
Maintain optimal hydration.	To replace losses caused by diarrhea.
Record I&O status every shift. Obtain parameters from health care provider for notification of output.	An example of a parameter established by health care provider for a dehydrated patient would be urinary output <30 ml/hr × 4 or hourly stools of specific volume amount.
Check weight daily.	To assess fluid status. With diarrhea, the concern is weight loss. For example, 1 kg/day could signal a loss of 1000 ml.
If patient is receiving a bolus feeding, switch to intermittent or continuous feeding.	Bolus feedings may contribute to dumping syndrome, which would result in increased diarrhea.
Use aseptic technique when handling feeding tube, enteral products, and feeding sets.	Bacteria can grow in feeding sets and on hands of caregiver and could cause diarrhea if allowed to be transported to patient.
Change all equipment per agency policy.	Same as above.
Refrigerate all opened products but discard after 24 hr. Date and time all products.	These products are potential growth media for bacteria and could cause diarrhea if the product is given to patient. All manufacturers state on their products to discard after opened for 24 hr and store in refrigerator.

●●● **Related NIC and NOC labels:** *NIC:* Diarrhea Management; Medication Management; Fluid Management; Fluid Monitoring *NOC:* Bowel Elimination; Hydration

Nursing Diagnosis:

Nausea

(or risk of same) *related to* underlying medical condition, too rapid infusion of enteral product, food intolerance, or medication administration

Desired Outcome: Nausea is decreased or absent with food intake.

INTERVENTIONS	RATIONALES
Give antiemetic as prescribed.	To decrease/eliminate nausea.
Offer food in small portions, six times per day.	Smaller meals are better tolerated than larger meals.
Give chewing gum or hard candies prn if permitted.	Providing some sugar to the system may stimulate the GI tract and decrease nausea.
Suggest that patient brush teeth and tongue q8h and prn.	A bad taste in the mouth may increase nausea in some individuals.
If odor of food induces nausea, remove it immediately.	To eliminate nausea caused by odor.
Reduce rate per minute of enteral formula infusion.	Nausea may be caused by increased infusion rate, which may result in delayed gastric emptying, overdistention, or constipation.

Continued

INTERVENTIONS	RATIONALES
If patient is receiving bolus infusion, change to intermittent or continuous.	Overdistention with a bolus infusion may cause or increase nausea, whereas a slower infusion rate with an intermittent or continuous infusion may be better tolerated.
If patient has nausea, inspect abdomen for distention and auscultate bowel sounds. Monitor for and record flatus and bowel movements. Notify health care provider of significant findings.	Absence of bowel sounds may signal ileus. Decreased bowel sounds may indicate need to decrease feeding and check stool output. Distention may appear either with ileus or with decreased motility. These signs would necessitate notifying health care provider for intervention.
If medically indicated, consider bowel suppository.	To stimulate intestinal tract. Nausea may occur secondary to constipation or decreased motility.
Monitor electrolyte levels, especially potassium.	Hypokalemia is associated with ileus and nausea.

●●● **Related NIC and NOC labels:** *NIC:* Nausea Management; Medication Management; Environmental Management: Comfort; Medication Administration *NOC:* Comfort Level; Nutritional Status: Food and Fluid Intake

Asthma

The prevalence of asthma and associated morbidity and mortality rates have risen over the past decade. Asthma is the leading cause of chronic illness in children and the most frequent admitting diagnosis in children's hospitals. Eleven percent of U.S. children under 18 yr of age, or 8.1 million children, have been diagnosed with asthma. The highest prevalence is in children 5-17 yr old. There is an increased incidence in boys and African-American children. Acute exacerbations of asthma account for a loss of >10 million school days and are responsible for more hospitalizations, restricted activity, and significant health care costs than any other pediatric chronic illness. The classification of asthma is based on severity and frequency of symptoms. Daily or maintenance treatment is based on the following:

- Step 1: Mild intermittent asthma
- Step 2: Mild persistent asthma
- Step 3: Moderate persistent asthma
- Step 4: Severe persistent asthma

Asthma is a chronic reversible (in most cases) obstructive airway disease characterized by inflammation and mucosal edema, increased sensitivity of the airways, and airway obstruction (bronchospasm and in some children, excessive, thick mucus). Increased inflammation causes increased sensitivity of the airways and is the most common feature of asthma. In 1999, 4657 Americans died from asthma.

HEALTH CARE SETTING

Primary care, with possible hospitalization resulting from severe acute attacks

ASSESSMENT

Common early warning signs: Breathing changes, sneezing, moodiness, headache, itchy/watery eyes, dark circles under eyes, easy fatigue, sore throat, trouble sleeping, chest or throat itchiness, downward trend in peak flow values, cough especially at night (hallmark symptom of asthma), slight tightness in chest.

Symptoms of acute episode: Coughing, shortness of breath, dyspnea, anxiety, apprehension, tightness in chest, and wheezing (primarily on expiration).

- *Severe asthma symptoms:* Severe coughing, shortness of breath, tightness in chest and/or wheezing, and difficulty talking or concentrating. The mucosal edema causes shortness of breath, tachypnea or bradypnea, hunched shoulders (posturing), suprasternal and intercostal retractions, cyanosis, increasing dyspnea, nasal flaring and use of accessory muscles, extreme anxiety, and apprehension.
- *Symptoms of severe respiratory distress and impending respiratory failure:* Profuse diaphoresis, sitting upright and refusing to lie down, suddenly becoming agitated or becoming quiet when previously agitated, decrease in or absence of wheezing.

Physical assessment: Chest has hyperresonance on percussion. Breath sounds are loud and coarse, with sonorous crackles throughout the lung fields. Prolonged expiration is noted. Coarse rhonchi may be heard, as well as generalized inspiratory and expiratory wheezing that becomes more high pitched as obstruction increases. With minimal obstruction, wheezing may be minimal or heard only on end expiration with auscultation. Breath sounds and crackles may become inaudible with severe obstruction or bronchospasm. Pulsus paradoxus (an abnormally large decrease in systolic blood pressure and pulse wave amplitude during inspiration) also may be noted because of lung hyperinflation.

Children with chronic asthma may develop a barrel chest with depressed diaphragm, elevated shoulders, and increased use of accessory muscles of respiration.

Caution: If symptoms are untreated or treated unsuccessfully, an acute asthma attack may progress to status asthmaticus, a severe unrelenting attack. Status asthmaticus is an acute, severe, and prolonged asthma attack in which respiratory distress continues despite vigorous therapeutic measures and may result in death.

DIAGNOSTIC TESTS

Pulse oximetry: Noninvasive method that will reveal decreased O_2 saturation (<93%-95%, depending on protocol of facility).

Arterial blood gas (ABG) values: Reveal status of oxygenation and acid-base balance. In severe asthma exacerbation with PaO_2 <60 mm Hg (on room air) and $PaCO_2$ ≥42 mmHg, child may have cyanosis and may progress to respiratory failure. ABGs are not tested very often in children except in intensive care unit (ICU) and with initial assessment.

Chest x-ray examination: To rule out pneumonia and assess for air trapping. It is also used to evaluate possible cardiomegaly secondary to pulmonary hypertension resulting from chronic obstruction. Typical findings in a child with significant asthma symptoms are hyperinflation, atelectasis, and flattened diaphragm.

Complete blood count (CBC): May show slight elevation during acute asthma, but white blood cell elevations >12,000/mm^3 or an increased percentage of band cells may indicate a respiratory infection. Eosinophils >500/mm^3 tend to suggest an allergic or inflammatory disorder.

Sputum: Gross examination may reveal increased viscosity or actual mucous plugs. Culture and sensitivity may reveal microorganisms if infection was the precipitating event. Cytologic examination will reveal elevated eosinophils, which is commonly associated with asthma.

Serum theophylline level: Important baseline indicator for patients who are receiving this therapy, although it is now considered a third-line agent and used infrequently. Current guidelines call for a serum concentration of 5-15 µg/ml.

Theophylline toxicity can occur with serum levels >20 µg/ml. Side effects include nausea, vomiting, headache, irritability, and insomnia. Early signs of toxicity are nausea, tachycardia, irritability, and seizures. Dysrhythmias occur at serum levels >30 µg/ml.

Pulmonary function tests: Provide an objective method of evaluating presence and degree of lung disease, as well as response to treatment, and usually can be performed reliably on children by 5 or 6 years of age. They typically show diminished maximal breathing capacity, tidal volume, and timed vital capacity.

Peak expiratory flow rate (PEFR): Assesses severity of asthma by measuring maximum flow of air that can be forcefully exhaled in 1 sec using peak flow meter (PFM). Each child's PEFR varies according to age, height, sex, and race. Once personal best value is established, it is recommended that it be done 1-2 times/day in children with moderate-to-severe persistent asthma. The child should measure the PEFR 3 times with at least 30 sec between each measurement; then record the highest reading. Maintaining a diary or log book is most beneficial and helps direct plan of care.

Skin testing: The 1997 revised guidelines and 2002 update issued by the National Asthma Education and Prevention Program Expert Panel through the National Heart, Lung and Blood Institute, National Institutes of Health recommend that all patients with persistent asthma be tested to determine sensitization to perennial allergens.

Nursing Diagnosis:

Ineffective Airway Clearance

related to bronchospasm, mucosal edema, and increased mucus production

Desired Outcomes: *Child with a significant asthma attack:* Within 48 hr of interventions/treatment, adventitious breath sounds, cough, and work of breathing (WOB) are decreased. Within 72 hr, RR returns to child's normal range, and retractions and nasal flaring disappear. *Child with a mild asthma attack:* Within 3 hr after interventions/treatment, adventitious breath sounds and cough are decreased, and retractions and nasal flaring are absent.

Note: Work of breathing (WOB) means ease or effort of breathing. Signs of increased WOB include nasal flaring, retractions, and use of accessory muscles.

INTERVENTIONS	RATIONALES
Assess respiratory status with initial assessment, with each VS check, and prn.	After establishing the baseline, changes can be detected quickly with subsequent assessments, enabling rapid intervention.
Administer nebulizer treatment/metered dose inhaler (MDI; usually albuterol) as prescribed.	Decreases bronchospasm/mucosal edema, thereby opening the airway and allowing more effective airway clearance.
Assess RR, HR, O_2 saturation, and breath sounds before and after each nebulizer treatment/MDI administration.	To determine child's status and effectiveness of medication in decreasing bronchospasm/mucosal edema and enabling more effective airway clearance.

Continued

INTERVENTIONS	RATIONALES
Hold albuterol treatment if HR is: >180 bpm (children 2 to 3 yr) >160 bpm (children 3 to 6 yr) >140 bpm (children 6 to 12 yr) >120 bpm (children >12 yr) Notify health care provider as directed.	Tachycardia is a major side effect of albuterol. When it is present, the health care provider needs to assess patient to ensure that side effects of medication do not outweigh the benefit of decreasing bronchospasm.
Position child in high Fowler's position and encourage deep breathing.	This will ensure that child has maximum lung expansion and that medication will be dispersed more effectively, thereby improving airway clearance.
Check PEFR in children >5 yr of age before and after each albuterol treatment using PFM.	To assess effectiveness of medication in decreasing bronchospasm and increasing effective airway clearance. For more information about PEFR, see "Diagnostic Tests" section.
Use a spacer or AeroChamber with administration of MDI. A mask may be required with a spacer in children <5 yr of age or anyone who is unable to seal lips effectively around mouthpiece.	Most effective methods of getting maximum amount of medication delivered to child.
Encourage deep breathing and effective cough q2h while awake.	To loosen and expectorate secretions (many young children cough up secretions and swallow them). This will lead to more effective airway clearance.
Teach children ≥7 yr old breathing exercises and controlled breathing.	To promote proper diaphragmatic breathing and improve chest wall mobility. Children younger than 7 are diaphragmatic breathers normally. Proper diaphragmatic breathing decreases WOB and improves airway clearance.
Administer other medications as prescribed (usually corticosteroids).	Corticosteroids decrease inflammation, thereby improving airway clearance. Antibiotics are only given if a bacterial infection is present.
Encourage maintenance fluids appropriate for child's weight.	To thin mucus and improve ability to expectorate it, which improves airway clearance.
Give child/family specific guidelines for hydration (maintenance fluids).	For example, a 2-yr-old child who needs 1200 ml/day and drinks from a 4-oz sippy cup, needs to drink 10 sippy cupfuls/day. Understanding appropriate care improves compliance and decreases symptoms.
Monitor and document I&O q4h.	Assessing I&O on a regular basis alerts one to inadequate intake or output before the child shows signs of dehydration. Dehydration thickens secretions and decreases airway clearance.
Assess hydration status q4h, including level of consciousness (LOC), anterior fontanel (if child is <2 yr old), abdominal skin turgor, and urine output.	Because of increased insensible water loss (owing to ↑ RR, ↑ metabolic rate, and ↑ secretions), child may still become dehydrated *even if* receiving maintenance fluids and having appropriate I&O. Ongoing assessment detects early changes and provides more prompt resolution of the problem. Dehydration thickens secretions and decreases airway clearance. Signs of dehydration include decreasing LOC, sunken fontanel, tented abdominal skin, and decreasing urine output.
Avoid iced fluids and caffeinated fluids.	May trigger bronchospasm.

●●● **Related NIC and NOC labels:** *NIC:* Respiratory Monitoring; Positioning; VS Monitoring; Cough Enhancement; Medication Administration: Inhalation; Fluid Monitoring *NOC:* Respiratory Status: Gas Exchange; Respiratory Status: Ventilation

Nursing Diagnosis:

Anxiety

related to illness, loss of control, and medical/nursing interventions

Desired Outcome: Following interventions/treatments, child/parents verbalize and demonstrate decreased anxiety.

INTERVENTIONS	RATIONALES
Explain all procedures/interventions performed on child (e.g., blood drawing, starting IV).	Knowledge often helps decrease anxiety.
Explain purpose of equipment used on child (HR monitor, O₂ and pulse oximeter, BP monitor). Use therapeutic play with equipment in children >3 yr old.	Increased understanding of equipment decreases fear of pain, which in turn will decrease anxiety. For example, put BP cuff on a doll or teddy bear or let child put cuff on you.
Provide a quiet room where child can be closely observed.	Increased stimuli increase anxiety.
Encourage parents to stay with child if possible.	To promote sense of security, which will decrease child's anxiety.
Avoid making parents feel guilty if they are unable to stay.	Parents are already anxious about child being ill and in hospital.
Keep parents informed of child's progress, including what is being done and why.	To decrease their anxiety. The child easily perceives parental anxiety.
Talk quietly and calmly to child in age-appropriate language. Reassure child that you are available and will be there to help.	Establishing rapport increases trust and decreases anxiety.
Encourage transitional objects (items from child's home).	Increases feeling of security and decreases anxiety.
Facilitate coordination of care.	To avoid disturbing child any more than necessary, which would otherwise increase anxiety level.

●●● **Related NIC and NOC labels:** *NIC:* Anxiety Reduction; Calming Technique; Presence; Therapeutic Play *NOC:* Anxiety Control

Nursing Diagnosis:

Interrupted Family Processes

related to child having a chronic illness

Desired Outcome: Within 1 mo of diagnosis, family provides a normal environment for the child and copes effectively with the symptoms, management, and effects of asthma.

INTERVENTIONS	RATIONALES
Teach parents to have realistic expectations toward child's asthma.	Having knowledge and knowing what to expect enable family to cope more effectively. Expectations will vary, depending on child's developmental age and severity of asthma.
Encourage parents and siblings to focus on child as a normal child who needs some lifestyle modifications.	Child needs to be the focus, not the disease. Normalizing the environment as much as possible promotes child as the focus.

Continued

INTERVENTIONS	RATIONALES
Reinforce to parents the importance of setting consistent behavior limits and not enabling secondary gain for asthma attack.	Discipline and guidelines are essential for all children to develop appropriate behavior.
Use every chance to reinforce understanding of asthma and its therapies.	Accurate knowledge enables family to cope more effectively with child's chronic illness.
Reinforce need to use PFM at least 1-2 times/day and implement child's asthma action plan.	Understanding importance of monitoring child's status enables family to cope more effectively and incorporate monitoring into daily routine, thereby promoting normalization and child's optimal health status.
Teach child/parents how to give respiratory treatments (nebulizer, MDI) correctly, using prescribed medication and administering it with proper technique.	Eliminates confusion about administration of correct medications and method of delivery, thereby improving ability to cope with managing a chronic illness.
Encourage family to contact school (nurse, teachers, coaches) to develop a 504 plan for child.	Promotes family's coping while facilitating child's improvement. A 504 plan makes accommodations in the school environment so that the child can function better and thereby learn more effectively. For example, a child who is allergic to grass will not be assigned to a classroom with windows that open near a field of grass when the grass is being mowed.
Refer family to appropriate support groups and community agencies.	To help child and family function and deal with chronic illness more effectively.

●●● **Related NIC and NOC labels:** *NIC:* Coping Enhancement; Family Support; Support Group
NOC: Family Coping

Nursing Diagnosis:

Deficient Knowledge:

Purpose, precautions, and potential side effects of prescribed medications

Desired Outcome: Following interventions/instructions, child/parents verbalize accurate information about prescribed medication.

INTERVENTIONS	RATIONALES
Teach Parents and Patients the Following:	
Long-term control medications	Taken daily to achieve and maintain control of persistent asthma.
Cromolyn sodium/nedocromil sodium	Antiallergic agent.
- Observe for and report rash, cough, bronchospasm, and nasal congestion. If used orally, be alert for headache or diarrhea. If Spinhaler is used, monitor for bronchospasm and pharyngeal irritation occurring with cromolyn.	Side effects.
- Decrease in asthma symptoms should occur after medication has been taken for 4-6 wk.	Therapeutic response may occur within 2-4 wk, but maximum response occurs in 4-6 wk.
- Protect cromolyn from direct light and heat. Store oral capsules in foil pouch until ready for use.	This drug is light- and heat-sensitive.
- Store nedocromil at room temperature; do not freeze.	This drug is temperature-sensitive.

Continued

INTERVENTIONS	RATIONALES
Inhaled corticosteroids, such as fluticasone (Flovent), beclomethasone (Vanceril), and flunisolide (AeroBid)	Treat inflammation.
- Rinse mouth and gargle with water after oral inhalation.	To prevent thrush (oral candidiasis).
- Administer using a spacer.	May enhance drug delivery of inhaled form and help decrease incidence of thrush.
- Monitor for and report ongoing cough, thrush, voice impairment, or difficulty in speaking.	If no improvement, health care provider may need to adjust medication dosage.
- Do not decrease dose or discontinue without consent of health care provider.	This is a maintenance medication, and child may have exacerbation of symptoms if it is decreased or discontinued inappropriately.
Oral corticosteroids, such as prednisolone and prednisone	Decrease inflammation.
- Monitor for and report mood changes, seizures, increased blood sugar, diarrhea, nausea, gastrointestinal (GI) bleeding (seen in emesis, stools), weight gain, and tissue swelling.	Side effects; dosage may need to be changed.
- Take cautiously with barbiturates, carbamazepine, phenytoin, rifampin, or isoniazid.	These medications may reduce effect of prednisone and increase risk for GI ulcer.
- Observe carefully if taking salicylates, toxoids, nonsteroidal antiinflammatory drugs (NSAIDs), or diuretics that are potassium depleting.	These drugs may increase risk for GI ulcer when taken with corticosteroids.
- Limit use of caffeine and alcohol.	May increase risk for GI ulcer.
- **Caution:** Avoid vaccination while taking prednisone.	Live virus vaccines increase risk of viral infection. Vaccines in general may have decreased effect.
- Do not change or discontinue dose without consent of health care provider.	Long-term steroid dosage needs to be decreased carefully in order to allow for gradual return of pituitary-adrenal axis functioning. Failure to do so can result in adrenal insufficiency.
Leukotriene modifiers such as montelukast (Singulair)	Antiasthmatics; decrease inflammation and bronchoconstriction.
- Be alert for and report headache, abdominal pain, stomach ache, fatigue, dizziness, cough, diarrhea, laryngitis, pharyngitis, nausea, ear ache, sinus discomfort, and viral infections.	Side effects.
- Use cautiously with phenobarbital.	Phenobarbital reduces action duration of Singulair.
Long acting beta$_2$-agonists such as salmeterol (Serevent)	Relax bronchial smooth muscle to relieve bronchospasm.
- Be alert for and report increased HR, tremors, palpitations, dizziness, headache, and nausea.	Side effects.
- Store canister at room temperature.	Therapeutic effect may decrease when canister is cold or hot.
- Use Serevent Diskus powder up to 6 wk after removing protective foil.	Serevent powder for inhalation is stable for 6 wk after removal from foil packet.
Methylxanthines such as aminophylline and theophylline (rarely used now)	Bronchodilators.
- Be alert for and report GI upset, GI reflux, diarrhea, vomiting, nausea, abdominal pain, nervousness, insomnia, agitation, dizziness, tremors, and increased pulse rate.	Most common side effects.
- Limit caffeine (e.g., caffeinated beverages and chocolate).	Excessive intake may increase risk of cardiovascular and central nervous system side effects.
- Limit intake of charcoal broiled foods.	Excessive intake may increase elimination/decrease effectiveness of medication.
- Check with health care provider or pharmacist before taking any other medications.	Numerous medications increase or decrease theophylline level.

Continued

INTERVENTIONS

RATIONALES

INTERVENTIONS	RATIONALES
Immediate-relief medications	To treat acute signs and symptoms and pretreat exercise-induced asthma.
Short-acting inhaled beta$_2$-agonists such as albuterol (Proventil or Ventolin) and metaproterenol (Alupent)	Bronchodilators.
- Be alert for and report increased HR, palpitations, tremor, insomnia, nervousness, nausea, and headache.	Side effects.
- If using an MDI, use with a tube spacer or chamber.	Increases drug efficiency.
- Limit caffeinated beverages if taking albuterol or metaproterenol.	May increase side effects of albuterol or metaproterenol.
Oral corticosteroids (also see under long-term control medication)	Decrease inflammation.
- Be alert for and report dizziness, headache, anxiety, GI discomfort, and cough.	Side effects.
- Shake inhaler canister well before use.	To mix well.
- Use spacer with MDI.	Increases drug efficiency.

●●● **Related NIC and NOC labels:** *NIC:* Teaching: Prescribed Medication *NOC:* Knowledge: Medication

Nursing Diagnosis:

Fatigue

related to hypoxia and increased WOB

Desired Outcome: Within 24 hr following treatment/interventions, child exhibits decreased fatigue as evidenced by less irritability and restlessness, improved sleeping pattern, and ability to perform usual activities.

INTERVENTIONS

RATIONALES

INTERVENTIONS	RATIONALES
Assess HR, RR, and WOB q4h for increases from child's normal. Report significant findings.	Recognizing and reporting changes promptly facilitates appropriate actions that resolve the problem and decrease likelihood of fatigue.
Monitor for signs of hypoxia.	Recognizing symptoms of hypoxia (restlessness, fatigue, irritability, tachycardia, dyspnea, change of LOC) promptly enables timely treatment and decreases fatigue.
Provide calm and restful environment.	Promotes rest and decreases stress, oxygen demand, and fatigue.
Consolidate care; organize nursing care to provide periods of uninterrupted rest and sleep.	To provide maximum rest and decrease oxygen expenditure.
Encourage parents' presence, especially with younger children.	Parents' presence decreases fear and anxiety, thereby decreasing O$_2$ consumption and fatigue.
Encourage quiet, age-appropriate play activities as child's condition improves. Ensure child's physical comfort.	Emotional and physical comfort increase sense of well-being, promote rest, and decrease oxygen expenditure and fatigue.

●●● **Related NIC and NOC labels:** *NIC:* Energy Management; Environmental Management
NOC: Energy Conservation

ADDITIONAL NURSING DIAGNOSES/ PROBLEMS:

"Cystic Fibrosis" for **Impaired Gas Exchange.** However, with asthma, be aware that oxygen saturation needs to be >93%-95%, depending on agency protocol.

p. 651

PATIENT-FAMILY TEACHING AND DISCHARGE PLANNING

When providing patient/family teaching, focus on sensory information, avoid giving excessive information, and initiate a visiting nurse referral for necessary follow-up teaching and assessment. Include verbal and written information about the following, ensuring that it is written at a level understandable to child/family:

✓What is asthma? Discuss definition, signs and symptoms, and pathophysiology.

✓Identification of specific triggers for child that can precipitate an attack and removal of as many as possible from environment. Asthma triggers vary for each child. Most common triggers of asthma are upper respiratory infection (URI), cigarette smoke, exercise, and weather changes. Other triggers unique to the environment are important (e.g., humid weather, frequent rainy days, local industry). Additional common triggers include pollens, dust mites, mold, cockroaches, rodents, and pet dander.

✓Importance of personal asthma action plan with green, yellow, and red zone values specific for child. This plan is set up by health care provider based on child's best score (PEFR). Zones are established similar to a stoplight. The green zone is a score 80%-100% of child's best score and with no symptoms present. The yellow zone is a score 50%-80% of the child's best score and signals caution: the child may need extra asthma medicine. Follow guidelines in child's personal asthma action plan. The red zone is a score that is below 50% of the child's best score and signals an emergency situation. Follow asthma action plan and call health care provider. A sample asthma action plan is available at http://asthma.nationaljewish.org.

✓Importance of knowing early warning signs before acute attack (e.g., fatigue, sneezing, sore throat, itchy/watery eyes, headache, slight tightness in chest, drop in PFM values). These differ for each child.

✓Medications, including drug name, route, purpose, type (controller: long-term management or short-acting immediate relief), dosage, precautions, drug/drug and food/drug interactions, and potential side effects.

✓Importance of taking medication at home and at school as directed. Medication in the original bottle/canister (with prescribing label) and written prescription from health care provider are needed for child to be able to take any medication at school.

✓Proper technique for using MDIs with spacer (chamber) or spacer with a mask (usually for child <5 yr old). Document adequate return demonstration. Remind family that over-the-counter (OTC) inhalers contain medications that can interfere with prescribed therapy. Instruct child/parent to contact health care provider before trying any OTC medications. Instruct child/parent in sequencing of inhalers; bronchodilator inhalers are used 15 min before administration of steroid inhaler.

✓Cleaning and care of equipment—nebulizer, MDI, or other medication delivery systems, including assessment of when canister is low or empty.

✓If child is taking oral corticosteroids while at home, instructions to ensure that he or she receives correct amount each day, especially if medication is going to be tapered.

✓Signs and symptoms of increased respiratory distress in children relating to age (e.g., an infant may have increased RR when sleeping, decreased interest in eating/drinking, nasal flaring, grunting, retractions). Other signs and symptoms include difficulty speaking in sentences, inability to walk short distances, hunched posture, and PFM values in red zone.

✓Correct PFM technique. Most children >5 yr old can use PFM. Document return demonstration before discharge. Child should check this rate at least daily and more often if rate is decreased. Child should keep a log to document PEFR.

✓Maintaining asthma symptom diary, especially for a child with frequent symptoms.

✓Importance of avoiding contact with infectious individuals, especially those with respiratory infection.

✓Recommendation that a child receive pneumococcal vaccination and annual influenza vaccination.

✓Importance of follow-up care on a regular basis (not just emergency room). Confirm date and time of next appointment.

✓Phone numbers to call should questions or concerns arise about therapy or disease.

✓When to call health care provider:
1. To refill medications
2. PEFR in yellow zone >24 hr or child has event such as coughing, wheezing, chest tightness, or shortness of breath
3. PEFR in red zone or child is in increased respiratory distress
4. Immediate reliever (albuterol) is needed more often than q4h
5. Reliever medication is not helping

✓When to call emergency medical services:
1. Child is in severe respiratory distress
2. Child is gray/blue
3. Child is unable to answer questions or seems confused

✓Importance of communication with child's school or day care regarding child's condition, need for medication, and activity level.

✓Legal rights of the child—Section 504 of Rehabilitation Act of 1973: Each student with a disability is entitled to accommodation needed to attend school and participate as fully as possible in school activities. This accommodation may be related to a medical condition or an education issue.

✓Guidelines for attendance, activity level, and exercise at school/day care.

✓Referral to community resources, such as the local and national American Lung Associations and camps for educational programs for children with asthma. Additional general information can be obtained by contacting:

American Lung Association
61 Broadway, 6th floor
New York, NY 10006
(800) 586-4872 or (212) 315-8700
www.lungusa.org/

Allergy & Asthma Network Mothers of Asthmatics (AANMA)
2751 Prosperity Avenue, Suite 150
Fairfax, VA. 22031-4397
(800) 878-4403 or (703) 641-9595
www.aanma.org/

Asthma and Allergy Foundation of America (AAFA)
1233 20th Street, NW, Suite 402
Washington, DC 20036
(800) 7-ASTHMA or (202) 466-7643
www.aafa.org/
Student Asthma Action Card and Child Care Asthma/
Allergy Action Card are available as free downloads (look under "Education Parents and Caregivers").

Samples of asthma diaries:
www.betterhealth4kids.com/asthmaschooldiary.pdf
www.betterhealth4kids.com/asthmababydiary.pdf

STARBRIGHT Foundation
1850 Sawtelle Boulevard, Suite 450
Los Angeles, CA 90025
(800) 315-2580 or (310) 479-1212
www.starbright.org
Asthma CD-ROM: education and adventure for children 7-15 yr old, available free

Attention Deficit–Hyperactivity Disorder

Attention deficit–hyperactivity disorder (ADHD) is a neurodevelopmental disorder involving developmentally inappropriate behavior. ADHD is the most commonly diagnosed mental health condition among children in the United States, affecting 4%-12% of all school age children. Although the exact etiology is unknown, it probably involves a combination of biologic, genetic, and psychologic factors. It is seen more often in children who have a family member with ADHD, particularly the father, brother, or uncle. Chromosomal or genetic abnormalities such as fragile X syndrome have been implicated. ADHD commonly occurs in association with oppositional disorder, conduct disorder, depression, anxiety disorder, and many developmental disorders, such as speech and language delays and learning disabilities. ADHD is 2-3 times more common in males than females. Approximately 50%-80% of children affected continue to demonstrate symptoms into adolescence, and 66% carry symptoms into adulthood. There is some belief that ADHD is not "outgrown" but that people learn to compensate.

HEALTH CARE SETTING

Primary care

ASSESSMENT

Includes standard history and physical examination, neurologic examination, family assessment, and school assessment.

Signs and symptoms: The behaviors exhibited are not unusual aspects of any child's behavior. The difference lies in the quality of motor activity and developmentally inappropriate inattention, impulsivity, and hyperactivity displayed. The symptoms vary with developmental age and may range from a few to numerous different symptoms. The core symptoms include inattention, hyperactivity, and impulsivity. Children may experience significant functional problems such as school difficulties, academic underachievement, troublesome interpersonal relationships with family members and peers, and low self-esteem.

Physical assessment: Physical examination includes vision and hearing screening and a detailed neurologic exam that will help rule out any severe neurologic disorders.

Guidelines for the Diagnosis of ADHD (published by the American Academy of Pediatrics in May 2000):

1. Use of specific criteria for the diagnosis using the *Diagnostic and Statistical Manual of Mental Health Disorders,* 4th edition (DSM-IV) criteria.
2. Importance of obtaining information concerning the child's symptoms/behavior in more than one setting (especially from school).
3. Evaluation for coexisting conditions that may make the diagnosis more difficult or complicate treatment planning.

Multidisciplinary evaluation including the primary pediatrician (and possibly a developmental pediatrician, pediatric neurologist, or pediatric psychiatrist), psychologist, pediatric/school nurse, classroom teacher, specialty teachers as appropriate, and the child's parents in order to obtain all perspectives of child's behavior.

Detailed history: Both medical and developmental history and descriptions of the child's behavior should be obtained from as many observers as possible. Traumatic experiences and psychiatric and other disorders are ruled out, including lead poisoning, seizures, partial hearing loss, psychosis, and witnessing sexual activity and/or violence.

Psychologic testing: Valuable in determining a variety of deficits and helpful in identifying the child's intelligence and achievement level.

Behavioral checklists and adaptive scales: Helpful in measuring social adaptive functioning in children with ADHD.

Diagnostic Tests: ADHD is a diagnosis of exclusion. There is no definitive test for ADHD.

Nursing Diagnosis:

Disturbed Thought Processes

related to inability to concentrate, control impulses, and organize thoughts in a manner appropriate for age and development

Desired Outcomes: Within 1 mo of this diagnosis, child completes activities of daily living (ADL) and cooperates in school setting. Within one semester, child shows improvement in academic activities.

INTERVENTIONS	RATIONALES
Encourage parents/teachers to provide a structured environment and consistency.	Offers opportunity for child to focus on areas that need improvement.
Promote ongoing communication between parents and teachers.	Consistency among family and teachers in reinforcing same guidelines improves child's ability to concentrate.
Encourage parents/teachers to decrease stimuli when concentration is important.	Children with ADHD are easily distracted by extraneous stimuli. Removing those stimuli should improve concentration. For example, parents/teachers should have child do homework in a quiet area without TV or radio on or sit in a quiet section of the classroom, not near an open door.
Advise parents to work with school in determining if child is eligible for care under Individuals with Disabilities Education Act (IDEA) and therefore an Individualized Education Plan (IEP) or for Section 504 eligibility.	Many parents are unaware of the rights of disabled children. Environmental accommodation and appropriate classroom placement help children with ADHD reach their maximum potential by concentrating better, controlling impulses, and improving organizational ability. For example, for a child with ADHD, the desk may be placed in the front and on the quieter side of the classroom, and the child may be given extra time to complete tests.

●●● **Related NIC and NOC labels:** *NIC:* Environmental Management *NOC:* Concentration

Nursing Diagnosis:

Self-Esteem Disturbance

related to negative responses from others regarding behavior

Desired Outcome: Within 1 mo of this diagnosis, child achieves at least one goal, lists strengths, and elicits fewer negative responses from others.

INTERVENTIONS	RATIONALES
Monitor child's interactions with others.	To determine existence/degree of negative responses from other people.
Reward positive behavior and provide limit setting as needed. Avoid negative comments and giving attention for negative behavior.	Positive reinforcement is an effective way to improve behavior and self-esteem.
Help child set goals that are age appropriate, realistic, and achievable. Set timetable to achieve step-by-step progress until child accomplishes overall goal.	Achieving goals increases self-esteem. For example, if child has difficulty completing assignments, divide the assignment into manageable tasks. For example, for an essay assignment: day 1, make outline; day 2, begin literature search; day 3, begin writing paper; day 4, finish paper and have someone review it; day 5, finalize paper.
Encourage child to make a list of his or her strengths. Teach self-questioning techniques (e.g., What am I doing? How is that going to affect others?). Encourage positive self-talk (e.g., I did a good job with that!). Provide feedback accordingly.	Encourages positive self-thought and builds self-esteem.

●●● **Related NIC and NOC labels:** *NIC:* Self-Esteem Enhancement; Counseling; Self-Awareness Enhancement *NOC:* Self-Esteem

Nursing Diagnosis:

Risk for Injury

related to increased activity level, limited judgment skills, and impulsivity

Desired Outcome: Child remains free from signs of injury.

INTERVENTIONS	RATIONALES
Reinforce to parents the importance of child using appropriate safety equipment/protective device (e.g., seat belt, bicycle helmet).	Using this equipment/device decreases likelihood of injury.
Encourage parents to model the use of appropriate safety equipment/protective devices.	Children are more likely to wear a seat belt or bicycle helmet if parents wear them also.
Encourage parents to set clear limits on where child may ride a bike or play and to offer choices from several safe areas child can go.	Clear, simple guidelines are easier for a child with ADHD to focus on and follow. Allowing child some choice improves compliance, which decreases likelihood of injury.
Encourage child's participation in active play rather than in passive activities (e.g., playing softball rather than playing video games).	Active play helps child grow physically and cognitively. It also helps the child with ADHD to redirect energy in a safe and effective manner, thus decreasing risk of injury.
Reinforce importance of parents monitoring child's activities frequently.	Adequate supervision decreases likelihood of injury.
Teach parents to reinforce positive behavior with feedback and intermittent rewards.	Encourages appropriate behavior and activity, thereby decreasing risk of injury.

●●● **Related NIC and NOC labels:** *NIC:* Environmental Management; Safety; Surveillance: Safety; Area Restriction; Parent Education: Childrearing Family *NOC:* Safety Behavior: Home Physical Environment

Nursing Diagnosis:

Deficient Knowledge:

Chronicity of ADHD and its treatment

Desired Outcome: Within 1 mo of this diagnosis, child/parents verbalize accurate understanding of the chronic condition of ADHD and possible treatments.

INTERVENTIONS	RATIONALES
Determine parents' and child's understanding of ADHD. As indicated, teach them about the disorder, including the fact that it is chronic.	This assessment enables development of an individualized teaching plan. Accurate knowledge about the condition facilitates their understanding of the need for treatment and ways to manage it realistically.
Discuss different treatment strategies.	Promotes understanding that no single treatment strategy is *the* answer and that there are multiple strategies that may help the child, such as medication, behavioral/psychosocial interventions (parent training and education, behavior modification, teacher training/proper classroom placement and management, counseling, psychotherapy), combined or multimodal treatment, and biofeedback.

●●● **Related NIC and NOC labels:** *NIC:* Teaching: Disease Process; Teaching: Procedure/Treatment; Parent Education: Childrearing Family *NOC:* Knowledge: Disease Process; Knowledge: Treatment Regimen

Nursing Diagnosis:

Deficient Knowledge:

Purpose, precautions, and potential side effects of prescribed medications

Desired Outcome: Within 1 wk of starting medication, child/parents verbalize accurate information about prescribed medications.

INTERVENTIONS	RATIONALES
Teach the Following to Parents/Patients:	
Stimulant medications: short, intermediate, and long-acting methylphenidate (Ritalin) and short, intermediate, and long-acting dextroamphetamine (Dexedrine)	Given to promote attentiveness and decrease restlessness by increasing dopamine and norepinephrine levels, which leads to stimulation of the inhibitory system of the central nervous system (CNS).
First-line treatment:	
• Be alert for and report decreased appetite, weight loss, stomach ache or headache, delayed sleep onset, jitteriness, increased crying or irritability, and social withdrawal.	Common side effects that may require either dosage adjustment or change in schedule.
• Monitor for and report tics (involuntary movements of a small group of muscles such as of the face).	Occur in 15%-30% of children and are usually transient.
• Monitor for and report child becoming overfocused while on medication or appearing dull or overly restricted.	Seen in children receiving too high a dose or who are overly sensitive. Decreasing dose usually resolves these problems.

Continued

INTERVENTIONS	RATIONALES
- Take the medication on an empty stomach 30-45 min before meals.	Absorption of methylphenidate is increased when taken with meals, with the exception of Concerta, a long-acting form.
- Do not crush, chew, or break sustained-release forms.	Action of medication will change and probably not be as effective.
- To avoid insomnia, take last daily dose 4-6 hr before bedtime.	Reduces potential for insomnia.
- Get all prescriptions filled at the same pharmacy or give a list of all current medications to every pharmacy used.	There are many drug interactions with these medications. An informed pharmacist can identify all potential interactions among medications. For example, methylphenidate may increase serum levels of tricyclic antidepressants, phenytoin, phenobarbital, and warfarin. Monoamine oxidase (MAO) inhibitors or general anesthetics potentiate methylphenidate.
- Limit caffeine and decongestants.	They are stimulants and can potentiate medications the child is receiving.
- Monitor height, weight, and blood pressure.	Suppression of growth may occur with long-term use, and it can increase blood pressure as well.
- Caution is necessary when taken by children with seizures.	May lower seizure threshold.
- Do not give with acidic foods, juices, or vitamin C.	May decrease oral absorption of amphetamines.
- Child may need periodic drug holiday (e.g., no medication during the summer) or periodic discontinuation.	To assess patient's requirement for medication, decrease tolerance, and limit suppression of linear growth and weight.
- Monitor for and report decreased impulsiveness, improved social interaction, and increased academic productivity and accuracy.	Indicates effectiveness of medication.

Antidepressants

Tricyclics. imipramine (Tofranil) and desipramine (Norpramin)	Block norepinephrine and serotonin at nerve endings and increase action of both substances in nerve cells.
Second-line treatment:	
- Child should have a baseline evaluation of blood pressure (standing and supine), electrocardiogram (ECG), and complete blood count (CBC) with reevaluation whenever dosages change.	Dysrhythmias, ECG changes, and hypotension (especially orthostatic) are possible. Blood dyscrasias also may occur. Baseline evaluation shows status when medication is initiated and enables comparison as therapy continues.
- Be alert for and report palpitations, blurred vision, constipation, dry mouth, sedation, urinary retention, dizziness, and drowsiness.	Common side effects, which may require dose adjustment. Hour of sleep (HS) dosing during first few weeks of therapy reduces sedation.
- Do not take/give with clonidine.	May result in hypertensive crisis.
- Get all prescriptions filled at the same pharmacy or give a list of all current medications to every pharmacy used.	These drugs interact with many medications. An informed pharmacist can identify all potential interactions among medications.
- Slowly decrease dosage per health care provider's guidelines; do not stop abruptly.	Abrupt discontinuation may cause nausea, vomiting, diarrhea, headache, trouble sleeping, vivid dreams, and irritability.
Bupropion (Wellbutrin)	Antidepressant; a dopamine-reuptake inhibitor whose mechanism of activity is not well understood.
- Be alert to and report CNS side effects such as seizures, agitation, headache, or tremors; weight change; dry mouth; nausea; or vomiting.	Major side effects. Dose adjustment may be required.
- Get all prescriptions filled at the same pharmacy or give a list of all current medications to every pharmacy used.	There are many drug interactions with this medication. An informed pharmacist can identify all potential interactions among medications. For example, many seizure medications decrease the clinical effect of bupropion, MAO inhibitors increase its toxicity, and many herbs such as kava kava and St. John's wort interact with it.

Continued

INTERVENTIONS	RATIONALES
- Administer doses in equally spaced time intervals.	To minimize risk of seizures.
- Implement frequent mouth rinses and good oral hygiene.	May minimize dry mouth.
- Be alert for mood changes.	Indication of effectiveness of medication.
Other Drug **Clonidine** (not listed with recommended medications by American Academy of Pediatrics but frequently used)	Inhibits presynaptic release of norepinephrine to act as a mood stabilizer.
- Be alert for and report dry mouth, dizziness, drowsiness, fatigue, constipation, anorexia, palpitations, and local skin reactions with patch.	Side effects; may necessitate change in dosage.
- Do not stop medication abruptly.	Patient will go through withdrawal symptoms.
- Monitor carefully if given with CNS depressants.	Additive sedation would occur if given with CNS depressants, including alcohol, antihistamines, opioid analgesics, and sedative/hypnotics.

●●● **Related NIC and NOC labels:** *NIC:* Teaching: Prescribed Medication *NOC:* Knowledge: Medication

Nursing Diagnosis:

Compromised Family Coping

related to need for constant and close supervision of the child, hyperactivity of the child, or the stigma associated with a child with impulsive or aggressive behavior

Desired Outcome: Within 1 wk of diagnosis, family members discuss child's needs and develop a plan to provide the necessary support.

INTERVENTIONS	RATIONALES
Assist family with problem-solving ways of managing child's behavior and needs.	Positive reinforcement, time-out, response cost, or token rewards are examples of effective behavioral techniques for children with ADHD.
Provide handouts for caregivers explaining behavioral management techniques.	Verbal and written guidelines promote understanding. Handouts increase consistency among caregivers and improve ability to meet child's needs.
Allow family to vent concerns and problems.	Discussing concerns increases ability to cope with the situation.
Assist in identifying community resources for support (e.g., many school systems have ADHD support groups, local Children and Adults with ADHD [CHADD] chapter).	Support groups often help families function and cope more effectively.
Encourage family to advocate for their child within the school system (IEP or 504 accommodation plan as appropriate).	This involvement/support by the family increases potential for child to function well/succeed.

●●● **Related NIC and NOC labels:** *NIC:* Active Listening; Coping Enhancement; Family Involvement Promotion; Family Support *NOC:* Caregiver Stressors; Family Coping

ADDITIONAL NURSING DIAGNOSES/ PROBLEMS:

"Psychosocial Support for the Patient's   p. 95
Family and Significant Others," for relevant
psychosocial care plans that would help
family members cope with ADHD

PATIENT-FAMILY TEACHING AND DISCHARGE PLANNING

The child with ADHD may have a wide variety of symptoms and treatment modalities. Providing support and information about the disease is essential because of the stigma associated with ADHD. When providing child/family teaching, focus on sensory information and avoid giving excessive information. Include verbal and written information about the following (ensure that written information is at a level the reader can understand):

✓ Clarification of myths and realities concerning ADHD: Child is not "bad," "lazy," or "stupid."

✓ Safety measures relative to developmental age, impulsivity, inattentiveness, and hyperactivity.

✓ Medications, including drug name, purpose, dosage, frequency, precautions, drug/drug and food/drug interactions, and potential side effects.

✓ Importance of taking medication as directed at home and school. Medication in the original pharmacy bottle and written prescription from health care provider are needed for child to be able to take medication at school.

✓ Importance of consistency, structure, and routine for the child with ADHD.

✓ Importance of collaboration of family, health care provider, and school for optimal outcome.

✓ Environmental manipulation and appropriate classroom placement, which increase child's ability to function optimally.

✓ Suggestions regarding house rules:
- Give clear, specific directions.
- Use positive rewards; don't punish.
- Implement contingency plan.

✓ Suggestions to help children with ADHD:
- Daily picture with schedule of activities and events
- Index cards with written steps or pictures
- Organized backpack and notebook
- Physical relaxation techniques
- Standing when needing to work at desk
- Two chairs (can move back and forth between them)
- Boundaries in classroom

- Provide *only* needed materials
- Include short, fast-paced tasks
- Soothing music, carpet, earplugs
- One step—student verbalizes step, student performs step, next step
- Positive self-talk and reinforcement practices

✓ Suggestions to facilitate communication between family and school, including daily written communication with teacher per behavior (gives better overall evaluation of effectiveness of medication/behavioral modification).

✓ Legal rights of the child
- Individuals with Disabilities Education Act (IDEA): Requires states to identify, diagnose, educate, and provide related services for children 3-21 years old.
- Individualized Education Plan (IEP): Multidisciplinary team designs this plan to facilitate special education and therapeutic strategies and goals for each eligible child. Parents need to be involved in this process.
- Section 504 of Rehabilitation Act of 1973: Each student with a disability is entitled to the accommodation needed to attend school and participate as fully as possible in school activities.

✓ Signs that indicate when to contact health care provider:
- Child appears very drowsy
- Child unable to concentrate after being on medication several weeks
- Child physically harms self or others
- No improvement seen in school performance over 1-2 mo

✓ Importance of follow-up care, including primary pediatrician and multidisciplinary team.

✓ Referral to community resources such as support groups, pediatricians who are comfortable dealing with ADHD, child psychologists, and local community services boards, including:

Children and Adults with Attention-Deficit/Hyperactivity Disorder (CHADD)
8181 Professional Place, Suite 201
Landover, MD 20785
(800) 233-4050 or (301) 306-7070
www.chadd.org/

National Information Center for Children and Youth with Disabilities (NICHCY)
PO Box 1492
Washington, DC 20013-1492
(800) 695-0285
www.nichcy.org/

Bronchiolitis

Bronchiolitis is an acute inflammation and obstruction of the bronchioles, the smallest, most distal sections of the lower respiratory tract. It rarely occurs in children >2 yr old and has a peak incidence between 2 and 6 mo of age. Bronchiolitis is one of the major causes of hospitalization in children <1 yr of age. Incidence is greatest in the winter and early spring.

Acute bronchiolitis is most often a viral infection, and 60%-90% of the time it is caused by the respiratory syncytial virus (RSV). RSV is highly contagious; about two thirds of infants are infected with RSV by 1 yr of age, and almost 100% are infected by the age of 2 yr. RSV is the leading cause of lower respiratory tract disease in infants and young children, causing approximately 125,000 hospitalizations annually. Most of these infants and young children can be cared for at home, but approximately 2% of those hospitalized with RSV bronchiolitis die from the disease.

HEALTH CARE SETTING
Primary care with possible hospitalization for respiratory distress

ASSESSMENT
Initially upper respiratory infection (URI) symptoms for 2 to 3 days: fever, rhinorrhea, and cough.

Acute respiratory distress: Expiratory wheezing, tachypnea with RR $\geq$60-80 breaths/min, nasal flaring, paroxysmal nonproductive cough, increased respiratory effort or work of breathing (WOB), cyanosis, retractions, difficulty feeding because of increased RR, irritability, lethargy.

Physical assessment: Auscultation of expiratory wheezing and crackles or rhonchi. Symptoms of dehydration may be present: decreased level of consciousness (LOC), sunken anterior fontanel (if <2 yr old), dry or sticky oral mucosa, decreased abdominal skin turgor, decreased urine output.

Risk factors for severe RSV bronchiolitis:
- Premature infants born at <35 wk gestation
- Chronic lung disease (CLD) or bronchopulmonary dysplasia (BPD)
- Congenital heart disease (CHD); mortality was once 50% but is now 5%
- Low socioeconomic status
- Weight <5 kg or birth weight <1500 g
- T-cell immunodeficiency

DIAGNOSTIC TESTS
Diagnosis may be made on the basis of history, physical examination, and chest radiography.

RSV washing on nasal or nasopharyngeal secretions: To identify cause of respiratory distress; detects RSV antigen.

Arterial blood gases (ABGs): May be done initially to determine presence/degree of hypoxemia and acid-base imbalance.

Pulse oximetry: Noninvasive method of monitoring oxygen saturation.

Complete blood count (CBC): May be normal or show mild lymphocytosis.

Chest x-ray examination: Usually shows hyperinflation with mild interstitial infiltrates, but segmental atelectasis occurs infrequently.

Nursing Diagnosis:

Impaired Gas Exchange

related to edema of the bronchiole mucosa and presence of increased mucus

Desired Outcome: Immediately following treatment/intervention, child attains O_2 saturation >92%. By discharge, child maintains O_2 saturation >92% on room air (unless child was O_2 dependent before the illness).

INTERVENTIONS	RATIONALES
Observe for signs and symptoms of hypoxia (restlessness, change in LOC, dyspnea). Remember that cyanosis is a late sign of hypoxia in children.	Ongoing observation results in early detection of problems and early intervention, thereby decreasing severity of the hypoxia if it occurs.
Assess respiratory status q2h: LOC, RR, breath sounds, signs of WOB (nasal flaring, retractions, use of accessory muscles), cough, and skin and mucus membrane color.	Early identification of signs of respiratory distress (decreased LOC, increased RR, adventitious or decreasing breath sounds, increased WOB, and pallor or bluish tint) ensures prompt intervention, which results in decreased severity of respiratory symptoms.
Monitor VS q2-4h and prn.	Hypoxia causes an increase in HR, RR, and BP. A drop in BP and decreasing RR may be signs of impending respiratory arrest.
Maintain continuous oximetry while child is on O_2 and document at least q2h.	Provides continuous monitoring of O_2 saturation and alerts nurse to changes.
Provide humidified O_2 via nasal cannula to maintain O_2 saturation >92%. Report to health care provider if O_2 saturation ≤92%.	Delivering oxygen increases oxygen to the tissues. Oxygen is drying to the nasal mucosa, and humidity liquefies mucus. O_2 saturation ≤92% may indicate deteriorating condition.
Position child for maximum ventilation (e.g., head elevated but without compression on diaphragm).	Children are diaphragmatic breathers until 7 yr of age. Preventing compression of the diaphragm improves breathing effort.
Use cardiorespiratory monitor for infant or young child at high risk for or with history of apnea.	Ensures quick detection of deterioration in status or apneic episode.
Consolidate care to provide maximum rest.	Oxygen needs decrease with decreased energy expenditure.
Provide a neutral thermal environment.	An environment in which the child does not need to use any energy to cool or warm self reduces O_2 demand.

●●● **Related NIC and NOC labels:** *NIC:* Oxygen Therapy; Energy Management; Positioning; Respiratory Monitoring; Vital Signs Monitoring *NOC:* Respiratory Status: Gas Exchange; Vital Signs Status

Nursing Diagnosis:

Ineffective Airway Clearance

related to increased mucosal edema and secretions secondary to respiratory infection

Desired Outcomes: Within 24 hr of treatment/intervention, child exhibits decreased RR and decreased WOB (use of accessory muscles, retractions, and nasal flaring). By discharge, child is able to manage respiratory secretions as evidenced by more normal RR and minimal WOB (nasal flaring, retractions, and use of accessory muscles).

INTERVENTIONS	RATIONALES
Assess respiratory status q2h: LOC, RR, breath sounds, signs of WOB (nasal flaring, retractions, use of accessory muscles), cough, and skin and mucous membrane color.	Ensures early identification of changes that might indicate increasing respiratory distress. See details in previous nursing diagnosis.
Administer racemic epinephrine or albuterol with handheld nebulizer (HHN), if prescribed.	To decrease mucosal edema, which will open the airway and decrease WOB. Racemic epinephrine is a specific type of epinephrine that is administered via nebulizer, generally for croup or bronchiolitis. Examples include Vaponefrin, MicroNefrin, and AsthmaNefrin.

Continued

INTERVENTIONS	RATIONALES
Assess HR, RR, O$_2$ saturation, and breath sounds before and after nebulizer treatment.	Monitors effectiveness of treatment and for its side effects (see next rationale).
Hold nebulizer treatment if HR is >230 bpm (≤1 yr) or >180 bpm (>1 yr). Notify health care provider accordingly.	Tachycardia is one of the main side effects of both medications. Side effects should not outweigh the benefit of improving airway clearance.
Instill saline nose drops, wait 1-2 min, and suction nares before feedings and prn.	Suctioning too often causes nasal edema if using bulb syringe. Suction before feedings to clear nares, which will improve intake, inasmuch as young infants are obligate nose breathers.

●●● **Related NIC and NOC labels:** *NIC:* Airway Suctioning; Vital Signs Monitoring; Respiratory Monitoring
NOC: Respiratory Status: Airway Patency; Respiratory Status: Gas Exchange

Nursing Diagnosis:

Deficient Fluid Volume

related to increased insensible loss (secondary to increased RR, fever, increased metabolic rate) and decreased intake

Desired Outcome: Within 4 hr following treatment, child has adequate fluid volume as evidenced by alertness and responsiveness, soft anterior fontanel (in child <2 yr), moist oral mucous membranes, good skin turgor, and normal urine output (UO; e.g., infant UO >2-3 ml/kg/hr, toddler and preschooler UO 2 ml/kg/hr, school-age UO >1-2 ml/kg/hr, and adolescent UO 0.5-1 ml/kg/hr).

INTERVENTIONS	RATIONALES
Ensure that child is receiving daily maintenance fluids based on his or her weight.	Daily maintenance fluid requirements need to be met in order for child to have adequate hydration. The smaller the child, the greater the percentage of body weight is water. To meet minimal fluid requirements, calculate volume needed based on child's weight: **Up to 10 kg: 100 ml/kg/24 hr = _____** **10-20 kg: 50 ml/kg/24 hr = _____** **>20 kg: 20 ml /kg/24 hr = _____** **= maintenance fluid requirement** *For example, child weighs 23 kg:* 10 kg × 100 ml/kg/24 hr = 1000 ml/24 hr 10 kg × 50 ml/kg/24 hr = 500 ml/24 hr 3 kg × 20 ml/kg/24 hr = 60 ml/24 hr 23 kg 1560 ml/24 hr Maintenance fluid requirement for child weighing 23 kg is 1560 ml/24 hr.

Continued

INTERVENTIONS	RATIONALES
Assess hydration status: LOC, anterior fontanel (in child <2 yr old), oral mucous membranes, abdominal skin turgor, urine output q4h.	Child may be receiving maintenance fluids but still be dehydrated because of increased insensible losses. Frequent assessment leads to early recognition of problems and quicker treatment. Deficient fluid volume may be evidenced by decreased LOC, sunken anterior fontanel, dry or sticky oral mucous membrane, tented abdominal skin, and decreased urinary output.
Monitor I&O q2h.	Enables earlier intervention if a deficit is noted.
Monitor daily weights, using same scale at the same time of day and without any clothing (including diaper).	Short-term weight changes are the most reliable measurement of fluid loss or gain.
Offer a variety of liquids frequently that child likes (e.g., frozen juices, Popsicles, Pedialyte, Ricelyte, formula).	Replaces measurable and insensible fluid losses and helps to liquefy secretions. Child is more likely to cooperate if offered preferred fluids.
Do not offer PO fluids if child's RR is >80 breaths/min while awake.	There is increased chance of aspiration when child is tachypneic.
Administer IV fluids as prescribed.	Child may not be able to take adequate oral fluid because of respiratory distress. Administering IV fluids ensures that child receives maintenance fluids.

●●● **Related NIC and NOC labels:** *NIC:* Fluid Management: Hypovolemia Management; Intravenous Therapy; Fluid Monitoring; Fever Treatment *NOC:* Hydration; Fluid Balance

ADDITIONAL NURSING DIAGNOSES/ PROBLEMS:

"Asthma" for **Anxiety** *related to* illness, loss of control, and medical/nursing interventions	p. 604
"Asthma" for **Fatigue** *related to* hypoxia and increased WOB	p. 607

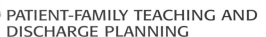

PATIENT-FAMILY TEACHING AND DISCHARGE PLANNING

When providing child/family teaching, focus on sensory information, avoid giving excessive information, and initiate a visiting nurse referral for necessary follow-up teaching and assessment as needed. Include verbal and written information about the following (ensure that written information is at a level the reader can understand):

✓ RSV bronchiolitis: definition, signs and symptoms, and basic pathophysiology.

✓ If child is on medications, drug name, route, purpose, type, dosage, precautions, drug/drug and drug/food interactions, and potential side effects.

✓ Despite having RSV bronchiolitis, the child can develop another RSV infection.

✓ Risk factors for developing RSV bronchiolitis:
- Exposure to tobacco smoke
- Day care attendance
- School-age siblings
- Crowded living conditions (two or more children in the same bedroom)
- Multiple births and/or premature infant born at <35 wk gestation
- Born within 6 mo of RSV season (November-April)
- Bottle-fed rather than breastfed

✓ Guidelines for preventing RSV infection:
- Good handwashing
- Keeping anyone with a fever or cold away from the child
- Avoiding secondhand smoke
- Avoiding crowds/day care

✓ Importance of checking hydration status at least several times a day when child is ill (i.e., the less the child weighs and the younger, the greater the percentage of body weight is water. Therefore, dehydration occurs much more quickly than it would in an older child or adult).
- Is the child alert and interactive? Child would not be as alert and interactive as normal if dehydrated.
- Check soft spot on top of the head (in children <2 yr old). If it is sunken, the child is dehydrated.
- Check inside the mouth, not the lips. If dry or sticky, the child is dehydrated.
- Pinch skin on the abdomen. If it sits up like a tent instead of falling down right away, the child is dehydrated.
- How many wet diapers does the child normally have a day? If the number of diapers is decreased or they are not as wet as usual, the child may be dehydrated.

✓How much should the child drink per day? Give parents information they can understand, such as an infant that weighs 9 kg needs 900 ml/day for maintenance fluids, which is 30 ounces. If the infant drinks from 4-oz bottles, he or she needs to take eight 4-oz bottles of fluid/day to get maintenance fluids.

✓Use of normal saline nose drops and bulb syringe to clear nares before feedings. An infant breathes primarily through the nose until 5-6 mo old, so if the nose is congested, he or she cannot breathe and therefore cannot drink or eat.

✓Continued prophylaxis against RSV with Synagis or Respigam if already receiving prophylaxis or per prescription (e.g., monthly IM or IV medication that gives passive immunity against RSV during RSV season, November through April).

✓Child may still have some signs and symptoms of RSV but may return to babysitter/day care if he or she doesn't have a fever and looks well after the follow-up visit to the health care provider.

✓Importance of follow-up care; typically follow-up appointment is made within 24-48 hr after discharge.

✓Phone number to call should questions or concerns arise about treatment or disease after discharge.

✓When to call health care provider:
- Fever increases
- Rate of breathing increases (>60 breaths/min)
- Nostrils flare out with each breath when child is resting (crying will cause this to happen when child isn't having breathing problems)
- Chest sinks in with each breath
- Child looks like he or she is working harder to breathe
- Lips turn gray or blue (cold can make lips look very pale and almost blue)
- Child exhibits signs of dehydration

✓Importance of infant/child receiving all routine childhood immunizations and rationale for giving immunizations.

✓Importance of cardiopulmonary resuscitation (CPR) and safety training.

✓Refer to community resources such as local and national American Lung Associations. Additional information can be obtained by contacting:

The American Lung Association
61 Broadway, 6th floor
New York, NY 10006
(800) 586-4872
http://www.lungusa.org/diseases/rsvfac.html (fact sheet on RSV)

Burns

Burn injuries represent one of the most painful and devastating traumas a person can experience. Fire and burn-related injuries are a leading cause of death from injury in children ages 1-14. Most burns in children are relatively minor and do not require hospitalization, but in 1999 an estimated 99,500 children ≤14 yr old were treated in hospital emergency rooms for burn-related injuries, 63% of which were thermal burns (hair curlers and curling irons, radiators, ovens and ranges, irons, gasoline, and fireworks being the most common causes).

The causative agent for burns varies depending on the child's developmental age. For instance, in children ≤4 yr old hospitalized with burn-related injuries, about 65% are treated for scald burns, with the highest incidence in children between 6 mo and 2 yr. In children over 8 yr old, flame burns involving liquids such as gasoline account for approximately 30% of burn-related injuries. Fires caused by children playing are the leading cause of residential fire-related death and injury in children ≤5 yr old.

Another source of burn injury is child abuse. About 10% of all child abuse cases are caused by burn injuries (e.g., immersion burns and cigarette burns). Approximately 10% of hospital admissions of children to burn units are the result of child abuse. The majority of child abuse burn victims are <2 yr old and almost always <10 yr old.

Factors affecting severity of the burn and seriousness of the injury:

1. Percentage of total body surface area (TBSA) burned: Use modified rule of nine for children (i.e., percentage of TBSA of head varies with age of child; at 1 yr old, it is 19%; at 5-9 yr old, it is 13%).
2. Burn depth:
   a. Superficial (first-degree) burn involves epidermis and heals in 5-10 days without scarring.
   b. Partial-thickness (second-degree) injury involves epidermis and varying degrees of the dermis. It may be superficial (usually healing in 14-21 days with variable scarring) or deep dermal (usually heals in 30 days to several months if no infection occurs and with extensive scarring).
   c. Full-thickness (third-degree) burn involves the epidermis and dermis and extends into the subcutaneous tissue. Nerve endings, sweat glands, and hair follicles are destroyed. It cannot reepithelialize and requires surgical excision and wound grafting.
   d. Fourth-degree is a full-thickness burn that involves underlying structures—muscles, fascia, and bones.
3. Wound location: Certain body areas carry a higher risk of complications and require specialized care (e.g., burns of the hand and feet and across joints can interfere growth and development because of scar formation).
4. Age of the child: For example, the very thin skin of a premature infant would take longer to heal and be damaged more easily than that of a healthy 3-yr-old.
5. Causative agent
6. Presence of respiratory involvement
7. General health of the child
8. Presence of concomitant injuries

Children most at risk:

- Children ≤4 yr old because of their natural curiosity and lack of awareness of danger are especially at risk for scald and contact burns and for sparkler injury.
- Children with disabilities related to developmental level or physical inability to get out of harm's way are especially at risk for scald and contact burns.
- Boys are at greater risk than girls.
- Children in homes without smoke detectors are at greatest risk for fires and fire-related death and injury.
- Males 10-14 yr old are at highest risk for fireworks-related injuries.

Differences in effects of burn injury in children:

- There is a higher mortality rate in very young children who have been severely burned compared to older children and adults with comparable burns.

625

- Lower temperatures and shorter exposure time can cause more severe burns in children than in adults because of the child's thinner skin.
- Larger body surface area as compared with adults puts severely burned children at increased risk for fluid and heat loss.
- The greater proportion of body fluid to mass in children increases risk of dehydration and cardiovascular problems because of less effective cardiovascular response to changing intravascular volume. The younger the child, the greater the percentage of total body weight is water and the greater his or her percentage of extracellular fluid (i.e., interstitial fluid surrounds the cell; intravascular fluid is within the blood vessels or plasma; and transcellular fluid such as spinal fluid and sweat).
- Because of smaller muscle mass and less body fat than adults, children are at increased risk for protein and calorie deficiency.
- The younger the child, the less mature the immune system and the greater the risk for infection.
- Extensive burns may result in delayed growth.
- Hypertrophic scarring is increased, and scar maturation is prolonged.

HEALTH CARE SETTING

Emergency department, with possible hospitalization for significant burns; some burns are treated in primary care and others at home

ASSESSMENT

Varies significantly depending on burn severity and seriousness of the injury.

Superficial burn (e.g., mild sunburn): Erythemic, moderate discomfort/pain, blanches with pressure, good capillary refill.

Partial-thickness burn:

- *Superficial:* Fluid-filled blisters, skin red to ivory with moist surfaces, considerable pain, blanches with pressure and refills.
- *Deep:* May or may not have fluid-filled blisters; blisters are often flat and dehydrated, making skin tissue-paper like; color is mottled, waxy white and with dry surface. Nerve endings are intact, so pain is severe on exposure to air or water.

Full-thickness burn: Varies in color from red to tan, waxy white, brown, or black. It does not blanch with pressure.

Edema is present. It has a dry, leathery appearance and lacks sensation because of destruction of nerve endings. However, because it is usually surrounded by superficial and partial-thickness burns that have intact nerve endings, adjacent areas likely will be painful.

Respiratory compromise: Upper airway edema related to injury starts within a few minutes, and the airway may occlude in minutes to a few hours, although it may be delayed up to 24-48 hr.

Respiratory distress: Abdominal breathing in a child >7 yr old (children are primarily abdominal breathers until that age), head bobbing with respiratory effort, nasal flaring, coughing, stridor, wheezing.

Burn shock: With severe burns (>15%-20% TBSA) a type of hypovolemic shock may occur with increased HR, increased RR, low BP, hypothermia, pallor, cyanosis, decreased level of consciousness (LOC), poor muscle tone.

Physical assessment: In addition to signs mentioned above, the examiner may notice singed nasal hairs and nasopharynx edema. It is also important to assess for other injuries such as fractures and internal injuries.

Complications:

- Pulmonary complications are the leading cause of death in thermal trauma: Inhalation injury, aspiration of gastric contents, bacterial pneumonia, pulmonary edema/insufficiency, and emboli.
- Wound sepsis: Disorientation is the first sign of overwhelming sepsis.
- Gastrointestinal complications: Impaired gastric and large bowel motility is common with burns >20% TBSA.
- Encephalopathy: Hallucinations, personality changes, delirium, seizures, and coma. Although encephalopathy is relatively common, full neurologic recovery usually occurs.

DIAGNOSTIC TESTS

Chemistries:

- **Fluid and electrolytes:** Deficits of fluid and sodium occur with burn shock.
- **Blood urea nitrogen (BUN) and creatinine:** Elevations may indicate renal failure.
- **Glucose:** May be elevated in young infants. Stress may cause either hypoglycemia or pseudodiabetes, resulting in elevated glucose levels.

Arterial blood gas level: To determine respiratory status; variations from normal may signal respiratory compromise.

Nursing Diagnoses:

Impaired Skin Integrity/Impaired Tissue Integrity

related to burn injury

Desired Outcomes: The skin/graft site heals without signs of infection (e.g., drainage, erythema, edema, or pain). Superficial burns heal within 5-10 days without scarring; deep partial-thickness burns heal within 30 days with varying degrees of scarring.

INTERVENTIONS	RATIONALES
Carefully clean wound and tissue immediately surrounding wound as prescribed.	Cautious cleansing is necessary to avoid damaging the epithelialization of granulating skin and decrease risk of infection.
Débride wound as prescribed.	To promote healing.
Apply ointment and/or dressings as prescribed using clean/ sterile technique.	Protects wound, decreases risk of infection, and promotes healing.
Minimize child scratching and picking at wound using methods appropriate for developmental age.	Promotes better wound healing and decreases scarring. Methods for developmental age include: - Young child: distraction and supervision - Older child: explanations of importance of not scratching, picking, or hitting wound
Offer high-calorie, high-protein meals and snacks, providing foods that the child likes.	Child has increased metabolism and catabolism because of burn injury and therefore needs increased calories and protein to promote positive nitrogen balance, which facilitates healing. Offering foods that the child likes increases likelihood of increased intake.
Perform active (or ensure passive) range-of-motion (ROM) exercises to affected joints as prescribed.	Promotes reabsorption of edema, prevents contracture formation, and improves healing.
Monitor child and wound/graft site/donor site q4h for signs and symptoms of infection	Ensures prompt recognition of problem, more rapid treatment, and maximum healing. Infection indicators include change in LOC, hypothermia or hyperthermia, odor, drainage, increased edema, increased erythema, and increased pain.
Administer vitamins and minerals (e.g., vitamins A, B, C, zinc, and iron) as prescribed.	These supplements facilitate wound healing and epithelialization.
Position for minimal stress/pressure on wound/graft.	Promotes healing and protects wound/graft. For example, do not allow child to lie on wound; use a cradle to keep sheets/blankets off the graft site.
Monitor graft q4h for evidence of hematoma, edema, or sloughing of graft; notify health care provider promptly if noted.	Early recognition of the problem and prompt treatment increase chance of saving the graft.
For more detailed information, see "Managing Wound Care," p. 583.	

●●● **Related NIC and NOC labels:** *NIC:* Wound Care; Infection Protection; Positioning; Medication Administration; Nutrition Management; Wound Irrigation; Skin Care: Topical Treatments *NOC:* Tissue Integrity: Skin & Mucous Membranes; Wound Healing: Secondary Intention

Nursing Diagnosis:

Acute Pain

related to thermal injuries and medical–surgical interventions

Desired Outcome: Within 30 min to 1 hr after treatment/intervention, child's pain level is decreased (≤2 on FACES scale or ≤4 on FLACC or numeric scale) or at a level acceptable to child.

INTERVENTIONS	RATIONALES
Establish pain scale appropriate for child's developmental level (e.g. FLACC, Wong-Baker FACES, or numeric scales).	Increases ability to accurately assess pain and degree of relief obtained.

Continued

INTERVENTIONS	RATIONALES
Assess level of pain q2-4h, as well as before and after pain medication administration (e.g., 1 hr after PO medications, 10-20 min after IV medications).	To detect early changes in pain level and assess effectiveness of pain medications.
Provide pain medications/non-pharmacologic pain relief measures around the clock on a regular basis, not prn.	Scheduled rather than prn pain relief provides better and more reliable pain control. Prolonged stimulation of pain receptors results in increased sensitivity to painful stimuli and will increase the amount of drug needed to relieve pain. Pain relief measures such as distraction; relaxation; repositioning; guided imagery; cutaneous stimulation such as massage, heat, or cold; and positive self-talk increase effectiveness of medication.
Explain how patient-controlled analgesia (PCA) works and that child cannot give self too much medication. Encourage child/parent to use PCA when needed if it is available. Reassure parent that addiction rarely occurs when medication is used to relieve pain.	Fear of addiction may decrease use of pain medication.
Premedicate child before painful procedures.	Pain medications given before painful procedures will help control pain. Time frame before procedure depends on route (e.g., 10-20 min IV and 1 hr PO).
Explain all procedures at developmental level appropriate for child.	Anxiety increases pain; knowing what to expect may decrease anxiety.

●●● **Related NIC and NOC labels:** *NIC:* Pain Management; Medication Management; Patient-Controlled Analgesia Assistance; Positioning; Distraction; Simple Relaxation Therapy; Simple Guided Imagery; Cutaneous Stimulation; Anxiety Reduction *NOC:* Comfort Level

Nursing Diagnosis:

Risk for Infection

related to loss of skin barrier/denuded skin, increased metabolic demands, altered nutritional status, invasive procedures/lines, and the hospital environment

Desired Outcome: Child exhibits wound healing without signs of burn wound infection (e.g., odor, drainage, increased erythema or edema, increased pain) or systemic infection (e.g., pneumonia or septicemia).

Note: *See interventions and rationales for impaired skin/tissue integrity plus the following:*

INTERVENTIONS	RATIONALES
Wash hands before and after working with child.	Handwashing is the best method of preventing nosocomial infection.
Use gloves as indicated, following standard precautions.	Provides additional level of protection for patient by reducing risk of contamination of open wounds by bare hands of caregivers. (Wearing gloves also protects caregiver from contact with patient's open wounds.)
Screen visitors for colds or other infectious illnesses before they enter child's room.	Child has altered immune response and is at greater risk for infection because of the following:

Continued

INTERVENTIONS	RATIONALES
	- Open wounds or denuded skin have lost the protective skin barrier and are potential entry sites for infection.
	- Decreased circulation to the burned area compromises the body's ability to fight infection at the tissue level because fewer leukocytes (white blood cells [WBCs], which act as scavengers and fight infection) are able to reach damaged tissue.
	- Mature neutrophils, the body's first line of defense against bacterial infection and severe stress, are decreased as immature neutrophils increase to digest products of burn injury.
Monitor VS q4h and notify health care provider of findings indicative of infection (e.g., temperature <36 or >38.5° C, HR >100 bpm, or RR >30 breaths/min, but will vary depending on age of child).	Early signs of infection/sepsis include tachycardia, tachypnea, and fever or hypothermia. Early recognition of abnormality enables prompt treatment and less serious infection.
Monitor LOC q4h.	Disorientation is one of the first signs of overwhelming sepsis/septic shock in burn patients.
Monitor for signs of pneumonia q4h (varies depending on age of child).	Early recognition facilitates prompt treatment and a less severe infection.
	- Infant: fever, restlessness, anxiety, grunting, nasal flaring, retractions, tachypnea, head bobbing
	- Child and adolescent: fever, chills, cough, chest pain, restlessness, anxiety, tachypnea
Position child with head elevated 15-30 degrees for 1-2 hr after meals.	Decreases incidence of aspiration of gastric contents, which could lead to aspiration pneumonia.
Depending on developmental age, ensure that child turns, coughs, and deep breathes or uses incentive spirometer q2h while awake. Younger children can blow bubbles or blow on a pinwheel.	Deep breathing expands alveoli and aids in mobilizing secretions to the airways, and coughing further mobilizes and clears the secretions to help prevent pneumonia.
Assess IV sites (peripheral or central access) q4h for signs of infection (e.g., erythema, warmth, edema).	There is potential for increased rate of infection because of child's altered immune response and because IV site is another entry site for bacteria.
For more information, see Appendix for "Infection Prevention and Control," p. 831.	

●●● **Related NIC and NOC labels:** *NIC:* Infection Protection; Respiratory Monitoring; Aspiration Precautions; Wound Care *NOC:* Immune Status; Infection Status; Wound Healing: Secondary Intention

Nursing Diagnosis:

Deficient Fluid Volume

related to fluid shift from intravascular to interstitial compartment, increased metabolic demands, and decreased intake

Desired Outcomes: Within 4 hr following intervention/treatment, child has adequate fluid volume as evidenced by normal LOC for child, moist oral mucous membranes, good abdominal skin turgor (on unaffected areas), and normal urine output (UO). For example, infant UO >2-3 ml/kg/hr, toddler and preschooler UO 2 ml/kg/hr, school-age UO 1-2 ml/kg/hr, and adolescent UO 0.5-1 ml/kg/hr.

INTERVENTIONS	RATIONALES
Administer IV fluids as prescribed.	Fluid resuscitation is required in children with burns >10% TBSA. Fluids help maintain general circulation to vital organs and capillary circulation to viable skin.
Once stabilized, ensure that child receives *at minimum* maintenance fluids based on his or her weight.	The smaller the child, the greater the percentage of body weight is water and the larger the percentage of extra-cellular fluid. Because of excess fluid loss from the burn injury and increased metabolic demands related to child's age and increased catecholamine release caused by burn stress, child probably will need more than maintenance fluids. First, use this formula to determine maintenance fluids: **Up to 10 kg: 100 ml/kg/24 hr = _____** **10-20 kg: 50 ml/kg/24hr = _____** **>20 kg: 20 ml/kg/24hr = _____** **= maintenance fluid requirement** *For example, child weighs 33 kg:* 10 kg × 100 ml/kg/24 hr = 1000 ml/24 hr 10 kg × 50 ml/kg/24 hr = 500 ml/24 hr 13 kg × 20 ml/kg/24 hr = 260 ml/24 hr ――――――――――――――――――――――― 33 kg 1760 ml/24 hr Maintenance fluid requirement for child weighing 33 kg is 1760 ml/24 hr. Remember that the child probably will need *more* than maintenance fluids.
Assess I&O q2h. Assess hydration status q4h: LOC, anterior fontanel (in child <2 yr old), oral mucous membranes, abdominal skin turgor, and urine output. **Note:** Edema may occur around the burn or from fluid shifts.	Child may be receiving maintenance fluids but still be dehydrated because of increased insensible water losses, especially in a child with burns. Frequent assessment leads to early detection of problems and quicker treatment. Signs of impaired hydration include decreasing LOC, sunken fontanel, dry and sticky oral mucous membranes, tenting of abdominal skin, and decreased UO.
Monitor VS, capillary refill, and LOC q4h for changes related to hypovolemia.	Hypovolemia may be present because of reduced circulating blood volume that occurs with plasma loss in burns. Tachycardia, changes in tissue perfusion (e.g., capillary refill >2 sec), and alteration in LOC are early signs of hypovolemic shock. BP will be normal initially because increased systemic vascular resistance helps to maintain it. However, perfusion with a normal BP may be inadequate to meet the body's demands. Therefore decreased BP can be a late sign of hypovolemia in children.
Monitor daily weights, using same scale at same time of day and with same amount of clothing (no clothes, including diaper in infants).	Short-term weight changes are the most reliable measurement of fluid loss or gain. Excessive weight gain indicates fluid retention, which could interfere with wound healing; weight loss could signal dehydration or excessive fluid loss, which also would interfere with wound healing.
Alert health care provider promptly to significant findings or changes.	To ensure timely treatment.

Disturbed Body Image

related to child's perception of altered appearance and mobility/skills

Desired Outcomes: Child receives emotional support from the onset of injury and discusses feelings related to change in appearance and mobility/skills after wound healing begins. Within 48-72 hr of this diagnosis, child relates at least one positive example of his or her appearance/abilities and expresses realistic expectations for the future.

INTERVENTIONS	RATIONALES
Ensure a positive attitude when caring for the child.	Shows acceptance and encourages expectation that child will get better.
Point out positive aspects of child's appearance/abilities. Ask child during subsequent care to give examples of positive aspects.	Positive reinforcement encourages child to focus on positive aspects rather than on deficits.
Encourage child to provide for developmentally appropriate self-care as much as his or her condition allows.	Enables child to focus on tasks that he or she can do and promotes positive self-image in the process.
Give honest answers to child and family regarding care and appearance.	Facilitates building of a trusting nurse-patient/family relationship and assists in developing realistic expectations.
Assess support systems and coping mechanisms used in previous stressful situations.	Mobilizes previous effective strategies to assist child in dealing with current altered appearance and mobility/skills.
Arrange for continued schooling, depending on age of child.	Decreases isolation and provides normalization, which may help self-image.
Promote peer contact if possible and prepare peers for child's appearance.	Facilitates acceptance and support.
Support appropriate adaptive behaviors.	Builds on strengths.
Encourage verbalization about feelings regarding appearance and changes in lifestyle.	Identifies child's concerns and anxieties, enabling nurse to provide more realistic feedback about appearance if appropriate and aids in working on coping strategies.
Point out evidence of healing.	Promotes sense of hope.
Discuss ways child can "cover-up" disfigurement, dressings, and pressure garments.	Facilitates coping. Examples include clothing (e.g., turtleneck sweaters, larger shirt than normal), wigs, makeup.
Assist child in devising a plan to address and cope with reactions of others.	Increases sense of control. Role playing may help child perfect this plan.
Facilitate transition back to day care, school, and home environment. Encourage communication of family and medical staff with other care providers, including school nurse and teachers.	Prepares other children and caregivers for change in child's appearance and encourages them to make transition a positive experience.

●●● **Related NIC and NOC labels:** *NIC:* Body Image Enhancement; Active Listening; Anxiety Reduction; Coping Enhancement; Emotional Support; Self-Awareness Enhancement; Support System Enhancement; Self-Modification Assistance *NOC:* Body Image

Nursing Diagnosis:

Imbalanced Nutrition: Less than body requirements

related to hypermetabolic state and decreased appetite

Desired Outcome: Within 1 wk of intervention/treatment, child exhibits adequate nutrition as evidenced by maintenance of or gaining weight.

INTERVENTIONS	RATIONALES
Provide high-calorie, high-protein meals and snacks, as well as foods high in vitamin C content.	Because of smaller muscle mass and less body fat than adults, children are at increased risk for protein and calorie deficiency. This diet provides positive nitrogen balance and nutrients needed for wound healing. Energy requirements increase according to size of the burn; caloric requirements may be 2 to 3 times normal because of increased metabolic rate. High-protein meals replace protein lost by exudation.
Ensure that child is receiving adequate nutrients. Discuss child's needs with health care provider.	If this cannot be accomplished orally, enteral or parenteral feedings may be necessary. Burns will not heal well without adequate nutrients.
Provide foods that the child likes and encourage child to feed self as much as possible.	Stimulates appetite and promotes cooperation.
Try to minimize anorexia in the following ways: - Offer small, frequent meals. - Make meal times pleasant with attractive meals, companionship, and no treatments or unpleasant interruptions.	Occurs in many children with burn injury. - Child may eat better with 4-5 small meals/day rather than 3 large meals. - Encourages eating if in a more "homelike" environment.
Maintain neutral thermal environment.	Caloric expenditure is minimized when child does not need to use energy to cool or heat body.
Monitor I&O q4h.	To ensure that child is receiving appropriate intake and has adequate output.
Monitor for hypoglycemia.	Can result from stress of injury as glycogen stores in liver are rapidly depleted.
Monitor for hyperglycemia.	Can occur because of mobilization of glucagon and decreased insulin production.
Ensure that child is having a normal stooling pattern. Monitor for constipation or diarrhea and notify health care provider if either occurs.	Constipation caused by decreased activity and intake could further affect intake because of discomfort and thus interfere with weight gain. Diarrhea would decrease weight as well.
Weigh weekly on the same scale at the same time of day with the same amount of clothing.	Consistency with weight measurements helps ensure more accurate results. Weight is a reliable indicator of nutritional status.

●●● **Related NIC and NOC labels:** *NIC:* Nutrition Monitoring; Enteral Tube Feeding; Nutrition Management; Weight Gain Assistance; Total Parenteral Nutrition Administration *NOC:* Nutritional Status; Nutritional Status: Nutrient Intake

ADDITIONAL NURSING DIAGNOSES/ PROBLEMS:

PATIENT-FAMILY TEACHING AND DISCHARGE PLANNING

When providing patient/family teaching, focus on sensory information, avoid giving excessive information, and initiate visiting nurse referral for necessary follow-up teaching and assessment. Include verbal and written information about the following (ensure that written information is at a level the reader can understand):

✓ Type of burn and normal healing time.

✓ Wound care as appropriate:

- Administering oral pain medication about 1 hr before wound care if needed

- Cleaning wound
- Applying ointment
- Applying dressing

✓ Treatment of pain (e.g., administering medication on a regular basis, which gives better control and assists healing process; use of nonmedication adjuncts such as distraction).

✓ Signs and symptoms of burn wound, graft site, or donor site infection:
- Purulent drainage or odor
- Increased redness or swelling
- Temperature >101.5° F

✓ Ways to prevent infection:
- Good handwashing before and after caring for wound
- Dressing changes performed in a clean area with good light
- Making sure that dressing stays clean and dry

✓ Methods of preventing scars and contractures:
- Wearing pressure garments as prescribed (usually 23 hr/day)
- Wearing splints as prescribed (over top of pressure garment)
- ROM exercises as prescribed and demonstrated by physical therapist (PT)
- Child performing as many activities of daily living (ADL) as possible (e.g., feeding self, combing hair, dressing self)

✓ Care of healing skin:
- May be dry: Apply lotion (cocoa butter is most often recommended) but avoid those containing alcohol or lanolin
- May be itchy: Use lotion, prescribed medication (e.g., Benadryl), distraction
- Bathing: Use lukewarm water and be gentle!
- Protect new skin over burned area
  - Wear comfortable clothing, not constrictive
  - Try to avoid hitting or bumping area
  - Protect from sun with clothing and sunscreen (SPF >15)
  - Do not stay out in cold weather; burned area is sensitive to cold

✓ If child is on any medications: drug name, route, purpose, type, dosage, precautions, drug/drug and drug/food interactions, and potential side effects.

✓ Demonstrate drawing up and administering medication and having family member perform return demonstration.

✓ Adjustment after burn injury, which is often prolonged and painful. Family and individual psychosocial support is important.

✓ Feelings that child may experience with reentry to school/society, which vary depending on developmental age and severity of burn: fear, anger, guilt, depression, withdrawal, altered body image, anticipating peer response.

✓ Potential for regression. This is normal after a stressful event.

✓ Developmentally related risks for burn injuries (see introductory data).

✓ Tips for childproofing the home:
- Set water heater thermostat at ≤120° F or install anti-scald devices in faucets and showerheads in buildings

where one does not have access to the water tank (e.g., apartment buildings).
- Water temperature of 120° takes 2.5 min for partial-thickness burn.
- Water temperature of 130° takes 15 sec for partial-thickness burn.
- Water temperature of 140° takes 2.5 sec for partial-thickness burn.

- The younger the child, the thinner the skin, and the quicker and more deeply the burn that occurs.
- Never leave a young child alone, especially in the kitchen or bathroom, even to answer the phone for a minute. Take the child with you.
- Turn pot handles toward back of the stove and use back burners when cooking.
- Cover stovetop knobs.
- Keep appliance cords out of child's vision and reach (e.g., coffee pot), especially if appliance contains hot food or liquid.
- Cover unused electrical outlets with appropriate outlet covers (not the ones that just plug in).
- Keep hot foods and liquids away from table and counter edges.
- Do not leave hot foods or liquids on a table with a tablecloth that child can reach.
- Never carry or hold child and hot food and/or beverage at the same time.
- Stress dangers of open flames; explain what "hot" means.
- Place protective cover in front of radiator, fireplace, or other heating element.
- Keep matches, gasoline, lighters, and all other flammable materials locked away and out of child's reach.
- Teach children how to STOP, DROP, AND ROLL if their clothes catch on fire and how to crawl to safety if a fire occurs in the building they are in.
- Over 6 mo old, apply sunscreen with SPF ≥15 when child is exposed to sunlight.

✓ Additional tips for preventing fire-related injuries:
- Install smoke detectors in home in every bedroom and on each level. Test them monthly and change batteries at least yearly. Having smoke detectors cuts the risk of dying in a fire by 50%.
- Have at least two multipurpose dry chemical fire extinguishers: one in the kitchen and one in workshop or area where potential sources of fire exist (e.g., water heater or furnace). Check monthly for signs of damage, corrosion, tampering, and leaks. Always call the fire department before using the fire extinguisher. Use the PASS method (Point, Aim at the base of the fire, Squeeze the handle, and Sweep from side to side).
- Set up a home emergency fire escape plan and have practice drills using escape plan at least quarterly. Include a meeting place outside the home in your plan.

✓ Nutritional needs (child needs increased calories and protein to heal well):

- Make pudding with Ensure instead of milk (increases calories).
- Eat small frequent meals or three meals with nutritious snacks between meals.
- Make mealtime a social, shared time. Turn off TV.
- Feed child when he or she is well rested.
- If receiving tube feeding: procedure for checking placement and administering feeding, checking residual, and recognizing and reporting problems.
- Vitamins that help skin heal: A and C (oranges, grapefruit, tomatoes, broccoli, and carrots).
- Protein promotes skin healing: meat, fish, eggs, peanut butter, chicken, and milk.

✓ Growth and development (realistic expectations of what child should be doing at different ages and encouragement of activities that promote normal growth and development).

✓ Importance of adequate fluid intake to promote healing (child should receive at least maintenance fluids or more per health care provider). How much should the child drink per day? Give parents information they can understand, such as an infant that weighs 9 kg needs 900 ml/day for maintenance fluids, which is 30 oz. If the infant drinks from 4-oz bottles, he or she needs to take eight 4-oz bottles of fluid/day to get maintenance fluids. An older child weighing 40 kg would need 1900 ml/day for maintenance fluids. If this child drinks from 12-oz glasses, he or she would need at least five and a half 12-oz glasses/day. These examples are only for maintenance fluids; child may need 1½-2 times maintenance fluids to stay well hydrated, depending on size and stage of healing of the burn injury.

✓ Importance of checking hydration status at least several times a day while the child is still healing from the burn. The less the child weighs and the younger he or she is, the greater the percentage of body weight is water. Therefore dehydration occurs much more quickly than it would in an older child or adult. The child may still be losing fluid from the burn and using more energy to heal, therefore using more fluid.

- Is the child alert and interactive? Child would not be as alert and interactive as normal if dehydrated.
- Check soft spot on top of the head (in children <2 yr old). If it is sunken in, the child may be dehydrated.
- Check inside the mouth, not the lips. If dry or sticky, the child is dehydrated.
- Pinch skin on the abdomen. If it sits up like a tent instead of falling down right away, the child is dehydrated.
- How many wet diapers does the child normally have a day or how many times does he or she normally void? If the number of diapers is decreased, they are not as wet as usual, or the child is voiding less often, he or she may be dehydrated.

✓ First-aid emergency care for burn injury: Put burned area under cool running water immediately, remove clothing, cover burned area loosely with bandage or clean cloth, seek medical assistance.

✓ Importance of follow-up care with health care provider, PT, and any other specialists involved.

✓ Phone numbers to call for health care provider, home health nurse, and PT should any questions or concerns about treatment or injury arise after discharge.

✓ When to call health care provider:

- If child is not eating well or showing signs of dehydration
- If there is unmanageable behavior at home or school
- If there are any signs of infection (e.g., healing burn area or donor site looks, feels, or smells different—red, warm, swollen, very tender to touch or there is foul smelling drainage)
- If there is itching that is not controlled with lotion or medication
- If the healing/healed area cracks open or splits
- If contracture occurs
- If child's temperature is >101.5° F
- If dressing change is painful despite giving pain medication as prescribed

✓ Referral to community resources, such as National SAFE KIDS Campaign, public health nurse, home health agencies, community support groups, camps for children with burns, psychologists, and financial counseling as appropriate. Additional general information can be obtained by contacting the following organizations:

National SAFE KIDS Campaign
1301 Pennsylvania Avenue, NW, Suite 1000
Washington, DC 20004
(202) 662-0600
www.safekids.org/

Shriners Hospitals Burn Prevention Tips
(800) 237-50055
www.shrinershq.org/Prevention/

Alisa Ann Ruch Burn Foundation
3600 Ocean View Boulevard #1
Glendale, CA 91208
(800) 242-BURN or (818) 249-2230
www.aarbf.org/
Burn survivor assistance; prevention materials

Phoenix Society for Burn Survivors
1840 Wealthy South East, Suite 215
East Grand Rapids, MI 49506
(800) 888-2876 or (616) 458-2773
www.phoenix-society.org/
Assistance locating local resources; listing of camps for children; "You Can Do It" video for teens

78

Cerebral Palsy

*C*erebral palsy is a term used to describe a group of chronic conditions affecting body movement and muscle coordination. It is caused by damage to one or more specific areas of the brain, which typically occurs before birth during fetal development but can occur during or shortly after birth—usually before age 5 yr. Cerebral palsy is the most common physical disability of childhood, and the incidence is 1.2-2.7 per 1000 live births with an increased incidence in premature or very low-birth-weight babies. It is nonprogressive, although secondary conditions (e.g., muscle spasticity) can develop and may remain the same, improve, or deteriorate. A child with cerebral palsy may have intellectual, perceptual, and language deficits.

A large number of factors may contribute to cerebral palsy, either singly or multifactorially. No identifiable cause is found in about 24% of patients. There are three main types of cerebral palsy, and there may be a mixture of types.

- **Spastic:** May involve one or both sides. Hypertonicity is present with poor control of posture, balance, and coordinated movements. The patient has difficulty with fine and gross motor skills.
- **Dyskinetic/athetoid:** Involuntary and uncontrolled body movement.
- **Ataxic:** Disturbed sense of balance and depth perception.
- **Mixed:** Combination of spasticity and athetosis.

HEALTH CARE SETTING

Primary care, with possible hospitalization for surgery or pneumonia

ASSESSMENT

Involves physical assessment along with a detailed health history. Ongoing developmental surveillance is important. Cerebral palsy is not usually diagnosed until 6-12 mo of age.

Signs and symptoms: Clinical manifestations vary tremendously from child to child. Some children may have a mild problem with ataxia, whereas some may be severely affected. The universal clinical manifestation is delayed gross motor development. Other common problems are abnormal motor performance, alterations of muscle tone (hypertonicity or hypotonicity), abnormal postures, reflex abnormalities, and numerous associated disabilities and problems, including intellectual impairment, attention deficit–hyperactivity disorder (ADHD), seizures, drooling, feeding and speech problems, orthopedic complications, increased incidence of dental problems, and visual and hearing problems.

Physical assessment: Involves evaluation of range of motion (ROM), muscle strength and tone, abnormal movements, and contractures.

DIAGNOSTIC TESTS

Primary method of diagnosis is neurologic examination with developmental screening and history.

Neuroimaging tests: To determine site of brain injury and provide clues to potential causes, as well as rule out slow growing brain tumors.

Cytologic studies: Genetic evaluation is done to determine if a progressive degenerative disease is present or symptoms are part of a syndrome.

Metabolic studies: To evaluate for metabolic defects (e.g., Guthrie blood test for phenylketonuria [PKU] or serum galactose levels for galactosemia).

Electroencephalogram (EEG): Can rule out seizure disorders or slowly growing brain tumor.

Electrolyte levels: To assess for and rule out electrolyte imbalance that may be causing symptoms.

Nursing Diagnosis:

Impaired Physical Mobility

related to neuromuscular impairment

Desired Outcome: Within 1 mo after intervention/treatment, child demonstrates improved mobility, and parents demonstrate correct use of splints/braces and physical therapy techniques.

INTERVENTIONS	RATIONALES
Encourage performance of developmental tasks such as sitting, crawling, and walking, as appropriate.	Helps to stretch and strengthen muscles.
Reinforce use of physical therapy exercises to strengthen and help muscle coordination.	Facilitates optimum muscular development.
Provide incentives to move.	Developmentally appropriate incentives (e.g., a mobile for an infant functioning at a 4-mo-old level) increase likelihood of child trying to move.
Encourage rest before locomotion activities.	Spasticity and abnormal posturing increase when child is tired. Being rested before attempting locomotion improves chance of accomplishing goal.
Incorporate play into mobility exercises.	This is the normal activity of a child and encourages cooperation.
Instruct parents in correct use of orthoses.	To help prevent contractures, protect skin, and maintain or improve function.
Encourage parents to be active in child's daily physical and occupational therapy.	Facilitates integration of therapy skills into child's activities of daily living (ADL) and promotes continuity of care.
Evaluate child's response to therapy on a regular basis.	Ongoing evaluation of effectiveness of current plan increases chance of success because modifications or changes can be made in a timely manner, as necessary.

●●● **Related NIC and NOC labels:** *NIC:* Body Mechanics Promotion; Energy Management; Exercise Promotion; Teaching: Prescribed Activity/Exercise *NOC:* Mobility Level

Nursing Diagnosis:

Bathing/Hygiene, Dressing/Grooming, Toileting Self-Care Deficits

related to neuromuscular impairment

Desired Outcome: Within 1 mo following intervention/treatment, child begins to assist with or perform ADL.

INTERVENTIONS	RATIONALES
Assess child's developmental and intellectual level.	Enables development of an individualized care plan for assisting child with ADL.
Encourage child to assist with care as much as possible, depending on developmental age and capabilities.	To facilitate child in performing optimum level of self-care.

Continued

INTERVENTIONS	RATIONALES
Encourage parents to have realistic expectations of what the child can do.	Likelihood of success is increased if child is given tasks that he or she can accomplish. For example, an 18-mo-old functioning at the level of a 6-mo-old would not be able to feed self with a spoon.
Use toys and activities that encourage maximum participation by child and improve motor and sensory function.	Improved fine motor control will enable child to accomplish more self-care tasks. For example, in a 5-yr-old with poor fine motor control, putting together large "pop beads" may be an appropriate activity.
Set a series of small goals for child to accomplish. Avoid undue pressure.	Child may be unable or not ready to accomplish final goal but may be able to complete one small task at a time (e.g., picking up brush, holding brush correctly, and then brushing hair).
Encourage use of adaptive clothing and utensils and consumption of finger foods.	Facilitates success in self-care. Examples include clothing that opens up in front with self-adhering closures rather than buttons, shoes with self-adhering straps rather than shoe strings, large spoons with padded handles, finger foods and foods that won't slide off the eating utensil.
Provide guidance for toilet training based on developmental age and physical/cognitive abilities.	This is a significant developmental milestone for families and one that causes the most problems in healthy children. Realistic expectations improve chances of child being successful. Methods of toilet training may need to be changed based on child's abilities. For example, a 4-yr-old functioning at the level of a 1-yr-old would not be physically or cognitively ready to be toilet trained.
Stress importance of good oral hygiene and regular dental care. Provide suggestions for how to accomplish this.	There is an increased incidence of dental caries in children with cerebral palsy because of improper dental hygiene (may result from spastic or clonic movements that cause gagging or biting down on toothbrush or from oral hyper-sensitivity), congenital enamel defects, high carbohydrate intake without proper brushing, dietary imbalance with poor nutritional intake, inadequate fluoride, and difficulty with mouth closure and drooling. Up to 90% of children with cerebral palsy have malocclusion as well. A child with gum overgrowth from seizure medications, for example, will have gums that bleed easily. Teeth should be brushed after every meal with a soft toothbrush, and child should see dentist q3-6mo for checkup and cleaning beginning at 2-3 yr old.

●●● **Related NIC and NOC labels:** *NIC:* Self-Care Assistance: Bathing/Hygiene; Self-Care Assistance: Dressing/Grooming; Self-Care Assistance: Feeding; Self-Care Assistance: Toileting *NOC:* Self-Care: Activities of Daily Living

Nursing Diagnosis:

Risk for Injury

related to physical disability, perceptual or cognitive impairment, seizures, and lack of preventative knowledge

Desired Outcomes: Child remains free from signs and symptoms of injury. Parents verbalize accurate knowledge about how to provide a safe environment for the child.

INTERVENTIONS	RATIONALES
Educate family about ways of childproofing the home based on child's developmental age.	Reduces child's risk for injury in the home. Examples include: - No furniture or tables with sharp edges - No scatter rugs or polished floors - Remove small or sharp objects from reach - Use a protective helmet for the child prone to falls
Teach family ways in which to institute seizure precautions as appropriate (they will vary depending on type, severity, and frequency of seizures).	To help prevent injury caused by seizures. General suggestions include: - Keep side rails raised when child is napping or sleeping (there are toddler side rails that can be used on beds at home) to keep child from falling out of bed with a seizure or from spastic movements or posturing. - Keep side rails and hard objects padded (e.g., bumper guards on side rails that can be secured well) to keep child from being injured during a seizure. - Do not pad bed side rails with pillows. Pillows can cause suffocation or slide out from under the side rail. - Ensure that child wears or carries medical identification describing his/her condition. Seizures can be confused with other medical conditions and may be misdiagnosed in an emergency.
Teach family how to secure child properly in wheelchair, positioning devices, and motor vehicle.	Decreases chance of injury by falling as a result of spasticity, posturing, or lack of muscular control. Instruction in proper ways to secure child based on system used by family is vital because there are many different systems used to secure children. General suggestions include: - Secure all straps and belts, ensuring that they fit snugly. - Put brakes on wheelchair when transferring child or while child is sitting in it. - Use appropriate child safety restraint system (based on developmental age, not just chronologic age) whenever child is in a motor vehicle.
Review with family safe, appropriate toys for developmental age and physical limitations.	No sharp, small, or easily shattered toys should be allowed for a child who may fall during a seizure or is prone to falling. Aspiration/choking on small toys occurs frequently in children who are developmentally <3 yr of age.

●●● **Related NIC and NOC labels:** *NIC:* Fall Prevention; Surveillance: Safety; Environmental Management; Seizure Precautions; Parent Education: Childrearing Family; Health Education NOC: Safety Behavior: Home Physical Environment; Safety Status: Physical Injury; Safety Status: Falls Occurrence

Nursing Diagnosis:

Impaired Verbal Communication

related to hearing loss, neuromuscular impairment, and difficulty with articulation

Desired Outcome: Within 1 mo of intervention/treatment, child's ability to communicate needs to caregivers improves.

INTERVENTIONS	RATIONALES
Coordinate with speech therapist if child has difficulty with articulation and/or feeding.	Early interventions maximize speech and feeding potential in children with poor control of oral musculature.
Reinforce importance of using speech therapy techniques, including nonverbal methods of communicating, jaw control, and appropriate feeding techniques.	To facilitate goals of speech therapy, which include improving communication and feeding ability, thereby decreasing child's frustration with inability to communicate or eat orally. Increased control of oral musculature improves ability to chew, swallow, and speak.
Speak slowly and clearly when talking with child.	Gives child time to understand speech.
Listen closely to what child says and ask him or her to repeat it if you cannot understand.	Ignoring or not listening to child increases frustrations with failure to communicate.
Use assistive devices such as pictures or flash cards.	Promotes child's communication ability and mutual understanding of what is being said.
Help family obtain assistive equipment for child.	Facilitates child's nonverbal communication. Examples include typewriter, communication board, and computer with voice synthesizer. These may be acquired through the school system or funded by Medicaid.

●●● **Related NIC and NOC labels:** *NIC:* Active Listening; Communication Enhancement: Hearing Deficit; Communication Enhancement: Speech Deficit; Communication Enhancement: Visual Deficit *NOC:* Communication Ability; Communication: Expressive Ability; Communication: Receptive Ability

Nursing Diagnosis:

Imbalanced Nutrition: Less than body requirements

related to chewing and/or swallowing difficulty and motor problems

Desired Outcome: Within 1 wk of intervention/treatment, child exhibits improved intake and maintains or gains weight.

INTERVENTIONS	RATIONALES
Provide high-calorie meals and snacks.	Child likely will need increased calories because of increased muscle activity (i.e., spasticity or dyskinetic movements).
Provide foods that child likes.	Stimulates appetite and promotes cooperation in eating.
Encourage child to feed self as much as possible.	Allowing child to try to feed self may increase intake by decreasing frustration of having no control over other matters.
Make meal times pleasant with no interruptions, a relaxed environment, attractive meals, eye contact, and conversation appropriate for child.	Encourages focusing on eating, thereby increasing intake.
Approach child with a greeting that alerts him or her that movement or a change in activity is going to occur.	To prevent a startle reflex, which interferes with ability to chew and swallow successfully.
Use the following aids and techniques to facilitate feeding; seek input from occupational/speech therapists.	Improves likelihood of adequate oral intake.
- Let child know that food is coming.	Prepares child for meal and increases likelihood of successful feeding.
- Put a bib on child.	Signal for child that it is mealtime.

Continued

INTERVENTIONS	RATIONALES
- Ensure proper positioning:	Decreases incidence of aspiration and gastroesophageal reflux (GER) and improves intake.
- Firmly support child through hips and trunk.	Provides a stable base for sitting up.
- Ensure that head and neck are in a midline, neutral position.	Prevents aspiration and allows better oral muscular control.
- Place spoon in middle of child's mouth, placing pressure on the tongue.	Prevents tonic bite reflex and tongue thrust.
- Sit in front of child.	Facilitates eye contact, conversation, and use of prescribed therapy techniques.
- Hold jaw with hand.	Promotes jaw control.
- If child has GER, position sitting up for 30 min to 1 hr after meal.	Decreases incidence of GER and ultimately improves intake.
- Make sure that food and liquid are the proper texture (e.g., pureed or bite size) and temperature for the child.	Some children aspirate when taking regular liquids (they need them to be thickened), and some children cannot chew.
Monitor I&O.	To ensure child is receiving adequate nutrients and has adequate output.
Weigh weekly on same scale, at same time of day, and with child wearing same clothing.	Consistency with weight measurements helps ensure more accurate results. Child is receiving adequate nutrients if maintaining or gaining weight (as long as weight gain is not excessive). If weight is decreasing, diet may need to be supplemented.
Ensure that child is receiving adequate nutrients. If child is unable to take sufficient nutrients orally, discuss child's needs with health care provider.	Because of difficulty swallowing and increased motor activity, some children are unable to take sufficient nutrients orally, necessitating enteral feedings, which do not require adequate swallowing.

●●● **Related NIC and NOC labels:** *NIC:* Nutrition Management; Nutritional Monitoring; Enteral Tube Feeding; Self-Care Assistance: Feeding; Feeding *NOC:* Nutritional Status; Nutritional Status: Food & Fluid Intake

ADDITIONAL NURSING DIAGNOSES/ PROBLEMS:

PATIENT-FAMILY TEACHING AND DISCHARGE PLANNING

When providing patient-family teaching, focus on sensory information and avoid giving excessive information. The child with cerebral palsy may have a wide range of symptoms with varying degrees of severity. Providing support, as well as information for cerebral palsy, is essential in dealing with a lifelong disabled child. Include verbal and written information (ensure that written information is at a level the reader can understand) about the following:

✔ Importance of the multidisciplinary team to evaluate and monitor child on a regular basis and involvement of early intervention programs/school for optimum outcome.

✔ Early intervention program with Individual Family Service Plan (IFSP) for children from birth to 3 yr old or Individualized Education Plan (IEP) for children 3-21 yr old.

✓Safety measures appropriate for physical disability and developmental level, including childproofing home.

✓Medications, including drug name, purpose, dosage, frequency, precautions, drug/drug and drug/food interactions, and potential side effects.

✓Importance of meticulous oral hygiene, especially if receiving seizure medication that causes gum overgrowth and gums to bleed easily (i.e., brush after each meal with a soft toothbrush and see dentist q3-6mo for cleaning and checkups beginning at 2-3 yr old).

✓Carrying a list of medications, dosage, and frequency. Both parents and child should carry this list.

✓Nutrition, including special formulas, foods, and devices/techniques to help child feed self.

✓Methods to facilitate communication.

✓Correct use and care of orthoses and adaptive equipment.

✓Seizure precautions and care during and after a seizure.

✓Routine immunizations, as well as pneumonococcal and yearly influenza vaccines.

✓List of phone numbers to call should questions or concerns arise about therapy or treatment plan.

✓Importance of finding respite care, such as family, friends, support group.

✓Referral to community resources, such as national and local Cerebral Palsy Association, local community services board, and any available respite care resources.

✓Additional information can be obtained from:

United Cerebral Palsy Association
1660 L Street NW, Suite 700
Washington, DC 20036-5602
(800) 872-5827 or (202) 776-0406
www.ucpa.org/

Exceptional Parent Magazine
"Parenting Your Child or Young Adult with a Disability or Special Healthcare Needs"
(800) 372-7368
www.eparent.com/

Child Abuse and Neglect

The problem of child abuse and neglect, formerly called "battered child syndrome," is now recognized as a serious threat to children in the United States. Approximately 3 million cases of suspected abuse/neglect are reported each year; 25%-33% of them are substantiated. Between 1000-2000 children die each year because of abuse and/or neglect. Many more children are left permanently disabled, and thousands of victims are overwhelmed by this trauma for the rest of their lives.

Child abuse and neglect occur in all cultural, ethnic, occupational, and socioeconomic groups. It is not usually a single event but rather a pattern of behavior that occurs over time. The following factors increase the likelihood of abuse or neglect occurring in families:

- **Parental characteristics:** Predisposition to maltreatment (perhaps having been victims themselves), substance abuse, lack of parenting skills, poor impulse control, and emotional immaturity.
- **Child characteristics:** Temperament, physical or cognitive disability that predisposes child to injury, chronic illness or disability, being born to unmarried parents, or hyperactivity.
- **Environmental characteristics:** Divorce, marital problems, financial strain, poor housing, isolation from support of families or friends.
- **Societal factors:** Increased violence, children viewed as property and not valued, physical methods of punishment, lack of willingness in community to become involved in family violence issues.

The highest incidence of child abuse and neglect occurs in children <3 yr old, with the rate declining as children get older (except for sexual abuse). Between 50% and 60% of victims suffer neglect, 20%-30% suffer physical abuse, and 10%-15%

are sexually abused. About a third of the victims experience more than one type of maltreatment. Terms include:

- **Child maltreatment:** A broad term that includes intentional physical abuse or neglect, emotional abuse or neglect, and sexual abuse (<18 yr old) usually by an adult caregiver, most often the parent.
- **Physical abuse:** The deliberate infliction of physical injury or pain. It may result from punching, beating, kicking, biting, bruising, shaking, or otherwise harming a child and can occur from overdiscipline or physical punishment.
- **Physical neglect:** Failure to provide basic necessities such as food, clothing, shelter, and a safe environment in which the child can grow and develop normally.
- **Emotional abuse:** Deliberate attempt to destroy or significantly impair self-esteem or competence by rejecting, ignoring, criticizing, isolating, or terrorizing the child. The most common form is verbal abuse or "belittling."
- **Emotional neglect:** Failure to meet the child's needs for affection, attention, and emotional support. The most common feature is absence of normal parent-child attachment and interaction.
- **Sexual abuse:** Contacts or interactions between a child and an adult for the adult's sexual gratification, with or without physical contact. It includes pedophilia and all forms of incest and rape. It also includes fondling, oral-genital contact, all forms of intercourse, exhibitionism, voyeurism, and involvement of children in the production of pornography. It is believed to be one of the most common but underreported crimes against children.
- **Medical care neglect:** Failure to provide needed treatment to infants or children who generally have life-threatening or serious medical conditions.
- **Munchausen syndrome by proxy:** Abuse inflicted on a child in which a parent (usually the mother) fabricates

symptoms and falsifies medical history or actually causes an illness that results in evaluation and treatment.

- **Shaken baby syndrome (SBS):** Caused by violent shaking of an infant or young child (usually <2 yr old), resulting in severe injury. It accounts for 10%–12% of all deaths from abuse and neglect. About a third die, a third have little or no sequelae, and another third suffer permanent physical damage (brain damage, blindness, paralysis, mental retardation, seizures).

HEALTH CARE SETTING

Primary care or emergency department with possible hospitalization resulting from complications

ASSESSMENT

Note: History is critical in making a diagnosis. Frequently in child abuse/neglect cases, the history is inconsistent with injury severity, or it changes during evaluation. It is essential that the nurse taking the history be nonjudgmental and report factual information. This is difficult to do at times, and collegial support is beneficial.

Physical abuse: Acts out violently against others; frightened of parents or caregivers; avoids changing clothes (e.g., in gym class); old, new, and multiple injuries; burn or restraint injuries; questionable bruises and welts; questionable burns (e.g., imprint or immersion); questionable fractures (e.g., spiral fracture); questionable lacerations or abrasions (e.g., human bite marks); or internal abdominal injuries.

Physical neglect: Consistently hungry; poor hygiene, or inappropriate dress for weather; consistently left without supervision; abandoned; begging or stealing for food; constant fatigue and listlessness; frequently absent or tardy for school; failure to gain weight or failure to thrive (FTT), developmentally delayed; assumes adult responsibility; given inappropriate food, drink or medication; reportedly ingests harmful substances.

Emotional abuse or neglect: Antisocial or destructive behavior; sleep disorders; habit disorders such as biting, head banging, rocking, or thumb sucking (in an older child); demanding behaviors; self-destructive, suicide attempt; overly adaptive behavior; emotional or intellectual developmental delays; speech disorders.

Sexual abuse: Recurrent abdominal pain; genital, urethral, or anal trauma; sexually transmitted diseases; recurrent urinary tract infections; enuresis (involuntary discharge of urine) or encopresis (incontinence of stool not caused by organic defect or illness); pregnancy; sleep disturbances (e.g., nightmares and night terrors); appetite disturbances (e.g., anorexia or bulimia); neurotic or conductive disorders; withdrawal, guilt, or depression; temper tantrums (in older children); aggressive behaviors; suicidal or runaway threats or behaviors; hysterical or conversion reactions; excessive masturbation; sexualized play in developmentally immature children; school problems; promiscuity; reluctance to change clothes.

Munchausen syndrome by proxy: Signs and symptoms only occur when the perpetrator (usually the mother) is present. Common presenting indicators include poisoning, seizures, apnea, bleeding, vomiting, diarrhea, fever, and even cardiopulmonary arrest.

SBS: Often there are no external signs of injury other than change in level of consciousness (LOC). The child may have history of poor feeding, vomiting, lethargy, and irritability occurring for several days or weeks. More severe shaking may cause brain damage, seizures, blindness, paralysis, and death. On ophthalmologic exam, retinal hemorrhages are seen. Anterior fontanel may be tense or full when infant is quiet.

DIAGNOSTIC TESTS

Radiographs of injured area or skeletal survey: Certain findings on x-ray examination are strong indicators of physical abuse. These include metaphyseal "corner" or "bucket handle" fractures of long bones in infants, spiral fractures of long bones in nonambulatory infants, and multiple fractures of ribs or long bones in varying stages of healing. These findings may help to distinguish abuse from osteogenesis imperfecta (an inherited condition marked by abnormally brittle bones that are subject to fracture).

Computed tomography (CT) or magnetic resonance imaging (MRI): May reveal subdural hematoma and subarachnoid hemorrhage, hallmark signs of SBS.

Bone scans: Detect soft tissue and bone trauma, especially in locating unseen fractures or bone injuries. For example, they can define rib fractures, which are difficult to assess because of overlying structures such as the heart, lungs, and liver.

Coagulation studies: Used in children with many bruises in different stages to differentiate abuse from a medical condition such as leukemia or bleeding or clotting disorders.

CBC: Helps rule out medical condition in child with FTT.

Forensic evaluation: In sexually abused children, it may be done to identify evidence such as semen or detect sexually transmitted disease.

Nursing Diagnosis:

Risk for Injury

related to family history of neglect or physical, emotional, or sexual abuse

Desired Outcome: Following intervention/treatment, child exhibits no further evidence of abuse or neglect.

INTERVENTIONS	RATIONALES
Assess child's physical and mental status.	A thorough evaluation should be done on all children in all health care settings. Abuse occurs in all cultural and socioeconomic groups and may not be the admitting diagnosis. - Note bruises, scars, or other signs of abuse. - Note unusual interactions or responses of child.
Observe interactions between child and family.	Signs of abuse or neglect may be detected in the way that child interacts with parents and other adults.
Obtain detailed history.	May detect pattern of injury or neglect or lack of correlation between history and severity of injury; or history may change as examination progresses.
Keep factual, detailed, objective records for documentation.	Medical records may be subpoenaed as evidence in court proceedings and therefore need to be as detailed and objective as possible. Being factual (i.e., no opinions, impressions, or interpretations) is imperative. - Physical condition (e.g., "Three small, well-delineated, circular lesions, approximately 3-5 mm in diameter and 1 mm in depth, dark purple-red, noted on sole of left foot"). - Pictures, which are most beneficial in documenting injuries, need to be dated and kept in patient's chart. - Child's behavioral response to parents, others, and environment (e.g., child with FTT often does not verbally or physically interact with anyone). - Specific comments of child, parents, or other family members. - Developmental age of child.
Use nonjudgmental, nonthreatening manner when interacting with child's parents.	Frequently it is unclear who actually abused the child. Child is more likely to be helped if parents trust staff. If parents feel alienated by staff, they may deny child access to care. Parents will be more receptive to teaching in a trusting environment.
Report all cases of suspected child abuse or neglect.	All 50 states consider health care workers mandatory reporters of child abuse/neglect.
Keep child in a safe environment in the hospital.	Suspected abuser may be restricted from visiting, or only certain individuals may be approved to visit.
Assist in removing child from unsafe situation (whether verbal or physical neglect or abuse is suspected). Report any suspicious behavior to Social Services in the hospital and Child Protective Services in the community.	Nurses are mandated reporters of suspected neglect or abuse in all 50 states.
Refer families to social agencies for assistance with finances, food, clothing, and health care.	To help ameliorate causes of neglect.
Collaborate with multidisciplinary health care team involved with case.	To provide continual evaluation of progress/status of child in hospital, foster care, or on return to home.
Help parents identify events that precipitate an abusive act and alternative ways to deal with release of anger (e.g., role playing).	To prevent further abuse for this child or siblings.

●●● **Related NIC and NOC labels:** *NIC:* Risk Identification; Abuse Protection Support: Child; Health Screening; Surveillance: Safety *NOC:* Parenting: Social Safety

Nursing Diagnosis:

Risk for Impaired Parenting

related to child's, caregiver's, or situational characteristics that precipitate child abuse or neglect

Desired Outcome: Within 1 wk following interventions, parents demonstrate more positive interactions with child and more appropriate parenting activities and verbalize accurate understanding of normal expectations for the child.

INTERVENTIONS	RATIONALES
Identify families at risk for abuse/neglect.	Identifying at-risk families is the first step in helping prevent abuse or neglect. Such families tend to have immature, single parents; parents who were abused as children; premature infant; child <3 yr old or with a chronic illness or disability; parental substance abuse.
Observe parents' interactions with child.	This is the best way to get realistic view of the relationship.
Assess parents' strengths and weaknesses, normal coping behaviors, and presence or absence of support systems.	Provides basis for developing an appropriate plan of care and making necessary referrals.
Demonstrate age-appropriate child-rearing practices, especially communication and discipline.	Parents may care for their child the way their parents cared for them and may not know age-appropriate child-rearing practices.
Teach alternative methods of discipline, such as rewards, time-out, consequences, and verbal disapproval.	Parents may not know any nonviolent methods of discipline.
Provide care for child until parent is ready to provide care.	Allows parents time to "relax" and observe age-appropriate care.
Encourage parents to participate in care of child. Reinforce positive behaviors.	Helps build self-esteem and confidence in parents to improve interactions.
Focus on positive aspects of child (e.g., "What beautiful eyes you have").	Parents may have negative view of child, and this gives them another perspective.
Teach family what to expect in terms of growth and development for their child—physical, psychosocial, and cognitive—through role modeling and having parents return demonstration.	Parents will incorporate information better if not "instructed" and feeling as though they are being criticized. This increases their knowledge and reinforces accurate expectations of what is normal for the child.
Also provide education about nutrition, care related to activities of daily living, routine well-child care, manifestations of illness, and importance of caring/loving attitude in dealing with children.	Increases realistic expectations and chance of positive parenting.
Convey nonjudgmental attitude of genuine concern.	Facilitates developing trust and respect and enables parents to observe and develop better methods of caring for child.
Refer family to appropriate social agencies to assist with financial support, adequate housing, employment, and so on.	To ameliorate risk factors of abuse/neglect.
Help identify support systems for parents such as extended family, neighbors, or support groups.	To decrease family stress and hence decrease risk of abuse/neglect.

●●● **Related NIC and NOC labels:** *NIC:* Abuse Protection Support: Child; Developmental Enhancement: Child; Risk Identification; Surveillance: Safety; Family Support; Self-Esteem Enhancement; Self-Modification Assistance; Support Group *NOC:* Parenting: Social Safety

Nursing Diagnoses:

Fear/Anxiety

related to maltreatment, powerlessness, and potential loss of parents

Desired Outcome: Within 72 hr following interventions, child verbalizes source of fear/anxiety and exhibits more interactivity and sociability and less withdrawal.

INTERVENTIONS	RATIONALES
Provide consistent caregivers and an age-appropriate safe environment.	To help relieve child's anxiety and provide a positive role model for family.
Reassure child about his or her personal safety.	Verbal reassurance increases sense of security.
Demonstrate acceptance of child but do not reinforce inappropriate behaviors.	Children need acceptance, as well as guidance regarding appropriate behaviors.
Support child in talking about family or stressful events.	Verbalization of fears/anxieties decreases their impact on child.
Do not ask too many questions.	This may upset child and interfere with other professionals' interrogations.
Encourage play, especially with family or dollhouse activity.	Play is the "work of the child" and may help reveal types of relationships perceived by child. This could include, for example, playing with dolls that represent father, mother, and siblings or drawing pictures of events. Child may tell story of events with dolls. Drawings often depict fears and reactions to experiences.
Incorporate therapeutic play into care activities if possible.	To help child cope with new, frightening experiences in a nonthreatening way. For example, have child check blood pressure on doll before checking it on child.
Treat child as you would other children, not as an "abused" victim.	This encourages child to interact with others rather than promoting isolation.
Offer choices whenever possible regarding clothing, diet, and other activities of daily living (ADL); recreation time; and socialization time.	Being allowed to make choices provides a sense of control and decreases sense of powerlessness, and hence anxiety.

●●● **Related NIC and NOC labels:** *NIC:* Anxiety Reduction; Active Listening; Coping Enhancement; Security Enhancement; Therapeutic Play; Abuse Protection Support *NOC:* Anxiety Control; Fear Control

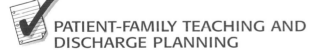

PATIENT-FAMILY TEACHING AND DISCHARGE PLANNING

When providing patient-family teaching, focus on sensory information, avoid giving excessive information, and initiate a visiting nurse referral for necessary follow-up teaching and assessment. Include verbal and written information about the following, ensuring that it is written at a level understandable to the child/family.

✓ Care related to any specific injury.

✓ Realistic expectations for individual child related to:
  • Growth and development (e.g., regression is normal after a child has been hospitalized or severely stressed)
  • Nutrition (e.g., toddler's food jags—may only want one food for every meal for several days)

✓ Guidelines based on developmental level:
  • Safety (e.g., preschooler does not understand danger of chasing a ball across the street)
  • Need for love and attention

✓ Methods of handling normal developmental problems that increase parent's stress level (e.g., toddler's negativism, temper tantrums, toilet training, and need for rituals and routines).

✓ Demonstration of care related to ADL; observe return demonstration by parents.

✓ Importance of regular well-child visits and provision of routine well-child care.

✓ Suggestions for nonviolent, age-appropriate methods of disciplining child (e.g., reward, time-out, consequences, and verbal disapproval).

✓Identifications of stressful situations for parents and ways to deal with them. For example, if an infant cries for prolonged periods, make sure that infant is clean and dry and is not uncomfortable, hungry, or ill; put infant in crib on his or her back and go out of the room. DO NOT SHAKE THE BABY. This can cause severe damage.

✓Review of situations/circumstances that precipitate abuse/violence and of methods to deal with anger constructively.

✓Importance of providing child with positive reinforcement of appropriate behavior to build self-esteem.

✓Teaching child the difference between "good touch" and "bad touch."

✓Name or place a child can go if being abused (e.g., neighborhood "safe house").

✓Suggestions for local support systems (e.g., extended family members, church members, neighbors).

✓Referrals to community resources, such as parenting classes, support groups, public health nurse, social worker, and financial counseling if appropriate. Additional general information can be obtained by contacting the following organizations:

Parents Anonymous, Inc.
675 West Foothill Boulevard, Suite 220
Claremont, CA 91711
(909) 621-6184
www.parentsanonymous.org/
Provides support and resources for overwhelmed families.

National Child Abuse Hotline
(800) 4-A-CHILD (1-800-422-4453)
www.childhelpusa.org/

Prevent Child Abuse America
200 South Michigan Avenue, 17th floor
Chicago, IL 60604-2404
(312) 663-3520
www.preventchildabuse.org/

Shaken Baby Alliance
P.O. Box 150734
Fort Worth, TX 76108
(877) 6-END-SBS (636-3727)
www.shakenbaby.com/

National Center on Shaken Baby Syndrome
2955 Harrison Boulevard, #102
Ogden, UT 84403
(888) 273-0071 or (801) 627-3399
www.dontshake.com/

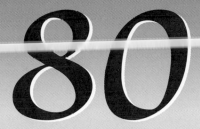

Cystic Fibrosis

Cystic fibrosis (CF) is a chronic, progressive multisystem disease in which there is a dysfunction of the exocrine (mucus-producing) glands. This results in abnormally thick secretions, causing obstruction of the small passageways of many organs. CF is an autosomal recessive hereditary disease with more than 500 gene mutations. This is why there is such a wide variation in clinical manifestations.

In the recent past, CF was described as the most common lethal genetic illness in white children. The median life expectancy has improved dramatically from 14 years in 1969 to 31 years in 1999. The CF Foundation no longer lists the median life expectancy because of earlier diagnosis, antibiotic therapy, improved nutritional management, and recent breakthroughs in treatment.

About 30,000 people in the United States have CF, and 63% are children. One in 31 Americans (1 in 28 Caucasians) is a carrier.

HEALTH CARE SETTING

Primary care, with possible hospitalization for CF exacerbation or other complications

ASSESSMENT

Initially involves overall appraisal, including monitoring general activity, physical findings, nutritional status, and chest x-ray examination.

Signs and symptoms: Vary widely, as does the severity of involvement of specific organ systems. Patients tend to have periods without acute symptoms and then periods with acute exacerbation of symptoms. The first clinical manifestation may be meconium ileus in a newborn, or the patient may not have symptoms for months or years.

Most of the usual symptoms are caused by the following:
- **Progressive chronic obstructive lung disease:** Initially wheezing and dry cough, progressing to paroxysmal cough that frequently causes posttussive emesis. Other signs include increased dyspnea, barrel chest, mild to severe clubbing of nail beds, cyanosis, and repeated pulmonary infections that cause scarring and bronchiectasis. Numerous complications such as pneumothorax and hemoptysis often occur.
- **Pancreatic enzyme deficiency** resulting from duct blockage (present in 80%-85% of children with CF): Stools that are frothy (bulky and large), foul smelling, fat containing (steatorrhea), and float (four *F*'s of CF); voracious appetite initially, progressing to loss of appetite late in the disease; weight loss, marked tissue wasting, protuberant abdomen with thin extremities, failure to thrive (FTT), anemia; and evidence of deficiency of fat-soluble vitamins (A, D, E, K). Complications include pancreatic fibrosis leading to glucose intolerance, diabetes mellitus, and pancreatitis.
- **Sweat gland dysfunction** resulting in increased sodium and chloride concentrations. Infant "tastes" salty and is more prone to dehydration.

Other gastrointestinal (GI) complications: Include intestinal obstruction in infants, distal intestinal obstruction syndrome (DIOS) in adolescents and adults, and rectal prolapse (occurs in 20%-25% of children with CF, usually <5 yr old).

Liver complications: Biliary cirrhosis and gallbladder dysfunction.

DIAGNOSTIC TESTS

CF has been called the "great imitator" because signs of chronic respiratory infection and FTT are symptoms of many other childhood conditions.

Pilocarpine iontophoresis (quantitative sweat chloride test): Production of sweat is stimulated with a special device, and the sweat is collected and measured. Diagnosis is made with sodium and chloride levels >60 mEq/L (levels of 40-60 are considered suggestive and should be repeated) and the presence of clinical symptoms or a family history of CF. Sweat test is not usually done before 4-6 wk of age because the infant has decreased sweat production until then.

Chest x-ray examination: Shows characteristic patchy atelectasis and chronic obstructive emphysema.

Pulmonary function tests (after 5-6 yr old): Assess degree of pulmonary disease and response to therapy and help distinguish between restrictive and obstructive pulmonary disease. In the presence of CF the test will show decreased vital capacity (VC) and tidal volume, increased airway resistance, increased residual volume, and decreased FEV1 (forced expiratory volume in 1 sec) and FEV_1/VC ratio.

Stool fat and/or enzyme analysis to determine pancreatic involvement: For digestive enzymes, stool must be fresh or frozen immediately. Trypsin (breaks down dietary proteins) is either absent or severely diminished in children with CF. For fat content (steatorrhea), stool is collected over 72 hr with documented and measured intake. The test will show significant increase in fat content because of malabsorption.

Complete blood count (CBC): Increased white blood cells (WBCs) with increased neutrophils on differential count will be present with infection.

Oximetry: Will reveal decreased oxygen saturation.

Sputum culture: For identification of infective organisms and sensitivity of these organisms. Many resistant organisms develop because of the frequency of respiratory infections.

Immunoreactive trypsinogen (IRT) test: Newborn screening test that can be done at the same time as phenylketonuria (PKU) and other screening tests. This test enables early detection and treatment of CF and is done several days after birth. If positive, it is confirmed by a mutation analysis (i.e., genetic testing). The combination of these two tests is sensitive 90%-100% of the time.

Deoxyribonucleic acid (DNA) analysis of chorionic villi or amniotic fluid: Can establish prenatal diagnosis.

Nursing Diagnosis:

Ineffective Airway Clearance

related to thick, tenacious mucus in airways

Desired Outcome: Immediately following treatment/interventions, child expectorates mucus and exhibits improved airway clearance as evidenced by improved breath sounds and HR and RR within child's normal limits.

INTERVENTIONS	RATIONALES
Assess HR, RR, and breath sounds.	To establish baseline data from which to compare later findings. With ineffective airway clearance, the child will have increased HR and RR. Breath sounds may be decreased with little air movement because of the blocked airway, or adventitious sounds may be increased because of mucus in the airway.
Assist with sputum expectoration:	
- Assess HR, RR, breath sounds, and O_2 saturation before nebulization and after chest physiotherapy.	Assessment before and after treatment monitors effectiveness of treatment.
- Position child in an upright sitting position, ensuring that he or she does not slouch.	This position facilitates maximum inhalation of medication and improves effectiveness of cough to clear secretions out of airways.
- Administer nebulization (albuterol) as prescribed 1 hr before or 2 hr after meals.	To open bronchi and loosen secretions. This treatment usually causes considerable coughing followed by expectoration of mucus and sometimes vomiting from excessive coughing. Scheduling in relation to meals is essential to provide maximum benefit of treatment and prevent interference with nutrient ingestion. Treatment before breakfast helps loosen secretions that built up overnight. Treatment before bedtime helps clear secretions that would otherwise provide a medium for bacterial growth.
- Perform chest physiotherapy after nebulizer treatment. Examples follow.	To loosen secretions, which will facilitate their expectoration. This treatment is performed at least 2-4 times/day for maintenance/routine daily care. Method used depends on age of child, effectiveness of technique, child's/parent's ability to perform/tolerate technique, and preference of child/parent.

Continued

INTERVENTIONS

RATIONALES

INTERVENTIONS	RATIONALES
- Chest percussion and postural drainage for 20-30 min.	Chest percussion loosens secretions, and postural drainage facilitates drainage of secretions so that they can be expectorated.
- Mucus clearance device (e.g., FLUTTER) used for 5-15 min.	This handheld pipelike device has a plastic mouthpiece on one end that child breathes into. On the other end of the pipe a stainless steel ball rests inside a plastic circular cone. Exhaling into the device vibrates the airways, thereby loosening mucus from the airway walls and accelerating airflow, which facilitates upward movement of mucus so that it can be more readily cleared. This device is very effective and gives child control because it can be used without assistance of others.
- Airway clearance system (e.g., The Vest).	This inflatable vest fits like a life jacket and is connected by tubes to a generator. The vest inflates and deflates rapidly, applying gentle pressure to the chest. It provides high-frequency chest wall oscillation to help loosen secretions and increase mucus expectoration.
- Suction as necessary.	For infants/young children or if there is a large volume of mucus, assistance may be needed to clear secretions from airway. However, child usually coughs sufficiently after nebulizer treatment and chest physiotherapy to clear secretions independently.
Ensure that child is receiving at least maintenance fluids.	Hydration thins and loosens secretions for easier expectoration.
Administer dornase alfa (Pulmozyme) as prescribed.	To thin mucus, which will facilitate expectoration.

●●● **Related NIC and NOC labels:** *NIC:* Airway Suctioning; Chest Physiotherapy; Positioning; Vital Signs Monitoring; Cough Enhancement; Medication Administration: Inhalation *NOC:* Respiratory Status: Gas Exchange; Respiratory Status: Airway Patency

Nursing Diagnosis:

Impaired Gas Exchange

related to airway obstruction secondary to air trapping in alveoli and airways narrowed by tenacious mucus

Desired Outcome: Within 2 hr following treatment/intervention, child has adequate gas exchange as evidenced by O_2 saturation >92% (or consistent with child's baseline).

INTERVENTIONS

RATIONALES

INTERVENTIONS	RATIONALES
Along with VS, assess respiratory status q2-4h, or more frequently as indicated by child's condition.	Increased HR and RR would occur with impaired gas exchange, as would chest retractions, increased work of breathing (WOB), nasal flaring, and use of accessory muscles of respiration. These are signs of respiratory distress necessitating prompt intervention/treatment.
Monitor for behavioral indicators of hypoxia.	Restlessness, mood changes, and/or change in level of consciousness (LOC) are early signs of O_2 deficiency.
Be alert to changes in child's skin color.	Cyanosis of the lips and nail beds is a late indicator of hypoxia and a signal of the need for prompt treatment/intervention.

Continued

INTERVENTIONS	RATIONALES
Position child in high Fowler's position and/or leaning forward.	For comfort and to promote optimal gas exchange by enabling maximal chest expansion.
Ensure continuous monitoring of pulse oximetry readings; report low value (usually ≤92%).	Decreased O_2 saturation can indicate need for initiation of/increased O_2.
Deliver O_2 along with humidity via most appropriate delivery system and at rate prescribed.	To ensure adequate oxygenation. Developmental age and flow rate determine most effective delivery system (e.g., nasal cannula for infants with liter flow rate <4). Humidity use replaces convective losses of moisture.
Monitor child on O_2 delivery closely.	O_2-induced CO_2 narcosis is a hazard of O_2 therapy in the child with chronic pulmonary disease. If O_2 saturation is consistently >96%, for example, it is likely that the flow rate can be decreased slowly by small increments.
Encourage games or physical exercise appropriate to child's condition (e.g., blowing bubbles or walking) but avoid overexertion.	Breathing more deeply facilitates clearing of mucus and improves oxygenation.
Provide neutral thermal environment for child.	A room temperature in which the body does not have to use any energy to stay warm or cool off enables child to use energy to grow or heal. With decreased energy demands, more O_2 is available to ensure these needs are met.

●●● **Related NIC and NOC labels:** *NIC:* Oxygen Therapy; Energy Management; Positioning; Respiratory Monitoring; Vital Signs Monitoring *NOC:* Respiratory Status: Gas Exchange; Vital Signs Status

Nursing Diagnosis:

Imbalanced Nutrition: Less than body requirements

related to decreased appetite (advanced disease) or increased metabolic requirements because of WOB, infection, and/or malabsorption

Desired Outcome: By discharge or within 7 days after treatment/intervention, patient maintains or gains weight and does not have more than 2 or 3 stools per day.

INTERVENTIONS	RATIONALES
Administer pancreatic enzymes with meals and snacks per health care provider's prescription if child has pancreatic insufficiency (80%-85% of children with CF).	Replacement of enzymes is necessary for proper digestion and absorption of nutrients. Failure to replace pancreatic enzymes would affect child's growth and ability to fight infection.
For young children unable to swallow a capsule, mix powder, granules, or contents of the capsule with a small amount of carbohydrate food.	Protein foods break down this enzyme and can burn mouths of infants and young children. Using smallest amount of food possible (e.g., 1-2 tsp of applesauce) helps ensure that child receives all the medication.
Do not administer with formula/milk in a bottle or cup.	Pancreatic enzymes curdle milk and formula. In addition, patient may not receive all the medication and may not take milk/formula in the future if he or she associates it with medication.

Continued

INTERVENTIONS

RATIONALES

INTERVENTIONS	RATIONALES
Monitor and document frequency and appearance of stools.	Pancreatic enzymes are adjusted to provide normal stooling (i.e., decreased enzymes given with constipation; increased enzymes given with frequent, bulky, foul-smelling stools that float). Normal stooling indicates decreased malabsorption.
Provide well-balanced, high-calorie, high-protein diet (usually 1.5-2 × recommended daily allowance [RDA]).	Only 80%-85% of nutrients are absorbed in children with CF who have GI involvement.
Provide adequate salt, especially with fever, hot weather, or exercise.	Patient is at risk for electrolyte imbalance (hyponatremia) because NaCl concentration in sweat of a child with CF is 2-5 × greater than that of a child without CF.
Administer fat-soluble vitamins in water-miscible form as prescribed.	To counteract malabsorption of fat-soluble vitamins (A, D, E, and K). Water miscible means it can be mixed in a suspension that will not separate. Examples of water-miscible forms of vitamins include Aquasol A and ADEK.
Administer iron preparations as prescribed.	Malabsorption can cause iron deficiency.
Administer supplemental tube feedings or total parenteral nutrition (TPN) as prescribed.	Measures described in previous interventions are not always effective in child exhibiting FTT.
Ensure daily weight measurements in the hospital and teach importance of weekly weight measurements at home.	Assesses effectiveness of nutritional interventions. If child is losing weight, he or she may not be receiving adequate nutrients or may not be absorbing nutrients properly.

●●● **Related NIC and NOC labels:** *NIC:* Nutrition Management; Medication Management; Nutrition Therapy; Sustenance Therapy; Enteral Tube Feeding; Total Parenteral Nutrition *NOC:* Nutritional Status: Nutrient Intake

Nursing Diagnosis:

Deficient Knowledge:

Purpose, precautions, and potential side effects of prescribed medications

Desired Outcome: Within 1 wk of diagnosis or change in medication, patient/parent verbalizes accurate information about prescribed medications.

INTERVENTIONS

RATIONALES

INTERVENTIONS	RATIONALES
Teach the Following to Patient/Parent for the Prescribed Drugs	
Aerosolized bronchodilators: albuterol	Help open the bronchi for easier expectoration of mucus.
	Route: nebulizer or metered-dose inhalers (MDIs)
- Be alert for and report palpitations, increased HR, chest pain, muscle tremors, dizziness, headache.	Side effects: may need dosage adjustment.
- Be alert for and report nervousness, central nervous system (CNS) stimulation, hyperactivity, and insomnia.	Side effects that occur more often in younger children than in adults.
- All above symptoms, as well as dry mouth, may occur with MDI. Notify prescriber if they persist.	Side effects.
- Limit caffeinated beverages.	May increase side effects.

Continued

INTERVENTIONS	RATIONALES
- Do not take with β-adrenergic blocking agents (e.g., propranolol), monoamine oxidase (MAO) inhibitors, tricyclic antidepressants.	Propranolol antagonizes action of albuterol. MAOIs potentiate sympathometic effects. Tricyclic antidepressants increase cardiovascular effects.
- Do not take with other sympathomimetics.	Albuterol increases cardiovascular effects.
- Rinse mouth with water following each inhalation of MDI.	Helps moisten dry mouth and throat.
Aerosolized antibiotics: tobramycin (Tobi)	To fight infection, which would cause increased symptoms.
- Be alert to and report hoarseness, shortness of breath, increased cough, pharyngitis, and hoarseness.	Side effects.
- Store in refrigerator. Date and time the drug when removing it from refrigerator.	Can only be used for 28 days when stored at room temperature.
- Do not use if cloudy or contains particles.	Signs that the medication is compromised.
- Protect from intense light.	Light adversely affects medicine.
- Do not take with dornase alfa (Pulmozyme).	When tobramycin and Pulmozyme are mixed, a precipitate may form.
- Take bronchodilator first, then chest physiotherapy, then other inhaled medications, and tobramycin last.	Most effective method of administration.
Aerosolized mucolytic enzymes: dornase alfa (Pulmozyme)	Thin secretions and optimally decrease number of pulmonary infections.
- Use with appropriate nebulizer system.	A nebulizer unit is available that is made specifically to administer this medication.
- Be alert to and report hoarseness, pharyngitis, laryngitis, rash, chest pain, and conjunctivitis.	Typically side effects are mild and subside within a few weeks.
- Do not dilute or mix with other drugs in nebulizer.	May deactivate the drug.
- Store in refrigerator and discard if unopened vials are subjected to room temperature for ≥24 hr.	Room temperature may deactivate medication.
- Protect from strong light. Discard if solution is cloudy or discolored.	Signs that the medication may be deactivated.
Pancreatic enzymes	Increase food and nutrient absorption.
- As prescribed, take with meals and snacks within 30 min of eating.	Promotes degradation and absorption of nutrients just consumed.
- If patient is an infant or young child, may open capsule and give in small amount of nonfat, nonprotein food (e.g., applesauce).	Protein foods break down this enzyme and can burn mouth in infant/young child.
- Do not mix with milk or formula.	Pancreatic enzymes curdle milk or formula.
- Do not chew microspheres or microtabs; swallow capsules or tablets whole.	Chewing or mouth retention before swallowing may cause mucosal irritation and stomatitis.
- Monitor stools for frequency and appearance.	Constipation or increased stooling (>3 stools/day) indicates need to adjust dosage.
- Do not take if allergic to pork or patient has acute or chronic pancreatitis.	Contraindications for use.
- Be alert for and report nausea, abdominal cramps, mouth irritation, sneezing, constipation, or diarrhea.	Side effects; may need dosage adjustment.
- Notify prescriber if patient is taking H_2 antagonists or gastric acid pump inhibitors (e.g., ranitidine, cimetidine, omeprazole).	These agents increase effectiveness of pancreatic enzymes; dosage adjustment may be needed.

Continued

INTERVENTIONS

RATIONALES

Vitamins/minerals	To supplement overall diet
- Take vitamins A, D, E, and K in water-miscible form as prescribed.	Water-miscible form enables absorption of fat-soluble vitamins.
Antibiotics—usually IV (e.g., ticarcillin, tobramycin)	To treat infections.
- Take as prescribed, usually for at least 10 days and often for several weeks.	Children with CF have frequent respiratory infections and often develop drug resistance. Antibiotics may need to be given for an extended time.
- Monitor for side effects specific to each individual antibiotic.	Side effects vary, depending on specific antibiotic.

●●● **Related NIC and NOC labels:** *NIC:* Teaching: Prescribed Medication *NOC:* Knowledge: Medication

ADDITIONAL NURSING DIAGNOSES/ PROBLEMS:

"Psychosocial Support " for relevant nursing diagnoses that pertain to patient's psychologic status in dealing with a chronic and potentially fatal illness   p. 81

"Psychosocial Support for the Patient's Family and Significant Others" for relevant nursing diagnoses for family members dealing with a chronic and potentially fatal illness in their loved one   p. 95

"Asthma" for:

Anxiety related to illness, loss of control, and medical/nursing interventions   p. 604

Interrupted Family Processes   p. 604

 PATIENT-FAMILY TEACHING AND DISCHARGE PLANNING

When providing child-family teaching, focus on sensory data, avoid excessive information, and initiate a visiting nurse referral for necessary follow-up assessment or teaching. Include verbal and written information about the following and ensure that written information is at a level the reader can understand:

✓ Basic information about disease process with emphasis on respiratory and GI components.

✓ Remission/maintenance and exacerbation aspects of this chronic disease process.

✓ Genetic transmission and screening for CF. Discuss autosomal recessive gene (both parents must at least carry the trait) and implications of this diagnosis on parents and siblings. Ensure that parents understand chance of future children having CF and need for screening of siblings.

✓ Diet, including rationale for increased calories and protein (usually two to three snacks/day).

✓ Administration of pancreatic enzymes with meals and snacks (usually a fractional dose given with snacks).

• If patient is an infant or young child, may mix contents of capsule, granules, or powder with a small amount of applesauce or other carbohydrate food.
• Do not chew or bite capsule or enteric-coated microspheres.
• Do not administer in bottle or cup with fluid.

✓ Need for salt replacement and free access for child to salt, especially during hot weather, fever, diarrhea, or vomiting.

✓ GI symptoms that signal malabsorption and inadequate enzyme replacement (e.g., bloating, abdominal cramping and distention, and diarrhea).

✓ Need to monitor stools (constipation indicates too much enzyme; frequent fatty loose stools indicate insufficient enzyme).

✓ Administration of nebulizer treatment and chest physiotherapy (i.e., chest percussion and postural drainage, mucus clearance device [e.g., FLUTTER] or a vest airway clearance system [e.g., The Vest]). Nebulizer treatment is done first (1 hr before or 2 hr after meals), followed by chest physiotherapy. Stress the importance of routine pulmonary toilet because thickened mucus is an ideal medium for bacterial growth, which causes pulmonary infections.

✓ Cleaning and care of equipment (e.g., nebulizer attachments for albuterol and Pulmozyme).

✓ Medications, including drug name, route, purpose, dosage, precautions, drug/drug and food/drug interactions, and potential adverse effects.

✓ Importance of taking medication at home and at school as directed. Medication in the original container (with prescribing label) and written prescription from health care provider are needed for child to be able take medication at school.

✓ Importance of regular medical follow-up care:
• Routine immunizations plus pneumococcal vaccinations and yearly influenza vaccination
• Prompt attention to infection (fever, increased coughing, green sputum)
• Regular visits with health care provider

✓ Team care approach, including pediatrician, school nurse and teachers, pulmonologist, or infectious disease physician.

✓ Realistic expectations for the child, especially concerning growth and development, participation in school activities and sports, and child's participation/responsibility for self care.

✓ Child's legal rights: Section 504 of Rehabilitation Act of 1973. Each student with a disability (physical or mental impairment) is entitled to accommodation in order to attend school and participate as fully as possible in school activities. A child with significant pulmonary involvement may need to be excused from class for 15-30 min after receiving a nebulizer treatment and chest physiotherapy because of excessive coughing and expectoration of mucus, or the class schedule might need to be rearranged to accommodate required treatment.

✓ Phone numbers to call should questions or concerns arise about therapy or disease after discharge.

✓ When to call health care provider:
  • Increased respiratory effort (e.g., increased RR, nasal flaring, retractions)
  • Excessive coughing and/or coughing up blood
  • Color change: pallor or cyanosis (blue around mouth or eyes)
  • Temperature increase >101.5° F lasting more than a few days or a low-grade fever lasting for a week or more
  • Weight loss
  • Abdominal pain or distention, with or without constipation

✓ Referral to community resources such as support groups, specialists working with children affected by CF, CF care center if available, and genetic counselors.

✓ Additional information can be obtained by contacting:

Cystic Fibrosis Foundation
6931 Arlington Road
Bethesda, MD 20814-3205
(800) Fight CF (344-4823) or (301) 951-4422
www.cff.org/

STARBRIGHT Foundation
1850 Sawtelle Boulevard, Suite 450
Los Angeles, CA 90025
(800) 315-2580 or (310) 479-1212
www.starbright.org

Information for FLUTTER mucus clearance device, high-calorie shakes, and pancreatic enzymes:
www.axcanscandipharm.com

Information for The Vest:
www.thevest.com

CareFirst for CF: Program to help ease financial burden of infants (includes children up to 2 years of age). Must be prescribed by health care provider.
www.axcan.com/en-us/carefirst.aspx

Comprehensive Care Program for CF: Provides additional support for CF patients by helping reduce cost of therapy (includes a certificate for a FLUTTER mucus clearance device).
www.axcan.com/en-us/cfdirect.aspx

Diabetes Mellitus in Children

Diabetes mellitus (DM) is the most common childhood endocrine disorder and one of the most costly chronic diseases of childhood. It is a disorder of carbohydrate metabolism marked by hyperglycemia and glycosuria, and it results from inadequate production or use of insulin. The major classifications seen in children are as follows:

- **Type 1 DM:** There is an absolute deficiency of insulin secretion resulting from destruction of beta cells, causing hyperglycemia and ketosis. This destruction is often an immune-mediated or related response. Previously it was called insulin-dependent DM (IDDM) or juvenile onset diabetes. Historically, this was the primary type of diabetes seen in children. Currently, approximately 30,000 Americans are diagnosed each year with type 1 DM, and about 13,000 are children. Incidence peaks during puberty (10-12 yr in girls and 12-14 yr in boys), although children have been diagnosed as young as 12 mo old. These children are dependent on insulin for survival and to prevent diabetic ketoacidosis (DKA). Even with insulin, type 1 diabetes shortens the life span by 15 yr.
- **Type 2 DM:** There is an insulin resistance with this type, so there is a relative, not absolute, insulin deficiency. Previously this was called non–insulin-dependent DM (NIDDM) or adult onset DM. In the 1990s there was an alarming epidemic of children developing type 2 DM. Children as young as 8 yr old with an average age of 13-14 yr old were being diagnosed. Currently, 8%-45% (depending on geographic location) of children newly diagnosed with diabetes have type 2 non–immune-related DM. Previously, only 2% of children were diagnosed with type 2 DM. Obesity is a strong risk factor for type 2 DM, and 1999 data noted that obesity currently affects about 20%-30% of children and adolescents in the United States

and is increasing. Sedentary lifestyle is another significant risk factor. There is also an increased risk of developing type 2 diabetes in African-American, Mexican-American, Asian-American, and Native-American populations.
- **Mature onset diabetes of youth (MODY):** This type involves impaired insulin secretion with minimal or no defects in insulin action, usually in individuals <25 yr old and symptomatic only with stress or infection.
- For information on other types, see the adult Diabetes Mellitus care plan, p. 399.

HEALTH CARE SETTING

Primary care, with possible hospital admission because of complications

ASSESSMENT

Signs and symptoms: These are the same as in the adult DM care plan except for the following:

Type 2 DM: Usually these children have hypertension, dyslipidemia, and acanthosis nigricans (hypertrophy or thickening of skin with gray, brown, or black pigmentation chiefly in axilla, other body folds, and sometimes on hands, elbows, and knees). Females may have vaginitis because of long-standing glycosuria. DKA also may occur in children and adolescents.

COMPLICATIONS

Potential for acute crisis: This is the same as in the adult DM care plan with the following addition:

- **Idiopathic cerebral edema** in resolving DKA: Occurs more often in children than in adults. The patient may have headache and lethargy or be asymptomatic. Symptoms can start with abrupt change in level of consciousness (LOC); pupils dilated, fixed, or unequal; papilledema; decorticate or decerebrate posturing; rapid progression to deep coma, respiratory arrest, or brain death (herniation of brain stem).

Long-term complications: Micro and macro complications are very aggressive in children with type 2 DM. They occur over a much shorter time frame than is usually seen in adults.

DIAGNOSTIC TESTS

In 2000, the American Diabetes Association (ADA) recommended that the same 1997 classification and diagnostic criteria that apply to adults with type 2 DM be applied to children and adolescents as well.

Fasting plasma glucose: Will reveal a value ≥126 mg/dl. Fasting is defined as no caloric intake for at least 8 hr. This is the recommended test for children, and it should be confirmed by a second positive test on another day.

- *Normal plasma glucose:* A value <110 mg/dl.
- *Impaired fasting glucose:* 110-126 mg/dl or impaired glucose tolerance if 2 hr postprandial plasma glucose is 140-200 mg/dl. Impaired fasting plasma glucose or impaired glucose tolerance should be monitored on a regular basis because approximately 25% of those affected will progress to diabetes (ADA, 1998).
- *Testing recommendations* (Report on Expert Committee on Diagnosis and Treatment of Diabetes Mellitus, Fall 1999) for type 2 DM:
  - Obesity: 85% of children are overweight or obese at diagnosis.
  - Two or more of the following risk factors:
    - Family history of type 2 DM in first- and second-degree relatives
    - Belonging to certain race/ethnic groups (Native-American, African-American, Mexican-American, Asian/South Pacific Islanders)
    - Signs of insulin resistance or conditions associated with insulin resistance (acanthosis nigricans, hypertension, dyslipidemias, polycystic ovarian syndrome)
  - If listed factors present, testing should be done:
    - Every year starting at age 10 or
    - At onset of puberty, if it occurs at a younger age
    - Preferred test is fasting plasma glucose

Two-hour postprandial plasma glucose: Will reveal a value ≥200 mg/dl during oral glucose tolerance test. It is not usually done in children.

Random plasma glucose: Symptoms of diabetes (polyuria, polydipsia, polyphagia, unexplained weight loss) and a fasting plasma glucose ≥200 mg/dl are diagnostic of diabetes.

Glycosylated hemoglobin or hemoglobin A1C (HbA$_1$C): Assesses control of blood glucose over preceding 2 to 3 mo. Normal range is 4%-7%. Range in children varies depending on age, with higher glucose levels allowed in younger children. Values differ depending on test done:
- Under 5 yr old: HbA$_1$C 7.5%-9.3%
- 5-11 yr old: HbA$_1$C <8.5%
- Adolescent: HbA$_1$C 7%-7.5%

Fasting lipid panel, if type 2 diabetes suspected: Dyslipidemia is frequently seen in children in type 2 DM and also needs to be treated. Values vary depending on age of child and if reference range is in conventional units or international units.

Basic metabolic panel (electrolytes, glucose, blood urea nitrogen [BUN], creatinine): Serum glucose will be elevated, usually >250 mg/dl. Sodium and potassium may be lost because of osmotic diuresis. The higher the glucose level, the greater the dehydration and loss of electrolytes. Serum potassium may be normal on admission, but after fluid and insulin administration, rapid return of potassium to the cells decreases serum potassium, which necessitates monitoring for cardiac dysrhythmias. BUN and creatinine likely will be elevated because of dehydration. Also, renal dysfunction occurs when serum glucose level rises to >600 mg/dl.

Thyroid-stimulating hormone (TSH) and thyroxine (T$_4$): Thyroid hormone increases gluconeogenesis (synthesis of glucose from noncarbohydrate sources such as amino acids and glycerol) and peripheral use of glucose. Elevated or decreased value would impact carbohydrate metabolism and therefore plasma glucose. Normal range varies for children depending on their age and type of reference units reported.

Ketones: Elevated when insulin is not available and the body starts to break down stored fats for energy. Ketone bodies are by-products of this fat breakdown, and they accumulate in the blood and urine. Normal range for children is 0 with the qualitative test and 0.5-3 mg/dl (conventional units) or 5-30 mg/L (international units) with the quantitative test.

Nursing Diagnosis:

Deficient Knowledge:

Meal planning and its relationship to blood glucose.

Desired Outcome: Within 48 hr after teaching, child/family demonstrates ability to perform meal planning based on blood glucose levels.

INTERVENTIONS	RATIONALES
Teach the action different foods (carbohydrates, fats, proteins) have on blood glucose level.	Facilitates understanding of need for adhering to prescribed diet. For example, carbohydrates raise blood sugar, and simple sugars raise blood sugar more rapidly. Fats and proteins have less immediate effect on blood sugar level.
Involve dietitian in developing and instructing child/family about prescribed meal plan.	Dietitian has expertise in designing a plan appropriate for child based on age, cultural background, preferences, and caloric needs. Including these variables in the meal plan increases knowledge, understanding, and hence likelihood of compliance.
Use handouts from dietitian and guidelines in diabetes book used by facility for diabetes education (see resources at end of care plan) to review prescribed diet.	Written and verbal explanations increase understanding and promote compliance.
As indicated, teach carbohydrate counting.	Understanding diet plan increases ability to continue this regimen at home and improves compliance as well. Counting grams of carbohydrate and matching them with amount of insulin is the diet used most often in children. A no-concentrated-sweets diet is another plan used in some facilities.
Review child's normal schedule and set up a schedule that includes time for blood glucose tests, medication, meals, and snacks.	Having a written schedule facilitates child's/family's adjustment to new routines. Meal plan is tailored to child and his or her activity level. Ongoing assessment enables change as necessary and/or a follow-up dietary consultation.
Assess weight on admission and daily thereafter (same time of day, same scales, same amount of clothing).	Whether child is maintaining or gaining weight may be an indicator of effectiveness of diet and treatment and/or compliance.
Identify ideal blood glucose levels for child based on age.	Diet and activity levels vary more in the younger child. Generally at <6 yr old, a child is more likely to have hypoglycemia and less likely to recognize early signs and symptoms, so blood glucose values are kept in a higher range. - Infants/toddler: 100-200 mg/dl - Child (<6 yr): 80-180 mg/dl - Older child or adolescent: 70-150 mg/dl
Instruct family to write meal plans for several days implementing use of prescribed foods.	Method of assessing and promoting family's understanding of diet instruction.
Provide scenarios for family when blood glucose is outside normal range and have them identify ways of adjusting diet, insulin, and/or exercise to get closer to blood glucose goal.	Facilitates development of problem-solving skills within family and assesses family's understanding of interaction among blood glucose, insulin, diet, and exercise.

●●● **Related NIC and NOC labels:** *NIC:* Teaching: Prescribed Diet; Nutrition Management
NOC: Knowledge: Diabetes Management

Nursing Diagnosis:

Deficient Knowledge:

Causes, signs and symptoms, and treatment of hypoglycemia or hyperglycemia

Desired Outcome: Immediately following teaching, child/family verbalizes accurate understanding of possible causes, signs and symptoms, and treatment of hypoglycemia and hyperglycemia.

INTERVENTIONS	RATIONALES
Define hypoglycemia for child and family.	Knowledge facilitates early recognition of problem, enabling prompt treatment. Hypoglycemia is defined as low blood glucose level (<60-70 mg/dl) that occurs rapidly with signs and symptoms noted within minutes to an hour. Hypoglycemia is a potential emergency and needs to be treated promptly.
Teach child and family causes of hypoglycemia.	Understanding causes of hypoglycemia optimally will help child/parent decrease occurrences. Causes include: - Too little food or not eating on time - Increased exercise/activity with no increased intake - Too much insulin
Teach child and family to recognize early and late signs and symptoms of hypoglycemia.	Signs and symptoms of hypoglycemia should prompt child or family to check blood glucose level. - Early signs occurring secondary to adrenaline release are trembling, tachycardia, sweating, headache, anxiety, and hunger. - Later signs and symptoms occurring secondary to cerebral glucose deficit are dizziness, personality/mood changes, slurred speech, loss of coordination, and decreased LOC. Some children may not show early symptoms of adrenaline release or if <6 yr old may not recognize early symptoms.
Teach child and family the best method of assessing and treating hypoglycemia.	Some signs and symptoms of hypoglycemia and hyperglycemia are difficult to distinguish from one another, but the treatments are different. It is essential to know which reaction a child is experiencing to treat it effectively. Measures include: - Check blood sugar to determine if child is hypoglycemic. - In the presence of hypoglycemia, give 15 g of readily absorbed carbohydrates such as 4 oz orange juice, 6 oz regular soda, 4 glucose tablets, or 6 Life-Savers. If blood glucose is not increased or the child is still having signs and symptoms of hypoglycemia in 15 min, repeat the treatment. This will elevate plasma glucose level and relieve symptoms of hypoglycemia. Understanding of appropriate initial treatment improves ability to treat hypoglycemia successfully. - If it is not time for a meal or snack within 1 hr, give complex carbohydrates and protein such as bread or crackers with peanut butter or cheese to sustain glucose level inasmuch as readily absorbed carbohydrates (fast-acting or simple sugars) will be out of the system in 45-60 min. Complex carbohydrates (e.g., crackers) take 2-3 hr and proteins (e.g., cheese or peanut butter) 3-4 hr to be metabolized. Knowledge of appropriate follow-up treatment and understanding necessity of this treatment improve ability to resolve situation successfully.
Teach strategies to prevent hypoglycemia by identifying pattern of activity or time of day that precedes reactions.	Knowledge of these patterns enables child/family to prevent or decrease incidence of hypoglycemia. For example, patient/parent should record in log/diary all unusual events or change in activity or diet to help identify patterns.
Teach care if child is unable to eat, drink, or swallow or is unconscious.	Knowing appropriate treatment improves outcome. - Administer glucagon (SC or IM) if available to raise blood glucose level when child is unable to drink or eat fast-acting carbohydrate.

Continued

INTERVENTIONS	RATIONALES
	- If glucagon is not available, position child on side and rub honey, corn syrup, or Cake Mate Gel inside the cheek. This position prevents aspiration, especially if giving glucagon, because vomiting may occur. Fast-acting/simple sugars are absorbed through the oral mucosa without danger of aspiration.
Define hyperglycemia.	To help differentiate between hyperglycemia and hypoglycemia. Knowledge enables recognition and discernment of which reaction child is experiencing. Hyperglycemia is defined as blood glucose levels higher than target range. Signs and symptoms appear within hours to several days.
Teach child and family causes of hyperglycemia.	Understanding situations that can result in hyperglycemia (e.g., increased food intake, too little insulin, decreased exercise, infection or illness, and emotional stress) can help child/family avoid such events.
Teach signs and symptoms of hyperglycemia.	Recognition of hyperglycemia enables earlier and more effective treatment and prevents development of DKA. Signs and symptoms include the three *P*'s (polydipsia, polyuria, polyphagia), fatigue, fruity-smelling breath, weight loss.
Teach treatment for hyperglycemia.	Interventions to prevent DKA through early treatment. These include: - If blood glucose level is >250 mg/dl, check urine for ketones. - If ketone results are trace to small, drink extra water and recheck for ketones in 2 hr. - If ketone results are medium to large, contact health care provider.
Teach patient to call health care provider if blood glucose is >250 mg/dl 3 times in a row.	Provider may need to adjust insulin.

●●● **Related NIC and NOC labels:** *NIC:* Hyperglycemia Management; Hypoglycemia Management
NOC: Knowledge: Diabetes Management

Nursing Diagnosis:

Deficient Knowledge:

Blood glucose monitoring

Desired Outcome: Within 48 hr of this diagnosis, child/family demonstrates and verbalizes accurate understanding of proper blood glucose monitoring and when to monitor for ketones.

INTERVENTIONS	RATIONALES
Discuss reasons for blood glucose testing.	Understanding purpose of performing tests facilitates compliance. Reasons for blood glucose testing include: - Allows child to relate "how I feel at this time" with actual blood glucose level. - Gives child/family some control.

Continued

INTERVENTIONS	RATIONALES
	- Enables understanding of effects of food, exercise, insulin, and/or stress.
	- Enables adjustments in insulin or diet.
Demonstrate correct use of Glucometer the child will use at home and proper technique for fingerstick.	There are many different models and strips available commercially. Each system functions a little differently, and it could be overwhelming having to learn a new system at home without assistance or guidance. General guidelines include:
	- Use side of finger, not tip. Sides of the fingers have fewer nerve endings and hurt less. In addition, using sides decreases loss of sense of touch in fingertips.
	- Clean hands with soap and warm water. Cleansing helps reduce risk of infection. Warm water facilitates circulation and hence blood flow.
	- Avoid regular use of alcohol to cleanse skin. Any trace of alcohol left on the skin will interfere with the chemical reaction involved in checking blood glucose. It is okay to use occasionally (e.g., at a picnic), but the finger must be dried carefully and the first drop of blood discarded. Repeated use of alcohol also can lead to thickening of the skin, making fingerstick more difficult and painful.
	- Hold hand down, not up, to facilitate blood flow.
Discuss when blood glucose testing should be done.	Knowledge and understanding facilitate compliance.
	- Normally before each meal and bedtime snack. Checking blood glucose on a regular basis and documenting findings help determine if adjustments need to be made in insulin/diet/exercise/medication by assessing pattern of blood glucose levels.
	- If sick, q4h. Risk of hyperglycemia is increased when the child is ill (e.g., with headache, fever, sore throat) or has an infection owing to stress on the body and increased energy demands. Stress causes the adrenal gland to produce more epinephrine, norepinephrine, and cortisol. These stress hormones are "anti-insulin" in their actions, so blood glucose increases and ketones are formed by the liver, breaking down fat stores for energy. As blood glucose increases, the three *P*'s occur, causing dehydration as well as nausea and vomiting owing to ketosis. Blood glucose testing will determine if changes need to be made in insulin and if health care provider should be contacted.
	- With hypoglycemic or hyperglycemic symptoms to identify which event is occurring and therefore facilitate proper treatment.
If blood glucose is >250 mg/dl or if child is ill, check urine for ketones with every void.	The body starts breaking down stored fats for energy because it cannot use blood glucose for energy. Ketone bodies are by-products of this fat breakdown and can lead to DKA if not controlled/treated.
Demonstrate use of diary or log to record blood glucose levels, ketones, insulin, dose diet, exercise, and any comments.	Provides good overview of how child is doing and assists health care provider in making adjustments based on pattern seen in log/diary.
Instruct child/family when to call health care provider per blood glucose levels or ketones.	Understanding when to call improves compliance and decreases complications such as DKA:

Continued

INTERVENTIONS	RATIONALES
	- Blood glucose >250 mg/dl 3 times in a row
	- Blood glucose <70 mg/dl twice in 1 wk
	- Ketones moderate or large

●●● **Related NIC and NOC labels:** *NIC:* Hyperglycemia Management; Hypoglycemia Management
NOC: Knowledge: Diabetes Management

ADDITIONAL NURSING DIAGNOSES/ PROBLEMS:

"Psychosocial Support"	p. 81
"Psychosocial Support for the Patient's Family and Significant Others" for **Interrupted Family Processes** and **Readiness for Enhanced Family Coping**	p. 95
Diabetes Mellitus" in the adult care plans for **Ineffective Peripheral, Cardiopulmonary, Renal, Cerebral, and GI Tissue Perfusion**	p. 401
Risk for Infection	p. 402
Impaired Skin Integrity	p. 403
Deficient Knowledge: Proper insulin administration and dietary precautions for promoting normoglycemia	p. 404
"Asthma" for **Anxiety** related to illness, loss of control, and medical/nursing interventions	p. 604
"Asthma" for **Interrupted Family Processes**	p. 604

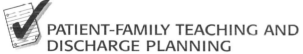

PATIENT-FAMILY TEACHING AND DISCHARGE PLANNING

Children with DM may have different classifications of DM with varying symptoms and complications. When providing patient-family teaching, focus on sensory information, avoid giving excessive information, and initiate a visiting nurse referral for necessary follow-up teaching and assessment. A part of initial assessment should include asking about existing knowledge of the disease, ability for self-care by child and/or family, and psychologic acceptance. Include verbal and written information (ensuring that written material is at a level the reader can understand) about the following:

✓ DM: definition, type child has, brief pathophysiology, characteristics of specific type.

✓ Major influences on blood sugar control: diet, exercise, insulin/oral medication, stress/infection.

✓ Diet prescribed for child (most often carbohydrate-counting or no-concentrated-sweets diet). The diet is also low

in fat and high in fiber to prevent or decrease problems with blood fats, especially cholesterol and triglycerides. Provide rationale for three meals and two to three snacks on a consistent schedule.

✓ Exercise/activity: lowers blood glucose, helps maintain normal cholesterol levels, increases circulation, and is an essential part of a child's life. If exercise is increased or has a different time frame than usual, it may be necessary to adjust diet (add 15-30 g carbohydrates for each 45-60 min of exercise), insulin, or oral medications.

✓ Stress or illness/infection: increases blood glucose level; therefore adjustments may be necessary in diet and/or insulin dosage.

✓ Insulin: type of insulin; characteristics of particular insulin, including onset, peak, and duration; dose prescribed; and dosing schedule.

- Have child/parent demonstrate drawing up each prescribed dose (e.g., lispro and NPH before breakfast, lispro before supper, and NPH at bedtime)
- Rotation of injection sites:
  - Insulin absorption varies by site (most rapidly in abdomen, then in the arms, in the hips, and slowest in the thighs).
  - Insulin absorption is affected by injection site. Massage after injection, exercise of injected limb, and body temperature increase the rate of absorption.
  - Use all spots in one site before you move on to another site or use the same site for every AM injection and the same site for every PM injection until all spots have been used (gives same absorption of insulin).
- Have child/parent administer insulin using proper technique.
- At least two people (one could be the child) need to know how to draw up and administer insulin.

✓ Other medications, including drug name, purpose, dosage, frequency, precautions, drug/drug and food/drug interactions, and potential side effects.

✓ Honeymoon phase or period: may occur a short time after diagnosis, usually within 2 to 8 wk, and usually lasts 1-3 mo, but may last up to a year. Insulin requirement decreases. The child is *not* cured. The insulin requirement will increase again.

✓ Acute complications of DM: hypoglycemia and hyperglycemia

- Possible causes
- Signs and symptoms
- Treatment

✓Long-term complications (avoid addressing for now if child has just been diagnosed): microvascular, macrovascular, joint contractures.

✓Blood glucose monitoring: See details in **Deficient Knowledge:** Blood glucose monitoring.

✓Sick-day plan of care
- Always give insulin.
- Check blood sugar at least q4h and urine ketones with each void. Document in log/diary.
- If small amount of ketones, increase fluid intake.
- If child does not feel like eating, then give fluids with sugar such as fruit juice, regular soda, and regular Jell-O, and broth-type soups (provides some electrolytes and extra fluid) unless blood sugar is >200 mg/dl. Then give diet fluids.
- Call health care provider or nurse educator if:
  - Nausea and vomiting
  - Fruity odor to breath
  - Deep, rapid respirations
  - Decreasing LOC
  - Moderate or high ketones in urine
  - Persistent hyperglycemia >250 mg/dl (3 times in a row)

✓Prevention of infection:
- Have good body hygiene with special attention to feet.
- Report any breaks in skin and treat promptly.
- Wear only properly fitting shoes and do not go barefooted.
- Get regular dental checkups.
- Need for pneumococcal and yearly influenza vaccines.

✓Importance of child wearing medical-alert necklace or bracelet (depending on age) and carrying a card that states child has diabetes, the type of diabetes, child's name, address, phone number, and health care provider's name and number.

✓Psychosocial adjustment:
- Reactions of child: shock, denial, and sadness
- Reaction of parents: grief reaction

✓Delegation of tasks to child, based on age (with supervision):
- Toddler/preschooler: Chooses and cleans finger for puncture; tries to identify word or phrase to describe feeling of hypoglycemia. Help choose food; give child a choice of appropriate options.
- School-age child: Performs finger puncture and blood glucose test. Pushes plunger down on insulin syringe after needle is inserted by parent or gives own injection. Performs ketone test on urine. Recognizes need to eat on time to avoid hypoglycemia. Verbalizes the treatment for hypoglycemia.
- Older school-age child: Records blood glucose values in log/dairy. May draw up and inject insulin. Knows meal plan. Can choose correct foods for snacks.
- Adolescent: Looks for patterns in blood glucose values. Recognizes when to test for ketones. Initiates treatment

for ketones (increased fluids). Can plan meals and snacks based on dietary plan. Can choose appropriate food at a party.

✓Coordination of care. Need to talk with school nurse and/or other adults who are in close contact with child (e.g., teachers, scout leaders, day care provider).

✓Legal rights of the child:
- Individuals with Disabilities Education Act (IDEA): Mandates federal government to provide funding to education agencies, state and local, to facilitate free and appropriate education to qualifying students with disabilities. This includes children with diabetes because diabetes can, at times, adversely affect school performance in some students. If this can be proved, school is then required to develop an Individualized Education Plan (IEP).
- IEP: Designed by multidisciplinary team to facilitate special education and therapeutic strategies and goals for each child. Child does not have to be in special education classes. Parents need to be involved in this process.
- Section 504 of Rehabilitation Act of 1973: Each student with a disability is entitled to accommodation in order to attend school and participate as fully as possible in school activities. This accommodation may be related to a medical condition or an education issue. For example, child may leave the classroom to use bathroom facilities without raising hand and will not be penalized for excessive absences from school that are caused by the diabetes. The 504 plan may include as many accommodations as necessary for child to function well at school. Composition of the 504 team may include teachers, school nurse, therapists (physical, occupational, or speech therapist), psychologist, and parents and child as appropriate for child's needs. Input from health care provider is vital.

✓Necessity of having health care provider's prescription form at school detailing guidelines for when to check blood sugar and administer medication or treatment for diabetes-related problems, as well as medications in the original container with prescribing label intact.

✓Goals of care for child with diabetes:
- Focus is on child with diabetes, *not* on the diabetic child.
- Child will have appropriate growth (height and weight).
- Child will have age-appropriate lifestyle (development).
- Child will have near normal HbA$_1$C (varies with age).
- Child will not have acute complications (hypoglycemia or hyperglycemia).
- Child will have minimal serious complications associated with long-term diabetes.
- Child will be able to perform age-appropriate self-care tasks.

✓Importance of follow-up care and regular visits to health care provider and any other specialists working with child, such as dietitian, physical therapist, or endocrinologist.

✓Phone numbers for family to call if any questions arise about therapy or disease after discharge.

✓ When to call health care provider:
- Increased blood sugar >250 mg/dl 3 times in a row
- More than two episodes of hypoglycemia per week
- Moderate-to-large amount of ketones in urine

✓ Diabetes camps, which are a fun way for children to learn more about their diabetes and feel less isolated. Listing is available at www.childrenwithdiabetes.com. (Under keyword search, type in "camp.")

✓ Referrals to community resources, such as local and national chapters of the American Diabetes Association and Juvenile Diabetes Foundation, public health nurses or home health nurse, diabetes nurse educator or endocrinologist, community teaching programs or support groups for children, diabetes camps, or other resources as necessary.

✓ See "Diabetes Mellitus," p. 406, for additional family teaching and discharge planning suggestions and resources.

✓ Additional resources include the following:

Children with Diabetes: online community for kids, families, and adults with diabetes. Sample 504 and IEP available. Rufus, the teddy bear with diabetes, is available here.
www.childrenwithdiabetes.com/index_cwd.htm

Juvenile Diabetes Research Foundation International (JDRF)
120 Wall Street
New York, NY 10005-4001
(800) 533-CURE (2873)
www.jdrf.org/

American Association of Diabetes Educators
100 West Monroe Street, Suite 400
Chicago, IL 60603
(800) 338-3633
www.aadenet.org/

Understanding Insulin-Dependent Diabetes, ed 10, 2002
H. Peter Chase, MD
Barbara Davis Center for Childhood Diabetes
Dept. of Pediatrics, University of Colorado Health Sciences Center
www.barbaradaviscenter.org.
To order, call (800) 695-2873 ($18.00)

An Instructional Aid on Insulin-Dependent Diabetes Mellitus, ed 12, 2003
Luther B. Travis, MD
Children's Diabetes Management Center
University of Texas Medical Branch
Galveston, TX
To order, call (512) 832-0611 ($21.50)

Carb Counting and Exchange Lists
Novo Nordisk Pharmaceuticals, Inc.
www.novonordisk-us.com
To order, call (800) 727-6500

STARBRIGHT Foundation
1850 Sawtelle Boulevard, Suite 450
Los Angeles, CA 90025
(800) 315-2580 or (310) 479-1212
www.starbright.org

82

Fractures in Children

Fractures are common childhood injuries and usually the result of trauma (falls, motor vehicle accidents, sports injuries, child abuse) or bone disease with abnormally fragile bones (osteogenesis imperfecta). Fractures usually result from increased mobility and immature understanding of potentially dangerous situations. Fractures in infancy are most often caused by trauma or child abuse.

Important variables that affect care of fractures in children as compared with adults:

- Children's bones heal faster than adults'; the younger the child, the faster the bone heals.
- Children's bones are softer than adults'; rather than breaking, they bend or buckle.
- Children's bones have a thicker periosteum and increased amount of immature bone.
- Children's bones have an open growth plate or epiphysis. Damage to the growth plate can interrupt and alter growth.
- Children usually only complain when something is wrong. Restlessness, extended periods of crying, and calling for the parent more than usual, as well as disuse of affected extremity or increased use of unaffected extremity after a fall or injury are signals that more investigation of the event is needed.

Most frequent types of fractures in children:

- **Bends or plastic deformation:** A child's flexible bone can be bent ≥45 degrees before breaking and remains bent when the force is removed. The ossification of bones begins at birth and continues until the child is 18-21 years old. The less ossified the bone, the more easily it bends. Thus, this type of injury occurs only in children, most often in the ulna and fibula.
- **Buckle or torus fracture:** Compression of the porus bone as a result of minimal angular trauma. It causes a bulge at the fracture site and occurs most often in young children, usually in the distal radius or ulna.

- **Greenstick:** Break occurs through the periosteum on one side of the bone but only bows or buckles the other side. It occurs most often in the forearm.
- **Complete fracture:** Break divides the bony fragments. The four types include spiral fracture (from rotational force, often associated with child abuse, especially in infants), oblique, transverse, and epiphyseal.

Most common fracture sites in children: Ulna, clavicle, tibia, and femur.

Most fractures are treated with closed reduction and immobility. Developmental age is key to the cause of injury (falls, motor vehicle accidents, sports) and type of fracture.

HEALTH CARE SETTING

Emergency department, with possible hospitalization

ASSESSMENT

Child's symptoms, trauma history (should match physical examination), and physical examination are all part of the assessment profile.

Signs and symptoms: Vary with location, severity, and type of injury. Pain or tenderness at site, decreased range of motion (ROM) or immobility, deformity at fracture site, crepitus, gross motion at injured site, edema, erythema, ecchymosis, muscle spasm, and inability to bear weight may be present.

Physical assessment: Assess for location of deformity, swelling, ecchymosis, and pain. Check VS and perform neurovascular assessment.

DIAGNOSTIC TESTS

X-ray examination: Most effective tool for determining type and location of a fracture. Much of the skeleton of infants and young children is composed of radiolucent growth cartilage that does not appear on radiographs. Observation of gross deformity and point tenderness may be more reliable in diagnosing extremity fractures than would an x-ray. X-rays of unaffected limb may be obtained for comparison. Radiography of the suspected limb fractures should include joint above and below with a minimum of two views. X-rays are also taken after fracture reduction and often during healing process to assess progress.

Computed tomography (CT) scans, magnetic resonance imaging (MRI), bone scan: May be needed to evaluate fracture in certain circumstances.

Nursing Diagnosis:

Acute Pain

related to fracture and other injury

Desired Outcome: Following treatment/intervention, child's report of pain/pain level is <2 on a 5-point scale (e.g., FACES scale) or <4 on a 10-point scale (e.g., numeric scale). Or child exhibits behavior consistent with pain <4 on a 10-point scale (e.g., FLACC scale).

INTERVENTIONS	RATIONALES
Establish a pain scale appropriate for child (FLACC, Wong-Baker FACES, Oucher, Poker Chip, numeric) and use it to assess pain before and after analgesia administration and at least q4h.	Helps determine degree of pain and effectiveness of pain medication.
Administer pain medication around the clock for first 24-48 hr or depending on severity of injury.	Decreases or prevents pain more effectively than when given prn. Prolonged stimulation of pain receptors results in increased sensitivity to painful stimuli and will increase the amount of drug required to relieve pain.
Position, align, and support affected body part.	Decreases tension on affected area, thereby decreasing pain.
Use nonpharmacologic pain control measures as appropriate for child depending on developmental age.	Adjuncts to pain medication. These include rocking, play, toys, music, distraction, relaxation techniques, humor, and massage.
Ice and elevate extremity, especially for first 48 hr.	Decreases edema, thereby decreasing pain.
Notify health care provider if relief from pain is not obtained 1 hr after PO pain medication was given and after using all above measures.	Medication may need to be adjusted for optimal pain control. It also may signify a fracture complication.

●●● **Related NIC and NOC labels:** *NIC:* Pain Management; Analgesic Administration; Humor; Positioning; Cold Application; Distraction; Simple Massage; Music Therapy *NOC:* Comfort Level; Pain Level

Nursing Diagnosis:

Ineffective Tissue Perfusion: Peripheral

related to edema or immobilization following fracture

Desired Outcome: Child's neurovascular checks are within normal limits within 48 hr of fracture as evidenced by digits that are warm and sensitive to touch, brisk capillary refill (≤2 sec), peripheral pulse amplitude >2+ on a 0-4+ scale, and minimal or decreased swelling in affected limb.

INTERVENTIONS	RATIONALES
Elevate extremity.	To prevent/decrease edema, thereby promoting tissue perfusion.
Apply ice first 48 hr.	Decreases edema, thereby promoting tissue perfusion.

Continued

INTERVENTIONS	RATIONALES
Perform neurovascular checks (color, sensation, pulses, warmth, swelling) qh for first 24 hr and then q2-4h. Use a measuring tape in millimeter increments to compare circumference of area distal to the injury to that of noninjured limb to determine amount of edema. Or, depending on size of child, you should be able to insert one or two fingers into the cast opening.	To determine presence of decreased peripheral tissue perfusion in the injured limb, which would be evidenced by darker or lighter color than opposite extremity, decreased sensation, decreased or absent pulse, skin cool to touch, and increased swelling distal to the injury.
Be alert to subjective and behavioral indicators of decreasing perfusion.	Complaints of constant or increasing pain (especially on passive movement of the digits) and numbness or tingling in the digits of the injured extremity are subjective indicators of decreasing perfusion. Constant crying or increasing irritability may be seen in young children.
Notify health care provider immediately if tissue perfusion deteriorates quickly from baseline.	Child may be developing or experiencing compartment syndrome, an emergency situation. For details, see "Fractures" in the adult care plans for **Risk for Peripheral Neurovascular Dysfunction** related to interruption of capillary blood flow secondary to increased pressure within the myofascial compartment, p. 542.
Encourage child to move digits.	Improves circulation, thereby decreasing edema and increasing tissue perfusion. **Note:** Inability to move digits is another sign of compartment syndrome.

●●● **Related NIC and NOC labels:** *NIC:* Neurologic Monitoring; Positioning; Circulatory Precautions
NOC: Tissue Perfusion: Peripheral

Nursing Diagnosis:

Risk for Impaired Skin Integrity

related to presence of immobilization device (bandages, splint, cast)

Desired Outcome: Child's skin remains intact while wearing immobilization device.

INTERVENTIONS	RATIONALES
Assess for erythema or irritation caused by the immobilization device q4h. - Check edges of immobilization device above and below fracture site. - If edges are rough, petal moleskin to smooth edges.	Ongoing assessment results in early detection and treatment, thereby decreasing risk of break in skin integrity.
Run hand over immobilization device to feel for indentations or "hot" spots q4h.	Indentation can cause skin breakdown/pressure. Hot spots (after cast has dried) may indicate an infection that might occur as a result of a break in skin integrity.
Feel around edges of immobilization device for tightness q4h.	Determines if cast/immobilization device fits appropriately and is not too tight or loose. Examiner should be able to insert fingers between cast and child's skin after it dries. If cast is too tight, it will cause pressure, which can result in decreased tissue perfusion and skin breakdown. If cast is too loose, it can rub on the skin and cause skin breakdown.

Continued

INTERVENTIONS	RATIONALES
Instruct child/family not to put powder or cornstarch under cast.	May cake and cause skin irritation and breakdown.
Suggest that family use cool air blown from fan or hair dryer to relieve itching or rub unaffected extremity.	Distraction techniques to keep child from itching or putting things inside cast to scratch and cause skin breakdown.
Caution child/family not to put anything inside cast to scratch skin.	Can cause skin breakdown or become lodged inside cast.
Encourage position changes q2-4h as appropriate.	Improves circulation by preventing prolonged pressure at same area.

●●● **Related NIC and NOC labels:** *NIC:* Pressure Management; Skin Surveillance; Cast Care: Maintenance; Positioning; Traction/Immobilization Care *NOC:* Tissue Integrity: Skin and Mucous Membranes

ADDITIONAL NURSING DIAGNOSES/ PROBLEMS:

"Prolonged Bedrest" for such care plans as **Risk for Activity Intolerance, Risk for Disuse Syndrome,** and **Constipation,** which occur with prolonged immobilization — p. 67

"Psychosocial Support" for such care plans as **Fear,** which child may experience as a result of injury and treatment — p. 86

"Psychosocial Support for Patient's Family and Significant Others" for such care plans as **Interrupted Family Processes,** which may occur with child's injury — p. 95

"Fractures" for care plans that discuss self-care deficits — p. 537

"Asthma" for **Anxiety** related to illness, loss of control, and medical/nursing interventions — p. 604

PATIENT-FAMILY TEACHING AND DISCHARGE PLANNING

When providing child-family teaching, focus on sensory data, avoid giving excessive information, and initiate a visiting nurse referral for necessary follow-up teaching as needed. All information should emphasize that which is developmentally appropriate for the child. Include written and verbal information about the following (ensuring that written information is at a level the reader can understand):

✓ Proper care of immobilization device. See **Risk for Impaired Skin Integrity,** earlier.

✓ Medications, including drug name, purpose, dosage, frequency, precautions, drug/drug and food/drug interactions, and potential adverse affects.

✓ Importance of taking medications at home and at school as directed. Medication in the original bottle (with prescribing label) and written prescription from health care provider are needed for child to be able to take medication at school.

✓ Legal rights of the child—Section 504 of Rehabilitation Act of 1973: Each student with a disability (whether temporary or permanent) is entitled to accommodation needed to attend school and participate as fully as possible in school activities. This accommodation may be related to a medical or an education issue. The 504 team for this child includes teachers, school nurse, possibly therapists, and parents and child, with input from health care provider. For example, a child with a long leg cast who has to go up and down steps to change classes would need accommodation—either staying in the same room all day, leaving one class early enough to be able to get to the next class, having someone else carry his or her books, or possibly having a teacher provide lessons at home. As many accommodations can be made as necessary for the child to be able to be successful in school.

✓ Adjustments needed for activities of daily living (ADL).

✓ Age-appropriate (developmental age, not just chronologic age) safety measures to help prevent further injuries:
- Childproof home and play area (include what is appropriate for *all* children in home).
- Avoid use of baby walkers, which are responsible for many injuries in infants.
- Proper use of protective equipment (e.g., car safety seats, bicycle helmets).
- Adaptation of child safety restraint system to accommodate cast/immobilization device.
- Importance of supervising young children while playing.
- Realistic expectations for child.

✓ When to call health care provider:
- Child complains of pain consistently in the same spot or pain seems to be getting worse.
- Child has tingling or numbness of toes or fingers.
- Child cannot feel something touching fingers or toes.
- Red or sore areas appear around cast edges.
- Child's fingers or toes are cold when in a warm environment.
- Child's nails stay pale when pressing on them and releasing pressure.

- Child's nails look blue even after elevating limb.
- Child's fingers or toes become very swollen several days after injury. Most swelling should occur in the first 48 hr.
- A foul smell comes from the cast.
- A "hot" spot is felt on the cast.
- Staining appears on the cast that was not there when child first came home. This could be an infected area or pressure sore.
- Child complains of constant itching that nothing helps.
- Cast is too tight or too loose.
- The cast starts to break down or fall apart or has indented areas. The cast may need to be reinforced or replaced to provide appropriate support for the injured area.
- Swelling after the first few days, pain, numbness, tingling, red marks or sores, and foul smell are serious signs of a problem. Talk with child's health care provider

immediately. If health care provider is unavailable, go to nearest emergency care facility.

✓ Importance of follow-up care.

✓ Referral to community resources for assistance as needed (e.g., in providing safe home environment and transport to accommodate cast/immobilization device). Additional information can be obtained by contacting the local children's hospital, Social Services, and the following organizations:

National SAFE KIDS Campaign
1301 Pennsylvania Avenue, NW, Suite 1000
Washington, DC 20004
(202) 662-0600
www.safekids.org/

Easter Seals
230 West Monroe, Suite 1800
Chicago, IL 60606-4802
(800) 221-6827 or (312) 726-6200
www.easter-seals.com/

Gastroenteritis

astroenteritis, one of the most common outpatient infectious diseases seen in children, is an inflammation of the stomach and intestines that accompanies numerous gastrointestinal (GI) disorders. Acute infectious gastroenteritis is caused by a variety of bacterial, viral, and parasitic pathogens. Rotavirus infection is the most common cause of gastroenteritis in infants and young children worldwide. Rotaviral gastroenteritis affects almost all children by the time they are 3 yr old, but it occurs most often between 3-24 mo of age.

Other common causes of infectious gastroenteritis include *Salmonella, Shigella,* and *Campylobacter* as the most common bacterial pathogens and *Giardia* and *Cryptosporidium* as the most common parasites. *Clostridium difficile* is the most common nosocomial source, and it occurs after antibiotic use.

HEALTH CARE SETTING

Primary care, with possible hospitalization depending on severity of illness

ASSESSMENT

Signs and symptoms vary widely depending on illness severity. Age, general health, and environment are factors that predispose children to gastroenteritis.

Signs and symptoms: Children usually present with some degree of the following:

- Fever
- Vomiting
- Diarrhea: Wide range of frequency and character (e.g., watery, bloody)
- Tenesmus: Painfully urgent but ineffectual attempt to urinate or defecate
- Abdominal pain
- Dehydration: Symptoms vary depending on degree of dehydration/water deficit
  - Minimal (<3%): No physical signs and symptoms, possibly increased thirst

- Mild (3%-5%): May have slight dryness of mucous membranes, thickened saliva, mild oliguria, and normal capillary refill time and be alert and consolable.
- Moderate (6%-9%): Dry lips and buccal mucosa, sunken eyes and fontanel, diminished or absent tears, decreased skin elasticity and turgor, oliguria, delayed capillary refill time, irritability, or listlessness.
- Severe (>10%): Moderate dehydration signs and symptoms, as well as signs of impending circulatory collapse (i.e., cool extremities, cyanosis, hypotension, tachycardia, thready pulse, capillary refill time >3 sec, grunting, lethargy, or coma).

Most often isotonic dehydration occurs:

- Infants and young children have a greater percentage of body weight that is water than adults (e.g., a newborn has 75%-80% of body weight that is water, and 40% of that is extracellular; a preschooler has 60%-65% of body weight that is water, and 30% of that is extracellular).
- Extracellular fluid is lost first with gastroenteritis.
- The younger the child, the more quickly dehydration occurs.
- Insensible water loss is also greater in infants and young children via skin and GI tract because of a proportionally greater body surface area in relation to body mass. Increased RR also increases insensible water loss.

The most serious consequences of gastroenteritis are dehydration, electrolyte imbalance, and malnutrition.

DIAGNOSTIC TESTS

History is important in determining source of gastroenteritis and if there is a need for any tests. In general, laboratory tests are not performed unless the child exhibits moderate-to-severe dehydration, appears toxic, and has abdominal pain or bloody stools.

Complete blood count (CBC): Hgb and Hct are elevated in dehydration. The differential will determine whether viral or bacterial infection is present. In a bacterial infection the white blood cell (WBC) count is elevated with increased polymorphonuclear leukocytes or neutrophils. In a viral infection the WBC count is slightly elevated with increased lymphocytes.

Serum electrolytes: To determine severity of electrolyte imbalance and type of fluid replacement necessary.

Creatinine and blood urea nitrogen (BUN): Elevated with dehydration but should return to normal with rehydration.

Blood culture: Obtained if child is acutely ill to help determine cause of illness.

Stool specimen: Examined if diarrhea lasts more than a few days to help determine cause.

Stool culture: Obtained if blood or mucus is present in stool, when symptoms are severe, or if there is history of travel to a developing country.

Stool for ova and parasites: May be used instead of culture because it is less expensive and often more reliable. A specimen is obtained 3 days in a row.

Nursing Diagnosis:

Deficient Fluid Volume

related to fluid loss secondary to fever, vomiting, diarrhea

Desired Outcome: Within 24 hr following intervention/treatment, the infant/child exhibits adequate hydration as evidenced by alertness and responsiveness, anterior fontanel soft and not sunken (in children <2 yr), moist oral mucous membranes, elastic abdominal skin turgor, and age-appropriate urine output (UO; i.e., infant 2-3 ml/kg/hr, toddler and preschooler 2 ml/kg/hr, school-age 1-2 ml/kg/hr, and adolescent 0.5-1 ml/kg/hr).

INTERVENTIONS	RATIONALES
Weigh child on admission and daily on the same scale, at same time of day, and wearing same amount of clothing (infants are weighed without any clothing). Notify health care provider if child is losing weight.	Consistency with weight measurements helps ensure more accurate results. Weight is a useful indicator of fluid balance. Weight loss indicates that child is not receiving adequate fluid replacement and adjustments need to be made.
Monitor VS q4h or more often if outside normal parameters. Report abnormalities to health care provider.	Dehydration can quickly lead to shock in infants and young children.
Do not measure temperatures rectally.	Rectal temperature measurements stimulate stooling, which can lead to dehydration.
Administer oral rehydration solution (ORS), for example, Pedialyte, Infalyte, Ricelyte, Rehydralyte.	To replace fluid volume in children with minimal-to-moderate dehydration.
	- To make it more palatable for child, may add 1 tsp presweetened sugar-free Kool-Aid to chilled 1-liter bottle of ORS or try flavored brands of these solutions.
	- Small amounts are given frequently, especially if child is vomiting (5 ml q1-2min or small volume, depending on child's age and weight, q10-20min). This is from the 1996 guideline issued by American Academy of Pediatrics for children 1 mo-5 yr to replace fluid and electrolytes, as well as glucose. This guideline states that fluid should be replaced in small frequent volumes, which are better tolerated.
Do not give clear liquids such as apple juice, soda, gelatin, or sports drinks.	Liquids with a large amount of simple sugars can exacerbate osmotic effects associated with diarrhea and vomiting.
Do not give tea or soda with caffeine.	Caffeine can perpetuate diarrhea.
Do not give chicken or beef broth.	Broths are high in salt and low in carbohydrates.
Administer and monitor IV fluids as prescribed for severe dehydration and vomiting.	If child is unable to take sufficient ORS, IV fluid and electrolyte replacement likely will be necessary.

Continued

INTERVENTIONS	RATIONALES
Assess hydration status q4h.	Although child may be receiving maintenance fluids, he or she may still be dehydrated because of diarrhea, vomiting, and/or insensible water losses. A dehydrated child is likely to exhibit decreasing level of consciousness (LOC), sunken fontanel, dry or sticky oral mucous membrane, tented abdominal skin, and decreasing urinary output.
Ensure that child has at least minimal UO but that output is not more than intake.	Shows adequate hydration.
After child is rehydrated, calculate maintenance fluids based on child's weight.	The smaller the child, the greater the percentage of body weight is water. To meet minimal fluid requirements, the necessary volume is calculated in the following way: **Up to 10 kg: 100 ml/kg/24 hr = _____** **10-20 kg: 50 ml/kg/24 hr =** **>20 kg: 20 ml/kg/24 hr = _____** **= maintenance fluid requirement** *For example, if child weighs 43 kg:* 10 kg × 100 ml/kg/24 hr = 1000 ml/24 hr 10 kg × 50 ml/kg/24 hr = 500 ml/24 hr 23 kg × 20 ml/kg/24 hr = 460 ml/24 hr 43 kg 1960 ml/24 hr Maintenance fluid requirement is 1960 ml/24 hr.
Ensure that child is receiving at least maintenance fluids.	Minimum amount of fluid needed on a daily basis to be well hydrated if there are no unusual fluid losses (e.g., fever, diarrhea, vomiting).
Administer medications as prescribed	For example, antibiotics to treat the bacterial pathogen causing the diarrhea.
After child is rehydrated, begin regular diet as tolerated.	Enteral nutrition stimulates renewal of intestinal cells, whereas fasting increases gut atrophy and permeability, which can contribute to dehydration. A regular diet is likely to comprise the following factors: low in fat, avoiding high concentrations of simple sugars, and encouraging complex carbohydrates such as starches. Examples of an appropriate diet include cereals, lean meats, yogurt, and cooked vegetables.
Instruct family members in providing ORS, monitoring I&O, and assessing for signs of dehydration.	To improve compliance and promote optimum results.

●●● **Related NIC and NOC labels:** *NIC:* Fluid/Electrolyte Management; Hypovolemia Management; Intravenous Therapy; Diarrhea Management; Vital Signs Monitoring *NOC:* Hydration

Nursing Diagnosis:

Risk for Impaired Skin Integrity

related to irritation caused by frequent stooling

Desired Outcome: Child's skin in perineal and perianal areas remains intact.

INTERVENTIONS	RATIONALES
Assess perineal and perianal areas for signs of irritation or excoriation with every diaper change.	The earlier the problem is detected, the sooner appropriate interventions can be made to ensure that skin remains intact.
Change diaper as soon as it becomes wet or soiled.	Helps keep skin clean and dry.
Cleanse buttocks gently (pat, do not rub) with water or immerse in tepid water to cleanse. Avoid using soap if possible.	Diarrheal stools are very irritating to the skin. Rubbing the skin every time the diaper is changed would irritate it further. Soap dries skin by removing normal moisturizing skin oils, thereby increasing potential for irritation and skin breakdown.
Do not use commercial baby wipes with alcohol or perfume or baby powder on irritated or excoriated skin.	All are painful to irritated skin.
If not contraindicated, apply protective ointments such as Vaseline, A&D, or zinc oxide when child is wearing a diaper.	To protect skin from irritation.
Leave diaper area open to air if possible (but not in the presence of explosive diarrhea). Reapply protective ointment before putting diaper on.	Facilitates drying and healing
Instruct family members in appropriate skin care methods.	Increases likelihood of family using these techniques at home.

●●● **Related NIC and NOC labels:** *NIC:* Skin Surveillance; Bathing; Skin Care: Topical Treatments; Diarrhea Management *NOC:* Tissue Integrity: Skin & Mucous Membranes

Nursing Diagnosis:

Risk for Infection

related to gastroenteritis and lack of knowledge about transmission prevention

Desired Outcome: Following intervention, family members and other children are free of indicators of gastroenteritis.

INTERVENTIONS	RATIONALES
Implement Standard Precautions as well as appropriate Expanded Precautions. For more information, see Appendix for "Infection Prevention and Control," p. 831.	Reduces risk of spreading infection. These include: - Good handwashing: Wash hands before and after working with child, even with appropriate gloving. - Wear gloves when changing diaper. - Wear other personal protective equipment (PPE) as designated by isolation guidelines.
Dispose of linen and other soiled items per hospital protocol.	To prevent spread of infection.
Apply diaper securely.	To prevent fecal spread.
Try to keep infants and small children from placing hands or objects in contaminated areas.	Gastroenteritis is mostly spread by the fecal-oral route. Infants and young children tend to put their hands in their mouths, and if their hands get into their diaper or stool, fecal-oral spread occurs.
Teach children, as appropriate, protective measures such as washing their hands after using the toilet.	To prevent spread of infection.
Instruct family members and visitors in protective measures, especially handwashing and not visiting other patients.	To reduce risk of spreading infection.

●●● **Related NIC and NOC labels:** *NIC:* Infection Control; Infection Prevention; Communicable Disease Management *NOC:* Infection Status

Nursing Diagnosis:

Imbalanced Nutrition: Less than body requirements

related to inadequate intake and fluid loss secondary to vomiting, diarrhea, and fever

Desired Outcome: Within 48-72 hr following intervention/treatment, child maintains or gains weight and exhibits no further vomiting or diarrhea.

INTERVENTIONS	RATIONALES
Assess weight on admission and daily (on same scale, at same time, wearing same clothing—no diaper on infants).	Measures child's progress in attaining adequate nutrition. Consistency with weight measurements helps ensure more accurate results.
If mother is breastfeeding, encourage her to continue along with giving ORS (if child has mild-to-moderate dehydration) as described in **Deficient Fluid Volume,** earlier.	Tends to reduce severity and duration of illness by maintaining normal intake so that child has adequate nutrition.
Avoid BRAT (bananas, rice, apples, and toast) diet.	These foods do not provide complete caloric and protein requirements. They provide excessive carbohydrates and, overall, are also low in electrolytes. Therefore the child does not get the needed nutrients.
Resume regular diet when child is rehydrated as described in **Deficient Fluid Volume,** earlier.	Enteral nutrition stimulates renewal of intestinal cells, whereas fasting increases gut atrophy and permeability.
Instruct family in appropriate diet.	To gain compliance with treatment plan.
Monitor response to feedings.	To assess feeding tolerance.
	- Some children have increased stooling with lactose-containing milk products.
	- Most children do well with lactose-containing milk products, especially if they are eating foods at the same time.
Give liquids at room temperature.	Cold liquids stimulate peristalsis and hence diarrhea.
Keep room as odor free as possible.	Minimizing unpleasant or strong (perfume/aftershave) odors increases interest in eating and feeling of well-being.
Provide oral hygiene.	Enhances sense of well-being and improves chances of child eating/drinking more.

●●● **Related NIC and NOC labels:** *NIC:* Diet Staging; Nutrient Intake; Teaching: Prescribed Diet; Sustenance Support; Fluid Monitoring; Lactation Counseling *NOC:* Nutritional Status; Nutritional Status: Food & Fluid Intake; Nutritional Status: Nutrient Intake

Additional Nursing Diagnoses/ Problems:

"Psychosocial Support for the Patient's Family and Significant Others" for:

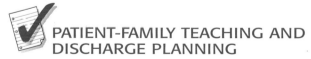

PATIENT-FAMILY TEACHING AND DISCHARGE PLANNING

When providing child-family teaching, focus on sensory information, avoid giving excessive information, and initiate a visiting nurse for follow-up teaching and assessment as needed. Include verbal and written information about the following (ensure that written material is at a level the reader can understand):

✓ Pathophysiology of gastroenteritis.

✓ Causes of gastroenteritis: If caused by improper food storage, address proper hygiene, formula or food preparation, handling and storage.

✓ Why gastroenteritis can be such a serious problem, especially for infants and young children:

- The younger the child, the greater the percentage of body weight that is water.
  - Premature infant: 85%-90% of body weight is water.
  - Full-term infant: 75%-80% of body weight is water.
  - Preschooler: 60%-65% of body weight is water.
  - Adolescents: 50%-55% of body weight is water.
- Therefore the younger the child, the quicker dehydration can occur (the child loses more fluid than is taken in).
- Problems that cause or increase severity of dehydration: fever, vomiting, diarrhea, not eating or drinking enough.

✓ Importance of checking hydration status q2-4h when child is ill with any of the above problems (the younger the child, the more often status is reassessed):

- Is the child alert and interactive? Child would not be as alert and interactive as normal if dehydrated.
- Check the soft spot on top of head in children <2 yr old: if it is sunken in, the child is dehydrated.
- No tears when crying in a child >6 mo old.
- Check inside the mouth, not the lips: if dry or sticky, the child is dehydrated.
- Pinch skin on the abdomen: if it sits up like a tent instead of falling down right away, the child is dehydrated.
- How many wet diapers does the child normally have per day? If the number is decreased or they are not as wet as normal, the child may be dehydrated.

✓ Contagious aspect of gastroenteritis. It is important to use good handwashing technique, especially after changing a diaper. Teach children that are old enough to wash their hands after they use the toilet.

✓ Feeding of child who has diarrhea:

- If child is breastfeeding, continue breastfeeding and supplement with ORS (e.g., Pedialyte, Infalyte, or Rehydralyte).
- If child is taking only formula or milk, it may not be necessary to stop that fluid as long as child is also taking ORS.
- 1 tsp presweetened sugar-free Kool-Aid can be added to a chilled 1-L bottle of ORS to improve taste or use flavored ORS.

✓ Feeding of child who is vomiting: Give small amounts of ORS frequently—amount varies depending on age and weight of child.

✓ Once child is rehydrated, begin regular diet as tolerated.

- Do not give BRAT (bananas, rice, apples, tea, or toast). This combination does not provide enough calories or protein.
- Use low-fat foods (no peanut butter, potato chips, or hot dogs).
- Give starchy foods such as cooked baby cereal, oatmeal, cream of wheat, rice, nonsugared cereals, noodles, potatoes, bread, and yogurt.
- Give fruits (not packed in syrup), vegetables without butter, and well-cooked chicken, fish, or lean meat.
- Avoid concentrated sweets such as candy or ice cream.
- Most children have no problems drinking formula or milk.

✓ Call health care provider when:

- There are signs of dehydration.
- There is blood or pus in the stool.
- The child has a fever.
- The vomiting or diarrhea lasts >8-24 hr (the younger the child, the earlier the health care provider should be called).
- Child is not drinking fluids or is less alert than usual.
- Child has abdominal pain >2 hr.
- Child is <6 mo old and is vomiting or has diarrhea.
- Diaper area is very red or irritated and getting worse.

✓ Change diaper frequently:

- Clean after stool with warm water. Pat skin; do not rub.
- Do not use soap if possible. If that is not possible, use mild, nonantiseptic soap.
- Do not use baby wipes containing alcohol or fragrances.
- Avoid powders and cornstarch, which trap fluid and get caked in creases.
- Leave skin open to air if irritated (but not in the presence of explosive diarrhea).
- Put protective ointment such as Vaseline, A&D, or zinc oxide on skin.

✓ Phone numbers to call should questions or concerns about treatment or disease arise after discharge.

✓ Importance of follow-up care.

✓ Referral to community resources as necessary.

84

Otitis Media

Otitis media is the most common reason for visits to the pediatrician in the first 3 yr of life, the leading cause of antibiotic use, and the most common cause of hearing loss in children. The highest incidence of otitis media occurs between 6 mo and 3 yr. There is growing evidence that many "ear infections" will resolve within 2-7 days without antibiotics. With the continuing problem of overdiagnosis and the increase in drug-resistant *Streptococcus pneumoniae* (believed to be the major cause of ear infections in young children), one of the objectives of Healthy People 2010 is to reduce the number and frequency of courses of antibiotics for ear infections in young children.

Otitis media includes several conditions ranging from acute to chronic with or without symptoms.

- **Otitis media (OM):** Inflammation of the middle ear.
- **Acute otitis media (AOM):** Middle ear infection with symptoms of acute illness (fever, pain, irritability) and full or bulging tympanic membrane (TM) under positive pressure that lasts ≤3 wk.
- **Otitis media with effusion (OME)** or serous otitis media: An inflammation of the middle ear without signs and symptoms of acute infection (other than reduced hearing), TM retracted or in neutral position under negative pressure or no pressure, and fluid in the middle ear space.
- **Chronic OM with effusion:** Middle ear effusion lasting >3 mo.

HEALTH CARE SETTING

Primary care; possible hospitalization if OM exacerbates a chronic condition

ASSESSMENT

Signs and symptoms: Vary depending on type of OM and age of child.

AOM:

- *Infant or young child:* fever; possible ear drainage; crying; irritable and fussy; may tug, rub, or hold affected ear; sleep disturbances; decreased appetite; rolling head side to side; difficult to comfort; possible difficulty hearing.
- *Older child:* fever, possible ear drainage, complaints of ear hurting, crying, irritable, lethargic, decreased appetite (chewing causes increased ear pain), possible difficulty hearing.

OME: Difficulty hearing, feeling of fullness/pressure in ear, tinnitus or popping sounds, mild balance disturbances.

Physical assessment

AOM: Pneumatic otoscopy reveals bulging, red, immobile TM (or decreased mobility of TM). Crying, removal of cerumen and thereby irritating the auditory canal, and fever can cause redness of the TM without infection being present. Postauricular and cervical lymph nodes may be enlarged.

OME: Pneumatic otoscopy may show a slightly injected, dull gray membrane, obscured landmarks; and fluid visible behind the TM. There is also decreased mobility of the TM.

DIAGNOSTIC TESTS

Pneumatic otoscopy: A pneumatic attachment to the otoscope enables health care provider to introduce puffs of air into the ear. The TM does not move as well with fluid behind it. This device improves diagnostic accuracy by assessing mobility of TM, as well as visualizing it.

Tympanometry: Method of providing information about possible presence of a middle ear effusion, including the actual pressures in the middle ear space. This is a quick and simple method of assessing TM mobility.

Tympanocentesis: Gold standard for diagnosis of AOM, although it is not routinely used because of cost, effort, and lack of availability. It involves removal of fluid from the middle ear to identify the bacteria causing the infection. It improves diagnostic accuracy, guides treatment by finding the causative pathogen, and avoids unnecessary medical or surgical intervention. It is especially useful in AOM unresponsive to antibiotics or recurrent AOM.

Culture and sensitivity: Not routinely done, but if drainage is present or tympanocentesis is performed, it helps guide treatment in finding causative pathogen and antibiotics to which it is sensitive.

Nursing Diagnosis:

Acute Pain

related to increased pressure in the middle ear secondary to presence of fluid and/or infection

Desired Outcome: Child is free from pain or has significantly decreased pain (e.g., <2 on Wong-Baker FACES scale or <4 on FLACC or a numeric scale) within 1-2 hr after intervention/treatment.

INTERVENTIONS	RATIONALES
Establish appropriate pain scale for child (FLACC, Wong-Baker FACES, or numeric scale) and assess pain level at least q4h.	A pain scale appropriate for child will enable accurate assessment of pain level and help evaluate relief obtained.
Administer antipyretics/analgesics on a regular basis, for example, q4-6h for a maximum of 5 doses/day.	Provides better control of fever and pain than on a prn basis.
Reassess pain level and/or temperature 1 hr after administering medication.	Evaluates effectiveness of pain relief measure.
Administer antibiotics, if prescribed.	Many cases of AOM resolve in 2-7 days without antibiotics.
Instruct parents to:	
- Administer correct dose of medication at correct time.	For optimal effectiveness of medication.
- Administer all doses (correct number/day and total number of doses prescribed).	Child may feel better after several days, and parents may stop giving medication.
- Store medications appropriately.	Many antibiotics have to be refrigerated.
Use localized comfort measures based on developmental age and that which provides maximal comfort for child.	What is comforting to an infant usually is not comforting to an adolescent. Every child has specific measures that are comforting to him or her.
- Apply warm compresses to affected ear or have child lie on affected ear on a heating pad on low setting, covered with a towel to protect child from potential burns.	
- Apply wrapped ice bag over affected ear to decrease edema and pressure.	
Administer analgesic otic drops if prescribed.	To relieve severe pain.
Position for comfort according to type of OM.	To decrease pressure on the TM.
- AOM: Position with affected ear in dependent position.	
- OME: Elevate head.	
Teach older children to open eustachian tube by yawning or performing Valsalva's maneuver.	Facilitates drainage of fluid from middle ear into the pharynx; decreases pressure on TM.

●●● **Related NIC and NOC labels:** *NIC:* Medication: Administration; Pain Management; Positioning; Heat/Cold Application; Teaching: Procedure/Treatment *NOC:* Comfort Level; Pain Control

Nursing Diagnosis:

Risk for Deficient Fluid Volume

related to losses associated with fever and decreased intake

Desired Outcome: Within 24 hr of intervention, child is alert and responsive, anterior fontanel is soft and not sunken (in child <2 yr), oral mucus membranes are moist, abdominal skin turgor is good, child has age/weight-appropriate urine output (e.g., infant 2-3 ml/kg/hr, toddler and preschool child 2 ml/kg/hr, school-age child 1-2 ml/kg/hr, and adolescent 0.5-1 ml/kg/hr), and child receives at least maintenance level fluids.

INTERVENTIONS	RATIONALES
Assess hydration status q4h, instruct parent how to do this, and explain its importance:	The younger the child is and the less he or she weighs, the greater the percentage of body weight that is water. The child can become dehydrated easily. Routinely assessing for dehydration in a child who is running a fever and/or has decreased intake facilitates rapid treatment to resolve dehydration. A child who is dehydrated may have decreasing LOC, sunken anterior fontanel (if <2 yr old), dry or sticky oral mucous membranes, tenting abdominal skin, and decreasing urine output.
Teach parents when to call health care provider regarding dehydration.	Facilitates parent's ability to detect a problem early, thereby ensuring quicker problem resolution. Parent should call under the following conditions: - Child not as alert as usual - Anterior fontanel sunken - Inside of mouth dry or sticky - Skin on abdomen stays up like a tent when pinched - Fewer wet diapers than usual/voiding less than usual
Calculate maintenance fluids for the child and teach family to provide this in terms that they can understand.	Specific information enables parents to ensure that their child receives correct fluid volume. For example, if the child weighs 15 kg, maintenance fluids are 1250 ml/day (42 oz), and if the child drinks from a 6-oz sippy cup, that child needs to drink at least 7 sippy cups of fluid a day. Calculation for minimum daily maintenance fluids: For the child weighing 15 kg. Up to 10 kg: 100 ml/kg/24 hr = 10 kg × 100 ml/kg/24 hr = 1000 ml/24 hr 10 – 20 kg: 50 ml/kg/24 hr = 5 kg × 50 ml/kg/24 hr = 250 ml/24 hr >20 kg: 20 ml/kg/hr = 15 kg 1250 ml/24 hr
Offer child small amounts of fluid at a time and soft food.	Sucking on a nipple or straw or chewing can increase ear pain.

●●● **Related NIC and NOC labels:** *NIC:* Hypovolemia Management; Fever Treatment; Fluid Monitoring
NOC: Hydration

Nursing Diagnosis:

Deficient Knowledge:

Disease process and prevention

Desired Outcome: Parents verbalize accurate understanding of disease process and ways to decrease/prevent future incidents of OM.

INTERVENTIONS	RATIONALES
Describe different types of OM and symptoms of each.	Knowledge and understanding improve compliance with treatment plan. - AOM: Infection of middle ear; fever, pain.

Continued

INTERVENTIONS	RATIONALES
	- OME: Inflammation of middle ear with fluid behind TM without signs of acute infection; feeling of fullness in ear, difficulty hearing.
Instruct parents about importance of giving full course of antibiotics if they are prescribed and having ear rechecked when medication is finished.	Adequate treatment of AOM requires full course of antibiotics. Ear rechecks assess effectiveness of treatment.
Discuss preventative feeding practices for infant.	Feeding practices that prevent OM in infants include the following: - Feed infant in an upright position: Facilitates drainage of middle ear. - Do not put infant in bed with a bottle: Increases incidence of ear infections. - Do not use pacifier after 1 yr old: Causes bacteria to reflux back up into the ear.
Avoid smoking around child.	Passive smoking increases incidence of OM.
Encourage gentle blowing of nose during upper respiratory infection (URI) rather than forceful nose blowing.	Decreases risk of transferring organisms from the eustachian tube to the middle ear.
Encourage blowing activities (e.g., bubbles, pinwheels) or chewing sugarless gum during a URI.	Helps to promote equalization of pressure in middle ear.
Explain prevention of ear pain during airplane travel.	Increased atmospheric pressure increases ear pain. - Health care provider may prescribe nasal mucosal shrinking spray if child has URI or chronic OME to decrease pressure on TM from edema. - Parent should offer bottle or pacifier to infant or give older child gum during descent to help equalize TM pressure.
Describe potential complications of OM.	Inadequate or noncompliance with treatment may result in the following: - Hearing loss - Perforated, scarred eardrum - Mastoiditis - Cholesteatoma (a cystic mass composed of epithelial cells and cholesterol that occurs as a result of chronic OM. It may occlude the middle ear, or enzymes produced by the cyst may destroy adjacent bones, including the ossicles.) - Intracranial infections such as meningitis

●●● **Related NIC and NOC labels:** *NIC:* Teaching: Procedure/Treatment; Teaching: Disease Process; Teaching: Prescribed Medication *NOC:* Knowledge: Illness Care; Knowledge: Disease Process

ADDITIONAL NURSING DIAGNOSES/ PROBLEMS:

"Psychosocial Support for the Patient's Family and Significant Others" for relevant psychosocial nursing diagnoses	p. 95
"Asthma" for **Anxiety**	p. 604

✓ PATIENT-FAMILY TEACHING AND DISCHARGE PLANNING

When providing child-family teaching, focus on sensory information and avoid giving excessive information. Include verbal and written information about the following, ensuring that written information is at a level the reader can understand:

✓ Types of ear infections, signs and symptoms, and treatment of each type.

✓ Importance of administering antibiotics as prescribed.
- Return demonstration of drawing up correct dose of medication and administering it to the child correctly.
- Use of a syringe or other calibrated device for administering medication to children.
- Administering doses at correct time each day and for total number of days prescribed.
- Teach five rights of medication administration:
  - Right child
  - Right medication
  - Right dose (i.e., right concentration and right amount of medication)
  - Right route (e.g., ear drops or oral medication)
  - Right time
- Correct storage of medication (e.g., some need to be refrigerated)

✓ Method of assessing pain in child and importance of administering analgesic for pain on a regular basis.

✓ Treating fever correctly:
- Discuss at what temperature antipyretic is needed.
- Explain that fever increases ear pain.

✓ If receiving otic drops, how to administer based on child's age:
- Child <3 yr old, pull ear lobe down and back.
- Child >3 yr old, pull pinna up and back.

✓ Prevention:
- Never give infant a bottle to drink while lying down.
- Keep infant upright during feeding.
- Breastfeed as long as possible.
- Avoid pacifiers after 1 yr of age.
- Do not smoke around child or take him or her where smoking occurs.
- If child has to go to day care, try to put with least number of children possible.
- Vaccinate child against pneumococcus infections.

✓ Signs and symptoms of dehydration:
- Child is not as alert and responsive as normal.
- Soft spot on top of head looks sunken (for children <2 yr).
- Inside of mouth (not lips) is dry or sticky rather than moist.
- Skin on abdomen sits up like a tent when pinched.
- Decreased number of wet diapers or same number but not as wet as normal for infant or young child or decreased number of voids/day in older child.

✓ Phone number to call should any questions arise about therapy or disease after office/emergency room visit.

✓ Importance of follow-up (e.g., many health care providers will do an ear recheck after child finishes medication).

✓ When to call health care provider:
- Fever or pain has not decreased after 48 hr while on antibiotics.
- Child is showing signs of dehydration.
- Child develops a stiff neck.
- Drainage present from child's ear canal.

✓ If child has had OME for >3 mo, he or she should have hearing evaluated.

✓ Referral to pediatric ear, nose, and throat (ENT) specialist if OM or OME is chronic.

Poisoning

Poisoning can result in death and is a leading cause of hospitalization in children. It may occur through ingestion, inhalation, or contact with skin or mucous membranes and is seen most often in children <5 yr old, with the greatest incidence in children <2 yr old. Curiosity and natural desire to put things in their mouths put younger children at greater risk for accidental poisoning. The most commonly ingested poisons in young children include cosmetics, household cleaning agents, and medications (prescription or over the counter). Inhalation of carbon monoxide is a common wintertime occurrence. Adolescents also have an increased incidence of hospitalization resulting from poisoning, but it is most often intentional and frequently involves inhaling substances (e.g., glues/adhesives, nail polish remover, paint thinner, air conditioning coolant) or ingesting alcohol or drugs (e.g., marijuana or ecstasy).

Eighty to ninety percent of all poisoning incidents occur in the home. Most homes have more than 500 toxic substances in them, and one third of these are in the kitchen. Improper storage of toxic substances is a major cause of poisoning in children.

Other risk factors besides developmental age include the following:

- Male children are more likely than females to be poisoned.
- Black children <5 yr have a poisoning death rate twice that of white children.
- Children are more likely to suffer from elevated blood levels of poison if they live in homes built before 1978.
- Children living in low-income communities or in large metropolitan areas are at greater risk.

HEALTH CARE SETTING
Emergency room with possible hospitalization

ASSESSMENT
Varies depending on source of the poisoning.

Gastrointestinal system: Nausea, vomiting, diarrhea, abdominal pain, anorexia.

Respiratory system: Depressed or labored respirations, unexplained cyanosis.

Circulatory system: Signs of shock, including increased, weak pulse; decreased BP; increased, shallow respirations; pallor; cool, clammy skin.

Central nervous system: Dizziness, overstimulation, sudden loss of consciousness, behavioral changes, seizures, stupor/lethargy, coma.

Integumentary system: Skin rashes; burns to mouth, esophagus, and stomach; eye inflammation; skin irritations; stains around the mouth; oral mucus membrane lesions.

Signs and symptoms specific to various poisons:

- **Acetaminophen ingestion** (included in many over-the-counter medications) is the most common drug ingestion in children. Symptoms occur in stages:
  - Stage 1 (first 24 hr): malaise, nausea, vomiting, sweating, pallor, and weakness, or the child may be asymptomatic.
  - Stage 2 (next 24-48 hr): decrease or disappearance of symptoms in stage 1 and right upper quadrant (RUQ) pain caused by liver damage and increase in liver enzymes.
  - Stage 3 (3-7 days): jaundice, liver necrosis, and possible death from hepatic failure.
  - Stage 4: occurs if the child does not die during the hepatic stage (stage 3) and involves gradual recovery.
- **Corrosive ingestion** (toilet and drain cleaners, bleach, ammonia, liquid dishwasher detergent, denture cleaner). Complaints of severe burning pain in mouth, throat, and stomach; whitish burns of mouth and pharynx with edema of lips, tongue, and pharynx; difficulty swallowing, which leads to drooling; respiratory distress; anxiety and agitation; and shock.
- **Hydrocarbon ingestion** (gasoline, kerosene, paint thinner, lamp oil, turpentine, lighter fluid, some furniture polishes). Gagging, choking, coughing; nausea, vomiting; characteristic petroleum breath odor; central nervous system (CNS) depression. Respiratory symptoms of pulmonary involvement include tachypnea, cyanosis, retractions, and grunting.

- **Lead ingestion** (paint chips from lead-based paint, lead-contaminated dust in home, soil contaminated with lead, lead solder used in plumbing and artwork, vinyl mini-blinds, improperly glazed pottery, and traditional/folk remedies). Symptoms may be vague with insidious onset. Children absorb 50% of the lead they ingest and deposit it in their growing bones. Adults only absorb 10% of lead ingested.
  - **Gastrointestinal:** anorexia, nausea, vomiting, and constipation.
  - **CNS:** *Low-dose exposure*—distractibility, impulsivity, hyperactivity, hearing impairment, mild intellectual deficits, loss of recently acquired developmental skills, and loss of coordination. *High-dose exposure*—lead encephalopathy may occur 4-6 wk following first symptoms. Mental retardation, severe ataxia, altered level of consciousness, paralysis, blindness, seizures, coma, and death all can occur.
  - **Cardiovascular:** hypertension, bradycardia.
  - **Hematologic:** anemia.
  - **Renal:** glycosuria, proteinuria, possible acute or chronic renal failure, and impaired calcium function.
- **Iron ingestion** (vitamin supplements with iron): one of most commonly ingested poisonous substances in

children. It occurs in stages ranging from the initial stage (0.5-6 hr after ingestion) with vomiting, hematemesis, bloody stools, and abdominal pain to the hepatic injury stage (48-96 hr after the ingestion) with seizures and coma. If the child survives, pyloric or duodenal stenosis or hepatic cirrhosis develops 2-4 wk after ingestion.
- **Carbon monoxide inhalation** (improperly ventilated heaters, wood stoves, and charcoal grills; poorly ventilated automobile).
  - *Low-level exposure:* Headache, stomach upset, and being tired (similar to early "flu" symptoms).
  - *High-level exposure:* Within minutes, cherry red lips and cheeks, altered level of consciousness (LOC), extreme dizziness, and coma. Cherry-red skin is a late sign most commonly noted in fatalities.

DIAGNOSTIC TESTS

History and physical examination help to determine tests necessary.

Serum levels: Blood levels of acetaminophen, salicylate, lead, and iron help determine if treatment with antidote is necessary.

Arterial blood gases: May be done if child is hypoventilating.

Serum carboxyhemoglobin level: To determine degree of carbon monoxide poisoning.

Nursing Diagnosis:

Risk for Poisoning

related to inadequate parental knowledge about poison prevention

Desired Outcomes: Child does not ingest, inhale, or touch potentially toxic substances. Immediately following teaching, parents verbalize accurate understanding of how to childproof all areas (home, babysitter's home, grandparent's home) in which child lives or plays.

INTERVENTIONS	RATIONALES
Based on child's developmental age, discuss ways in which child might be exposed to poisons.	Understanding developmentally appropriate behavior enables parents to childproof home more effectively. For example, a 1-yr-old puts everything in the mouth but is not climbing yet, so any potential poison the child could reach while crawling or standing should be secured out of his or her reach.
Going room-by-room, discuss areas that need to be child-proofed, with special emphasis on kitchen, storage areas, and bathroom.	Many poisonings involve household cleaners or medications. Knowledge of childproofing each area decreases risk of exposure to potentially toxic substances.
Review all materials in home environment that could be poisonous.	Parents may not be aware of all the potentially poisonous substances in their home. Increased awareness likely will decrease child's exposure to poisonous substances, including the following:
	- Household cleaners, disinfectants
	- Cosmetics
	- Insecticides
	- Mouthwash with alcohol in it

Continued

INTERVENTIONS	RATIONALES
	- Alcohol (beverages or rubbing alcohol)
	- Liquid dishwasher detergent
	- Foreign bodies and toys, such as bubble-blowing solution
	- Arts, crafts, and office supplies, such as pen and ink
	- Toxic plants
	- Hydrocarbons
	- Prescription and nonprescription medications
Describe ways to childproof home to prevent poisoning.	Guidelines enhance parents' ability to effectively and efficiently childproof home against poisoning. Examples include:
	- Put childproof locks on all kitchen, bathroom, and storage room cabinets.
	- Make sure all poisonous products are out of reach in locked cabinets.
	- Avoid having poisonous plants (e.g., azaleas, dumb cane [dieffenbachia], mistletoe) in the home or yard where children play.
	- Do not leave purse/briefcase sitting out that contains medication, cosmetics, or pens.
	- Buy medications with child-resistant caps.
	- Do not store poisonous substances in food containers; store them in the original container.
	- Throw away all old medications and other potential poisons that are no longer being used; flush medications down the toilet. Dispose of other poisons out of child's reach (i.e., if poison is discarded in the kitchen trash can and the child can reach the can, it was not disposed "out of child's reach"). Guidelines for disposing of hazardous household waste are available from the EPA at www.epa.gov/epaoswer/non-hw/muncpl/hhw.htm and from Earth 911 at www.earth911.org (this website provides closest locations for disposal of hazardous materials).
	- Hang or install a carbon monoxide detector on each level of the home on which bedrooms are located.
	- If home was built before 1978, have it tested for lead-based paint.
Discuss these general guidelines to prevent poisoning.	
- Stay alert when using poisonous household products.	Poisoning by ingestion or inhalation can occur in a matter of seconds.
- Never refer to medicine or vitamins as "candy."	Child may think it is harmless or tastes good.
- Do not take medicine in front of young children.	Toddlers and preschoolers often imitate adult behavior.
Reinforce importance of informing family/friends of above guidelines.	Even with home childproofed by parents, visitors may bring potentially poisonous substances into the home (e.g., grandmother may visit and leave purse containing medicine bottle on the floor).
Encourage parents to childproof all residences/facilities visited by child.	Child may be safe at home but not at day care or grandparents' home.

●●● **Related NIC and NOC labels:** *NIC:* Parent Education: Childrearing Family; Environmental Management: Safety; Surveillance: Safety *NOC:* Safety Behavior: Home Physical Environment; Safety Behavior: Personal; Safety Status: Physical Injury

Nursing Diagnosis:

Deficient Knowledge:

First aid for toxic ingestion/inhalation/exposure in accidental poisoning

Desired Outcome: Immediately following teaching, parents verbalize accurate knowledge of steps to take if accidental poisoning occurs.

INTERVENTIONS	RATIONALES
Teach Parents the Following:	
Post Poison Control Center (PCC) number on all phones. Also have emergency medical services (EMS) and pediatrician's number readily available.	It is vital to call PCC for possible ingestion of a toxic substance before administering any antidote to ensure correct treatment is implemented.
Have syrup of ipecac available and stored in a secured area.	To be used for gastric decontamination by inducing vomiting.
If syrup of ipecac is in the child's home, babysitter's home, or any other facility in which the child is cared for, it should be disposed of safely.	The American Academy of Pediatrics believes that ipecac should no longer be used routinely in the home as a poison treatment strategy and that any ipecac in the home should be disposed of safely (*Pediatrics* 112(5):1182-1185, November 2003).
Only administer ipecac with instructions from PCC, emergency room, or health care provider.	Ipecac causes vomiting, which may be contraindicated in some circumstances.
Review immediate action response if a child is poisoned.	To decrease absorption and provide appropriate treatment. Immediate actions include the following:
	- If swallowed, remove any remaining poison from mouth. Call PCC immediately.
	- If poison is on the skin, remove contaminated clothing right away without touching poison and rinse skin with running water. Wash skin with soap and water and rinse well. Call PCC immediately.
	- If poison is in the eye, flush the eye with lukewarm-to-cool water for a full 15 min. Call PCC immediately.
	- If poison is inhaled, move child to fresh air right away. Call PCC.
Discuss specific information parent should give to PCC.	Specific information enables PCC to direct treatment more appropriately. This should include:
	- Child's weight and age.
	- Time poisoning occurred.
	- Amount ingested.
	- Name of poison, if possible. If medicine bottle or container is available, have it on hand when speaking with PCC.

●●● **Related NIC and NOC labels:** *NIC:* Health Education; Teaching: Procedure/Treatment *NOC:* Knowledge: Child Safety; Knowledge: Health Resources; Knowledge: Illness Care; Knowledge: Treatment Regimen

ADDITIONAL NURSING DIAGNOSES/ PROBLEMS:

"Psychosocial Support for the Patient's   p. 95
Family and Significant Others" for such
nursing diagnoses as **Compromised
Family Coping** and **Fear** for family
whose child is being seen in emergency
room or is hospitalized for life-threatening
condition

"Bronchiolitis" for **Deficient Fluid Volume.**   p. 621
Child will be dehydrated related to
effects of ingested substances, treatment
for poisoning, or decreased fluid intake.

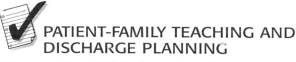

PATIENT-FAMILY TEACHING AND DISCHARGE PLANNING

When providing child-family teaching, focus on sensory information, avoid giving excessive information, and initiate a visiting nurse referral for necessary follow-up teaching or to assess safety of home. Include verbal and written information about the following (ensure that written information is at a level the reader can understand):

✓ Contributing factors to potential for poisoning for each child:
- Developmental age of child (e.g., cognitive, physical, and psychosocial)
- Environmental factors
- Behavioral problems
- Level of supervision

✓ Poison prevention tips:
- Keep all poisonous products out of reach in cabinets locked with safety locks.
- Know what household products are poisonous or potentially poisonous.
- Be careful and alert when using poisonous household products.
- Regularly discard old medications and other potential poisons in a safe manner.
- Keep all products in their original containers.
- Remember that many cosmetics and personal products may be poisonous (e.g., after-shave, cologne, hair spray, fingernail polish remover). Be sure to store them out of child's reach and where child cannot climb to get them.

- Buy products with child-resistant tops.
- Make sure that poisonous plants are not in the house or yard where child plays.
- Put a carbon monoxide detector on each level of the home where bedrooms are located.
- Keep all medications (prescription and nonprescription) in labeled containers and locked in a cabinet (none in purse or briefcase or on a counter or dresser).
- If home was built before 1978, have it tested for lead-based paint.
- Review sources of lead poisoning besides paint.
- Keep alcoholic beverages out of child's reach.

✓ Importance of having PCC, EMS, and health care provider's phone number posted by all phones. Also have home address and nearest intersection available in case babysitter or other family member needs to call EMS.

✓ Necessity of close supervision of infants and young children.

✓ Anticipatory guidance for next milestones child will achieve and childproofing for each age, including for all children in family (i.e., what is safe for a 6-mo-old is not safe for a 2-yr-old). Childproof all residences in which child stays. Reassess safety/childproofing frequently.

✓ Referrals to community resources, such as local and National Safe Kids Organization, safety experts, stores with a variety of materials to help childproof a home. Additional information can be obtained by contacting the following organizations:

National SAFE KIDS Campaign
1301 Pennsylvania Avenue, NW, Suite 1000
Washington, DC 20004
(202) 662-0600
www.safekids.org/

Nationwide Poison Control Center (PCC) number
(800) 222-1222

✓ Resources for disposal of hazardous household material:
- EPA at www.epa.gov/epaoswer/non-hw/muncpl/hhw.htm
- Earth 911 at www.earth911.org/ (lists closest location according to zip code for disposing of hazardous material)

86

Sickle Cell Pain Crisis

Sickle cell disease comprises a group of hereditary blood disorders in which hemoglobin S (Hb S) is the dominant hemoglobin. Hemoglobin S (sickle hemoglobin) replaces normal adult hemoglobin (Hb A). Hb S differs from Hb A in the substitution of one amino acid (valine) for another (glutamine). Under conditions of dehydration, acidosis, hypoxia, and temperature elevations, Hb S changes its molecular structure and forms a crescent- or sickle-shaped red blood cell (RBC). This causes the cardinal clinical features of chronic hemolytic anemia and vaso-occlusion, which result from obstruction caused by the sickled RBCs and increased RBC destruction. In most instances the sickling response is reversible under conditions of adequate hydration and oxygenation. After repeated cycles of sickling and unsickling, the RBC remains in the sickled form. The most common form of sickle cell disease is hemoglobin SS disease.

The inheritance pattern is autosomal recessive (both parents must at least have the sickle cell trait). If both parents have the sickle cell trait, there is a 25% chance that each child will have sickle cell disease, a 25% chance that each child will have neither the trait nor the disease, and a 50% chance that each child will have the trait. Therefore a child may be asymptomatic (except under rare circumstances) with the trait or have varying degrees of symptoms with the disease. Sickle cell disease is among the most prevalent of genetic diseases in the United States, predominantly affecting African American, African/Hispanic-Caribbean, and South American people.

Pain is the leading cause of emergency department visits and hospitalizations. It can occur as early as age 6 mo and unpredictably throughout a lifetime. There is considerable variation in the severity, frequency, and types of pain among and within affected individuals.

HEALTH CARE SETTING

Primary care with possible hospitalization for infections or pain crisis

ASSESSMENT

Signs and symptoms: Generally do not appear in infants before 4-6 mo of age because of high levels of fetal hemoglobin. Pain is the hallmark manifestation and is caused by vaso-occlusion. Types of pain states include acute painful event, acute hand-foot syndrome (dactylitis—usually seen in children between 6 mo and 2 yr old), acute joint inflammation, acute chest syndrome (a common cause of mortality manifesting as chest pain, fever, pneumonia-like cough, and anemia), splenic sequestration (enlarged spleen with sudden drop in hemoglobin —can be life threatening), intrahepatic sickling or hepatic sequestration, abdominal and intraabdominal pain, priapism, and avascular necrosis of the femur or humerus. Stroke is another form of vaso-occlusive event and has a high rate of recurrence. Overwhelming infection/sepsis is the leading cause of death in young children with sickle cell disease.

Physical assessment: History and physical, including character, location, severity, and duration of pain, as well as at-home treatment. Information should be obtained about methods used in the past to treat pain crises effectively. Initial pain assessment should be done and repeated before and after analgesia.

DIAGNOSTIC TESTS

Hemoglobin electrophoresis, isoelectric focusing, and high-performance liquid chromatography: Enable definitive diagnosis of sickle cell disease.

Complete blood count (CBC) with retic: May show increased white blood cells (WBCs) with infection. The life span of the normal RBC is decreased from 120 days to 10-14 days, so bone marrow compensates with increased production.

Retic count gives an indication of RBC production by the bone marrow.

Blood culture: Infection may have triggered crisis. Sepsis is the leading cause of death in children <5 yr old.

Chest x-ray examination: Helps differentiate between acute chest syndrome and pneumonia.

Basic metabolic panel (if signs and symptoms of dehydration are present): Helps assess degree of dehydration and need for electrolyte replacement.

Oximetry: Noninvasive method that will reveal decreased O_2 saturation if it is present.

Nursing Diagnosis:

Acute Pain

related to tissue anoxia secondary to vaso-occlusion

Desired Outcomes: For mild-to-moderate pain, child states or demonstrates that pain has decreased within $1-1\frac{1}{2}$ hr of receiving oral medication. For severe pain, child states or demonstrates that pain has decreased within 24 hr of intervention/treatment. Pain is <2 on a 5-point scale such as Wong-Baker FACES scale or <4 on a 10-point scale such as FLACC or numeric scale.

INTERVENTIONS	RATIONALES
Establish pain scale appropriate for child (FLACC, Wong-Baker FACES, Oucher, Poker Chip, or numeric) and use it before and after analgesic is administered (within 10-30 min after IV medication administration and within $1-1\frac{1}{2}$ hr after oral medication administration). Assess pain level q 2-4 hr unless on continuous infusion of pain medication – then assess q hr.	Monitors degree of pain and effectiveness of pain medication.
Plan schedule of pain medication around the clock, not prn.	Uses lower total amounts of medication with better control. Prolonged stimulation of pain receptors results in increased sensitivity to painful stimuli and will increase the amount of drug required to relieve pain.
Do *not* administer meperidine (Demerol).	Increases risk of normeperidine-induced seizures, *especially* in a child with sickle cell disease.
Carefully apply warmth to affected area.	May be soothing to child, but it should be done judiciously because ischemic tissue is fragile.
Do *not* apply cold compresses.	Cold promotes sickling and vasoconstriction.
Assess hydration status q4h (level of consciousness [LOC], anterior fontanel if <2 yr old, oral mucous membranes, abdominal skin turgor, and urine output).	To detect and prevent/treat dehydration, which causes vaso-occlusion/pain. A child who is dehydrated may exhibit decreased LOC, sunken anterior fontanel (if <2 yr old), dry or sticky oral mucous membranes, tented abdominal skin, and decreased urine output.
Use nonpharmacologic pain control measures as appropriate for child.	Optimally, comfort measures will distract child from the pain and augment effects of pharmacologic measures. Examples include distraction (watching TV or playing games), deep breathing, relaxation exercises, music, touch, imagery, and massage.

●●● **Related NIC and NOC labels:** *NIC:* Medication Management; Analgesic Administration; Presence; Simple Relaxation Therapy; Distraction; Heat Application; Music Therapy; Simple Massage; Simple Guided Imagery *NOC:* Comfort Level; Pain: Disruptive Effects

Nursing Diagnosis:

Deficient Knowledge:

Precautions and side effects of prescribed medications

Desired Outcome: Child/family verbalizes accurate information about prescribed medications, including precautions and side effects.

INTERVENTIONS	RATIONALES
Teach Child/Parent the Following, Depending on Prescribed Medication:	
Morphine sulfate (administered in hospital)	Opioid analgesic.
Purpose of monitoring child for level of sedation, pain relief obtained, O$_2$ saturation, and respiratory and cardiac status.	To evaluate effectiveness of medication and possible need to adjust dosage. Morphine can cause respiratory depression, and if it occurs, O$_2$ saturation would decrease along with respiratory rate.
Need to monitor for dizziness, drowsiness, itching, nausea, vomiting, constipation, urinary retention, and low blood pressure. Parent/child should notify staff or health care provider if any of these symptoms occur.	Side effects. May indicate need to change dosage of medication or medication itself or to provide additional medication, such as diphenhydramine for itching or an antiemetic for nausea.
Reassure child/parents that analgesics, including opioids, are medically indicated, and high doses may be needed to relieve pain.	There is confusion about the issues of pain control and drug dependence. Children rarely become addicted, and needless suffering may occur as a result of unnecessary fears.
Acetaminophen with codeine	Central analgesic/antipyretic with added narcotic.
Monitor for and report palpitations, dizziness, drowsiness, itching, nausea, vomiting, cramping, low blood pressure, and constipation, as well as excessive sedation and respiratory depression.	Side effects; may indicate need to adjust or change medication.
Assess if pain has decreased within 1-1½ hr of oral administration. If child has no relief after several doses of pain medication, parent should notify health care provider.	Evaluates effectiveness of medication as this is the time of peak action. If there is no relief after several doses, health care provider may increase dosage.
Ibuprofen	Augments pain control when administered with morphine or acetaminophen with codeine.
Be alert to and report dizziness, drowsiness, and heartburn.	Side effects; may indicate need for health care provider to adjust dosage or change medication.
Administer with food or milk.	Decreases gastrointestinal (GI) upset.
Folic acid	Enhances bone marrow's ability to produce new blood cells.
Penicillin	Prophylactic antibiotic. Overwhelming infection/sepsis is the leading cause of death in young children with sickle cell disease.
Importance of daily administration as prescribed at least until child is 5-6 yr old.	Reduces morbidity risks associated with pneumococcal septicemia. It may need to be continued for a longer period if child has experienced invasive pneumococcal infection, has not received pneumococcal immunizations, is on a hypertransfusion program, or is anatomically asplenic.
Monitor for and report rash, nausea, vomiting, diarrhea, black hairy tongue, and hypersensitivity reactions. Call 911 promptly if anaphylaxis occurs.	Side effects; may indicate need for health care provider to adjust dosage or change medication.
Administer/take with water on an empty stomach 1 hr before meals or 2 hr after meals; may give with food to decrease GI upset.	Food or milk may decrease absorption.

Continued

INTERVENTIONS	RATIONALES
Docusate	Stool softener
Administer when child is taking analgesics.	Analgesics may cause constipation.
If using in liquid form, administer with a small amount of milk, fruit juice, or infant formula.	Masks the bitter taste.
Ensure that child is receiving 1.5-2 × maintenance fluids unless pulmonary symptoms exist. For calculation of maintenance fluids, see "Bronchiolitis," p. 621, for **Deficient Fluid Volume.**	Facilitates effectiveness of docusate and provides adequate hydration for child with sickle cell pain crisis.
Monitor for and report rash, diarrhea, abdominal cramping, or throat irritation.	Side effects; health care provider may need to adjust dosage or change medication.
Acetaminophen	Analgesic.
Administer immediately for mild complaint of pain or discomfort.	Prevents pain crisis.
Monitor for and report rash.	Side effect; may indicate need for health care provider to adjust dosage or change medication.
Ensure that child is receiving therapeutic dose of acetaminophen.	To provide effective pain relief while avoiding hepatic necrosis.

●●● **Related NIC and NOC labels:** *NIC:* Teaching: Prescribed Medication; Analgesic Administration; Pain Management *NOC:* Knowledge: Medication

Nursing Diagnosis:

Ineffective Tissue Perfusion: Cardiopulmonary and cerebral

related to vaso-occlusion and anemia

Desired Outcomes: Within 2 hr following treatment/intervention, child's oxygen saturation is maintained at ≥95% or at level prescribed by health care provider. There is no evidence of long-term complications from lack of oxygen.

INTERVENTIONS	RATIONALES
Assess respiratory status and mental status q2-4h and prn	Frequent assessment ensures early detection of changes in respiratory status. Tachypnea and increased work of breathing (WOB) are early signs of hypoxia. LOC is a good indicator of oxygen perfusion to the brain.
Monitor pulse oximetry continuously.	Noninvasive method of assessing oxygen saturation and noting changes promptly.
Administer oxygen as prescribed to keep oxygen saturation levels at ≥95% or at level appropriate for individual child.	Delivering oxygen when child is hypoxic eases WOB. However, it does not reverse the sickling process, and long-term use can depress bone marrow activity and increase the anemia.
Encourage use of incentive spirometry q2h while awake in older children. For younger children, have them blow bubbles, blow on a pinwheel to make it spin, or blow a crumpled piece of paper across the bedside table.	Deep breathing facilitates lung expansion and decreases incidence of acute chest syndrome.
Elevate head of bed (HOB) to a comfortable level for the child.	Facilitates chest expansion by decreasing pressure on the diaphragm.
Administer packed RBCs as prescribed.	Improves tissue perfusion by correcting anemia.

●●● **Related NIC and NOC labels:** *NIC:* Oxygen Therapy; Respiratory Monitoring; Positioning; Blood Products Administration *NOC:* Tissue Perfusion: Pulmonary; Tissue Perfusion: Cerebral

Nursing Diagnosis:

Deficient Knowledge

Sickle cell disease, measures to avoid vaso-occlusive crisis, home management to prevent severe pain crisis, and the genetics that could result in having other children with this disease

Desired Outcome: Within 48 hr following teaching, child/family verbalizes accurate understanding of the disease process, especially pain crisis and appropriate treatment, and the genetics of disease transmission.

INTERVENTIONS	RATIONALES
Instruct older child/family in basic information about sickle cell disease and measures to minimize sickling.	Improves understanding of disease process and promotes compliance with plan of care, for example, taking prescribed medications such as penicillin and folic acid on a regular basis, staying up to date on immunizations, and avoiding precipitating factors (i.e., dehydration, exposure to individuals who are ill with infections, extreme temperatures, high elevations, excessive physical activity).
Encourage child/family to obtain medical alert bracelet/necklace and inform significant health professionals/school personnel of diagnosis.	Helps ensure prompt and appropriate treatment.
Explain signs of developing pain crisis, its significance, and importance of prompt treatment.	Knowledge about the signs of pain crisis and its significance optimally will result in prompt reporting and treatment, which may avoid a severe vaso-occlusive crisis. For example, in an infant or toddler, a combination of unusual behaviors such as inconsolability, decreased appetite, unexplained crying, and rapid breathing may indicate discomfort or pain. Older children may complain of mild discomfort or aching.
Discuss home treatment for mild/early symptoms of pain crisis.	To decrease severity of pain crisis by early/prompt treatment (e.g., resting, increasing fluid intake to 1.5-2 × maintenance fluids, and administering pain medication)
Discuss transmission of disease and refer for genetic counseling as indicated.	Enables family to make informed reproductive decisions. See discussion in introductory data.
Encourage family members to be advocates for the child in the hospital, during appointments with the health care provider, and in day care or school setting (e.g., Individualized Education Plan [IEP] or 504 plan at school). Reinforce that they know the child best and understand what is normal or abnormal in relationship to the child.	Family members may be hesitant to ask questions or advocate for the child; however, they are the best resource. Encouraging advocacy increases likelihood that child will receive the best care and facilitates optimal development.
Supply family with information about support groups, local/national sickle cell organizations, and resources for additional information.	Support systems likely will improve knowledge base about disease process and therapeutics involved.
Encourage family to have child receive follow-up visits at a sickle cell clinic on a regular basis.	Promotes continuity and quality of care.

●●● **Related NIC and NOC labels:** *NIC:* Teaching: Disease Process; Risk Identification; Parent Education: Childrearing Family *NOC:* Knowledge: Treatment Regimen; Knowledge: Disease Process; Knowledge: Illness Care

ADDITIONAL NURSING DIAGNOSES/ PROBLEMS:

Constipation can occur as a result of narcotic analgesics and decreased mobility. See "Prolonged Bedrest" for **Constipation.**	p. 75
"Psychosocial Support" for **Anticipatory Grieving** related to potentially fatal diagnosis.	p. 88
"Psychosocial Support for Patient's Family and Significant Others"	p. 95
"Asthma" for **Anxiety** related to illness, loss of control, and medical/nursing interventions	p. 604
"Asthma" for **Interrupted Family Processes** related to having a child with a chronic illness	p. 604
"Bronchiolitis" for **Deficient Fluid Volume** (however, child with sickle cell pain crisis needs 1.5-2 × maintenance, unless pulmonary symptoms – then only maintenance fluids)	p. 621
Appendix for "Infection Prevention and Control." Overwhelming infection/sepsis is the leading cause of death in young children with sickle cell disease.	p. 831

PATIENT-FAMILY TEACHING AND DISCHARGE PLANNING

When providing patient-family teaching, focus on sensory information. Avoid giving excessive instructions and institute a visiting nurse referral as necessary for follow-up teaching and assessment. Include verbal and written information about the following (ensure written information is at a level the reader can understand):

✓Basic pathophysiology about sickle disease and pain crisis.

✓Cause of pain, including precipitating factors (e.g., dehydration, infection, fever, hot or cold temperatures, high elevations, excessive physical activity) and importance of avoiding same.

✓Avoiding exposure to individuals who are ill with infections (e.g., do not go in crowded areas during flu season). Overwhelming infection/sepsis is the leading cause of death in young children with sickle cell disease.

✓Importance of maintaining adequate oral intake to prevent dehydration and thereby prevent clumping of Hb S.

✓Signs and symptoms of early pain crisis and treatment (i.e., rest, increase fluids to 1.5-2 × maintenance, and administer acetaminophen or ibuprofen first. If no relief, try prescription pain medication from the health care provider).

✓Maintaining a pain diary, which may be beneficial in finding precipitating factors and effective pain control measures. The most effective treatment in an emergency department also should be included in the event that child is seen in another hospital.

✓Medications, including drug name, route, purpose, dosage, precautions, drug/drug and food/drug interactions, and potential side effects.

✓Importance of taking medications at home and school as directed. Medication in the original bottle (with prescribing label) and written prescription from health care provider are needed for child to be able to take any medication at school.

✓Nonpharmacologic methods to relieve pain:
- Psychologic strategies: distraction, imagery, education/teaching, and hypnotherapy
- Behavioral strategies: deep breathing, relaxation exercises, self-hypnosis, biofeedback, and behavior modification
- Physical strategies: careful application of heat to painful area, massage, and mild exercise, if tolerated

✓Frequent urination, which is normal with increased fluids; enuresis may occur as a result.

✓When to contact physician:
- Temperature ≥101° F
- Severe pain not relieved by prescribed pain medication (usually acetaminophen with codeine)
- Child is pale, lethargic, irritable, or dehydrated
- Vomiting and/or diarrhea lasting more than a day
- Shortness of breath or other acute pulmonary symptoms

✓Coordination of care. Parents should discuss child's illness and needs with school nurse and other adults who are in close contact with child (e.g., teachers, scout leaders, day care providers).

✓Legal rights of the child:
- Individuals with Disabilities Education Act (IDEA): Mandates federal government to provide funding to education agencies for free and appropriate education to qualifying students with disabilities, including children with sickle cell disease if the disease adversely affects school performance. School is then required to develop an Individualized Education Plan (IEP).
- IEP: A multidisciplinary team designs this plan to facilitate special education and therapeutic strategies and goals for each child. Child does not have to be in special education classes. Parents need to be involved in this process.
- Section 504 of Rehabilitation Act of 1973: Each student with a disability (physical or mental impairment) is entitled to accommodation to attend school and participate as fully as possible in school activities. This accommodation may be related to a medical condition or an educational issue. For example, child may leave the classroom to use bathroom facilities without raising his or her hand and will not be penalized for excessive absences from school that are caused by sickle cell disease. The 504 Plan may include as many accommodations as necessary for child to function well.

✓Importance of ongoing health care management with health care provider experienced in dealing with sickle cell disease to identify and manage chronic complications:
- Receiving childhood immunizations at the appropriate age, especially pneumococcal and yearly flu vaccine

- Prompt attention to symptoms of infection (e.g., fever, sore throat)
- Regular visits with health care provider, not just when ill

✓Phone numbers to call should questions or concerns arise about therapy or disease after discharge.

✓Additional general information can be obtained by contacting the following organizations:

The Sickle Cell Information Center
P.O. Box 109
Grady Memorial Hospital
80 Jessie Hill Jr. Drive SE
Atlanta, GA 30303
(404) 616-3572
www.scinfo.org

Sickle Cell Disease Association of America
200 Corporate Point, Suite 495
Culver City, CA 90203-8727
(800) 421-8453 or (310) 216-6363
www.sicklecelldisease.org

Guideline for Management of Acute and Chronic Pain in Sickle Cell Disease
American Pain Society
4700 West Lake Avenue
Glenview, IL 60025-1485
(847) 375-4715
www.ampainsoc.org

STARBRIGHT Foundation
1850 Sawtelle Boulevard, Suite 450
Los Angeles, CA 90025
(800) 315-2580 or (310) 479-1212
www.starbright.org

Starbright Explorer Series (no charge for CD-ROMs):
"Spotlight on IVs" recommended for children 6-10 yr old
"The Sickle Cell Slime-O-Rama Game" recommended for children 6-14 yr old
"Blood Tests: Exploring Our Incredible Blood" recommended for children 10-15 yr old
"Medical Imaging: Welcome to the Radiology Center" recommended for children 6-10 yr old

Bleeding in Pregnancy

Bleeding in pregnancy can be minor to life threatening. Causes include implantation bleeding (bleeding after the embryo implants in the endometrium), blighted ovum (ovum does not develop because of chromosomal abnormalities of the sperm or egg), severe chromosomal abnormalities, ectopic pregnancy (implantation outside of the uterus), threatened abortion (confirmed pregnancy with vaginal bleeding), incomplete abortion (retention of some products of conception [POC]), missed abortion (fetus has died but is retained with the placenta in the uterus), inevitable spontaneous abortion (ruptured membranes or POC passed at onset of bleeding before 20 wk gestation), complete spontaneous abortion (bleeding and cramping followed by passing of tissue or POC before 20 wk gestation, followed by a marked decrease in cramping and bleeding), gestational trophoblastic disease (includes hydatidiform mole [molar pregnancy] and gestational trophoblastic tumors), cervicitis, cervical polyps, cervical dysplasia (such as cervical carcinoma), hyperemia of the cervix, incompetent cervix (painless dilation of the cervix), maternal bleeding disorders, placenta previa (abnormally implanted placenta that covers or partially covers the cervix), placental abruption (premature separation from the uterine wall of a normally implanted placenta), uterine rupture (may be seen after a previous classical cesarean), cervical dilation, postcoital bleeding, and sexual assault.

HEALTH CARE SETTING

Primary care; acute care (emergency room or inpatient setting) if surgical intervention is deemed necessary

ASSESSMENT

Bleeding in the first trimester is not uncommon, inasmuch as some women are not aware they are pregnant. The bleeding can range from light pink spotting to brown discharge (indicating old blood) to bleeding like a heavy menses and may or may not be accompanied by abdominal pain. It can result in significant emotional changes from relief, concern, and ambivalence to fear. Bleeding in the second and third trimesters is of significant concern because it can affect maternal/fetal morbidity and mortality.

Early pregnancy symptoms: Amenorrhea, breast tenderness, fatigue, abdominal bloating, nausea, and vomiting. With a missed spontaneous abortion, these symptoms may no longer be present when vaginal bleeding begins.

Vaginal bleeding:
- **First trimester vaginal bleeding** may be light pink, bright red, or dark brown spotting (noticed when the woman wipes her perineum or on her underpants); like a heavy menses; or bright red and saturating pads. Some women pass blood clots with or without tissue. Light vaginal spotting may be an early indication of an ectopic pregnancy or threatened abortion.
- **Second and third trimester vaginal bleeding** may be light pink, bright red, or dark brown spotting (noticed when the woman wipes her perineum or on her underpants); like a heavy menses; or bright red and saturating pads. Some women pass blood clots. Any vaginal bleeding in the second and third trimesters requires immediate evaluation and may indicate placenta previa, abruptio placentae, or antepartum rupture of a scarred uterus in patients with previous cesarean section.

Vaginal discharge (other than bleeding): If an infection is present the woman may note a change in her vaginal discharge before the bleeding episode. Discharge may range from thick white and clumpy to thin white, yellow, or green with or without a foul odor.

Abdominal pain: Pain from uterine cramping may or may not be present and can range from mild to severe. In the presence of placental abruption or uterine rupture, abdominal pain is often severe, although not always. With uterine rupture the pain may be absent to moderate or localized, and the abdomen may be tender. With placenta previa there is usually no abdominal pain. With ectopic pregnancy the pain may be vague and achy to sharp and colicky, may be unilateral or bilateral, and may be accompanied by nausea, vomiting, and diarrhea.

Back pain: May or may not be present with vaginal bleeding, depending on the cause. When present, it is usually described as low (lumbar), dull, and aching and may radiate around the hips and down the thighs. With abruption the back pain may be mild to severe.

Passage of POC: Normally in the first trimester the POC appear as grainy, granular tissue that looks more like clotted blood. Some women state their bleeding and abdominal pain decrease significantly after the passage of POC.

Cardiovascular: Dizziness, lightheadedness, syncope, shortness of breath, or tachycardia if significant blood loss has occurred.

Signs—fetal: Decreased or absent fetal movement (gestation appropriate) may be present with fetal compromise or demise.

Physical assessment: Vaginal bleeding can occur at any time during pregnancy and be of varying degrees depending on its cause. Some bleeding episodes resolve on their own, and the pregnancy will continue; others lead to the spontaneous abortion of the fetus, demise of the neonate, and possible serious consequences for the mother. Maternal VS may be within normal limits or show postural changes (drop in BP with rise in HR, indicating fluid depletion). The woman also may be anxious, irritable, and apprehensive with significant blood loss.

Abdominal examination: Abdominal tenderness with palpation will be present with an ectopic pregnancy, placental abruption, and uterine rupture. Fetal heart tones (FHTs) may be auscultated at the appropriate gestational age or be absent in the presence of fetal demise. Uterine contractions may be palpable, depending on gestational age.

Risk factors: Previous history of spontaneous abortion, ectopic pregnancy, cervical polyps and other cervical lesions (cervical dysplasia), incompetent cervix, bleeding in pregnancy (postpartum hemorrhage), placenta previa, molar pregnancy, or uterine myomas/leiomyomata (fibroids or smooth muscle cell tumors). Other risk factors include luteal phase defect (inadequate progesterone production by a poorly functioning corpus luteum), structural abnormalities of the uterus, antiphospholipid syndrome (autoimmune syndrome that may be associated with recurrent spontaneous abortion), chromosomal abnormalities, smoking, substance abuse (especially cocaine use), vaginal infections, abdominal trauma, previous history of abruption, and use of some chemotherapy drugs.

DIAGNOSTIC TESTS

Rapid qualitative urine pregnancy test: Tests for the presence of human chorionic gonadotropin (hCG), which may be detected after implantation is complete/8-10 days after conception. A pregnancy can be diagnosed even before a menstrual period has been missed.

Serial serum qualitative and quantitative pregnancy test: Tests for the presence of hCG. After implantation is complete, hCG is detectable in serum (8-11 days after conception). Normally serum concentration of hCG doubles every 1-2 days and is helpful in determining gestational age with rising numbers or a spontaneous abortion with declining numbers.

Obstetric ultrasound: Done abdominally, transvaginally, or translabially. It detects the presence of a viable pregnancy or a fetus without cardiac activity. It locates the pregnancy as either intrauterine or ectopic and evaluates presence of a gestational sac, whether it contains a fetus or is empty, and gestational age. It also locates the position of the placenta and fetus, number of fetuses, presence of subchorionic hemorrhage (bleeding beneath the outer membrane that contains blood vessels), and abruption.

Complete blood count: May be within normal limits unless there has been significant blood loss and anemia is present. An elevated white blood cell (WBC) count is suggestive of an intrauterine infection.

Blood Rh factor and antibody screen: Results will indicate the mother's Rh factor as either positive or negative and if there are antibodies present. Rh-negative women with negative antibodies will need Rh immune globulin (RhoGAM) administered for prevention of Rh sensitization of subsequent pregnancies.

Kleihauer-Betke test: Tests for the presence of fetal cells in the maternal circulation that can be seen after fetomaternal bleeding (e.g., occurring with abdominal trauma).

Speculum examination: To examine the cervix for the presence of dilation, effacement, or evidence of POC at the cervical os or within the vaginal vault or for polyps, cervical friability, lacerations, or lesions that would contribute to the bleeding. Cultures may be taken at this time. Caution is used when performing a speculum examination on a woman with known placenta previa who has vaginal bleeding in her second or third trimester. Speculum examination also enables assessment for rupture of amniotic membranes using Nitrazine paper and ferning (microscopic crystallization of amniotic fluid when allowed to air dry on a glass slide).

Fetal monitoring: Before gestational viability, monitoring of uterine tone may be done only to elicit uterine contractions. It is used in the second and third trimesters to check for fetal well-being by eliciting FHTs and uterine tone (contractions). Normally, a reactive fetal heart rate tracing may be seen after 32 wk gestation and as early as 27 wk gestation, depending on fetal central nervous system (CNS) development. It includes a minimum of 20 min of tracing that shows a fetal heart rate baseline between 120-160 bpm and at least two accelerations that must rise at least 15 bpm and last at least 15 sec from onset to return to baseline. With maternal hemorrhage, as in placenta previa or abruptio placentae, fetal oxygenation is compromised because of maternal hypotension, decrease in placental surface area, and uterine hyperactivity. Nonreassuring fetal heart rate patterns that may be seen with bleeding may include the following: late decelerations, progressively severe variable decelerations, tachycardia, loss of variability, recurrent prolonged decelerations, and sinusoidal tracing. In the presence of an acute abruptio placentae, there is a rapid deceleration of the fetal heart rate, which can indicate imminent fetal demise.

- *Late decelerations:* Gradual onset, U shaped, start at the peak of contraction and return to baseline gradually. Generally the tracings descend 30-40 bpm below baseline. The cause is a temporary interruption of uteroplacental perfusion during peak of contractions.

- *Variable decelerations:* Onset and resolution are sharp and abrupt. Size, shape, depth, duration, and timing vary in relation to a contraction. The cause is a temporary compression of the umbilical cord.

- *Sinusoidal tracing:* A repetitive, small, wavelike pattern of the fetal heart rate. The cause is fetal anemia.

Nursing Diagnosis:

Deficient Knowledge:

Effects of bleeding on self, pregnancy, and fetus

Desired Outcome: Immediately following teaching, patient and significant other verbalize accurate knowledge about the effects of bleeding on the patient, pregnancy, and fetus and comply with the treatments accordingly.

INTERVENTIONS	RATIONALES
Inform patient and significant other what bleeding may indicate and the effect it can have on the pregnancy, mother, and fetus.	Knowledgeable patients are more likely to comply with therapy (e.g., bedrest, frequent clinic visits, no intercourse, stopping work, and possible hospitalizations or surgery) and understand consequences of noncompliance. Bleeding plays a major role in maternal/fetal morbidity and mortality, depending on cause and gestational age at the time of occurrence.
Teach patient the signs and symptoms of bleeding, depending on her trimester.	Patient will understand that vaginal bleeding or abdominal pain in the presence of amenorrhea or a positive pregnancy test requires evaluation and that there is increased risk for maternal/fetal morbidity and mortality if bleeding occurs under these conditions. See descriptions under Assessment, earlier.
Explain that when a miscarriage is occurring there is nothing that can be done to prevent it.	More than 50% of first and second trimester spontaneous abortions occur because of chromosomal abnormalities. Understanding this may alleviate some feelings of anguish or guilt about embryo/fetus nonsurvival.
Teach patient how to palpate contractions that may accompany vaginal bleeding (gestation appropriate).	Palpation and awareness of contractions enable patient to be an active participant in her health care. Timely reporting of contractions to her health care provider can play a significant role in affecting outcome.
	To palpate contractions, the patient lies comfortably on her side. She spreads her fingers apart and places one hand on the left side and the other on the right side of her abdomen. She will palpate the abdomen using her fingertips. When the uterus is relaxed, the abdomen should feel soft. In the presence of a contraction, the uterus should feel hard, tight, or firm under her fingertips. She then times the duration of the contraction from the beginning of one contraction to the beginning of the next. Any number of contractions, combined with vaginal bleeding, necessitates immediate evaluation and can prove ominous in the second and third trimesters. Contractions can increase the severity of vaginal bleeding with placenta previa and abruptio

Continued

INTERVENTIONS	RATIONALES
	placentae. Duration of the contraction may or may not be an indication of contraction intensity. It is believed that the longer the contraction in true labor the more effective it is in progressing dilation and effacement.
Teach fetal movement counts.	Fetal movement counts are a good first-line indicator of fetal well-being and are performed as follows, beginning at 28 wk gestation: Patient lies on her side and counts "distinct fetal movements" (hiccups do not count) daily; 10 movements within a 2-hr period are reassuring. After counting 10 movements, the count is discontinued. Fewer than 10 movements signals need for fetal nonstress testing.
Teach signs and symptoms of maternal complications with vaginal bleeding.	Promotes understanding of the need to seek medical attention in a timely manner if indicators such as saturating >1 pad/hr, passing golf-ball-size clots, dizziness, lightheadedness, syncope, shortness of breath, and tachycardia occur.
Explain how to save POC if requested by health care provider.	Proper storage and transport aids in cytologic and pathologic evaluation. Each laboratory has specific requirements for transport and should be contacted accordingly.
For patients in the second and third trimesters, explain home management of placenta previa or chronic abruption and its purpose. Teach patient to decrease physical activity and avoid intercourse and insertion of anything into the vagina, including tampons.	Although some patients with placenta previa may not experience vaginal bleeding during pregnancy, vaginal bleeding with placenta previa or abruptio placentae can be serious. Patients can exsanguinate rapidly. In some patients, increased physical activity, including lifting, may decrease uterine perfusion, which increases risk of placental abruption. Intercourse and use of tampons increase risk of bleeding in the presence of placenta previa and its location over the cervical os.
Caution against sexual foreplay.	The uterine contractility that can occur in sexual foreplay (breast stimulation, oral or digital stimulation) promotes release of prostaglandins, which cause uterine contractions and hence increase risk of bleeding.

●●● **Related NIC and NOC labels:** *NIC:* Teaching: Disease Process; Health Education; High-Risk Pregnancy Care *NOC:* Knowledge: Pregnancy

Nursing Diagnosis:

Acute Pain

related to uterine cramping and backache that may be associated with vaginal bleeding in pregnancy

Desired Outcome: Patient reports the pain in a timely manner for appropriate evaluation and treatment and within 1-2 hr after intervention states that pain is at an acceptable level (≤4 on a 0-10 scale).

INTERVENTIONS	RATIONALES
Evaluate patient's level of abdominal pain/uterine cramping using a scale of 0-10, with 10 being the worst pain she has ever had.	Each patient experiences levels of pain differently. Baseline assessment will enable proper analgesia and help determine relief of pain obtained after subsequent evaluation.

Continued

INTERVENTIONS	**RATIONALES**
Evaluate location and duration of pain.	Location and duration of the pain may signal different problems. For example, pain/aching under the scapula may indicate blood in the peritoneum, a sign of a ruptured ectopic pregnancy/internal bleeding.
Administer pain medications if their use is not contraindicated.	To provide pain relief. In some situations, however, pain is a useful indicator of a potential problem, such as a ruptured ectopic pregnancy, in which masking of symptoms is not desirable.
Provide emotional support.	Aids in decreasing anxiety, which also may decrease the level of pain.

●●● **Related NIC and NOC labels:** *NIC:* Pain Management; Emotional Support; Medication Administration
NOC: Comfort Level; Pain Control

Nursing Diagnosis:

Anticipatory Grieving

related to the potential loss of the pregnancy

Desired Outcome. Within 24 hr of this diagnosis, patient and significant other verbalize their feelings and identify and begin to use support systems to aid them in the grief process.

INTERVENTIONS	**RATIONALES**
Encourage patient and significant other to verbalize their feelings and concerns regarding potential or definite (e.g., ectopic) loss of the pregnancy.	Validates their feelings and conveys the message that grief is a normal and expected reaction to the potential or actual loss of the fetus. It also enables the nurse to intervene in the event of misperceptions about the bleeding.
Assess and accept patient's behavioral response.	Reactions such as disbelief, denial, guilt, anger, and depression are normal reactions to grief.
Teach the five stages of grief and explain that there is no specific time frame in which to go through this process.	Enables patient and family members to understand their stage in the grief process. Stages include (1) shock and numbness; (2) denial and searching-yearning; (3) anger, guilt, and sense of failure; (4) depression and disorganization; and (5) resolution.
Clarify misconceptions about the potential risk for fetal loss with vaginal bleeding.	Although they play a major role in fetal mortality, not all bleeding episodes in pregnancy lead to fetal loss. The gestational age at which the bleeding occurs and the amount of vaginal bleeding play a significant role in the outcome. This information will help the patient process information regarding bleeding in pregnancy appropriately while not being given false hope.
Involve Social Services in the care of the patient. If such services are not available, refer to a community support group if one exists.	If patient is placed on bedrest either at home or in the hospital, the social worker will evaluate for psychologic/social/spiritual concerns and provide written material and appropriate resources and referrals for support groups.

●●● **Related NIC and NOC labels:** *NIC:* Coping Enhancement; Grief Work Facilitation: Perinatal Death; Support Group; Anxiety Reduction *NOC:* Coping; Grief Resolution

Nursing Diagnosis:

Deficient Knowledge:

Purpose and potential side effects of prescribed medications

Desired Outcome: Immediately following teaching, patient and family verbalize accurate understanding of the risks and benefits of medications used.

INTERVENTIONS	RATIONALES
Teach the following about patient's prescribed medications:	A knowledgeable patient is more likely to comply with therapy, identify and report side effects, and recognize and report precautions that might preclude use of the prescribed drug.
Prostaglandin synthesis inhibitors *Ibuprofen*	Inhibit prostaglandin synthesis, thereby decreasing myometrial contractility/pain from cramping. Administration: oral.
Be alert for and report nausea, vomiting, heartburn, diarrhea, constipation, and abdominal cramps.	Common side effects. If these symptoms persist, the medication may need to be changed, dose adjusted, or discontinued.
Take the medication with food.	Decreases gastrointestinal (GI) side effects.
Precaution for patients with a history of GI ulcers.	May cause GI bleeding.
Not recommended for use in patients who are taking warfarin or heparin.	Further increases risk of bleeding.
Opioid analgesics *Percocet, Vicodin*	Alter processes in the CNS that affect pain perception. Used for mild to moderately severe pain. Administration: oral.
Be alert for and report nausea and vomiting.	Common side effects. If these symptoms persevere, the medication may need to be discontinued or changed.
Be alert for dizziness, lightheadedness, and weakness.	Common side effects. Patient needs to use caution for activities that require alertness if these indicators occur.
Precautions are necessary for patients taking other CNS depressants, monoamine oxidase (MAO) inhibitors, or tricyclic antidepressants.	These drugs may potentiate CNS side effects of opioid analgesics.
Prophylactic antibiotics	Prevent and reduce effects of infection and maternal morbidity. The type of antibiotic used varies and may include but is not limited to the following: ampicillins, gentamicin, and cephalosporins.
Follow complete course for all prescribed medications and take them on time.	To prevent development of antibiotic resistance and maintain a constant level of medication in the bloodstream.
Be alert for and report excessive and explosive diarrhea.	*Clostridium difficile* is a potentially serious side effect of antibiotic therapy in which the normal flora of the bowel are reduced and the anaerobic organism, *C. difficile,* multiplies and produces toxins causing severe diarrhea. This reaction necessitates discontinuation of the antibiotic and laboratory evaluation of a stool sample.
Uterotonics *Prostaglandin suppository (Prostin E2)*	Used to produce myometrial contractions to evacuate the gravid uterus in a missed abortion after 12 wk gestation or intrauterine fetal death up to 28 wk.

Continued

INTERVENTIONS	RATIONALES
	Administration: vaginally in the hospital setting. IV administration avoided.
Use not recommended with other uterotonic drugs or in patients with history of a previous classical (vertical) uterine incision.	May cause uterine rupture.
Be alert for and report nausea, vomiting, diarrhea, headache, fever, chills, backache, and dizziness.	Adverse reactions. Administration of antiemetics, analgesics, and antipyretics before administering prostaglandin may prevent or reduce these side effects.
Methylergonovine and oxytocin (Methergine and Pitocin)	Increase uterine contractility and decrease uterine/vaginal bleeding after spontaneous abortion or after dilation and curettage for missed abortion.
	Administration: IV, IM, and PO after surgical procedures or delivery of fetus/neonate.
Methergine is avoided in a patient with hypertension, whether chronic or preeclamptic.	There is risk for sudden hypertension and stroke.
Carboprost (Hemabate, 15-methyl-prostaglandin F2-alpha).	Augments effects of uterotonics for postoperative/postpartum vaginal bleeding.
	Administration: deep IM.
Be alert for and report fever, hypertension, nausea, vomiting, diarrhea, and flushing.	Common side effects. Because this drug is usually given in an emergent situation, premedication to reduce these side effects is usually not done.
Intravenous infusions of crystalloid fluids	Crystalloids form true solutions and are capable of passing through a semipermeable membrane. They are used as a volume expander after significant blood loss.
Be alert for shortness of breath, increased pulse rate, and sacral and lower extremity edema.	Signs of fluid overload.
IV blood and blood products	Used for blood loss/volume replacement.
Packed red blood cells (RBCs)	Packed RBCs are the most effective way to increase oxygen carrying capacity to the anemic patient after significant blood loss.
Platelets	Necessary for the initial phase of hemostasis and used in patients with disseminated intravascular coagulation (DIC), massive hemorrhage, severe preeclampsia, and idiopathic thrombocytopenic purpura (ITP).
Clotting factors (cryoprecipitate)	Clotting factors (cryoprecipitate) are the precipitate from warmed fresh frozen plasma, which contains clotting factors such as factor VIII, factor XIII, fibrinogen, and Von Willebrand's factor and is used to treat hypofibrinogenemia.
Whole blood	Although its use is discouraged and in some blood centers has been discontinued, it may be delivered in obstetric emergencies when there is a need to replace >4000 ml volume loss.
Be alert for and report severe anxiety, flushing, chest or back pain, fever, shortness of breath, dizziness, and increased pulse rate.	Signs of a transfusion reaction, which is life threatening and must be reported promptly for immediate intervention.
Rh-immune globulin (human) *RhoGAM*	Prevents hemolytic disease as long as the mother has not already been sensitized by the presence of Rh-positive antibodies in her bloodstream.

Continued

INTERVENTIONS	RATIONALES
	Administration: IM only to nonsensitized Rh-negative women after bleeding any time during the pregnancy, after spontaneous abortion, and after delivery. It is recommended that this drug be given within 72 hr of the bleeding episode.
Patient may note discomfort at the site of injection.	Common side effect.

●●● **Related NIC and NOC labels:** *NIC:* Teaching: Prescribed Medication; Prenatal Care
NOC: Knowledge: Medication

ADDITIONAL NURSING DIAGNOSES/ PROBLEMS:

PATIENT-FAMILY TEACHING AND DISCHARGE PLANNING

Bleeding in pregnancy is an emotionally charged situation that requires both physical and psychologic assessment. Include verbal and written information about the following:

✔Importance of reporting vaginal bleeding to the health care provider in a timely manner.

✔Importance of compliance with prescribed health care and ready access to hospital and family/social support.

✔Medications, including drug name, purpose, dosage, frequency, precautions, drug/drug and food/drug interactions, and potential side effects.

✔Fetal movement counts (gestation appropriate).

✔Palpation of contractions (gestation appropriate).

✔Importance of complying with intercourse restrictions.

✔Measures that help with constipation, which occurs frequently in pregnancy and is exacerbated by bedrest.

✔Compliance with scheduled prenatal visits.

✔Referral to local and national support organizations, including:

Sidelines, a national support organization for women and their families experiencing complicated pregnancies:
Sidelines High Risk Pregnancy Support National Office
P.O. Box 1808
Laguna Beach, CA 92652
(888) 447-4754
www.sidelines.org/

SHARE, a national support group for parents who have experienced loss through miscarriage, stillbirth, or newborn death:
SHARE Pregnancy & Infant Loss Support, Inc.
National SHARE Office
St. Joseph Health Center
300 First Capitol Drive
St. Charles, MO 63301-2893
(800) 821-6819 or (636) 947-6164
www.nationalshareoffice.com/

Cervical Incompetence

Diagnosis of cervical incompetence is made when there is an obstetric history of recurrent, passive, and painless dilation and/or effacement of the cervix in the second or early third trimester in the absence of contractions, bleeding, infection, ruptured membranes, or fetal anomalies. This may lead to preterm premature rupture of membranes (PPROM) and preterm delivery with the possibility of fetal demise.

HEALTH CARE SETTING

Primary care (outpatient obstetric clinic, perinatal high-risk clinic) or acute care (inpatient antepartum unit)

ASSESSMENT

Evaluating cervical incompetence in a patient with no previous history can be difficult. Patient may present at a routine clinic visit having acute cervical changes and complaining of vague symptoms (e.g., backache, pelvic pressure) that can be common in pregnancy.

Pelvic pressure: Patient complains of a sensation of pelvic fullness or heaviness that may or may not have been present previously during the pregnancy. Some patients relate a sensation of vaginal fullness such as that of having a large tampon in the vagina.

Increased vaginal discharge: An increase in vaginal discharge is a normal process in pregnancy. Normal vaginal discharge can be clear, white, or light yellow and thin to thick in consistency. The patient with incompetent cervix may not note a change in consistency but a change in color such as light pink, blood-tinged, or tan. These are symptoms of possible cervical dilation as the surface vessels of the cervix break and bleed.

Backache: Although this is a very common complaint in pregnancy, any woman with a history of cervical incompetence who complains of new-onset backache needs to be evaluated for cervical changes, especially if she describes backache as low lumbar/sacral in position, deep tissue in nature, or as a dull aching sensation that may radiate around the hips to the lower abdomen/pelvic area and down the thighs.

Contractions: Uterine tightening/contractions begin in the first trimester as the uterus enlarges and continue throughout the pregnancy. These contractions are considered Braxton-Hicks and occur at irregular intervals, usually are painless, and do not change the cervix. Some women complain of a lower pelvic aching sensation that may be detected by palpation or uterine monitoring. However, any woman with a history of cervical incompetence who complains of new-onset contractions needs to be evaluated for cervical changes.

Cervical changes: Reduced cervical competence may be congenital or acquired. The cervix may dilate and then efface or efface and then dilate. Funneling of the cervix may be seen. This occurs when the internal cervical os dilates and the external os remains closed. It appears as a funnel shape when seen on ultrasound. Protrusion or bulging of the amniotic membranes may be visible through the cervical os. A normal cervical length is ≥3.5 cm.

Complications—fetal: Prematurity and fetal/neonatal death may occur.

Physical assessment: Normally, cervical incompetence is asymptomatic until signs of significant cervical change are present. With advanced cervical dilation, PPROM may occur, increasing fetal morbidity and mortality.

Risk factors: Previous history of incompetent cervix or preterm birth, previous cervical trauma, cervical conization (a cone-shaped portion of the cervix is removed in the presence of cervical dysplasia), cervical biopsy, cervical length <3.5 cm, congenital structural anomalies, extensive cervical dilation as occurs in second-trimester pregnancy terminations, cervical laceration(s) at the time of a previous vaginal delivery, diethylstilbestrol (DES) exposure.

DIAGNOSTIC TESTS

Transvaginal or translabial ultrasound: Assessment to determine cervical length. Diagnostic ultrasound criteria of incompetent cervix include a total cervical length between 2 and 2.5 cm, accompanied by funneling of the internal cervical os.

Obstetric ultrasound: Confirms gestational age, position of the placenta and fetus, number of fetuses, amniotic fluid volume index, presence of funneling and fetal anomalies and measures cervical length and dilation. Serial ultrasound examinations can monitor the cervix for any changes. Ultrasound does not replace digital cervical exams.

Digital cervical examination: A gentle digital exam of the cervix is done to evaluate the cervix for dilation, effacement, position (anterior/posterior), and consistency (firm/soft). Protrusion or bulging of the amniotic membranes through the cervical os (funneling) may be detected at this time. Of note, cervical change in the mid-to-late second trimester of 1-2 cm dilation has been seen in women who have not progressed to preterm labor and/or delivery.

Urinalysis for microscopy: Urinary tract infection (UTI) is associated with preterm labor. It is not a cause of incompetent cervix but should be ruled out as a cofactor. If bacteria are present, including group B streptococci, antibiotic therapy should be initiated.

Antepartum fetal monitoring: Before gestation of viability (i.e., <25 wk) the patient may be monitored for the presence and frequency of contractions using only the tocodynamometer. A documentation of fetal heart tones (FHTs) is necessary with each tracing. Once viability is reached, both the transducer and tocodynamometer are used.

Complete blood count with differential: Helps rule out chorioamnionitis, a bacterial infection of the fetal membranes. If present, white blood cells (WBCs) will be elevated.

Nursing Diagnosis:

Deficient Knowledge:

Effects of incompetent cervix on self, the pregnancy, and fetus and the treatment and expected outcome

Desired Outcome: Immediately following teaching, patient and significant other verbalize accurate knowledge about the effects of an incompetent cervix on the pregnancy and fetus and comply with the treatment(s) accordingly.

INTERVENTIONS	RATIONALES
Explain to patient and significant other the effects an incompetent cervix may have on the mother, pregnancy, and fetus.	Information helps patients comply with treatments and understand possible consequences of noncompliance. Incompetent cervix may result in preterm delivery and fetal/neonatal morbidity or mortality.
Explain treatment options such as cervical cerclage placement.	A cerclage involves placement of a purse-string suture through the cervix to hold it closed until threat of miscarriage has passed. It is usually removed at around 35 wk gestation. The success of the cerclage is related to the dilation of the cervix (best when <2 cm) at the time of the procedure. The patient may be required to decrease physical activity or go on bedrest, decrease work hours or stop work, and avoid vaginal intercourse. She is also at risk for infection and failed cerclage.
Teach signs and symptoms that may indicate cervical change and importance of reporting them promptly.	A knowledgeable patient will likely report symptoms (pelvic pressure; increased vaginal discharge; pink, bloody, or tan vaginal discharge; backache; or contractions) promptly. See introductory information for detailed signs and symptoms of cervical incompetence. The earlier cervical incompetence is diagnosed, the better the chance for placing a cerclage, prolonging the pregnancy, and decreasing fetal morbidity and mortality.

Continued

INTERVENTIONS	RATIONALES
Teach daily fetal movement counts.	Fetal movement counts are a good first-line indicator of fetal well-being and are performed as follows beginning at 28 wk gestation: The patient lies on her side and counts "distinct fetal movements" (hiccups do not count) daily; 10 movements within a 2-hr period is reassuring. After detecting 10 movements, the count is discontinued. Fewer than 10 movements indicates need for fetal nonstress testing.
Teach patient how to palpate contractions.	Palpation and awareness of contractions enable patient to be an active participant in her health care. Timely reporting of contractions to her health care provider can play a significant role in affecting outcome. To palpate contractions, the patient lies comfortably on her side. She spreads her fingers apart and places one hand on the left side and the other on the right side of her abdomen. She will palpate the abdomen using her fingertips. When the uterus is relaxed, the abdomen should feel soft. In the presence of a contraction, the uterus will feel hard, tight, or firm under her fingertips. She then times the duration of the contraction from the beginning of one contraction to the beginning of the next. Contractions will vary in frequency and duration. If the patient experiences 4-6 contractions/hr for 1-2 hr, she should call her health care provider for further evaluation. Contractions may place tension on the cervical cerclage, cause bleeding of the cervix at the suture insertion sites, and dilate or cause funneling of the cervix above the cerclage.
	Duration of the contraction may or may not be an indication of contraction intensity. It is believed that the longer the contraction in true labor, the more effective it is in progressing dilation and effacement.
Question patient at each prenatal visit starting at the beginning of the second trimester if she is experiencing any cervical symptoms that may indicate cervical change. Encourage patient to report any "vague" or "subtle" symptoms no matter what time of day or night. Provide patient with written instructions and phone numbers to call accordingly.	Early recognition and reporting of cervical changes (e.g., light menstrual-like cramps, pelvic heaviness, sharp pains in the vagina or cervix, change in vaginal odor or discharge) may lead to better fetal outcome.
Instruct patient to drink at least six 8-oz glasses of water/day (48-64 fluid oz).	Patients with incompetent cervix may also experience preterm labor. The uterus is a muscle and will respond to dehydration by cramping/contracting. Adequate hydration is a preventative measure.

●●● **Related NIC and NOC labels:** *NIC:* High-risk Pregnancy Care; Disease Process *NOC:* Knowledge: Pregnancy; Disease Process

Nursing Diagnosis:

Ineffective Coping

related to adjustment in lifestyle to provide an optimal outcome for the pregnancy and fetus or lack of support from family, friends, and community

Desired Outcome: Within 24 hr of this diagnosis, patient begins to modify her lifestyle or behavior to provide the best pregnancy outcome for herself and the fetus.

INTERVENTIONS	RATIONALES
Assess patient's perceptions and comprehension of current health status regarding cervical incompetence.	Evaluation of perception and comprehension enables development of an individualized care plan.
Help patient identify or develop a support system.	Many people benefit from the aid and reduction of stress from outside support systems in helping them cope.
Arrange community referrals, as appropriate.	Support in the home environment promotes healthier adaptations and may avert crises.
Affirm that the necessary lifestyle adjustment (e.g., no work, bedrest, no intercourse), while it may seem austere, is for a limited time.	Facilitates acceptance of outside support and assistance. It also reconfirms that by not making lifestyle changes, activities that cause increased pressure on an incompetent cervix with or without a cerclage increase risk of cervical dilation, preterm delivery, and possible fetal/neonatal demise.
Provide referral sources for support groups, written material, Internet chat groups, or home help if the patient is on home bedrest or hospitalization. Also, involve Social Services in care of the patient as needed.	Communicating with others who have experienced similar circumstances may aid in developing coping mechanisms.
Offer emotional support when patient verbalizes her concerns.	Validates patient's concerns and may help her cope better.
Help patient identify previous methods of coping with life problems. Help patient focus on positive coping methods.	How patient has handled problems in the past may be a reliable predictor of how she will cope with current problems.

●●● **Related NIC and NOC labels:** *NIC:* Coping Enhancement; Emotional Support; Support System Enhancement *NOC:* Coping

Nursing Diagnosis:

Caregiver Role Strain

related to care significant other, family member, or support person needs to provide not only for the patient but possibly for other children in order for patient to remain compliant with treatments

Desired Outcome: Within 24 hr of this diagnosis, caregiver and patient verbalize their concerns/ frustrations about caregiving responsibilities, identify at least one other support person, and recognize at least one change that would make their jobs easier.

INTERVENTIONS	RATIONALES
Encourage caregiver to relate feelings and concerns regarding added responsibilities. Help caregiver clarify the responsibilities with patient and other family members.	Validates caregiver's concerns and helps him or her understand if expectations are realistic.
Involve Social Services in support of caregiver as needed in helping to establish a plan for time-outs.	Provides caregiver with visible goals and coping mechanisms.
Encourage caregiver to identify which activities would benefit from outside assistance and assist in identifying sources of help (e.g., family members, friends, neighbors, church members).	Confirms caregiver's need to seek help. During times of stress, caregivers may know they need help, but may not know where to look for it.
Affirm that added caregiving responsibilities are for a limited time.	Facilitates acceptance of outside support and assistance and may make current added responsibilities more tolerable.

●●● **Related NIC and NOC labels:** *NIC:* Coping Enhancement; Respite Care; Support System Enhancement; Behavior Modification *NOC:* Caregiver Well-Being; Role Performance

Nursing Diagnosis:

Risk for Impaired Parent/Infant Attachment

related to disruption for bonding or interactive process secondary to fetal health risks

Desired Outcome: Patient and significant other verbalize their concerns regarding potential
barriers to the parental bonding process.

INTERVENTIONS	RATIONALES
Encourage patient and significant other to verbalize concerns regarding the potential delay or loss in the bonding process.	Provides an opportunity for assessment, confirmation, and/or validation of their feelings.
If a loss occurs, allow patient and significant other time with the infant if they so desire (will depend on the appropriateness of the gestational age).	Validates their experience of loss and assists in transitioning to the grieving process.

●●● **Related NIC and NOC labels:** *NIC:* Emotional Support; Coping Enhancement; Family Involvement
Promotion *NOC:* Parent-Infant Attachment

Nursing Diagnosis:

Anticipatory Grieving

related to potential loss of the fetus secondary to cervical incompetence

Desired Outcome: Patient and significant other verbalize their feelings and identify and use
support systems to aid them in the grief process as needed.

INTERVENTIONS	RATIONALES
Encourage patient and significant other to verbalize their feelings and concerns regarding the potential for loss of their baby.	Validates concerns and conveys message that grief is a normal and expected reaction to the loss of a baby.
As appropriate, clarify misconceptions about the potential risk for fetal loss with incompetent cervix.	Allows patient and significant other to process the information regarding incompetent cervix appropriately while not providing false hope.
Assess and accept patient's behavioral response.	Disbelief, denial, guilt, anger, and depression are normal reactions to grief.
Teach the five stages of grief and explain that there is no specific time frame in which to go through the process.	Enables patient and family members to understand their stage of the grief process. Stages include (1) shock and numbness (2) denial and searching-yearning; (3) anger, guilt, and sense of failure; (4) depression and disorganization; and (5) resolution.
Involve Social Services when available and needed or when a loss is perceived or present.	Can provide resources and appropriate referral services for individual counseling, support groups for bereaved parents and grandparents, and guidance through the disposition of the fetus/neonate.
If a loss occurs, provide patient and family with support if they decide to see and hold the baby (gestation appropriate) and place appropriate items in a memory/keepsake box.	To assist with the grieving process. Items such as footprints and lock of hair may be tucked away and not looked at right away, but it may help them to know they are there.

●●● **Related NIC and NOC labels:** *NIC:* Coping Enhancement; Grief Work Facilitation: Perinatal Death;
Emotional Support; Hope Instillation; Support System Enhancement *NOC:* Coping

Nursing Diagnosis:

Sexual Dysfunction

related to inability to have sexual (penile-vaginal, digital-vaginal) intercourse during the pregnancy

Desired Outcome: Immediately following teaching, patient and partner verbalize accurate understanding of the effect that intercourse may have on an incompetent cervix and the reason for abstinence.

INTERVENTIONS	RATIONALES
Teach patient and her partner the effect that sexual foreplay or sexual intercourse may have on cervical incompetence. Explain that sexual intercourse may increase uterine contractions and promote cervical changes.	Knowledge promotes patient/partner compliance. Increased uterine activity is not uncommon after sexual intercourse. It may be caused by breast stimulation, female orgasm, or prostaglandin in male ejaculate.
Encourage patient and significant other to verbalize feelings and anxieties about sexual abstinence or having to use alternative methods (nothing per vagina) for sexual gratification. Develop strategies with patient and significant other.	Promotes knowledge of ways to achieve sexual satisfaction while understanding need to monitor uterine activity (cramping/ contractions) in response to the alternatives used (e.g., kissing, touching).

●●● **Related NIC and NOC labels:** *NIC:* Sexual Counseling; Anxiety Reduction *NOC:* Sexual Functioning

Nursing Diagnosis:

Deficient Knowledge:

Risks and benefits for cervical cerclage placement

Desired Outcome: Patient and significant other relate accurate understanding of the risks and benefits of the placement of a cervical cerclage.

INTERVENTIONS	RATIONALES
Inform patient and family of the risks and benefits of a cerclage.	Information helps them make an informed decision about cervical cerclage placement.
	A cerclage is usually placed early in the second trimester when the threat of a first trimester spontaneous abortion has passed. Risks include infection, cervical injury, displacement of the cerclage, PPROM, preterm labor, and preterm delivery. The benefit is a more likely continuation of the pregnancy.
Instruct patient in postoperative activities that should be avoided.	A knowledgeable patient likely will comply with limitations. These include avoidance of intercourse, prolonged (>90 min) standing, heavy lifting, and insertion of anything (including tampons) into the vagina.

●●● **Related NIC and NOC labels:** *NIC:* Teaching: Procedure/Treatment; Anxiety Reduction *NOC:* Knowledge: Treatment Procedure

ADDITIONAL NURSING DIAGNOSES/ PROBLEMS:

PATIENT-FAMILY TEACHING AND DISCHARGE PLANNING

Include verbal and written information about the following:

✔ Potential risk factors for cervical incompetence that may be present at the initial prenatal visit.

✔ Monitoring for signs and symptoms that may indicate cervical changes (increased vaginal discharge, light pink, blood-tinged, or tan).

✔ Palpation of contractions.

✔ Promptly reporting signs of UTI.

✔ Importance of adequate oral hydration.

✔ Compliance with scheduled prenatal visits. Confirm date and time of next visit.

✔ Measures for coping with muscle pain, back pain, and muscle weakness that can be present with prolonged bedrest.

✔ Measures that help with constipation, which occurs frequently in pregnancy and is exacerbated by bedrest.

✔ Importance of complying with restrictions on intercourse, heavy lifting, or prolonged (>90 min) standing.

✔ Medications, including drug name, purpose, dosage, frequency, drug/drug and food/drug interactions, precautions, potential drug reactions, and side effects.

✔ Guidelines for checking maternal pulse rate before dosing while taking terbutaline (a premature labor inhibitor).

✔ Fetal movement counts.

✔ Referral to national and local support organizations, including:

Sidelines, a national support organization for women and their families experiencing complicated pregnancies:
Sidelines High Risk Pregnancy Support National Office
P.O. Box 1808
Laguna Beach, CA 92652
(888) 447-4754
www.sidelines.org/

SHARE, a national support group for parents who have experienced loss through miscarriage, stillbirth, or newborn death:
SHARE Pregnancy & Infant Loss Support, Inc.
National SHARE Office
St. Joseph Health Center
300 First Capitol Drive
St. Charles, MO 63301-2893
(800) 821-6819 or (636) 947-6164
www.nationalshareoffice.com/

Diabetes in Pregnancy

Diabetes mellitus (DM) is classified as either type 1 or type 2. Type 1 (insulin-deficient diabetes) is usually characterized by onset at an early age (present before pregnancy) requiring insulin injections to avoid ketoacidosis (a state of increased hepatic glucose production and decreased or absent tissue disposal of glucose that results in hyperglycemia). Type 2 (insulin-resistant diabetes) includes gestational diabetes mellitus (GDM). GDM is a carbohydrate intolerance that has its onset or is first recognized during pregnancy. There is a 50% risk of GDM turning to chronic DM within 5 yr after diagnosis if no lifestyle changes are made. Both types of diabetes pose significant risks to maternal/fetal morbidity and mortality.

HEALTH CARE SETTING

Primary care (outpatient obstetric clinic, high-risk perinatal clinic); or acute care (inpatient) when starting or adjusting insulin.

ASSESSMENT

Every pregnant woman should be screened for GDM by obtaining history, clinical risk factors, or serum glucose levels. Patients with low risk factors (age <25 yr, not a member of an ethnic group at risk for developing type 2 diabetes, body mass index [BMI] <25, no previous history of abnormal glucose tolerance, no previous history of adverse obstetric outcomes that are usually associated with GDM, and no known diabetes in a first-degree relative [mother, father, siblings]) may not need the traditional glucose tolerance test. Only 10% of the pregnant population would fall into this category, and 3% of women with GDM would not have been diagnosed using this method. Therefore many providers prefer to screen all of their patients using the 1-hr glucose tolerance test.

Type 1 DM: Increased risk of abnormal embryogenesis (growth, differentiation, and organization of fetal cellular components), spontaneous abortion, sacral agenesis or caudal dysplasia (absence or deformity of the sacrum), pyelonephritis, preterm labor/birth, polyhydramnios (abnormally high level of amniotic fluid), preeclampsia, ketoacidosis, cesarean section, fetal hypoxia, stillbirth, fetal macrosomia (birth weight ≥4000 g) or intrauterine growth restriction, birth trauma (e.g., shoulder dystocia because of macrosomia), congenital anomalies (ventral septal defect, transposition of the great vessels, anencephaly (absence of neural tissue in the cranium), open spina bifida (a defect in the closure of the neural tube), holoprosencephaly (absence of midline cerebral structures because of the incomplete division of the forebrain), respiratory distress syndrome (RDS), and neonatal hypoglycemia.

Type 2 DM/GDM: Increased risk of macrosomia or intrauterine growth restriction (depending on extent of the maternal illness and glycemic control), preeclampsia, ketoacidosis, cesarean section, hypoxia, RDS, stillbirth, birth trauma, and neonatal hypoglycemia.

Note: During pregnancy the classic symptoms of diabetes (polydipsia, polyphagia, and polyuria) cannot be used as diagnostic tools because they are normal changes of pregnancy.

Renal-urinary: Glucosuria is not a reliable sign of diabetes during pregnancy because of a lowered renal threshold that occurs at that time. If glucose (≥+1) appears consistently (≥2 times) in the urine, however, the patient needs to be evaluated for GDM.

Neurologic: Frequent headaches, fatigue, and drowsiness may be present as a result of maternal insulin resistance. Retinopathy is commonly seen in woman with type 1 DM (preexisting disease) caused by abnormal vasculature, capillary rupture, or hemorrhage within the retina.

Cardiovascular: In patients with long-term diabetes, deterioration of glomerular function can lead to hypertension and superimposed preeclampsia. These women can also develop arteriosclerosis.

Other symptoms: Pregnant women with diabetes are at an increased risk of developing preeclampsia. See additional symptoms in "Preeclampsia," p. 747.

Complications—fetal:
- Miscarriage/fetal death
- Embryonic growth delay
- Congenital malformations, especially cardiac and skeletal
- Hypertrophic and congestive cardiomyopathy
- Fetal macrosomia (gigantism)
- Hypoglycemia
- Respiratory distress syndrome
- Hyperbilirubinemia
- Hypocalcemia
- Intrauterine growth restriction

Risk factors: Family history of DM, previous history of GDM, previous macrosomic infant, previous unexplained stillbirth, poor obstetric outcome, polyhydramnios (past or present), excessive weight gain or obesity, history of congenital anomalies in offspring, chronic hypertension, recurrent infections including vaginal monilial, recurrent glucosuria, and age >30. There is also increased risk for GDM among African Americans, Hispanics, Native Americans, Asians, and South Pacific Islanders.

DIAGNOSTIC TESTS

One-hour glucose screening: Performed between wk 24-28 of the pregnancy or earlier, even at the initial prenatal visit. If results are negative in an earlier test, the test is repeated between 24-28 wk in the pregnancy if patient meets risk factors (discussed earlier). This test requires the patient to drink a 50-g glucose load, followed in 1 hr by venous plasma measurement. A value ≥140 mg/dl is considered abnormal and indicates need for the 3-hr 100-g oral glucose tolerance test. When a 1-hr value is ≥190 mg/dl, a fasting glucose should be done before proceeding to the 3-hr test. If the fasting value is ≥95 mg/dl, the patient is treated for GDM.

Three-hour glucose tolerance test: After fasting for 8-12 hr and abstaining from smoking, a fasting blood sugar is drawn after which the patient drinks 100-g glucose load followed by serum venous plasma measurements at 1, 2, and 3 hr. Two of the four values need to be abnormal to make the diagnosis of GDM. There are two diagnostic criteria for diagnosing GDM, depending on medical facility preference. They are as follows.

National Diabetes Data Group	Carpenter and Coustan
Fasting: 105	Fasting: 95
1–hr: 190	1–hr: 180
2–hr: 165	2–hr: 155
3–hr: 145	3–hr: 140

Glycosylated hemoglobin (HbA₁C): Reflects the average blood sugar levels for the 2-3 mo period before the test. Values may be increased in iron deficient anemia and decreased in pregnancy. Levels <7% are desired in pregnancy.

Home glucose monitoring: The patient at home performs glucose monitoring (obtaining whole blood from a fingerstick) at given intervals prescribed by the health care provider. Normal values during pregnancy are fasting blood sugar (FBS) <95 mg/dl and 2-hr pp ≤120 mg/dl. Patients with poor glucose control will have FBS well above 90-95 mg/dl and 2-hr postprandial (pp) well above 120 mg/dl. Careful regulation of maternal glucose levels during pregnancy leads to decreased maternal/fetal compromise and better outcomes.

Renal function studies: Normally during pregnancy creatinine clearance is increased, but it is decreased in GDM because of deterioration in glomerular function. A 24-hr urinalysis for protein is recommended early in the pregnancy that can be used as a comparison later if renal function worsens.

Obstetric ultrasound: A screening ultrasound and fetal cardiac echo are done at around 20 wk gestation to check for fetal anomalies inasmuch as incidence is increased in fetuses of mothers with diabetes. Further ultrasounds may be done at 2-4 wk intervals to monitor fetal growth, placental function, amniotic fluid levels, and fetal position and check for presence of polyhydramnios (excess amniotic fluid).

Antepartum fetal monitoring: Patients with GDM who are diet controlled and at low risk for intrauterine death do not routinely require antepartum fetal heart rate testing unless they have hypertension, history of prior stillbirth, or current fetal macrosomia. Any of these conditions would necessitate weekly to twice weekly testing starting at 32 wk (or sooner if necessary) to monitor fetal well-being.

Nursing Diagnosis:

Deficient Knowledge:

Effects of diabetes on self, pregnancy, and fetus

Desired Outcome: Immediately following teaching, patient verbalizes accurate knowledge about the effects of diabetes on self, the pregnancy, and fetus and complies with the treatment accordingly.

INTERVENTIONS	RATIONALES
Explain to patient and significant other the effects diabetes may have on the mother, pregnancy, and fetus.	An informed patient is more likely to comply with the therapeutic plan (e.g., frequent blood sugar checks, frequent clinic visits, insulin injections, dietary monitoring) and understand possible problems associated with type 1 DM and GDM or consequences of noncompliance.
Encourage compliance with prenatal appointments, testing, and dietary regimen.	Pregnant women with type 1 DM are at increased risk for maternal/fetal morbidity and mortality. Fetal death, preeclampsia, renal disease, cardiac disease, and retinopathy are possible. Women with GDM are at increased risk for fetal macrosomia and preeclampsia, especially when they are not compliant with the therapeutic plan. There is a 50% risk of GDM turning to chronic DM within 5 yr after diagnosis if no lifestyle changes are made.
Inform patient about probable increased need for insulin to manage glycemic control during the pregnancy.	The body's insulin requirements increase as the pregnancy advances. Insulin therapy should be considered when nutritional therapy fails to keep 1-hr pp <130-140 mg/dl, 2-hr pp <120 mg/dl, or fasting glucose <95 mg/dl.
For patients with GDM, arrange for one-on-one teaching with a diabetes educator for the following: how to check blood sugars with a Glucometer, how to document blood sugars, and importance of exercise during pregnancy.	A one-on-one session with a diabetes educator experienced with GDM enables an opportunity for questions/interactions and greater patient comprehension.
Teach patient and significant other signs and symptoms of hypoglycemia, hyperglycemia, diabetic ketoacidosis, and insulin shock. For more information, see "Diabetes Mellitus," p. 399, and "Diabetic Ketoacidosis," p. 409.	A knowledgeable patient likely will report these symptoms promptly. During pregnancy the goal is for lower blood sugar levels than when not pregnant. Therefore the patient is more likely to experience hypoglycemia than hyperglycemia.
Develop a sick-day plan with the patient.	Helps maintain adequate glycemic control. For example, patient should do the following: - Check blood sugar and urine for ketones q2-4h during illness. Maintain normal insulin schedule. - Maintain normal meals when possible. Drink plenty of water and/or calorie-free liquids if unable to maintain solid foods. Consume a minimum of 150 g of carbohydrates per day, taken in small amounts over 24 hr. - Call provider if temperature is ≥101° F (38.3° C), ketone level is moderate to high, or if vomiting and unable to keep anything down. Patient may need to be hospitalized for IV fluids and regulation of blood sugar. In diabetes associated with pregnancy, early detection of ketones is critical to fetal mortality because ketoacidosis is a significant factor that contributes to intrauterine death.
Encourage patient to maintain or initiate an exercise program.	Exercise improves cardiopulmonary fitness and may improve glucose metabolism.
Teach daily fetal movement counts.	Fetal movement counts are a good first-line indicator of fetal well-being and are performed as follows, beginning at 28 wk gestation: Patient lies on her side and counts "distinct fetal movements" (hiccups do not count) daily; 10 movements within a 2-hr period is reassuring. After 10 movements are noted, the count is discontinued. Fewer than 10 movements indicates need for fetal nonstress testing.

●●● **Related NIC and NOC labels:** *NIC:* Teaching: Disease Process; Hyperglycemia Management; Hypoglycemia Management; Nutrition Management *NOC:* Knowledge: Diabetes Management

Nursing Diagnosis:

Fear

related to effects of GDM on self, pregnancy, and fetus; potential complications; and insulin injections.

Desired Outcomes: Immediately following interventions, patient and significant other express fears and concerns. Within 24 hr of interventions, patient reports feeling greater psychologic comfort, understanding of the effects of diabetes on the pregnancy, and confidence in administering insulin if needed.

INTERVENTIONS	RATIONALES
Encourage and support patient and significant other in verbalizing their fears and concerns.	Validates their fears/concerns and enables development of an individualized care plan.
Acknowledge patient's fears.	Acknowledging feelings in an empathetic manner encourages communication, which optimally will reduce fear. For example, "I understand that giving yourself injections frightens you, but it is necessary to control your blood sugar."
When appropriate and if available, involve Social Services in patient management. Provide patient with a list of support groups available for patients with GDM.	Social Services can provide individual counseling and information on referrals, support groups, and Internet chat groups for patients with GDM. Some support groups are listed at the end of this care plan.
Encourage patient to ask questions and become as knowledgeable as possible about her condition and treatment.	Increasing knowledge levels about appropriate dietary intake and blood sugar control reduces/eliminates fear of the unknown and affords a sense of control.
Teach patient appropriate techniques for checking blood sugar, documenting results, and drawing up, injecting, and storing insulin (see "Diabetes Mellitus," p. 399, for individuals who are not pregnant).	Provides opportunity to assess and validate patient's knowledge and fears. Knowledge likely will help decrease fear of self-administration of insulin and aid in compliance with treatments.

●●● **Related NIC and NOC labels:** *NIC:* Active Listening; Anxiety Reduction; Support System Enhancement; Teaching: Procedure *NOC:* Fear Control

Nursing Diagnosis:

Anxiety

related to actual or perceived threat to self or fetus secondary to the effects diabetes may have on the pregnancy

Desired Outcome: Within 1-2 hr of intervention, patient states that her anxiety has lessened or resolved, and she describes appropriate coping mechanisms in managing the anxiety.

INTERVENTIONS	RATIONALES
Engage in honest communication with patient; provide empathetic understanding. Listen closely.	To establish an atmosphere that allows free expression.
Be alert for verbal and nonverbal cues about patient's anxiety level.	Aids in providing appropriate assistance and support. Levels of anxiety include: - *Mild:* restlessness, irritability, increased questions, focusing on the environment.

Continued

INTERVENTIONS	RATIONALES
	- *Moderate:* inattentiveness, expressions of concern, narrowed perceptions, insomnia, increased HR.
	- *Severe:* expression of feelings of doom, rapid speech, tremors, poor eye contact. Patient may be preoccupied with the past or unable to understand the present and may have tachycardia, nausea, and hyperventilation.
	- *Panic:* inability to concentrate or communicate, distortion of reality, increased motor activity, vomiting, tachypnea.
Explain that patients with poor glycemic control or who need to initiate first-time insulin use usually are admitted to the hospital for teaching and monitoring.	Offers potential of a supportive environment that aids in decreasing anxiety and increasing patient confidence.
Encourage patient to communicate cause of anxiety, for example, dietary changes, failure to maintain adequate glycemic control, checking blood sugars, insulin injections.	Helps determine patient's knowledge of diabetes in pregnancy and ways in which patient teaching can alleviate anxiety.
Provide reassurance and a safe, quiet environment for patient to relax.	An anxious person has difficulty learning.
Assess at each appointment if patient has enough supplies to maintain self-care.	Having adequate supplies (e.g., Glucometer, test strips, lancets, record book, insulin, syringes, alcohol wipes, sharps disposal box) on hand may increase compliance and decrease anxiety.
Encourage patient to attend diabetes classes and support groups for patients with diabetes.	Talking with others who have or are experiencing diabetes in pregnancy aids in establishing outside support resources. Some support groups are listed at the end of this care plan.
Inform patient with GDM that although she has diabetes associated with the pregnancy, this does not mean she will have lifelong diabetes.	Having this information may alleviate anxiety and increase compliance with therapeutic plan.
However, advise her that if she has other risk factors such as a first-line relative with history of type 1 or type 2 DM, obesity, and diet high in carbohydrates and fats, these factors can increase risk for developing chronic DM during the next 10-15 yr.	Identifies some factors over which she has control, which optimally will decrease anxiety and encourage weight loss, dietary control, and exercise postpartum to prevent future development of chronic DM.

●●● **Related NIC and NOC labels:** *NIC:* Anxiety Reduction; Active Listening; Environmental Management; Support Group *NOC:* Anxiety Control

Nursing Diagnosis:

Imbalanced Nutrition: Less or more than body requirements

related to inability to follow prescribed dietary regimen for effective glycemic control

Desired Outcome: Patient follows prescribed dietary regimen.

INTERVENTIONS	RATIONALES
Assess patient's cultural habits surrounding diet (foods she can and cannot eat, who shops, who cooks).	Working within cultural habits aids in dietary compliance. For example, there may be high carbohydrate consumption, depending on cultural group: rice for Asian women; tortillas and rice for Hispanic women; and breads and pasta for non-Hispanic white women.

Continued

INTERVENTIONS	RATIONALES
Arrange for a meeting with a nutritionist who specializes in diabetes in pregnancy.	A nutritionist is trained to answer questions regarding specific foods and meal plans that are appropriate for glycemic control and can act as a resource person for the patient. Nutritional interventions should achieve normal glucose levels and avoid ketosis while maintaining appropriate nutrition and weight gain in pregnancy.
Encourage patient to keep a daily dietary log.	Provides quick reference to compare blood sugars and foods eaten.
Praise patient when blood sugars are within normal limits.	Encourages patient to follow the prescribed dietary regimen. Good glycemic control reduces incidence of maternal and fetal morbidity and mortality.
Inform patient of the risks to self and fetus associated with poor glycemic control related to dietary noncompliance.	Knowledge aids in patient compliance. Dietary noncompliance can result in miscarriage, fetal anomalies, fetal macrosomia and increased risk of shoulder dystocia with a vaginal delivery, and increased potential for cesarean delivery.
Teach patient to monitor urine for ketones.	Ketones are weak acids produced when blood sugar is poorly controlled and the body burns fat instead of sugar for energy. Moderate to large (2-4+) ketones may signal ketoacidosis, which necessitates immediate evaluation. If untreated, prolonged ketoacidosis can result in fetal brain damage.
Develop a "sick-day plan" with patient.	See discussion in **Deficient Knowledge:** Effects of diabetes on self, pregnancy, and fetus, earlier.

●●● **Related NIC and NOC labels:** *NIC:* Nutritional Counseling; Teaching: Prescribed Diet
NOC: Nutritional Status: Nutrient Intake

Nursing Diagnosis:

Deficient Knowledge:

Benefits and potential side effects of prescribed medications used to treat GDM

Desired Outcome: Immediately following teaching, patient and significant other verbalize accurate understanding of the risks and benefits of medications used during the pregnancy to treat diabetes.

INTERVENTIONS	RATIONALES
Sulfonylureas: second-generation	Lower blood glucose by stimulating release of insulin from the pancreas.
Glyburide (Micronase, DiaBeta, Euglucon)	This is currently the only oral glycemic agent shown to be safe and effective in GDM. There is concern for teratogenicity with other oral agents. Diabetes itself is teratogenic, making it difficult to determine effects of the oral agents from those of the disease. Most patients with type 1 DM who have been managed on oral agents are changed to insulin during the pregnancy. Administration: oral.

Continued

INTERVENTIONS	**RATIONALES**
Teach patient to be alert for and report shakiness, sweating, nervousness, headache, and blood sugar level <60 mg/dl.	Signs of hypoglycemia.
Teach patient to be alert for and report blurred vision.	Side effect caused by fluctuation in blood glucose levels.
Stress importance of monitoring blood glucose levels as directed.	Helps detect hypoglycemia or hyperglycemia promptly. The usual routine in pregnancy is to monitor blood glucose fasting (first thing in the morning before breakfast or taking medications), 2 hr after eating, at hs, and when glucose levels have been low or high. Poor glycemic control when taking the oral agent necessitates initiation of insulin.
Teach patient to be alert for and report nausea, epigastric fullness, and heartburn.	Adverse reactions. If these reactions occur consistently, patient may require dose adjustment or be started on insulin—whichever maintains glycemic control.
Caution patients taking nonsteroidal antiinflammatory drugs (NSAIDs) and β-adrenergic blocking agents to notify health care provider before taking sulfonylureas.	Hypoglycemic reaction may be potentiated by these medications.
Insulin *Regular Humalog and lispro (rapid acting), NPH (intermediate acting), glargine (long acting)*	Parenteral blood glucose–lowering agents that regulate glucose metabolism. Lispro has a more rapid onset of action than regular insulin and does not cross the placenta.
	Administration: SC or by insulin pump. Some patients may be started on SC insulin as an outpatient. This choice is individualized based on patient compliance and comprehension of insulin therapy (drawing up insulin, injecting accurately, and timing doses). Inpatient setting is required for initial teaching for how to use the pump, including monitoring of glucose levels and making necessary insulin dose adjustments.
Teach patient to be alert for and report shakiness, sweating, nervousness, headache, and low blood sugar levels.	Signs of hypoglycemia, a potential side effect. Some patients may be symptomatic between 60-70 mg/dl and others not until 50-60 mg/dl (or lower)
Teach patient to be alert for and report blurred vision.	Side effect secondary to fluctuations in blood glucose levels.
Stress importance of monitoring blood glucose levels as directed.	Aids in prompt identification of hypoglycemic reactions.
Caution patients taking NSAIDs, salicylates, and β-adrenergic blocking agents to notify their health care provider.	Insulin requirements may be decreased when also taking drugs with hypoglycemic activity. β-Blockers may mask the symptoms of hypoglycemia.
Caution patient taking terbutaline to notify health care provider.	This drug may alter glucose metabolism. Terbutaline is used to decrease uterine myometrial activity (contractions).

●●● **Related NIC and NOC labels:** *NIC:* Teaching: Prescribed Medication; Hyperglycemia Management; Hypoglycemia Management *NOC:* Knowledge: Medication

ADDITIONAL NURSING DIAGNOSES/ PROBLEMS:

"Psychosocial Support" for relevant nursing diagnoses such as **Ineffective Coping**   p. 87

"Psychosocial Support for the Patient's Family and Significant Others" for such nursing diagnoses as **Compromised Family Coping**   p. 97

"Diabetes Mellitus" for additional information   p. 399

"Diabetic Ketoacidosis" for additional information   p. 409

"Mastitis" for **Anxiety**   p. 734

PATIENT-FAMILY TEACHING AND DISCHARGE PLANNING

Patients with GDM require close monitoring for maternal and fetal well-being. Education is the key to making the pregnancy a success. When providing patient-family teaching, avoid giving excessive information. Part of the initial assessment should include asking about existing knowledge of the disease, ability for self-management, and psychologic acceptance. Include written and verbal information about the following:

✓ Recommended glucose levels in pregnancy: Fasting 60-90 mg/dl; before lunch, dinner, or hs snack 60-105 mg/dl; 2-hr pp ≤120 mg/dl.

✓ Reminder that stress from illness or infection can increase insulin requirements.

✓ Recognizing warning signs of both hyperglycemia and simple and advanced hypoglycemia and insulin shock, treatment, and factors that contribute to both conditions.

- *Hypoglycemia:* Possible causes are too much insulin, too little food, not eating on time, vomiting, and too much exercise. (See next three items for treatment options.)

- *Hyperglycemia:* Possible causes include not enough insulin or increased insulin resistance (as seen with advancing gestational age), too much food, stress of illness, emotional stress, and decreased exercise. Patient should call health care provider for treatment, which may include increasing insulin dose and/or self-administering an insulin bolus.

Review "Diabetes Mellitus," p. 399, for further information.

✓ Foods to treat hypoglycemia such as 4-oz orange juice, 4-oz milk, 4-oz cola drink (not diet cola), 3-4 pieces of hard candy, 3-4 sugar cubes, 2-3 glucose tablets.

✓ How and when to take glucose tablets. Keep glucose tablets with you when away from home and available food sources. Instruct patient to use glucose tablets if becoming shaky, nauseated, nervous, headachy, drowsy, and diaphoretic and blood sugar is ≤60 mg/dl.

✓ When to call for emergency services. With advanced hypoglycemia (blood sugar 20-50 mg/dl) the patient may not be the person calling in an emergency situation; this information needs to be communicated to significant other and family members as well.

✓ Importance of carrying an identification card or wearing a bracelet or necklace that identifies patient as having diabetes in case of emergency. For patients with GDM the necklace or bracelet may be obtained at a local pharmacy. If the patient has preexisting diabetes, the above information may be obtained by contacting the following organization: Medic Alert Foundation, 323 Colorado Avenue, Turlock, CA 96382, (209) 668-3333.

✓ Importance of compliance with prescribed health care and ready access to hospital and family/social support.

✓ Parameters and guidelines for blood sugar levels as recommended by health care provider.

✓ Nutritional regimen as recommended by health care provider. Adequate nutrition and controlled calories are essential to maintaining normoglycemia and appropriate fetal growth.

✓ Medications, including drug name, purpose, dosage, frequency, precautions, administration, food/drug and drug/drug interactions, and potential side effects.

✓ How to monitor urine for ketones.

✓ Fetal movement counts (gestational age appropriate).

✓ Referrals to local and national support organizations, including:

American Diabetes Association (ADA)
1660 Duke Street
Alexandria, VA 22314
(800) 232-3472
www.diabetes.org

Sidelines, a national support organization for women and their families experiencing complicated pregnancies: Sidelines High Risk Pregnancy Support National Office
P.O. Box 1808
Laguna Beach, CA 92652
(888) 447-4754
www.sidelines.org

Joslin Diabetes Center
Director, Joslin Clinic
1 Joslin Place
Boston, MA 02215
(617) 732-2501
www.joslin.harvard.edu

90

Hyperemesis Gravidarum

Nausea and vomiting are common symptoms of unknown cause in the first trimester of pregnancy. Hyperemesis is excessive vomiting in pregnancy that can interfere with hydration, electrolytes, acid base balance, and nutritional status and may last throughout the entire pregnancy. Theories regarding cause include rising estrogen and human chorionic gonadotropin levels, relaxation of the smooth muscles of the abdomen caused by an increase in progesterone, decrease in motilin levels, and psychogenic factors.

HEALTH CARE SETTING

Some hyperemesis patients may be treated on an outpatient basis with home IV infusion therapy given to replace fluids and electrolytes, or some may receive total parenteral nutrition. Others require hospitalization.

ASSESSMENT

Patients with nausea and vomiting in pregnancy who can no longer retain solids or liquids need to be evaluated for dehydration, weight loss, and electrolyte imbalances. They may exhibit a low-grade fever, weakness, dry skin, and poor skin turgor. Patients may appear extremely fatigued and listless with cracked, dry lips and may have lost 5%–10% of total body weight; be constipated as a result of dehydration; and have a markedly decreased urinary output with ketonemia (presence of ketones in the blood). Women with diabetes who have hyperemesis need to be monitored closely to maintain glycemic control and avoid ketoacidosis. See "Diabetes in Pregnancy," p. 715.

Gastrointestinal: Gastrointestinal motility is reduced because of increased progesterone and decreased motilin levels. "Normal" nausea and vomiting of pregnancy usually has an onset between 4-6 wk, peaks at about 12 wk, and optimally resolves at around 20 wk. Nausea and vomiting with hyper-

emesis may extend beyond this period, possibly throughout the entire pregnancy.

Fluid and electrolyte imbalance: With the inability to maintain adequate fluids for hydration and solids for fuel, the body experiences an imbalance of the elements necessary for health maintenance, which can lead to maternal ketosis.

Cardiopulmonary: The patient may experience one or all of the following: tachycardia, hypotension, postural changes, and tachypnea.

Renal: Possible presence of oliguria and ketonuria.

Complications—fetal: With prolonged dehydration and maternal weight loss, fetal intrauterine growth restriction (IUGR) and low birth weight may be seen.

Physical assessment: The pregnant patient with hyperemesis looks and is ill, appearing extremely fatigued and pale. A thorough assessment is needed to rule out other causes of severe nausea and vomiting, such as gastroenteritis, cholecystitis, pyelonephritis, gastrointestinal (GI) ulcers, or a molar pregnancy (intrauterine neoplastic mass of grapelike enlarged chorionic villi).

Risk factors: Previous history of hyperemesis, molar pregnancy, multiple gestation, emotional/psychologic stress, gastroesophageal reflux, primigravida, uncontrolled thyroid disease, increased body weight/obesity.

DIAGNOSTIC TESTS

Liver enzymes: Slight elevations of aspartate aminotransferase (AST) and alanine aminotransferase (ALT), which reverse with IV fluid hydration, adequate nutrition, and cessation of vomiting.

Complete blood count (CBC): With dehydration, there likely will be evidence of hemoconcentration (i.e., elevated red blood cell [RBC] and Hct levels).

Serum chemistry: Azotemia (increased blood urea nitrogen [BUN]) is seen with salt and water depletion. Serum creatinine will be elevated because of changes in renal function caused by the dehydration. Hyponatremia and hypokalemia also may be present because of fluid loss.

Urine chemistry: The urine may be "dipped" (or sent for microscopy) for the presence of ketones, which are seen in dehydration/prolonged vomiting.

Obstetric ultrasound: Ultrasound is used to evaluate a normal intrauterine pregnancy vs. a molar pregnancy, presence of multiple gestation, and fetal growth for IUGR and amniotic fluid volume/amniotic fluid index (AFI).

Nursing Diagnosis:

Anxiety

related to actual or perceived threat to self and fetus because of inadequate nutritional status

Desired Outcome: Within 1-2 hr of intervention, patient verbalizes her anxieties, assesses her support system(s), and uses appropriate coping mechanisms for management.

INTERVENTIONS	RATIONALES
Engage in honest communication with patient; provide empathetic understanding. Listen closely.	To establish an atmosphere that allows free expression.
Encourage patient to communicate cause(s) of her anxiety.	Aids in developing a care plan specific to patient's needs, such as whether home or hospital treatment will be more helpful. Examples of causes that may be contributing to patient's anxiety include weight loss, frustration with constant nausea and vomiting, ambivalence about the pregnancy, lack of support from significant other and family, and inability to care for self or others.
	Patients with severe nausea and vomiting who demonstrate changes in laboratory values and weight loss should be admitted to the hospital for hydration, nutritional supplementation, medications, and monitoring of weight loss or gain. This will provide a supportive environment that aids in decreasing anxiety and increasing patient comfort.
Be alert for verbal and nonverbal cues about patient's anxiety level.	Aids in providing appropriate assistance and support.
	Levels of anxiety include:
	- *Mild:* restlessness, irritability, increased questions, focusing on the environment.
	- *Moderate:* inattentiveness, expressions of concern, narrowed perceptions, insomnia, increased HR.
	- *Severe:* expression of feelings of doom, rapid speech, tremors, and poor eye contact. Patient may be preoccupied with the past or unable to understand the present and may have tachycardia, increased nausea and vomiting, and hyperventilation.
	- *Panic:* inability to concentrate or communicate, distortion of reality, increased motor activity, increased vomiting and tachypnea.
Involve assistance of Social Services when available.	Provides counseling, support, and resources for written material and Internet chat groups with others who have experienced similar circumstances.

Continued

INTERVENTIONS	RATIONALES
Involve assistance of a psychologist as needed.	Enables evaluation for possible psychologic factors that may be contributing to the anxiety and hyperemesis.
Encourage patient to obtain as much rest as possible.	Enhances coping mechanisms by decreasing physical and psychologic stress.

●●● **Related NIC and NOC labels:** *NIC:* Anxiety Reduction; Active Listening; Coping Enhancement; Counseling *NOC:* Anxiety Control; Coping

Nursing Diagnosis:

Imbalanced Nutrition: Less than body requirements

related to inability to ingest and maintain sufficient calories secondary to the nausea and vomiting of hyperemesis gravidarum

Desired Outcome: Within 1 wk of this diagnosis, patient increases her nutritional intake and demonstrates improvement in her acid–base balance and electrolyte and nutritional status.

INTERVENTIONS	RATIONALES
Suggest frequent small meals, six or more per day.	Helps reduce feeling of a distended stomach and hence the potential for nausea and vomiting.
Suggest eating meals with the highest protein/calorie intake when the nausea is the least problematic, possibly after taking medication for nausea and vomiting.	The meal providing the most nutrition would be consumed at the time the patient is most likely to retain it.
Suggest that patient use high-protein supplemental drinks.	Liquids may be easier to tolerate than solid foods.
Suggest that patient avoid food odors and foods that are greasy, highly spiced, rich, or overly sweet.	Prevents stimulating the gag reflex or increasing acid reflux. However, because some patients prefer salty and spicy foods, patient should try anything that is appealing and that she believes she will be able to keep down.
Administer IV hydration as needed.	Aids in resolving dehydration and improving electrolyte balance.
Administer parenteral nutrition as needed. Secure assistance of the hyperalimentation team to manage patient's parenteral nutrition.	To improve nutritional status and thereby help ensure adequate fetal growth.
Encourage patient to take approximately 100 ml of liquid between meals and avoid fluids with meals.	Prevents dehydration between meals and overdistention of the stomach during meals, allowing more space for caloric foods.
Encourage patient to stay upright for 2 hr after eating.	Prevents esophageal spasms that can be caused by reflux of acid and food into the esophagus. Gravity aids in facilitating movement of food through the esophagus to the stomach and into the small intestine.

●●● **Related NIC and NOC labels:** *NIC:* Fluid Management; Intravenous Therapy; Total Parenteral Nutrition Administration; Sustenance Support *NOC:* Nutritional Status: Food & Fluid Intake

Nursing Diagnosis:

Ineffective Coping

related to loss of control over maintaining adequate nutritional intake because of the nausea and vomiting of pregnancy

Desired Outcome: Within the 24-hr period after this diagnosis is made, patient verbalizes her concerns, fears, strengths, and weaknesses and identifies personal coping mechanisms and support systems.

INTERVENTIONS	RATIONALES
Assess patient's perceptions and ability to understand current health status.	Evaluation of patient's perceptions and comprehension level enables development of an individualized care plan.
Establish honest and empathetic communication with patient.	To promote effective therapeutic communication. For example, "Please tell me what I can do to help you through this difficult time in your pregnancy."
Help patient identify previous methods of coping with life problems.	How patient has handled problems in the past may be a reliable predictor of how she will cope with current problems.
Identify patient's support systems. If possible, observe their interaction with the patient.	Knowing the family unit's strengths and weaknesses aids in planning patient's care and, optimally, reducing stress and promoting effective coping.
Enlist assistance from social workers, nutritional services, and spiritual care as needed.	To provide emotional support, education, and appropriate referrals as needed.
Teach patient how to effectively use her time when she feels well (e.g., performing activities of daily living [ADL] or running errands).	Provides patient with some sense of control over her situation.
Teach possible treatment methods for hyperemesis.	Knowledge that there are viable treatments aids in improving coping mechanisms and treatment compliance. For examples of treatments, see next care plan.

●●● **Related NIC and NOC labels:** *NIC:* Coping Enhancement; Support System Enhancement; Emotional Support *NOC:* Coping

Nursing Diagnosis:

Deficient Knowledge:

Effects hyperemesis has on self, the pregnancy, and fetus and the treatment and expected outcome

Desired Outcome: Immediately following teaching, patient and significant other verbalize accurate knowledge about hyperemesis, its treatment, and the expected outcome.

INTERVENTIONS	RATIONALES
Explain to patient and family the effect hyperemesis has on the patient and the fetus.	Hyperemesis causes decreased maternal-fetal placental transfer of nutrients and IUGR. Information helps patient comply with treatments and understand possible consequences of noncompliance.
Explain the various treatment options.	Treatments may include IV hydration, medications (IV, IM, PO), total parenteral nutrition, home care, and hospitalization.

Continued

INTERVENTIONS	RATIONALES
	Explanation of treatment options aids patient and provider in deciding on a care plan that is most beneficial to patient and fetus.
Teach signs and symptoms that may indicate worsening hyperemesis and dehydration.	A knowledgeable patient likely will report symptoms (inability to keep solids or liquids down for previous 12 hr, dizziness, extreme fatigue, poor skin turgor, caramel-colored urine, and weight loss) promptly. Early evaluation and treatment may decrease severity of symptoms.
Explain expected outcome that adequate fluid and nutritional intake will have on fetal development: increases maternal-fetal placental transfer of nutrients and ensures intrauterine fetal growth.	Reinforces need for patient compliance with possible hospitalization or home infusion, IV fluids, or parenteral nutrition.
Encourage patient to avoid brushing her teeth within 1-2 hr after meals or on arising in the morning.	Stimulates the gag reflex and aggravates vomiting in women who are pregnant.
Encourage good oral hygiene.	Prevents dental decay that may accompany contact with the acids present in emesis and for some may help decrease nausea. For example, patient may use mouthwash and brush and floss teeth when she feels the least nauseated.

●●● **Related NIC and NOC labels:** *NIC:* Teaching: Disease Process; Teaching: Procedure/Treatment *NOC:* Knowledge: Disease Process; Knowledge: Treatment Procedures

Nursing Diagnosis:

Deficient Knowledge:

Purpose, potential side effects, and safety of prescribed medications used during hyperemesis gravidarum

Desired Outcome: Immediately following teaching, patient verbalizes accurate understanding of the risks, benefits, and precautions of medications used during pregnancy in the treatment of hyperemesis.

INTERVENTIONS	RATIONALES
Teach the following about patient's prescribed medications:	A knowledgeable patient is more likely to comply with therapy, identify and report side effects, and recognize and report precautions that might preclude use of the prescribed drug.
Metoclopramide hydrochloride (Reglan)	Antiemetic that works on the chemoreceptor trigger zone in the brain to decrease nausea and vomiting. Helps move food through the GI tract, counteracting the effects of progesterone produced in the pregnancy that slow down the GI tract.
	Administration: PO/IM/IV.
	May be given as outpatient or inpatient.
Be alert for and report twitching of the eyelids or muscles surrounding the eyes, hands, or legs.	Extrapyramidal reactions seen with high IV doses.
Be alert for and report involuntary repetitious movements of the muscles of the face, limbs, and trunk.	This is a sign of tardive dyskinesia (a syndrome of potentially irreversible involuntary repetitious movements) and a serious side effect seen with long-term use.

Continued

INTERVENTIONS	RATIONALES
Be alert for and report drowsiness, agitation, seizures, hallucinations, lactation, constipation, and diarrhea.	Common side effects.
Caution is necessary in patients with seizure disorders.	This drug may lower the seizure threshold.
Caution is necessary in patients taking this medication with sedatives, narcotics, and tranquilizers.	Additive sedative effects may occur.
Promethazine (Phenergan)	Antiemetic/antihistamine/tranquilizer.
	Administration: PO/IV/IM/rectal.
	It is not administered SC because it may cause chemical irritation and necrotic lesions at site of injection. Infiltration when given IV can cause the same symptoms seen with SC administration.
Be alert for and report sedation, blurred vision, fatigue, ringing in the ears, nervousness, insomnia, and tremors.	Common side effects. Patient should avoid activities that require alertness until the drug's effect on the central nervous system (CNS) is known.
Precautions are needed for patients taking other CNS depressants such as opioids.	Drug interactions can occur, necessitating a lower dose of opioids.
Be alert for and report involuntary movements and decreased BP.	Extrapyramidal reactions (involuntary movements) and hypotension are seen with rapid IV administration.
Be alert for and report dry mouth and blurred vision.	Anticholinergic side effects.
Caution is necessary in patients taking monoamine oxidase (MAO) inhibitors.	Drug interaction can occur, causing increased incidence of extrapyramidal reactions.
Prochlorperazine (Compazine)	Antiemetic.
	Administration: PO/IM/IV/rectal.
Be alert for and report blurred vision, fatigue, ringing in the ears, nervousness, insomnia, and tremors.	Common CNS side effects. Patient should avoid activities that require alertness until the drug's effect on the CNS is known.
Precautions are needed for patients taking other CNS depressants such as narcotics.	Drug interactions can occur, necessitating decreasing the opioid dose by half.
Be alert for and report involuntary movements and decreased BP.	Extrapyramidal reactions and hypotension are seen with IV administration.
Be alert for and report heart palpitations, seizures, dry mouth, constipation, and urinary retention.	Less common side effects.
Ondansetron (Zofran)	Antiemetic.
	Administration: PO/IM/IV.
Be alert for and report pain, redness, and burning at the site of injection.	Local reaction with IM injection or IV infiltration.
Be alert for and report headache, fever, constipation, and diarrhea.	Common side effects.
Be alert for and report involuntary movements.	Extrapyramidal reactions are rare CNS side effects.
Be alert for and report rapid heart rate, dizziness, feeling faint, and chest pain.	Rare cardiac side effects.
Caution is necessary in patients with liver disease.	Liver clearance of this drug is reduced in patients with hepatic impairment.
Doxylamine (Unisom Nighttime Sleep Aid)	Antihistamine
	May be used as an antiemetic with mild symptoms of nausea and vomiting caused by pregnancy.

Continued

INTERVENTIONS	RATIONALES
	Administration: PO.
	Often used in combination with pyridoxine (Vitamin B$_6$).
Be alert for and report sedation.	Common side effect. Patient needs to avoid activities that require alertness until the drug's effect on the CNS is known.

●●● **Related NIC and NOC labels:** *NIC:* Teaching: Prescribed Medication *NOC:* Knowledge: Medication

ADDITIONAL NURSING DIAGNOSES/ PROBLEMS:

"Prolonged Bedrest" for relevant nursing diagnoses   p. 67

(The patient may be on self-imposed bedrest for comfort reasons.)

"Psychosocial Support" for relevant nursing diagnoses such as:

Anxiety   p. 82

Disturbed Sleep Pattern   p. 86

Social Isolation   p. 91

Disturbed Body Image   p. 92

"Psychosocial Support for the Patient's Family and Significant Others" for relevant nursing diagnoses such as:
Interrupted Family Processes   p. 95

"Cervical Incompetence" for **Caregiver Role Strain**   p. 710

✔ PATIENT-FAMILY TEACHING AND DISCHARGE PLANNING

Include verbal and written information about the following:

✓ Possible causes and effect hyperemesis has on the pregnancy and fetus.

✓ Signs and symptoms patient should report to her health care provider.

✓ Treatment of hyperemesis.

✓ Importance of attaining as much rest as possible.

✓ Nutritional options that would be most beneficial to patient.

✓ Importance of eating small, frequent meals during the day.

✓ Importance of oral hydration.

✓ Importance of avoiding lying down or reclining for 2 hr after eating.

✓ If parenteral nutrition is needed, the importance of maintaining insertion site and reporting any signs of site infection and pump malfunction.

✓ Importance of frequent clinic visits if being monitored on an outpatient basis and the date and time of next clinic visit.

✓ Importance of informing health care provider of any physical and emotional changes that may exacerbate the hyperemesis.

✓ Medications, including drug name, purpose, dosage, frequency, precautions, potential drug/drug and food/drug interactions, and potential side effects.

✓ Referral to local and national support organizations, including:

Sidelines, a national support organization for women and their families experiencing complicated pregnancies: Sidelines High Risk Pregnancy Support National Office
P.O. Box 1808
Laguna Beach, CA 92652
(888) 447-4754
www.sidelines.org/

Mastitis, Postpartum

Mastitis is an infection of the breast connective tissue (usually unilateral), and it occurs during lactation. It may be caused by transmission of bacteria (*Staphylococcus aureus, Streptococcus viridans,* group A and B streptococci, *Haemophilus influenzae,* and *Haemophilus parainfluenzae*) from the infant's oropharynx and nose into the breast through abrasions and fissures that develop during breastfeeding, a clogged milk duct, milk stasis as a result of incomplete breast emptying, infrequent nursing, or weaning. The breast is painful; a hard, warm, tender lump may be palpable; and erythema may be present.

HEALTH CARE SETTING

Patients may be treated in primary care on an outpatient basis with oral antibiotics.

ASSESSMENT

The onset of mastitis is usually sudden and seen between 2-3 wk postpartum or several months postpartum when weaning. When treated early with antibiotics, symptoms usually resolve within 24-48 hr. If symptoms do not resolve with adequate treatment, the patient should be referred to a breast specialist. On rare occasions, septic or toxic shock may occur and become a threat to maternal mortality.

Signs and symptoms—maternal:
- Lobular, V-shaped, streaking cellulitis of the periglandular connective tissue (a sunburn-like rash/erythema)
- Nipple abrasions, cracking, or fissures
- Localized breast pain, tenderness, and engorgement
- Temperature may be ≥101° F (38.3° C)
- Generalized malaise (flulike symptoms)
- Breast abscess may be present

Thrush vs. mastitis—maternal: Thrush is caused by the organism *Candida albicans,* a fungus that thrives in breast milk and is seen on the nipples, in milk ducts, and in the neonate's oropharynx. Symptoms may be misinterpreted as mastitis. The mother may complain of prolonged or sudden onset of sore nipples; sharp shooting/stabbing pains from the nipple up into the breast tissue;

and cracked, pink, crusty, red and often itchy nipples and areola. Thrush is more likely to occur after the mother has been treated with antibiotics. If thrush is present, both the mother and neonate need to be treated at the same time to prevent reinfection. Milk expressed during a thrush outbreak should not be saved and frozen. Freezing deactivates the yeast but does not kill it.

Signs and symptoms for thrush—neonate/infant: Thrush (demonstrated by the presence of white patches on the inside of the mouth, cheeks, or tongue) is caused by maternal antibiotic administration. Baby may refuse to eat because the mouth is sore. In some instances the baby may be without symptoms even if the mother has thrush on her nipples.

Physical assessment: Patient usually complains of having an aching sensation, extreme discomfort, and tenderness in one breast. She may state that she is unable to wear her bra or touch her breast because of the pain and that her nipples are either cracked, bleeding, or both. The breast may be engorged, warm to the touch, edematous, and erythematous (looks like a sunburn). Mastitis symptoms are usually accompanied by flulike symptoms: headache, anorexia, fatigue, myalgias, fevers (≥101° F [38.3° C]), and tachycardia.

Risk factors: Ductal abnormalities, poor handwashing, interruption of regular nursing, chronic nipple fissures or cracking, recurrent mastitis resulting from inadequate antibiotic therapy, failure to empty breasts adequately.

DIAGNOSTIC TESTS

Diagnostic tests are limited for mastitis. Typically diagnosis is made by symptoms and objective findings.

Cultures: Culture and microscopic analysis of secreted breast milk for bacteria and leukocyte count. An infection usually will result in a leukocyte count >1 million/ml and a bacteria count >1000/ml.

Ultrasound of the breast with or without a biopsy: When another pathologic condition is suspected or a breast mass is palpable yet symptoms may not be consistent with mastitis, an ultrasound of the breast should be done. If an abscess is seen, it may be incised and drained under ultrasound guidance and the fluid cultured.

Nursing Diagnosis:

Deficient Knowledge:

Potential for mastitis

Desired Outcome: Immediately following teaching, patient verbalizes accurate understanding of the early signs and symptoms of mastitis and ultimately obtains antibiotic coverage and assistance with comfort measures during the healing process if mastitis occurs.

INTERVENTIONS	RATIONALES
Teach signs and symptoms of mastitis before patient is discharged from the hospital.	A knowledgeable patient likely will report these symptoms promptly and obtain the necessary antibiotic coverage. See "Signs and symptoms—maternal" in the introductory data.
Teach the cause of mastitis and importance of completing the course of antibiotics.	Aids in patient compliance and assists in decreasing likelihood of reinfection. Causes of mastitis are discussed in the introductory material.
In the event of mastitis, teach patient the following interventions:	
- Wear a supportive bra, preferably without underwires.	Provides support to the breast and helps to decrease pain from tissue swelling.
- Take pain medications (i.e., ibuprofen, acetaminophen) as needed.	Promotes patient comfort, compliance, and continuation of nursing. Ibuprofen and acetaminophen are approved for use during breastfeeding by the American Academy of Pediatrics.
- Apply warm compresses or soak the breast in warm water before nursing. (Some patients will prefer cold compresses for comfort.)	Promotes patient comfort, "let down" effect, and continuation of nursing.
- Nurse frequently, including from the affected breast.	Aids in decreasing pressure on the affected breast and promotes adequate drainage from clogged milk ducts. It is necessary for the patient to empty the affected breast completely at each feeding, either by nursing or pumping.
- Vary positions of the breast when nursing.	Facilitates emptying of all ducts.
- Get plenty of rest and proper fluid and nutrition intake.	Promotes the healing process.

●●● **Related NIC and NOC labels:** *NIC:* Health Education; Postpartal Care *NOC:* Knowledge: Postpartum

Nursing Diagnosis:

Risk for Ineffective Breastfeeding

related to interruption in breastfeeding caused by pain secondary to infection

Desired Outcome: Patient adequately produces milk with minimal discomfort by pumping or continued breastfeeding during resolution of the breast infection.

INTERVENTIONS	RATIONALES
Encourage patient to verbalize her concerns about breastfeeding.	Enables evaluation of obstacles patient may have in producing adequate milk supply.
Encourage patient to continue nursing during mastitis.	Continuation of nursing on the affected breast promotes healing by preventing milk stasis. The infection will not be passed on to the infant.

Continued

INTERVENTIONS	RATIONALES
Teach patient preventive measures against acquiring mastitis and preventing reinfection.	Provides patient with some measures she can control as needed. These measures include breast hygiene, early interventions for nipple cracking and bleeding (appropriate infant latching, using lanolin on nipples, avoiding soap or alcohol on nipples, air drying nipples after nursing, and using comfortable nursing positions), good handwashing, avoiding long periods between nursing, and trial of various positions to promote emptying.
Teach patient how to use a breast pump (manual and electric), manual expression, and storage of milk.	Measures that aid in success of producing/sustaining milk and reducing risk of mastitis or reinfection.
Help patient choose which breast-pumping measure to use, based on need and expense.	When the patient needs to pump on an occasional basis, manual (hand-operated) pumps may be effective and are less costly than an electric pump. If the patient has limited time, large milk volume, or the baby is in the hospital, an electric pump is more likely to satisfy her needs. An electric pump also has a suck-release cycle that is closer to that of baby's. Pumps may be purchased or rented. Patient also may ask to borrow a breast pump (electric only) from friends or family.
Teach patient to bathe daily and keep breasts clean and to wash hands before pumping. Advise patient that after each use to wash all parts of the breast pump that come in contact with milk in warm soapy water.	Decreases risk of transmitting bacteria to the breasts and infant.
Teach patient that after pumping to place the milk in a clean plastic container or a disposable bottle bag and secure with a clean rubber band.	Plastic is better than glass because some of the immune factors in breast milk stick to glass.
Teach patient to label the milk with date and time.	Labeling enables use of the oldest milk first.
Advise patient to place several small bags in one large plastic bag before putting them in the freezer.	Prevents the small bags from sticking to the freezer shelf and tearing.
Provide guidelines for storing her milk in the refrigerator or freezer.	Safe and appropriate storage reduces the possibility of bacterial contamination. - Refrigerator: 34-40° F (1-2° C) for up to 48 hr after pumping or thawing. - Freezer, within the refrigerator: 20-28° F (−7 to −2° C) for up to 3 wk. - Freezer with a separate door: 5-15° F (−15 to −9° C) for up to 3 mo. - Deep freezer: 0° F or below (18° C) for up to 6 mo.
Provide patient with support of lactation specialists (e.g., hospital-based certified lactation consultants, outside support groups available in her home area, and Internet sites dedicated to lactation).	Promotes success of breastfeeding and enables interaction with women who have experienced the challenges and rewards of breastfeeding.

●●● **Related NIC and NOC labels:** *NIC:* Lactation Counseling; Anxiety Reduction; Skin Care: Topical Treatments; Positioning *NOC:* Breastfeeding Establishment: Maternal

Nursing Diagnosis:

Anxiety

related to not producing an adequate milk supply or stopping breastfeeding before desired date

Desired Outcome: Patient verbalizes her anxieties and fears and identifies/uses appropriate coping mechanisms in managing her anxiety.

INTERVENTIONS	RATIONALES
Engage in honest communication with patient; provide empathetic understanding. Listen closely.	Establishes an atmosphere that enables free expression.
Encourage patient to verbalize the cause of her anxiety (e.g., fear of pain, fatigue, inadequate milk supply, transmission of infection to infant, medications).	Validates her concerns and aids in identifying areas that would benefit from patient teaching.
Encourage patient to relax during breastfeeding. Teach her relaxation techniques such as deep breathing, taking a warm shower before feeding, and feeding in a comfortable/quiet environment.	Oxytocin is critical to milk ejection during lactation. Its release can be inhibited by fear, pain, tension, and anxiety.
Identify patient's support systems and help her formulate a plan for acquiring assistance with her responsibilities during the time of her infection. Inform her that the infection is for a limited time only.	Validates importance of acquiring adequate rest during the time of infection and helps her identify and accept outside support.

●●● **Related NIC and NOC labels:** *NIC:* Anxiety Reduction; Simple Relaxation Therapy; Environmental Management *NOC:* Anxiety Control

Nursing Diagnosis:

Risk for Impaired Parenting

related to decrease in frequency of nursing secondary to the pain of mastitis or fear of infecting the infant

Desired Outcome: Within 24 hr of this diagnosis, patient verbalizes her concerns regarding the parental bonding process and barriers present resulting from the mastitis and expresses her satisfaction with the bonding achieved.

INTERVENTIONS	RATIONALES
Teach patient how to intervene to reduce pain in mastitis. See **Deficient Knowledge,** earlier.	Reducing pain optimally will increase the frequency, production, and continuation of breastfeeding.
Reassure patient that she is able to continue to breastfeed even from the affected breast, or if an abscess is present she would empty the breast by using a pump.	Helps alleviate mother's fear of passing an infection to the infant.
Support patient if she decides to discontinue breastfeeding.	Bottle feeding also can promote the parental bonding process.
Provide patient with support via lactation specialists. See **Risk for Ineffective Breastfeeding,** earlier.	Aids in success of continuing breastfeeding or helps with the decision to discontinue nursing after all avenues have been explored.

●●● **Related NIC and NOC labels:** *NIC:* Breastfeeding Assistance; Parent Education: Infant *NOC:* Parenting

Nursing Diagnosis:

Deficient Knowledge

Prescribed medications and their safety with breastfeeding

Desired Outcome: Immediately following teaching, patient verbalizes accurate understanding about the benefits, safety issues, side effects, and importance of completing the course of medications prescribed.

INTERVENTIONS	RATIONALES
Teach the following about patient's prescribed medications:	A knowledgeable patient is more likely to comply with therapy, identify and report side effects, and recognize and report precautions that might preclude use of the prescribed drug.
Antimicrobials	
Dicloxacillin (Dynapen)	Drug of choice for penicillin-resistant staphylococci.
	Administration: oral route.
Caution: Patients with penicillin allergy should avoid this drug.	Cross-sensitivity with penicillins is possible. Serious and possible fatal reactions can occur.
Teach patient to be alert for and report nausea, vomiting, and diarrhea.	Possible side effects.
Caution patient to follow complete course for all prescribed medications and take them on time.	To reduce risk of reinfection, prevent development of antibiotic resistance, and maintain a constant level of medication in the bloodstream.
Teach patient to be alert for and report excessive and explosive diarrhea.	*Clostridium difficile* is a potentially serious side effect in which the normal flora of the bowel are reduced by antibiotic therapy and the anaerobic organism *C. difficile* multiplies and produces its toxins, causing severe diarrhea. This necessitates discontinuation of the antibiotic and laboratory evaluation of a stool sample.
Advise patient to be alert for and report a rash and pruritus.	Possible allergic reaction.
Caution use of this drug with erythromycin.	Erythromycin may interfere with the bactericidal effects of penicillin.
Erythromycin (Eryc, E-mycin)	Drug of choice for patients with penicillin allergy.
	Administration: oral.
Teach patient to be alert for and report abdominal pain, nausea, vomiting, and diarrhea.	Possible side effects.
Caution patient to follow complete course for all prescribed medications and take them on time.	To reduce risk of reinfection, prevent development of antibiotic resistance, and maintain a constant level of medication in the bloodstream.
Advise patient to be alert for and report excessive and explosive diarrhea.	See discussion with *C. difficile,* earlier.
Teach patient to be alert for and report a rash and pruritus.	Possible allergic reaction.
Caution use of this drug in patients with hepatic disease.	Erythromycin is excreted by the liver.
Vancomycin (Vancocin)	Used if a methicillin-resistant staphylococcus is suspected.
	Administration: oral.
Teach patient to be alert for and report nausea, vomiting, and diarrhea.	Possible side effects.

Continued

INTERVENTIONS	RATIONALES
Advise patient to be alert for and report excessive and explosive diarrhea.	See discussion with *C. difficile,* earlier.
Teach patient to be alert for and report a rash and pruritus.	Possible allergic reaction.
Cephalexin (Keflex, Keftab)	Cross-sensitivity with penicillin is possible.
	Severe reactions including anaphylaxis can occur with both drugs.
	Administration: oral.
Teach patient to be alert for and report nausea, vomiting, and diarrhea.	Possible side effects.
Caution patient to follow complete course for all prescribed medications and take them on time.	To reduce risk of reinfection, prevent development of antibiotic resistance, and maintain a constant level of medication in the bloodstream.
Advise patient to be alert for and report excessive and explosive diarrhea.	See discussion with *C. difficile,* earlier.
Teach patient to be alert for and report stomach upset and abdominal pain.	Adverse reactions.
Analgesics and antipyretics	Aid in decreasing breast pain and reducing fever.
Ibuprofen (Motrin, Advil, Nuprin, Rufen):	Administration: oral.
Teach patient to be alert for nausea and gastrointestinal (GI) upset. Advise taking this medication with food.	Side effect; taking it with food may alleviate this problem.
Caution patient to be alert for and report wheezing, shortness of breath, hives, swelling of the face, and irregular heartbeat.	Severe allergic reactions.
Caution use in patients allergic to aspirin.	Does not contain aspirin but may cause allergic reactions in patients also allergic to aspirin.
Caution use in patients with a history of GI ulcers.	May cause GI bleeding.
Acetaminophen (Tylenol)	Aids in decreasing breast pain and reducing fever.
	Administration: oral.
Advise that aspirin is *not* recommended in the breastfeeding mother.	Kernicterus, an abnormal toxic accumulation of bilirubin in central nervous system (CNS) tissues caused by hyper-bilirubinemia, may occur in the infant because of breakdown products from aspirin that compete for bilirubin binding sites.

●●● **Related NIC and NOC labels:** *NIC:* Teaching: Prescribed Medication *NOC:* Knowledge: Medication

ADDITIONAL NURSING DIAGNOSES/ PROBLEMS:

"Psychosocial Support" for such nursing diagnoses as:	p. 81
Disturbed Sleep Pattern	p. 86
Disturbed Body Image	p. 92

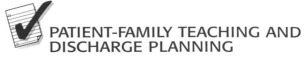

PATIENT-FAMILY TEACHING AND DISCHARGE PLANNING

Include verbal and written information about the following:
✔ Cause of mastitis and the rationale for using antibiotics.
✔ Importance of early reporting of signs and symptoms of mastitis.

✓Signs of a breast abscess and the need for immediate evaluation.

✓Frequent feedings or use of the breast pump to prevent milk stasis and provide some comfort from engorgement.

✓Importance of good handwashing and breast hygiene.

✓Applying warm moist packs to affected breast or taking a warm shower before feeding or pumping.

✓Importance of rest and adequate fluid and nutrient intake.

✓Wearing a supportive, nonconstrictive nursing bra.

✓Proper weaning techniques if mother decides to wean the infant.

✓Medications, including drug name, purpose, dosage, frequency, precautions, drug/drug and food/drug interactions, potential drug reactions, and side effects.

✓Referrals to local and national lactation support groups, including:

La Leche League International, a support group providing national and local assistance and education to mothers who are breastfeeding:
La Leche League International
1400 N. Meacham Road
Schaumburg, IL 60183-4840
(800) LALECHE
www.lalecheleague.org

92

Postpartum Wound Infection

*A*bdominal wound infection after cesarean section is not uncommon and can be caused by endogenous or exogenous bacteria. The incidence increases when amniotic membranes have been ruptured for ≥6 hours before delivery. Two determining factors are the amount of bacterial contamination present and resistance of the patient in warding off infection. *Episiotomy infections* can occur but are less common. Sepsis (septic shock), though rare, is associated with *Staphylococcus aureus* at the wound site. A patient who persistently has a fever and does not respond to multiple antibiotic therapies may have *septic pelvic thrombophlebitis.* Patients with this condition do not generally appear ill and may have minimal to no pain. The only variance is the wide swing in temperature. These patients are treated with SC heparin and normally have rapid improvement within 48-72 hours. This condition occurs more often after cesarean section than after vaginal birth. Prompt evaluation and treatment of these infections help alleviate need for lengthy hospitalizations and home therapy.

HEALTH CARE SETTING

Primary care (outpatient clinic), acute care (hospital), or home care

ASSESSMENT

Early-onset infections occur within the first 48 hr after surgery and are seen as a discoloration of the skin surrounding the incision (cellulitis) and fever. This should be caught early with daily inspection of the wound site or episiotomy while the patient is in the hospital. Late-onset infections are usually seen 6-8 days after surgery. Indicators include fever and a swollen, erythematous, and draining wound.

Cardiopulmonary: Tachycardia, hypotension, tachypnea, or syncope may be seen in the acutely ill patient when sepsis is present.

Fever: Temperature may be ≥101° F (38.3° C). With mild infection the patient may remain afebrile. Headache and overall "body aches" may accompany fever.

Chills: Patient may feel she cannot get warm even in the presence of an elevated temperature. Body shakes may accompany the chills. An overall flulike feeling may be present.

Malaise: A feeling of uneasiness, general discomfort, and fatigue may be present.

Pain: Pain may be present with light or deep external palpation of the abdomen or bimanual palpation of the uterus. Cervical motion tenderness (CMT) on bimanual exam also may be present with a uterine infection. With an episiotomy infection, pain may be localized (throbbing, aching, or sharp) and deep tissue in nature. Some women complain of a sensation of vaginal pressure or "fullness."

Vaginal discharge: With an episiotomy infection, discharge may be purulent, and it may be foul smelling if endometritis (intrauterine infection) coexists with the infected episiotomy.

Abdominal surgical incision: In early-onset infection, the skin around the incision is erythematous and warm to the touch. In late-onset infection, the incision is swollen and erythematous. If the wound is not already open and draining bloody, serosanguineous, or purulent discharge, it may be probed with a cotton-tipped applicator to promote drainage. Dehiscence may or may not have occurred.

Episiotomy or perineal laceration: Localized edema, erythema, and exudate. Dehiscence of the episiotomy may or may not have occurred. Any episiotomy, whether infected or not, causes interruption of tissue integrity that can lead to stress incontinence, pelvic floor prolapse, anal incontinence, and pelvic floor muscle dysfunction.

Complications—neonatal: If the maternal infection is caused by an antepartum uterine infection (chorioamnionitis), the neonate is at increased risk for infection or sepsis and should be monitored carefully. When the infection appears within the first week of life and most likely within the first 48 hr of life, rapid deterioration and a high mortality rate are possible for the neonate.

Physical assessment: Not every patient with a wound infection looks or feels acutely ill. Some mild infections, such as cellulitis, respond well to early oral antibiotic coverage. Others will require IV antibiotic administration, wound debridement, or daily wound packing that allows the open incision to heal from the inside out via secondary intention (tissue granulation) or possible secondary wound closure including use of retention sutures and extended hospitalization. Early assessment and treatment are critical in reducing maternal morbidity/ mortality. Sepsis is rare but can occur.

Risk factors: Advanced maternal age, type 1 diabetes, low socioeconomic status, positive group B streptococci culture, malnutrition, obesity, anemia, prolonged preoperative hospitalization, extended duration of ruptured membranes before delivery, long labor, frequent vaginal exams during labor, corticosteroid therapy, immunosuppressed state, duration of the surgery (cesarean section or postpartum tubal ligation), razor shaving the operative site, use of electrosurgical knife, use of open drains (e.g., Penrose), closure technique (suture vs. staples), and emergency surgery (e.g., fetal distress).

DIAGNOSTIC TESTS

Complete blood count (CBC) with differential: Leukocytes (white blood cells [WBCs]) will be elevated in the presence of an infection. The differential lists the five types of leukocytes, which all perform a special function. The type of leukocyte elevation will depend on the type of infection present (e.g., monocytes = severe infection by phagocytosis; lymphocytes = viral infections).

Blood cultures: During acute febrile illness, blood cultures identify the source of bacteria causing the infection, and sensitivity analysis determines the most effective antibiotic coverage.

Gram stain and culture of foul-smelling lochia: Helps in identifying clostridia, anaerobes, and *Chlamydia* and indicates the sensitivity analysis for the most effective antibiotic to use.

Urinalysis for microscopy: Detects presence of a urinary tract infection (UTI), which can be seen postoperatively after removal of an indwelling urinary catheter.

Pelvic ultrasound: Detects and locates possible abscesses and hematomas.

Computed tomography (CT) scan/magnetic resonance imaging (MRI): In patients who do not respond to antibiotic coverage and have a negative ultrasound exam, this study can detect obscure pelvic abscesses and pelvic thrombi.

Nursing Diagnosis:

Deficient Knowledge:

Effects of postpartum wound infection (either abdominal or episiotomy) on self and neonate and the importance of following the treatment course

Desired Outcome: Immediately following teaching, patient and significant other verbalize accurate knowledge about the effects of postpartum wound infections on the patient and neonate and the treatment involved.

INTERVENTIONS	RATIONALES
Teach patient, significant other, and family about the effect a postpartum wound infection may have on the mother and neonate and the likely treatments for the infection.	Information helps patient comply with treatments, report symptoms in a timely manner, and understand consequences of noncompliance. Effects an infection may have on the mother include pain, fever, chills, wound dehiscence, sepsis, and increased morbidity/mortality. For the neonate, effects include fever and possible rapid deterioration and increased morbidity/mortality. Likely treatments include IV antibiotics and fluids, wound packing, secondary wound closure, and possible lengthy hospitalization or home treatments.
Teach signs and symptoms of worsening wound infection.	A knowledgeable patient will be more likely to report these symptoms (increasing fever, foul-smelling vaginal discharge, spreading abdominal cellulitis, severe pain, vaginal bleeding, wound drainage) in a timely manner. Early evaluation and treatment result in decreased maternal morbidity.

Continued

INTERVENTIONS	**RATIONALES**
Explain potential for complications with wound infections.	Explanation of potential complications (e.g., cellulitis, seroma, hematoma, dehiscence, secondary closure, necrotizing fasciitis, bacteremia, and disseminated intravascular coagulation) provides knowledge that optimally will promote compliance with the therapeutic regimen.
Explain treatment options such as daily wound packing or secondary wound closure and IV or PO antibiotics in treating the infection and decreasing risk for further infection.	Once the acute infection has been treated with antibiotics, the patient may be treated at home. If a secondary wound closure is done, it requires readmittance to the hospital (or an extended stay if the infection occurs before hospital discharge). Daily wound care consists of inspecting, irrigating, debridement, packing, and applying dressings. (See "Managing Wound Care," p. 583, for more information.)
Explain to patient and partner that intercourse is not recommended during the process of wound healing, especially in the presence of wound dehiscence.	Usually intercourse is not recommended until 6 wk postpartum. This time frame allows the cervix to close, bleeding to stop, and incisions to heal without risk of introducing bacteria and potential for infection or further infection.

●●● **Related NIC and NOC labels:** *NIC:* Teaching: Individual; Infection Control; Teaching: Procedure/Treatment *NOC:* Knowledge: Illness Care

Nursing Diagnosis:

Impaired Skin Integrity

related to wound infection and/or dehiscence

Desired Outcome: Patient's wound heals within an acceptable time frame (2-3 wk).

INTERVENTIONS	**RATIONALES**
Teach patient how to monitor abdominal surgical site or episiotomy for suture integrity and signs and symptoms of infection.	A knowledgeable patient is likely to report infection indicators promptly. Prompt medical intervention reduces maternal morbidity and possibly hospitalization and length of treatment. - *Abdominal surgical site:* redness surrounding incision, abdomen warm to touch, drainage from incision, wound dehiscence (incision partially or fully open), and evisceration (protrusion of an organ, usually bowel, through open surgical wound). - *Episiotomy:* extreme pain in any position but especially sitting, foul vaginal odor in the absence of abdominal tenderness, drainage of pus, or dehiscence of sutures. Patient should use a mirror for self-examination or ask a family member to examine her perineum.
Assess patient's and significant other's level of acceptance/confidence in caring for the wound on an outpatient basis.	Evaluates comfort level for home wound care. Subsequent teaching/reassurance, if need is determined, will provide an opportunity for patient to take control of her own care.
As needed, provide patient with a home nursing care referral.	Decreases stress when patient or family members are unable to care for the wound because of work commitments or uneasiness in self-management of a surgical wound. Home care enables patient to be home and decreases medical costs.

Continued

INTERVENTIONS	RATIONALES
Teach patient or significant other aseptic techniques in caring for the wound, such as thorough handwashing, wearing gloves (nonsterile acceptable), disposing of soiled dressings in plastic bags, maintaining a clean field for irrigation and packing, and alternatives to tapes for holding dressings in place. See Appendix for "Infection Prevention and Control," p. 831, for more information.	Decreases risk of introducing additional microorganisms into the wound. Dressings with body fluids are considered hazardous waste. Tape can cause skin reactions and break down sensitive tissue.
Encourage patient to eat a well-balanced diet that includes protein, carbohydrates, fruits, vegetables, and adequate fluid intake.	Adequate diet provides nutrients and a positive nitrogen state, which in turn promote wound healing. Adequate hydration also promotes wound healing.
Encourage patient to keep medical appointments.	Compliance with appointments enables evaluation of the wound's healing process and changes in care as needed.
Provide patient with abdominal support/binder after a cesarean section or bilateral tubal ligation.	Provides support and decreases stretching/tension on muscles/surrounding tissue of the wound to promote healing.

●●● **Related NIC and NOC labels:** *NIC:* Incision Site Care; Perineal Care; Wound Irrigation; Wound Care; Skin Care: Topical Treatments; Nutrition Management; Infection Protection *NOC:* Tissue Integrity: Skin & Mucous Membranes

Nursing Diagnosis:

Ineffective Coping

related to needed adjustment in lifestyle to provide an optimal environment for wound healing or lack of support from family, friends, and community

Desired Outcome: Optimally within 24 hr of this diagnosis, patient modifies her lifestyle or behavior to promote wound healing.

INTERVENTIONS	RATIONALES
Assess patient's perceptions and ability to understand current health status.	Evaluation of patient's perceptions and comprehension enables development of an individualized care plan.
Establish empathetic communication with patient.	To promote effective therapeutic communication. For example, "I know this is difficult to deal with while caring for a newborn. Tell me what I can do to help you."
Help patient identify previous methods of coping with life problems.	How patient has handled problems in the past may be a reliable predictor of how she will cope with current problems.
Help patient identify or develop a support system.	Many people benefit from outside support systems in helping them cope. Patient may need assistance with personal and homemaking tasks in order to modify her lifestyle so that wound healing can occur.
Arrange community referrals such as visiting nurse service, as appropriate.	Support in the home environment is likely to promote healthier adaptations.
Affirm that lifestyle adjustment (e.g., increased rest, dressing changes, frequent clinic visits, taking medications) is for a limited time.	Facilitates acceptance of outside support and assistance while reinforcing understanding of the healing process of an infected wound.

Continued

INTERVENTIONS

RATIONALES

Explain diagnostic tests (e.g., blood work to monitor for further infection, ultrasound to check for abscess) and procedures (e.g., wound packing, secondary wound closure).	Explanations of what to expect enable patient to initiate her coping mechanisms.

●●● **Related NIC and NOC labels:** *NIC:* Coping Enhancement; Counseling; Support System Enhancement; Behavior Modification; Health Education *NOC:* Coping; Role Performance

Nursing Diagnosis:

Deficient Knowledge:

Purpose for and potential side effects of prescribed medications used to treat wound infections

Desired Outcome: Immediately following teaching, patient and family verbalize accurate understanding of the risks and benefits of medications used in treating postpartum wound infections.

INTERVENTIONS

RATIONALES

Teach the following about patient's prescribed drugs:	A knowledgeable patient is more likely to comply with therapy, identify and report side effects, and recognize and report precautions that might preclude use of the prescribed drug.
Antimicrobials	May be used as a perioperative prophylaxis, treating wound cellulitis/infection.
Cephalosporins: cefazolin (Ancef, Kefzol), cefoxitin (Mefoxin), cefotetan (Cefotan), cefoperazone (Cefobid), cephalexin (Keflex)	Administration: IV, PO, IM.
Teach patients who are breastfeeding that this drug will be present in low concentrations in breast milk.	Patients can breastfeed without it causing a problem to the infant.
Explain caution necessary for patients with sensitivity to penicillins.	Cross-sensitivity with penicillins is possible. Serious and possible fatal reactions can occur.
Teach importance of following complete course for all prescribed medications and taking them on time.	To reduce risk of reinfection, prevent development of antibiotic resistance, and maintain a constant level of medication in the bloodstream.
Teach patient to be alert for and report diarrhea, nausea, vomiting, stomach cramps, and anorexia.	Possible side effects.
Advise patient to be alert for and report excessive and explosive diarrhea.	*Clostridium difficile* is a potentially serious side effect in which the normal flora of the bowel are reduced by antibiotic therapy and the anaerobic organism *C. difficile* multiplies and produces its toxins, causing severe diarrhea. This problem necessitates discontinuation of the antibiotic and laboratory evaluation of a stool sample.
Caution patient to be alert for a rash and pruritus.	Possible allergic reactions.
Penicillins: penicillin, amoxicillin, amoxicillin/clavulanate potassium (Augmentin), ampicillin-sulbactam (Unasyn)	Treat infections. Administration: IV/IM/PO. Breastfeeding: OK with amoxicillin.
Caution patient that the drug is not to be used if allergic to penicillins.	Serious and possible fatal reactions can occur.

Continued

INTERVENTIONS	RATIONALES
Caution use in patients with a sensitivity to cephalosporins.	Possible cross-sensitivity can lead to serious and sometimes fatal reactions.
Advise patient to follow complete course for all prescribed medications and take them on time.	To reduce risk of reinfection, prevent development of antibiotic resistance, and maintain a constant level of medication in the bloodstream.
Teach patient to be alert for and report nausea, indigestion, and vomiting.	Possible side effects.
Teach patient to monitor for and report itching, rash, and shortness of breath.	May signal an allergic reaction.
Teach patient to be alert for and report excessive and explosive diarrhea.	See discussion of *C. difficile,* earlier.
Aminoglycosides: gentamicin (Garamycin)	Used in the treatment of infections.
	It is not administered during pregnancy because it crosses the placenta and can cause total irreversible bilateral congenital deafness.
	Breastfeeding: unknown.
	Administration: IM/IV.
Teach patient to be alert for and report lethargy, confusion, respiratory depression, visual disturbances, depression, weight loss, hypotension or hypertension, decreased appetite, rash, itching, headache, nausea, vomiting, and hearing loss.	Potential adverse and allergic reactions.
Teach patient to be alert for and report excessive and explosive diarrhea.	See discussion about *C. difficile,* earlier.
Caution use in patients with neuromuscular disorders.	May lead to neurotoxicity.
Caution use in patients with impaired renal function.	May lead to nephrotoxicity.
Other antimicrobials	Used in the treatment of infections.
Clindamycin (Cleocin)	Breastfeeding: not recommended.
	Administration: IV/IM/PO.
Teach patient to monitor for and report itching and rash.	Possible allergic reactions.
Teach patient to be alert for and report diarrhea, nausea, vomiting, stomach cramps, and anorexia.	Possible adverse reactions.
Advise patient to follow complete course for all prescribed medications and take them on time.	To reduce risk of reinfection, prevent development of antibiotic resistance, and maintain a constant level of medication in the bloodstream.
Advise patient to be alert for and report excessive and explosive diarrhea.	See discussion about *C. difficile,* earlier.
Caution use in patients with a history of colitis.	May exacerbate the colitis.
Teach patient to be alert for and report redness, swelling, and pain at IV insertion site.	Thrombophlebitis can occur after IV infusion of clindamycin.
Caution use in patients with renal disease.	Injectable drug is potentially nephrotoxic.
Analgesics	
Meperidine (Demerol)	Opiate analgesic used in the treatment of moderate-to-severe pain.
	Breastfeeding: not recommended.
	Administration: IM/IV (poor oral absorption/efficacy).

Continued

INTERVENTIONS	RATIONALES
Teach patient to be alert for and report dry mouth, blurring vision, and dizziness.	Side effects.
Teach patient to be alert for and report itching and rash.	Possible allergic reactions.
Caution patient to be alert for and report weakness, headache, restlessness, agitation, hallucinations, and disorientation.	Adverse reactions.
Advise patient to be alert for and report shortness of breath.	Adverse reaction. May indicate overdose.
Caution patient to arise slowly from a supine position or have assistance with ambulating after receiving this medication. Caution patient to avoid activities that require alertness until the drug's effect on the central nervous system (CNS) is known.	Meperidine is a CNS depressant. It may impair mental and/or physical abilities and cause hypotension. Drowsiness is a common side effect.
Caution use with other CNS depressants.	Can potentiate the CNS effects.
Morphine	Opioid used in the treatment of moderate-to-severe pain.
	Breastfeeding: generally accepted as safe.
	Administration: IV/IM/PO.
Teach patient to be alert for and report itching and rash.	Possible allergic reactions.
Teach patient to be alert for and report weakness, headache, restlessness, agitation, hallucinations, and disorientation.	Adverse reactions.
Teach patient to be alert for and report shortness of breath.	Adverse reaction. May indicate overdose.
Caution patient to arise slowly from a supine position or have assistance with ambulating after receiving this medication. Caution patient to avoid activities that require alertness until the drug's effect on the CNS is known.	Morphine is a CNS depressant. It may impair mental and/or physical abilities and cause hypotension. Drowsiness is a common side effect.
Caution use with other CNS depressants.	Can potentiate CNS effects.
Caution use in patients with seizure disorder.	Seizures may result from high doses.
Caution use in patients with renal/hepatic insufficiency.	Active metabolite may accumulate and potentiate the sedative effects.
Oxycodone with acetaminophen *(Percocet) and hydrocodone with acetaminophen (Vicodin)*	Narcotic analgesics used to treat moderate to moderately severe pain.
	Administration: oral.
Teach patient to be alert for and report itching, rash, nausea, and vomiting.	Possible allergic reactions.
Teach patient to be alert for and report dizziness and headache.	Common adverse reactions.
Teach patient to be alert for and report shortness of breath.	Adverse reaction. May indicate overdose.
Caution patient to arise slowly from a supine position or have assistance with ambulating after taking this medication.	These drugs are CNS depressants. They may impair mental and/or physical abilities and cause hypotension.
Caution patient to avoid activities that require alertness until the drug's effect on the CNS is known.	Drowsiness is a common side effect.
Anticoagulant *Heparin*	Inhibits reaction that leads to clotting of blood and formation of fibrin clots. It is used in treating septic pelvic thrombophlebitis.
	Administration: SC/IV. IM not recommended.
Teach patient to be alert for and report increase in vaginal bleeding (saturating one regular-size sanitary pad/hr and/or passing golf-ball–sized clots).	Hemorrhage can occur at any site in patients receiving heparin.

Continued

INTERVENTIONS	RATIONALES
Caution patient about using aspirin or aspirin-containing products and nonsteroidal antiinflammatory drugs (NSAIDs; e.g., ibuprofen) or NSAID-containing products while taking heparin.	Aspirin and NSAIDs are platelet aggregation (clotting) inhibitors that can lead to increased bleeding.
Inform patient that bleeding and bruising at the site of injection is not unusual.	Heparin can lead to bleeding and bruising. The tendency for bleeding at the injection site will necessitate prolonged compression over injection site.
Teach patient to be alert for and report redness, pain, swelling, and firmness at injection site.	Local irritation that may indicate injection site cellulitis.
Advise patient to take a calcium supplement while receiving heparin.	Heparin affects bone density and may lead to osteoporosis.

●●● **Related NIC and NOC labels:** *NIC:* Teaching: Prescribed Medication *NOC:* Knowledge: Medication

ADDITIONAL NURSING DIAGNOSES/ PROBLEMS:

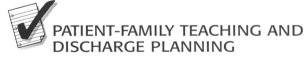

PATIENT-FAMILY TEACHING AND DISCHARGE PLANNING

Wound infections place a great deal of strain on the patient and family dynamics. Any form of information or patient education that can be provided optimally will decrease the level of anxiety. Referral to a wound care specialist may be necessary at any time during the assessment/healing process. Include verbal and written information about the following:

✓ Signs and symptoms of a wound infection.

✓ Wound care (cleansing, packing, and dressing); instructions will vary depending on facility and provider preference. Check with health care provider for specific instructions. Also see care plans in "Managing Wound Care," p. 583.

✓ Good handwashing.

✓ Where to obtain dressing materials for home care (prescriptions for supplies that may be acquired via a pharmacy or medical supply store).

✓ Importance of adequate rest, nutrition, and oral hydration for effective wound healing.

✓ Importance of compliance with prescribed health care regimen and ready access to hospital and family/social support.

✓ Medications, including drug name, purpose, dosage, frequency, precautions, drug/drug and food/drug interactions, potential drug reactions, and side effects.

✓ Referral to local and national support organizations, including:

> Sidelines, a national support organization for women and their families experiencing complicated pregnancies: Sidelines High Risk Pregnancy Support National Office
> P.O. Box 1808
> Laguna Beach, CA 92652
> (888) 447-4754
> www.sidelines.org/

93

Preeclampsia

Preeclampsia, characterized primarily by the onset of acute hypertension, is a multiorgan disease process with onset usually after 20 wk of gestation except in the case of gestational trophoblastic disease (includes hydatidiform mole and gestational trophoblastic tumors). Preeclampsia can affect the cardiovascular, neurologic, renal, hepatic, and hematologic systems. The cause is unknown, and clinical manifestations can be mild to severe, thereby affecting maternal/fetal morbidity and mortality.

Individuals with severe preeclampsia (BP >160 mm Hg systolic or ≥110 mm Hg diastolic on at least two occasions 6 hr apart with patient on bedrest) may show evidence of HELLP syndrome (*h*emolysis of red blood cells, *e*levated *l*iver enzymes, and *l*ow *p*latelet count). HELLP syndrome may be present even in the absence of severe hypertension and is most common in Caucasian women. HELLP syndrome can occur at any time during the second and third trimesters.

HEALTH CARE SETTING

Primary care, including obstetric or high-risk perinatal clinic, or acute care antepartum/intrapartum unit

ASSESSMENT

Preeclampsia is one of the most common medical complications in pregnancy. It may have a gradual or rapid onset depending on the organ system involved.

HELLP syndrome: Epigastric or right upper quadrant (RUQ) pain, nausea and vomiting, body aches, malaise, edema, and weight gain. Some of these symptoms overlap with preeclampsia; therefore laboratory values become the deciding diagnostic factor.

Cardiovascular: Normally during pregnancy, plasma volume and cardiac output increase approximately 40%. Blood pressure ≥140/90 mm Hg on at least two occasions taken a minimum of 4 hr apart, along with proteinuria (see Renal), are diagnostic of preeclampsia.

Vasospasm is a major pathophysiologic change of this disease process, along with activation of the coagulation system and

abnormal hemostasis, and plays a major role in end-organ effects. It results in increased peripheral vascular resistance with decreased perfusion to tissues and vital organs. Maternal signs and symptoms vary depending on which blood vessels are affected.

Neurologic: *Hyperreflexia* with or without clonus (abnormal pattern of rapidly alternating involuntary contraction and relaxation of skeletal muscle) reflects the effects of the disease on upper motor neurons and central nervous system (CNS). Although deep tendon reflexes (DTRs) may be increased before a seizure, seizures can occur without hyperreflexia.

Headaches, typically frontal or occipital and unrelieved by analgesics, usually are related to vasoconstriction, cerebral edema, or cerebral ischemia.

Other cerebral symptoms may include dizziness, drowsiness, and tinnitus.

Visual disturbances usually are described as flashing lights, "seeing spots," "floaters," blurring of vision, diplopia, or scotomata (an area of depressed vision within the visual field surrounded by an area of less depressed or of normal vision). Occasionally, blindness may result. These symptoms are the result of retinal arteriolar spasm, ischemia, and edema or, on rare occasion, retinal detachment.

Eclampsia: Presence of convulsions (seizures) or coma that is not related to other cerebral conditions and occurs in the presence of the signs and symptoms of preeclampsia. The seizures may occur antepartum, intrapartum, or postpartum (usually within 48 hr). Other associated symptoms are presence of ≥2+ proteinuria, headache, visual disturbances, and RUQ pain. The cause of seizure activity during preeclampsia is not known.

Renal: Sodium retention leads to nondependent edema of the face, hands, and lower extremities. Edema also may be caused by damage to the endothelial lining of the blood vessels, which enables fluid to leak into the interstitial space. Vasospasm and glomerular capillary endothelial swelling lead to a reduction in the glomerular filtration rate. Protein concentrations of 0.1 g/L in two random urine specimens collected 4 hr apart or 0.3 g in a 24-hr period are indicative of preeclampsia.

Hepatic: Epigastric/RUQ pain may occur because of stretching of the hepatic capsule as a result of hepatic edema or hemorrhage. This causes feelings of indigestion or heartburn that are unrelieved with antacids. Nausea and vomiting may be seen.

Complications—fetal:

- **Intrauterine growth restriction (IUGR):** An abnormally restricted symmetric or asymmetric growth of the fetus.
- **Oligohydramnios:** Abnormally low volume of amniotic fluid.
- **Risk of placental abruption:** Premature separation of a normally situated placenta from the wall of the uterus.
- **Risk of preterm delivery** (often iatrogenic): Delivery before 37 wk gestation.

Physical assessment:

- Rapid weight gain ≥5 lb in 1 wk with generalized edema or edema of the face, hands, and lower extremities (edema need not be present to make the diagnosis of preeclampsia)
- Gradual or rapid increase in BP prenatally, antenatally, and postpartum
- Headache, mental confusion, hyperreflexia, epigastric pain (substernal that may radiate to the right side and back), nausea and vomiting, and shortness of breath
- Decreased fetal movement
- Proteinuria

Risk factors: Nulliparity (status of a woman who has not given birth to a viable infant), African-American race, history of preeclampsia, renal disease, diabetes mellitus, age >40, family history of preeclampsia (mother/sister), chronic hypertension, thrombophilias (antiphospholipid syndrome, proteins C and S, antithrombin deficiency, factor V Leiden), multiple gestation, obesity, gestational trophoblastic disease (molar pregnancy).

DIAGNOSTIC TESTS

Complete blood count (CBC): May be within normal limits unless anemia is present or there is evidence of hemoconcentration in which the Hct rises and the platelets drop.

Liver function tests: In mild preeclampsia, serum aspartate aminotransferase (AST; serum glutamic-oxaloacetic transaminase [SGOT]) and serum alanine aminotransferase (ALT; serum glutamic-pyruvic transaminase [SGPT]) are usually within normal limits or slightly elevated. In severe preeclampsia and HELLP syndrome, SGOT will be increased.

Coagulation studies: The most common hematologic abnormality in preeclampsia is thrombocytopenia (platelet count <150,000 mm^3). The degree to which platelets are decreased is indicative of disease severity and is dependent on coexistence of abruptio placentae. The platelet count, fibrinogen, prothrombin time (PT), and partial thromboplastin time (PTT) are usually normal in mild preeclampsia or begin to show a slight decline in values.

Urine/renal function studies: Proteinuria is present in preeclampsia with a minimum of 300 mg in a 24-hr urine analysis. Proteinuria, along with hypertension, is an indicator of fetal risk. In mild preeclampsia, blood urea nitrogen (BUN) and creatinine are usually within normal limits to slightly elevated. Uric acid is the most sensitive indicator and increases as the severity of preeclampsia increases. In severe preeclampsia with HELLP syndrome, the BUN and creatinine are significantly elevated.

Obstetric ultrasound: May be prescribed q2-3wk to follow fetal growth trend in a case of mild preeclampsia that is being monitored closely. IUGR can become evident with significant uteroplacental insufficiency caused by vasospasm.

Antepartum fetal monitoring: Weekly to twice weekly fetal nonstress testing is done to monitor fetal well-being. This also may include weekly amniotic fluid index (AFI) checks and biophysical profiles (BPPs).

Nursing Diagnosis:

Deficient Knowledge:

Effects of preeclampsia on patient, the pregnancy, and fetus

Desired Outcome: Immediately after teaching, patient and significant other verbalize accurate knowledge about the effects of preeclampsia on the patient, pregnancy, and fetus and comply with the treatment accordingly.

INTERVENTIONS	RATIONALES
Inform patient and family/significant other about the effect preeclampsia may have on the pregnancy, mother, and fetus.	An informed patient is likely to be more compliant with the prescribed therapy and understand the consequences of noncompliance. Examples of effects preeclampsia may have on the pregnancy, mother, and fetus include uteroplacental insufficiency (alteration in uteroplacental blood flow

Continued

INTERVENTIONS	RATIONALES
	and oxygenation), IUGR (abnormally restricted symmetric or asymmetric growth of the fetus), oligohydramnios (abnormally low volume of amniotic fluid), preterm delivery (delivery before 37 wk gestation), and placental abruption (premature separation of a normally situated placenta from the wall of the uterus). Likely therapies include bedrest, taking medications, stopping work, frequent clinic visits, and possible lengthy hospitalizations.
Teach patient to lie on either her right or left side when on bedrest and avoid the supine position.	Increases uteroplacental blood flow and oxygenation to the fetus by eliminating compression of the maternal aorta by the enlarging uterus and fetus.
Teach daily fetal movement counts.	Fetal movement counts are a good first-line indicator of fetal well-being and are performed beginning at 28 wk gestation, as follows: Patient lies on her side and counts "distinct fetal movements" (hiccups do not count) daily; 10 movements within a 2-hr period is reassuring. After 10 movements are counted, the assessment is discontinued. Fewer than 10 movements indicates need for fetal nonstress testing.
Teach patient how to palpate contractions.	Palpation and awareness of contractions enable patient to be an active participant in her health care. Timely reporting of contractions to her health care provider can play a significant role in affecting outcome.
	To palpate contractions, the patient lies comfortably on her side. She spreads her fingers apart and places one hand on the left side and the other on the right side of her abdomen. She will palpate the abdomen using her fingertips. When the uterus is relaxed, the abdomen should feel soft. In the presence of a contraction, the uterus will feel hard, tight, or firm under her fingertips. She then times the duration of the contraction from the beginning of one contraction to the beginning of the next. Contractions will vary in frequency and duration. See "Preterm Labor," p. 755, if contractions occur at <35 wk gestation. Contractions in a patient with preexisting preeclampsia can raise maternal BP even higher and therefore requires close monitoring. If the patient experiences 4-6 painful contractions over a 1-2-hr period, she needs to call her primary provider for evaluation.
	Duration of the contraction may or may not be an indication of contraction intensity. It is believed that the longer the contraction in true labor, the more effective it is in progressing dilation and effacement.
Teach signs and symptoms that indicate worsening preeclampsia.	Onset of preeclampsia may be slow with minimal symptoms or rapid with severe symptoms. A knowledgeable patient will likely report these symptoms promptly, including headache; visual changes such as blurred vision, spots, or flashing lights; epigastric/RUQ pain; nausea; vomiting; rapid weight gain ($\geq$5 lb/wk); increasing edema (face, hands, feet); and decreased fetal movements (see above).
Explain that urine and blood work will be evaluated on a daily basis, especially if patient is hospitalized.	To monitor for worsening preeclampsia or onset of HELLP syndrome. The following values are diagnostic: - Oliguria: $\leq$400 ml in 24 hr - Urinary dipstick for protein: $\geq$3+ - Total urine protein: $\geq$5 g/24 hr

Continued

INTERVENTIONS	RATIONALES
	- Hct: >35% - Platelet count: <150,000/mm^3 - Serum creatinine: ≥0.9 mg/dl - Serum uric acid: ≥6.6 mg/dl - Creatinine clearance: ≥100 ml/min - AST (GOT): >50 U/L - ALT (GPT): >50 U/L Platelets: The following classes are used to predict rapidity of recovery postpartum, maternal-perinatal outcome, and need for plasmapheresis. - Class I platelets: <50,000/mm^3—Patient is at extreme risk for hemorrhage, is unable to receive regional anesthesia (e.g., epidural, spinal, caudal), and may require plasmapheresis. - Class II platelets: 50,000-100,000/mm^3—Patient is at a moderately increased risk for hemorrhage and, at the anesthesiologist's discretion, may not be able to receive regional anesthesia. - Class III platelets: 100,000-150,000/mm^3—Patient is at risk of increased postpartum bleeding but should be able to receive regional anesthesia.
With the diagnosis of severe preeclampsia (including HELLP syndrome), inform patient of the seriousness of the diagnosis and that conservative management (e.g., stopping work and home bedrest) is not usually effective.	Development of severe preeclampsia is an indication to proceed with delivery. Severe preeclampsia increases need for maternal blood transfusions and risk for renal failure, pulmonary edema, ascites (abnormal intraperitoneal accumulation of fluid), pleural effusions (abnormal accumulation of fluid in the intrapleural spaces of the lungs), hepatic rupture, placenta abruption, and disseminated intravascular coagulation (hypercoagulability followed by a deficiency in clotting). Explanation aids the family in understanding the possibility of an early delivery and mode of management.

●●● **Related NIC and NOC labels:** *NIC:* Teaching: Individual; Teaching: Procedure/Treatment; High-Risk Pregnancy Care *NOC:* Knowledge: Illness Care; Knowledge: Pregnancy

Nursing Diagnosis:

Ineffective Coping

related to needed adjustment in lifestyle to provide an optimal outcome for the pregnancy and fetus or lack of support from family, friends, and community

Desired Outcome: Within 24 hr of this diagnosis, patient modifies her lifestyle or behavior to provide the best pregnancy outcome for both herself and the fetus.

INTERVENTIONS	RATIONALES
Assess patient's perceptions and ability to understand current health status.	Evaluation of patient's comprehension and perceptions enables development of an individualized care plan.
Help patient identify support systems (e.g., family members, neighbors, church members, co-workers). Observe their interaction with the patient.	Understanding strengths and weaknesses of patient's support systems will aid in planning patient's overall care; eliciting support from available and positive support systems optimally will help reduce patient's stress and facilitate coping.
Affirm that lifestyle adjustments (e.g., bedrest and cessation of work, cooking, cleaning, shopping), while austere, are for a limited time.	Facilitates acceptance of outside support and assistance and reconfirms for patient that activities could increase her blood pressure, as well as risk of maternal/fetal morbidity and mortality.
Provide patient with referral sources for support groups, written material, Internet chat groups, or home help if patient is on home bedrest or hospitalization is required. Involve Social Services in the care of patient if indicated.	Talking with others who have experienced similar circumstances may aid in developing coping mechanisms.

●●● **Related NIC and NOC labels:** *NIC:* Coping Enhancement; Support Group Enhancement
NOC: Coping

Nursing Diagnosis:

Caregiver Role Strain

related to care the significant other, family member, or support person needs to provide not only to the patient but possibly to other children in order for the patient to remain compliant and thereby prolong the gestational period

Desired Outcome: Within 24 hr of this diagnosis, caregiver verbalizes concerns/frustrations about caregiving responsibilities, identifies at least one other support person, and recognizes at least one change that would make his or her job easier.

INTERVENTIONS	RATIONALES
Encourage caregiver to relate feelings and concerns regarding added responsibilities. Help caregiver clarify responsibilities with patient and other family members.	Validates caregiver's concerns and helps him or her understand if expectations are realistic.
Encourage caregiver to identify which activities would benefit from outside assistance.	Confirms caregiver's need to seek help and facilitates that help.
Involve Social Services in support of the caregiver establishing a plan for time-outs or for referrals to community support groups.	Confirms need to seek help and provides caregiver with coping mechanisms. During times of stress, caregivers may know they need help but may not know where to find it.

●●● **Related NIC and NOC labels:** *NIC:* Caregiver Support; Respite Care; Coping Enhancement
NOC: Caregiver Well-Being

Nursing Diagnosis:

Deficient Knowledge:

Purpose and potential side effects of prescribed medications

Desired Outcome: Immediately following teaching, patient and family verbalize accurate understanding of the risks and benefits of medications used during the pregnancy to aid in treatment of preeclampsia.

INTERVENTIONS	RATIONALES
Teach the following about patient's prescribed medications:	A knowledgeable patient is more likely to comply with therapy, identify and report side effects, and recognize and report precautions that might preclude use of the prescribed drug.
Magnesium sulfate (MgSO$_4$)	Used to decrease the CNS irritability seen with preeclampsia in preventing seizure activity. Therapeutic level is 4-8 mg/dl.
	Administration: IV. It is never used with nifedipine because their combined use could lead to pulmonary edema.
	Used on an inpatient basis only.
Teach patient to be alert for and report headaches, hot flashes, nausea, vomiting, and dizziness.	Common side effects.
Teach patient to be alert for and report shortness of breath, coughing, and lethargy.	Pulmonary edema is a serious side effect of this drug. For this reason, it is used with caution in patients who have received large amount of IV fluid hydration.
Explain that BP, HR, RR, DTRs, urinary output, and level of consciousness will be monitored at frequent intervals.	This drug has potentially serious side effects. Levels outside therapeutic range can cause toxicity:
	- Loss of DTRs: 9-12 mg/dl
	- Respiratory arrest: >15 mg/dl
	- Cardiac arrest: >25-30 mg/dl
Advise patient that use is contraindicated in maternal renal failure and hypocalcemia, and serum values of calcium will be monitored.	MgSO$_4$ is excreted via the kidneys; therefore increases in maternal serum magnesium may result in maternal hypocalcemia because magnesium opposes the action of calcium in the body.
Calcium channel blocker *Nifedipine (Procardia)*	Vasodilates and reduces peripheral resistance of the blood vessels without reducing cardiac output. Usually it is used to treat the chronic hypertension present before onset of preeclampsia. No adverse maternal/fetal side effects have been reported.
	Administration: oral route.
	May be used on an outpatient basis.
	It is never used in combination with MgSO$_4$ because their combined use could lead to pulmonary edema.
Teach patient to be alert for and report lightheadedness and dizziness. Instruct patient to rise slowly from a supine position.	There is potential for hypotension with this drug.
Explain that patient may notice transient headaches and flushing for the first few days of taking this drug.	Common side effects.
Advise that this drug is used with caution in patients with hepatic disease.	Nifedipine is primarily metabolized and excreted by the liver; therefore with hepatic disease these two processes may be delayed, causing an increase in serum nifedipine levels.
β-Blockers *Labetalol (Normodyne) and atenolol (Tenormin)*	These drugs decrease blood pressure and maternal heart rate without significantly decreasing cardiac output. Usually they are used to treat chronic hypertension present before onset of preeclampsia.
	Administration: oral route. May be given IV on an inpatient basis only.
Advise that patient may notice transient paresthesias or scalp tingling.	Possible mild side effects seen at onset of treatment.

Continued

INTERVENTIONS	RATIONALES
Teach patient to be alert for and report dizziness, fatigue, nausea, vomiting, and shortness of breath.	Adverse reactions.
Caution patients with diabetes of need for vigilance regarding checking blood glucose levels when taking these drugs.	These drugs reduce the release of insulin in response to hyperglycemia.
Advise patients with bronchial asthma and systemic lupus erythematosus (SLE) of the need to use caution when taking these drugs.	These drugs may exacerbate symptoms of asthma and SLE.
Advise patients taking tricyclic antidepressants of the need to use caution when taking β-blockers.	β-Blockers may cause tremors when used along with tricyclic antidepressants.
Teach importance of serial ultrasounds to monitor fetal growth when taking this drug.	These drugs have been associated with fetal growth restriction.
Antenatal glucocorticoids *Betamethasone or dexamethasone*	Aid in reducing effects of respiratory distress syndrome (RDS), intraventricular hemorrhage, and necrotizing enterocolitis on preterm neonate when preterm delivery is anticipated. These drugs also accelerate maturation of fetal organs, including cardiovascular, and the central nervous system. Administration: - Betamethasone: two doses of 12 mg given 24 hr apart. - Dexamethasone: four doses of 6 mg given 12 hr apart. They are usually administered when a preterm delivery is anticipated and after gestation of viability (25 wk). Maximum benefit is 48 hr after administration.
Explain that patients with diabetes need to monitor glucose levels and inform provider of abnormal levels: fasting >90 mg/dl, 2 hr pp >120 mg/dl, and hs >120 mg/dl.	A side effect of these drugs is impaired glucose tolerance. Women with borderline gestational diabetes may develop true gestational diabetes. A rise in blood glucose is usually seen for approximately 48-96 hr after administration, and it may require IV insulin.
Aspirin *Low-dose aspirin (81 mg)*	During pregnancy it decreases platelet aggregation and increases vasodilation. It is given to women with autoimmune disease to prevent fetal wastage. Its use as a preventative for preeclampsia is controversial. Administration: oral.
Teach patient to be alert for and report nausea, vomiting, and epigastric pain.	Possible side effects. However, they are also symptoms of worsening preeclampsia.
Advise of the need for caution in patients with a history of gastrointestinal (GI) ulcers.	Aspirin may cause GI bleeding.

●●● **Related NIC and NOC labels:** *NIC:* Teaching: Prescribed Medication *NOC:* Knowledge: Medication

Nursing Diagnosis:

Risk for Impaired Parent/Infant Attachment

related to disruption for bonding or interactive process secondary to maternal/fetal health risks

Desired Outcome: Within 24 hr of this diagnosis, patient and family members verbalize their concerns regarding the parental bonding process and barriers present and participate in care of mother and infant when possible.

INTERVENTIONS	RATIONALES
Encourage patient and family to verbalize feelings and concerns regarding the labor, delivery, and postpartum experience and the effect it will have on parental bonding.	Provides an opportunity for reassessment, confirmation, and validation of patient's/family's feelings and concerns.
If the infant is in the neonatal intensive care unit (NICU) and the mother is unable to visit because of her medical condition, arrange for significant other or family to visit and provide her with updates on baby's condition and items such as photos and footprints.	Provides for one form of maternal bonding.
Encourage mother to speak with her infant's caregivers for updates.	Enables her to participate in care and well-being of her infant.
When possible, encourage mother to visit NICU as soon as possible.	Promotes the bonding process.
Assist mother with breast pumping.	Enables bonding process and fetal nutrition.
If it is necessary for the infant to be transferred to another facility, provide opportunity for parents and family to see and touch the infant before transport.	Assists in the bonding process.

●●● **Related NIC and NOC labels:** *NIC:* Attachment Promotion; Anticipatory Guidance; Breastfeeding Assistance; Family Involvement Promotion *NOC:* Parent-Infant Attachment

ADDITIONAL NURSING DIAGNOSES/ PROBLEMS:

"Prolonged Bedrest" as indicated	p. 67
"Psychosocial Support" for **Anxiety**	p. 82
"Psychosocial Support for the Patient's Family and Significant Others" for **Interrupted Family Processes**	p. 95

PATIENT-FAMILY TEACHING AND DISCHARGE PLANNING

Preeclampsia is a progressive disease in which monitoring for maternal and fetal changes is of critical importance. Include verbal and written information about the following:

✔ Signs and symptoms of worsening preeclampsia (headache, increased edema, oliguria, RUQ pain, decreased fetal movement, nausea, and vomiting) and importance of contacting health care provider promptly should they occur.

✔ Seizure precautions.

✔ Medications, including drug name, purpose, dosage, frequency, precautions, potential drug/drug and food/drug interactions, potential drug reactions, and side effects.

✔ Importance of compliance with prescribed health care and ready access to hospital and family/social support.

✔ Parameters and guidelines for home bedrest.

✔ Measures that help with constipation, which occurs frequently in pregnancy and can be exacerbated with bedrest.

✔ Measures for coping with muscle pain, back pain, and muscle weakness that can be present with prolonged bedrest.

✔ Fetal movement counts.

✔ Referrals to national and local support agencies, including:

Sidelines, a national support organization for women and their families experiencing complicated pregnancies: Sidelines High Risk Pregnancy Support National Office
P.O. Box 1808
Laguna Beach, CA 92652
(888) 447-4754
www.sidelines.org/

SHARE, a national support group for parents who have experienced loss through miscarriage, stillbirth, or newborn death:
SHARE Pregnancy & Infant Loss Support, Inc.
National SHARE Office
St. Joseph Health Center
300 First Capitol Drive
St. Charles, MO 63301-2893
(800) 821-6819 or (636) 947-6164
www.nationalshareoffice.com/

Preterm Labor

Preterm labor (PTL) is labor occurring after 20 wk gestation and before completion of the 37th wk. Preterm labor leading to preterm delivery plays a major role in neonatal morbidity and mortality, although infants born at >34 wk gestation usually do fine, barring major preexisting medical complications. PTL is a major medical concern. Spontaneous labor involves a series of interactions among hormones, enzymes, and cells between the fetus and mother. It is unclear if the mechanisms associated with labor in a term pregnancy are the same as those with PTL. Surviving preterm infants may suffer from neurodevelopmental handicaps, chronic respiratory disease, and long-term mental and physical impairment.

HEALTH CARE SETTING

Some patients may be managed via primary care on an outpatient basis with frequent clinic evaluation or in a high-risk perinatal clinic. Others may receive acute care in an inpatient antepartum setting.

ASSESSMENT

Symptoms may range from the obvious to subtle—from light menstrual-like cramping to strong palpable contractions. There may be an increase in normal vaginal discharge, low dull backache to an intense aching that may radiate to the hips and down the thighs, and no bleeding to light pink vaginal spotting or bright red vaginal bleeding. The mother may feel that the baby is "balling up" in her abdomen and describe a "heavy" feeling in the perineum or pelvic pressure. Many symptoms of PTL do not cause pain, and it does not present in the same way as labor at term.

Contractions/uterine tightening: As the pregnancy progresses, so does the frequency of uterine activity. Uterine tightening/contractions begin in the first trimester as the uterus enlarges and continue throughout the pregnancy. These contractions are considered Braxton-Hicks and occur at irregular intervals, usually are painless, and do not change the cervix. PTL is diagnosed when uterine contractions are persistent and accompanied by cervical change, either dilation or effacement.

Backache: Although this is a very common complaint in pregnancy, any woman with a history of preterm labor/delivery who complains of new-onset backache needs to be evaluated for cervical changes, especially if she describes the backache as low lumbar/sacral in position, deep tissue in nature, or a dull aching sensation that radiates around the hips to the lower abdomen/pelvic area and down the thighs.

Pelvic pressure: May be described as "heaviness" or a sensation of "fullness," either constant or intermittent. The mother may state that she feels the "baby has dropped."

Abdominal cramping: Gastrointestinal (GI) symptoms such as increased flatus or diarrhea may be present. The abdomen may be tender to palpate, as is seen with chorioamnionitis (inflammatory reaction in the amniotic membranes caused by bacteria or virus).

Vaginal discharge: An increase in vaginal discharge is normal during pregnancy. It can be clear, thick, or thin and "milky white" or light yellow. It may become watery in nature as with preterm premature ruptured membranes (PPROM) or bloody as with placental abruption or when the cervix dilates and its surface vessels break. A foul odor may indicate an infection.

Fever: Temperature may range from 98.6° F (37° C) to ≥101° F (38.3° C) if an infection is present.

General complaints: Other symptoms may include a feeling of unease and body aches. The woman may state, "I just feel different."

Physical assessment: Even with vague symptoms, cervical changes may be taking place. Therefore it is important not to underestimate reported symptoms. Early evaluation and treatment are critical in attempting to stop PTL and preventing fetal morbidity and mortality.

Risk factors: Abdominal surgery during current pregnancy, chronic urinary tract infections (UTIs), polyhydramnios (excess amniotic fluid), poor weight gain after 20 wk, prepregnancy weight <100 lb, multiple gestation, previous preterm delivery, smoking, substance abuse, poor prenatal care, uterine/cervical anomalies, cervical incompetence, maternal infection, age <18 or >35, history of cervical conization, low socioeconomic status, non-Caucasian, the patient herself a preterm infant, strenuous work, previous second trimester abortion, uterine infections, abruptio placentae, psychologic stress, and domestic violence leading to physical or emotional abuse.

Complications—fetal:
- Preterm delivery
- Respiratory distress syndrome (RDS)
- Patent ductus arteriosus (PDA; an abnormal opening between the pulmonary artery and aorta)
- Intraventricular hemorrhage (IVH)
- Sepsis
- Necrotizing enterocolitis (ischemic, inflammatory bowel disorder that can lead to perforation and peritonitis)
- Hyperbilirubinemia
- Hypoglycemia
- Impaired/immature immunologic system
- Neonatal death

DIAGNOSTIC TESTS

External uterine and fetal monitoring: External uterine monitoring is done to evaluate fetal well-being and the presence, frequency, and duration of uterine contractions. Abnormal fetal heart rate patterns (decreased variability, moderate-to-severe variable decelerations and late decelerations) are suggestive of fetal compromise, which uteroplacental insufficiency, umbilical cord compression, cord prolapse or infection can cause. This is an important diagnostic tool because some women are not aware of contractions when they are clearly documented on monitoring.

Urinalysis for microscopy: UTIs are associated with PTL. A clean catch urine specimen should be obtained when attempting to rule out PTL, even when the patient is asymptomatic. When a UTI is present, antibiotic therapy will be initiated.

Cervical evaluation: Digital cervical examinations are done to evaluate cervical dilation (centimeters [cm] dilated), effacement (percentage of thinning), consistency (e.g., soft, firm), and position (e.g., anterior vs. posterior position in the vaginal vault) to confirm the diagnosis of PTL. During a nonsterile speculum exam, cultures may be done to evaluate for the presence of *Chlamydia trachomatis,* herpes simplex virus, group B streptococci, *Gardnerella vaginalis,* and other anaerobes.

Sterile speculum exam to rule out rupture of membranes: This exam is not routinely done in patients with PTL; it is performed only if there is reason to suspect that membranes may have ruptured. A sterile speculum is inserted into the vagina to visualize leaking of amniotic fluid coming from the cervical os or observe pooling of amniotic fluid in the vagina. Vaginal fluid pH is tested with nitrazine paper. A positive test is noted when the paper turns from yellow to blue (the pH is >6.0). False-positive results can be seen in the presence of semen, blood, vaginal infections, or alkaline antiseptics. Vaginal fluid is examined under the microscope for the presence of a ferning pattern that amniotic fluid makes when it dries on a slide. A digital exam of the cervix is not recommended in a patient with suspected PPROM who is not in labor because of the risk of introducing an infection.

Ultrasound: Abdominal ultrasound is used to confirm gestational age, calculate amniotic fluid index (AFI) and biophysical profile (BPP), rule out multiple gestation, and determine placental location and fetal presentation. Transvaginal or translabial ultrasound is used to evaluate cervical length, dilation, effacement, and the presence of funneling (see discussion in "Cervical Incompetence") of the internal cervical os. The shorter the cervix, the greater the risk of PTL. The shortest acceptable cervical length is 3 cm. A cervical length of ≤2.5 cm is associated with increased PTL risk. Cervical length determination by ultrasound should not take the place of digital exams.

Fetal fibronectin enzyme immunoassay: Fetal fibronectin (fFN) is an extracellular matrix protein, a gluelike substance that is present between fetal membranes and the uterine decidua. It is usually seen after 37 wk gestation. Its presence between 22-37 wk may have a predictive value for pending PTL. It is obtained from secretions present in the posterior vaginal vault, but only if the amniotic membranes are intact, cervical dilation is <3 cm, and the gestational age is between 24-35 wk. This test is best used as a negative predictor. In other words, if fFN is not present between 22 and 37 wk gestation, chances are great the woman will not deliver prematurely.

Amniocentesis: To determine fetal lung maturity as a predictor for fetal RDS, as well as to check for chorioamnionitis.

Nursing Diagnosis:

Deficient Knowledge:

Effects of preterm labor on self and the fetus

Desired Outcome: Patient and significant other verbalize accurate knowledge about the effects of preterm labor on the patient, pregnancy, and fetus and comply with the treatment accordingly.

INTERVENTIONS	RATIONALES
Inform patient and significant other about treatments for PTL and the effects preterm labor and delivery can have on the fetus.	Information about the effects preterm labor and delivery can have on the fetus (i.e., RDS, hypoglycemia, IVH, sepsis, necrotizing enterocolitis, hyperbilirubinemia, and neonatal death) is likely to promote compliance with treatments (e.g., bedrest, adequate hydration, decreasing activity, stopping work, frequent clinic visits, no intercourse, taking medications, possible lengthy hospitalizations).
Explain importance of access to a specialized facility.	Delivering a preterm infant at a facility with perinatal and neonatal specialists and neonatal intensive care unit (NICU) provides the greatest opportunity for infant survival.
Teach signs and symptoms of PTL to *all* pregnant women.	An informed patient likely will report these symptoms promptly. See introductory information for detailed signs and symptoms of preterm labor. Barring the presence of chorioamnionitis, the earlier PTL is diagnosed, the better the chance for prolonging the pregnancy and decreasing fetal morbidity and mortality.
Question patient at each prenatal visit, starting at the beginning of the second trimester, if she is experiencing any signs or symptoms of preterm labor/contractions.	Early recognition of PTL (see signs and symptoms in the introductory data) may lead to prolonging the gestational period and decreasing fetal morbidity and mortality.
Encourage patient to report even vague or subtle symptoms no matter the time of day or night. Provide written instructions and phone numbers to call should concerns or changes arise.	Uterine contractions may be painless. Fewer than 50% of patients in PTL are aware of their contractions. Incidence of PTL is approximately 10%, and preterm birth accounts for almost 85% of all neonatal mortality not caused by congenital anomalies (Chin, 2001).
Teach daily fetal movement counts.	Fetal movement counts done twice a day are a good first-line indicator of fetal well-being and are performed as follows, beginning at 28 wk gestation: Patient lies on her side and counts "distinct fetal movements" (hiccups do not count); 10 movements within a 2-hr period is considered reassuring. After 10 movements are discerned, the count is discontinued. Fewer than 10 movements in a 2-hr period signals need for fetal nonstress testing.
Teach patient how to palpate contractions.	Timely reporting of preterm contractions to her health care provider can play a significant role in affecting outcome. Palpation and awareness of contractions enable patient to be an active participant in her health care.
	To palpate contractions, the patient lies comfortably on her side. She spreads her fingers apart and places one hand on the left side and the other on the right side of her abdomen. She will palpate the abdomen using her fingertips. When the uterus is relaxed, the abdomen should feel soft. In the presence of a contraction, the uterus should feel hard, tight, or firm under her fingertips. She then times the duration of the contraction from the beginning of one contraction to the beginning of the next. Contractions will vary in frequency and duration. If the patient experiences 4-6 contractions for 1-2 hr, she needs to call her primary provider. Contractions may be mild to severe in intensity and difficult for a gravida I (first pregnancy) mother to discern as PTL.
Instruct patient to drink at least six 8-oz glasses of water per day (48-64 fluid oz).	The uterus is a muscle and will respond to dehydration by cramping/contracting. Adequate oral hydration is a preventative measure for PTL.

Continued

INTERVENTIONS	RATIONALES
Teach patient and her partner the effect that sexual foreplay or intercourse may have on PTL. Advise patient to avoid all forms of sexual stimulation.	To promote patient/partner understanding and compliance. Sexual intercourse may increase uterine contractions and promote cervical change. Increased uterine activity also may be caused by breast stimulation, female orgasm, and prostaglandin in male ejaculate.

●●● **Related NIC and NOC labels:** *NIC:* Teaching: Individual; Teaching: Disease Process; High-Risk Pregnancy Care *NOC:* Knowledge: Medication; Knowledge: Pregnancy

Nursing Diagnosis:

Ineffective Coping

related to adjustment in lifestyle to provide an optimal environment for the fetus or lack of support from family, friends, and community

Desired Outcome: Within the 24-hr period after this diagnosis is made, patient verbalizes feelings and identifies strengths and coping behaviors to provide the best pregnancy outcome for herself and fetus.

INTERVENTIONS	RATIONALES
Assess patient's perceptions and ability to understand current health status regarding PTL.	Evaluation of patient's perceptions and comprehension enables development of an individualized care plan.
Provide referral sources for support groups, written material, Internet chat groups, or home help if patient is on home bedrest or hospitalization. Involve Social Services in care of patient as needed.	Communicating with or learning about others who have experienced similar circumstances may aid in the development of positive coping mechanisms.
Help patient identify or develop a support system.	Having a support system will aid in patient's overall care and reduction of stress to promote positive coping behaviors.
Arrange community referrals as appropriate or at the request of the patient.	Support in the home environment promotes healthier adaptations and may avert crises.
Offer realistic hope for continuing the pregnancy to a safe gestation. Help patient and family develop realistic expectations for the future if a preterm delivery occurs and to identify support persons or systems that will assist them with planning for the future.	Fosters realistic expectations about a preterm neonate's health status (in the absence of congenital anomalies) and promotes adaptation to possible changes in family dynamics.
Teach patient and family that hospitalization and medical interventions in preventing a preterm birth may not always be effective or wise.	Medications, bedrest, and hydration are not always successful in stopping PTL. In some instances an early delivery may be in the best interest of the mother, fetus, or both, as would be the case in the presence of infection, nonreassuring fetal heart rate tracings, severe oligohydramnios (abnormally low amount of amniotic fluid), anhydramnios (no amniotic fluid), and congenital anomalies.
Affirm that lifestyle adjustment (e.g., no work, bedrest, no intercourse) is for a limited time.	Facilitates acceptance of outside support and assistance and reinforces knowledge that routine or increased activity with PTL may increase risk of cervical change and possible preterm delivery.

●●● **Related NIC and NOC labels:** *NIC:* Coping Enhancement; Anxiety Reduction; Counseling; Emotional Support; Support System Enhancement; Family Involvement Enhancement *NOC:* Coping; Social Support

Nursing Diagnosis:

Caregiver Role Strain

related to the care significant other, family member, or support person needs to provide not only to the patient but possibly to other family members in order for patient to remain compliant and prolong the gestational period

Desired Outcome: Within 24 hr from this diagnosis, caregiver verbalizes concerns/frustrations about caregiving responsibilities, identifies at least one other support person, and recognizes at least one change that would make his or her job easier.

INTERVENTIONS	RATIONALES
Encourage caregiver and patient to relate their feelings and concerns regarding their roles.	Validates concerns and helps them understand if expectations are realistic.
Acknowledge caregiver's role in patient care; identify and praise strengths.	Reinforces positive ways of dealing with current health crisis and promotes a sense of involvement and appreciation.
Involve social services in support of the caregiver in helping establish a plan for time-outs.	Provides caregiver with a weekly visible goal and coping mechanisms and validates need to seek help.
Provide patient and caregiver with status reports on effectiveness of patient's bedrest, decreased activity, stopping work, or inability to participate in routine household activities.	Reassuring patient and caregiver that the support and assistance are positively affecting patient's health likely will promote more of the same.
Affirm that this is for a limited time.	Facilitates patient's and caregiver's acceptance in receiving and giving support and assistance.
Encourage diversional activities (e.g., time alone away from home or hospital and other children) and interaction with support persons or systems outside the family.	Promoting respite enhances coping and assists family members in remaining focused and supportive of patient. For example, "I know this must be a difficult time and you want to stay with your wife, but I will call you if any changes occur."

●●● **Related NIC and NOC labels:** *NIC:* Caregiver Support; Coping Enhancement; Respite Care; Family Involvement Promotion; Support System Enhancement *NOC:* Caregiver Lifestyle Disruption; Caregiver Well-Being

Nursing Diagnosis:

Constipation

related to decreased peristalsis secondary to immobility, stress, lack of exercise, and prolonged bedrest

Desired Outcome: Patient has normal bowel movements and minimal discomfort from gas and hard stooling within 2-3 days of interventions, thereby reducing the risk of preterm contractions.

INTERVENTIONS	RATIONALES
Identify patient's normal bowel status and whether she requires laxatives or stool softeners on a routine basis.	Enables patient assessment and identifies if constipation is playing a role in PTL. Constipation is a normal symptom of pregnancy because the descending colon vies for space with the uterus as it enlarges and because progesterone, one of the hormones produced in pregnancy, decreases gastric motility. However, in a patient prone to PTL who is on bedrest, constipation can be exacerbated because of the decrease in peristalsis associated with inactivity.

Continued

INTERVENTIONS	RATIONALES
Explain effects of constipation in a patient prone to PTL.	Constipation or gastric irritability can increase uterine irritability in the form of contractions. This would increase risk of PTL.
Encourage daily intake of at least 8-10 glasses of water/day and increasing dietary fiber or adding a fiber laxative or stool softener to her daily regimen.	To provide bulk and aid in keeping the stool soft.

●●● **Related NIC and NOC labels:** *NIC:* Constipation Management; Fluid Management *NOC:* Bowel Elimination; Hydration; Symptom Control

Nursing Diagnosis:

Risk for Impaired Parent/Infant Attachment

related to disruption for bonding or interactive process secondary to maternal/fetal health risks

Desired Outcome: Patient and family members verbalize their concerns regarding the parental bonding process and barriers present and participate in the care of both mother and infant when possible.

INTERVENTIONS	RATIONALES
Encourage mother and family to take a guided tour of the NICU (time permitting) if a preterm delivery is expected or necessary.	Decreases fear of the unknown and facilitates questions and answers.
Encourage patient and family to verbalize feelings and concerns regarding the labor, delivery, and postpartum experience.	Provides for an opportunity of reassessment, confirmation, and/or validation of their concerns and feelings.
When possible, encourage mother to visit baby in NICU as soon as possible after the delivery. Provide the mother with written information on care provided in the NICU.	Promotes the bonding process, encourages communication with baby's care providers, and provides an opportunity to have questions answered.
Encourage mother to breastfeed or express milk for later feeding of the infant.	In the preterm infant, it is not always possible or recommended to feed at the breast. However, either method promotes psychologic benefits for the mother by involving her in the infant's daily care and reinforcing importance her breast milk has to the health of her infant.
Explain benefits of breast milk to preterm infant.	For the preterm infant, breast milk decreases incidences of infectious complications and metabolic disturbances. Maternal antibodies in breast milk also promote immunologic health inasmuch as the infant's immune system is immature.
	Infants fed breast milk will gain the same weight at the same rate as if they were fed formula. Breast milk also helps establish nonpathogenic bacterial flora in the newborn intestinal tract and stimulates passage of stool.
If mother chooses to breastfeed by expressing milk for later infant feeding, assist her with breast pump operation and arrange for rental of a breast pump for home use as needed.	See "Mastitis, Postpartum" care plan, p. 731, for breast pump teaching interventions.
If it is necessary for the infant to be transferred to another facility, provide the opportunity for parents and family to see and touch the infant before transport.	Assists in the bonding process. Some facilities transport the mother along with the preterm infant.

●●● **Related NIC and NOC labels:** *NIC:* Attachment Promotion; Environmental Management: Attachment Process; Breastfeeding; Assistance Infant Care; Family Involvement Promotion *NOC:* Parent-Infant Attachment

Nursing Diagnosis:

Ineffective Breastfeeding

related to interruption in the normal process resulting from a premature and/or ill infant

Desired Outcome: Patient produces breast milk using a breast pump or makes an informed decision regarding which method of feeding most benefits the infant's needs and her own emotional/physical state of well-being.

INTERVENTIONS	RATIONALES
Encourage mother to verbalize her concerns.	Validates her concerns and evaluates possible obstacles preventing her from producing adequate milk supply.
Teach patient the physical process of lactation after birth.	Assists in decreasing her anxiety about "not having enough milk" and helps her understand the importance of breast stimulation via actual breastfeeding or pumping.
	Delivery of the placenta causes a fall in progesterone and a rise in prolactin, the hormone that stimulates lactogenesis (milk production). Prolactin is released from the anterior pituitary gland during breastfeeding, which in turn stimulates milk production. Oxytocin is released from the posterior pituitary gland at the same time and causes the milk ejection reflex, or milk "let down." During the course of breastfeeding, these hormones are released and regulated on a supply and demand basis.
Provide support to the mother through lactation specialists available within the hospital or as outside consultants.	Lactation instructors assist the mother in proper use of a breast pump or in actual infant breastfeeding, positioning the infant for comfort and ease of nursing, and use of various breast shields as needed and teach how to manage engorgement, inverted or flat nipples, milk supply problems, plugged ducts, sore nipples, and infant sucking problems.
Teach use of a breast pump and manual expression, storage, and transport of milk.	Aids in the success of producing milk and the safety of its storage. For details, see "Mastitis, Postpartum" care plan, p. 731.
Teach importance of adequate oral hydration, nutrition, and rest.	Adequate maternal caloric intake, oral hydration, and rest help meet the periods of increased demand for breast milk during infant's growth spurts and maintain a consistent supply of breast milk.
See previous nursing diagnosis for other interventions and details.	

●●● **Related NIC and NOC labels:** *NIC:* Breastfeeding Assistance; Lactation Counseling; Fluid Management; Nutritional Counseling *NOC:* Breastfeeding Establishment: Maternal

Nursing Diagnosis:

Deficient Knowledge:

Purpose and potential side effects of prescribed medications

Desired Outcome: Immediately following teaching, patient and family relate accurate understanding of the risks and benefits of medications used during the pregnancy to aid in managing PTL.

INTERVENTIONS	RATIONALES
Teach patient and family the following about prescribed fluids and medications:	A knowledgeable patient is more likely to comply with therapy, identify and report side effects, and recognize and report precautions that might preclude use of the prescribed drug.
Intravenous fluid hydration	In the dehydrated patient, IV fluids may be useful in treating PTL. They have not been shown to be beneficial in treating the hydrated patient.
Type of IV fluids varies among providers.	
Caution is necessary when used with tocolytic drugs.	IV fluid overload can lead to pulmonary edema when used with tocolytic drugs. A tocolytic drug is any agent used to suppress PTL. Examples include indomethacin (Indocin), magnesium sulfate (MgSO$_4$), nifedipine (Procardia), and terbutaline (Brethine).
Prostaglandin synthesis inhibitor	Inhibits prostaglandin synthesis, thereby decreasing myometrial contractility (contractions).
Ibuprofen	Administration: Oral.
Be alert for and report nausea and vomiting, heartburn, diarrhea, constipation, and abdominal cramps.	Common side effects. If these symptoms persist, the medication may need to be changed, dose adjusted, or discontinued.
Avoid use of this drug after 34-35 wk.	This drug can decrease amniotic fluid volume (oligohydramnios) and prevent closure of PDA (an abnormal opening between the pulmonary artery and aorta).
Caution is necessary for patients with gastrointestinal (GI) ulcers and renal disease.	May cause gastric bleeding, fluid retention, and renal toxicity.
Take these drugs with food.	Decreases GI side effects.
Avoid use if taking warfarin or heparin.	Increases risk of bleeding.
Indomethacin (short-term use only)	Inhibits prostaglandin synthesis, thereby decreasing myometrial contractility (contractions). Used as a second- or third-line agent for tocolysis (an agent that suppresses uterine contractions).
	Pregnancy: safety unknown or controversial.
	Not used for more than 48 hr.
	Administration: oral or rectal suppository.
Be alert for and report nausea and vomiting, drowsiness, dizziness, depression, psychosis, and headaches.	Possible maternal side effects. If these symptoms occur, the medication should be discontinued.
Take this medication with food.	Decreases GI symptoms.
Avoid taking this drug after 34-35 wk.	This drug can decrease amniotic fluid volume (oligohydramnios) and prevent closure of PDA (an abnormal opening between the pulmonary artery and aorta).
Avoid this drug if also taking warfarin or heparin.	May increase risk of bleeding.
Caution is necessary in patients with asthma.	May exacerbate asthmatic symptoms.
Caution is necessary in patients with renal disease.	May cause renal toxicity.
Calcium channel blocker	Inhibits smooth muscle contractility, thus decreasing or eliminating uterine contractions.
Nifedipine	Administration: oral route.
	No adverse maternal/fetal effects have been reported.
	May be used on an outpatient basis.
	It is never used with MgSO$_4$ because their combined use could lead to pulmonary edema.
Patient may notice transient headaches and flushing for the first 24-72 hr of taking this drug.	Common side effects; not life threatening; symptoms resolve after this time.

Continued

INTERVENTIONS	RATIONALES
Rise slowly from a supine position.	There is potential for hypotension (especially in a normotensive woman).
Be alert for and report nausea, flushing, and nervousness.	Common side effects. If these symptoms persist, the dose of the medication may need to be changed or dose adjusted.
Caution is necessary for patients with hepatic disease.	Nifedipine is primarily metabolized and excreted by the liver; therefore with hepatic disease these two processes may be delayed, causing an increase in serum nifedipine levels.
Caution is necessary for patients taking cimetidine (Tagamet).	Causes increase in peak nifedipine plasma levels (higher drug concentration).
β-Adrenergic agonist	Decreases uterine myometrial activity (contractions).
Terbutaline (Brethine)	Administration: IM, SC, PO.
Be alert for and report rapid heart rate, restlessness, agitation, nausea, and vomiting.	Common side effects. If these symptoms persist, the dose of the medication may need to be changed or discontinued.
Be alert for and report shortness of breath.	There is potential for pulmonary edema, which is the most common maternal side effect and can occur between 30-60 hr after IV administration of the first dose.
Rise slowly from a supine position.	There is potential for hypotension with this drug.
This drug is contraindicated with maternal cardiac dysrhythmias, diabetes mellitus, maternal cardiac disease, uncontrolled hypertension, and thyrotoxicosis (Graves' disease/hyperthyroidism).	Significant cardiac side effects are seen in patients without cardiac disease who take this drug.
Magnesium sulfate (MgSO$_4$)	Decreases uterine myometrial activity (contractions) at a therapeutic serum magnesium level of 4-8 mg/dl.
	Administration: IV infusion.
	Used on an inpatient basis only.
	It is never used with nifedipine because their combined use could lead to pulmonary edema.
Be alert for and report headaches, hot flashes, nausea, vomiting, and dizziness.	Common side effects.
Be alert for and report shortness of breath, coughing, and lethargy.	Pulmonary edema is a serious side effect that can occur in patients taking this drug who have received large amounts of IV fluid hydration.
BP, HR, RR, deep tendon reflexes (DTRs), and urinary output will be monitored at frequent intervals.	This drug has potentially serious side effects. Levels outside therapeutic range can cause toxicity:
	- Loss of DTRs: 9-12 mg/dl
	- Respiratory arrest: >15 mg/dl
	- Cardiac arrest: >25-30 mg/dl
Use is contraindicated with maternal renal failure and hypocalcemia.	MgSO$_4$ is excreted via the kidneys; increases in maternal serum magnesium can result in maternal hypocalcemia because magnesium opposes the action of calcium in the body.
Antenatal glucocorticoid	Aids in reducing the effects of RDS, IVH, and necrotizing enterocolitis on preterm neonate. It also accelerates the maturation of the central nervous system and fetal organs, including cardiovascular. It is usually administered when a preterm delivery is anticipated after the gestation of viability. Maximum benefit is 48 hr after administration.
Betamethasone or dexamethasone	
	Administration: IM.

Continued

INTERVENTIONS	RATIONALES
	- Betamethasone: two doses of 12 mg given 24 hr apart.
	- Dexamethasone: four doses of 6 mg given 12 hr apart.
Be alert for and report signs of infection (elevated temperature, chills, body aches) and elevated maternal glucose levels.	Possible side effects of this medication are reduced maternal-fetal resistance to infection, impaired glucose tolerance (people with borderline gestational diabetes may develop true gestational diabetes), and suppression of maternal or neonatal adrenal function. Usually a rise in blood glucose is seen for approximately 48-96 hr after administration, and it may require IV insulin. Individuals with diabetes need to monitor glucose levels closely and inform provider of abnormal levels (fasting >90 mg/dl, 2-hr pp >120 mg/dl, and hs >120 mg/dl) and decrease in fetal movement.

●●● **Related NIC and NOC labels:** *NIC:* Teaching: Prescribed Medication *NOC:* Knowledge: Medication

ADDITIONAL NURSING DIAGNOSES/ PROBLEMS:

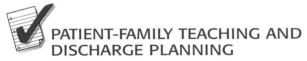

PATIENT-FAMILY TEACHING AND DISCHARGE PLANNING

Preterm labor and birth can have lifelong effects on the child and family. Early diagnosis and treatment are imperative. Educating each patient about signs and symptoms of PTL should be a part of every woman's prenatal care. Include verbal and written information about the following:

✓Potential risk factors for PTL that may be present early in prenatal care.

✓Signs and symptoms of PTL.

✓Palpation of contractions.

✓Promptly reporting any signs of UTI.

✓Importance of adequate oral hydration during the pregnancy.

✓Importance of compliance with routine prenatal care.

✓Medications, including drug name, purpose, dosage, frequency, drug/drug and food/drug interactions, precautions, potential drug reactions, and potential side effects.

✓Measures that help with constipation, which occurs frequently in pregnancy and can be exacerbated with bedrest.

✓Measures for coping with muscle pain, back pain, and muscle weakness that can be present with prolonged bedrest.

✓Fetal movement counts.

✓Referral to local and national support organizations, including:

Sidelines, a national support organization for women and their families experiencing complicated pregnancies: Sidelines High Risk Pregnancy Support National Office
P.O. Box 1808
Laguna Beach, CA 92652
(888) 447-4754
www.sidelines.org/

SHARE, a national support group for parents who have experienced loss through miscarriage, stillbirth, or newborn death:
SHARE Pregnancy & Infant Loss Support, Inc.
National SHARE Office
St. Joseph Health Center
300 First Capitol Drive
St. Charles, MO 63301-2893
(800) 821-6819 or (636) 947-6164
www.nationalshareoffice.com/

La Leche League
1400 North Meacham Road
Schaumburg, IL 60173-4808
(847) 519-7730
www.lalecheleague.org/

95

Preterm Premature Rupture of Membranes

Preterm premature rupture of membranes (PPROM) is the leakage of amniotic fluid before the 37th week of gestation. The balance of amniotic fluid is maintained by the production of fetal lung fluid and urine and is reabsorbed by fetal swallowing. The fetal lungs secrete approximately 300-400 ml/day at term. Fetal urine is the main source of amniotic fluid, with an output averaging 400-1200 ml/day at term. Amniotic fluid volume at term has a wide range from approximately 500-1500 ml. Amniotic fluid provides an environment that protects the fetus from trauma and injury, provides even distribution of temperature, and enables a medium in which the fetus can move. It also plays a major role in fetal development of the lungs and kidneys. Although its cause is unknown, PPROM plays a major factor in the morbidity and mortality of the neonate, depending on gestational age. The risk for a preterm birth is high. The majority of patients with PPROM deliver from within 24 hr to 2 wk of onset.

HEALTH CARE SETTING

The woman may be evaluated in the health care provider's clinic and then managed by obstetricians or perinatologists as an outpatient or inpatient, depending on week of gestation. Hospital sites may vary depending on gestational age and ability of the hospital to provide care for a high-risk pregnancy and neonate. Some patients with PPROM before gestational viability (25 weeks) may be managed at home.

ASSESSMENT

Patients may have difficulty determining presence of ruptured membranes, and symptoms may be obvious or subtle. Some women liken the sensation of leaking amniotic fluid to that of leaking urine. Therein lies the difficulty in determining PPROM from subjective data alone and the necessity of hands-on evaluation. On some occasions, leakage of amniotic fluid may stop, or it may reaccumulate without signs of infection.

Vaginal discharge: Patient may experience a "sudden gush" or sensation that something "popped" followed by a constant slow leakage of clear, watery fluid from the vagina. The fluid may be blood-tinged or meconium-stained. Patient may state that her underwear is wet or that she needs to wear a sanitary pad. Vaginal bleeding may accompany PPROM and range from light pink spotting to bleeding as with a heavy menses.

Backache: May or may not be present with PPROM. In the presence of infection, the patient may complain of a low lumbar/sacral pain that is deep tissue in nature or a dull, aching sensation that may radiate around the hips to the lower abdomen/pelvic area. If abruptio placentae is present with PPROM, the back pain may be mild to severe.

Abdominal pain/cramping or uterine cramping/contractions: There may be a feeling of pelvic pressure or fullness or menstrual-like cramping or contractions. Some women state that their thighs ache when experiencing uterine cramping. In the presence of infection, the patient may complain of abdominal/uterine tenderness or pain. If abruptio placentae accompanies PPROM, the pain may be mild to severe.

Fever: May occur in the presence of an infection and be ≥101° F (38.3° C).

Complications—fetal: The risk to the fetus depends on the gestational age at the time of PPROM, the severity of

PPROM (the amount of amniotic fluid remaining, if any), and the presence of infection.

- Prematurity
- Fetal infections/sepsis
- Hypoxia and asphyxia caused by umbilical cord compression/prolapse
- Fetal deformities with PPROM at an early gestational age (i.e., hypoplastic lungs)
- Amniotic band syndrome (an abnormal condition characterized by development of fibrous bands within the uterus that entangle the fetus, leading to deformities in fetal structure and function)
- Abruptio placentae
- Fetal death

Physical assessment: In most cases the cause of PPROM is unknown and there is no forewarning. Therefore it is important to evaluate changes in vaginal discharge. A timely diagnosis of PPROM is critical to optimum fetal outcome.

Risk factors: Genital tract infections such as *Chlamydia trachomatis,* gonorrhea, bacterial vaginosis, or trichomoniasis; low socioeconomic status; smoking; multiple gestation; incompetent cervix (painless cervical dilation before term without contractions); previous history of PPROM; diethylstilbestrol (DES) exposure; amniocentesis; chorionic villi sampling (CVS); coitus; group B streptococci; poor nutrition; bleeding in pregnancy; polyhydramnios (excess of amniotic fluid); cervical cerclage (a suture used for holding the cervix closed during a pregnancy); previous cervical laceration or surgery; placental abruption (abnormal separation of the placenta from the wall of the uterus before delivery); chorioamnionitis (intraamniotic infection); history of midtrimester pregnancy loss; cocaine use; hypertension; diabetes; and Ehlers-Danlos syndrome (a group of heritable connective tissue diseases).

DIAGNOSTIC TESTS

External uterine and fetal monitoring: External uterine monitoring is done to evaluate fetal well-being and presence, frequency, and duration of uterine contractions. Abnormal fetal heart rate patterns (decreased variability, moderate-to-severe variable decelerations, and late decelerations) are suggestive of fetal compromise, which can be caused by umbilical cord compression, cord prolapse, or infection that can accompany PPROM.

Sterile speculum exam: A sterile speculum is inserted into the vagina to visualize leaking of amniotic fluid coming from the cervical os or pooling of amniotic fluid in the vagina. This fluid is tested with Nitrazine paper. If positive for amniotic fluid, the paper will turn from yellow to dark blue, and the pH will be >6.0. False-positive results may be seen in the presence of semen, blood, vaginal infections, or alkaline antiseptics. Using a cotton swab, a sample of vaginal fluid is taken from the posterior vaginal fornix (the posterior space below the cervix) and examined under the microscope for the presence of a ferning pattern that amniotic fluid makes when it dries on a slide. A digital exam of the cervix is not recommended in a patient with suspected PPROM who is not in labor because of the risk of introducing an infection.

Obstetric ultrasound: Abdominal ultrasound is used to confirm gestational age, calculate amniotic fluid index (AFI) and biophysical profile (BPP), rule out multiple gestation, and determine placental location and fetal presentation. A normal value for the AFI is between 10-20 ml of amniotic fluid. A normal rating on the BPP is 6-8 out of 10.

Amniocentesis: Transabdominal aspiration of remaining amniotic fluid to test for fetal lung maturity and the presence of chorioamnionitis.

Intrauterine dye test: Done only if other tests are inconclusive in determining PPROM or to document that the membranes have sealed over. Resealing is rare, but it can occur. Under ultrasound guidance a diluted solution of indigo carmine dye is inserted with a spinal needle transabdominally into the uterus. The patient is observed for passage of blue fluid from the vagina that would indicate rupture of membranes.

Blood Rh factor and antibody screen: This test should be a part of the routine prenatal screening. In patients with no prenatal care who have PPROM, this laboratory test needs to be performed on admittance to determine need for Rh-immune globulin in an Rh-negative patient.

Nursing Diagnosis:

Deficient Knowledge:

Signs and symptoms of PPROM, its effects on the pregnancy and fetus, and guidelines to follow for an optimal outcome

Desired Outcome: Immediately following teaching, patient and significant other verbalize accurate knowledge about the effects of PPROM on the patient and fetus, as well as its signs and symptoms and treatment guidelines for an optimal outcome.

INTERVENTIONS	RATIONALES
Teach patient and significant other signs and symptoms of PPROM and chorioamnionitis (intraamniotic infection), which may be present after PPROM.	A knowledgeable patient likely will report symptoms promptly and understand consequences of noncompliance. PPROM plays a major factor in the morbidity and mortality of the neonate, depending on gestational age. See introductory information for signs and symptoms of PPROM. Indicators of chorioamnionitis include abdominal pain, uterine tenderness, fever, chills, foul vaginal odor, and contractions.
Inform patient and significant other about the effects PPROM can have on patient and fetus.	Information facilitates compliance with treatments. Amniotic fluid is critical to fetal development. PPROM increases risk of preterm delivery and neonatal pulmonary hypoplasia. PPROM also increases risk of chorioamnionitis (see above symptoms) for the mother and subsequently poses a postpartum risk of endometritis (inflammation of the endometrial lining of the uterus) following delivery. Maternal death from sepsis is rare, but it can occur.
Discuss risks/benefits of conservative management (delaying delivery and monitoring mother for signs of infection and fetus for signs of distress) vs. active delivery with the possibility of a preterm infant with respiratory distress syndrome (RDS), infection, and neonatal death but enabling ability to monitor and support baby more safely in an extrauterine environment.	When there are no signs of maternal infection or cervical change and the intrauterine environment is safe for both mother and fetus, conservative management may buy time for fetal lung maturation. In the presence of a uterine infection, however, labor should not be stopped. Treating the mother postpartum and the fetus in an extrauterine environment improves maternal/fetal well-being.
Teach daily fetal movement counts.	Fetal movement counts are a good first-line indicator of fetal well-being and are performed as follows, beginning at 28 wk gestation: Patient lies on her side and counts "distinct fetal movement" (hiccups do not count) daily; 10 movements within a 2-hr period is reassuring. After 10 movements, the count is discontinued. Fewer than 10 movements indicates need for fetal nonstress testing.
Teach patient palpation of contractions, which may accompany PPROM (gestation appropriate).	A knowledgeable patient likely will report an increase in contractions promptly: for a singleton pregnancy, ≥4 contractions/hr; for a multiple pregnancy, ≥6 contractions/hr. Palpation and awareness of contractions enable patient to be an active participant in her health care. Timely reporting of contractions can play a significant role in optimum maternal/fetal outcome. Although contraction frequency alone is insufficient in diagnosing preterm labor, it can serve as a helpful guideline.
	Patient lies comfortably on her side. She will spread her fingers apart and place one hand on the left side and the other on the right side of the abdomen. Palpation is done with the fingertips of both hands. When the uterus is relaxed, the abdomen should feel soft. When a contraction occurs, the uterus will feel hard, tight, or firm under the fingertips. She will time the duration from the beginning of one contraction to the beginning of the next. Duration of the contraction may or may not be an indication of contraction intensity. It is believed that the longer the contraction in true labor, the more effective it is in progressing dilation and effacement.

●●● **Related NIC and NOC labels:** *NIC:* Teaching: Disease Process; Teaching: Individual; High-Risk Pregnancy Care; Prenatal Care *NOC:* Knowledge: Illness Care; Knowledge: Pregnancy

Nursing Diagnosis:

Ineffective Coping

related to health crisis, sense of vulnerability, inadequate support systems, and needed adjustment in lifestyle to provide an optimal environment for the fetus and prolong the gestational period

Desired Outcome: Within 24 hr of this diagnosis, patient verbalizes feelings, identifies strengths, exhibits positive coping behaviors, and modifies her lifestyle to provide the best pregnancy outcome for her fetus.

INTERVENTIONS	RATIONALES
Assess patient's perceptions and ability to understand current health status of herself and fetus.	Evaluation of patient's comprehension enables development of an individualized care plan.
Help patient identify previous methods of coping with life problems.	How patient has handled problems in the past may be a reliable predictor of how she will cope with current problems.
Provide patient with resources for support groups, written information, Internet chat groups, or home helpers.	Talking with others who have experienced similar circumstances may aid in development of coping mechanisms. A home helper, for example, likely will decrease pressure on patient and thereby promote coping abilities.
Affirm that lifestyle adjustments and need for support systems will be necessary only for a limited time.	This knowledge may facilitate acceptance of outside support and assistance and facilitate coping accordingly.
Acknowledge patient's cultural beliefs regarding coping during pregnancy.	Shows respect for patient and a willingness to understand and work with her emotional state and coping skills. You might ask, "In your home country a high-risk pregnancy must be very difficult to deal with. Could you tell me how you and your family are coping with this pregnancy?"
	Different cultures perceive pregnancy in various ways. Some patients come from countries in which maternal/fetal mortality rate is high and daily survival is the major focus. Their method of coping may be emotional detachment from the fetus. The current pregnancy may not seem as important as the children and family that are already at home and need care. In the Hmong culture, for example, women and their families do not appear to bond with their infant after birth. They believe to do so would be prideful and welcome evil spirits who would take the infant away (infant death).
Involve assistance of Social Services when available.	To provide counseling and make recommendations for referrals.
Provide patient and family with information regarding effectiveness of hospitalization bedrest vs. home bedrest.	Helps patient and her health care provider decide the best method of management. Before gestation of viability (25 wk), when fetal survival rates are lower, home management of bedrest in the absence of signs of maternal/fetal infection may be assumed. Patients undergoing home bedrest must be able to remain in bed in alternating side-lying positions (occasionally sitting up propped with pillows) and avoid doing housework, laundry, cooking, or shopping. The side-lying position improves uteroplacental blood flow and oxygenation, which in turn improves the chance of reaccumulation of amniotic fluid. After gestation of viability (when fetal survival rates are higher), hospitalization is usually recommended to monitor for signs of maternal/fetal infection, fetal distress, preterm labor, and worsening

Continued

INTERVENTIONS	RATIONALES
	oligohydramnios (abnormally low volume of amniotic fluid) or anhydramnios (absence of amniotic fluid).
	Both home management and hospitalization may require outside assistance to care for family members or pets at home.
Encourage patient and family to verbalize their concerns in a supportive environment.	Helps alleviate stress, anxiety, and misconceptions. See **Anxiety,** p. 82.

●●● **Related NIC and NOC labels:** *NIC:* Coping Enhancement; Counseling; Support Group; Support System Enhancement; Family Involvement Promotion *NOC:* Coping; Role Performance

Nursing Diagnosis:

Deficient Knowledge:

Purpose and potential side effects of prescribed medications for managing PPROM

Desired Outcome: Immediately following teaching, patient and family relate accurate understanding of the risks and benefits of medications used to manage PPROM.

INTERVENTIONS	RATIONALES
Teach the following about patient's prescribed medications:	A knowledgeable patient is more likely to comply with therapy, identify and report side effects, and recognize and report precautions that might preclude use of the prescribed drug.
Antenatal glucocorticoids *Betamethasone or dexamethasone*	Aid in reducing effects of RDS, intraventricular hemorrhage, and necrotizing enterocolitis on preterm neonate when delivery is anticipated to be preterm and after the gestation of viability. It also accelerates maturation of the central nervous system (CNS) and fetal organs, including cardiovascular. Administration: - Betamethasone: two doses of 12 mg given 24 hr apart. - Dexamethasone: four doses of 6 mg given 12 hr apart. Maximum benefit is 48 hr after administration.
Be alert and report signs of infection (elevated fever, chills, body aches), decrease in fetal movement (gestation appropriate), and elevated maternal glucose levels in patients with diabetes.	Possible side effects of medication include reduced maternal-fetal resistance to infection, impaired glucose tolerance (people with borderline gestational diabetes may develop true gestational diabetes), and suppression of maternal or neonatal adrenal function. Usually a rise in blood glucose is seen for approximately 48-96 hr after administration, and it may necessitate IV insulin.
Prophylactic antibiotics The type of antibiotic used varies and may include but is not limited to the following: ampicillin, erythromycin, gentamicin, and cephalosporins.	Prevent or reduce effects of maternal-fetal infections. These antibiotics may reduce morbidity and prolong the pregnancy.
Caution patient to follow complete course for all prescribed medications and take them on time.	To prevent development of antibiotic resistance and maintain a constant level of medication in the bloodstream.

Continued

INTERVENTIONS	RATIONALES
Teach patient to be alert for and report excessive and explosive diarrhea.	*Clostridium difficile* is a potentially serious side effect in which the normal flora of the bowel are reduced by antibiotic therapy and the anaerobic organism *C. difficile* multiplies and produces its toxins, causing severe diarrhea. This problem necessitates discontinuation of the antibiotic and laboratory evaluation of a stool sample.
Magnesium sulfate (MgSO$_4$)	Decreases uterine myometrial activity (contractions) at a therapeutic serum magnesium level of 4-8 mg/dl.
	Administration: IV. It is never used with nifedipine because their combined use could lead to pulmonary edema.
	Used on an inpatient basis only.
Teach patient to be alert for and report headaches, hot flashes, nausea, vomiting, and dizziness.	Common side effects.
Explain that this drug is used with caution in patients who have received large amounts of IV fluid hydration. Patient should be alert for and report shortness of breath, coughing, and lethargy.	Pulmonary edema is a serious side effect.
Advise patient that BP, HR, RR, deep tendon reflexes (DTRs) and urinary output will be monitored at frequent intervals.	Levels outside the therapeutic range of this drug can cause toxicity:
	- Loss of DTRs: 9-12 mg/dl
	- Respiratory arrest: >15 mg/dl
	- Cardiac arrest: >25-30 mg/dl
Caution patient that use is contraindicated in maternal renal failure and hypocalcemia.	MgSO$_4$ is excreted via the kidneys; therefore increases in maternal serum magnesium may result in maternal hypocalcemia.
Calcium channel blocker	Inhibits smooth muscle contractility, thereby decreasing or eliminating uterine contractions.
Nifedipine	No adverse maternal/fetal side effects have been reported.
	Administration: oral route.
	May be used on an outpatient basis. It is never to be used with MgSO$_4$ because their combined use could lead to pulmonary edema.
Teach patient to be alert for and report lightheadedness and dizziness. Instruct patient to rise slowly from a supine position.	There is potential for hypotension with this drug.
Explain that patient may notice transient headaches and flushing for the first few days of taking this drug.	Common side effect.
Caution patients with hepatic disease about using this drug.	Nifedipine is primarily metabolized and excreted by the liver; therefore with hepatic disease these two processes may be delayed, causing an increase in serum nifedipine levels.
β-Adrenergic agonists	Decrease uterine myometrial activity (contractions). With PPROM this drug is used only on a short-term basis (between 24-26 wk) to allow for the antenatal glucocorticoids (see above) and antibiotics to become effective.
Terbutaline (Brethine)	Administration: SQ, IM, PO.
	May be used on an outpatient basis.
Teach patient to be alert for increased heart rate, restlessness, nervousness, tremor (shaking hands), nausea, and vomiting.	Common side effects. They are usually transient in nature and do not require intervention.

Continued

INTERVENTIONS	RATIONALES
Teach patient to be alert for and report shortness of breath and chest pain.	May signal pulmonary edema and myocardial ischemia, conditions that would warrant discontinuation of the medication.
Advise patient to rise slowly from a supine position.	There is potential for hypotension.
Explain that the drug is contraindicated in patients with maternal cardiac dysrhythmias, diabetes mellitus, and maternal cardiac disease.	Has significant cardiac side effects in patients without cardiac disease and can increase maternal blood sugar.
Rh-immune globulin (human) *RhoGAM*	Prevents hemolytic disease as long as the mother has not already been sensitized by the presence of Rh-positive antibodies in her bloodstream. Administration: IM only to nonsensitized Rh-negative women after bleeding any time during the pregnancy, after spontaneous abortion, or after delivery. Recommended administration is within 72 hr after the bleeding episode.
Advise that patient may note discomfort at the site of injection.	Common side effect.

●●● **Related NIC and NOC labels:** *NIC:* Teaching: Prescribed Medication *NOC:* Knowledge: Medication

Nursing Diagnosis:

Deficient Knowledge:

Muscle weakness, back pain, and decreased circulation that can occur with prolonged bedrest

Desired Outcome: Within 24 hr of this diagnosis, patient verbalizes understanding of and demonstrates measures to reduce or relieve back pain and improve circulation.

INTERVENTIONS	RATIONALES
Teach patient to recognize signs and symptoms of back pain related to bedrest vs. back pain associated with contraction activity.	A knowledgeable patient optimally will discern the different causes of back pain and report these symptoms accordingly. Back pain related to bedrest is usually thoracic to lumbar in position and superficial in nature and will be improved by position change or massage to promote circulation. Back pain related to contraction activity is usually lumbar/sacral in position and deep tissue in nature, and it may radiate to the hips and low abdominal/pelvic area. Position change and massage may decrease intensity.
Teach patient the probable causes of muscle pain, weakness, and back pain.	Aids in patient understanding and optimally in compliance with management. For example, probable causes include lack of use of certain muscles, delay in change of positioning, increasing weight of the uterus, and dehydration, which can lead to the buildup of lactic acid in the muscles and cause pain.
Teach patient leg exercises for period in which she is on bedrest.	Leg exercises promote peripheral tissue perfusion and decrease risk of deep vein thrombosis (DVT) and muscle wasting. Calf-pumping (ankle dorsiflexion–plantar flexion) and ankle-circling exercises are examples of leg exercises. Patient should repeat each movement 10 times, performing each exercise hourly during extended periods of immobility, provided patient is free of symptoms of DVT. Passive and active range-of-motion (ROM) exercises are other options.

Continued

INTERVENTIONS	RATIONALES
Encourage patient to change positions frequently in bed, from alternating side-lying positions to sitting propped up with pillows. Teach patient to use pillows between knees to prevent pressure on the back.	Changing position at frequent intervals (i.e., q2h) promotes circulation and decreases pressure and hence discomfort on tissues, joints, and muscles. Pillows provide support and decrease strain on muscles and promote comfort.
Caution patient to *avoid* the supine position.	The supine position places pressure on the aorta by the enlarging fetus. This could result in a vasovagal response, which would decrease maternal blood pressure and cause diaphoresis, nausea, dizziness, and decreased uteroplacental perfusion.
Provide patient with referral for physical or massage therapy for back pain related to prolonged bedrest.	Professional interventions likely will aid in promoting circulation and patient comfort.

●●● **Related NIC and NOC labels:** *NIC:* Teaching: Individual; Teaching: Disease Process; High-Risk Pregnancy Care *NOC:* Knowledge: Disease Process; Knowledge: Pregnancy

Nursing Diagnosis:

Anticipatory Grieving

related to potential fetal loss secondary to PPROM

Desired Outcome: Patient and significant other verbalize their feelings and identify and use support systems to aid them in the grief process within 24 hr of this diagnosis.

INTERVENTIONS	RATIONALES
Encourage patient and significant other to verbalize their feelings and concerns regarding the potential for loss of their baby.	Validates concerns and conveys message that grief is a normal and expected reaction to the potential loss of a baby.
Assess and accept patient's behavioral response.	Disbelief, denial, guilt, anger, and depression are normal reactions to grief.
Teach patient the stages of grief and explain that there is no specific time frame in which to go through the process.	Enables patient to understand where she or her family members may be in the grief process. Stages include (1) shock and numbness; (2) denial and searching-yearning; (3) anger, guilt, and sense of failure; (4) depression and disorganization; and (5) resolution.
Clarify misconceptions about the potential risk for fetal loss with PPROM.	Allows patient and significant other to process the information regarding PPROM appropriately while not providing false hope. The gestational age at which the PPROM occurs plays a significant role in the outcome. The earlier the gestational age at delivery, the higher the risk of fetal loss. A gestational age of 25 wk is considered viable, but with each passing day and week, there is better opportunity for fetal survival and decreased morbidity barring preexisting fetal complications such as cardiac, respiratory, and CNS problems.
If available, involve Social Services when a loss is perceived or present.	To provide resources and referrals for individual counseling and support groups for bereaved parents and grandparents, which may help the participants feel less isolated. Social Services also can guide the family through the disposition of the infant should the death occur.

Continued

INTERVENTIONS	RATIONALES
If a loss occurs, provide patient and family with support if they decide to see and hold the baby and place appropriate items in a memory/keepsake box.	Assists with the grieving process by enabling parents/grandparents to spend time with and affirm their baby. Such items as footprints and a lock of hair may be tucked away and not looked at right away, but it may help to know they are there.

●●● **Related NIC and NOC labels:** *NIC:* Coping Enhancement; Grief Work Facilitation: Perinatal Death; Anxiety Reduction; Emotional Support; Family Support; Support Group Enhancement; Hope Instillation
NOC: Coping; Family Coping; Grief Resolution

ADDITIONAL NURSING DIAGNOSES/ PROBLEMS:

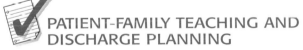

PATIENT-FAMILY TEACHING AND DISCHARGE PLANNING

PPROM is potentially life threatening to the fetus, depending on the gestational age at the time of occurrence. When pro-symptoms of PPROM and the importance of patient compliance in hopes of decreasing fetal morbidity and mortality. Include verbal and written information about the following:

✓ Signs and symptoms of ruptured membranes and the importance of contacting health care provider in a timely manner.

✓ Signs and symptoms of preterm labor (see p. 755) because it may precede or follow PPROM.

✓ Palpation of contractions.

✓ Importance of compliance with prenatal care.

✓ Potential risk factors for PPROM that may be present early in the pregnancy.

✓ Measures for muscle pain, back pain, and muscle weakness that can be present with prolonged bedrest. See **Deficient Knowledge**, earlier.

✓ Measures that help with constipation, which occurs frequently in pregnancy and can be exacerbated with bedrest.

✓ Availability of Social Services and spiritual care.

✓ Medications, including drug name, purpose, dosage, frequency, precautions, potential drug/drug and food/drug interactions, and potential side effects.

✓ Fetal movement counts.

✓ Referral to local and national support organizations, including:

Sidelines, a national support organization for women and their families experiencing complicated pregnancies: Sidelines High Risk Pregnancy Support National Office P.O. Box 1808 Laguna Beach, CA 92652 (888) 447-4754 www.sidelines.org/

SHARE, a national support group for parents who have experienced loss through miscarriage, stillbirth, or newborn death: SHARE Pregnancy & Infant Loss Support, Inc. National SHARE Office St. Joseph Health Center 300 First Capitol Drive St. Charles, MO 63301-2893 (800) 821-6819 or (636) 947-6164 www.nationalshareoffice.com/

96

Anxiety Disorders

*A*nxiety is a diffuse response to a vague threat, as opposed to fear, which is an acute response to a clear-cut external threat. Anxiety often precedes significant changes, for example, beginning new employment. When it is prolonged or excessive, crippling physical or psychologic symptoms may develop. The anxiety disorders are a group of conditions characterized by anxiety symptoms and behavioral efforts to avoid these symptoms. They are the most common psychiatric disorders in the United States, affecting more than 23 million people. Acute anxiety creates physical sensations of arousal (fight or flight), an emotional state of fear or panic, decreased cognitive problem-solving ability, and altered spiritual state with hopelessness. Anxiety is considered abnormal when reasons for it are not evident or when manifestations are excessive in intensity and duration. Psychologic *stress* refers to the response of an individual appraising the environment and concluding that it exceeds his or her resources and jeopardizes well-being. Some stressors are universal, whereas others are person specific because of highly individual interpretations of events.

Anxiety is always part of the stress response and has four levels, ranging from mild to panic. Normally, a person experiencing mild-to-moderate anxiety uses voluntary behaviors called coping skills, that is, distraction, deliberate avoidance, and information seeking. Another common response is use of unconscious defense mechanisms, including repression, suppression, projection, introjection, reaction formation, undoing, displacement, denial, and regression. If stress continues at an unbearable level or if the individual lacks sufficient biologic mechanisms for coping, an anxiety disorder may develop. There are eight major categories:

Generalized anxiety disorder: Characterized by excessive, uncontrollable worrying over a period of at least 6 mo. Symptoms include motor tension (trembling; shakiness; muscle tension, aches, soreness; easy fatigue), autonomic hyperactivity (shortness of breath, palpitations, sweating, dry mouth, dizziness, nausea, diarrhea, frequent urination), and scanning behavior (feeling on edge, having an exaggerated startle response, difficulty concentrating, sleep disturbance, irritability).

Panic disorder: Characterized by a specific period of intense fear or discomfort with at least four of the following symptoms: palpitations or pounding heart, sweating, trembling or shaking, sensations of smothering or difficulty breathing, feeling of choking, chest pain, nausea, feeling dizzy or faint, feeling of unreality or losing control, numbness, and chills or flushes.

Phobias: Characterized by a persistent and severe fear of a clearly identifiable object or situation despite awareness that the fear is unreasonable. There are two types, specific and social. Specific phobias are subdivided into five types: animals, natural environment (e.g., lightening), blood injection-injury type, situational (e.g., flying), and other (situations that could lead to choking or contracting an illness). Social phobia relates to profound fear of social or performance situations in which embarrassment could occur.

Obsessive-compulsive disorder (OCD): Characterized by a preoccupation with recurrent, ritualistic thoughts or actions. Obsessions are persistent thoughts, ideas, impulses, or images that are intrusive and cause marked anxiety. Compulsions are repetitive acts that follow an obsession, performed according to strict rules, and aimed at decreasing the feeling of distress.

Posttraumatic stress disorder (PTSD): Results from a pathologic response to a devastating event. The person continues to reexperience the event through intrusive thoughts or nightmares. Memories of the trauma occur randomly, or symptoms may emerge when the person is exposed to situations that resemble or symbolize the original trauma. Fear and persistent states of arousal lead to difficulty falling asleep or remaining asleep. Hypervigilance with an exaggerated startle response may occur, resulting in problems concentrating and completing tasks. The duration of the symptoms is at least 1 mo, and the syndrome may emerge many months after the event. On the other hand, some victims may have no memories of the trauma for a period of time. They may complain of feeling detached or separate from others and lose the ability to enjoy pleasurable events, reflecting "psychic numbing." In both cases, anger, sadness, rage, depression, or stoicism may be demonstrated.

Acute stress disorder: Like PTSD, the problem begins with exposure to a traumatic event, with a response of intense fear, helplessness, or horror. In addition, the person shows dissociative symptoms, that is, subjective sense of numbing, feeling "in a daze," depersonalization, or amnesia and clearly tries to avoid stimuli that arouse recollection of the trauma. But just like PTSD, the victim reexperiences the trauma and shows functional impairment in social, occupational, and problem-solving skills. The key difference is that this syndrome occurs within 4 wk of the traumatic event and only lasts 2 days to 4 wk.

Anxiety disorder caused by medical condition: May be characterized by severe anxiety, panic attacks, or obsessions or compulsions, but the cause is clearly related to a medical problem, excluding delirium. History, physical examination, and laboratory findings support a specific diagnosis, for example, hypoglycemia, pheochromocytoma, thyroid disease.

Anxiety disorder not otherwise specified: Describes individuals with significant anxiety or phobic avoidance but not enough symptoms to meet the criteria for a particular anxiety or adjustment disorder diagnosis. The patient may show a mixed anxiety-depressive picture or demonstrate social phobic symptoms related to having another medical problem, for example, Parkinson's disease, or present with insufficient data to rule out a general medical condition or substance abuse.

HEALTH CARE SETTING

Depends on the type of anxiety disorder. Primary (outpatient) care is likely for most categories, and possibly emergency department care for panic disorders. If the patient has developed panic disorder with agoraphobia, psychiatric home care may be the best care option. Some patients may be hospitalized for physiologic problems.

ASSESSMENT

Physical indicators: Dry mouth, elevated vital signs, diarrhea, increased urination, nausea, diaphoresis, hyperventilation, fatigue, insomnia, sexual dysfunction, irritability, tenseness.

Emotional indicators: Fear, sense of impending doom, helplessness, insecurity, low self-confidence, anger, guilt.

Cognitive indicators: Mild anxiety produces increased awareness and problem-solving skills. Higher levels produce narrowed perceptual field, missed details, diminished problem-solving skills, and deteriorated logical thinking.

Social indicators: Marital and parental functioning may be adversely affected by anxiety and therefore should be assessed.

Spiritual indicators: Patient may exhibit hopelessness, feeling of being cut off from God, anger at God for allowing anxiety.

Suicidality: Suicide assessment is critical with anxious patients, especially those with panic disorder. For patients suffering dual diagnoses of depression and substance abuse or even other anxiety disorders, risk of self-injury is even greater. Suicidal assessment includes questions to determine presence of suicidal ideation and the lethality of any plan. Essential questions to ask include:

- Have you thought of hurting yourself?
- Are you presently thinking about hurting yourself?
- If you have been thinking about suicide, do you have a plan?
- What is the plan?
- Have you thought about what life would be like if you were no longer a part of it?

A previous history of suicide attempts combined with depression places the patient at high risk in the present. A patient whose depression is lifting is at higher risk for suicide than a severely depressed individual. The improvement may result in an increase in energy. This increased energy is not enough to make the patient feel well or hopeful, but it is enough to carry out a suicidal plan.

DIAGNOSTIC TESTS

There is no specific diagnostic test for anxiety disorders. The diagnosis of anxiety is made through history, interview of patient and family, and observation of verbal and nonverbal behaviors. A number of effective scales are available to quantify the degree of anxiety, such as The Yale-Brown Obsessive Scale, the Maudsley Obsessional-Compulsive Inventory, The Leyton Obsessional Inventory, Hamilton Rating Scale for Anxiety, Panic Attack Cognitions Questionnaire, State-Trait Anxiety Inventory, Sheehan Patient Rated Anxiety Inventory, and the Beck Anxiety Inventory.

Nursing Diagnosis:

Deficient Knowledge:

Causes, signs and symptoms, and treatment of anxiety or specific anxiety disorder

Desired Outcome: By discharge (if inpatient) or after 2 wk of outpatient treatment, patient and/or significant other verbalize accurate information about at least two of the possible causes of anxiety, four of the signs and symptoms of the specific anxiety disorder, and the available treatment options.

INTERVENTIONS

RATIONALES

INTERVENTIONS	RATIONALES
Inform patient and significant other that anxiety disorders are physiologic disorders caused by the interplay of many factors, such as stress, imbalance in brain chemistry, psychodynamic factors, faulty learning, and genetics.	Many people who suffer from anxiety disorders accept that they are just "nervous worriers" and lack the knowledge that anxiety disorders represent a complex interplay of treatable biologic, genetic, and environmental factors.
Inform patient and significant other about the holistic nature of anxiety, which produces physical, emotional, cognitive, social, and spiritual symptoms.	Many people believe that anxiety equates with nervousness and fail to recognize the many other signs and symptoms that make this a holistic disorder.
Inform patient and significant other that anxiety disorders are treatable.	Medications are usually indicated for treatment of these disorders and may include antidepressants and anxiolytics or a combination of medications. In addition, other interventions are useful, including dietary interventions (e.g., elimination of caffeinated products), breath control, exercise program, relaxation techniques, and psychologic interventions (i.e., distraction, positive self-talk, psychoeducation, exposure therapy, systematic desensitization, implosive therapy, social interventions, cognitive therapy, stress and time management interventions).

●●● **Related NIC and NOC labels:** *NIC:* Teaching: Individual; Teaching: Procedure/Treatment; Teaching: Disease Process *NOC:* Knowledge: Illness Care

Nursing Diagnosis:

Anxiety

related to recurring panic attacks

Desired Outcome: Within 24 hr of treatment/intervention, patient verbalizes methods for dealing with panic attacks and understanding that panic attacks are not life threatening and that they are time limited and demonstrates this knowledge accordingly.

INTERVENTIONS

RATIONALES

INTERVENTIONS	RATIONALES
Administer medication as prescribed for panic attacks.	Panic attacks are neurobiologic events that respond to medications.
Teach patient to reduce or eliminate dietary substances that may promote anxiety and panic, such as caffeine, food coloring, and monosodium glutamate (MSG).	Caffeine increases feelings of anxiety. However, caffeine withdrawal symptoms also can stimulate panic. Therefore the plan should include focus on reducing consumption first, followed by elimination from the diet. Some individuals are sensitive to food colorings and MSG. This sensitivity is experienced as increased anxiety.
Teach patient relaxation techniques; assist with practicing imagery, deep breathing, progressive relaxation, and use of relaxation tapes. See **Health-Seeking Behaviors:** Relaxation technique effective for stress reduction and control, p. 183.	Relaxation is effective in reducing anxiety. The patient's ability to master relaxation techniques provides a sense of control and enhances self-care ability.

Continued

INTERVENTIONS	RATIONALES
Stay with patient during panic attacks. Use short, simple directions. Encourage patient to use relaxation, remind patient that attack is time limited, and reduce environmental stimulation. REMAIN CALM.	During a panic attack, ability to refocus is limited. The patient needs reassurance that he or she is not dying and that this will pass. Therefore it is important that the nurse remain calm and not respond to patient's anxiety with anxiety.

●●● **Related NIC and NOC labels:** *NIC:* Anxiety Reduction; Behavior Management; Calming Technique; Medication Administration; Presence; Simple Relaxation Therapy; Simple Guided Imagery; Progressive Muscle Relaxation *NOC:* Anxiety Control

Nursing Diagnosis:

Social Isolation

related to agoraphobia

Desired Outcome: By discharge (if inpatient) or after 4 wk of outpatient treatment, patient demonstrates behavior consistent with increased social interaction.

INTERVENTIONS	RATIONALES
Assist patient in graded exposure plan to gradually increase independent functions and interactions with others.	Gradual exposure is effective in treating agoraphobia.
Assist patient with practicing relaxation techniques.	Relaxation helps to mitigate impending panic attacks.
Discuss alternatives for social interaction.	Patient may need assistance with developing activity plans.

●●● **Related NIC and NOC labels:** *NIC:* Socialization Enhancement; Coping Enhancement *NOC:* Well-Being; Social Support; Social Involvement

Nursing Diagnosis:

Ineffective Coping

related to anxiety

Desired Outcome: Within 24 hr of intervention/treatment, patient identifies ineffective coping behaviors and consequences, expresses feelings appropriately, identifies options and uses resources effectively, and uses effective problem-solving techniques.

INTERVENTIONS	RATIONALES
Identify previous methods of coping with life problems.	How patient has handled problems in the past is a reliable predictor of how current problems will be handled.
Determine use of substances (alcohol, other drugs, smoking and eating patterns).	Patient may have used substances as coping mechanisms to control anxiety. This pattern can interfere with ability to deal with the current situation.

Continued

INTERVENTIONS	RATIONALES
Provide information regarding different ways to deal with situations that promote anxious feelings, for example, identification and appropriate expression of feelings and problem-solving skills.	Provides patient with opportunity to learn new coping skills.
Role-play and rehearse new skills.	Promotes skill acquisition in a nonthreatening environment.
Encourage and support patient in evaluating lifestyle and identifying activities and stresses of family, work, and social situations.	Enables patient to examine areas of life that may contribute to anxiety and make decisions about how to engender changes gradually without adding undue anxiety.
Assist patient with identifying some short- and long-term goals focused on making life changes and decreasing anxiety.	Helps provide direction in making necessary changes.
Teach patient how to break responsibilities into manageable units.	Small steps enhance success and avoid the anxiety that comes from facing a huge task and feeling overwhelmed.
Suggest incorporating stress management techniques (e.g., relaxation) into normal day.	Encourages patient to take care of self, take control, and decrease stress.
Teach importance of balance in life.	A life out of balance adds tremendously to stress and anxiety. Changes such as getting adequate sleep, nutrition, exercise, quiet time, work time, family time, and spiritual time enhance quality of life, decrease anxiety, and increase sense of power and control.
Refer to outside resources, including support groups, psychotherapy, religious resources, and community recreation resources.	Many people benefit from the support of other people and resources to help keep life in balance and monitor stress level.

●●● **Related NIC and NOC labels:** *NIC:* Coping Enhancement; Decision-Making Support; Anxiety Reduction; Sleep Enhancement; Support Group; Spiritual Support; Simple Relaxation Therapy; Mutual Goal Setting; Behavior Modification *NOC:* Coping

Nursing Diagnosis:

Compromised Family Coping

related to family disorganization and role changes

Desired Outcome: Within 24 hr of this diagnosis, family members identify resources within themselves to deal with situation; interact appropriately with patient, providing support and assistance as needed; recognize own needs for support; seek assistance; and use resources effectively.

INTERVENTIONS	RATIONALES
Assess level of information available to and understood by family.	Lack of understanding about patient's anxiety disorder can lead to unhealthy interaction patterns and contribute to anxiety felt by family members.
Identify role of patient and discuss how illness has changed the family organization.	The patient's disability (e.g., resulting in inability to go to work or maintain the household) interferes with performance of usual family role and can substantially contribute to family stress and disorganization.
Help family identify other factors besides patient's illness that affect ability to provide support to each other.	This takes focus off of the patient as "the problem" and helps family members examine each of their individual responsibilities and behaviors.

Continued

INTERVENTIONS	RATIONALES
Discuss reasons for patient's behaviors.	This helps the family understand and accept behaviors that may be very difficult to handle.
Help family and patient recognize to whom the problem belongs and who is responsible for resolution of the problem.	This promotes self-responsibility for owning and fixing a problem. The individual with the problem can seek support and ask for help, but it is not the responsibility of the family to rescue that person or to solve the person's problem.
Teach the family constructive problem-solving skills.	This helps the family learn new ways to deal with conflicts and reduce anxiety-provoking situations.
Refer family to appropriate community resources.	Family may need additional assistance (e.g., from counselors, psychotherapy, Social Services, financial advisors, and spiritual advisor) to work through family issues and remain intact.

●●● **Related NIC and NOC labels:** *NIC:* Coping Enhancement; Support Group; Family Integrity Promotion; Role Enhancement; Spiritual Support; Normalization Promotion *NOC:* Family Coping; Family Normalization

Nursing Diagnosis:

Deficient Knowledge:

Prescribed medications, their purpose, and their potential side effects

Desired Outcome: By discharge (if inpatient) or after 4 wk of outpatient treatment, the patient verbalizes accurate information about the prescribed medications and their side effects.

INTERVENTIONS	RATIONALES
Teach the physiologic action of anxiolytics and/or antidepressants and how they alleviate symptoms of patient's anxiety disorder.	Anxiety disorders are neurobiologic occurrences that respond to both anxiolytics and antidepressants. Many people who suffer from anxiety are fearful of taking medication because they fear drug dependence and view taking it as a sign of weakness.
Explain importance of taking medication as prescribed.	These medications require certain blood levels to be therapeutic; therefore patient needs to take them at the dose and time interval prescribed.
Teach the side effect profile and its management of the patient's prescribed drugs that follow:	The anxiolytic medications, as well as each class of antidepressants, carry specific side-effect profiles. Knowledge about expected side effects, ways to manage these side effects, and how long these side effects last is important for ensuring compliance.
Tricyclic antidepressants: amitriptyline (Elavil), desipramine (Norpramin), doxepin (Sinequan), imipramine (Tofranil), nortriptyline (Pamelor), protriptyline (Vivactil), and trimipramine (Surmontil)	Imipramine and desipramine are very effective in anxiety disorders and are used in higher doses than would be used for depressive disorders.
Monitor for anticholinergic effects, sedation, decreased blood pressure, and weight gain.	Common side effects.
Drink at least 8 glasses of water a day and add high-fiber foods to diet.	Combats constipation, a potential anticholinergic effect.

Continued

INTERVENTIONS	**RATIONALES**
Rise from sitting position slowly. Discuss risks of falling related to dizziness associated with hypotension.	Orthostatic hypotension is a potential side effect.
Suck on sugar-free candy or mints or use sugar-free chewing gum.	Combats dry mouth, a potential anticholinergic effect.
Establish sleep routine and regular exercise.	Combats feelings of fatigue associated with these drugs.
Limit intake of refined sugars and carbohydrates.	Combats weight gain and controls carbohydrate cravings.
Be aware of seizure potential.	Tricyclic antidepressants lower the seizure threshold. Caution is needed with patients with epilepsy or other seizure disorder.
Be alert for and report signs of cardiac toxicity. Patients >40 yr of age need an electroencephalogram (EEG) evaluation before treatment and periodically thereafter.	These drugs may decrease vagal influence on the heart secondary to muscarinic blockade and by acting directly on bundle of His to slow conduction. Both effects increase risk of dysrhythmias.
Possible drug interactions.	The combination of tricyclics with monoamine oxidase (MAO) inhibitors can cause severe hypertension. The combination of tricyclics with central nervous system (CNS) depressants, such as alcohol, antihistamines, opioids, and barbiturates, can cause severe CNS depression. Because of the anticholinergic effects of tricyclics, any other anticholinergic drug, including over-the-counter antihistamines and sleeping aids, should be avoided.
MAO inhibitors: isocarboxazid (Marplan), phenelzine (Nardil), and tranylcypromine (Parnate)	Phenelzine and tranylcypromine are used in anxiety disorders in doses higher than those for treating depressive disorders and are useful for patients who have not responded to other drugs.
There is potential for mild sedation and hypotension.	Common side effects
MAO inhibitor restrictions.	MAO inhibitors combined with dietary tyramine can cause a life-threatening hypertensive crisis. Dietary restrictions include avocados; fermented bean curd; fermented soybean; soybean paste; figs; bananas; fermented, smoked, or aged meats; liver; bologna, pepperoni, and salami; dried, cured, fermented, or smoked fish; practically all cheeses; yeast extract; some imported beers; Chianti wine; protein dietary supplements; soups that contain protein extract; shrimp paste; and soy sauce. Large amounts of chocolate, fava beans, ginseng, and caffeine may cause a reaction.
Possible drug interactions and the need to avoid all prescription and over-the-counter drugs unless health care provider has specifically approved them.	MAO inhibitors can interact with many drugs to cause potentially serious results. Use of ephedrine or amphetamines can lead to hypertensive crisis. The interaction of tricyclic antidepressants with MAO inhibitors is discussed above. Selective serotonin reuptake inhibitors (SSRIs) should not be used with MAO inhibitors. Antihypertensive drugs combined with MAO inhibitors may result in excessive lowering of blood pressure. MAO inhibitors with meperidine (Demerol) can cause hyperpyrexia (excessive elevation of temperature).
SSRIs: fluoxetine (Prozac), fluvoxamine maleate (Luvox), sertraline (Zoloft), paroxetine (Paxil), and citalopram (Celexa)	SSRIs are helpful not only for patients with obsessive-compulsive symptoms but for patients with panic and anxiety disorders as well.
Be alert for nausea, headache, nervousness, insomnia, anxiety, agitation, sexual dysfunction, dizziness, fatigue, rash, diarrhea, excessive sweating, and anorexia with weight loss.	Reported side effects. Because these drugs increase anxiety, it is recommended that treatment be started at very low doses and increased gradually.

Continued

INTERVENTIONS	RATIONALES
Possible drug interactions.	Interaction with MAO inhibitors can cause serotonin syndrome, a potentially life-threatening event. Symptoms include anxiety, diaphoresis, rigidity, hyperthermia, autonomic hyperactivity, and coma. Because of this possibility, MAO inhibitors should be withdrawn at least 14 days before starting an SSRI, and when an SSRI is discontinued, at least 5 wk should elapse before an MAO inhibitor is given.
Benzodiazepines: diazepam (Valium), chlordiazepoxide (Librium), clorazepate (Tranxene), prazepam (Centrax), flurazepam (Dalmane), lorazepam (Ativan), oxazepam (Serax), temazepam (Restoril), triazolam (Halcion), alprazolam (Xanax), halazepam (Paxipam), and clonazepam (Klonopin)	All except for alprazolam are used for generalized anxiety disorder. Alprazolam is used for panic disorder.
Explain that drowsiness, impairment of intellectual function, impairment of memory, ataxia, and reduced motor coordination can occur.	Common side effects that subside as tolerance to drug develops.
For patients who use these medications for sleep, there may daytime fatigue, drowsiness, and cognitive impairments that can continue while person is awake.	Common side effects that subside as tolerance to drug develops.
A gradual tapering is recommended when being taken off the drug.	Abrupt discontinuation of the benzodiazepines can result in a recurrence of target symptoms such as anxiety.
Nausea, vomiting, impaired appetite, dry mouth, and constipation may occur.	These are gastrointestinal (GI) symptoms associated with this drug.
Take the drug with food.	Taking the drug with food may ease GI distress.
Monitor for worsening of depression symptoms.	This effect may occur in patients who are both depressed and anxious.
Older adults should take the smallest possible therapeutic dose.	Older adults taking this drug are at increased risk for incontinence, memory disturbances, dizziness, and falls.
Pregnant women and nursing mothers should avoid using benzodiazepines.	Benzodiazepines are excreted in breast milk of nursing mothers. They also cross the placenta and are associated with increased risk of certain birth defects.
Decrease or stop smoking altogether.	Nicotine decreases effectiveness of benzodiazepines.
Nonbenzodiazepines: buspirone	Buspirone is indicated in treatment of generalized anxiety disorder. It does not add to depression, so it is a good choice when anxiety and depression coexist. It is not effective in treating other anxiety disorders.
Take buspirone on a continual dosing schedule tid.	Buspirone has a short half-life.
Cardiac patients should avoid this drug.	Buspirone can cause digoxin toxicity.
This drug can cause liver and kidney toxicity. Patients with kidney or liver impairment must be monitored for this adverse effect.	Buspirone is metabolized in the liver and excreted predominantly by the kidneys.
Be alert for dizziness, drowsiness, nausea, excitement, and headache.	Common side effects.

●●● **Related NIC and NOC labels:** *NIC:* Teaching: Prescribed Medication *NOC:* Knowledge: Medication

ADDITIONAL NURSING DIAGNOSES/ PROBLEMS:

"Major Depression" for:

Hopelessness   p. 805

Risk for Suicide   p. 806

Self-Esteem Disturbance   p. 808

PATIENT-FAMILY TEACHING AND DISCHARGE PLANNING

The patient with an anxiety disorder experiences a wide variety of symptoms that affect ability to learn and retain information. Teaching must be geared to a time when medication has begun to calm the person and improve abilities to concentrate and learn; otherwise, it is wasted effort. Verbal teaching should be simple and supplemented with reading materials to which the patient and/or significant other and family can refer at a later time. Ensure that follow-up treatment is scheduled and that patient and/or significant other and family understand need to get prescriptions filled and to take medication as prescribed. Psychiatric home care might be a valuable part of the discharge planning to facilitate compliance with the discharge plan. In addition, provide verbal and written information about the following issues:

✓ Medications, including drug name, purpose, dosage, frequency, precautions, drug/drug and food/drug interactions, and potential side effects.

✓ Thought-stopping techniques to deal with negativism.

✓ Importance of maintaining a healthy lifestyle—balanced diet, minimal to no caffeine, decrease or stop smoking, exercise and regular adequate sleep patterns—for remaining in remission.

✓ Importance of continuing medication use long after depressive symptoms have gone.

✓ Importance of social support and strategies to obtain it.

✓ Importance of using constructive coping skills to deal with stress.

✓ Importance of using relaxation techniques to minimize stress.

✓ Importance of maintaining or achieving spiritual well-being.

✓ Importance of follow-up care, including day treatment programs, appointments with psychiatrist and therapists, and vocational rehabilitation program if indicated.

✓ Referrals to community resources for support and education. Additional information can be obtained by contacting the following organizations:

Anxiety Disorders Association of America (ADAA)
11900 Parklawn Drive, Suite 100
Rockville, MD 20852
(301) 231-9350
www.adaa.org/

National Alliance for the Mentally Ill (NAMI)
200 North Glebe Road, Suite 1015
Arlington, VA 22203-3754
(800) 950 6264
www.nimh.nih.gov/anxiety/panicmenu.cfm

National Institute of Mental Health (NIMH) Panic Disorder Education Program
Room 7c-02
5600 Fishers Lane
Rockville, MD 20857
(800) 64 PANIC
www.nimh.gov/anxiety/anxiety/panic/index.htm

97

Bipolar Disorder (Manic Component)

Bipolar disorder is a mood disorder characterized by episodes of major depression and mania or hypomania. (See the care plan on "Major Depression," p. 803, for specifics regarding depression.) *Mania* is characterized by a period in which there is a dramatic change in mood; the individual is either elated and expansive or irritable. For the diagnosis to be made, this change in mood must last 1 wk (less if hospitalization is required). At least three other symptoms from the following list must be present: inflated self-esteem or grandiosity, decreased need for sleep, pressured speech, flight of ideas, distractibility, increased involvement in goal-directed activities or psychomotor agitation, and overinvolvement in pleasurable activities with potentially damaging consequences, for example, hypersexuality, impulsive spending, and reckless and dangerous behavior.

Hypomania is characterized by at least 4 days of abnormally and persistently elevated, expansive, or irritable mood accompanied by at least three additional symptoms seen in a manic episode.

About 25% of the first episodes of bipolar disorder occur before age 20. Hormonal factors may account for a greater rate of rapid cycling (meaning highs and lows in a short period) by women, but, in general, women and men are equally affected with this disorder. There is no difference in prevalence rates by race or ethnicity. Bipolar disorder is a chronic, relapsing, and episodic disease. In individuals ≥40 yr of age who experience a first episode of mania, it is most likely related to medical conditions such as substance abuse or a cerebrovascular disorder. About 50% of bipolar patients have concurrent substance abuse disorders. Theories that explain causation of bipolar disorder include disorders in brain function or structure, sleep deprivation, and genetic factors.

HEALTH CARE SETTING

Primary (outpatient) care for most patients, except for those who are at high risk for suicide, represent a danger to others, or are experiencing a psychotic mania. Acute care (inpatient) stays are brief and focus on restabilization. Patients with bipolar disorder require long-term medication management, intensive psychosocial support to function within the community, and possibly individual, group, and family therapy.

ASSESSMENT

Similar to depression, the assessment of mania involves much more than an assessment of mood. This is a holistic disorder that results in changes in self-attitude (feelings of self-worth), as well as vital sense (sense of physical well-being) and spiritual sense. Depression diminishes self-worth, self-attitude, and vital sense, whereas mania increases these perceptions.

Feelings, attitudes, and knowledge: During manic episodes, patients express inflated views of themselves. Many manic patients state that they enjoyed being high and because of this refused medications. After the mania has subsided, the patient is confronted with the consequences of behaviors and actions engaged in while manic. Being faced with the reality of those behaviors and their consequences produces negative feelings expressed as shame, humiliation, denial, anger, fear of experiencing a relapse, fear of passing the disorder onto children, and fear of completing the bipolar cycle with an episode of depression.

Elevated mood or irritability: Patients may be excessively cheerful and unusually elated or display irritability over the smallest matters. This irritability increases when others attempt to reason with them. A manic person may display a haughty or superior attitude toward others. He or she may display overt anger, particularly if his or her requests or behaviors are curtailed.

Increased self-attitude: Patients may express and act in unusually optimistic fashion, engaging in behaviors that reflect poor judgment. The manic person is overconfident and energetic. Unfortunately the excess energy is channeled into inappropriate, dangerous, or indiscreet behaviors. A normally conservative person may engage in sexual indiscretions or speak in overly critical or judgmental terms, often at inappropriate times and about sensitive subjects.

Increased vital sense: The person with mania has increased energy and may appear tireless in the face of physical and mental efforts that would greatly tax unaffected individuals. He or she may feel completely refreshed after only a few minutes or hours of sleep.

Spiritual issues: Bipolar disorder mania carries with it many negative experiences—such as marital and family problems, divorce, legal difficulties, financial ruin, and unemployment—that contribute to the downward spiral of self-appraisals. Bipolar disorder can lead to a crisis in faith in self, others, life, and ultimately God. This loss of faith and hope contributes significantly to the risk of suicide.

Additional signs: Manic individuals may experience a voracious appetite or may be too busy to eat. A change in sleep pattern is characteristic of mania, with many individuals feeling less need for sleep, so sleep is usually decreased. An increase in sexual interest and activity is characteristic of manic individuals.

Suicidality: Suicide assessment is critical with manic patients. The presence of psychotic thinking, hyperactivity, impulsiveness, and possible substance abuse increases suicide risk significantly. It is important to ask questions to determine the presence of suicidal ideation and the lethality of any plan. Essential questions to ask include:

- Have you thought of hurting yourself?
- Are you presently thinking about hurting yourself?
- If you have been thinking about suicide, do you have a plan? What is the plan?
- Have you thought about what life would be like if you were no longer a part of it?

A previous history of suicide attempts places the patient at high risk for attempting suicide.

DIAGNOSTIC TESTS

There are no diagnostic tests to diagnose bipolar disorder-mania. Diagnosis is made through history, interview of patient and family, and observation of verbal and nonverbal behaviors. The Young Mania Scale is an effective instrument to quantify the degree of mania.

Nursing Diagnosis:

Deficient Knowledge:

Causes, signs and symptoms, and treatment of bipolar disorder mania

Desired Outcome: Within 24 hr of teaching, patient and/or significant other verbalize accurate information about at least two possible causes of bipolar disorder, four signs and symptoms of the disorder, and available treatment options.

INTERVENTIONS	RATIONALES
Inform patient and significant other that bipolar disorder is a physiologic disorder caused by the interplay of many factors, such as imbalance in brain function and structure, sleep deprivation, psychodynamic factors, and genetics.	Providing education about the physical basis for the disorder increases understanding and acceptance and decreases blaming behavior.
Inform patient and significant other that there are treatments available for bipolar disorder.	Medications are essential to stabilize and maintain mood. However, they are not enough. Comprehensive treatment involves intensive outpatient programs, frequent office visits, crisis telephone calls, family involvement, and psychosocial interventions including psychoeducation, suicide prevention, psychotherapy for depression, and limit setting in mania and hypomania. Management of bipolar disorders is a lifelong commitment.

●●● **Related NIC and NOC labels:** *NIC:* Teaching: Individual; Teaching: Procedure/Treatment
NOC: Knowledge: Illness Care

Nursing Diagnosis:

Risk for Other-Directed Violence

related to manic excitement

Desired Outcome: By the time of discharge from an inpatient setting, patient demonstrates self-control and decreased hyperactivity.

INTERVENTIONS	RATIONALES
Decrease environmental stimuli, avoid exposure to situations of predictable high stimulation, and remove patient from area if he or she becomes agitated.	Patient may be unable to focus attention on relevant stimuli and will be reacting/responding to all environmental stimuli.
Continually evaluate patient's response to frustration or difficult situations.	Enables early intervention and helps patient manage situation independently, if possible.
Ensure that environment is safe. Remove objects that could be dangerous and rearrange room to decrease environmental risks to prevent accidental/purposeful injury to self or others.	Hyperactive behavior and grandiose thinking can lead to destructive actions with possible harm to self or others.
Intervene at earliest signs of agitation. Use direct verbal interventions prompting appropriate behavior, redirect or remove patient from difficult situation, establish voluntary time-out or move to a quiet room, use physical control (e.g., hold patient).	Early intervention assists patient in regaining control, defuses a difficult situation, prevents violence, and enables treatment to continue in least restrictive manner.
Until patient is calm, avoid analyzing or problem solving regarding prevention of violence or collecting information about precipitating events or provoking stimuli.	Any questioning will only add to agitation. Analyze and problem solve when patient is calm.
Communicate rationale for taking action using a concrete, direct, and simple approach.	People are unable to process complicated communication when they are agitated or upset.
When patient is ready to leave quiet area or time-out location, allow gradual reentry to area of greater stimulation.	Patient has diminished tolerance for environmental stimuli; gradual reentry fosters coping skills.
Do not argue with patient who verbalizes put-downs or unrealistic or grandiose ideas.	Arguing only increases agitation and reinforces undesirable behavior.
Ignore and minimize attention given to bizarre dress or use of profanity, while placing clear limits on destructive behavior.	Avoids reinforcing negative behavior while providing controls for potentially dangerous behavior.
Avoid unnecessary delay of gratification when patient makes a request. If refusal is necessary, make sure that rationale is given in nonjudgmental and concrete manner.	Patients in a hyperactive state do not tolerate waiting or delays that add to frustration or agitation level. Any unnecessary delays could trigger aggressive behavior.
Offer alternatives when available.	This uses patient's distractibility to decrease the frustration of having request refused. For example, "I don't have any soda. Would you like a glass of juice?"
When patient is less agitated and labile, provide information about alternative problem-solving strategies.	When calm, patient is able to hear and retain information.
When patient is calm, help to examine the antecedents/precipitants to agitation.	Promotes early recognition of developing problem, enabling patient to plan for alternative responses and intervene in a timely fashion.
Collaborate with patient to identify alternative behaviors that are acceptable to both patient and staff. Role-play how to use these behaviors if appropriate.	Patient is more apt to follow through if the alternatives are mutually agreed on. This practice enables patient to "try on" new behaviors while calm and ready to learn.
Give positive reinforcement when patient attempts to deal with difficult situations without violence.	Praise increases patient's sense of success and increases likelihood that desired behaviors will be repeated.

Continued

INTERVENTIONS	RATIONALES
Administer the following medications as prescribed:	
Antimanic medications: lithium carbonate (Lithobid, Eskalith), divalproex sodium (Depakote), or carbamazepine (Tegretol)	Lithium is the drug of choice for mania and is indicated for alleviation of hyperactive symptoms. Some patients are lithium nonresponders and may need either divalproex or carbamazepine.
Antipsychotic medications: chlorpromazine (Thorazine), haloperidol (Haldol), or clonazepam (Klonopin), a benzodiazepine	These drugs are useful in decreasing extreme hyperactivity and improving an accompanying thought disorder until therapeutic level of lithium is achieved or when lithium is ineffective.
Provide restraint or seclusion per agency policy.	May be necessary for brief periods to protect patient, staff, and others.
Prepare patient for electroconvulsive therapy (ECT) if indicated.	In severely manic episode, ECT may be necessary.

●●● **Related NIC and NOC labels:** *NIC:* Environmental Management: Safety; Behavior Management; Counseling; Impulse Control Training; Medication Management; Physical Restraint; Seclusion *NOC:* Impulse Control

Nursing Diagnosis:

Imbalanced Nutrition: Less than body requirements

related to inadequate intake in relation to metabolic expenditures

Desired Outcome: Immediately following interventions, patient displays increased attention to eating behaviors.

INTERVENTIONS	RATIONALES
Establish a baseline regarding nutritional and fluid intake, as well as activity level.	Necessary to quantify deficits, needs, and progress toward goals.
Weigh patient daily.	Another form of quantification that provides information about therapeutic needs and effectiveness of interventions.
Serve meals in a setting with minimal distractions.	Encourages patient to focus on eating and prevents other distractions from interfering with food intake.
Stay with patient during mealtime, even if this means walking with patient.	Provides support and encouragement for patient to take in adequate nutrition and does not set unrealistic expectation that patient must sit during mealtime.
Provide finger foods, snacks, and juices.	Recognizes that patient will most likely eat small frequent meals on the move and allows a reasonable accommodation for this behavior.
Enable patient to choose food when he or she is able to make choices.	Encouraging choices before patient is ready may add to confusion. However, if patient is able to handle choices, this increases sense of control.
Refer to dietitian as indicated.	It may be useful to involve an expert in determining patient's nutritional needs and the most appropriate options for meeting these needs.
Administer vitamins and mineral supplements as prescribed.	Corrects dietary deficiencies and improves nutritional status.

●●● **Related NIC and NOC labels:** *NIC:* Nutrition Management: Nutritional Monitoring *NOC:* Nutritional Status

Nursing Diagnosis:

Self-Care Deficit

related to impulsivity and lack of concern

Desired Outcome: Immediately following interventions, patient performs self-care activities within level of ability.

INTERVENTIONS	RATIONALES
Assess current level of functioning; reevaluate daily.	Patient's abilities for self-care may change daily. This information is needed to plan or modify care.
Provide physical assistance, supervision and simple directions, reminders, encouragement, and support as needed.	Helps patient focus on task. Provide only required assistance to foster independence.
If possible, use patient's clothing and toiletries.	Patient may have been disorganized entering the hospital or was hospitalized as an emergency measure, so own belongings were left at home. Having own clothes and supplies supports autonomy and self-esteem.
As appropriate, limit choices regarding clothing.	During periods of extreme hyperactivity and distractibility, patient may be unable to make appropriate choices or to care for personal belongings.
Monitor patient's ability to manage money and valuables, as well as other personal effects.	Manic patients may give away possessions, spend money extravagantly, or become involved in grandiose plans, necessitating intervention.
Intervene to protect patient from own impassivity and exploitation from others.	Protects patient from negative consequences of impulsiveness
As condition improves, set goals to establish minimum standards for self-care, for example, take a bath every other day.	Promotes idea that patient is responsible for self and enhances sense of self-worth.

●●● **Related NIC and NOC labels:** *NIC:* Self-Care Assistance; Self-Responsibility Facilitation; Behavior Modification *NOC:* Self-Care: Activities of Daily Living

Nursing Diagnosis:

Deficient Knowledge:

Medication use, including purpose and potential side effects of prescribed medications

Desired Outcome: Immediately following teaching interventions, patient verbalizes accurate information about the prescribed medications.

INTERVENTIONS	RATIONALES
Teach physiologic action of mood stabilizers.	Bipolar disorder mania responds to mood stabilizers, with lithium carbonate being the drug of choice
Teach importance of taking medication as prescribed and the need for follow-up blood tests to monitor drug serum level.	The medication requires certain blood levels to be therapeutic, and therefore patient needs to take it at the dose and time interval prescribed. The scheduled serum evaluations ensure that the medication level remains within therapeutic range.

Continued

INTERVENTIONS	RATIONALES
Antimanic drugs for adults: lithium carbonate (Lithobid, Eskalith, Duralith) or lithium citrate (Cibalith)	Lithium provides mood stability and prevents dangerous highs and despairing lows experienced in bipolar disorder.
Teach Patient the Following:	
Monitor for swelling of feet or hands, fine hand tremor, mild diarrhea, muscle weakness, fatigue, memory and concentration difficulties, metallic taste, nausea or abdominal discomfort, polydipsia, polyuria,	Common side effects.
Importance of monitoring I&O, Na^+ intake, and weight and how to elevate legs when sitting or lying down.	Interventions for edema of feet and hands.
Importance of notifying health care provider if urinary output decreases.	May be sign of increasing serum level of lithium.
Tremors worsen when patient is anxious. Patient should notify prescriber if tremors interfere with work.	A drug that interferes with work may result in compliance issues. Smaller, more frequent doses may help.
Take lithium with meals and replace fluids lost with diarrhea.	Interventions for mild diarrhea.
Notify prescriber if diarrhea becomes severe.	Prescriber may need to change patient's medication.
If they occur, muscle weakness, fatigue, and memory and concentration difficulties are short lasting. Patient should avoid driving or operating hazardous equipment during this period and should use reminders and cues for memory.	Interventions for muscle weakness, fatigue, and memory and concentration difficulties.
Notify prescriber if muscle weakness, fatigue, and memory and concentration problems become severe.	Prescriber may change patient's medication.
Use sugarless candies or throat lozenges and engage in frequent oral hygiene.	Interventions for metallic taste.
Take medication with meals.	Intervention for nausea or abdominal discomfort.
Drinking large amounts of fluids is a normal mechanism for coping with the side effect of increased urine.	Reassurance for polydipsia.
Have laboratory work done as prescribed.	To ensure that serum drug level is maintained between 0.6 and 1.2 mEq/L. Usually once stabilization is achieved, laboratory work is done q1-2 wk during first 2 mo and q3-6 mo during long-term maintenance.
Avoid alcohol or other central nervous system (CNS) depressant drugs.	May increase serum lithium level.
Notify prescriber if pregnant or planning to become pregnant. Do not breastfeed while taking this medication.	Safe use during pregnancy and breastfeeding has not been established.
Notify prescriber before taking any other prescription or over-the-counter (OTC) medication.	Many other drugs interact with lithium to either increase or decrease the serum level.
Do not abruptly discontinue.	This could lead to exacerbation of manic symptoms.
Antiseizure medications with mood-stabilizing effects: divalproex sodium or valproic acid (Depakote or Depakene) and carbamazepine (Tegretol)	These medications are generally used when lithium does not work or when side effects from lithium are intolerable to patient.
Teach patient to be alert for anorexia, nausea, vomiting, drowsiness (most common), and tremor.	Common side effects.

●●● **Related NIC and NOC labels:** *NIC:* Teaching: Prescribed Medication *NOC:* Knowledge: Medication

ADDITIONAL NURSING DIAGNOSES/ PROBLEMS:

"Major Depression" for:

Hopelessness	p. 805
Risk for Suicide	p. 806
Self-Esteem Disturbance	p. 808

PATIENT-FAMILY TEACHING AND DISCHARGE PLANNING

The patient with a bipolar disorder mania experiences a wide variety of symptoms that affect the ability to learn and retain information. Teaching must be geared to a time when medication has begun to decrease hyperactive symptoms and improve abilities to concentrate and learn; otherwise, it is a wasted effort. Verbal teaching should be simple and supplemented with reading materials the patient and/or significant other and family can refer to at a later time. Ensure that follow-up treatment is scheduled and that patient and/or significant other and family understand need to get prescriptions filled and importance of taking medication as prescribed. Consider whether or not patient has transportation available to get to follow-up treatment. Psychiatric home care might be a valuable part of the discharge planning to facilitate compliance with the discharge plan. In addition, provide patient and/or significant other/ family with verbal and written information about the following issues:

✓ Medications, including drug name, purpose, dosage, frequency, precautions, drug/drug and food/drug interactions, and potential side effects.

✓ Importance of laboratory follow-up tests for serum lithium levels.

✓ Importance of maintaining a healthy lifestyle—balanced diet, minimal to no caffeine or alcohol, exercise, and regular adequate sleep patterns—to ensure remaining in remission.

✓ Importance of continuing medication use probably for a lifetime.

✓ Importance of social support and strategies for obtaining it.

✓ Importance of using community follow-up resources, for example, psychiatrist, psychiatric nurse, intensive outpatient, support groups, family counseling.

✓ Importance of maintaining or achieving spiritual well-being.

✓ Referrals to community resources for support and education. Additional information can be obtained by contacting the following organizations:

Depression and Related Affective Disorders Association (DRADA)
Meyer 3-181
600 North Wolfe Street
Baltimore, MD 21287-7381
(410) 955-4647 (Baltimore)
(202) 955-5800 (Washington, DC)
www.drada.org/

This nonprofit organization is composed of individuals with mood disorders, family members, and mental health professionals. It offers information, education, referral, and support services to people nationwide. DRADA sponsors a nationally renowned training program for group leaders.

Depression Awareness, Recognition, and Treatment Program (D/ART)
5600 Fisher's Lane, Suite 10-85
Rockville, MD 20857
(301) 443-4140
Fax: (301) 443-4045

D/ART is a national self-help clearinghouse. It provides a list of resources throughout the United States that can help in networking and providing consultative assistance.

98

Dementia— Alzheimer's Type

Dementia is a chronic cognitive disorder that is part of a category of psychiatric disorders classified as *Delirium, Dementia, and other Cognitive Disorders*. These disorders are divided into two categories: *Acute Cognitive Disorders,* which includes delirium, and *Chronic Cognitive Disorders,* which includes the various types of dementia. There are five types of dementia: primary, dementia with extrapyramidal symptoms (EPS), dementia resulting from brain lesions, vascular dementia, and dementia associated with other physical conditions.

The most common form is Alzheimer's disease, a primary dementia accounting for 60%-80% of dementia cases, and it is the focus of this care plan. Although Alzheimer's disease is age related, it does not represent the normal process of aging. It occurs with distinctive brain lesions without any known physiologic basis. The brain lesions are neurofibrillary tangles and neuritic plaques that take up space in the brain, replacing normal tissue in the cell body of the neuron. There are multiple theories to explain the occurrence of Alzheimer's disease, including genetic transmission, a decrease in acetyl choline, beta-amyloid activity, impact of head injury, ministrokes, lack of estrogen, immunologic factors, effects of a slow-acting virus, and environmental factors.

Alzheimer's disease affects more than 4 million people, making it the most common neuropsychiatric illness in older adults. The actual course of the disorder follows a predictable pattern of early, middle, and late stages, each displaying characteristic behaviors and requiring a different focus of treatment. The early stage is frequently referred to as the amnestic stage, the middle stage as the dementia stage, and the late stage as the vegetative stage. As the disease progresses, patients lose control over their bladder and bowel functions and later over swallowing. Seizures are common. Death inevitably occurs as a result of neurologic complications imposed by the brain lesions.

Alzheimer's disease represents the clinical prototype for chronic cognitive disorders. The care required by the Alzheimer's patient, especially in the middle and late stages of the disorder, is essentially the same care required by all dementia patients regardless of type. The cognitive symptoms of dementia involve serious memory impairment, as well as significant alterations in language and perceptual acuity and abilities to abstract, problem solve, and make appropriate judgments. Patients ultimately experience loss of all memory and aphasia (loss of meaningful verbal communication). Noncognitive behavioral symptoms can be just as profound. These include significant personality changes, purposeless movements, agitation and aggression, overreaction to situations, irritating behavior, and emotional disinhibition.

HEALTH CARE SETTING

In the early stage of Alzheimer's disease, care takes place in the home and primary care setting. By the end of the early stage of the disease, additional services such as home care and use of adult day care are needed to maintain the patient at home. At the end of the early stage and moving into the middle stage, the decision regarding where to place the patient begins. Patient is generally moved into residential care in the middle stage, and during the late stage, care is provided in a skilled nursing facility.

ASSESSMENT

Psychiatric assessment

Involves assessment of primary and secondary psychiatric manifestations of Alzheimer's disease and differential diagnosis from psychosis, depression, anxiety, and phobias.

Family history: Dementing illness, psychiatric disease, neurologic disease, substance abuse.

Social history: Education, past level of functioning per occupational history, close relationships, current living situation.

Medical history: All past and present medical illnesses, past surgeries, past trauma especially to the head, allergies, and medication.

Psychiatric history: Psychotic illness, depressive illness, other psychiatric illnesses, psychiatric symptoms, past and current treatments, hospitalizations, suicide, violence.

Present illness: Length of cognitive loss and degree of memory loss:

- Is short-term memory loss so significant that patient is no longer able to remember activities of daily living (ADL)?
- Other presenting problems, physical symptoms, functional deficits, psychiatric symptoms.
- Personality changes, including low tolerance for normal frustrations, oversensitivity to remarks of others, lack of initiative, decreased attention span, diminished emotional presence, emotional lability, restlessness.
- Difficulty with word finding and comprehension; thought blocking.

Mental status examination: Appearance, behavior, speech, mood, hallucinations, delusions, anxiety, phobias, cognition, insight and judgment, behavioral disturbances such as agitation, combativeness, screaming, catastrophic reactions.

Physical assessment

Psychomotor functioning: Difficulty carrying out new or complex motor tasks is apparent in the early stages; difficulty carrying out activities such as dressing, eating, and walking becomes apparent in the middle stages. Unsteadiness of gait and a listing posture pose a significant risk for falls during the middle stages. In addition, marked psychomotor agitation is common. Restlessness, agitation, and aimless pacing replace normal motion.

Nutrition and elimination: Eating difficulties may present in early stages. Patient may forget that he or she has just eaten, exhibit lax table manners, fail to know it is mealtime without prompting, experience changes in taste and appetite, express denial of hunger or need to eat, and experience weight loss. As disease progresses, patient does not respond to need for elimination, and this necessitates the caregiver planning regular bathroom breaks. Constipation and incontinence of urine and feces become problems.

Activity and rest: Fatigue increases severity of symptoms, especially as evening approaches. Patient may reverse days and nights, with wakefulness and aimless wandering at night and disturbance of sleep rhythms. Patient may be content to sit and watch others. Main activity may be hoarding inanimate objects, hiding articles, wandering, or engaging in repetitive motions.

Hygiene: As disease progresses, so does dependence on caregiver to meet basic hygiene needs. Appearance may be disheveled, and patient may have body odor. Clothing may be inappropriate for situation or weather conditions. Patient may forget to go to the bathroom and the steps involved in toileting.

Social assessment: Patient may ignore rules of social conduct and exhibit inappropriate behavior. Speech may be fragmented; family roles may be altered/reversed as patient becomes more dependent.

Spiritual assessment

An assessment of patient's faith tradition, practices, level of commitment, and connection to a faith community is critical. In the early stage of Alzheimer's disease the patient may have full awareness of the journey that lies ahead, and spirituality may offer support and comfort in ways that nothing else can. As the disease progresses and deficits become greater, it is difficult to assess the patient's spiritual needs. However, because long-term memory remains intact long after the short-term memory is gone, patient may still be comforted by spiritual traditions such as worship services, prayers, and hymns that are a vivid part of his or her history. Moreover, care of the Alzheimer's patient is so demanding that spiritual needs of the caregiver must be assessed and support provided. A faith community may provide invaluable assistance in the actual care of the patient, providing caregiver with respite and help with day-to-day activities.

DIAGNOSTIC TESTS

Obtaining an accurate differential diagnosis of dementia is essential. Alzheimer's disease is basically a rule-out disorder; that is, the diagnosis is made after family history, laboratory tests, and brain imaging eliminate other disorders with similar cognitive deficits. Sources of information needed to make a differential diagnosis of dementia include a full neurologic assessment, laboratory tests to rule out metabolic factors, and family history of patient's past behavior and symptom progression. Mini-Mental State Examination and functional assessment of ADL provide necessary information. A computed tomography (CT) scan identifies structural deficits. Brain imaging with positron emission tomography (PET) provides the clinician with information about changes in the metabolic activity and neurochemical characteristics associated with dementia. Typically testing of patients in the early stage of Alzheimer's disease reveals a normal electroencephalogram (EEG), CT, and magnetic resonance imaging (MRI), and generally laboratory tests are within normal range. Comprehensive psychiatric assessment provides additional information.

Nursing Diagnosis:
Deficient Knowledge:

Disease progression and care of the dementia patient

Desired Outcome: By the time the diagnosis of Alzheimer's disease is confirmed, significant other/family relay accurate information about the course of the disease and the role they will play in the care of their loved one.

INTERVENTIONS	RATIONALES
Provide significant other/family information about the staging of the disease and changes to expect in their loved one.	The significant other and family play integral roles in the care of their loved one. Initially they are the informants, providing information that facilitates diagnosis; they move into role of advocate, then primary caregivers, and finally patient supporter. Staging is discussed in introductory data.
Provide information regarding educational resources, such as *The Thirty-Six Hour Day* (1999) by Mace and Rabins, and support groups.	The cited book presents a compilation of family experiences with the disorder at different stages. Although there are other helpful books, this one remains the definitive resource for family caregivers. Support groups for family members offer an ongoing, practical socioeducational source, even in the early stage. They provide a safe place to explore issues such as whether or not the patient should stop driving; should other people be told about the diagnosis; should the patient wear an ID bracelet or carry a card indicating a dementia diagnosis; how does the healthy spouse handle the sexual desires of the affected spouse when the unaffected spouse no longer feels as though he or she has an adult relationship anymore.
Coach the family to use all their senses and past memories in talking with their loved one.	Families feel more comfortable and are more likely to continue to interact with patient if they know that reduced animation in patient's face is part of the disease; conversation may have noticeable pauses with less spontaneous speech; conversations should be short and simple; reassuring the patient decreases overconcern about minor matters; touch continues to be important; and sharing important memories from the past helps maintain links to the patient even if the response is minimal.
Teach about safety issues.	Safety issues become the responsibility of the caregiver early in the disorder. The Alzheimer's patient needs room to pace and fails to notice scatter rugs, spills on the floor, and changes in floor elevations, which make falls more likely. Other safety concerns deal with wandering, turning on stove and forgetting, and using toxic substances inappropriately.
Provide information about legal matters.	Decisions about durable power of attorney need to be decided in the early stage of the disease when the patient is still competent. Legal counsel may be desirable for decisions regarding financial matters.
Provide information about health care resources.	The job of the family caregiver is overwhelming. Family members need to consider use of adult day care centers and varieties of respite care, even in the early stage of the illness. Use of home health services also may be of assistance to the caregiver.
Teach strategies to deal with behavioral issues such as wandering, rummaging, incontinence, difficulty following directions, and profound memory loss.	The more knowledge the family has regarding strategies to deal with these various behaviors, the better they will be able to care for the patient.

●●● **Related NIC and NOC labels:** *NIC:* Teaching: Disease Process; Teaching: Procedure/Treatment
NOC: Knowledge: Illness Care; Knowledge: Disease Process

Nursing Diagnosis:

Risk for Injury

related to impaired judgment and inability to recognize danger in the environment

Desired Outcome: Patient remains free of signs and symptoms of injury.

INTERVENTIONS	RATIONALES
Assess degree of impairment in patient's ability. Assist caregiver to identify the following risks and potential hazards that may cause harm in patient's environment and the necessary interventions that must be made to ensure patient's safety.	Patients with impulsive behavior are at increased risk for harm because they are less able to control their own behaviors. Patients may have visual/perceptual deficits that increase risk of falls. Caregivers need heightened awareness of potential risks in the environment and need to take appropriate action.
Eliminate or minimize identified environmental risks.	Because a person with a cognitive deficit is unable to take responsibility for basic safety needs, the caregiver must eliminate as many risks as possible: take knobs off of stove, remove scatter rugs, place a safety gate at the top and bottom of stairs, and make sure doors to outside are locked.
Routinely monitor patient's behavior. Initiate interventions to prevent negative behaviors from escalating.	Close observation of patient's behavior allows early identification of problematic behaviors (e.g., increasing agitation) and enables early intervention.
Use distraction or redirection of patient's attention when agitated or dangerous behavior such as climbing out of bed occurs.	Using patient's distractibility avoids confrontation and maintains safety.
Ensure that patient wears an ID bracelet providing name, phone number, and diagnosis. Do not allow patient to have access to stairways or exits.	Because of memory deficits and confusion, these patients may not be able to provide this basic identifying information. The ID bracelet facilitates patient's safe return.
Ensure that doors to outside are locked. Make sure there is supervision and/or activities if patient is regularly awake at night.	Taking appropriate preventative measures facilitates safety without constant supervision. Activities keep patient occupied and limit wandering.
Ensure that patient is dressed appropriately for weather/physical environment and individual need.	Patients with cognitive disorders many times experience seasonal disorientation. In addition, Alzheimer's disease affects the hypothalamic gland, making the person feel cold. The patient is not able to make appropriate choices regarding dress.
Inspect patient's skin during care activities.	Identification of rashes, lacerations, and areas of ecchymosis enables necessary treatment and signals need for closer monitoring and protective interventions.
Attend to nonverbal expression of physiologic discomfort.	Patient may lack ability to express needs clearly but may give clue of a problem by grimacing, sweating, doubling over, or panting.
Monitor for medication side effects; signs of overmedication, for example, gastrointestinal (GI) upset; extrapyramidal symptoms; and orthostatic hypotension.	Drugs easily build up to toxic levels in older adults, and patient may not be able to report any signs or symptoms that would indicate drug toxicity.

●●● **Related NIC and NOC labels:** *NIC:* Environmental Management: Safety; Surveillance: Safety; Fire-Setting Precautions; Risk Identification; Security Enhancement; Fall Prevention *NOC:* Safety Behavior: Home Physical Environment; Safety Status: Falls Occurrence

Nursing Diagnosis:

Disturbed Thought Processes

related to physiologic changes secondary to progressive course of Alzheimer's disease

Desired Outcome: Patient remains calm and displays fewer undesirable behaviors.

INTERVENTIONS	RATIONALES
Provide a predictable environment with orientation cues.	A calm environment with scheduled activities, adequate lighting, low noise level, calendars, clocks, and frequent verbal orientation helps maintain patient's sense of calm and security.
Always address patient by name.	Patients may respond to own name long after they no longer recognize their significant others. Names are an integral part of self-identity; using a person's name is a part of reality orientation.
Communicate with patient using a low voice, slow speech, and eye contact.	Deliberate communication techniques such as these increase patient's attention and chance for comprehension. Calm begets calm.
Break directions into a simple step-by-step process, giving one direction at a time and using simple and clear words.	As disease progresses, patient's ability to comprehend complex directions and interactions diminishes greatly. Simplicity is the key to effective communication.
Encourage patient's response, allow pauses in interaction, and use open-ended comments and phrases.	These interventions invite a verbal response.
Listen carefully to the content of patient's speech even if it is incomprehensible.	The patient may be having difficulty processing and decoding messages. However, listeners need to continue to show interest and encouragement to keep communication going.
Offer interpretations regarding patient's statements, meanings, and words. If patient struggles to find a word, supply the word if possible.	Assisting patient in processing words promotes continuing communication efforts and decreases frustration.
Avoid negative comments, taking argumentative stands, confrontations, and criticism.	These aggressive responses only serve to increase frustration, agitation, and inappropriate behaviors. Cognitively impaired patients have no internal controls over their thinking and communications.
Engage patient in conversation about real events and real people.	Patients who are encouraged and allowed to ruminate about people and events that are not real will experience greater disorientation.
Monitor for presence of hallucinations. Observe patient for verbal and nonverbal cues of responding to hallucinations. Validate patient's hallucinatory experiences.	Validating that patient is hearing voices allows some discussion of fears associated with the experience and permits assurance that the experience is part of the illness.
Allow patient to hoard safe objects.	Provides patient with a sense of security.
Provide useful and productive outlets for patient to engage in repetitive activities, for example, folding and unfolding laundry, collecting junk mail, dusting and sweeping floors.	Acknowledges that repetitive activities are a normal expression of illness but channels these activities in a way that increases patient's self-esteem and may decrease restlessness.

●●● **Related NIC and NOC labels:** *NIC:* Dementia Management: Hallucination Management; Anxiety Reduction; Environmental Management: Safety; Active Listening *NOC:* Distorted Thought Control

Nursing Diagnosis:

Disturbed Sensory Perceptions: Visual or auditory

related to altered sensory reception, transmission, and/or integration

Desired Outcomes: Patient demonstrates improved response to stimuli. Caregiver identifies and controls external factors that contribute to sensory/perceptual disturbances.

INTERVENTIONS	RATIONALES
Encourage use of assistive devices, corrective lenses, and hearing aids.	Provides enhancement of sensory input and reduces misinterpretation of stimuli.
Ensure that interpersonal communication and environment are geared to reality orientation.	Reality cues (e.g., calendars, clocks, notes, cards, signs, seasonal cues) are necessary in the environment. Interpersonal communication must include verbal reminders of time, place, and person in order to reduce confusion and promote coping with frustrating struggles of misperception and being disoriented and confused. Visual clues provide concrete reminders that promote recognition and may help with memory gaps, increasing independence.
Ensure that environment is quiet, calm, and visually nondistracting.	These qualities help to avoid visual/auditory overload.
Provide touch to patient in a caring way.	Touch enhances perception of self and body boundaries, as well as communicates caring.
Involve patient in activities that enable use of remaining skills.	Activities such as folding laundry, clearing the table, and watering plants provide outlets for patient that support dignity and provide pleasure and satisfaction.
Use reminiscence therapy with props such as photo albums, old music, historic events, and mementos. Encourage patient to talk about memories and feelings attached to these items.	Aids in preservation of self by recalling past accomplishments and events, increases patient's sense of security, and encourages sharing that keeps patient linked to others socially.
Encourage intellectual activity such as word games, discussion of current events, and story telling.	Provides patient with normalcy and connection to others and the world and stimulates remaining cognitive abilities.
Advise caregiver to facilitate spiritual activities, including Bible study, participation in worship services, singing hymns, visitation by clergy or church members, or televised church services.	Spiritual needs remain important. There is no certainty that because cognitive decline occurs, spirituality in anyway declines in awareness and importance.
Suggest that caregiver accompany patient on short outings in the car, taking walks, and going shopping.	Decreases sense of isolation, increases physical stamina, and provides sensory pleasure.
Advise caregiver to involve patient in social activities as tolerated.	Social activities involving crafts, family parties, socialization groups at day care center, and involvement with pets help maintain some level of social contact and sensory pleasure.

●●● **Related NIC and NOC labels:** *NIC:* Dementia Management; Environmental Management; Reminiscence Therapy; Surveillance: Safety; Reality Orientation; Communication Enhancement: Visual Deficit; Recreation Therapy; Communication Enhancement: Hearing Deficit *NOC:* Cognitive Orientation; Distorted Thought Control

Nursing Diagnosis:

Anticipatory Grieving

related to awareness on part of patient and significant other/family that something is seriously wrong as changes in memory and behaviors are increasingly evident

Desired Outcome: Patient and family discuss loss and participate in planning for the future.

INTERVENTIONS	RATIONALES
Encourage patient and family to discuss feelings associated with anticipated losses.	Conveys message that grief is a normal and expected reaction to the diagnosis of Alzheimer's disease.
Acknowledge expressions of anger and statements of despair and hopelessness, such as, "I and my family would be better off if I were dead."	Feelings of anger may be patient's way of dealing with underlying feelings of despair. Despairing and hopeless statements may be indicative of suicidal ideation. These should be explored and appropriate action taken to protect patient from self-directed violence (see **Risk for Suicide**, p. 806, in "Major Depression").
Provide honest answers and do not give false reassurances or gloomy predictions.	Honesty promotes a trusting relationship and open communication. False reassurances or predictions of gloom are not helpful.
Discuss with patient and significant other/family ways they can plan for the future.	Participation in problem solving increases patient's and family's sense of control.
Emphasize that this is a disease in which research is active and ongoing, as well as the possibility the disease will progress slowly.	Real hope may exist for the future.
Assist patient/significant other/family to identify strengths they see in themselves, each other, and in available support systems.	Emphasizes that there are supports and resources to help work through grief.

●●● **Related NIC and NOC labels.** *NIC:* Coping Enhancement; Anticipatory Guidance; Caregiver Support; Family Support; Hope Instillation; Support System Enhancements; Decision-Making Support
NOC: Coping; Family Coping; Psychosocial Adjustment: Life Change

Nursing Diagnosis:

Risk for Caregiver Role Strain

related to severity of patient's illness, duration of care required, and complexity and number of caregiving tasks required

Desired Outcome: Caregiver exhibits behaviors consistent with a healthy lifestyle.

INTERVENTIONS	RATIONALES
Assess caregiver's physical/emotional/spiritual condition and the caregiving demands that are present.	Helps to determine individual care needs of caregiver.
Determine caregiver's level of responsibility, involvement in, and anticipated duration of care involved.	Helps caregiver realistically assess what is involved in a commitment to providing care.
Identify strengths of caregiver and patient.	Identifies positive aspects of each so that they may be incorporated into daily activities.

Continued

INTERVENTIONS	RATIONALES
Encourage caregiver to discuss personal perspective and views about situation.	Allows venting of concerns and provides opportunity for validation and acceptance of caregiver's issues.
Explore available supports and resources.	Enables evaluation of adequacy of current resources. For example, "What is currently used? Is it effective? What else is needed?"
Encourage and offer to facilitate family conference to develop plan for family involvement in care activities.	The more people that are involved in care, the less risk that one person will become overwhelmed.
Identify additional resources, including financial, legal, and respite care.	These issues of concern can add to the burden of caregiving if not resolved.
Identify equipment needs/resources and other environmental adaptations.	Appropriate equipment and environmental modifications promote patient safety and ease the care burden on the primary caregiver.
Teach caregiver/family techniques and strategies to deal with acting out and disoriented behaviors, as well as incontinence and other physical challenges.	Increases sense of control and competency of caregiver and family.
Teach caregiver the importance of continuing own activities.	Risk of caregiver burden, burnout, and stress is greatly diminished if caregiver takes time for self, for example, continuing a hobby, pursuing social activities, and taking care of personal needs.
Encourage and help caregiver/family to plan for changes that may be necessary, such as home care services, use of adult day care, and eventual placement in a long-term facility.	Planning is essential for these eventualities. As the disease progresses, the burden of care outstrips the resources of the caregiver.

●●● **Related NIC and NOC labels:** *NIC:* Caregiver Support; Coping Enhancement; Respite Care; Decision-Making Support; Family Support; Support System Enhancement; Family Involvement Promotion; Home Maintenance Assistance; Anticipatory Guidance *NOC:* Caregiver Lifestyle Disruption; Caregiver Well-Being

Nursing Diagnosis:

Deficient Knowledge:

Rationale, potential side effects, and interventions for side effects of prescribed medications

Desired Outcome: Immediately following teaching, caregiver and/or family verbalize accurate information about the rationale for use of certain medications, their common side effects, and methods for dealing with those side effects.

INTERVENTIONS	RATIONALES
Describe the physiologic action of cholinesterase inhibitors and how they improve cognition.	The two approved cholinesterase inhibitors, tacrine (Cognex) and donepezil (Aricept), do not cure Alzheimer's disease. Instead, they slow cognitive decline by slowing breakdown of acetylcholine released by intact cholinergic neurons. Tacrine was the first drug of this kind to be approved. Donepezil is a second-generation cholinesterase inhibitor.
Advise patient, caregiver, and family that these drugs will return patient's function to the level that was present 6-12 mo before the medication was started.	This is a significant improvement and may delay nursing home placement for as much as a year.

Continued

INTERVENTIONS	**RATIONALES**
Teach the side-effect profile of the specific prescribed medication and methods for dealing with those effects.	Knowledge about expected side effects and adverse effects is important for enhancing compliance.
Donepezil HCl (Aricept)	
Be alert for headache, fatigue, dizziness, confusion, nausea, vomiting, diarrhea, upset stomach, poor appetite, abdominal pain, rhinitis, and skin rash.	Common side effects, which if they become severe, should be reported to prescriber for possible decrease in dosage or gradual discontinuation.
Take drug exactly as prescribed around the clock and on an empty stomach.	Specific patient/family education.
If GI upset occurs, administer with meals.	A full stomach may decrease gastric upset.
Maintain appointments for regular blood work and medical follow-up while adjusting to drug.	This is especially important if patient has preexisting medical conditions, such as renal, liver, or cardiac disease, because these drugs may affect these organs.
Do not abruptly discontinue drug.	Can cause cognitive disorder.
Avoid use in pregnancy.	Safety not established.
Caution is necessary for patients with renal and hepatic disease, seizures, sick sinus syndrome, and GI bleeding.	Can worsen these conditions.
Avoid concomitant use with nonsteroidal antiinflammatory drugs (NSAIDs).	May increase effects and risk of toxicity.
Concomitant use with anticholinergic agents may decrease effect.	The action of donepezil is to inhibit action of cholinesterase, thus elevating acetylcholine levels in the cortex.
Tacrine (Cognex)	
Be alert for GI symptoms including diarrhea, nausea, and abdominal discomfort; polyuria; and increased sweating.	Common side effects.
Effectiveness of drug depends on taking it at regular intervals, as directed.	Specific patient/family education.
Notify provider about severity of side effects and any change in severity or emergence of new events.	May necessitate change in dose or medication.
Do not abruptly discontinue.	Can cause decline in cognitive function.
Give with food if GI symptoms are severe.	Reduces severity of side effects; however, it also decreases bioavailability of drug.
The drug should be used with caution if patient already has abnormal liver function tests.	The drug may cause liver damage.
The drug should be used with caution in patient with bladder outlet obstruction, asthma, sick sinus syndrome, cardiovascular disease, asthma, or peptic ulcer.	Taking the drug can worsen these conditions.
See care plans for "Major Depression," p. 803, "Anxiety Disorders," p. 775, and "Schizophrenia," p. 813, for a review of antidepressants, anxiolytics, and antipsychotic medications.	Patients with Alzheimer's disease may also suffer from co-occurring depression, anxiety, and psychosis.

●●● **Related NIC and NOC labels:** *NIC:* Teaching: Prescribed Medication *NOC:* Knowledge: Medication

ADDITIONAL NURSING DIAGNOSES/ PROBLEMS:

PATIENT-FAMILY TEACHING AND DISCHARGE PLANNING

The patient with dementia—Alzheimer's type progresses through predictable stages, each with characteristic symptoms and behaviors that directly affect the ability to effectively process and use new information. As the disease progresses, the patient requires increasing amounts of physical care, and the caregiver/family require information and support. Dementia is a family disease.

As soon as the diagnosis is made, education of the family begins. They need information on the nature and expected progress of the disease and use of memory triggers; establishment of a schedule for basic activities, such as bathing, toileting, meals, and naps; monitoring for intake and output, weight, and skin status; recognition of nonverbal indications of needs and problems; use of redirection and distraction to reduce difficult behaviors; identification of new symptoms or changes; physical and mental activities; necessary environmental modifications, safety measures, and legal issues; sources of information and support; and community resources for caregiving assistance and respite.

Teaching must be geared to a time when medication has begun to lift mood and clear thinking processes; otherwise, it is a wasted effort. Verbal teaching should be simple and supplemented with reading materials the patient and/or significant other and family can refer to at a later time. Ensure that follow-up treatment is scheduled and that patient and/or significant other and family understand the need to get prescriptions filled and to take medication as prescribed. Consider whether or not patient has transportation available to get to follow-up treatment. Psychiatric home care might be a valuable part of the discharge planning to facilitate compliance with the discharge plan. In addition, provide patient and/or significant other/ family with verbal and written information about the following issues:

✓ Nature and expected course of Alzheimer's disease.

✓ Medications, including drug name, purpose, dosage, frequency, precautions, drug/drug and food/drug interactions, and potential side effects.

✓ Strategies to deal with difficult behaviors.

✓ Strategies to maintain patient safety.

✓ Importance of self-care for the caregiver.

✓ Importance of using all available supports to aid in caregiving.

✓ Importance of caregiver and family engaging in honest expression of feelings and confronting negative emotions.

✓ Importance of caregiver using relaxation techniques to minimize stress.

✓ Importance of maintaining or achieving spiritual well-being for patient and caregiver.

✓ Referrals to community resources for support and education. Additional information can be obtained by contacting the following organizations:

Alzheimer's Association
919 North Michigan Avenue, Suite 1000
Chicago, IL 60611
(800) 272-3900
www.alz.org
Provides a 24-hour hotline, free publications, and information for local chapters. *Worship Services for People with Alzheimer's Disease and Their Families: A Handbook* is also available through this organization.

American Association of Retired Persons (AARP)
601 E. Street, NW
Washington, DC 20049
www.aarp.org
Advocacy group for elderly; also provides (for a reasonable fee) training materials associated with reminiscence therapy.

National Institute on Aging (NIA)
Public Information Office
Federal Building
Room 5C27, Building 3
9000 Rockville Parkway
Bethesda, MD 20892
www.nia.nih.gov
Alzheimer's Disease Education and Reference Center (ADEAR) is available through NIA.

99

Major Depression

Major depression is one of the mood disorders, a category of disorders characterized by profound sadness or apathy, irritability, or elation. These disorders rank among the most serious and poorly diagnosed and treated of the health problems in the United States. Major depression is defined as an illness characterized by either depression or the loss of interest in nearly all activities. The symptoms must be present for at least 2 wk. At least four other symptoms must be present from the following list: changes in appetite or weight, sleep, and psychomotor activity; feelings of worthlessness and guilt; difficulty concentrating or making decisions; and recurrent thoughts of death or suicidal ideation, plans, or attempts.

Major depression affects emotional, cognitive, behavioral, and spiritual dimensions. Depression may range from mild-to-moderate states to severe states with or without psychotic features. Major depression can begin at any age, although it usually begins in the mid-20s and 30s. The risk factors for depression include prior history of depression, family history of depression, prior suicide attempts, female gender, age of onset <40 yr of age, postpartum period, medical comorbidity, lack of social support, stressful life events, personal history of sexual abuse, and current substance abuse. There are many theories to explain causation of depression. Research supports influence of the following factors: sleep disturbance; effects of pharmacologic substances, including many of the antihypertensive, steroidal, cardiovascular, and antipsychotic medications; neuronal factors that involve injury or malfunction of the brain, such as stroke, Parkinson's disease, and deficiencies in neurotransmitters; endocrinologic factors, such as thyroid dysfunction; genetic factors; and psychodynamic factors.

HEALTH CARE SETTING

Primarily primary care settings, that is, offices of private psychiatrist, psychologist, or psychiatric nurse practitioner or clinics with occasional brief acute care hospitalization for very severe depression, especially if there is serious suicide threat.

ASSESSMENT

The assessment of major depression involves much more than an assessment of mood. It is a holistic disorder that results in changes in self-attitude (feelings of self-worth), as well as vital sense (sense of physical well-being) and spiritual sense.

Feelings, attitudes, and knowledge: Negative feelings expressed include sadness, lack of joy and happiness about anything, shame, humiliation, fear of reprisals if others find out about depression, denial, anger, fear of experiencing a relapse, and fear of passing the disorder on to children.

Signs of low mood: Withdrawal from activities that once provided pleasure, as well as from social interactions; negativism expressed in excessive skepticism and stubborn resistance to suggestions, orders, or instructions from others; and unhappiness expressed in persistent sadness or frequent crying.

Signs of lowered self-attitude: Self-deprecating, guilty, or self-blaming comments are common, as well as expressions of hopelessness.

Signs of decreased vital sense: A depressed person may neglect personal appearance or let assignments, tasks, and projects slide. Decreased energy is very common, with the depressed person complaining of fatigue and difficulty getting activities started, especially in the early morning hours. A decreased ability to concentrate makes it difficult for individuals to think through a problem. The inability to make choices becomes apparent even with simple decisions that were previously made routinely.

Spiritual Issues: Depression carries with it many negative experiences, such as marital and family problems, divorce, and unemployment, which contribute to the downward spiral of self-appraisals. Depression can lead to a crisis in faith in self, others, life, and ultimately God. This loss of faith and hope contributes significantly to the risk of suicide.

Additional signs: Some depressed individuals experience decreased appetite leading to weight loss. Others experience an increase in appetite and weight. A change in sleep pattern is characteristic of depression, with many depressed individuals awakening in the early morning hours between 2 AM and 6 AM, whereas others experience a need for excessive sleep and have difficulty awakening. A decline in sexual interest and activity is characteristic of depressed individuals.

Suicidality: Suicide assessment is critical with depressed patients and includes questions to determine the presence of suicidal ideation and the lethality of any plan. Essential questions to ask include:

- Have you thought of hurting yourself?
- Are you presently thinking about hurting yourself?
- If you have been thinking about suicide, do you have a plan?
- What is the plan?
- Have you thought about what life would be like if you were no longer a part of it?

A previous history of suicide attempts combined with depression places the patient at high risk in the present for attempting suicide. A patient whose depression is lifting is at higher risk for suicide than a severely depressed individual. The improvement may result in an increase in energy. This increased energy is not enough to make the patient feel good or hopeful, but it is enough to carry out a suicidal plan.

DIAGNOSTIC TESTS

Although there are physical changes such as abnormal sleep electroencephalograms (EEGs) that coincide with sleep disturbances, sleep EEGs are not used to diagnose depression. The diagnosis of depression is made through history, interview of patient and family, and observation of verbal and nonverbal behaviors. A number of effective scales are available to quantify the degree of depression, such as the Zung Self-Rating Depression Scale, the Beck Depression Inventory, and the Geriatric Depression Scale.

Nursing Diagnosis:

Deficient Knowledge:

Causes, signs and symptoms, and treatment of depression

Desired Outcome: By discharge (if inpatient) or after 4 wk of outpatient treatment, patient and significant other verbalize accurate information about at least two of the possible causes of depression, four of the signs and symptoms of depression, and use of medications, psychotherapy, and/or electroconvulsive therapy (ECT) as treatment.

INTERVENTIONS	RATIONALES
Inform patient and significant other that depression is a physiologic disorder caused by the interplay of many factors such as stress, loss, imbalance in brain chemistry, and genetics.	Many people believe that depression is caused by character weakness. This belief contributes to the stigma experienced by the person suffering with depression and interferes with seeking treatment.
Inform patient and significant other about the major symptoms of depression.	Many people believe depression equates with sadness and fail to recognize the many other signs and symptoms that make this a holistic disorder. These include sadness, loss of interest in normal activities, plus at least four of the following: changes in appetite or weight, sleep, or psychomotor activity; feelings of worthlessness and guilt; difficulty concentrating or making decisions; recurrent thoughts of death or suicidal ideation, plans, or attempts. If the depressed individual displays sadness through irritability, the conclusion that depression is present may be missed, and consequently, necessary treatment may be delayed or avoided entirely.
Inform patient and significant other that depression is treatable.	Medications are usually indicated for treatment. They do not solve the stressors or problems that may have precipitated the depression, but they provide the energy to deal with these issues. Antidepressants or psychotherapy or a combination of both generally relieves the symptoms of depression in weeks.

Continued

INTERVENTIONS	RATIONALES
Inform patient and significant other about electroconvulsive therapy (ECT) if this is appropriate.	Many antidepressant drugs take ≥3 wk to lift the mood. In the meantime, ECT may be used to achieve more rapid results and may provide necessary protection for the suicidal patient. Patient and significant other/family may fear ECT. This intervention provides an opportunity for education that presents ECT as a positive treatment alternative.

●●● **Related NIC and NOC labels:** *NIC:* Teaching: Disease Process; Teaching: Procedures/Treatment
NOC: Knowledge: Illness Care; Knowledge: Disease Process

Nursing Diagnosis:

Hopelessness

related to losses, stresses, and basic symptoms of depression

Desired Outcome: By discharge (if inpatient) or by the end of 4 wk of outpatient treatment, patient verbalizes feelings and acceptance of life situations over which he or she has no control, demonstrates independent problem-solving techniques to take control over life, and does not demonstrate or verbalize suicidality.

INTERVENTIONS	RATIONALES
Identify unhealthy behaviors used to cope with feelings.	Patient may have tried to overcome feelings of hopelessness with harmful and ineffective behaviors (e.g., withdrawal, substance abuse, avoidance) Recognizing these behaviors provides an opportunity for change.
Encourage patient to identify and verbalize feelings and perceptions.	The process of identifying feelings that underlie and drive behaviors enables patients to begin taking control of their lives.
Identify individual signs of hopelessness.	Helps to focus attention on areas of individual need. These signs may include decreased physical activity and social withdrawal.
Express hope to patient in a low-key manner.	Patient may feel hopeless, but it is helpful to hear positive expressions from others.
Help patient identify areas of life that are under his or her control.	Patient's emotional state may interfere with problem solving. Assistance may be required to identify areas that are under his or her control and to have clarity about options for taking control.
Encourage patient to assume responsibility for own self-care, for example, setting realistic goals, scheduling activities, and making independent decisions.	Helping patient set realistic goals increases feelings of control and provides satisfaction when goals are achieved, thereby decreasing feelings of hopelessness.
Help patient identify areas of life situation that are not within his or her ability to control. Discuss feelings associated with this lack of control.	Patient needs to recognize and resolve feelings associated with inability to control certain life situations before acceptance can be achieved and hopefulness becomes possible
Encourage patient to examine spiritual supports that may provide hope.	Many people find that spiritual beliefs and practices are a great source of hope.
Conduct a suicide assessment to determine level of suicide risk.	High risk will necessitate hospitalization.

Continued

INTERVENTIONS	RATIONALES
Ask patient to enter into a "No Harm Contract" whereby he or she makes a commitment not to harm self.	Unwillingness to enter into a "No Harm Contract" is indication for hospitalization. The rationale for the contract is that people usually honor commitments they make. In addition, agreeing with a nurse or physician not to harm self communicates an awareness that the nurse and/or physician cares about patient's safety.
Administer antidepressant medication or teach importance of taking medication as prescribed (for additional interventions, see **Risk for Suicide,** next).	Suicidal thinking is a symptom of depression that is ameliorated through appropriate medication.

●●● **Related NIC and NOC labels:** *NIC:* Crisis Intervention; Hope Installation; Spiritual Support; Suicide Prevention; Decision-Making Support; Patient Contracting; Self-Modification Assistance
NOC: Mood Equilibrium; Decision Making; Depression Control

Nursing Diagnosis:

Risk for Suicide

related to depressed mood and feelings of worthlessness

Desired Outcome: By discharge (if inpatient) or by the end of 4 wk (if outpatient), patient expresses and demonstrates that he or she is free of suicidal thinking.

INTERVENTIONS	RATIONALES
Complete an initial suicide assessment (see specific questions under "Assessment").	The degree of hopelessness expressed by the patient is important in assessing risk for suicide. The more the patient has thought out the plan, the greater the risk. Risk for suicide is increased if the patient has a history of a previous attempt or there is family history of suicide and depression. Patients who display impulsive behaviors are more likely to attempt suicide without giving clues. Patients who are experiencing psychotic thinking, especially when there are "voices" that encourage self-harm, are at great risk. Use of alcohol/substance abuse in the presence of any of the above risk factors increases the overall risk for a suicide attempt. A high risk for suicide should prompt hospitalization.
Reassess for suicidality, especially during times of change.	Changes such as patient's mood improving, medication regimen being altered, discharge planning being initiated, and increasing withdrawal are all signals to reassess suicidality. Suicide risk is greatest in the first few weeks after treatment is begun. The patient may be feeling a little better but not well enough to feel hopeful and may have regained enough energy to actually act on what seemed to be just suicidal thoughts.
Ask patient to enter into a "No Harm Contract" whereby he or she makes a commitment not to harm self.	This contract is signed by patient and nurse. It may also include other information such as telephone numbers of crisis hotlines, police, or other emergency personnel for patient to call if suicidal thinking becomes more intense and patient doubts his or her ability to honor the "No Harm

Continued

INTERVENTIONS	RATIONALES
	Contract." Unwillingness to enter into a "No Harm Contract" is indication for hospitalization. The rationale for the contract is that people usually honor commitments they make. In addition, agreeing with a nurse or physician not to harm self communicates an awareness that the nurse and/or physician care about patient's safety.
Administer antidepressant medication or instruct patient regarding importance of taking medication as prescribed.	Suicidal thinking is a symptom of depression that is ameliorated through appropriate medication.
Teach significant other safety precautions and to be alert for changes in patient's behavior and/or verbalization that would indicate an increase in suicidal thinking.	Using available support provides a safety net for patient and communicates that he or she is not alone but that others are concerned and involved in care.
If patient is hospitalized:	
Monitor q15min for moderate risk or provide constant one-on-one observation for serious risk. Place in room close to nurses' station. Do not assign to a single room. Accompany patient to all off-unit activities. Ask patient to remain in view of staff at all times.	Providing close observation may prevent suicidal attempts.
Remove items such as belts, scarves, razor blades, shoe laces, scissors—anything that could be used for self-harm. Check all items brought into unit by patients. Instruct family members to avoid bringing into the unit any hazardous items.	Provides environmental safety and removes potential suicide weapons.
Provide supervision when patient is in bathroom—door must remain open with staff member outside.	It is important to remove all opportunities to engage in self-harmful behaviors.
Make sure that patient swallows medications that are administered.	Prevents saving up medications to overdose or discarding and not taking.
Ensure that nursing rounds are made at frequent but irregular intervals, especially at times that are predictably busy for the staff, that is, change of shift, toward early morning.	It is important that staff surveillance not be predictable; otherwise, patient would be able to identify a possible suicide time. In addition, it is essential to maintain awareness of patient's location at all times.
Routinely check environment for hazards and ensure environmental safety.	Minimizing opportunities for self-harm (e.g., keeping doors, windows, and access to stairways and roof locked and monitoring cleaning chemical and repair supplies) is an ongoing concern requiring constant vigilance.

●●● **Related NIC and NOC labels:** *NIC:* Area Restriction; Behavior Management: Self-Harm; Environmental Management: Safety; Patient Contracting; Risk Identification; Security Enhancement; Surveillance: Safety; Suicide Prevention *NOC:* Impulse Control; Suicide Self-Restraint

Nursing Diagnosis:

Dysfunctional Grieving

related to actual or perceived loss

Desired Outcome: By discharge (if inpatient) or by the end of 4 wk of outpatient treatment, patient demonstrates progress in dealing with stages of grief at own pace, participates in work/self-care activities at own pace, and verbalizes a sense of progress toward resolution of grief and hope for the future.

INTERVENTIONS	RATIONALES
Assess losses that have occurred in the patient's life. Discuss the meaning these losses have had for patient.	Many people deny the importance/impact of a loss. They fail to recognize, acknowledge, or talk about their pain and act as if everything is fine. This, then, has a cumulative effect on the individual. Denial requires physical and psychic energy. When individuals become clinically depressed, they likely do so in a physically and emotionally depleted state.
Discuss cultural practices and religious beliefs and ways in which patient has dealt with past losses.	Cultural practices and religious beliefs influence how people express and accept the grieving process.
Encourage patient to identify and verbalize feelings and examine the relationship between feelings and event/stressor.	Verbalizing feelings in a nonthreatening environment can help patient deal with unrecognized/unresolved issues that may be contributing to depression. It also helps patient connect the response (feeling) to the stressor or precipitating event.
Discuss healthy ways to identify and cope with underlying feelings of hurt, rejection, and anger.	This helps expand patient's repertoire of coping strategies. The presentation of choices for behaving differently can often decrease feeling of being stuck.
If indicated, tell stories of how others have coped with similar situations.	This not only provides possible solutions but also suggests that the problem is manageable.
Teach normal stages of grief and acknowledge the reality of associated feelings, that is, guilt, anger, powerlessness.	Helps patient realize the normalcy of feelings and may alleviate some of the guilt generated by these feelings.
Assist patient with naming the problem, identifying need to address the problem differently, and fully describing all aspects of the problem.	Before patient can agree to change, he or she needs clarity about what the problem is.
Help patient identify and recognize early signs of depression and plan ways to alleviate these signs. Assist with formulating a plan that recognizes need for outside support if symptoms continue and/or worsen.	This actively involves patient and conveys the message that patient is not powerless but rather options are available.

●●● **Related NIC and NOC labels:** *NIC:* Coping Enhancement; Counseling; Grief Work Facilitation; Emotional Support; Support System Enhancement; Active Listening *NOC:* Coping; Grief Resolution

Nursing Diagnosis:

Self-Esteem Disturbance

related to the negative self-appraisal that is symptomatic of depression

Desired Outcome: By discharge (if inpatient) or after 4 wk of outpatient treatment, patient demonstrates behaviors consistent with increased self-esteem.

INTERVENTIONS	RATIONALES
Encourage patient to engage in self-care grooming activities.	Attending to grooming is often an initial step in feeling better about oneself.
Provide positive reinforcement for all observable accomplishments.	Patients with low self-esteem do not benefit from flattery or insincere praise. Honest, positive feedback enhances self-esteem.
Encourage patient to participate in simple recreational activities or art projects, proceeding to more complex activities in a group setting.	Initially patient may be too overwhelmed to engage in activities that involve more than one person.

Continued

INTERVENTIONS	RATIONALES
If patient persists in negativism about self, place a limit on length of time you will listen to negativity.	Time limits allow patient a safe time and place to vent negative feelings and demonstrate thought stopping, the conscious interruption of negative thoughts. For example, agree to 10 min of negativity followed by 10 min of positive comments.
Teach thought-stopping techniques.	Many depressed people engage in self-critical thinking and need to be taught to consciously stop that type of thinking and substitute positive thinking in its place.
Explore patient's personal strengths and suggest making a list to use as a reminder when negative thoughts return.	Having a written list to review can help patient during difficult times.

●●● **Related NIC and NOC labels:** *NIC:* Self-Esteem Enhancement; Cognitive Restructuring; Self-Awareness Enhancement; Socialization Enhancement *NOC:* Self-Esteem

Nursing Diagnosis:

Deficient Knowledge:

Medication use in depression, including potential side effects

Desired Outcome: By discharge (if inpatient) or after 4 wk of outpatient treatment, patient verbalizes accurate information about prescribed medications and their potential side effects.

INTERVENTIONS	RATIONALES
Teach physiologic action of antidepressant and how it alleviates symptoms of depression.	Many depressed patients resist taking medications because they fear becoming "addicted" to the drug. However, the antidepressants are not addictive drugs. Providing the patient with information about the drug's physiologic action helps with compliance.
Caution patient about importance of taking medication at pre-scribed dose and time interval.	These medications require certain blood levels to be therapeutic; therefore patient needs to take the medication at the dose and time prescribed.
Teach the side-effect profile of the specific prescribed medica-tion, including interventions to combat these effects, for the following drugs.	Each class of antidepressants carries with it a specific side-effect profile. Knowledge about expected side effects, ways to manage these side effects, and the length of time these side effects last is important in ensuring compliance.
Tricyclic antidepressants: amitriptyline (Elavil), desipramine (Norpramin), doxepin (Sinequan), imipramine (Tofranil), nortriptyline (Pamelor), protriptyline (Vivactil), and trim-ipramine (Surmontil)	These older antidepressant medications are effective in decreasing signs and symptoms of depression but can produce some troublesome side effects, such as anticholin-ergic effects, fatigue, weight gain, and orthostatic changes.
Potential for anticholinergic effects, sedation, hypotension, and weight gain.	Common side effects.
Drink at least 8 glasses of water a day and add high-fiber foods to diet.	Combats constipation, an anticholinergic effect.
Rise from a sitting position slowly.	Orthostatic hypotension is a potential side effect.
Suck on sugar-free candy or mints or use sugar-free chewing gum.	Combats dry mouth, an anticholinergic effect.
Establish sleep routine and regular exercise.	Combats feelings of fatigue.

Continued

INTERVENTIONS	RATIONALES
Limit refined sugars and carbohydrates.	Combats weight gain and controls carbohydrate cravings.
Patients with seizure history need to be monitored for seizures.	Tricyclics lower the seizure threshold.
Signs of cardiac toxicity. Patients >40 yr of age need an EEG evaluation before treatment and periodically thereafter.	These drugs may decrease the vagal influence on the heart secondary to muscarinic blockade and by acting directly on bundle of His to slow conduction. Both effects increase risk of dysrhythmias.
Possible drug interactions.	The combination of tricyclics with monoamine oxidase (MAO) inhibitors can cause severe hypertension. The combination of tricyclics with central nervous system (CNS) depressants such as alcohol, antihistamines, opioids, and barbiturates can cause severe CNS depression. Because of the anticholinergic effects of tricyclics, any other anticholinergic drug, including over-the-counter antihistamines and sleeping aids, should be avoided.
MAO inhibitors: isocarboxazid (Marplan), phenelzine (Nardil), and tranylcypromine (Parnate)	MAO inhibitors are used when patient has not responded to other antidepressants.
Potential for mild sedation and hypotension.	Common side effects.
MAO inhibitor restrictions.	MAO inhibitors combined with dietary tyramine can cause a life-threatening hypertensive crisis. Dietary restrictions include avocados; fermented bean curd; fermented soybean; soybean paste; figs; bananas; fermented, smoked, or aged meats; liver; bologna, pepperoni, and salami; dried, cured, fermented, or smoked fish; practically all cheeses; yeast extract; some imported beers; Chianti wine; protein dietary supplements; soups that contain protein extract; shrimp paste; and soy sauce. Large amounts of chocolate, fava beans, ginseng, and caffeine may cause a reaction.
Possible drug interactions and need to avoid all prescription and over-the-counter drugs unless they have been specifically approved by provider.	MAO inhibitors can interact with many drugs to cause potentially serious results. Use of ephedrine or amphetamines can lead to hypertensive crisis. The interaction of tricyclic antidepressants with MAO inhibitors is discussed above. Selective serotonin reuptake inhibitors (SSRIs) should not be used with MAO inhibitors (see rationale, below). Antihypertensive drugs combined with MAO inhibitors may result in excessive lowering of blood pressure. MAO inhibitors with meperidine (Demerol) can cause hyperpyrexia (excessive elevation of temperature).
SSRIs: fluoxetine (Prozac), fluvoxamine maleate (Luvox), sertraline HCl (Zoloft), paroxetine (Paxil), and citalopram (Celexa)	SSRIs are as effective as tricyclic antidepressants but have a better safety profile and are better tolerated.
Potential for nausea, headache, nervousness, insomnia, anxiety, agitation, sexual dysfunction, dizziness, fatigue, rash, diarrhea, excessive sweating, and anorexia with weight loss.	Reported side effects.
Possible drug interactions.	Interaction with MAO inhibitors can cause serotonin syndrome, a potentially life-threatening event. Symptoms include anxiety, diaphoresis, rigidity, hyperthermia, autonomic hyperactivity, and coma. Because of this possibility, MAO inhibitors should be withdrawn at least 14 days before starting an SSRI, and when an SSRI is discontinued, at least 5 wk should elapse before an MAO inhibitor is given.
Dual mechanism drugs: venlafaxine (Effexor) and nefazodone HCl (Serzone)	These drugs inhibit both norepinephrine and serotonin uptake and are used when tricyclics and SSRIs fail to improve symptoms.

Continued

INTERVENTIONS	RATIONALES
Potential for nausea, somnolence, dizziness, dry mouth, and sweating.	Common side effects.
Importance of frequent BP measurements for patients taking venlafaxine.	Venlafaxine causes an increase in BP in doses >200 mg/day.
Miscellaneous antidepressants: trazodone (Desyrel), amoxapine (Asendin), bupropion (Wellbutrin), and maprotiline (Ludiomil)	
Potential for anticholinergic effects (except trazodone), sedation, hypotension, and risks of falling related to dizziness associated with hypotension.	Common side effects.
Risk for seizures.	Risk is moderate with trazodone and increases with amoxapine, bupropion, and maprotiline.
Risk of cardiac toxicity. Patients >40 yr of age need an EEG evaluation before treatment and periodically thereafter.	Risk is minimal with amoxapine, bupropion, and trazodone. There is significant risk with maprotiline.

●●● **Related NIC and NOC labels:** *NIC:* Teaching: Prescribed Medication *NOC:* Knowledge: Medication

ADDITIONAL NURSING DIAGNOSES/ PROBLEMS:

"Anxiety" for **Social Isolation**	p. 778
"Bipolar Disorder" for:	
Imbalanced Nutrition: Less than body requirements	p. 788
Self-Care Deficit	p. 789
"Substance Abuse" for **Interrupted Family Processes**	p. 822

PATIENT-FAMILY TEACHING AND DISCHARGE PLANNING

The patient with major depression experiences a wide variety of symptoms that affect the ability to learn and retain information. Teaching must be geared to a time when medication has begun to lift mood and clear thinking processes; otherwise, it is a wasted effort. Verbal teaching should be simple and supplemented with reading materials the patient and/or significant other and family can refer to at a later time. Ensure that follow-up treatment is scheduled and that patient and/or significant other and family understand the need to get prescriptions filled and importance of taking medication as prescribed. Consider whether or not patient has transportation available to get to follow-up treatment. Psychiatric home care might be a valuable part of the discharge planning to facilitate compliance with the discharge plan. In addition, provide patient and/or significant other/family verbal and written information about the following issues:

✓ Remission/exacerbation aspects of depression.

✓ Medications, including drug name, purpose, dosage, frequency, precautions, drug/drug and food/drug interactions, and potential side effects.

✓ Thought-stopping techniques for dealing with negativism.

✓ Importance of maintaining a healthy lifestyle—balanced diet, exercise, and regular adequate sleep patterns—to facilitate remaining in remission.

✓ Importance of continuing medication use long after depressive symptoms have gone.

✓ Importance of social support and strategies for obtaining it.

✓ Importance of using constructive coping skills to deal with stress.

✓ Importance of honest expression of feelings and confronting of negative emotions.

✓ Importance of using relaxation techniques to minimize stress.

✓ Importance of maintaining or achieving spiritual well-being.

✓ Importance of follow-up care, including day treatment programs, appointments with psychiatrist and therapists, and vocational rehabilitation program if indicated.

✓ Referrals to community resources for support and education. Additional information can be obtained by contacting the following organizations:

Depression and Related Affective Disorders Association (DRADA)
Meyer 3-181
600 North Wolfe Street
Baltimore, MD 21287-7381

(410) 955-4647 (Baltimore)
(202) 955-5800 (Washington D.C.)
www.drada.org/
This nonprofit organization is composed of individuals with mood disorders, family members, and mental health professionals. It offers information, education, referral, and support services to people nationwide. DRADA sponsors a nationally renowned training program for group leaders.

Depression Awareness, Recognition, and Treatment Program (D/ART)
5600 Fisher's Lane, Suite 10-85
Rockville, MD 20857
(301) 443-4140
Fax: (301) 443-4045
D/ART is a national self-help clearinghouse. It provides a list of resources throughout the United States that can help in networking and providing consultative assistance.

100

Schizophrenia

Schizophrenia is a neurobiologic disorder of the brain categorized as a thought disorder with disturbances in thinking, feeling, perceiving, and relating to others and the environment. Schizophrenia is a mixture of both positive and negative symptoms that are present for a significant part of a 1-mo period but with continuous signs of disturbance persisting for at least 6 mo. Positive symptoms are those that exist but should not be present including delusions, hallucinations, thought disorder, disorganized speech, and disorganized or catatonic behavior. Negative symptoms refer to behaviors that should be present but are not, including restriction or flattening in the range and intensity of emotion, reduced fluency and productivity of thought and speech, withdrawal and inability to initiate and persist in goal-directed activity, and inability to experience pleasure. Schizophrenia is considered the most disabling of the major mental disorders, with an estimated 2 million Americans afflicted. Risk factors include being unmarried and <45 years of age for both men and women, having been the product of a difficult birth during the winter, and living in an industrialized urban area as a member of the lower socioeconomic class. Theories of causation include genetics, infectious autoimmune factors, neuroanatomic changes, the dopamine hypothesis, and psychologic factors. There are several subtypes of schizophrenia, including paranoid, disorganized, catatonic, undifferentiated, and residual.

HEALTH CARE SETTING

Most patients with schizophrenia receive treatment across a variety of settings, including inpatient and partial hospitalization, day treatment, psychiatric home care, and crisis stabilization. Community services include assertive community treatment, outpatient therapy, case management, and psychosocial rehabilitation.

ASSESSMENT

Schizophrenia affects all aspects of a person's being. How the individual looks, feels, thinks, interacts with others, and moves in the world are all drastically affected by this disorder. A thorough assessment focuses not only on the bizarre behaviors characteristic of the disease but on the whole person—his or her physical, emotional, social, and spiritual dimensions.

Biologic: A thorough history and physical are essential to rule out medical illness or substance abuse that could cause the psychiatric symptoms. It is essential to screen for comorbid treatable medical illnesses. People with schizophrenia have a higher mortality rate from physical illness and often have smoking-related illnesses such as emphysema and other pulmonary and cardiac disorders. The patient may appear awkward and uncoordinated, with poor motor skills and abnormalities in eye tracking. It is important before any medications are begun to have a baseline regarding abnormal movements. Use of a standardized assessment of abnormal movement disorders such as the Abnormal Involuntary Movement Scale (AIMS) or the Simpson-Angus Rating Scale is recommended.

Psychologic: Many patients report prodromal symptoms of tension and nervousness, lack of interest in eating, difficulty concentrating, disturbed sleep, decreased enjoyment and loss of interest, restlessness, forgetfulness, depression, social withdrawal from friends, feeling that others are laughing at them, feeling bad for no reason, thinking about religion more, hearing voices or seeing things, and feeling too excited. Most of these symptoms are negative ones.

Appearance: Patient may appear in bizarre and eccentric dress, be disheveled, and have poor hygiene.

Objective behaviors: Patient may display stereotypy (idiosyncratic, repetitive, purposeless movements), echopraxia (involuntary imitation of another's movements), and waxy flexibility (posture held in odd or unusual fixed position for extended periods). Patient may display altered mood states ranging from heightened emotional activity to severely limited emotional responses. Affect, the outward expression of mood, may be described as flat, blunted, or full range, or it may be described as inappropriate. Other common emotional symptoms include affective lability, ambivalence, and apathy.

Delusions: Delusions are beliefs that are held despite clear contradictory evidence. Sometimes they are nonbizarre and plausible; at other times the delusions expressed are bizarre, implausible, and not derived from ordinary life experiences. Delusions of persecution are the most common type. Delusions of grandeur are also commonly expressed. Ideas of reference are delusional ideas in which these patients believe actions of others are directed toward them. It is important to assess content of the delusion; the degree of conviction with which the delusion is held; how extensively other aspects of patient's life are incorporated into the delusion; the degree of internal consistency, organization, and logic evidenced in the delusion; and the impact exerted on patient's life by this delusion.

Hallucinations: A hallucination is an alteration in sensory stimulation. Although hallucinations can be experienced in all sensory modalities, auditory hallucinations are the most frequent in schizophrenia. Patients may not spontaneously share their hallucinations, and in order to assess for them, nurses may need to rely on observations of the patient's behavior, including pauses in a conversation during which the patient seems to be preoccupied or appears to be listening to someone other than the interviewer, looking toward the perceived source of a voice, or responding to the voices in some manner.

Disorganized communication: Both speech content and patterns are important to assess. Abrupt shifts in conversational focus are typical of disorganized communication and are referred to as loose association. The most severe shifts may occur after only one or two words, and this is referred to as word salad; a less severe shift may occur after one or two phrases, and this is referred to as flight of ideas; the least severe shift in the focus occurs when a new topic is repeatedly suggested and pursued from the current topic, and this is referred to as tangentiality. In addition to these abrupt shifts from one topic to another, the person with schizophrenia experiences thought blocking in which thoughts and psychic activity unexpectedly cease. Language may be difficult to understand and may begin to serve as a tool of self-expression rather than a tool of communication. Sometimes the person creates completely new words, referred to as neologisms.

Cognitive impairments: Although cognitive impairments vary widely from patient to patient, several problems are consistent across most patients, and these include hypervigilance (increased and sustained attention on external stimuli over an extended time), a diminished ability to distinguish relevant from irrelevant stimuli, familiar cues going unrecognized or being improperly interpreted, and diminished information processing leading to inappropriate or illogical conclusions from available observations and information.

- *Memory and orientation:* Individuals with schizophrenia display impairments in memory and abstract thinking. Although orientation to time, place, and person remains relatively intact unless the person is preoccupied with delusions and hallucinations, all aspects of memory are affected in schizophrenia. Patients experience diminished ability to recall within seconds newly learned information. Short- and long-term memory are affected.
- *Insight and judgment:* Insight and judgment depend on cognitive functions that are frequently impaired in people with schizophrenia.

Social issues: As the disorder progresses, individuals become increasingly socially isolated. People with schizophrenia have difficulty connecting with others on a one-to-one basis. Emotional blunting, inability to form emotional attachments, problems with face and affect recognition, inability to recall past interactions, problems making decisions and using appropriate judgment in difficult situations, and poverty of speech and language all serve to separate and isolate the individual.

Spiritual issues: Persons with schizophrenia may experience delusions and hallucinations with religious content, and some health care providers tend to dismiss all religious verbalizations as psychotic expressions. However, the contrary is true. Religion and spirituality can be a source of comfort to patients dealing with a terrible disease. It is important to assess religious commitment, religious practices, and spiritual issues such as the meaning of the illness to the individual, the role of God, and sources of hope and support.

Suicidality: Suicide assessment is critical in schizophrenia. The presence of psychotic thinking and command hallucinations, coupled with possible substance abuse, increases the suicide risk significantly. It is important to ask questions to determine the presence of suicidal ideation and the lethality of any plan. Essential questions to ask include:

- Have you thought of hurting yourself?
- Are you presently thinking about hurting yourself?
- If you have been thinking about suicide, do you have a plan? What is the plan?
- Have you thought about what life would be like if you were no longer a part of it?

DIAGNOSTIC TESTS

There are no specific tests to diagnose schizophrenia. Diagnosis is made using the diagnostic criteria put forth in *The Diagnostic and Statistical Manual IV* (American Psychiatric Association, 1994) through history, interview of patient and family, and observation of verbal and nonverbal behaviors. There are several reliable rating scales that are useful in the diagnosis of schizophrenia. These include the Scale for the Assessment of Negative Symptoms (SANS), Scale for the Assessment of Positive Symptoms (SAPS), Abnormal Involuntary Movement Scale (AIMS), Brief Psychiatric Rating Scale (BPRS), Simpson-Angus Rating Scale.

Nursing Diagnosis:

Deficient Knowledge:

Causes, signs and symptoms, and treatment of schizophrenia

Desired Outcome: Before discharge from care facility or after 4 wk of outpatient treatment, patient and/or significant other verbalize accurate information about at least two of the possible causes of schizophrenia, four of the signs and symptoms of the disorder, and the available treatment options.

INTERVENTIONS	RATIONALES
Explain that schizophrenia is a physiologic disorder caused by the interplay of many factors such as stress, genetics, infectious-autoimmune factors, neuroanatomic changes, the dopamine hypothesis, and psychologic factors.	Providing education about the physical basis for the disorder increases understanding and acceptance and decreases blaming behavior.
Inform patient and significant other that there are treatments available for schizophrenia.	Medications are essential to stabilize and maintain patients with schizophrenia. They decrease psychotic thinking, hallucinations, and delusions. Some, but not all, drugs target negative symptoms. However, medications are not enough. Comprehensive treatment involves inpatient and partial hospitalization, day treatment, psychiatric home care, and crisis stabilization. Community services include assertive community treatment, outpatient therapy, case management, and psychosocial rehabilitation.

●●● **Related NIC and NOC labels:** *NIC:* Teaching, Disease Process; Teaching: Procedure/Treatment
NOC: Knowledge: Illness Care; Knowledge: Disease Process

Nursing Diagnosis:

Disturbed Sensory Perception: Auditory

related to disturbance in thought and perception

Desired Outcome: Before discharge from care facility or after 4 wk of outpatient treatment, patient defines and tests reality, eliminating the occurrence of hallucinations.

INTERVENTIONS	RATIONALES
Evaluate and observe for hallucinations. Redirect back to reality by distracting patient with conversation.	Early assessment enables evaluation of patient's responses to hallucinations and how much time patient focuses on them. It also enables the nurse to assess if hallucinations place patient or others at risk and permits early intervention to protect patient, as well as others.
Ask what the voices are telling the patient.	It is essential to know if "voices" are command hallucinations that tell the patient to harm self or others. This question also communicates that the nurse does not hear the voices while at the same time validates presence of the voices in patient's reality.
Assure patient that you will provide safety for him or her regardless of what the voices say will happen.	This provides an anchor to reality and decreases patient's fear that harm will occur based on what the voices say.

Continued

INTERVENTIONS	RATIONALES
Avoid touching the patient.	Distortion of reality may lead patient to misinterpret physical touch, which along with excessive environmental stimuli can increase anxiety and precipitate hallucinations or aggressive response.
Determine when anxiety increases. Stay with patient to ensure safety.	Increasing anxiety often precedes hallucinations.
Administer antipsychotic medications as prescribed.	Antipsychotic medications reduce psychotic symptoms, including hallucinations.
Assist patient with increasing social interaction gradually, starting first with one-on-one interaction and progressing to small groups. Be available in a consistent, no-demand, supportive relationship.	Social isolation and lack of interpersonal relationships contribute to use of hallucinations as a substitute for human interaction. A slow, gradual approach to interaction with others based on reality enables some desensitization because interpersonal contacts often precipitate anxiety.
Investigate with patient sources of stress and explain the relationship of anxiety and stress to hallucinations.	Providing information about the relationship of anxiety and stress to hallucinations gives the patient increased control over the occurrence of hallucinations.
Teach patient to verbalize fears and describe methods for managing anxiety and stress constructively.	Verbalization of fears is one method of reducing anxiety. Alternative methods may also prove effective.

●●● **Related NIC and NOC labels:** *NIC:* Hallucination Management; Reality Orientation; Active Listening; Environmental Management; Anxiety Reduction *NOC:* Distorted Thought Control

Nursing Diagnosis:

Deficient Knowledge:

Medications used in schizophrenia, including purpose and potential side effects

Desired Outcome: Before discharge from care facility or after 4 wk of outpatient treatment, patient verbalizes accurate information about the prescribed medications.

INTERVENTIONS	RATIONALES
Teach patient about the physiologic action of antipsychotic medications.	Antipsychotics work by blocking dopamine receptors. People with schizophrenia appear to have excessive dopamine levels. Blocking dopamine decreases hallucinations, delusions, and confusion and improves disorganized speech, behavior, and perceptions.
Teach the Following Side-effect Profiles of the Specific Prescribed Medication, as Well as Interventions to Mitigate the Effects.	A knowledgeable patient is likely to report adverse symptoms and know how to intervene properly for others, which optimally will promote compliance.
Traditional antipsychotics: chlorpromazine (Thorazine), thioridazine (Mellaril), mesoridazine (Serentil), acetophenazine (Tindal), loxapine (Loxitane), molindone (Moban), perphenazine (Trilafon), trifluoperazine (Stelazine), thiothixene (Navane), fluphenazine (Prolixin), haloperidol (Haldol), and pimozide (Orap)	Traditional antipsychotics block all dopamine receptors in the central nervous system (CNS) and can produce serious movement disorders, referred to as extrapyramidal side effects (EPS).
Explain that sedation, orthostatic hypotension, and anticholinergic effects that can occur.	Common side effects of traditional antipsychotic drugs.

Continued

INTERVENTIONS	RATIONALES
Teach the patient to be alert for EPS, including acute dystonia (impaired muscle tone), parkinsonism, akathisia (restlessness, agitation), and tardive dyskinesia (involuntary movements of the face, trunk, and limbs) using the AIMS.	These are adverse effects of traditional antipsychotic drugs, with tardive dyskinesia being the most serious. Use of AIMS enables objective quantification of changes in movements and permits early intervention before the appearance of tardive dyskinesia.
Explain the potential for neuroleptic malignant syndrome (NMS).	This is an idiosyncratic hypersensitivity to antipsychotics that is believed to affect the body's thermoregulatory mechanism. It is a rare but serious reaction that carries with it a 4% risk of mortality.
Caution patient that there is a risk for seizures.	Antipsychotics can reduce seizure threshold and should be used with caution for patients with epilepsy or other seizure disorder.
Teach the importance of avoiding all drugs with anticholinergic actions, including antihistamines and specific over-the-counter sleeping aids.	Drugs with anticholinergic properties intensify the anticholinergic responses to antipsychotic drugs, including dry mouth, constipation, blurred vision, urinary hesitancy, and tachycardia.
Explain the importance of avoiding alcohol and other drugs with CNS-depressant actions, for example, antihistamines, opioids, and barbiturates.	Antipsychotics can intensify CNS depression caused by other drugs.
For patients taking Thorazine, triflupromazine (Vesprin), Serentil, Mellaril, Tindal, Prolixin, Trilafon, or Stelazine, teach the importance of avoiding excessive exposure to sunlight, using sunscreen, and wearing protective clothing.	These drugs belong to the phenothiazine class that causes sensitization of the skin to ultraviolet light, thus increasing the chance of severe sunburn.
Teach the patient that sexual dysfunction is a possible side effect and should be reported to the prescriber.	It is important that the patient not just stop the medication but rather report it so that the prescriber can intervene accordingly.
Atypical antipsychotic agents: clozapine (Clozaril), risperidone (Risperdal), olanzapine (Zyprexa), and quetiapine (Seroquel)	Atypical antipsychotics are more selective in blocking specific dopamine receptors. Because of this, they have less risk of EPS.
Teach Patients the Following:	
Patients taking clozapine should be alert for drowsiness and sedation, hypersalivation, tachycardia, constipation, and postural hypotension.	Common side effects of clozapine.
Patients taking clozapine need weekly hematologic monitoring for first 6 mo of treatment, and after 6 mo, monitoring is biweekly. Advise patient that clozapine will not be dispensed if the weekly or biweekly blood test is not done.	Agranulocytosis occurs in 1%-2% of patients, with an overall risk of death of about 1 in 5000. Agranulocytosis usually occurs in the first 6 mo.
Patients taking clozapine, especially those with seizure disorder, are at risk for seizures.	Generalized tonic-clonic seizures occur in 3% of patients taking clozapine, and the risk is dose related, with higher incidence in patients receiving doses >600 mg. Patients who have experienced a seizure should be warned not to drive a car or participate in other potentially hazardous activities while on this medication.
Patient taking clozapine should avoid drugs that can suppress bone marrow function such as carbamazepine (Tegretol) and many cancer drugs. Cimetidine and erythromycin increase levels of clozapine, leading to toxicity. Smoking, Tegretol, and phenytoin can decrease levels of clozapine, diminishing its efficacy.	These are drug interactions that can occur with clozapine.
Patients taking risperidone are at risk for insomnia, agitation, anxiety, constipation, nausea, dyspepsia and vomiting, dizziness, and sedation.	Common side effects of risperidone.

Continued

INTERVENTIONS	RATIONALES
Patients taking risperidone should be alert for EPS.	Adverse effect that is dose related (reported in doses >10 mg/day).
Patients taking olanzapine should be alert for headache, insomnia, constipation, weight gain, akathisia, and tremor.	Common side effects of olanzapine.
Patients taking quetiapine should be alert for headache, somnolence, constipation, and weight gain.	Common side effects of quetiapine.

●●● **Related NIC and NOC labels:** *NIC:* Teaching: Prescribed Medication *NOC:* Knowledge: Medication

ADDITIONAL NURSING DIAGNOSES/ PROBLEMS:

"Anxiety Disorders" for **Ineffective**   p. 779
    Coping: Compromised family coping

"Bipolar Disorder" for **Self-Care Deficit**   p. 789

"Major Depression" for:
   Hopelessness   p. 805
   Risk for Suicide   p. 806
   Self-Esteem Disturbance   p. 808

PATIENT-FAMILY TEACHING AND DISCHARGE PLANNING

The patient with schizophrenia experiences a wide variety of symptoms that affect the ability to learn and retain information. Teaching must be geared to a time when medication has begun to decrease the psychotic symptoms, thoughts are more organized, and communication is more effective. Verbal teaching should be simple and supplemented with reading materials that the patient and/or significant other and family can refer to at a later time.

Most patients with schizophrenia experience memory deficits, so retention of new information does not come easily. Repetition and attention to clarity and simplicity of teaching approaches and materials facilitate learning. Ensure that follow-up treatment is scheduled and that patient and/or significant other and family understand the need to get prescriptions filled and to take medication as prescribed. Consider whether or not patient has transportation available to get to follow-up treatment. Psychiatric home care might be a valuable part of the discharge planning to facilitate compliance with the discharge plan. In addition, provide patient and/or significant other/family with verbal and written information about the following issues:

✓ Medications, including drug name, purpose, dosage, frequency, precautions, drug/drug and food/drug interactions, and potential side effects.

✓ Importance of laboratory follow-up tests if patient is taking Clozaril.

✓ Importance of maintaining a healthy lifestyle—balanced diet, minimal to no caffeine or alcohol, exercise, and regular adequate sleep patterns—to facilitate remaining in remission.

✓ Importance of continuing medication use probably for a lifetime.

✓ Importance of social support and strategies to obtain it.

✓ Importance of using community follow-up resources, for example, psychiatrist, psychiatric nurse, intensive outpatient, support groups, family counseling, psychosocial programs including club houses, and other patient-run support groups.

✓ Importance of following up with medical care, as well as psychiatric care.

✓ Importance of maintaining or achieving spiritual well-being.

✓ Referrals to community resources for support and education. Additional information can be obtained by contacting the following organizations:

Person to Person (free Consumer and Family Support Service)
P.O. Box 21510
Boulder, CO 80308-4510
(800) 376-8282
Provides free educational and support services for people taking Risperdal (risperidone). Developed by Janssen Pharmaceutic Inc., Titusville, NJ 08560.

Lilly Cares Patient Assistance Program
Eli Lilly and Company
Lilly Corporate Center
Indianapolis, IN 46285
(800) 545-6962
Designed to assist providers, patients, and patient care-givers through reimbursement support and through temporary provision of Zyprexa and other drugs at no charge to eligible patients.

National Alliance for the Mentally Ill (NAMI)
Colonial Place Three
2107 Wilson Boulevard, Suite 300
Arlington, VA 22201
(800) 950-NAMI [6264] or (703) 524-7600
www.nami.org

Contact NAMI chapter in local state for information and schedule or contact national office of NAMI.

The NAMI Family to Family Education Program is a 12-session comprehensive course for families of people with serious mental illnesses.

Living with Schizophrenia

A two-session education program presented by consumers to other consumers.

Mental Illness Education Project, Inc.
P.O. Box 470813
Brookline Village, MA 02447
(800) 343-5540 or (617) 562-1111
www.miepvideos.org/
New videotape for families and mental health professionals entitled, "Families Coping with Mental Illness"

MedicAlert Foundation
2323 Colorado Avenue
Turlock, CA 95382
(888) 633-4298 or (209) 668-3333
www.medicalert.org
A simple tool to ensure that people with schizophrenia receive proper care in an emergency room or to help family members find a loved one who has stopped taking medication and is experiencing behavioral problems in public. To order a Medic Alert bracelet or necklace costs

$35.00 for a 1-year membership with stainless steel medallion. MedicAlert also has a program for people who cannot afford the fees.

National Institute of Mental Health
NIMH Public Inquiries
6001 Executive Boulevard
Room 8184, MSC 9663
Bethesda, MD 20892-9663
(301) 443-4513
www.nimh.nih.gov/
Booklet prepared by the Schizophrenia Research Branch, NIMH entitled, "Schizophrenia: Questions and Answers" (DHHS Publication No. ADM 90-1457).

National Alliance for Research on Schizophrenia and Depression (NARSAD)
60 Cutter Mill Road, Suite 404
Great Neck, NY 11021
(800) 829-8289 or (516) 829-0091
www.narsad.org/

Schizophrenia Society of Canada
75 The Donway West, Suite 814
Don Mills, ON M3C 2E9
(416) 445-8204
www.schizophrenia.ca/

Substance Abuse Disorders

Substance abuse is one of the major health issues in the United States. The connection between substance use and social and health problems is well documented and includes such issues as an increase in illegal and violent activities associated with the sale and distribution of illegal drugs, major health problems including the spread of human immunodeficiency virus (HIV) and other communicable diseases among IV drug users, developmental problems of babies born to addicted mothers, the epidemic of "crack babies," fetal alcohol syndrome babies, low-birth-weight babies, and the increase in domestic violence and child abuse/neglect. Deaths caused by motor vehicular accidents are directly linked to alcohol consumption. In addition, there are a full range of medical complications that are a direct result of alcohol dependence, including cardiovascular, respiratory, hematologic, nervous, digestive, endocrine, metabolic, skin, musculoskeletal, and genitourinary problems, as well as nutritional deficiencies.

The *Diagnostic and Statistical Manual IV (DSM-IV)* defines a substance abuse disorder as the nontherapeutic use of psychoactive agents or illicit use of a prescribed drug on a regular, binge, or episodic basis. The distinction between substance abuse and substance dependence is that the latter involves physical dependence and withdrawal symptoms. The rationale for classifying psychoactive substance disorders within a generic category of either substance use or substance dependence relates to commonalities in psychologic behavior patterns across drug classifications. Knowing the specific drug(s) abused is essential for treating toxicity and withdrawal. However, it is the outcome of psychoactive drug use, shared in common by all drug classifications, that is most likely to account for the problems associated with the disorder. These properties include acute and chronic structural and functional changes in the brain associated with drug intake; variable effects on the person

taking the drugs; the concepts of dependence, tolerance, and reinforcing properties that are unique characteristics of most psychoactive substances and are not found in other pharmacologic classifications; and the concepts of recovery and relapse prevention after cessation of drug intake.

HEALTH CARE SETTING

Treatment of substance abuse disorders occurs over the full range of the health care continuum. Acute detoxification usually takes place in an acute care facility. However, long-term care takes place in various community settings, including support groups like Alcoholics Anonymous (AA), Narcotics Anonymous (NA), outpatient therapy, vocational supports, and family therapy.

ASSESSMENT (ALCOHOLISM)

Assessment focuses on alcoholism because it constitutes the most frequently used and abused psychoactive substance in the United States.

Major symptoms supportive of a diagnosis of alcohol dependency:

- Withdrawal symptoms and significant interference with psychosocial functioning in family and job relationships.
- Tolerance, as evidenced by ability to consume the equivalent of a fifth of liquor or having a blood alcohol level ≥100 dl.
- Indiscriminate or regular drinking despite social or medical contraindications.
- Arrests for driving while under the influence of alcohol.

Assessment interview: Family history, history of drug use, and a description of behavior patterns described above. It is important to ask about preexisting mental disorders, metabolic conditions, cardiac and gas exchange problems, prescribed medications, and head injuries, all of which have symptoms that sometimes mimic acute intoxication or withdrawal symptoms.

Psychologic symptoms and behavior patterns: Patient uses denial to insist that she or he does not have a problem despite concrete evidence to the contrary. Rationalization appears in the form of self-imposed rules that explain the person's drinking habits as legitimate. Statements may be made such as, "I only drink on weekends" or "I limit myself to a beer, none of the hard stuff for me." Projection is evidenced in the blaming of external forces for stimulating the need to drink, for example, a nagging wife or a stressful job. Blackouts occur when there is a neuronal irritability that erases the alcoholic's memory of self-destructive behaviors while under the influence.

Physical indicators/examination:

- **Activity/rest:** Difficulty sleeping, not feeling well rested.
- **Cardiovascular:** Peripheral pulses weak, irregular or rapid; hypertension common in early withdrawal stage from alcohol but may become labile and progress to hypotension as withdrawal progresses; tachycardia common in early withdrawal; numerous dysrhythmias may be identified; other abnormalities depend on underlying heart disease/concurrent drug use.
- **Elimination:** Diarrhea, varied bowel sounds resulting from gastric complications such as gastric hemorrhage or distention.
- **Nutrition and fluid intake:** Nausea, vomiting, and food intolerance; difficulty chewing and swallowing food; muscle wasting; dry, dull hair; swollen salivary glands, inflamed buccal cavity, capillary fragility (malnutrition); possible generalized tissue edema resulting from protein deficiency; gastric distention, ascites, liver enlargement (seen in cirrhosis with long term use).
- **Pain/discomfort:** Possible constant upper abdominal pain and tenderness radiating to the back (pancreatic inflammation).
- **Respiration:** History of smoking; recurrent/chronic respiratory problems; tachypnea (with hyperactive state of alcohol withdrawal); diminished breath sounds.
- **Neurosensory:** Internal shakes, headache, dizziness, blurred vision, blackouts.
- **Psychiatric:** Possible dual diagnoses, for example, paranoid schizophrenia, bipolar disorder, major depression.
- **Level of consciousness/orientation:** Confusion, stupor, hyperactivity, distorted thought processes, slurred/incoherent speech.

- **Affect/mood/behavior:** May be fearful, anxious, easily startled, inappropriate, irritable, physically/verbally abusive, depressed, or paranoid.

Withdrawal assessment:

- **Stage I:** Mild. Temperature, pulse, respirations (TPR), and systolic blood pressure (SBP) elevated; slight diaphoresis; oriented × 3; mild anxiety and restlessness; restless sleep; hand tremors; decreased appetite; nausea.
- **Stage II:** Moderate. Pulse 100-120 bpm; increased temperature; increased SBP; obvious diaphoresis; intermittent confusion; transient visual and auditory hallucinations, primarily at night; increased anxiety and motor restlessness; insomnia; nightmares; nausea, vomiting, anorexia.
- **Stage III:** Severe. Pulse 120-140 bpm; increased temperature; increased diastolic blood pressure (DBP) and SBP; marked diaphoresis; marked disorientation and confusion; frightening visual, auditory, and tactile hallucinations; illusions (misinterpretation of objects); delusions; delirium tremens; disturbances in consciousness; agitation, panic states; inability to sleep; gross uncontrollable tremors; convulsions; inability to ingest any oral fluids or foods.

Safety assessment: History of recurrent accidents, such as falls, fractures, lacerations, burns, blackouts, or automobile accidents.

Suicidal assessment: Alcoholic suicide attempts may be as much as 30% higher than the national average.

Social assessment: Dysfunctional family system; problems in current relationships; frequent sick days off work/school; history of arrests because of fighting with others, disorderly conduct, or automobile accidents.

Spiritual assessment: It is important to assess for spiritual beliefs, practices, faith tradition, and commitment to that tradition. Many alcoholics and others addicted to substances find recovery through the spiritual model of AA and NA. Spiritual beliefs may provide the anchor that prevents an addicted individual from turning to suicide as a way out.

DIAGNOSTIC TESTS

Blood alcohol and drug levels can be obtained. However, diagnosis is generally made through interview history and physical examination. The diagnosis is made by confirmation of the presence of the four major symptoms of alcoholism listed above. Two of the most common assessment tools used to establish a definitive diagnosis are the Michigan Alcohol Screening Test (MAST) and the CAGE-AID questionnaire.

Nursing Diagnosis:

Interrupted Family Processes

related to long-term pattern of alcoholism and use of denial, rationalization, and projection

Desired Outcome: Before patient is discharged from care facility or after 4 wk if patient is outpatient, family members verbalize the dysfunctional behavioral dynamics present within the family system, the difference between caring and enabling, and the available services and treatment options that would help them.

INTERVENTIONS	**RATIONALES**
Provide family members with an opportunity to discuss their experiences of living with the disabling effects of alcoholism.	Allows validation of their experience and encourages open discussion of problem.
Educate family members about the effects of alcoholism on the family system.	Enables recognition that the dynamics in their family, although dysfunctional, is a predictable response to having a family member addicted to alcohol. It also encourages engagement in realistic appraisal of family's dynamics.
Provide family members with a list of services and treatment options available.	Provides validation that the dysfunction within the family is serious and requires support of professionals to correct the patterns.
Define the term *enabling* for family members. Encourage each of them to identify at least one time when he or she enabled the patient. Offer family members alternative choices to enabling behaviors. Have them practice what they will do and say when a situation arises.	It is important to reframe helping behavior as enabling behavior in order for family members to recognize the pattern. It is also important for them to realize that changing these patterns requires practice and feedback. During times of anxiety, it is normal to fall back on previous patterns of behaving.
Encourage the couple to consider marital therapy to begin to discuss regrets and resentments that have occurred as a result of alcoholism.	After many years of denial, it is important to begin to talk about feelings that have been buried. This process should be undertaken with a professional who can act as a mediator and teach the couple how to communicate without blaming, a common dynamic in a marriage affected by alcoholism.
Explain how roles have changed within the family as a result of alcoholism.	Teaching may have to be repeated frequently based on family's readiness to learn. Alcoholism produces dramatic role shifts that families are unaware of when they are in the midst of the problem. Presenting this emotionally charged information in a concrete, didactic manner increases family members' ability to hear.
Encourage family members to tell one another their needs and that caring about them is different from enabling.	Social and emotional isolation and denial of needs are common in alcoholic families. Enabling behaviors are frequently intended to be caring.
Encourage family to attend an Al-Anon meeting.	Significant change will require long-term commitment and support.

●●● **Related NIC and NOC labels:** *NIC:* Coping Enhancement; Family Support; Counseling; Family Therapy; Support Group; Support Group Enhancement; Role Enhancement; Behavior Modification
NOC: Family Coping; Family Functioning

Nursing Diagnosis:

Ineffective Denial

related to minimization of the symptoms and effects of alcoholism

Desired Outcome: Before discharge from care facility or after 4 wk if patient is outpatient, patient acknowledges that his or her drinking is out of control and his or her life has become unmanageable.

INTERVENTIONS	**RATIONALES**
Encourage patient to self-admit to an alcohol treatment program.	Self-admittance is preferred because the element of denial has been addressed to a certain degree.
Assure patient that alcoholism is a physiologic problem and not a moral one.	Demonstrates a nonjudgmental attitude; it is easier to accept treatment for an illness than it is for what may be perceived as a moral weakness or flaw.

Continued

INTERVENTIONS	RATIONALES
Encourage patient to compile a written list of the deleterious consequences of excessive alcohol use experienced over the time he or she has been drinking. Ask patient to show the list to another nurse or peer.	These interventions help break through the process of denial.
Ask patient to compile a list of situations that influenced excessive drinking and discuss ways to respond to these situations that do not involve drinking.	To help avoid relapse, it is important to know which situations triggered excessive drinking in the past.

●●● **Related NIC and NOC labels:** *NIC:* Counseling; Decision-Making Support; Self-Awareness Enhancement; Self-Responsibility Facilitation; Behavior Modification *NOC:* Acceptance: Health Status; Symptom Control

Nursing Diagnosis:

Risk for Injury

related to altered cerebral function (with risk for seizures) secondary to alcohol withdrawal

Desired Outcome: Patient does not exhibit evidence of physical injuries caused by alcohol withdrawal.

INTERVENTIONS	RATIONALES
Identify stage of alcohol withdrawal and severity of symptoms. Monitor VS, gait and motor coordination, and presence and severity of tremors, mental status, electrolyte status, and seizure activity.	The greater the severity of symptoms, the more likely the patient will experience increasing disorientation, confusion, and restlessness. As the withdrawal moves from stage I (mild) to stage III (severe), the risk for a fall or injury increases significantly.
Monitor for seizure activity; institute seizure precautions: bed in lowest position with side rails padded, oral airway at the bedside.	Withdrawal seizures usually occur within 48 hr following last drink.
Keep communication simple.	As disease progresses, patient's ability to comprehend complex directions and interactions diminishes greatly. Simplicity is the key to effective communication.
Stay with patient and provide emotional support and encouragement.	Risk of seizures is higher if patient is alone and has no one to keep him or her grounded in reality.
Continue to orient patient to surroundings and call light.	As blood alcohol level drops, disorientation increases and can last several days.
Maintain a calm, quiet environment.	Controlling the amount of external stimulation and keeping it at a minimal level promotes calm in the patient.
Administer IV/PO fluids with caution as indicated.	Careful fluid replacement corrects dehydration and facilitates renal clearance of toxins. Excessive alcohol use damages the cardiac muscle and/or conduction system. Overhydration poses significant risk to cardiac functioning.
Administer medications as prescribed and be alert for side effects. Benzodiazepines: clonazepam (Klonopin), diazepam (Valium), or chlordiazepoxide (Librium)	These medications are commonly used to control neuronal activity as alcohol is detoxified from the body. Either IV or PO route is preferred. These drugs produce muscle relaxation,

Continued

INTERVENTIONS

RATIONALES

INTERVENTIONS	RATIONALES
	which is effective in controlling the "shakes," trembling, and ataxic movements. They are usually initiated at a high dose and tapered and discontinued within 96 hr. They must be used cautiously in patients with hepatic disease because they are metabolized by the liver.
Oxazepam (Serax)	Serax may be the drug of choice for patients with liver disease. Although it does not produce quite the dramatic effects of controlling withdrawal symptoms, it has a shorter half-life, so is safer in the presence of hepatic disease.
Phenobarbital	Highly effective in suppressing withdrawal symptoms and is an effective anticonvulsant. Use must be monitored to prevent exacerbation of respiratory depression.

●●● **Related NIC and NOC labels:** *NIC:* Surveillance: Safety; Environmental Management: Safety; Risk Identification; Seizure Management *NOC:* Safety Status: Physical Injury

Nursing Diagnosis:

Disturbed Sensory Perceptions: Visual, auditory, or tactile

related to sudden cessation of alcohol consumption

Desired Outcome: Optimally, hallucinations do not occur, but if they do, patient's response is calm and controlled.

INTERVENTIONS	RATIONALES
Assess level of consciousness (LOC) and ability to communicate and respond to stimuli and commands.	Speech may be slurred, confused, or garbled. Response to commands may indicate inability to concentrate, impaired judgment, or muscle coordination deficits.
Monitor for disorientation, hyperactivity, confusion, restlessness, irritability, and sleeplessness.	Sleeplessness is common with loss of sedating effect of alcohol "nightcap." Sleep deprivation aggravates disorientation and confusion. Hyperactivity related to central nervous system (CNS) disturbances may show rapid escalation. Progression of these symptoms may signal impending hallucinations (common in stage II of alcohol withdrawal) or delirium tremens (seen in stage III of alcohol withdrawal).
Monitor for onset of hallucinations. Document as auditory, visual, or tactile.	Auditory hallucinations can be very frightening and threatening to the patient. Visual hallucinations include insects, animals, or faces of friends or enemies. The patient may yell for help from perceived threat. A tactile hallucination may include, for example, the sense that insects are crawling under the skin.
If hallucinations occur, stay with patient and speak in a calm, reassuring voice. Reassure patient that the voices and visions are not real and that he or she is safe.	Calm begets calm.
Turn off radio and/or TV; regulate lighting.	Reduces external stimuli when patient is hyperactive. Some patients become more agitated in a darkened room; others respond better to a quiet, darkened room.

Continued

INTERVENTIONS	RATIONALES
Maintain consistency in care providers as much as possible; try to remain with patient as much as possible.	Consistency promotes a sense of security; being with patient reduces fear.
Make sure environment is safe: bed in lowest position, bed rails padded, call light within reach, articles removed that could harm patient, doors in full open position, ongoing patient monitoring.	In addition to hallucinations, patient may experience reality distortion that could produce fear or suicidal ideation. Protection from self-harm is essential.
Administer medications as prescribed: see previous care plan.	May be necessary to provide calming effect and decrease symptoms of withdrawal.

●●● **Related NIC and NOC labels:** *NIC:* Hallucination Management; Anxiety Reduction; Medication Management; Environmental Management; Reality Orientation; Substance Use Treatment *NOC:* Cognitive Orientation

Nursing Diagnosis:

Imbalanced Nutrition: Less than body requirements

related to poor dietary intake

Desired Outcome: Within 24 hr of this diagnosis, patient verbalizes accurate understanding of the effects of alcohol and reduced dietary intake on nutritional status and demonstrates nutritional intake adequate for his or her needs.

INTERVENTIONS	RATIONALES
Assess for abdominal distention, tenderness, and presence and quality of bowel sounds.	Excessive alcohol intake may irritate gastric mucosa and result in epigastric pain and hyperactive bowel sounds. Other more serious gastrointestinal (GI) effects may occur secondary to hepatitis and cirrhosis.
Note presence of nausea/vomiting and diarrhea.	These signs are frequently among the first indicators of alcohol withdrawal and may interfere with establishing adequate nutritional intake.
Assess patient's ability to feed self.	A number of factors, including tremors, mental status changes, and hallucinations, may interfere with independent feeding and signal need for assistance.
Provide small, easily digested, and frequent feedings/snacks as desired; increase as tolerated.	Small feedings may enhance intake and toleration of nutrients by limiting gastric distress. As appetite and ability to tolerate food increase, adjustments are made to diet to ensure that adequate calories and nutrition are supplied for tissue repair and healing and restoration of energy and vitality.
Review liver function tests.	Liver function status influences choice of diet and need for/effectiveness of supplemental therapy.
Refer to dietitian as indicated.	Expert advice may be necessary to coordinate patient's nutritional regimen.
Provide diet high in protein with about 50% of calories supplied by carbohydrates.	Provides for energy needs and tissue healing while stabilizing blood sugar levels.

Continued

INTERVENTIONS	RATIONALES
Administer medications as prescribed:	
- Antacids, antiemetics, and antidiarrheals	These medications reduce gastric irritation.
- Thiamine and vitamins	All substance abusers should receive thiamine and vitamins because most have these deficiencies.
Keep patient NPO if indicated.	May be necessary to reduce gastric/pancreatic stimulation in presence of GI bleeding or excessive vomiting.

●●● **Related NIC and NOC labels:** *NIC:* Nutrition Monitoring; Self-Care Assistance: Feeding; Nutritional Counseling; Medication Management; Laboratory Data Interpretation *NOC:* Nutritional Status: Food and Fluid Intake; Nutritional Status: Nutrient Intake

Nursing Diagnosis:

Deficient Knowledge:

Prescribed medications, rationale for use, and potential side effects

Desired Outcome: Patient verbalizes accurate information about prescribed medication, including rationale for use and common side effects.

INTERVENTIONS	RATIONALES
Teach patient about the two medications that are sometimes used as adjuncts to alcohol dependence treatment:	
Disulfiram (Antabuse)	An agonist medication used as a deterrent to impulsive drinking.
Teach risks of drinking while taking Antabuse: severe nausea, vomiting, hypotension, headache, cardiovascular collapse, heart palpitations, seizures, or death.	Response of taking alcohol while on Antabuse.
Inform patient both verbally and in writing of serious side effects that occur when ingesting alcohol or other substances containing alcohol such as cough syrups or cold remedies.	Potential side effects are so serious that informed consent is essential.
Teach patient:	Required patient teaching.
- Do not take any form of alcohol (beer, wine, liquor, vinegars, cough medicines, sauces, aftershave lotions, liniments, or cologne). Doing so may cause a severe, even life-threatening reaction.	
- Take the drug daily (at bedtime if it produces fatigue or dizziness). Crush or mix tablet with liquid if necessary.	
- Wear or carry medical identification with you at all times to alert any medical emergency personnel that you are taking Antabuse.	
- Keep appointments for follow-up laboratory tests.	Disulfiram may worsen coexisting conditions such as diabetes mellitus, hypothyroidism, chronic and acute nephritis, and hepatic disease. It also increases prothrombin time. When these conditions exist, blood sugar monitoring, kidney and liver function tests, thyroid tests, and prothrombin times need scheduled follow-up evaluations.

Continued

INTERVENTIONS	RATIONALES
- The metallic aftertaste is temporary and will disappear after the drug is discontinued.	
- Avoid driving or performing tasks that require alertness if drowsiness, fatigue, or blurred vision occurs.	
Naltrexone (Trexan)	A narcotic antagonist originally used as a treatment for heroin abuse but has now been approved for treatment of alcoholism. The drug reduces the cravings for alcohol.
Teach patient about its adverse effects: difficulty sleeping, anxiety, nervousness, headache, low energy, abdominal pain, cramps, nausea, vomiting, delayed ejaculations, decreased potency, skin rash, chills, increased thirst, and joint and muscle pain.	Common adverse effects that should be reported to prescriber.
Teach patient:	Required patient teaching.
- This drug will make it easier for you not to drink and also block the effects of narcotics.	
- Wear a medical identification tag to alert emergency medical personnel that you are taking this drug.	
- Avoid use of heroin or other opiate drugs.	Small doses may have no effect, but large doses can cause death/serious injury or coma.
- Report any signs and symptoms of adverse effects.	
- Notify other health professionals that you are taking this drug.	
- Keep appointments for follow-up blood tests and treatment program.	

●●● **Related NIC and NOC labels:** *NIC:* Teaching: Prescribed Medication *NOC:* Knowledge: Medication

ADDITIONAL NURSING DIAGNOSES/ PROBLEMS:

PATIENT-FAMILY TEACHING AND DISCHARGE PLANNING

The patient with a substance abuse disorder suffers from a problem that can and will affect every area of his/her life. To remain free of substances, the patient will probably require lifelong support through AA or NA. The patient and family need to recognize that substance abuse disorders become family problems and professional counseling may be necessary and that alcoholism is a relentlessly progressive disease with profound medical, psychologic, social, and spiritual implications. Provide patient and family with verbal and written information about the following issues:

✓ Nature and expected course of alcoholism/substance abuse disorder.

✓ Medications, including drug name, purpose, dosage, frequency, precautions, drug/drug and food/drug interactions, and potential side effects.

✓ Withdrawal process—what to expect.

✓ Nutrition issues.

✓ Emergency measures.

✓ Importance of social support and strategies to obtain it; importance of changing social support if that support promotes drug use.

✔ Importance of using relaxation techniques to minimize stress.

✔ Importance of maintaining or achieving spiritual well-being.

✔ Importance of lifestyle issues such as benefits of exercise.

✔ Importance of group support for continued healing through AA or NA. Additional information can be obtained by contacting the following organizations:

National Clearinghouse for Alcohol and Drug Information (NCADI)
Prevline: Prevention Online
(800) 729-6686
www.health.org/

National Institute on Alcohol Abuse and Alcoholism (NIAAA)
6000 Executive Boulevard – Willco Building
Bethesda, MD 20892-7003
www.niaaa.nih.gov/

National Institute on Drug Abuse (NIDA)
National Institutes of Health
6001 Executive Boulevard, Room 5213
Bethesda, MD 20892-9561
(301) 443-1124
www.nida.nih.gov/

Online Alcoholics Anonymous (AA) Recovery Resources
www.recovery.org/aa/

Research Institute on Addictions
1021 Main Street
Buffalo, NY 14203-1016
(716) 887-2566
www.ria.org/

Appendix

Infection Prevention and Control

For several decades, infection prevention and control have focused on the use of barriers (e.g., gloves, gowns, masks) to interrupt transmission of organisms among and between patients and health care workers. These barriers are a major component of various systems of transmission precautions.

SYSTEMS OF TRANSMISSION PRECAUTIONS

Many different systems of transmission precautions have been used in hospitals over the years and were called *isolation precautions* until the most recent revision (2004) by the Centers for Disease Control and Prevention (CDC). The change in wording is to reflect clearly the purpose of these techniques and procedures, which is to interrupt transmission of organisms. The revised guideline adheres to four guiding principles: (1) to respond to challenges and needs not identified in the previous guideline; (2) to emphasize standard precautions as the essential foundation for preventing transmission of infectious agents in all health care settings; (3) to be epidemiologically sound and, whenever possible, evidence based; and (4) to be useful to persons delivering care in a variety of health care settings. The 2004 guideline contains two tiers of precautions (Table A-1): **Standard Precautions,** which are designed for the care of all patients in any health care setting, regardless of diagnosis or presumed infection status, and **Expanded Precautions,** which are used for patients known to be or suspected of being infected or colonized with epidemiologically important pathogens that can be transmitted by airborne or droplet transmission or by contact with dry skin or contaminated surfaces. A new type of Expanded Precautions has also been added, the Protective Environment, which is specifically for patients receiving hematopoietic stem cell transplantation (HSCT) who are at particular risk for infections with airborne fungi.

The 2004 guideline replaces the 1996 guideline for isolation precautions in hospitals. The 1996 Standard Precautions system synthesized the major features of Universal Precautions and Body Substance Isolation and applied to (1) blood; (2) all body fluids, secretions, and excretions, except sweat, regardless of

whether they contain visible blood; (3) nonintact skin; and (4) mucous membranes. In addition, Standard Precautions were designed to reduce risks of transmission of microorganisms from both recognized and unrecognized sources of infectious agents. The 2004 guideline continues these same principles of Standard Precautions and applies them to a broader range of situations and care settings. The 1996 Transmission-Based Precautions were designed for patients documented to be or suspected of being infected or colonized with organisms transmitted by the airborne route, by droplets, and by contact where extra precautions were necessary to interrupt transmission. The term *Expanded Precautions* replaces the term *Transmission Based Precautions* and modifies the 1996 guideline consistent with new information about mechanisms of transmission of epidemiologically important organisms. As always, the CDC offers hospitals and other types of health care settings the option of modifying the recommendations according to their needs and circumstances and as directed by federal, state, or local regulations. For example, the Occupational Safety and Health Administration's (OSHA's) Bloodborne Pathogens Standard (1991) is still operable, and all facilities are required to comply with its provisions. The CDC's 2004 Standard Precautions incorporate all requirements of the OSHA Bloodborne Pathogens Standard.

EXPANDED PRECAUTIONS FOR PATIENTS WITH PULMONARY OR LARYNGEAL TUBERCULOSIS

Airborne Infection Isolation Precautions are for persons diagnosed with or suspected of having pulmonary or laryngeal tuberculosis (TB) that can be transmitted to others via the airborne route. These guidelines focus on early identification and treatment of persons with a diagnosis or suspected diagnosis of active TB. In addition, the CDC defines requirements for special ventilation and use of respiratory protection masks that provide better filtration and a tighter fit than standard surgical masks. Masks of this type are called *particulate respirators (PRs),* and the specific type of PR for TB protection is called

TABLE **A-1**   Recommendations for Transmission Precautions in Health Care Settings, 2004*

	STANDARD PRECAUTIONS	EXPANDED PRECAUTIONS: AIRBORNE INFECTION ISOLATION	EXPANDED PRECAUTIONS: DROPLET	EXPANDED PRECAUTIONS: CONTACT	EXPANDED PRECAUTIONS: PROTECTIVE ENVIRON- MENT
When to use	For the care of all patients in all health care settings.	For patients known or suspected to be infected with microorganisms transmitted person-to-person by airborne droplet nuclei that remain suspended in the air and that can be dispersed widely by air currents.	For patients known or suspected to be infected with microorganisms transmitted by droplets that can be generated by the patient during coughing, sneezing, talking, or the performance of procedures.	For patients known or suspected of being infected or colonized with specific epidemiologically important organisms that can be transmitted by direct or indirect contact when there is evidence that standard precautions and hand hygiene are not effective in preventing health care–associated transmission (see Guideline for specific organisms to which Contact Precautions apply).	For allogeneic hematopoietic stem cell transplantation (HSCT) patients to minimize fungal spore counts in the air.
Hand hygiene 1. If hands are not visibly soiled, use an alcohol-based, waterless antiseptic agent. 2. When hands are dirty or contaminated with proteinaceous material, wash with soap and water.	Practice hand hygiene after touching blood, body fluids, secretions, excretions, and contaminated items, whether or not gloves are worn. Use hand hygiene immediately after gloves are removed, between patient contacts, and when otherwise indicated in *Hand Hygiene Guideline* (2002). Decontaminate hands after contact with inanimate objects (including medical equipment) in the immediate vicinity of the patient.				

Continued

TABLE A-1 Recommendations for Transmission Precautions in Health Care Settings, 2004*—cont'd

	STANDARD PRECAUTIONS	EXPANDED PRECAUTIONS: AIRBORNE INFECTION ISOLATION	EXPANDED PRECAUTIONS: DROPLET	EXPANDED PRECAUTIONS: CONTACT	EXPANDED PRECAUTIONS PROTECTIVE ENVIRON-MENT
Gloves	Wear gloves when it can be reasonably anticipated that contact with blood or other potentially infectious materials, mucous membranes, nonintact skin, or potentially colonized intact skin will occur. For purposes of preventing transmission of infectious agents, the choice of glove type (e.g., latex, vinyl, nitrile) is determined by permeability factors. Remove gloves after caring for patient. Do not wear the same pair of gloves for the care of more than one patient and do not wash gloves between patients. Change gloves during patient care if moving from a contaminated body site to a clean body site.			Wear gloves as indicated according to Standard Precautions and whenever touching the patient's intact skin and the patient's environment and articles, including medical equipment, computer keyboards, bed rails, etc. Remove gloves before leaving the patient's room and practice hand hygiene immediately. After glove removal and hand hygiene, ensure that hands do not touch surfaces or items in the patient's room to avoid transfer of microorganisms to other patients or surfaces or articles.	
Mask, eye protection, face shield	Wear a mask and eye protection or a face shield to protect mucous membranes of the eyes, nose, and mouth during procedures that are likely to generate splashes or sprays.	Wear respiratory protection (N95 respirator) when entering the room or home of a patient with known or suspected infectious pulmonary tuberculosis.	Wear a mask and eye protection when working within 3 ft of the patient.		Place a mask on patients when they leave the protective environment for diagnostic tests or treatments elsewhere in the facility to prevent inhalation of respirable particles and reaerosolization of

Continued

TABLE A-1 Recommendations for Transmission Precautions in Health Care Settings, 2004*—cont'd

	STANDARD PRECAUTIONS	EXPANDED PRECAUTIONS: AIRBORNE INFECTION ISOLATION	EXPANDED PRECAUTIONS: DROPLET	EXPANDED PRECAUTIONS: CONTACT	EXPANDED PRECAUTIONS: PROTECTIVE ENVIRONMENT
		Persons susceptible to measles (rubella), varicella (chickenpox), or smallpox should not enter the room of these patients if other immune caregivers are available. If susceptible persons must enter these rooms, respiratory protection should be used.			exhaled particles. Consult infection control professional for appropriate type of mask.
Gowns	Wear a gown to protect skin and prevent soiling of clothing during procedures and patient care activities that are likely to generate splashes or sprays of blood, body fluids, secretions, or excretions. Wear a gown for direct patient contact if patient has uncontained secretions, excretions, or wound drainage and contamination is likely to occur. Remove gown before leaving patient's environment.			Wear gowns as indicated according to Standard Precautions and whenever anticipating that the caregiver's clothing will have direct contact with the patient, environmental surfaces, or items in the patient's room. Remove gown before leaving patient's environment. After gown removal, ensure that clothing does not contact environmental surfaces.	
Patient placement	Consider potential for transmission of infectious agents when making patient placement decisions.	Inpatient or residential setting: Place patient in a private room that has monitored negative pressure ventilation, adequate numbers of air changes, and appropriate discharge	Maintain spatial separation of at least 3 ft between the infected patient and other patients and visitors. This may be more easily achieved using a private room. When a private	Place the patient in a private room to reduce the risk of transmission of epidemiologically important organisms. When a private room is not available, place the patient in a	Place allogeneic HSCT patients in a protective environment that includes appropriate environmental controls to reduce the risk of transmission of environmental

Continued

TABLE A-1 Recommendations for Transmission Precautions in Health Care Settings, 2004*—cont'd

	STANDARD PRECAUTIONS	EXPANDED PRECAUTIONS: AIRBORNE INFECTION ISOLATION	EXPANDED PRECAUTIONS: DROPLET	EXPANDED PRECAUTIONS: CONTACT	EXPANDED PRECAUTIONS: PROTECTIVE ENVIRONMENT
		of air outdoors or filtered before recirculation. Keep the door closed and the patient in the room. If an appropriate private room is not available, consult infection control professional for alternatives.	room is not available, patients with the same active infection may be in the same room (cohorting). Special air handling and ventilation are not necessary, and the room may remain open.	room with patient(s) colonized or infected with the same organism. When these options are not available, consult infection control professional for alternatives.	fungi. Consult infection control professional for details.
Patient transport		Limit movement and transport of the patient to essential purposes only. If transport or movement is necessary, minimize patient dispersal of droplet nuclei by placing a surgical mask on the patient. If patient has a viral infection that can be transmitted via the airborne route, cover patient to prevent aerosolization of virus from skin lesions that are not crusted.	Limit movement and transport of the patient to essential purposes only.	Limit movement and transport of the patient from the room to essential purposes only. If the patient is transported out of the room, ensure precautions are maintained to minimize the risk of transmission of microorganisms to other patients and contamination of environmental surfaces or equipment.	
Patient care equipment	Handle used patient care equipment in a manner that prevents skin and mucous membrane exposures, contamination of clothing, and transfer of microorganisms to other patients and environments.			Manage patient care equipment according to Standard Precautions. Note: Additional procedures may be indicated in outbreak situations.	

Continued

TABLE **A-1** Recommendations for Transmission Precautions in Health Care Settings, 2004*—cont'd

	STANDARD PRECAUTIONS	EXPANDED PRECAUTIONS: AIRBORNE INFECTION ISOLATION	EXPANDED PRECAUTIONS: DROPLET	EXPANDED PRECAUTIONS: CONTACT	EXPANDED PRECAUTIONS: PROTECTIVE ENVIRON-MENT
Care of the environment	Keep environmental surfaces visibly clean on a regular basis and as spills occur.			Clean the environment according to Standard Precautions. Note: Additional procedures may be indicated in outbreak situations.	
Textiles, laundry	Handle, transport, and process used linen in a manner that prevents skin and mucous membrane exposures and contamination of clothing and that avoids transfer of microorganisms to other patients and environments.				

Modified from Strausbaugh L, Jackson M, Rhinehart E, Siegel J, and the Healthcare Infection Control Practices Advisory Committee (HICPAC): *Guideline to prevent transmission of infectious agents in healthcare settings.* To be published by the Centers for Disease Control and Prevention, early 2004.
*Note: *This table was developed when this publication was in draft form; therefore the final version may differ slightly from what is published here.*

an N95 respirator. This type of respiratory protection is also appropriate for susceptible persons caring for patients known or suspected of having measles (rubeola), varicella (chickenpox), or smallpox. Of course, the best protection for any of the vaccine-preventable infectious diseases is for all caregivers to be immunized; then respiratory protection masks are not necessary.

MANAGEMENT OF DEVICES AND PROCEDURES TO REDUCE RISK OF NOSOCOMIAL INFECTION

Use of barriers is but one of many strategies that can reduce the risk of nosocomial infection among patients and personnel. In fact, studies from the CDC show that significant gains can be made in reducing infection risks by focusing on the management of devices and procedures commonly used in patient care. For example, many patients need intravascular devices that deliver therapeutic medications, but they are put at risk for site infections and bacteremias when these devices are used. It is well known that rotating the access site at appropriate intervals reduces these risks to the patient, and catheter materials that are more "vein friendly" also reduce trauma to the vascular system. In addition, use of needles to deliver medications and fluids to patients through these intravascular devices can put the health care worker at risk for puncture injury. Needleless or needle-free IV access devices are used to access line ports so that it is not necessary to use needles once the intravascular catheter has entered the vascular system. Thus the use of newer and safer intravascular devices and procedures can benefit both the patient and health care worker by reducing their risk of nosocomial infection. Research studies of interventions to reduce nosocomial infection risks are published in general and specialty journals and presented at professional meetings each year. Infection control practitioners and hospital epidemiologists use these studies to make recommendations about changes in nursing and medical practice. The Joint Commission on Accreditation of Healthcare Organizations (JCAHO) requires that all accredited facilities have a person qualified to provide infection surveillance, prevention, and control services. The national associations for these professionals are the Association for Professionals in Infection Control and Epidemiology, Inc. (APIC), which publishes the *American Journal of Infection Control,* and the Society for Healthcare Epidemiology of America (SHEA), which publishes the journal *Infection Control and Hospital Epidemiology.*

Appendix

Normal Laboratory Values

TABLE **A-2**   **Complete Blood Count (CBC)**

	ADULT NORMAL VALUES* (TRADITIONAL—U.S.)	SI ADULT NORMAL VALUES* (INTERNATIONAL SYSTEM)
Hemoglobin (Hgb)	Male: 14-18 g/dl Female: 12-16 g/dl	Male: 135-170 g/L Female: 120-160 g/L
Hematocrit (Hct)	Male: 40%-54% Female: 37%-47%	Male: 0.400-0.500 L/L Female: 0.370-0.490 L/L
Red blood cell (RBC) count	Male: 4.5-6.0 million/mm^3 Female: 4.0-5.5 million/mm^3	Male: 4.50-6.00×10^{12}/L Female: 4.00-5.50×10^{12}/L
RBC indices		
Mean corpuscular volume	80-95 μm^3	80-100 fl
Mean corpuscular hemoglobin	27-31 pg	27-31 pg
Mean corpuscular hemoglobin concentration	32-36 g/dl	320-360 g/L
White blood cell (WBC) count	4500-11,000/mm^3	4.0-11.0×10^9/L
Neutrophils	54%-75%	2.5-7.5×10^9/L
Band neutrophils	3%-8%	2% +/–4
Lymphocytes	20%-40%	1.0-4.0×10^9/L
Monocytes	2%-8%	0-1.0×10^9/L
Eosinophils	1%-4%	0-0.7×10^9/L
Basophils	0.5%-1.0%	0-0.3×10^9/L
Platelet count	150,000-400,000/mm^3	150-400×10^9/L

*Normal values may vary significantly with different laboratory methods of testing.

TABLE **A-3**   Serum, Plasma, and Whole Blood Chemistry

	ADULT NORMAL VALUES★ (TRADITIONAL—US)	SI ADULT NORMAL VALUES★ (INTERNATIONAL SYSTEM)
Adrenocorticotropic hormone (ACTH)	8-10 AM <100 pg/ml	0-16 pmol/L
Antidiuretic hormone (ADH; vasopressin)	1-5 pg/ml	0-10 ng/L
Albumin	3.5-5.0 g/dl	35-50 g/L
Aldosterone	Male: 6-22 ng/dl Female: 4-31 ng/dl	140-415 pmol/L
Alanine aminotransferase (ALT)	5-35 IU/L	Male: <40 IU/L Female: <31 IU/L
Ammonia	15-110 µg/dl	35-80 µmol/L
Amylase	60-180 Somogyi U/dl	<125 U/L
Aspartate aminotransferase (AST)	8-20 U/L (values slightly higher in older adults than in younger adults and slightly lower in females than in males)	Male: <37 IU/L Female: <31 IU/L
Bicarbonate	22-26 mEq/L	22-26 mEq/L
Bilirubin	Total: 0.3-1.4 mg/dl	Total: 2-17 µmol/L
Blood gases, arterial		
pH	7.35-7.45	7.35-7.45
$Paco_2$	35-45 mm Hg	35-45 mm Hg
Pao_2	80-100 mm Hg	80-100 mm Hg
O_2 saturation (Sao_2)	95%-99%	95%-99%
Blood urea nitrogen (BUN)	6-20 mg/dl	3.0-7.0 mmol/L
CA-125 cancer marker	0-35U/ml	0-35 U/mol
Calcitonin	<100 pg/ml	0-100 ng/L
Calcium	8.5-10.5 mg/dl; 4.3-5.3 mEq/L	2.2-2.6 mmol/L
Carcinoembryonic antigen (CEA)	<5 ng/ml	0-4.6 µg/l
Chloride (Cl⁻)	95-108 mEq/L	95-108 mmol/L
Cortisol		
8-10 AM	5-25 µg/dl	140-500 nmol/L
4 PM-midnight	2-18 µg/dl	83-441 nmol/L
CO_2 content (total CO_2)	22-28 mEq/L	22-30 mmol/L
Creatinine	0.6-1.5 mg/dl	50-110 mmol/L
Creatinine clearance	Male: 107-141 ml/min Female: 87-132 ml/min	1.5-2.2 ml/sec
Creatinine phosphokinase (CPK)	Male: 55-170 U/L Female: 30-135 U/L	Male: 130-150 IU/L Female: 20-115 IU/L
CPK isoenzyme (MB)	5% total CPK activity	<5% total CPK activity
Erythrocyte sedimentation rate (ESR) Westergren method	0-10 mm/hr Male: up to 15 mm/hr Female: up to 20 mm/hr	
Fibrin split products (FSPs, FDPs)	<10 µg/ml	<400 µg/L
Folic acid (folate)	5-20 µg/ml	3.4-47 nmol/L
Follicle-stimulating hormone (FSH, follitropin)		
Adult female		Follicular <16 IU/L
	Premenopausal 4-30 mIU/ml	Luteal <12 IU/L
	Postmenopausal 40-250 mIU/ml	Postmenopausal 23-167 IU/L
Adult male	4-25 mIU/ml	<18 IU/L
Globulins, total	1.5-3.5 g/dl	27-36 g/L
Glucose, fasting	True glucose: 60-120 mg/dl All sugars: 80-120 mg/dl	4.0-6.0 mmol/L

Continued

TABLE A-3   Serum, Plasma, and Whole Blood Chemistry—cont'd

	ADULT NORMAL VALUES* (TRADITIONAL—US)	SI ADULT NORMAL VALUES* (INTERNATIONAL SYSTEM)
Glucose, random	<145 mg/dl	
Glucose tolerance, oral		
Fasting:	60-120 mg/dl	3.3-6.0 mmol/L
1 hr:	<165 mg/dl	3.3-11.1 mmol/L
2 hr:	<120 mg/dl	3.3-7.8 mmol/L
Glycosylated hemoglobin (glycohemoglobin [GHb])	4%-8%	0.040-0.066
Growth hormone (GH)	<10 ng/ml	0-7 μg/L
Insulin	11-240 μU/ml	Fasting: 0-215 pmol/L
	4-24 μU/ml	
Iron	Total: 60-200 μg/dl	10-30 μmol/L
Iron	Male, average: 125 μg/dl	
	Female, average: 100 μg/dl	
	Older adult: 60-80 μg/dl	
Total iron-binding capacity	25-420 μg/dl	45-80 μmol/L
Ketone bodies	2-4 μg/dl	Negative
Lactic acid	Arterial: 0.5-1.6 mEq/L	0.5-2.0 mmol/L
	Venous: 1.5-2.2 mEq/L	
Lactic dehydrogenase	45-90 U/L	100-250 IU/L
Lipase	0-110 U/L	0-110 U/L
Magnesium	1.8-3.0 mg/dl	0.7-1.1 mmol/L
Osmolality	280-300 mOsm/kg H_2O	280-300 mmol/kg
Parathyroid hormone	<2000 pg/ml	1.0-5.5 pmol/L
Partial thromboplastin time (PTT)	60-70 sec	25.5-35.0 sec
On anticoagulant therapy	1.5-2.5 × control value	
Phosphatase, acid	0-1.1 U/ml (Bodansky)	Total: 0-6 U/L
	1-4 U/ml (King-Armstrong)	
	0.13-0.63 U/ml (Bessey-Lowery)	
Phosphatase, alkaline	1.5-4.5 U/dl (Bodansky)	30-110 U/L
	4-13 U/dl (King-Armstrong)	
	0.8-2.3 U/ml (Bessey-Lowery)	
Phosphorus	2.5-4.5 mg/dl; 1.7-2.6 mEq/L	0.80-1.45 mmol/L
Potassium (K^+)	3.5-5.0 mEq/L	3.5-5.0 mmol/L
Prolactin	2-15 ng/ml	Male: 0-5 μg/L
		Female: 0-20 μg/L
Prothrombin time (PT)	11-12.5 sec	INR: 0.81-1.2
Renin		
Normal sodium intake		
Supine	4-6 hr: 0.5-1.6 ng/ml/hr	Overnight or 6 hr: 6.4-23.8 ng/L/sec
Sitting	4 hr: 1.8-3.6 ng/ml/hr	2 hr: 9.3-43.4 ng/L/sec
Sitting		2 hr plus diuretic: 12.3-80.5 ng/L/sec
Low sodium intake		
Supine	4-6 hr: 2.2-4.4 ng/ml/hr	Overnight or 6 hr: <10.2 ng/L/sec
Sitting	4 hr: 4.0-8.1 ng/ml/hr	2 hr: 5.8-20.2 ng/L/sec
Reticulocyte count	0.5%-2% of total erythrocytes	40-80 × 10^9/L
Reticulocyte index	1.0	1.0
Sodium (Na^+)	137-147 mEq/L	137-147 mmol/L

Continued

TABLE **A-3**   Serum, Plasma, and Whole Blood Chemistry—cont'd

	ADULT NORMAL VALUES* (TRADITIONAL—US)	SI ADULT NORMAL VALUES* (INTERNATIONAL SYSTEM)
Thyroid screen		
Free thyroxine-index (FTI)	0.9-2.4 ng/dl	
Free thyroxine (free T_4)		12-22 pmol/L
Thyroid-stimulating hormone	2-10 mU/L	0.27-4.2 µmol/L
Thyroxine-binding prealbumin	20-30 mg/dl	
Triiodothyronine (T_3)	110-230 ng/dl	1.2-3.2 nmol/L
Thyroxine uptake (T uptake)		0.75-1.25 nmol/L
Transferrin	200-400 mg/dl	1.7-3.9 g/L
Urea clearance, serum/24 hr urine		
Maximum	64-99 ml/min	64-99 ml/min
Standard	41-65 ml/min	41-65 ml/min
Uric acid	Male: 2.0-7.5 mg/dl	<450 µmol/L
	Female: 2.0-6.5 mg/dl	<360 µmol/L

*Normal values may vary significantly with different laboratory methods of testing.

TABLE **A-4**   Urine Chemistry

	ADULT NORMAL VALUES* (TRADITIONAL—U.S.)	SI ADULT NORMAL VALUES* (INTERNATIONAL SYSTEM)
Albumin		
Random	Negative	Negative
24 hr	10-150 mg	150 mg
Amylase	Mayo clinic method: 10-80 U/hr	Random 350 U/L
	Somogyi mehod: 26-950 U/24 hr	24 hr: 440 U/d
Bilirubin (random)	Negative	Negative
Calcium (Ca++)		
Random	1+; <40 mg/dl	
24 hr	50-300 mg	2.5-6.3 mmol/L
Creatine (24 hr)	Male: 20-26 mg/kg	7.0-22 mmol/d
	Female: 14-22 mg/kg	
Creatine clearance	Male: 107-141 ml/min/1.73 m^2	1.5-2.2 ml/sec
	Female: 87-132 ml/min/1.73 m^2	
Glucose		
Random	Negative	Negative
24 hr	130 mg	
Ketone (random)	Negative	Negative
Microalbumin		
Random		<20 ml/L
Night collection		7 +/− 2 µg/min
24 hr		10 +/− 3 mg/d
Microalbumin/creatine ratio		
Male		<2.0 mg/mmol
Female		<2.8 mg/mmol
Osmolality		
Random	350-700 mOsm/kg H$_2$O	
24 hr	300-900 mOsm/kg H$_2$O	
Physiologic range	50-1400 mOsm/kg H$_2$O	
pH	4.6-8.0	4.6-8.0
Phosphorus (24 hr)	0.9-1.3 g; 0.2-0.6 mEq/L	16.1-48.4 mmol/d
Protein		
Random	Negative: 2-8 mg/dl	Negative
24 hr	40-150 mg	150 mg/d
Sodium (Na+)		
Random	50-130 mEq/L	
24 hr	40-220 mEq/L	50-150 mmol/d
Specific gravity		
Random	1.010-1.020	1.003-1.035
After fluid restriction	1.025-1.035	
Sugar (random)	Negative	Negative
Urea clearance (24 hr)		
Maximum	64-99 ml/min	64-99 ml/min
Standard	41-65 ml/min	41-65 ml/min

*Normal values may vary significantly with different laboratory methods of testing.

Bibliography

BIBLIOGRAPHY

Part 1: Medical-Surgical Nursing Care Plans

General Care Plans

Ackley BJ, Ladwig GB: *Nursing diagnosis handbook: a guide to planning care,* ed 5, St Louis, 2002, Mosby.

Acute Pain Management Guideline Panel: *Acute pain management: operative or medical procedures and trauma—clinical practices guideline,* AHCPR pub no 92-0032, Rockville, Md, 1992, Agency for Health Care Policy and Research, Public Health Service, U.S. Department of Health and Human Services.

Agency for Health Care Policy and Research: *Clinical practice guideline: management of cancer pain,* AHCPR pub no 94-0592, Rockville, Md, 1994, U.S. Department of Health and Human Services, Public Health Service, Agency for Health Care Policy and Research.

American Association of Cardiovascular and Pulmonary Rehabilitation: *Guidelines for cardiac rehabilitation programs,* ed 3, Champaign, Ill, 1999, Human Kinetic Books.

American College of Sports Medicine: *Guidelines for exercise testing and prescription,* ed 6, Philadelphia, 2000, Lippincott Williams & Wilkins.

American Pain Society: *Principles of analgesic use in the treatment of acute and cancer pain,* ed 4, Glenview, Ill, 1999, The Society.

American Pharmaceutical Association (Semla T et al, editors): *Geriatric dosage handbook,* ed 4, Hudson, Ohio, 1998, Lexicomp.

Baas LS: Prolonged bedrest. In Swearingen PL: *Manual of medical-surgical nursing care,* ed 5, St Louis, 2003, Mosby.

Bailes B: Perioperative care of the elderly surgical patient, *AORN* 72(2):186-206, 2000.

Borg GV: Psychophysical basis of perceived exertion, *Med Sci Sports Exerc* 14:377-381, 1982.

Brimacombe J et al: Two cases of naloxone-induced pulmonary edema: the possible use of phentolamine in management, *Anaesth Intensive Care* 19(4):578-580, 1991.

Caron PA: Cancer care. In Swearingen PL: *Manual of medical-surgical nursing care,* ed 5, St Louis, 2003, Mosby.

Caron PA: Psychosocial support. In Swearingen PL: *Manual of medical-surgical nursing care,* ed 5, St Louis, 2003, Mosby.

Caron PA: Psychosocial support for the patient's family and significant others. In Swearingen PL: *Manual of medical-surgical nursing care,* ed 5, St Louis, 2003, Mosby.

Chan D, Brennan N: Delirium: making the diagnosis, improving the prognosis, *Geriatrics* 54(3):28-42, 1999.

Clark P: Details on demand: consumers, cancer information, and the Internet, *Clin J Oncol Nurs* 5(1):19-24, 2001.

DeStoutz ND, Stiefel F: Assessment and management of reversible delirium: delirium in cancer patients. In Portenoy R, Bruera E, editors: *Topics in palliative care,* vol 1, New York, 1997, Oxford University Press.

DiGeronimo C: Perioperative care. In Swearingen PL: *Manual of medical-surgical nursing care,* ed 5, St Louis, 2003, Mosby.

Doyle D, Hanks GWC, MacDonald N: *Oxford textbook of palliative medicine,* ed 2, Oxford, England, 1998, Oxford University Press.

Ferrell BR, Coyle N: *Textbook of palliative nursing,* Oxford, England, 2001, Oxford University Press.

Fishman M et al: *Cancer chemotherapy guidelines and recommendations for practice,* ed 2, Pittsburgh, 1999, Oncology Nursing Press.

Five Wishes—An Advanced Directives Document available from the Commission on Aging with Dignity: (888) 5-WISHES or www.agingwithdignity.org.

Goodlin SJ et al: Death in the hospital, *Arch Intern Med* 158(14):1570-1572, 1998.

Hall G, Wakefield B: Confusion: what to do when the clouds roll in, *Nursing* 26(7):32-37, 1996.

Hoskin PJ, Hanks GW: Opioid agonist-antagonist drugs in acute and chronic pain states, *Drugs* 4(41):326-344, 1991.

Institute of Medicine: *Approaching death: improving care at the end of life,* Washington, DC, 1997, National Academy Press.

Jansen PR: Older adult care. In Swearingen PL: *Manual of medical-surgical nursing care,* ed 5, St Louis, 2003, Mosby.

Johnson M et al: *Nursing diagnoses, outcomes, and interventions: NANDA, NOC, and NIC linkages,* St Louis, 2001, Mosby.

Joint Commission on Accreditation of Healthcare Organizations: *JCAHO Pain Standards, Comprehensive Accreditation Manual for Hospitals,* Joint Commission Resources, 2002.

Kirkwood J: *Current cancer therapeutics,* ed 3, Philadelphia, 1998, Churchill Livingstone.

Letizia M, Shenk J, Jones TD: Intermittent subcutaneous injections for symptom control in hospice care: a retrospective investigation, *Hospice J* 15(2):1-11, 2000.

Logan P: *Principles of practice for the acute care nurse practitioner,* Boston, 1999, Prentice Hall.

Matteson M et al: *Gerontological nursing: concepts and practice,* ed 2, Philadelphia, 1997, WB Saunders.

McCaffrey M, Pasero C: *Pain: clinical manual,* ed 2, St Louis, 1999, Mosby.

Mroz IB: Pain. In Swearingen PL: *Manual of medical-surgical nursing care,* ed 5, St Louis, 2003, Mosby.

North American Nursing Diagnosis Association: *Nursing diagnoses: definitions and classification 2003-2004,* Philadelphia, 2003, NANDA International.

Occupational Safety and Health Administration: Controlling occupational exposure to hazardous drugs, OSHA Instruction CPL 2-2.20B, Washington, DC, 1995, Occupational Safety and Health Administration.

Pals J: Clinical triggers for detection of fever and dehydration: implications for long term care, *J Gerontol Nurs* 21(4):13-19, 1995.

Pasero C, McCaffrey M: Preventing and managing opioid induced respiratory depression, *Am J Nurs* 94(4):25-31, 1994.

Resnick N: Geriatric medicine. In Tierney L et al, editors: *Current medical diagnosis and treatment,* ed 3, Stamford, Conn, 1997, Appleton & Lange.

Roth AJ, Brietbart W: Psychiatric emergencies in terminally ill cancer patients. In Cherney NI, Foley KM, editors: *Pain and palliative care,* Philadelphia, 1996, WB Saunders.

Schuster JL: Delirium, confusion, and agitation at the end of life, *J Pall Med* 1(2):177-186, 1998.

Sharp J: The Internet: changing the way cancer survivors obtain information, *Cancer Pract* 7(5):266-269, 1999.

Sharp J: The Internet: changing the way cancer survivors receive support, *Cancer Pract* 8(3):145-147, 2000.

Van Ort S, Phillips L: Nursing interventions to promote functional feeding, *J Gerontol Nurs* 21(10):6-14, 1995.

Varricchio C: *A cancer source book for nurses,* ed 7, Sudbury, Mass, 1997, Jones & Bartlett.

Waller A, Caroline NL: *Handbook of palliative care in cancer,* ed 2, Boston, 2000, Butterworth-Heinemann.

Wallis M: Looking at depression through bifocal lenses, *Nursing* 30(9):58-61, 2000.

Whedon MB, Stephany TM: End-of-life care. In Swearingen PL: *Manual of medical-surgical nursing care,* ed 5, St Louis, 2003, Mosby.

World Health Organization Expert Committee: *Cancer pain relief and palliative care,* Geneva, Switzerland, 1990, World Health Organization, p 11.

World Health Organization: *Cancer pain relief: a guide to opioid availability, cancer pain relief, and palliative care,* ed 2, Report of the WHO Expert Committee Technical Report Series No. 804, Geneva, Switzerland, 1996, World Health Organization.

Yarbro C et al, editors: *Cancer nursing: principles and practice,* ed 5, Sudbury, Mass, 2000, Jones & Bartlett.

Respiratory Care Plans

Ackley BJ, Ladwig GB: *Nursing diagnosis handbook: a guide to planning care,* ed 5, St Louis, 2002, Mosby.

Arcasoy SM, Kreit JV: Thrombolytic therapy of pulmonary embolism: a comprehensive review of current evidence, *Chest* 115(6):1695-1707, 1999.

Baum GL et al: *Textbook of pulmonary diseases,* ed 6, Philadelphia, 1998, Lippincott-Raven.

Benayoun S, Ernst P, Suissa S: The impact of combined inhaled bronchodilator therapy in the treatment of COPD, *Chest* 119(1):85-92, 2001.

Bennett CL et al: Delays in tuberculosis isolation and suspicion among persons hospitalized with HIV-related pneumonia, *Chest* 117(1):110-116, 2000.

Blank-Reid C, Reid PC: Taking the tension out of traumatic pneumothoraxes, *Nursing* 29(4):41-47, 1999.

Boutotte JM: Keeping TB in check, *Nursing* 29(3):35-40, 1999.

Carroll P: Exploring chest drain options, *RN* 63(10):50-58, 2000.

Centers for Disease Control and Prevention: *Guidelines for prevention of nosocomial pneumonia,* Atlanta, 1997, Department of Health and Human Services.

Centers for Disease Control and Prevention: *Core curriculum on tuberculosis,* ed 4, Atlanta, 2000, Department of Health and Human Services.

Christie F: Pulmonary embolism, *Am J Nurs* 98(11):36-37, 1998.

Church V: DVT & PE, *Nursing* 30(2):35-44, 2000.

Contival C: Taking precautions against tuberculosis, *Am J Nurs* 98(11):16A-B, 1998.

Feldman C: Pneumonia in the elderly, *Clin Chest Med* 20(3):563-573, 1999.

Ferguson GT: Update on pharmacologic therapy for chronic obstructive pulmonary disease, *Clin Chest Med* 21(4):723-738, 2000.

Friedman LN: *Tuberculosis: current concepts and treatment,* ed 2, Boca Raton, Fla, 2000, CRC Press.

Gibbar-Clements TR et al: The challenge of warfarin therapy, *Am J Nurs* 100(3):38-40, 2000.

Goll CA: Respiratory disorders. In Swearingen PL: *Manual of medical-surgical nursing care,* ed 5, St Louis, 2003, Mosby.

Goode CJ, Piedalue F: Evidence-based clinical practice, *J Nurs Admin* 29(6):15-21, 1999.

Horne C, Derrico D: Mastering ABGs, *Am J Nurs* 99(8):26-32, 1999.

Johnson M et al: *Nursing diagnoses, outcomes, and interventions: NANDA, NOC, and NIC linkages,* St Louis, 2001, Mosby.

Kollef MH et al: Mechanical ventilation with or without daily changes of in-line suction catheters, *Am J Respir Crit Care Med* 156(2):466-472, 1997.

Monroe BS, Warner D: Intrapleural fibrinolytic therapy for complicated pleural effusions, *Crit Care Nurse* 18(6):73-80, 1998.

North American Nursing Diagnosis Association: *Nursing diagnoses: definitions and classification 2003-2004,* Philadelphia, 2003, NANDA International

Oertel LB: Monitoring warfarin therapy: how the INR keeps your patient safe, *Nursing* 29(11):41-45, 1999.

Reid E: Pulmonary embolism: an overview of treatment and nursing issues, *Br J Nurs* 8(20):1373-1378, 1999.

Stamm AM: Ventilator associated pneumonia and the frequency of circuit changes, *Am J Infect Control* 26(1):71-73, 1998.

Sutton PM, Nicas M, Harrison RJ: Tuberculosis isolation: comparison of written procedure and actual practices in three California hospitals, *Infect Control Hosp Epidemiol* 21(1):28-32, 2000.

Willeke K, Qian Y: Tuberculosis control through respirator wear: performance of National Institute for Occupational Safety and health-regulated respirators, *Am J Infect Control* 26(2):139-142, 1998.

Cardiovascular Care Plans

Ackley BJ, Ladwig GB: *Nursing diagnosis handbook: a guide to planning care,* ed 5, St Louis, 2002, Mosby.

Baird MS: Acute coronary syndromes. In Swearingen PL, Keen, JH, editors: *Manual of critical care nursing: nursing interventions and collaborative management,* ed 4, St Louis, 2001, Mosby.

Bernstein AD et al: The NASPE/BPEG generic pacemaker code for antibradyarrhythmia and adaptive rate pacing and antitachyarrhythmia devices, *Pacing Clin Electrophysiol* 10:794-799, 1987.

Cheever KH, Kitzes BK, Genthner D: Epoprostenol therapy for primary pulmonary hypertension, *Crit Care Nurse* 19(4):20-27, 1999.

Deelstra MW, Blue JM: Cardiovascular disorders. In Swearingen PL: *Manual of medical-surgical nursing care,* ed 5, St Louis, 2003, Mosby.

De Winter RJ et al: Value of myoglobin, troponin T, and CK-MB mass in ruling out an acute myocardial infarction in the emergency room, *Circulation* 92(12):3401-3407, 1995.

Durack D: Infective endocarditis. In Alexander RW, editor: *Hurst's the heart,* ed 9, New York, 1998, McGraw-Hill.

The EPIC Investigators: Use of a monoclonal antibody directed against the platelet glycoprotein IIb/IIIa receptor in high risk coronary angioplasty, *N Engl J Med* 330:949-955, 1994.

Fisher ML et al: Beneficial effects of metoprolol in heart failure associated with coronary artery disease: a randomized trial, *J Am Coll Cardiol* 23:943-950, 1994.

Fuster V et al: Primary pulmonary hypertension: natural history and the importance of thrombosis, *Circulation* 70:580-585, 1984.

Gylys K, Gold M: Acute coronary syndromes: new developments in pharmacological treatment strategies, *Crit Care Nurse (suppl)* pp 3-16, April 2000.

Johnson M et al: *Nursing diagnoses, outcomes, and interventions: NANDA, NOC, and NIC linkages,* St Louis, 2001, Mosby.

Murphy M, Berding CB: Use of measurements of myoglobin and cardiac troponins in the diagnosis of acute myocardial infarction, *Crit Care Nurse* 19(1):58-66, 1999.

North American Nursing Diagnosis Association: *Nursing diagnoses: definitions and classification 2003-2004,* Philadelphia, 2003, NANDA International.

Packer M et al: The effect of carvedilol on morbidity and mortality in patients with chronic heart failure, *N Engl J Med* 334:1349-1355, 1996.

Rich S, Kaufmann E, Levy PS: The effect of high doses of calcium-channel blockers on survival in primary pulmonary hypertension, *N Engl J Med* 327:76-81, 1992.

Woods SL, Froelicher ES, Motzer SA, editors: *Cardiac nursing,* ed 4, Philadelphia, 2000, Lippincott Williams & Wilkins.

Renal-Urinary Care Plans

Ackley BJ, Ladwig GB: *Nursing diagnosis handbook: a guide to planning care,* ed 5, St Louis, 2002, Mosby.

Bott M, Jansen PR: Renal-urinary disorders. In Swearingen PL: *Manual of medical-surgical nursing care,* ed 5, St Louis, 2003, Mosby.

Chow R: Benign prostatic hyperplasia: patient evaluation and relief of obstructive symptoms, *Geriatrics* 56(3):33-38, 2001.

Churchill DN: Clinical practice guidelines for initiation of dialysis, *J Am Soc Nephrol* 10(S13):S289-S291, 1999.

Danotovich GM, editor: *Handbook of kidney transplantation,* ed 3, Philadelphia, 2001, Lippincott Williams & Wilkins.

Gray M: Urinary diversions: perspectives on nursing care, *Perspectives* 2(2), 2000.

Jansen PR: Reproductive disorders. In Swearingen PL: *Manual of medical-surgical nursing care,* ed 5, St Louis, 2003, Mosby.

Jindal KK: Clinical practice guidelines for vascular access, *J Am Soc Nephrol* 10(S13):S297-S305, 1999.

Johnson M et al: *Nursing diagnoses, outcomes, and interventions: NANDA, NOC, and NIC linkages,* St Louis, 2001, Mosby.

Johnson S: From incontinence to confidence, *Am J Nurs* 100(2):69-76, 2000.

Kelly M: Chronic renal failure, *Am J Nurs* 96(1):36-27, 1996.

Kelly M: Acute renal failure, *Am J Nurs* 97(3):32-33, 1997.

Little C: Renovascular hypertension, *Am J Nurs* 100(2):46-51, 2000.

Llach F, Nikaktar B: Methods of controlling hyperphosphatemia in patients with chronic renal failure, *Curr Opin Nephrol Hypertens* 2:365-371, 1993.

Logham-Adham M: Phosphate binders for control of phosphate retention in chronic renal failure, *Pediatr Nephrol* 13:701-708, 1999.

MacDonald J: Dialysis (part 1): continuous ambulatory peritoneal dialysis, *Nurs Stand* 11(22):48-55, 1997.

McCarthy JT: A practical approach to the management of patients with chronic renal failure, *Mayo Clin Proc* 74(3):269-273, 1999.

McConnell J: *Benign prostatic hyperplasia: diagnosis and treatment,* Clinical Practice Guideline 8 AHCPR, Rockville, Md, 1994, U.S. Department of Health & Human Services.

Miller C: Update on treatments for urinary incontinence, *Geriatr Nurs* 19(2):109-110, 1998.

Nichol J et al: Efficacy and safety of finasteride therapy for benign prostatic hyperplasia: results of a 2-year randomized controlled trial (the PROSPECT study), *CMAJ* 155(9):1251-1259, 1996.

North American Nursing Diagnosis Association: *Nursing diagnoses: definitions and classification 2003-2004,* Philadelphia, 2003, NANDA International.

Ormandy P: Dialysis (part 2): haemodialysis, *Nurs Stand* 11(23):48-56, 1997.

Parker J, editor: *Contemporary nephrology,* ed 3, Pitman, NJ, 1998, American Nephrology Nurses' Association.

Sosa-Guerrero S, Gomez N: Dealing with end-stage renal disease, *Am J Nurs* 97(10):44-51, 1997.

Steinman TI: Kidney protection: how to prevent or delay chronic renal failure, *Geriatrics* 51(8):28-35, 1996.

Tanagho E, McAnich J: *Smith's general urology,* ed 15, New York, 2000, Lange.

Thompson J: A practical ostomy guide, part 1, *RN* 63(11):61-66, 2000.

Toffelmire EB: Clinical practice guidelines for the management of anemia coexistent with chronic renal failure, *J Am Soc Nephrol* 10(S13):S292-S296, 1999.

Yucha CB, Shapiro JI: Acute renal failure: recognition and prevention, *Lippincotts Prim Care Pract* 1(4):388-398, 1997.

Neurologic Care Plans

Ackley BJ, Ladwig GB: *Nursing diagnosis handbook: a guide to planning care,* ed 5, St Louis, 2002, Mosby.

Bederson JB, chair: *AHA scientific statement: recommendations for the management of patients with unruptured intracranial aneurysm—a statement for healthcare professionals from the Stroke Council of the American Heart Association,* Dallas, 2000, American Heart Association.

Brewer T, Therrien B: Minor brain injury: new insights for early nursing care, *J Neurosci Nurs* 32(6):311-317, 2000.

Browne TR, Holmes GL: *Handbook of epilepsy,* Philadelphia, 2000, Lippincott Williams & Wilkins.

Bryant G: When spinal cord injury affects the bowel, *RN* 63(2):29, 2000.

Caplan LR: *Caplan's stroke: a clinical approach,* ed 3, Boston, 2000, Butterworth-Heinemann.

Confavreux C: Relapses and progression of disability in multiple sclerosis, *New Engl J Med* 343(20):1430-1438, 2000.

Cooper PR, Golfinos JG, editors: *Head injury,* ed 4, New York, 2000, McGraw-Hill.

Davis PM: *Steps to follow: the comprehensive treatment of patients with hemiplegia,* ed 2, Berlin, 2000, Springer-Verlag Heidelberg.

Devinsky O: Patients with refractory seizures, *New Engl J Med* 340(20):1565-1570, 1999.

Gilbert K: An algorithm for diagnosis and treatment of status epilepticus in adults, *J Neurosci Nurs* 31(1):27-36, 1999.

Henson L: Identifying and overcoming barriers to providing sexuality information in the clinical setting, *Rehabil Nurs* 24(4):148-151, 1999.

Herndon CM, Young K, Herndon AD: Parkinson's disease revisited, *J Neurosci Nurs* 32(4):216-221, 2000.

Hickey J: *Clinical practice of neurological and neurosurgical nursing,* ed 4, Philadelphia, 1997, Lippincott Raven.

Hutton JT, editor: *Caring for the Parkinson patient: a practical guide,* New York, 1999, Prometheus Books.

Johnson M et al: *Nursing diagnoses, outcomes, and interventions: NANDA, NOC, and NIC linkages,* St Louis, 2001, Mosby.

Joy JE, Johnston RB Jr, editors: *Multiple sclerosis: current status and strategies for the future,* Washington, DC, 2001, National Academy Press.

Kallenbach AM, Rosenblum J: Carotid endarterectomy: creating the pathway to 1-day stay, *Crit Care Nurse* 20(4):23-36, 2000.

Lavasik D, Kerr ME, Alexander S: Traumatic brain injury research: a review of clinical studies, *Crit Care Nurs Q* 23(4):24-41, 2001.

Lehrich JR, Sheon RP: Treatment of low back pain: initial approach, *UpToDate* 8(1), 2000.

Lehrich JR, Sheon RP: Treatment of low back pain unresponsive to conservative management, *UpToDate* 8(1), 2000.

Leppik IE, Baringer JR: Selecting treatment in patients with epilepsy, *Hosp Pract* 35(5):35-52, 2000.

Linsenmeyer T, chair: *Acute management of autonomic dysreflexia: adults with spinal cord injury presenting to healthcare facilities,* Consortium for Spinal Cord Medicine Clinical Practice Guidelines (online text www.pva.org), Washington, DC, 1998, Paralyzed Veterans of America.

Margolis S, Kostuik JJ: *Johns Hopkins white papers 2000: low back pain and osteoporosis,* Baltimore, 2000, Johns Hopkins Medical Institute.

Mehta N, Levin M: Management and prevention of meningococcal disease, *Hosp Pract* 35(8):75-86, 2000.

Mitcho K, Yanko JR: Acute care management of spinal cord injuries, *Crit Care Nurs Q* 22(2):60-79, 1999.

Myers F: Meningitis: the fears, the facts, *RN* 63(11):52-57, 2000.

Nausieda P, Bock G, Dowling GA: *Parkinson's disease: what you and your family should know,* Miami, 1999, National Parkinson Foundation.

Neatherlin JS: Head trauma in the older adult population, *Crit Care Nurs Q* 23(3):49-57, 2000.

North American Nursing Diagnosis Association: *Nursing diagnoses: definitions and classification 2003-2004,* Philadelphia, 2003, NANDA International.

Noseworthy JH et al: Multiple sclerosis, *New Engl J Med* 343(13):938-952, 2000.

Oliveira-Filho J, Koroshetz WJ: Acute evaluation and management of ischemic stroke-I, *UpToDate* 8(1), 2000.

Oliveira-Filho J, Koroshetz WJ: Acute evaluation and management of ischemic stroke-II, *UpToDate* 8(1), 2000.

Salmen JPS: *The Do-able renewable home: making your home fit your needs,* Washington, DC, 1998, AARP.

Schacter SC: Management of chronic epilepsy, *UpToDate* 8(1), 2000.

Schacter SC: Pharmacology of antiepileptic drugs, *UpToDate* 8(1), 2000.

Seland TP, chair: *Urinary dysfunction and multiple sclerosis: evidence-based management strategies for urinary dysfunction in multiple sclerosis,* Multiple Sclerosis Council for Clinical Practice Guidelines (online text www.pva.org), Washington, DC, 1999, Paralyzed Veterans of America.

Sims M, Whiting J: Pin-site care, *Nurs Times* 96(48):46, 2000.

Stecker MM: Management of status epilepticus, *UpToDate* 8(1), 2000.

Swift CM: Neurologic disorders. In Swearingen PL: *Manual of medical-surgical nursing care,* ed 5, St Louis, 2003, Mosby.

Tarsy D: Treatment of advanced Parkinson's disease, *UpToDate* 8(1), 2000.

Tate J, Tasota FJ: Looking at lumbar puncture in adults, *Nurs* 24(11):91, 2000.

Travers PL: Autonomic dysreflexia: a clinical rehabilitation problem, *Rehabil Nurs* 24(1):19-23, 1999.

Travers PL: Poststroke dysphagia: implications for nurses, *Rehabil Nurs* 24(2):69-73, 1999.

Weeks SK, Hubbartt E, Michaels TK: Keys to bowel success, *Rehabil Nurs* 25(2):66-60, 2000.

Winkelman C: Effect of backrest position on intracranial and cerebral perfusion pressures in traumatically brain-injured adults, *Am J Crit Care* 9(6):373-380, 2000.

Wong FWH: Prevention of secondary brain injury, *Crit Care Nurse* 20(5):18-27, 2000.

Worsham TL: Easing the course of Guillain-Barré syndrome, *RN* 63(3):46-50, 2000.

Wyllie E: *The treatment of epilepsy: principle and practice,* ed 3, Baltimore, 2001, Lippincott Williams & Wilkins.

Endocrine Care Plans

Ackley BJ, Ladwig GB: *Nursing diagnosis handbook: a guide to planning care,* ed 5, St Louis, 2002, Mosby.

Adlin V: Subclinical hypothyroidism: deciding when to treat, *Am Fam Phys* 557(4):776-780, 1998.

Bailes BK: Hyperthyroidism in elderly patients, *AORN J* 69(1):254-256, 258, 1999.

Baird MS: Endocrine disorders. In Swearingen PL: *Manual of medical-surgical nursing care,* ed 5, St Louis, 2003, Mosby.

Bell SJ, Forse RA: Nutritional management of hypoglycemia, *Diabetes Educ* 25(1):41-47, 1999.

Bolli GB: Hypoglycemia unawareness, *Diabetes Metab* 23(suppl 3):29-35, Sept 1997.

Bolli GB: How to ameliorate the problem of hypoglycemia in intensive as well as non-intensive treatment of type 1 diabetes, *Diabetes Care* (suppl 2):B43-52, March 1999.

Deletter EA et al: Medicolegal implications of hidden thyroid dysfunction: a study of two cases, *Med Sci Law* 40(3):251-257, 2000.

Ezzone SA: SIADH, *Clin J Oncol Nurs* 3(4):187-188, 1999.

Fisken RA: Severe diabetic ketoacidosis: the need for large doses of insulin, *Diabet Med* 16(4):347-350, 1999.

Freeland BS: Emergency: diabetic ketoacidosis, *Am J Nurs* 98(8):52, 1998.

Goldsmith C: Hypothyroidism, *Am J Nurs* 99(6):42-43, 1999.

Grinslade S, Buck EA: Diabetic ketoacidosis: implications for the medical-surgical nurse, *Medsurg Nurs* 8(1):37-45, 1999.

Johnson M et al: *Nursing diagnoses, outcomes, and interventions: NANDA, NOC, and NIC linkages,* St Louis, 2001, Mosby.

Keenan AM: Syndrome of inappropriate secretion of antidiuretic hormone in malignancy, *Semin Oncol Nurs* 15(3):160-167, 1999.

Konick-McMahan J: Riding out a diabetic emergency, *Nursing* 29(9):34-39, quiz 40, 1999.

Lewis R: Diabetic emergencies part 1: hypoglycemia, *Accid Emerg Nurs* 7(4):190-196, 1999.

Meiner SE: Delegation can be miscalculated, *Geriatr Nurs* 20(2):100, 105, 1999.

Miller J: Management of diabetic ketoacidosis, *J Emerg Nurs* 25(6):514-519, 1999.

North American Nursing Diagnosis Association: *Nursing diagnoses: definitions and classification 2003-2004,* Philadelphia, 2003, NANDA International.

Robertson RP: Prevention of recurrent hypoglycemia in type 1 diabetes by pancreas transplantation, *Acta Diabetol* 36(1-2):3-9, 1999.

Shelton BK: Hypothyroidism in cancer patients, *Nurse Pract Forum* 9(3):185-191, 1998.

Singh RK, Perros P, Frier BM: Hospital management of diabetic ketoacidosis: are clinical guidelines implemented effectively? *Diabet Med* 14(6):482-486, 1997.

Slover-Zipf J: Hypoglycemia treatment, *Am J Nurs* 99(10):14, 1999.

Gastrointestinal Care Plans

Ackley BJ, Ladwig GB: *Nursing diagnosis handbook: a guide to planning care,* ed 5, St Louis, 2002, Mosby.

Bass M: Fluid and electrolyte management of ascites in patients with cirrhosis, *Crit Care Nurs Clin North Am* 10(4):459-467, 1998.

Broadwell DC, Jackson BS: *Principles of ostomy care,* St Louis, 1982, Mosby.

Friedman LS: Liver, biliary tract and pancreas. In Tierney LM et al, editors: *Current medical diagnosis and treatment 2001,* ed 40, New York, 2001, McGraw-Hill.

Goff K, Adrien LM: Gastrointestinal disorders. In Swearingen PL: *Manual of medical-surgical nursing care,* ed 5, St Louis, 2003, Mosby.

Goodwin H, Holmes J, Wisner D: Abdominal ultrasound examination in pregnant blunt trauma patients, *J Trauma Inj Infect Crit Care* 50(4):689-693, 2001.

Hayes K: Challenges in emergency care: the geriatric patient, *J Emerg Nurs* 26(5):430-435, 2000.

Heppell J, Kelly KA: Surgical treatment of inflammatory bowel disease. In Yamada T, editor: *Textbook of gastroenterology,* ed 3, Philadelphia, 1999, Lippincott Williams & Wilkins.

Hirsch MG: Gastrointestinal system. In Thompson JM et al, editors: *Mosby's clinical nursing,* ed 5, St Louis, 2002, Mosby.

Johnson M et al: *Nursing diagnoses, outcomes, and interventions: NANDA, NOC, and NIC linkages,* St Louis, 2001, Mosby.

Krumberger J: What is the most current recommendation for analgesic agents and pain management in patients with pancreatitis and other obstructive gastrointestinal (GI) disorders? *Crit Care Nurs Clin North Am* 19(2):110-112, 1999.

Lankisch PG et al, editors: Acute and chronic pancreatitis. In *Surgical Clinics of North America,* Philadelphia, 1999, WB Saunders.

Levins T: The use of ultrasound in blunt trauma, *J Emerg Nurs* 26(1):15-19, 2000.

McQuaid KR: Alimentary tract. In Tierney LM et al, editors: *Current medical diagnosis and treatment 2001,* ed 40, New York, 2001, McGraw-Hill.

North American Nursing Diagnosis Association: *Nursing diagnoses: definitions and classification 2003-2004,* Philadelphia, 2003, NANDA International.

Shweiki E et al: Assessing the true risk of abdominal injury in hospitalized rib fracture patients, *J Trauma Inj Infect Crit Care* 50(4):604-688, 2001.

Stenson WF: Inflammatory bowel disease. In Yamada T, editor: *Textbook of gastroenterology,* ed 3, Philadelphia, 1999, Lippincott Williams & Wilkins.

Wound, Ostomy and Continence Nurses Society: *Guidelines for management: caring for a patient with a continent diversion,* Laguna Beach, Calif, 1996, WOCN.

Wound, Ostomy and Continence Nurses Society: *Guidelines for management: caring for a patient with an ostomy,* Laguna Beach, Calif, 1998, WOCN.

Hematologic Care Plans

Ackley BJ, Ladwig GB: Nursing *diagnosis handbook: a guide to planning care,* ed 5, St Louis, 2002, Mosby.

American Association of Blood Banks, America's Blood Centers, and American Red Cross: *Circular of information for the use of human blood and blood components,* rev Aug 2000.

Horne MM, Heitz UE: *Pocket guide to fluid, electrolyte, and acid-base balance,* ed 4, St Louis, 2001, Mosby.

Johnson M et al: *Nursing diagnoses, outcomes, and interventions: NANDA, NOC, and NIC linkages,* St Louis, 2001, Mosby.

Knoop T: Polycythemia vera, *Semin Oncol Nurs* 12(1):70-77, 1996.

Krantz SB: Pathogenesis and treatment of anemia of chronic disease, *Am J Med* Sci 307:353-359, 1994.

Levi M et al: Novel approaches to the management of disseminated intravascular coagulation, *Crit Care Med* 28(9):20-24, 2000.

Lewis SM, Heitkemper MM, Dirksen SR: *Medical-surgical nursing: assessment and management of clinical problems,* ed 6, St Louis, 2004, Mosby.

North American Nursing Diagnosis Association: *Nursing diagnoses: definitions and classification 2003-2004,* Philadelphia, 2003, NANDA International.

Vanet SM: Hematologic disorders. In Swearingen PL: *Manual of medical-surgical nursing care,* ed 5, St Louis, 2003, Mosby.

Wright S, Finical J: Beyond leeches: therapeutic phlebotomy today, *Am J Nurs* 100(7):56, 2000.

Musculoskeletal Care Plans

Ackley BJ, Ladwig GB: *Nursing diagnosis handbook: a guide to planning care,* ed 5, St Louis, 2002, Mosby.

Altizer LL: Degenerative disorders. In Maher AB et al, editors: *Orthopaedic nursing,* ed 3, Philadelphia, 2002, WB Saunders.

Anderson LP, Dale KG: Infections in total joint replacements, *Orthop Nurs* 17(1):7-12, 1998.

Beck BR, Shoemaker MR: Osteoporosis: understanding key risk factors and therapeutic options, *Phys Sports Med* 28(2):69-70, 73-74, 76-78, 2000.

Brewster N, Lewis P: Joint replacement for arthritis, *Austral Fam Phys* 27(1/2):2-3, 25-27, 1998.

Bryant GG: Modalities for immobilization. In Maher AB et al, editors: *Orthopaedic nursing,* ed 3, Philadelphia, 2002, WB Saunders.

Carter G: Harvesting and implanting allograft bone, *AORN J* 70(4):659-660, 662-670, 672-676, 1999.

Cefalu CA, Waddell DS: Viscosupplementation: treatment alternative for osteoarthritis of the knee, *Geriatrics* 54(10):51-57, 1999.

Dougherty C: Musculoskeletal transplant, *Crit Care Nurs Q* 21(2):55-63, 1998.

Ehde DM et al: Chronic phantom sensations, phantom pain, residual limb pain, and other regional pain after lower limb amputation, *Arch Phys Med Rehab* 81(8):1039-1044, 2000.

Fetrow CW, Avila JR: *Professional's handbook of complementary and alternative medicines,* Springhouse, Pa, 1999, Springhouse Corp.

Fitzpatrick MC: The psychologic assessment and psychosocial recovery of the patient with an amputation, *Clin Orthop* 361:98-107, 1999.

Herzberg MA: *Osteoporosis independent study,* Pitman, NJ, 1997, NAON.

Hoover TJ, Siefert JA: Soft tissue complications of orthopedic emergencies, *Emerg Med Clin North Am* 18(1):115-139, 2000.

Horstman J: *The Arthritis Foundation's guide to alternative therapies,* Atlanta, 1999, Arthritis Foundation.

Hunt AH: Metabolic conditions. In Maher AB et al, editors: *Orthopaedic nursing,* ed 3, Philadelphia, 2002, WB Saunders.

Johnson M et al: *Nursing diagnoses, outcomes, and interventions: NANDA, NOC, and NIC linkages,* St Louis, 2001, Mosby.

Kee CC: Osteoarthritis: manageable scourge of aging, *Nurs Clin North Am* 35(1):199-207, 2000.

Messer SP et al: Long-term exercise and its effects on balance in older osteoarthritic adults: result from the Fitness, Arthritis, and Seniors Trial (FAST), *J Am Geriatr Soc* 48(2):131-138, 1999.

Neitzel JJ et al: Improving pain management after total joint replacement surgery, *Orthop Nurs* 18(4):37-45, 64, 1999.

North American Nursing Diagnosis Association: *Nursing diagnoses: definitions and classification 2003-2004,* Philadelphia, 2003, NANDA International.

Roberts D: Introduction to bone: structure and function, fractures and osteoporosis. In Ceccio CM et al: *An introduction to orthopaedic nursing,* ed 2, Pitman, NJ, 1999, NAON.

Roberts D: Management of clients with musculoskeletal trauma or overuse. In Black JM et al, editors: *Medical-surgical nursing: clinical management for positive outcomes,* ed 6, Philadelphia, 2001, WB Saunders.

Roberts D: Arthritic and connective tissue disorders. In Schoen D, editor: *Core curriculum for orthopaedic nursing,* ed 4, Pitman, NJ, 2001, NAON.

Roberts D, Lappe J: Management of clients with musculoskeletal disorders. In Black JM et al, editors: *Medical-surgical nursing: clinical management for positive outcomes,* ed 6, Philadelphia, 2001, WB Saunders.

Roberts D: Musculoskeletal disorders. In Swearingen PL: *Manual of medical-surgical nursing care,* ed 5, St Louis, 2003, Mosby.

Sharkey NA, Williams NI, Guerin JB: The role of exercise in the prevention and treatment of osteoporosis and osteoarthritis, *Nurs Clin North Am* 35(1):209-221, 2000.

Snyder PE: Fractures. In Maher AB et al, editors: *Orthopaedic nursing,* ed 3, Philadelphia, 2002, WB Saunders.

Whittington CF: Exercise- and sports-related disorders. In Maher AB et al, editors: *Orthopaedic nursing,* ed 2, Philadelphia, 1998, WB Saunders.

Williamson V: Amputation. In Maher AB et al, editors: *Orthopaedic nursing,* ed 3, Philadelphia, 2002, WB Saunders.

Special Needs Care Plans

Ackley BJ, Ladwig GB: *Nursing diagnosis handbook: a guide to planning care,* ed 5, St Louis, 2002, Mosby.

Arnold N, Watterworth B: Wound strategy: can nurses apply classroom education in the clinical setting? *Ostomy Wound Manage* 41(5):40-44, 1995.

A.S.P.E.N. Board of Directors: Guidelines for the use of parenteral and enteral nutrition in adult and pediatric patients, *J Parenter Enteral Nutr* 17(4):1SA-25SA, 1993.

Centers for Disease Control and Prevention: *Prevention and treatment of tuberculosis among patients infected with HIV: principles of therapy and revised recommendations,* Atlanta, 1998, CDC.

Centers for Disease Control and Prevention: *Public health service guidelines for the management of health-care worker exposures to HIV and recommendations for post-exposure prophylaxis,* Atlanta, 1998, CDC.

Centers for Disease Control and Prevention: *Guidelines for the use of antiretroviral agents in HIV-infected adults and adolescents,* Atlanta, 2001, CDC.

Eisenberg P: Gastrostomy and jejunostomy tubes, *RN* 57(11):54-59, 1994.

Eisenberg P: Feeding formulas, *RN* 57(12):46-52, 1994.

Eisenberg P: Nasoenteral tubes, *RN* 57(10):62-69, 1994.

Eisenberg P et al: Abrupt discontinuation of cycled parenteral nutrition is safe, *Dis Colon Rectum* 38:933-939, 1995.

Eisenberg PG: Providing nutritional support. In Swearingen PL: *Manual of medical-surgical nursing care,* ed 5, St Louis, 2003, Mosby.

Fischer JE, editor: *Nutrition and metabolism in the surgical patient,* ed 2, New York, 1996, Little, Brown.

Frank L: Making a difference: HIV treatment adherence, *Pitt Center AIDS Res Newslett* 4(6):8-9, 1998.

Frank L: Prisons and public health: emerging issues in HIV treatment adherence, *J Assoc Nurses AIDS Care* 10(6):24-32, 1999.

Frank L: Caring for patients with human immunodeficiency virus disease. In Swearingen PL: *Manual of medical-surgical nursing care,* ed 5, St Louis, 2003, Mosby.

Frank L, Miramontes H: *Health care provider curriculum on HIV treatment adherence,* Rockville, Md, 1998, U.S. Department of Health and Human Services, HIV/AIDS Bureau, National AETC Program.

Gianino S, St John R: Nutritional assessment of the patient in the intensive care unit, *Crit Care Nurs Clin North Am* 5(1):1-16, 1993.

Gianino S, Seltzer R, Eisenberg P: The ABCs of TPN, *RN* 59(2):42-47, 1996.

Gottschlich MM, editor: *The science and practice of nutrition support: a case-based core curriculum,* Dubuque, Iowa, 2001, Kendall/Hunt.

1998 Guidelines for the treatment of sexually transmitted disease, *MMWR* Jan 23, 1998.

Hoppe B: Central venous catheter-related infections: pathogenesis, predictors, and prevention, *Heart Lung* 24(4):333-339, 1995.

Johnson M et al: *Nursing diagnoses, outcomes, and interventions: NANDA, NOC, and NIC linkages,* St Louis, 2001, Mosby.

McClave SA et al: Use of residual volume as a marker for enteral feeding intolerance: prospective blinded comparison with physical examination and radiographic findings, *J Parenter Enteral Nutr* 16(2):99-105, 1992.

National Pressure Ulcer Advisory Panel: New stage I definition, *Adv Wound Care* 11(2):59, 1998.

North American Nursing Diagnosis Association: *Nursing diagnoses: definitions and classification 2003-2004,* Philadelphia, 2003, NANDA International.

Panel on the Treatment of Pressure Ulcers: *Treatment of pressure ulcers: clinical practice guideline,* no 15, pub no 95-0652, Rockville, Md, 1994, U.S. Department of Health and Human Services, Agency for Health Care Policy Research.

Public Health Service Task Force: *Recommendations for the use of antiretroviral drugs in pregnant HIV-infected women for maternal health and intervention to reduce perinatal HIV-1 transmission in the United States,* Rockville, Md, 2001, U.S. Department of Health and Human Services.

Recommendations for prevention and control of hepatitis C virus (HVC) infection and HCV-related chronic disease, *MMWR* Oct 16, 1998.

Rombeau JL, Rolandelli RH, editors: *Clinical nutrition: parenteral nutrition,* ed 3, Philadelphia, 2001, WB Saunders.

Ropka ME, Williams AB: *HIV nursing and symptom management,* Sudbury, Mass, 1998, Jones & Bartlett.

Stotts NA: Impaired wound healing. In Keene JH, Swearingen PL, editors: *Mosby's critical care consultant,* St Louis, 1997, Mosby.

Stotts NA, Arnold N: Managing wound care. In Swearingen PL: *Manual of medical-surgical nursing care,* ed 5, St Louis, 2003, Mosby.

Ungvarski PJ, Flaskerud JH: *HIV/AIDS: a guide to primary care management,* ed 4, Philadelphia, 1999, WB Saunders.

Part 2: Pediatric Nursing Care Plans

American Academy of Pediatrics: Diagnosis and evaluation of the child with attention-deficit/hyperactivity disorder (AC0002), *Pediatrics* 105(5):1158-1170, 2000.

American Academy of Pediatrics: Clinical practice guideline: treatment of the school-aged child with attention-deficit/hyperactivity disorder, *Pediatrics* 108(4):1033-1042, 2001.

American Lung Association Epidemiology & Statistics Unit, Best Practices and Programs Services: *Trends in asthma morbidity and mortality,* Table 1, 2002.

American Pain Society: *Guidelines for the management of acute and chronic pain in sickle cell disease,* no 1, 1999.

Betz CL: Use of 504 plans for children and youth with disabilities: nursing applications, *Pediatr Nurs* 27(4):347-352, 2001.

Bowden VR, Dickey SB, Greenberg CS: *Children and their families: the continuum of care,* Philadelphia, 1998, WB Saunders.

Brosnan CA, Upchurch S, Schreiner B: Type 2 diabetes in children and adolescents: an emerging disease, *J Pediatr Health Care* 15(4):187-193, 2001.

Castiglia PT: Growth and development: shaken baby syndrome, *J Pediatr Health Care* 15(2):78-80, 2001.

Centers for Disease Control and Prevention: Summary of health statistics for US children: national health interview survey, 1997, *Vital and Health Statistics,* series 10, 203:3, 2002.

Chase HP: *Understanding insulin dependent diabetes,* ed 10, Denver, 2002, Barbara Davis Center for Childhood Diabetes at Denver.

Corrarino JE et al: The cool kids: a community effort to reduce scald burns in children, *MCN* 25(1):10-16, 2000.

Elkin MK, Perry AG, Potter PA: *Nursing interventions and clinical skills,* ed 3, St. Louis, 2004, Mosby.

Ellmers K, Criddle LM: Cystic fibrosis, *RN* 65(9):61-68, 2002.

Gallagher C: Childhood asthma: tools that help parents manage it, *Am J Nurs* 102(8):71-83, 2002.

Gunn VL, Nechyba C: *The Harriet Lane handbook: a manual for pediatric house officers,* ed 16, St Louis, 2002, Mosby.

Hockenberry MJ: *Wong's clinical manual of pediatric nursing,* ed 6, St Louis, 2004, Mosby.

Hockenberry MJ et al, editors: *Wong's nursing care of infants and children,* ed 7, St Louis, 2003, Mosby.

James SR, Ashwill JW, Droske SC: *Nursing care of children: principles and practices,* ed 2, Philadelphia, 2002, WB Saunders.

Meleski DD: Families with chronically ill children, *AJN* 102(5):47-54, 2002.

Merkel SI et al: The FLACC: a behavioral scale for scoring postoperative pain in young children, *Pediatr Nurs* 23(3):293-297, 1997.

Mulryan K, Cathers P, Fagin A: Combating abuse, part II: protecting the child, *Nursing 2000* 30(7):39-43, 2000.

National Asthma Education and Prevention Program's Guidelines for the Diagnosis And Management Of Asthma: Updates on Selected Topics 2002 on National Heart, Lung, and Blood Institute website, accessed at www.nhlbi.nih.gov/guidelines/asthma/index.htm.

Nettina SM, editor: *The Lippincott manual of nursing practice,* ed 7, Philadelphia, 2001, Lippincott.

Pagana KD, Pagana TJ: *Mosby's diagnostic and laboratory test reference,* ed 6, St Louis, 2003, Mosby.

Ruiz EK: Diabetes update: type 2 diabetes in children, *RN* 64(10):44-48, 2001.

Sieberry CK, Iannone R, editors: *The Harriet Lane handbook: a manual for pediatric house officers,* ed 15, St Louis, 2000, Mosby.

Taketoma CK, Hodding JH, Kraus DM: *Pediatric dosage handbook,* ed 10, Cleveland, 2003-2004, American Pharmaceutical Association, Lexi-Comp.

Travis LB: *An instructional aid on insulin-dependent diabetes mellitus,* ed 12, Austin, 2003, Designer's Ink.

Part 3: Maternity Nursing Care Plans

Blackburn ST, Loper DL: *Maternal, fetal and neonatal physiology: a clinical perspective,* ed 2, Philadelphia, 2003, WB Saunders.

Carpenito LJ: *Handbook of nursing diagnosis,* ed 8, Philadelphia, 1999, Lippincott.

Chin HG: *On call obstetrics and gynecology,* ed 2, Philadelphia, 2001, WB Saunders.

Creasy RK, Resnik T: *Maternal-fetal medicine,* ed 4, Philadelphia, 1999, WB Saunders.

Cunningham PC et al: *Williams obstetrics,* ed 20, Stamford, Conn, 1997, Appleton & Lange.

Davis DL: *Empty cradle, broken heart: surviving the death of your baby,* Golden, Colorado, 1999, Fulcrum Publishing.

Fischbach F: *Manual of laboratory and diagnostic tests,* ed 5, Philadelphia, 1996, Lippincott.

Gabbe SG, Niebyl JR, Simpson JL, editors: *Pocket companion to obstetrics, normal and problem pregnancies,* ed 3, New York, 1999, Churchill Livingstone.

Gabbe SG, Niebyl JR, Simpson JL, editors: *Obstetrics: normal and problem pregnancies,* ed 4, New York, 2002, Churchill Livingstone.

Maloni, JA: Preventing preterm birth: evidence-based interventions shift toward prevention, Lifelines, Association of Woman's Health, *Obstetrics and Neonatal Nurses* 4(4):26-31, 2002.

Mandeville LK, Troiano NH: *High-risk and critical care intrapartum nursing,* ed 2, Philadelphia, 1999, Lippincott.

Star WL et al: *Ambulatory obstetrics,* ed 3, San Francisco, 1999, UCSF Nursing Press.

Swenson DE: *Telephone triage for the obstetric patient: a nursing guide,* Philadelphia, 2001, WB Saunders.

Tarascon pocket pharmacopoeia 2002 deluxe edition, Loma Linda, 2002, Tarascon Publishing.

Part 4: Psychiatric Nursing Care Plans

Allen K: Essential concepts of addiction for general nursing practice, *Nurs Clin North Am* 33(1):1-13, 1998.

Allender JA, Rector CL: *Readings in gerontological nursing,* Philadelphia, 1998, Lippincott Williams & Wilkins.

American Psychiatric Association: *Diagnostic and statistical manual of mental disorders,* ed 4, Washington, DC, 2000, American Psychiatric Association.

Ballenger JC et al: Consensus statement on generalized anxiety disorder, *J Clin Psychiatry* 62(11):53-58, 2001.

Beck A et al: *Cognitive theory of depression,* New York, 1979, Guilford Press.

Beck C: Teetering on the edge: a substantive theory of postpartum depression, *Nurs Res* 42(1):42-47, 1993

Berkman LF: Which influences cognitive function: living alone or being alone? *Lancet* 355(15):1291, 2000.

Calarco M, Krone K: An integrated nursing model of depressive behavior in adults: theory and implications for practice, *Nurs Clin North Am* 26(3):573-583, 1991.

Carson VB: *Spiritual dimensions of nursing practice,* Philadelphia, 1989, WB Saunders.

Carson VB: Spirituality and depression: smooth sailing, *DRADA Newsletter* Jan:34, 1994.

Carson VB: *Mental health nursing: the nurse patient journey,* Philadelphia, 2000, WB Saunders.

DeHert M, Mckenzie K, Peuskens J: Risk factors for suicide in young people suffering from schizophrenia: a long-term follow-up study, *Schizophr Res* 47:127 134, 2001.

Depression in primary care: detection and diagnosis, *Clinical Practice Guideline* 1(5), 1993. Rockville, U.S. Department of Health and Human Services, Public Health Service, Agency for Health Care Policy and Research, AHCPR Publication No 93-0550.

Dowling C: *You mean I don't have to feel this way? New help for depression, anxiety, and addiction,* New York, 1993, Bantam Books.

Eliopoulos C: *Manual of gerontologic nursing,* St Louis, 1999, Mosby.

Goodwin F, Jamison K: *Manic-depressive illness,* New York, 1990, Oxford University Press.

Greenberg P, Stiglin L, Finkelstein S: The economic burden of depression, *J Clin Psychiatry* 54 (11):406-418, 1993.

Herlz MI et al: American Psychiatric Association: practice guideline for the treatment of patients with schizophrenia, *Am J Psychiatry* 154(suppl):1-63, 1997.

Hollon S D, Shelton RC, Loosen PT: Cognitive therapy in relation to pharmacotherapy in depression, *J Consulting Psychology* 59:88-99, 1991.

Jacob BL: Serotonin, motor activity and depression-related disorders, *Am Sci* 82:456-463, 1994.

Jamison K: *Touched with fire: manic-depressive illness and the artistic temperament,* New York, 1993, The Free Press.

Jones P, Meleis A: Health is empowerment, *Adv Nurs Sci* 15(13):113, 1993.

Keck PE, Strakowski SM, McElry SL: The efficacy of atypical antipsychotics in the treatment of depressive symptoms, hostility, and suicidality in patients with schizophrenia, *J Clin Psychiatry* 61(suppl):4-9, 2000.

Kranzier HR: Medications for alcohol dependence-new vistas, *JAMA* 264(23/30):1016, 2000.

Mace NL, Rabins PV: *The 36-hour day,* ed 3, Baltimore, 1999, Johns Hopkins University Press.

Markey BT, Stone JB: An alcohol and drug education program for nurses, *AORN J* 66:845-853, 1997.

Miller AL et al: Texas Algorithm Project (TMAP) schizophrenia algorithms, *J Clin Psychiatry* 60(10):649-657, 1999.

Mondimore F: *Depression: the mood disease,* Baltimore, 1993, The Johns Hopkins University Press.

Morris J: Dementia, *Curr Pract Med* 2:621-626, 1999.

Neese J: Depression in the general hospital, *Nurs Clin North Am* 26(3):613-621, 1991.

Norbeck J et al: Social support needs of family caregivers of psychiatric patients from three age groups, *Nurs Res* 40(4):208-213, 1991.

Patterson CJS et al: The recognition, assessment, and management of dementing disorders: conclusions from the Canadian Conference on Dementia, *CMAJ* 160:1-21, 1999.

Preston JD: *Depression and anxiety management,* Oakland, 2001, New Harbinger Publications (audio cassette).

Preston JD: *You can beat depression,* ed 3, San Luis Obispo, 2001, Impact Publishers.

Preston JD, Johnson JR. *Clinical psychopharmacology made ridiculously simple,* Miami, 2000, Med Master Inc.

Preston JD, O'Neal JH, Talaga M: *Handbook of clinical psychopharmacology for therapists,* ed 2, Oakland, 2000, New Harbinger Publications.

Schoenbeck S, Trujillo-Stanley J, Lokken M: Helping the patient and their family understand depression, *J Pract Nurs* Sept:35-38, 1992.

Story M, Anderson G: Assessment and treatment strategies for depressive disorders commonly encountered in primary care settings, *Nurse Practitioner* June:25-36, 1992.

Terry M, Anderson G: Assessment and treatment strategy for depressive disorders encountered in psychiatric care centers, *Nurse Practitioner* 17(6):34, 1992.

Weaver AJ, Preston JD, Jerome L: *Counseling troubled teens and their families, a resource for pastors and religious care givers,* Nashville, 1999, Abingdon Press.

Withnow R: *Sharing the journey: support groups and America's new quest for community,* New York, 1994, The Free Press.

Zacharias S et al: Development of an alcohol withdrawal clinical pathway: an interdisciplinary process, *J Nurs Care Quality* 12(3):9-18, 1998.

Appendix

Boyce JM, Pittet D: Guideline for hand hygiene in health-care settings: recommendations of the Healthcare Infection Control Practices Advisory Committee and the HICPAC/SHEA/APIC/IDSA Hand Hygiene Task Force, *Infect Control Hosp Epidemiol* 23(12 suppl):S3-40, 2002.

Department of Labor, Occupational Safety and Health Administration: Occupational exposure to bloodborne pathogens: final rule, 29 CRF, part 1910:1030, *Federal Register* 56:64003-64182, December 6, 1991.

Garner JS and the Hospital Infection Control Practices Advisory Committee (HICPAC), Centers for Disease Control Practices and Prevention: Guidelines for isolation precautions in hospitals, *Infect Control Hosp Epidemiol* 17(1):53-80, 1996.

Jackson MM: Infection prevention and control. In Swearingen PL: *Manual of medical-surgical nursing care,* ed 5, St Louis, 2003, Mosby.

Strausbaugh L, Jackson M, Rhinehart E, Siegel J, and the Healthcare Infection Control Practices Advisory Committee (HICPAC): *Guideline to prevent transmission of infectious agents in healthcare settings.* (To be published early 2004.)

Index

A

AA Recovery Resources, Online. *See* Alcoholics Anonymous (AA) Recovery Resources, Online.
AAFA. *See* Asthma & Allergy Network Mothers of Asthmatics (AANMA).
AANMA. *See* Asthma & Allergy Network Mothers of Asthmatics (AANMA).
AARP. *See* American Association of Retired Persons (AARP).
Abdomen, pooling of fluids in, pancreatitis and, 490-491
Abdominal aneurysm, 161-163
Abdominal computed tomography, appendicitis and, 449
Abdominal cramping
    preterm labor and, 755
    preterm premature rupture of membranes and, 765
Abdominal distention, perioperative care and, 53-54
Abdominal examination, bleeding in pregnancy and, 700
Abdominal pain
    bleeding in pregnancy and, 700
    peritonitis and, 503
    preterm premature rupture of membranes and, 765
Abdominal plain films, ulcerative colitis and, 508
Abdominal surgical incision, postpartum wound infection and, 739
Abdominal trauma, 439-447
    acute pain, 441-442
    additional nursing diagnoses/problems and, 447
    assessment of, 439-440
    deficient fluid volume, 440-441
    diagnostic tests for, 440
    health care setting and, 439
    imbalanced nutrition, less than body requirements, 446
    impaired tissue integrity, 445
    ineffective breathing pattern, 443-444
    ineffective gastrointestinal tissue perfusion, 444-445
    nursing diagnoses and interventions for, 440-447
    patient-family teaching and discharge planning for, 447
    post-trauma syndrome, 446-447
    risk for impaired skin integrity, 445
    risk for infection, 442-443
Abdominal ultrasound
    appendicitis and, 449
    preterm labor and, 756
Abdominal wound infection after cesarean section, 739

Abdominal x-ray examination
    appendicitis and, 449
    pancreatitis and, 490
    peritonitis and, 501
Abduction wedge, total hip arthroplasty and, 565
ABGs. *See* Arterial blood gases (ABGs).
ABI. *See* Ankle-brachial index (ABI).
Ablation, radio frequency, radio frequency, dysrhythmias and conduction disturbances and, 193
Abnormal Involuntary Movement Scale (AIMS), schizophrenia and, 813, 814
Abscess, appendicitis and, 450
Absence seizures, generalized, 375
Abuse
    child. *See* Child abuse and neglect.
    emotional, 643-648
    physical, 643-648
    sexual, 643-648
    substance. *See* Substance abuse disorders.
Accelerated rejection, renal transplant recipient and, 262
Accident, cerebrovascular. *See* Cerebrovascular accident (CVA).
Acetaminophen
    with codeine, sickle cell pain crisis and, 693
    hydrocodone with, postpartum wound infection and, 745
    oxycodone with, postpartum wound infection and, 745
    postpartum mastitis and, 736
    sickle cell pain crisis and, 694
Acetaminophen ingestion, 685
Acetone, diabetic ketoacidosis and, 409
Acetophenazine, schizophrenia and, 816-817
Acid phosphatase, intervertebral disk disease and, 350
Acid-fast bacilli (AFB), pulmonary tuberculosis and, 159
Acid-fast stains
    pneumonia and, 141
    pulmonary tuberculosis and, 159
Acidosis, metabolic. *See* Metabolic acidosis.
Acnelike reaction, cancer care and, 34
Acquired immunodeficiency syndrome (AIDS), 569-582
ACS. *See* American Cancer Society (ACS).
Actinomycin D, cancer care and, 12-13
Activity
    alcohol dependency and, 822
    dementia-Alzheimer's type and, 794
Activity intolerance
    cancer care and, 15-16
    chronic renal failure and, 244-245
    coronary heart disease and, 181-182
    Crohn's disease and, 469-470

Activity intolerance—cont'd
    emphysema and, 136-137
    HIV infection and, 577
    hypothyroidism and, 427
    myocardial infarction and, 206-207
    pulmonary hypertension and, 213
    related to generalized weakness and bedrest secondary to cardiac surgery, 176-177
    related to imbalance between oxygen supply and demand secondary to decreased oxygen-carrying capacity of blood because of anemia, 519-520
    risk for
        cancer care and, 3-4
        prolonged bedrest and, 67-69
Acute appendicitis with perforation, 449
Acute bronchiolitis, 619
Acute cognitive disorders, 793
Acute confusion, benign prostatic hypertrophy and, 237-238
Acute crisis, potential for, diabetes mellitus and, 657-658
Acute hepatic failure, 483
Acute leukemia, 2
Acute otitis media (AOM), 679
Acute pain, 41-45
    abdominal trauma and, 441-442
    appendicitis and, 451
    benign prostatic hypertrophy and, 234-235
    cancer care and, 10, 41-45
    coronary heart disease and, 180-181
    Crohn's disease and, 468-469
    fractures and, 541
    gallstones and, 454-455
    Guillain-Barré syndrome and, 333
    HIV infection and, 576
    hyperthyroidism and, 422-423
    myocardial infarction and, 204-205
    neurologic disorders and, 307-308
    osteoarthritis and, 546-547
    otitis media and, 680
    peritonitis and, 502
    pneumothorax/hemothorax and, 150-151
    polycythemia and, 521-522
    related to amputation surgery and postoperative phantom limb sensation, 533-534
    related to fracture and other injury, 668
    related to headache, photophobia, and neck stiffness secondary to meningitis, 315-316
    related to headaches secondary to head injury, 343
    related to inflammatory process caused by thrombus formation, 218-219
    related to inflammatory process of pancreas, 491-492

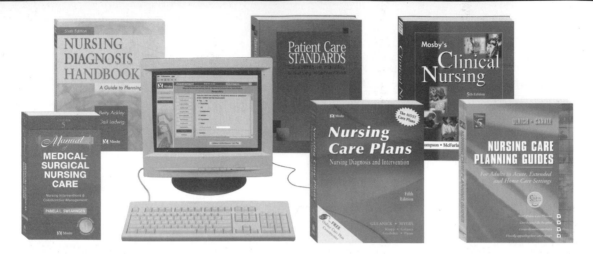